HYPERTENSION

Principles and Practice

HYPERTENSION

Principles and Practice

Edited by

Edouard J. Battegay
University Hospital Basel
Basel, Switzerland

Gregory Y. H. Lip
City Hospital
Birmingham, United Kingdom

George L. Bakris
Rush University Medical Center
Chicago, Illinois, U.S.A.

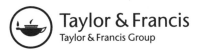

Taylor & Francis
Taylor & Francis Group

Boca Raton   London   New York   Singapore

Published in 2005 by
Taylor & Francis Group
6000 Broken Sound Parkway NW, Suite 300
Boca Raton, FL 33487-2742

International Standard Book Number-10: 0-8247-2855-6 (Hardcover)
International Standard Book Number-13: 978-0-8247-2855-7 (Hardcover)

Library of Congress Cataloging-in-Publication Data

Catalog record is available from the Library of Congress

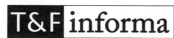

Taylor & Francis Group is the Academic Division of T&F Informa plc.

Visit the Taylor & Francis Web site at
http://www.taylorandfrancis.com

Preface

A wealth of information has accumulated on the subject of hypertension, and the number of publications dedicated to topics in this field of study continues to increase. It has become nearly impossible for medical professionals to absorb all of the diverse information and to gather the information into a coherent theoretical concept and practical approach to treating the disease, even for those of us who are actively involved in this research specialty on a daily basis. It becomes a still greater challenge for the many health care providers whose primary focus is clinical practice or for scientists who are doing research in basic science but whose work is relevant to the subject of hypertension.

Our goal for *Hypertension: Principles and Practice* has been to compile and present information about the most relevant underlying principles of hypertension and apply them to clinical practice. It takes facets of basic research and applies these concepts to bedside management. This concomitant emphasis on principles and practice confers a novel and distinctive quality to the book.

This reference is designed for use by primary care physicians, cardiologists, endocrinologists, nephrologists, vascular specialists, hypertension specialists, pharmacologists, scientists, nurses, students, and others, who want to obtain accurate, comprehensive, and up-to-date information on all aspects of hypertension in an attractive and easily readable format. The editors, contributors, and publisher envision this book as a new international platform for up-to-date information for the interested reader.

KEY FEATURES OF THE BOOK INCLUDE:

- A concomitant emphasis on principles and practice. Emphasis on the clinical aspects and patient management as well as on the molecular, biological, physiological, pathophysiological, and pharmacological aspects of hypertension.
- Authoritative, up-to-date, accurate, and evidence-based information.
- Organization to permit interconnection of various disciplines.
- Keypoints and summary sections at the beginning of each chapter to assist the reader in locating specific information of interest and in gaining an understanding of the scope of research in hypertension.
- Illustrations, algorithms, tables, and charts to clarify key data and relationships.
- Content provided by distinguished, well-established authors, drawn from all disciplines and from different areas of the world to ensure comprehensive and balanced international coverage.

The editors and publisher have worked intensively to give this book, written by many distinct authors, the tenor of one voice. Still, not all overlaps have been eliminated. Furthermore, we would like this book to evolve further and invite you, the reader, to provide us with feedback to prepare future editions.

Acknowledgments are due to Claudia Weiss, Basel (Switzerland), who skillfully and energetically organized the administrative processes required for the editing of the book. Without Claudia, the book would not have seen the light of the day. Many thanks are also due to our technical writer, Sigrid Strom and her colleagues, Seattle, Washington (USA), who expertly worked on so many distinct manuscripts to give them a common voice. The editors gratefully acknowledge the prompt and thoughtful support from Geoffrey Greenwood, the Acquisitions Editor at Taylor & Francis Group, who originally approached us to prepare this book.

Finally, we hope that *Hypertension: Principles and Practice* will serve our many hypertension patients by supporting their health care providers with a useful and comprehensive source of accurate information and education for daily use.

Edouard J. Battegay, MD
Gregory Y. H. Lip, MD
George L. Bakris, MD

Contents

Part E: Secondary Hypertension

Contributors

Brett Alyson Ange *Department of Epidemiology, Johns Hopkins Bloomberg School of Public Health, Baltimore, Maryland, USA*

Lawrence J. Appel *Department of Medicine, Epidemiology and International Health (Human Nutrition), Johns Hopkins Medical Institutions, Baltimore, Maryland, USA*

Ganesh Arunachalam *Clinical Pharmacology and Barts and the London Genome Centre, William Harvey Research Institute, St. Bartholomew's Hospital, London, UK*

George L. Bakris *Department of Preventive Medicine, Rush University Medical Center, Chicago, Illinois, USA*

Edouard J. Battegay *Medical Outpatient Department, University Hospital Basel, Basel, Switzerland*

D. Gareth Beevers *University Department of Medicine, Birmingham, UK*

Christopher J. Bulpitt *Division of Medicine, Imperial College School of Medicine, London, UK*

Michel Burnier *Service of Nephrology, CHUV, Lausanne, Switzerland*

Marc De Buyzere *Department of Cardiovascular Diseases, Ghent University Hospital, Ghent, Belgium*

Francesco P. Cappuccio *Department of Community Health Sciences, St. George's Hospital Medical School, London, UK*

Mark J. Caulfield *Clinical Pharmacology and Barts and the London Genome Centre, William Harvey Research Institute, St. Bartholomew's Hospital, London, UK*

Marco Centola *Dipartimento di Medicina Clinica, Università di Milano-Bicocca, Milano, Italy; Università di Pavia, Pavia, Italy, and Clinica Medica II, IRCCS S. Matteo, Centro Interuniversitario di Fisiologia Clinica e Ipertensione, Milano, Italy*

Dave C. Y. Chua *Department of Preventive Medicine, Rush University Medical Center, Chicago, Illinois, USA*

Denis L. Clement *Department of Cardiovascular Diseases, Ghent University Hospital, Ghent, Belgium*

Niall S. Colwell *Department Clinical Pharmacology, University College Cork, Cork, Ireland*

Veronique A. Cornelissen *Department of Molecular and Cardiovascular Research, University of K.U. Leuven, Leuven, Belgium*

Cheryl R. Dennison   *The Johns Hopkins University School of Nursing, Baltimore, Maryland, USA*

Hossam El-Gendi   *University Department of Medicine, City Hospital, Birmingham, UK*

William J. Elliott   *Department of Preventive Medicine, Rush University Medical Center, Chicago, Illinois, USA*

Stefan T. Engelter   *Neurological Clinic and Stroke Unit, University Hospital Basel, Basel, Switzerland*

Robert H. Fagard   *Department of Molecular and Cardiovascular Research, University of K.U. Leuven, Leuven, Belgium*

Bonita Falkner   *Department of Medicine and Pediatrics, Thomas Jefferson University, Philadelphia, Pennsylvania, USA*

Alberto U. Ferrari   *Dipartimento di Medicina Clinica, Università di Milano-Bicocca, Milano, Italy; Università di Pavia, Pavia, Italy, and Clinica Medica II, IRCCS S. Matteo, Centro Interuniversitario di Fisiologia Clinica e Ipertensione, Milano, Italy*

Gabriela B. Gomez   *Department of Community Health Sciences, St. George's Hospital Medical School, London, UK*

Joey P. Granger   *Department of Physiology and Biophysics, University of Mississippi Medical Center, Jackson, Mississippi, USA*

Guido Grassi   *Università Milano-Bicocca, Ospedale San Gerardo, Monza (Milano), Centro Interuniversitario di Fisiologia Clinica e Ipertensione, Milano, Italy*

John E. Hall   *Department of Physiology and Biophysics, University of Mississippi Medical Center, Jackson, Mississippi, USA*

Donna S. Hanes   *Division of Nephrology, Department of Medicine, University of Maryland Medical System, Baltimore, Maryland, USA*

Jiang He   *Tulane University School of Public Health and Tropical Medicine, New Orleans, Louisiana, USA*

Martha N. Hill   *The Johns Hopkins University School of Nursing, Baltimore, Maryland, USA*

John Kevin Hix   *Department of Nephrology and Hypertension, The Cleveland Clinic Foundation, Cleveland, Ohio, USA*

Elly Den Hond   *Studiecördinatiecentrum, Departmentvoor Moleculair en Cardiovasculair Onderzoek, Katholieke Universiteit Leuven, Leuven, Belgium*

Jonathan Hulme   *Department of Anesthesia & Intensive Care, University of Birmingham, Birmingham, UK*

Rok Humar   *Department of Research, University Hospital Basel, Basel, Switzerland*

Sabih M. Huq   *Clinical Pharmacology and Barts and the London Genome Centre, William Harvey Research Institute, St. Bartholomew's Hospital, London, UK*

Gilbert R. Kaufmann   *Medical Outpatient Department (Poliklinik), University Hospital Basel, Basel, Switzerland*

Kin-L. Kong   *University of Birmingham, Birmingham, UK*

Lawrence R. Krakoff   *Mount Sinai School of Medicine, New York, New York and Englewood Hospital and Medical Center, Englewood, New Jersey, USA*

Gregory Y. H. Lip   *University Department of Medicine, City Hospital, Birmingham, UK*

Peck-Lin Lip   *The Birmingham and Midland Eye Centre and City Hospital, Birmingham, UK*

Ted Lo   *University Department of Medicine, City Hospital, Birmingham, UK*

Thomas F. Lüscher   *Department of Cardiology, University Hospital, Zürich, Switzerland*

Robert J. MacFadyen   *University Department of Medicine and Department of Cardiology, City Hospital, Birmingham, UK*

Marc Maillard   *Service of Nephrology, CHUV, Lausanne, Switzerland*

Giuseppe Mancia   *Università Milano-Bicocca, Ospedale San Gerardo, Monza (Milano), Centro Interuniversitario di Fisiologia Clinica e Ipertensione, Milano, Italy*

Barry J. Materson *Department of Medicine, University of Miami School of Medicine, Miami, Florida, USA*

Lucia Mazzolai *Department of Angiology, Centre Hospitalier Universitaire Vaudois (CHUV), Lausanne, Switzerland*

Samy I. McFarlane *Department of Medicine, SUNY Downstate and Kings County Hospital Center, Brooklyn, New York, USA*

Trefor Morgan *Department of Physiology, University of Melbourne, Melbourne and Hypertension Clinic, Austin Health, Heidelberg, Australia*

Beat Mueller *Division of Endocrinology, Diabetes, and Clinical Nutrition, University Hospital, Basel, Switzerland*

Patricia B. Munroe *Clinical Pharmacology and Barts and the London Genome Centre, William Harvey Research Institute, St. Bartholomew's Hospital, London, UK*

Paul Muntner *Department of Epidemiology, Tulane University School of Public Health and Tropical Medicine, New Orleans, Louisiana, USA*

Michael B. Murphy *Department of Pharmacology and Therapeutics, University College Cork, Cork, Ireland*

Matthew T. Naughton *Department of Medicine, Monash University, Melbourne, Victoria, Australia*

Tim Nawrot *Studiecördinatiecentrum, Laboratorium Hypertensie, Departmentvoor Moleculair en Cardiovasculair Onderzoek, Katholieke Universiteit Leuven, Leuven, Belgium*

Stephen J. Newhouse *Clinical Pharmacology and Barts and the London Genome Centre, William Harvey Research Institute, St. Bartholomew's Hospital, London, UK*

Reto Nüesch *Outpatient Department of Internal Medicine, University Hospital Basel, Basel, Switzerland*

Maria I. Nunes *Division of Medicine, Imperial College School of Medicine, London, UK*

Jürg Nussberger *Department of Angiology, Centre Hospitalier Universitaire Vaudois (CHUV), Lausanne, Switzerland*

Stefano Perlini *Dipartimento di Medicina Clinica, Università di Milano-Bicocca, Milano, Italy; Università di Pavia, Pavia, Italy, and Centro Interuniversitario di Fisiologia Clinica e Ipertensione, Milano, Italy*

Richard A. Preston *Department of Clinical Medicine, University of Miami School of Medicine, Miami, Florida, USA*

Brian N. C. Prichard *University College London, London, UK*

Thompson G. Robinson *Department of Cardiovascular Science, University Hospitals of Leicester NHS Trust, Leicester, UK*

Therese Resink *Department of Research, University Hospital Basel, Basel, Switzerland*

Luis Miguel Ruilope *Hypertension Unit, Hospital 12 de Octubre, Madrid, Spain*

Thomas Rutledge *Department of Psychiatry, University of San Diego, San Diego, California, USA*

Michel E. Safar *Hôpital Hôtel-Dieu, Paris, France*

Julián Segura *Hypertension Unit, Hospital 12 de Octubre, Madrid, Spain*

Bansari Shah *University of Illinois/Christ Hospital, Chicago, Illinois, USA*

Alexander M. M. Shepherd *Department of Medicine and Pharmacology, University of Texas Health Sciences Center at San Antonio, San Antonio, Texas, USA*

Domenic A. Sica *Division of Nephrology, Virginia Commonwealth University, Richmond, Virginia, USA*

Ellen R. T. Silveira *Division of Medicine, Imperial College School of Medicine, London, UK*

James R. Sowers *Department of Medicine, University of Missouri and VA Medical Center, Columbia, Missouri, USA*

Lukas E. Spieker *Department of Cardiology, University Hospital, Zürich, Switzerland*

Jan A. Staessen   *Studiecördinatiecentrum, Laboratorium Hypertensie, Departmenívoor Moleculair en Cardiovasculair Onderzoek, Katholieke Universiteit Leuven, Leuven, Belgium*

Sameer N. Stas   *Department of Medicine, SUNY Downstate and Kings County Hospital Center, Brooklyn, New York, USA*

Sandra J. Taler   *Division of Nephrology and Hypertension, Mayo Clinic College of Medicine, Rochester, Minnesota, USA*

Lutgarde Thijs   *Studiecördinatiecentrum, Laboratorium Hypertensie, Departmenívoor Moleculair en Cardiovasculair Onderzoek, Katholieke Universiteit Leuven, Leuven, Belgium*

Jason G. Umans   *Department of Medicine, Obstetrics and Gynecology, and the General Clinical Research Center, Georgetown University Medical Center, and MedStar Research Institute, Washington, District of Columbia, USA*

Ronald G. Victor   *Divisions of Hypertension and Cardiology, University of Texas Southwestern Medical Center, Dallas, Texas, USA*

Donald G. Vidt   *Department of Nephrology and Hypertension, The Cleveland Clinic Foundation, Cleveland, Ohio, USA*

Wanpen Vongpatanasin   *Divisions of Hypertension and Cardiology, University of Texas Southwestern Medical Center, Dallas, Texas, USA*

Matthew R. Weir   *Division of Nephrology, Department of Medicine, University of Maryland Medical System, Baltimore, Maryland, USA*

Paul K. Whelton   *Tulane University School of Public Health and Tropical Medicine, New Orleans, Louisiana, USA*

Mohammed Youshauddin   *Department of Preventive Medicine, Rush University Medical Center, Chicago, Illinois, USA*

Andreas Zeller   *Medical Outpatient Department, University Hospital Basel, Basel, Switzerland*

Lukas Zimmerli   *Medical Outpatient Department, University Hospital, Basel, Switzerland*

Pieter A. van Zwieten   *Universiteit van Amsterdam, Amsterdam, The Netherlands*

Part A: History, Definitions, and Epidemiology

1

History of Hypertension

LAWRENCE R. KRAKOFF

Mount Sinai School of Medicine, New York, New York and Englewood Hospital and Medical Center, Englewood, New Jersey, USA

KEYPOINTS

- Before 1967, hypertension became well defined, but without an effective treatment.
- Since 1967 effective and highly beneficial drug treatment has evolved.
- Recent advances have been made in characterizing both high risk hypertensive phenotypes and specific causative genetic mutations.
- Computer technology for characterization of daily average blood pressure and its variation has made a major clinical contribution to care of hypertensives.

SUMMARY

The history of hypertension can be divided into two eras: the pretreatment era (before 1967) when the pathology and pathophysiology of hypertension were defined and the treatment era which established the benefit of drug therapy for hypertension. Clinical trials and meta-analyses have firmly established to extraordinary value of modern antihypertensive treatment. Advances in genetics have led to full characterization of several rare causes of hypertension. Progress in the technology of blood pressure measurement, specifically 24 h blood pressure monitoring has substantially improved the diagnosis of hypertension and the risk of average blood pressure for cardiovascular disease.

I. INTRODUCTION

Hypertension, as a specific concept, entered the language of medicine in the 19th and early 20th centuries. *Hypertension*, high arterial pressure, was associated initially with chronic renal disease and only later recognized as a more widespread trait in healthy individuals that was a predictor of cardiovascular disease and renal disease.

During the first 120 years of hypertension research (from the 1840s to 1965) basic and clinical research defined the following:

- Many of the mechanisms that increase arterial pressure.
- The natural history of untreated hypertension from normal health to cardiovascular disease.
- Many causes of secondary hypertension.
- Set the stage for recognizing potential therapy through drug treatment.
- Effective drugs first became available in the 1950s.

This chapter selectively summarizes the history of hypertension over the past 40 years. The focus is on the major advances in therapy as expressed in the randomized clinical trials. The early trials established unequivocally that drug therapy of hypertension is highly effective in the prevention of fatal and nonfatal cardiovascular disease. However, only a few drug classes were available in the 1950s. Since then, innovative research in pharmacology has provided several valuable drug classes with unique therapeutic properties and fewer adverse reactions. Long-acting formulations for once-daily administration have been introduced to enhance adherence to drug treatment regimens. During the past decade, the results of clinical trials suggest that some antihypertensive drugs prevent cardiovascular disease, independent of their effect in reducing blood pressure. Recent progress in the science of hypertension includes the following:

- Recognition of systolic hypertension as a target for beneficial treatment.
- Definition of the *metabolic syndrome*, which associates the risk of increased blood pressure with insulin resistance and with the deleterious patterns of lipid metabolism.
- Complete genetic characterization of several rare forms of secondary hypertension.
- Recognition of new regulators of vascular control.
- Modern technology that is miniaturized and computerized for measurement of blood pressure outside the clinic (ambulatory blood pressure monitoring), which may soon become the gold standard for clinical assessment.

Overall, the recent history of hypertension is one of extraordinary progress in translating basic and clinical science to highly effective medical therapy, with reduction of the cardiovascular disease burden in the developed world.

II. THE PRETREATMENT ERA

Hypertension, defined as increased systemic arterial blood pressure, is now widely accepted as a correctable cause of

cardiovascular and renal diseases. The treatment of hypertension through the prescription of antihypertensive drugs has become an integral and necessary part of modern medical therapy. This contemporary view of hypertension was not always recognized by medical science. In fact, drug treatment for hypertension was considered as a poorly conceived therapeutic adventure with more potential for harm than benefit, until the availability of decisive clinical trials in the 1960s and 1970s.

In 1964, Sir George Pickering (Fig. 1.1) described, in elegant and comprehensive detail, the history of hypertension as a concept in medicine, from its original description as Bright's disease until his own chapter was written in the early 1960s (1). Pickering's own research established that high arterial pressure was a widely distributed finding, best interpreted as a multifactorial trait that was unlikely to be due to a small number of genetic or environmental causes (2).

A more recent monograph describes many of the historical features of hypertension from various perspectives (3). This account and Pickering's chapter summarize nearly all of the relevant clinical descriptions, epidemiology, pathology, and pathophysiology that provided a scientific rationale for the progress was to follow. Several of the important milestones for the early history of hypertension, as identified by Pickering and Postel-Vinay, are listed in Table 1.1.

Many of the mechanisms that were suspected of being factors in hypertension were defined. In addition, it had become evident that hypertension, especially very high diastolic arterial pressure, was strongly associated with the development of cerebral hemorrhage, acute pulmonary

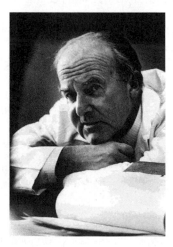

Figure 1.1 Sir George Pickering, one of the first researchers to recognize that hypertension is a trait, rather than a specific disease. His insights regarding the distribution of blood pressure in populations and in families dispelled the idea of simple genetic or environmental causes of hypertension and led to recognition of the multifactorial nature of essential hypertension.

Table 1.1 Important Discoveries for Hypertension Before the Era of Treatment

Discovery	Date and who made discovery
Bright's disease that linked arterial hypertension to renal pathology and left ventricular hypertrophy	1844, Bright
Initial measurement of arterial pressure and description of essential hypertension (without Bright's disease)	1874, Mahomed
Discovery of renin	1898, Tigerstet
Discovery of adrenalin	1895, Oliver and Schafer
Secondary hypertension—pheochromocytoma	1912, Pick
Histopathology of hypertension and arterial disease, malignant and benign nephrosclerosis	1914, Volhard and Fahr
Secondary hypertension—Cushing's syndrome	1932, Cushing
Role of renal artery stenosis, reno-vascular hypertension in experimental animals	1934, Goldblatt
Secondary hypertension—Conn's syndrome	1955, Conn
Noradrenaline, the sympathetic neurotransmitter	1955, Von Euler
Angiotensin II, the active peptide of the renin system	1955, Peart
Aldosterone	1953, Simpson et al.
Link between renin and aldosterone	1958–1960, Gross, Davis, Genest, Laragh
Role of structural change in arterioles	1970s, Folkow

Source: Pickering (1) and Postel-Vinay (69).

edema, hypertensive encephalopathy, and a form of rapidly progressive renal failure which is a result of malignant (fibrinoid) nephrosclerosis. A dramatic example of the devastating course of untreated severe hypertension is provided by the medical description of the final years of the American President, Franklin D. Roosevelt, who died "unexpectedly" of a cerebral hemorrhage in April 1945. He was hypertensive for many years, but in the months preceding his death, a rapid and relentless increase in his pressure was recorded, with systolic blood pressure measurements well above 200 mmHg. A writer has speculated that Roosevelt, a heavy smoker, may have had atherosclerotic renal artery stenosis as the cause of his accelerated course (4). There was no effective or trusted treatment available in the 1940s for severe hypertension, nor was there widespread knowledge of renal artery stenosis. Tests to detect renovascular hypertension and the use

of unilateral nephrectomy, as an attempted cure for this condition, were not reported until the 1950s (5).

Advances in the pharmacology of drugs that lower systemic arterial pressure paralleled or followed discoveries in the pathophysiology of hypertension. The approximate dates, when various classes of antihypertensive drugs were discovered or became available, for clinical assessment are shown in Table 1.2. It is notable that by 1965, several effective and reasonably tolerable drugs, representing distinct drug classes, were available for implementation in controlled trials. This table also shows the drugs and dates of discovery that would become incorporated in modern antihypertensive drug therapy and in the important clinical trials conducted in the years to come.

The natural history of severe hypertension (diastolic pressures >130 mmHg) and malignant hypertension was well known and recognized by the 1950s, so aggressive and high-risk treatments to lower arterial pressure were assessed openly in small series and seemed to promise benefit. The therapies that were studied included the use of the drugs that were then available, such as ganglionic blocking agents; and a surgical approach, the thoracolumbar sympathectomy. In selected cases, where renal artery stenosis could be established, unilateral nephrectomy or renal artery bypass surgery were undertaken. Although an occasional patient responded surprisingly well to these interventions, there remained enough skepticism, on the basis of bad outcomes and theoretical considerations, to prevent acceptance that treatment of

Table 1.2 Discovery of the Antihypertensive Drug Classes

Drug class or type	Date of discovery or characterization
Reserpine, a central and peripheral catecholamine depletory	1931
Thiazide-type diuretics	1958
Hydralazine, a primary arteriolar vasodilator	1950s
Guanethidine	1950s
Spironolactone	1957
Methyldopa	1960
Beta-receptor blockers (e.g., propranolol)	1973
Central alpha$_2$ agonists (e.g., clonidine)	1970s
Alpha$_1$ receptor blockers (e.g., prazosin)	1975
ACE inhibitors (e.g., captopril)	1977
Calcium channel blockers (e.g., verapamil and nifedipine)	1977
Angiotensin receptor blockers (e.g., losartan)	1993

Source: Oates (77).

severe hypertension would be beneficial on a more wide-spread basis. Less severe hypertension was associated with cardiovascular disease at this time, but causal relationships were unclear. Did hypertension cause atherosclerotic vascular pathology? Or did the pathology cause hypertension? There were some who predicted that lowering blood pressure with drugs might worsen the outlook rather than improve it.

This chapter summarizes the history of hypertension, as a target for therapy, and for selected recent advances. Owing to restrictions on the length of the chapter, not every important discovery has been included, nor have the topics selected been developed in great detail. Rather this is a limited survey that will hopefully prompt others to consider the rich and diverse history of hypertension and related cardiovascular disease that needs to be explained in detail.

III. EARLY CLINICAL TRIALS 1967–1990, DIASTOLIC HYPERTENSION

Skepticism in the 1960s that antihypertensive treatment could be beneficial for most hypertensive patients was countered, conceptually, by the emergence of a set of relatively safe drugs that lowered blood pressure and might therefore be tested for effectiveness in preventing cardiovascular disease by treating hypertension, itself. These considerations set the stage for a rigidly controlled, blinded, and randomized clinical trial, conducted within the Veterans Administration hospital system of the United States which compared a placebo with active antihypertensive medications. Largely designed and supervised by Edward Fries (Fig. 1.2), the Veterans Administration trial for treatment of severe hypertension

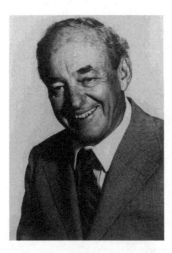

Figure 1.2 Edward Freis, the founder of randomized clinical trials for the treatment of hypertension. Dr. Fries' bold and innovative use of the placebo-controlled trial demonstrated the value of antihypertensive drug therapy with outstanding scientific rigor.

(diastolic pressures ≥115 mmHg) caused an irreversible increase in optimism concerning active treatment. Within 2 years after starting the trial, the group receiving the active drug treatment that lowered pressure had a highly significant reduction in occurrence of strokes, aortic dissection, and progression to the malignant phase of hypertension, when compared with the group that received the placebo. Physicians now knew that drug therapy could prevent death and disability for relatively asymptomatic patients who were at very high risk for fatal or devastating cardiovascular disease (6). Shortly thereafter, a second Veterans' Administration trial that used a similar design and similar medications, but included patients with diastolic pressures in the range of 90–114 mmHg, once again clearly demonstrated the benefit of antihypertensive drug therapy, especially for patients with a diastolic blood pressure ≥105 mmHg (7,8). The antihypertensive drugs employed in these pioneering trials were reserpine, chlorthazide, hydralazine, and guanethidine, and they were most often administered together in varying combinations.

By 1975, the treatment of hypertension by using drug therapy that was directed to the reduction of arterial pressure had passed the test for a "proof of principle". Antihypertensive drug treatment lowered blood pressure and prevented fatal and nonfatal events that were clearly identified as complications of very high blood pressure. Epidemiologists had already recognized that less severe hypertension, defined as diastolic pressures in the range 90–105 mmHg, was associated with the development of cardiovascular disease, especially coronary heart disease and thrombotic stroke. However, patients with these events often had, as the presumed basis for their outcomes, atherosclerosis of the large arteries. The role of hypertension as a cause of atherosclerosis and its thrombotic complications was less certain than its mere association or predictive value. Would antihypertensive drug treatment alter the course of events in those patients with blood pressures above normal, but whose blood pressures were not in the range studied by the Veterans Administration trials? This question was posed by the designers of randomized clinical trials in the United States (9,10), Europe (11–13), and Australia (14). Although they differed in many respects, all of these trials used the diastolic blood pressure as the entry criterion and focused on stroke as the primary outcome measure. However, coronary heart disease (fatal or nonfatal myocardial infarction) was considered, as well. One study that focused on older patients, those ≥60 years of age at entry, was conducted in Europe. A diastolic pressure >90 mmHg was required for entry. The results clearly showed the value of antihypertensive drug treatment for prevention of fatal cardiovascular disease when compared with placebo (12). Some trials that enrolled younger patients with milder hypertension were inconclusive (9,11). In contrast, trials that enrolled middle-aged and elderly patients (some of whom already had cardiovascular disease or other risk factors at entry) tended to demonstrate the value of active drug treatment when compared with a placebo or no treatment (13,14). A large trial, the High Blood Pressure Detection and Follow-up Program (HDFP), was conducted as a multi-center collaboration in the United States. HDFP was designed to compare active drug treatment in special clinics with treatment in usual care as then available in local community practices (15). Those patients randomized to the special clinics, which provided free medication and active follow-up, had lower pressures after treatment when compared with those assigned to the usual community-based care. Patients in the special clinics also had a highly significant reduction in fatal and nonfatal cardiovascular disease, especially stroke, when compared with patients who were treated in the usual care groups (10,16).

By 1990, meta-analyses of the combined evidence from the various trials that were published in the 1970s and 1980s strongly supported the conclusion that the reduction of diastolic pressure by using drug treatment unequivocally prevented stroke by nearly 40%, whether the stroke was a result of cerebral hemorrhage or a result of a thrombotic event. Fatal coronary heart disease was also prevented, but to a lesser extent when compared with strokes, about 15% (17). The antihypertensive drugs that were used in these trials were often the same as those used in the Veterans' Administration trials: reserpine, chlorthiazide, and hydralazine. Methyldopa had become available by the end of the 1960s and was often included in the active therapies in these trials. The beta-blockers appeared in the 1970s and gradually became incorporated into active therapy, eventually replacing methyldopa as the second step when added to a thiazide-type diuretic (13).

IV. CLINICAL TRIALS SINCE 1990, SYSTOLIC HYPERTENSION

In the 1980s, a shift in cardiovascular epidemiology occurred with the recognition that for those over the age 50, systolic blood pressure is a more accurate predictor of future cardiovascular disease and, therefore, a target for therapy (18–20). High systolic blood pressure in the absence of a diastolic pressure >90 mmHg (*isolated systolic hypertension*) had once been considered an inevitable part of the aging process as a result of the stiffening of the large arteries. By the end of the 1980s, enough evidence had accumulated to support a clinical trial to test the hypothesis that the lowering of systolic pressure in older patients with isolated systolic hypertension might be beneficial in the prevention of stroke and, perhaps, in the prevention of ischemic heart disease, as well. Two

large, randomized and placebo-controlled clinical trials were conducted to test the hypothesis—one in the United States and the other in Europe. Taken together, the results of both the Systolic Hypertension in the Elderly Program (SHEP) trial (21) and the Systolic Hypertension in Europe (Syst-Eur) trial (22) strongly supported the conclusion that antihypertensive drug treatment which lowers systolic pressure is highly effective for the prevention of fatal and nonfatal stroke and ischemic heart disease in patients >60 years of age with isolated or predominantly systolic hypertension. This conclusion was further strengthened by a meta-analysis that included older and smaller trials together with the SHEP and Syst-Eur studies (23). The larger SHEP trial also reported, for the first time, that antihypertensive therapy, beginning with a diuretic agent, could prevent the onset of congestive heart failure (24).

V. INTERPRETATION OF TRIALS

Cardiovascular epidemiology has long recognized that the probability of future cardiovascular disease occurring in patients, particularly ischemic or coronary heart disease, is multifactorial. The *absolute* risk of cardiovascular disease for a given patient varies substantially depending on the person's age, blood pressure levels, and presence or absence of diabetes, the lipid patterns, a history of smoking or nonsmoking, and other predictors (25,26). The *relative* benefit of reducing blood pressure, however, seems to be somewhat uniform and independent of other risk factors (27). Considered together, these two concepts predict that a reduction of blood pressure in patients at low absolute risk means that many people must be treated to benefit a single patient, but that a relatively small number must be treated to benefit one patient when the absolute risk is high (28). Calculation of the "number needed to treat" (NNT) is a useful concept for comparing different strategies in different risk groups for arriving at priorities in deciding how treatment might be allocated. The results of the SHEP trial (21) imply that active treatment of 30–40 hypertensive patients (not an unusual number for a single physician to see during 1 week of practice) for a duration of 5 years will prevent one fatal or nonfatal stroke. Such calculations combined with analyses of cost-effectiveness may be the guide for optimal decision-making strategies in the future.

VI. COMPARISON OF STRATEGIES IN TRIALS SINCE 1990

Beginning in the 1970s and accelerating into the 1980s and 1990s, the pharmacology of antihypertensive and cardiovascular drugs expanded in several ways. Beta receptor blockers became recognized as having cardio-protective effects for ischemic heart disease and were assessed for having added effectiveness to prevent ischemic cardiac disease in hypertensives with inconsistent results reported from various trials and analyses (13,29–32).

Discovery and initial clinical evaluation of the angiotensin-converting enzyme (ACE) inhibitors, calcium channel entry blockers, and, later, the angiotensin II type-1 receptor blockers defined new classes of antihypertensive drugs, each with unique pharmacologic actions. Long-acting, once-a-day, formulations became available in all drug classes, with the potential to improve adherence to treatment.

The availability of different and effective therapeutic pathways for treatment of hypertension led to several conjectures that various drug classes would differ in their effect on cardiovascular disease somewhat independent of their effect on lowering blood pressure. Clinical observations had associated circulating renin with cardiovascular disease in hypertensive patients (33,34). Blocking the renin–angiotensin system might then be beneficial for preventing cardiovascular disease as treatment of hypertension. ACE inhibitors, which act by reducing the formation of angiotensin II, became available for trial to test that concept and were effective for severe hypertension (35). The first controlled trials evaluating ACE inhibitors for preventing cardiovascular disease were not, however, conducted in hypertension. Instead, the value of ACE inhibition, on the basis of trial results, emerged as a treatment for heart failure (36), for impaired left ventricular function after myocardial infarction (37), and for treatment of diabetic nephropathy in type-1 diabetics (38).

Development of angiotensin II type-1 receptor antagonists stimulated the design of trials to explore blockade of the renin–angiotensin system by receptor blockade rather than by inhibition of the ACE. Apart from treatment of hypertension [see Losartan Intervention For Endpoint (LIFE) trial], the angiotensin receptor blockers have been shown to be effective for preventing the progression of nephropathy in type-2 diabetes nephropathy in several trials (39–41). The prevention of cardiovascular disease for this group by angiotensin receptor blockers is less certain (42). Angiotensin receptor blockers are effective for treatment of congestive heart failure (43).

Recent trials that use the now available antihypertensive drug classes can be divided into two groups according to their focus for treatment. Some trials are directed to the treatment of hypertension, *per se*, with a reduction of blood pressure as the only basis for comparison of outcomes. Other trials use antihypertensive drugs in patients with overall high cardiovascular risk. The question these trials pose is whether drugs reduce cardiovascular disease independent of a reduction in blood pressure that may (or may not) occur in those whose pressure is in the normal range or minimally elevated, but are also at risk for other reasons. Some of the recently conducted trials that typify these two different goals are summarized in Table 1.3.

The first five trials listed in Table 1.3 [Hypertension Optimal Treatment, HOT (44); Nordic Diltiazem, NORDIL (45); International Nifedipine GITS Study of Intervention as a Goal in Hypertension Treatment, INSIGHT (46); LIFE (47); Australian National Blood Pressure Study 2, ANBP2 (48)], all focus on participants with definite hypertension at entry. Other criteria are

Table 1.3　Selected Recent Trials Classified by Their Major Target (Hypertension or Overall Cardiovascular Risk)

Trial (Reference)	Design/results	Target population
HOT (44)	Different goals for pressure reduction with felodipine as starting drug	Hypertensive patients
NORDIL (45)	Compares diltiazem with old therapy: diuretic and beta blocker. No difference found.	Hypertensive patients
INSIGHT (46)	Compares nifedipine GITS with a thiazide-amiloride combination. No difference found	Hypertensive patients
LIFE (47)	Compares atenolol with losartan (β-blocker vs. ARB). Results favor losartan, primarily due to difference in stroke outcome.	Hypertensive patients with left ventricular hypertrophy
ANBP2 (48)	Compares thiazide type diuretics with ACE inhibitors, as initial treatment. Slightly favors ACE inhibitors, especially for men.	Elderly hypertensive patients studied in open practice setting. Limited to whites of European background.
HOPE (50)	ACE inhibitor (ramipril) vs. placebo in a largely normotensives population. Definitely better outcome for the group give ACE inhibitor.	Patients at high risk due to age and multiple risk factors
ALLHAT (51)	As initial therapy, chlorthalidone (thiazide-type diuretic) equal or superior to lisinopril or amlodipine.	Patients with mild hypertension and high risk due to multiple risk factors
EUROPA (49)	Similar design to HOPE. Outcomes favor the ACE inhibitor perindopril.	Patients at high risk due to coronary heart disease

included for increased predicted risk, such as older age or, notably,the requirement for left ventricular hypertrophy (by ECG) in LIFE. All five of these trials compare two different active drug therapies. Thus, these trials are fairly similar to older trials with the primary focus on the treatment of hypertension itself.

Three recent trials, Heart Outcomes Prevention Evaluation Study (HOPE), Antihypertensive and Lipid-Lowering Treatment to Prevent Heart Attack Trial (ALLHAT), and European Trial on Reduction of Cardiac Events with Perinopril in Stable Coronary Artery Disease (EUROPA), rather than enrolling participants with definite hypertension (≥ 160 mmHg systolic pressure), instead recruited subjects >55 years of age with a high risk for future cardiovascular disease on the basis of several traits in various combinations: hypertension, smoking history, diabetes, evidence of coronary or peripheral arterial disease, or left ventricular hypertrophy. ALLHAT recruited hypertensives who were ≥ 55 years and whose blood pressures were 140 mmHg systolic or 90 mmHg diastolic (or who were already in treatment for hypertension), together with diabetes, or target organ damage that would predict a high likelihood of coronary heart disease within the near future. On the basis of average baseline pressures, ALLHAT included many with blood pressures $<140/90$ mmHg. HOPE and EUROPA recruited those with a moderate to high risk for future cardiovascular disease with or without hypertension. Thus, these three trials diverge from a focus on treatment of hypertension only by reduction of blood pressure and test the hypothesis that certain drug classes reduce cardiovascular morbidity and mortality apart from a substantial reduction in pressure. For HOPE and EUROPA, an ACE inhibitor was highly effective when compared with a placebo (49,50). The results of ALLHAT are more difficult to interpret. There were differences in control of pressure among the three treatment groups, best control for the diuretic cohort and least good for the ACE inhibitor cohort (51). For the primary outcome, fatal or nonfatal myocardial infarction, those initially treated with the diuretic, or the ACE inhibitor, or the calcium blocker, had equal event rates despite the small differences in blood pressure control observed in comparing the groups. Stroke rates, however, were lower for those treated with either the diuretic or the calcium blocker, when compared with the ACE inhibitor. Development of heart failure was prevented more often for those treated initially with the diuretic or the ACE inhibitor when compared with those treated initially with a calcium blocker. Some researchers have concluded that the most effective and least costly initial therapy in ALLHAT was the diuretic (chlorthalidone), and they have recommended that all hypertensive patients be placed on a thiazide-type agent as the initial therapy (51,52).

Overall results of these trials are provided in several meta-analyses with somewhat differing conclusions (52–54). The main issue for continuing controversy is whether *all of the benefit* that is a result of antihypertensive drug therapy, regardless of drug class, is due *only* to reduction of blood pressure or whether some of the benefit is due to the pharmacologic actions of various individual drug classes that are independent of their effects on blood pressure. When the history of hypertension is written in the future, perhaps this controversy will be resolved.

VII. NEW HYPERTENSIVE "PHENOTYPES"

Prior to the 1980s, cardiovascular epidemiology had identified risk factors for cardiovascular disease as distinct from each other and separately contributing to risk, namely hypertension, smoking, diabetes, and elevated cholesterol, the tetrad defined so clearly by the Framingham study (20) (Fig. 1.3). Within the past decade, there has been recognition that hypertension is often found in clusters of individuals who also have a distinct pattern of metabolic traits (55): for example, resistance to the action of insulin associated with normal or impaired glucose tolerance or type-2 diabetes, and abnormal serum lipid patterns with low HDL cholesterol fraction and increased serum triglyceride concentration. Most often these individuals are overweight, and there may be patterns of familial association. The excess weight in these individuals is "central," expressed as a large waist or high waist–hip ratio. Patients with "metabolic" syndrome have a significantly higher risk of cardiovascular disease when compared with

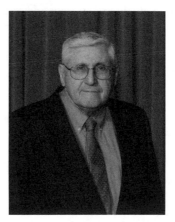

Figure 1.3 William Kannel, one of the leading investigators for the Framingham study. He and his colleagues defined the importance of systolic blood pressure, especially in older patients, as a crucial risk factor for cardiovascular disease. These observations set the stage for the clinical trials of treating systolic hypertension. The results confirmed the epidemiologic hypothesis that lowering systolic pressure would be beneficial.

patients without the syndrome (56). In addition, patients with the metabolic syndrome are more likely to progress to the onset of type-2 diabetes (57).

Recent clinical description also has identified a link between hypertension and a frequent correlate of overweight, the sleep–apnea syndrome (58,59). These two phenotypes strengthen the link between hypertension, overweight, and cardiovascular risk through two distinct pathways. The relationship between these prevalent phenotypes and specific genetic patterns remains uncertain at this time. However, this issue is being actively explored.

VIII. NEW HYPERTENSIVE "GENOTYPES"

Specific forms of familial hypertension, such as adult polycystic kidney disease, have long been recognized in the medical literature. However, the past decade has seen the molecular characterization of several forms of secondary hypertension with definition of the specific mutations, their gene products, and resultant pathophysiology. The first entity to be so defined was the syndrome of glucocorticoid-remediable hypertension, that is, a result of the presence of a chimeric gene that combines a regulatory site that is responsive to ACTH and the aldosterone synthase site (60). Subsequent reports have defined the gain of function mutation in the epithelial sodium transport channel associated with Liddle's syndrome and other forms of hypertension because of rare, but specific mutations (61). These observations have led to explorations of target genes in more usual forms of hypertension with some promising, if preliminary, reports. An increased frequency of a gain of function mutation for the amiloride-sensitive sodium channel has been reported in black hypertensive patients who live in UK with a favorable response to treatment with amiloride (62). Assessment of the Framingham study population has led to an increased frequency in hypertensives of a mutation in the WNK kinase system that is linked to the distal tubular site of chloride reabsorption and thiazide action (63).

IX. NEW MECHANISMS

Since the 1970s, several new mechanisms for control of arterial resistance have been defined. The importance of endothelial cell function has been revealed as these cells control vascular resistance through the nitric oxide system and production of endothelin. Endothelin receptor blockers have been defined and are being assessed for the treatment of cardiovascular disease. Endothelin receptor antagonism is effective for the treatment of pulmonary hypertension (64). Blood pressure reduction has been observed during treatment of systemic hypertension with bosentan, an endothelin antagonist (65). Natriuretic

peptides, originating in cardiac tissue and from other sources, have been characterized. Potentiation of the natriuretic peptides through inhibition of their metabolizing endopeptidases has been explored as a treatment for hypertension, when combined with ACE inhibition and is highly effective (66). However, the first drug with these combined actions to be assessed in clinic trials, omapatrilat, has been found to have excessive adverse effects (angioneurotic edema) and was not approved for release by regulatory agencies (67,68).

X. NEW TECHNOLOGIES FOR MEASURING BLOOD PRESSURE

Most physicians rely on the measurement of arterial pressure made with equipment and methods that have barely changed since the first part of the 20th century, when the insights provided by Riva-Rocci and Korotkoff led to the use of the mercury manometer and stethoscope (69). In the 1940s, Ayman and Goldshine suggested that measurements of blood pressure at home might be valuable for assessment of patients. It remained for Perloff et al. (70) (Fig. 1.4) to develop a wearable recording device for reliable measurement of ambulatory blood pressure during the day. A prospective survey using this device demonstrated that daytime average ambulatory blood pressures were superior to clinic pressures for prediction of future cardiovascular disease.

Fully automated devices for measuring blood pressure throughout the entire day were developed by the 1980s. The use of these devices characterized patterns of blood pressure in relation to usual activities such as sleep, exercise, or work (71) (Fig. 1.5). It was shown that the presence of a doctor, by itself, could temporarily raise blood pressure, either in the hospital or in a clinic (72,73).

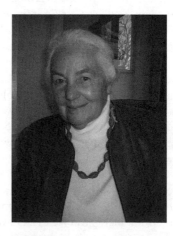

Figure 1.4 Dorothy Perloff, pioneer in the study of ambulatory blood pressure measurement and its importance in the diagnosis of hypertension.

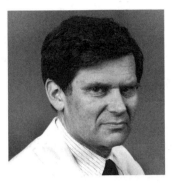

Figure 1.5 Dr. Pickering and his colleagues extended and expanded the foundation set by Dr. Perloff for the importance of 24 h ambulatory blood pressure and home blood pressure. His extensive investigations and presentations led to the widespread recognition of White Coat Hypertension and the value of average daily pressure for prognosis and treatment.

Groups of patients who had hypertension in the clinic but normal pressures at home or during their usual activities were identified; this is now called *white coat* hypertension (74). In general, those with white coat hypertension (also called isolated "office hypertension" or "clinic hypertension") were found to have less target organ damage, particularly less left ventricular hypertrophy, than those with established hypertension. Additional prospective studies have been conducted which confirm Perloff's original observation that ambulatory blood pressure measurements are superior to clinic blood pressure measurements for predicting future cardiovascular disease (75,76). As ambulatory monitoring becomes more available for clinical application, it may become the gold standard for the diagnosis of hypertension.

XI. CONCLUSIONS

The history of hypertension as a clinical entity and as a cardiovascular risk factor is an example of one of the success stories of modern medicine and demonstrates that the arduous clinical research of initial description with the unraveling of the pathology and mechanisms can lead to beneficial therapy, provided there is also the development of suitable, effective, and safe therapy. For hypertension, progress in pharmacology coupled with the conduct of randomized clinical trials has achieved an astonishingly consistent record of benefit. The continuing science of hypertension has advanced to new phases with the exploration of better methodologies for measuring blood pressure itself and the definition of new patterns that vary from descriptive phenotypes to genetic disorders, defined at the level of specific mutations. There is reason to be optimistic about the future for hypertension as the

lessons of the trials are translated into more widespread and appropriate treatment and the current basic science relevant to this field is, in time, translated into better care for the very large number of those with high blood pressure.

REFERENCES

1. Pickering G. Systemic arterial hypertension. In: Fishman AP, Richards DW, eds. Circulation of the Blood: Men and Ideas. New York: Oxford University Press, 1964:487–541.
2. Pickering G. The Nature of Essential Hypertension. New York: Grune and Stratton, 1961.
3. Postel-Vinay N, ed. A Century of Arterial Hypertension 1896–1996. New York: John Wiley & Sons/IMOTHEP, 1996.
4. Messerli FH. This day 50 years ago. N Engl J Med 1995; 332:1038–1039.
5. Berliner RW, Bricker NS, Gifford RW Jr, Hoobler SW, Kincaid-Smith P, Maxwell M, McCormack LJ, Meaney TF, Shapiro AP, Dustan HP. Renal arterial stenosis and parenchymal diseases. In: Page IH, McCubbin JW, eds. Renal Hypertension. Chicago: Year Book Medical Publishers, 1968:306–349.
6. Veterans Administration Cooperative Study Group on Antihypertensive Agents. Effects of treatment on morbidity in hypertension: results in patients with diastolic blood pressures averaging 115 through 129 mmHg. JAMA 1967; 202:1028–1034.
7. Veterans Administration Cooperative Study Group on Antihypertensive Agents. Effects of treatment on morbidity in hypertension: II. Results in patients with diastolic blood pressure averaging 90 through 114 mmHg. JAMA 1970; 213:1143–1152.
8. Veterans Administration Cooperative Study Group on Antihypertensive Agents. Effects of treatment on morbidity in hypertension: III. Influence of age, diastolic pressure, and prior cardiovascular disease; further analysis of side effects. JAMA 1972; 45:991–1004.
9. Smith WMcF. Treatment of mild hypertension: results of a ten-year intervention trial. Circ Res 1977; 40:I98–I105.
10. Hypertension Detection and Follow-up Program. Cooperative Group. Five-year findings of the hypertension detection and follow-up program: I. Reduction in mortality of persons with high blood pressure, including mild hypertension. JAMA 1979; 242:2562–2571.
11. Helgeland A. Treatment of mild hypertension: a five year controlled drug trial. Am J Med 1980; 69:725–732.
12. Amery A, Birkenhager W, Brixko P, Bulpitt C, Clement D, Deruyttere M, deSchaepdryver A, Dollery C, Fagard R, Forette F, Forte J, Hamdy R, Henry JF, Joossens JV, Leonetti G, Lund-Johansen P, O'Malley K, Petrie J, Strasser T, Tuomilehto J, Williams B. Mortality and morbidity results from the European Working Party on High Blood Pressure in the Elderly Trial. Lancet 1985; 1:1349–1354.

13. Medical Research Council Working Party. MRC trial of treatment of mild hypertension: principal results. BMJ 1985; 291:97–104.

14. Report by the Management Committee. The Australian therapeutic trial in mild hypertension. Lancet 1980; 1:1261–1267.

15. Hypertension Detection and Follow-up Program Cooperative Group. Blood pressure studies in 14 communities: a two-stage screen of hypertension. JAMA 1977; 237:2385–2391.

16. Hypertension Detection and Follow-up Program Cooperative Group. The effect of treatment on mortality in "mild" hypertension: results of the Hypertension Detection and Follow-up Program. New Engl J Med 1982; 307:976–980.

17. Collins R, Peto R, MacMahon S, Hebert P, Fiebach NH, Eberlein KA, Godwin J, Qizilbash N, Taylor JO, Hennekens CH. Blood pressure, stroke, and coronary heart disease. Part 2, short-term reductions in blood pressure: overview of randomized drug trials in their epidemiological context. Lancet 1990; 335:827–838.

18. Lichtenstein MJ, Shipley MJ, Rose G. Systolic and diastolic blood pressure as predictors of coronary heart mortality in the Whitehall study. BMJ 1985; 291:243–245.

19. Rabkin SW, Matthewson AL, Tate RB. Predicting risk of ischemic heart disease and cerebrovascular disease from systolic and diastolic blood pressures. Ann Int Med 1978; 88:342–345.

20. Castelli WP. Epidemiology of coronary heart disease: the Framingham study. Am J Med 1984; 76:4–12.

21. SHEP Cooperative Research Group. Prevention of stroke by antihypertensive drug treatment in older persons with isolated systolic hypertension: final results of the Systolic Hypertension in the Elderly Program SHEP. JAMA 1991; 265:3255–3264.

22. Staessen JA, Fagard R, Thijs L, Celis H, Arabidze G, Birkenhager WH, Bulpitt CJ, de Leeuw PW, Dollery CT, Fletcher AE, Forette F, Leonetti G, Nachev C, O'Brien ET, Rosenfeld J, Rodicio JL, Tuomilehto J, Zanchetti A, and for the Systolic Hypertension in Europe (Sys-Eur) Trial Investigators: randomized double-blind comparison of placebo and active treatment for older patients with isolated systolic hypertension. Lancet 1997; 350:757–764.

23. Staessen J, Gasowski J, Wang JG, Thijs L, Hond ED, Boissel JP, Coope J, Ekbom T, Gueyffier F, Liu L, Kerlikowske K, Pocock S, Fagard R. Risks of untreated and treated isolated systolic hypertension in the elderly: meta-analysis of outcome trials. Lancet 2000; 355:865–872.

24. Kostis JB, Davis BR, Cutler J, Grimm R, Berge KG, Cohen JD, Lacy CR, Perry HM Jr, Blaufox MD, Wassertheil-Smoller S, Black HR, Schron E, Berkson DM, Curb JD, Smith M, McDonald R, Applegate WB, and for the SHEP Cooperative Research Group. Prevention of heart failure by antihypertensive drug treatment in older persons with isolated systolic hypertension. JAMA 1997; 278:212–216.

25. Alderman MH. Blood pressure management: individualized treatment based on absolute risk and the potential for benefit. Ann Intern Med 1993; 119:329–335.

26. Ferruci L, Furberg CD, Penninx BWJH, Di Bari M, Williamson JD, Guralnick JM, Chen JG, Applegate WB, Pahor M. Treatment of isolated systolic hypertension is most effective in older patients with high-risk profile. Circulation 2001; 104:1923–1926.

27. MacMahon S, Neal B, Rodgers A. Blood pressure lowering for the primary and secondary prevention of coronary and cerebrovascular disease. Schweiz Med Wochenschr 1995; 125:2479–2486.

28. Cook RJ, Sackett DL. The number needed to treat: a clinically useful measure of treatment effect. BMJ 1995; 310:452–454.

29. Wilhelmsen L, Berglund G, Elmfeldt D, Fitzsimons T, Holzgreve H, Hosie J, Hornkvist P-E, Pennert K, Tuomilehto J, Wedel H. Beta-blockers versus diuretics in hypertensive men: main results from the HAPPHY trial. J Hypertens 1987; 5:561–572.

30. Psaty BM, Koepsell TD, LoGerfo JP, Wagner EH, Inui TS. Beta-blockers and primary prevention of coronary heart disease in patients with hypertension. JAMA 1989; 261:2087–2094.

31. Wikstrand J, Warnold I, Tuomilehto J, Olsson G, Barber HJ, Eliasson K, Elmfeldt D, Jastrup B, Karatzas NB, Leer J, Marchetta F, Ragnarsson J, Robitaille N-M, Valkova L, Wesseling H, Berglund G. Metoprolol versus thiazide diuretics in hypertension. Hypertension 1991; 17:579–588.

32. Messerli FH, Grossman E, Goldbourt U. Are beta-blockers efficacious as first-line therapy for hypertension in the elderly? A systematic review. JAMA 1998; 279:1903–1907.

33. Brunner HR, Laragh JH, Baer L et al. Essential hypertension: renin, and aldosterone, heart attack and stroke. New Engl J Med 1972; 286:441–449.

34. Alderman MH, Madhavan S, Ooi WL, Cohen H, Sealey JE, Laragh JH. Association of the renin–sodium profile with the risk of myocardial infarction in patients with hypertension. New Engl J Med 1991; 324:1098–1104.

35. Tifft CP, Gavras H, Kershaw GR, Gavras I, Brunner HR, Liang C-S, Chobanian AV. Converting enzyme inhibition in hypertensive emergencies. Ann Int Med 1979; 90:43–46.

36. The CONSENSUS Trial Study Group. Effects of enalapril on mortality in severe congestive heart failure: results of the Cooperative North Scandinavian Enalapril Survival Study (CONSENSUS). New Engl J Med 1987; 316:1429–1435.

37. Pfeffer MA, Braunwald E, Moye LA, Basta L, Brown EJ Jr, Cuddy TE, Davis BR, Geltman EM, Goldman S, Flaker GC, Klein M, Lamas GA, Packer M, Rouleau J, Rouleau JL, Rutherford J, Wertheimer JH, Hawkins CM, and SAVE Investigators. Effect of captopril on mortality and morbidity in patients with left ventricular dysfunction after myocardial infarction: results of the survival and ventricular enlargement trial. New Engl J Med 1992; 327:669–677.

38. Lewis EJ, Hunsicker LG, Bain RP, Rohde RD, and for the Collaborative Study Group. The effect of angiotensin-converting-enzyme inhibition on diabetic nephropathy. New Engl J Med 1993; 329:1456–1462.

39. Lewis EJ, Hunsicker LG, Clarke WR, Berl T, Pohl M, Lewis JB, Ritz E, Atkins RC, Rohde RD, Raz I, and for the Collaborative Study Group. Renoprotective effect of

the angiotensin-receptor antagonist irbesartan in patients with nephropathy due to type-2 diabetes. N Engl J Med 2001; 345:851–860.

40. Brenner BM, Cooper ME, de Zeeuw D, Keane WF, Mitch WE, Parving H-H, Remuzzi G, Snapinn SM, Zhang Z, Shahinfar S, and for the REENAL Study Investigators. Effects of losartan on renal and cardiovascular outcomes in patients with type-2 diabetes and nephropathy. N Engl J Med 2001; 345:861–869.

41. Parving H-H, Lehnert H, Brochner-Mortensen J, Gomis R, Andersen S, Arner P, and for the Irbesartan in Patients with Type-2 Diabetes and Microalbuminuria Study Group. The effect of irbesartan on the development of diabetic nephropathy in patients with type-2 diabetes. N Engl J Med 2001; 345:870–878.

42. Berl T, Hunsicker LG, Lewis JB, Pfeffer MA, Porush JG, Rouleau J-L, Drury PL, Esmatjes E, Hricik D, Parikh CR, Raz I, Vanhille P, Wiegmann TB, Wolfe BM, Locatelli F, Goldhaber SZ, Lewis EJ, and for the Collaborative Study Group. Cardiovascular outcomes in the irbesartan diabetic nephropathy trial of patients with type-2 diabetes and overt nephropathy. Ann Intern Med 2003; 138:542–549.

43. Pfeffer MA, Swedberg K, Granger CB, Held P, McMurray JJV, Michelson EL, Olofsson B, Ostergren J, Yusuf S, and for the CHARM Investigators and Committees. Effects of candesartan on mortality and morbidity in patients with chronic heart failure: the CHARM-Overall programme. Lancet 2003; 362:759–766.

44. Hansson L, Zanchetti A, Carruthers G, Dahlof B, Elmfeldt D, Julius S, Menard J, Rahn KH, Wedel H, Westerling S, and for the Hot Study Group. Effects of intensive blood-pressure lowering and low-dose aspirin in patients with hypertension: principal results of the Hypertension Optimal Treatment (HOT) randomized trial. Lancet 1998; 351:1755–1762.

45. Hansson L, Hedner T, Lund-Johansen P, Kjeldsen SE, Lindholm LH, Syvertsen J-O, Lanke J, de Faire U, Dahlof B, Karlberg BE, and for the NORDIL Study Group. Randomized trial of effects of calcium antagonists compared with diuretics and β-blockers on cardiovascular morbidity and mortality in hypertension: the Nordic Diltiazem (NORDIL) Study. Lancet 2000; 356:359–365.

46. Brown MJ, Palmer CR, Castaigne A, de Leeuw P, Mancia G, Rosenthal T, Ruilope LM. Morbidity and mortality in patients randomised to double-blind treatment with a long-acting calcium-channel blocker or diuretic in the International Nifedipine GITS study: Intervention as a Goal in Hypertension Treatment (INSIGHT). Lancet 2000; 356:366–372.

47. Dahlof B, Devereux RB, Kjeldsen SE, Julius S, Beevers G, de Faire U, Fyhrquist F, Ibsen H, Kristiansson K, Lederballe-Pedersen O, Lindholm LH, Nieminen MS, Omvik P, Oparil S, Wedel H, and for the LIFE study group. Cardiovascular morbidity and mortality in the Losartan Intervention For Endpoint reduction in hypertension (LIFE): a randomised trial against atenolol. Lancet 2002; 359:995–1003.

48. Wing LMH, Reid CM, Ryan P, Beilin LJ, Brown MA, Jennings GLR, Johnston C, McNeil JJ, Macdonald G, Marley JE, Morgan TO, West MJ, and for the Second Australian National Blood Pressure Study Group. A comparison of outcomes with angiotensin-converting enzyme inhibitors and diuretics for hypertension in the elderly. N Engl J Med 2003; 348:583–592.

49. The European trial on reduction of cardiac events with Perindopril in stable Coronary Artery Disease Investigators. Efficacy of perindopril in reduction of cardiovascular events among patients with stable coronary disease: randomised, double-blind, placebo-controlled, multicentre trial (the EUROPA study). Lancet 2003; 362:788.

50. The Heart Outcomes Prevention Evaluation Study Investigators. Effects of an angiotensin-converting-enzyme inhibitor, ramipril, on death from cardiovascular causes, myocardial infarction, and stroke in high-risk patients. N Engl J Med 2000; 342:145–153.

51. The ALLHAT Officers and Coordinators for the ALLHAT Collaborative Research Group. Major outcomes in high-risk hypertensive patients randomized to angiotensin-converting enzyme inhibitor or calcium channel blocker vs diuretic. The Antihypertensive and Lipid-Lowering Treatment to Prevent Heart Attack Trial (ALLHAT). JAMA 2002; 288:2981–2997.

52. Furberg CD, Psaty BM, Pahor M, Alderman MH. Clinical implications of recent findings from the Antihypertensive and Lipid-Lowering Treatment to Prevent Heart Attack Trial (ALLHAT) and other studies of hypertension. Ann Intern Med 2002; 135:1074–1078.

53. Psaty BM, Lumley T, Furberg CD, Schellenbaum G, Pahor M, Alderman MH, Weiss NS. Health outcomes associated with various antihypertensive therapies used as first line agents: a network meta-analysis. JAMA 2003; 289:2534–2544.

54. Staessen JA, Wang J-G, Thijs L. Cardiovascular prevention and blood pressure reduction: a quantitative overview updated until March 2003. J Hypertens 2003; 21:1055–1076.

55. Reaven GM, Lithell H, Landsberg L. Hypertension and associated metabolic abnormalities—the role of insulin resistance and the sympathoadrenal system. New Engl J Med 1997; 334:374–381.

56. Lakka HM, Laaksonen DE, Lakka TA, Niskanen LK, Kumpusalo E, Tuomilehto J, Salonen JT. The metabolic syndrome and total and cardiovascular disease mortality in middle-aged men. JAMA 2002; 288:2709–2716

57. Meigs JB. The metabolic syndrome. BMJ 2003; 327:61–62.

58. Nieto FJ, Young TB, Lind BK, Shahar E, Samet J, Redline S, D'Agostino RB, Newman AB, Lebowitz MD, Pickering TG, and for the Sleep Hearth Health Study. Association of sleep-disordered breathing, sleep apnea, and hypertension in a large community-based study. JAMA 2000; 284:1829–1836.

59. Egan BM. Insulin resistance and the sympathetic nervous system. Curr Hypertens Rep 2003; 5:247–254.

60. Lifton RP, Dluhy RG, Powers M, Rich GM, Cook S, Ulick S, Lalouel J-M. A chimaeric 11 beta-hydroxylase/aldosterone synthase gene causes glucocorticoid-remediable aldosteronism and human hypertension. Nature 1992; 355:262–265.

61. Karet FE, Lifton RP. Mutations contributing to human blood pressure variation. Recent Prog Horm Res 1997; 52:263–276.

62. Baker EH, Duggal A, Dong Y, Ireson NJ, Wood M, Markandu ND, MacGregor GA. Amiloride, a specific drug for hypertension in black people with T594M variant. Hypertension 2002; 40:13–17.

63. Wilson FH, Disse-Nicodeme S, Choat KA, Ishikawa K, Nelson-Williams C, Desitter I, Gunel M, Milford DV, Lipkin GW, Achard J-M, Feeley MP, Dussol B, Berland Y, Unwin RJ, Mayan H, Simon DB, Farfel Z, Jeunemaitre X, Lifton RP. Human hypertension caused by mutations in WNK kinases. Science 2001; 293:1107–1112.

64. Rich S, McLaughlin VV. Endothelin receptor blockers in cardiovascular disease. Circulation 2003; 108:2184–2190.

65. Krum H, Viskoper R, Lacourciere Y, Budde M, Charlon V, and for the Bosentan Hypertension Investigators. The effect of an endothelin-receptor antagonist, bosentan, on blood pressure in patients with essential hypertension. N Engl J Med 1998; 338:784–790.

66. Kostis JB, Cobbe S, Johnston C, Ford I, Murphy M, Weber MA, Black HR, Plouin PF, Levy D, Mancia G, Larochelle P, Kolloch RE, Alderman M, Ruilope LM, Dahlof B, Flack JM, Wolf R. Design of the Omapatrilat in Persons with Enhanced Risk of Atherosclerotic events (OPERA) trial. Am J Hypertens 2002; 15:193–198.

67. Company News. Bristol-Myers drug rejected by government panel. New York Times, 20 July 2002, 3.

68. Coats AJ. Omapatrilat—the story of Overture and Octave. Int J Cardiol 2002; 86:1–4.

69. Postel-Vinay N, ed. Measuring blood pressure. A Century of Arterial Hypertension. New York: John Wiley & Sons/ IMOTHP, 1996:15–30.

70. Perloff D, Sokolow M, Cowan R. The prognostic value of ambulatory blood pressures. JAMA 1983; 249:2792–2798.

71. Pickering TG, Harshfield GA, Kleinert HD, Blank S, Laragh JH. Blood pressure during normal daily activities, sleep, and exercise. JAMA 1982; 247:992–996.

72. Simons RJ, Baily RG, Zelis R, Zwillich CW. The physiologic and psychologic effects of the bedside presentation. New Engl J Med 1989; 321:1273–1275.

73. Mancia G, Bertinieri G, Grassi G, Pomidossi G, Ferrari A, Gregorini L, Zanchetti A. Effects of blood pressure measurement by the doctor on patient's blood pressure and heart rate. Lancet 1983; 2:695–698.

74. Pickering TG, James GD, Boddie C, Harshfield GA, Blank S, Laragh JH. How common is white coat hypertension? JAMA 1988; 259:225–228.

75. Verdecchia P, Porcellati C, Schillaci G, Borgioni C, Ciucci A, Battistelli M, Guerrieri M, Gatteschi C, Zampi I, Santucci A, Santucci C, Reboldi G. Ambulatory blood pressure: an independent predictor of prognosis in essential hypertension. Hypertension 1994; 24:793–801.

76. Clement D, De Buyzere M, De Bacqer DA, de Leeuw PW, Duprez DA, Fagard RH, Gheeraert PJ, Missault LH, Braun JJ, Six RO, Van der Niepen P, O'Brien E, and for the Office versus Ambulatory Pressure Study Investigators. Prognostic value of ambulatory blood-pressure recordings in patients with treated hypertension. N Engl J Med 2003; 348:2407–2415.

77. Oates JA. Antihypertensive agents and the drug therapy of hypertension. In: Hardman JG, Limbird LE, Gilman AG, eds. Goodman and Gilman's The Pharmacological Basis of Therapeutics. New York: McGraw Hill, 1996: 780–808.

2

Definition and Classification of Hypertension

GIUSEPPE MANCIA, GUIDO GRASSI

Università Milano-Bicocca, Ospedale San Gerardo, Monza (Milano), Centro Interuniversitario di Fisiologia Clinica e Ipertensione, Milano, Italy

KEYPOINTS

- Operational definition of hypertension is based on values indicated by Guidelines.
- Differences exist between European and American Guidelines on blood pressure normality and abnormality.
- Classification of hypertension is based on disease evaluation, magnitude of blood pressure increase as well as on etiology.
- An useful classification based on evaluation of global cardiovascular risk is that proposed by the European Society of Hypertension/European Society of Cardiology Guidelines on hypertension.

SUMMARY

This chapter will provide conceptual as well as practical definitions of hypertension, the latter being based on the 2003 Guidelines on diagnosis and treatment of the hypertension issued by European and American Institutions. A further issue addressed in the present chapter is represented by the classification of the hypertensive state, with particular emphasis on the methodologies employed to evaluate blood pressure values as well as on the assessment of the overall cardiovascular risk profile.

I. INTRODUCTION

The purpose of this chapter is to describe the classification of hypertension according to a number of different parameters, which include not only the primary hemodynamic variable on which the definition of the disease itself is based (i.e., blood pressure values), but also concomitant risk factors and the overall risk profile of the patient. Particular emphasis is given to the classifications that are proposed by various international scientific organizations, as well as to a more practical definition that is based on different approaches for assessing clinical and ambulatory blood pressures.

II. DEVELOPING A DEFINITION

Arterial hypertension is an example of a medical concept that is more difficult to define than might be assumed at first glance. From a purely semantic point of view, the definition of hypertension can be stated as either the pathological condition (the so-called *conceptual definition*) or a numerical entity (the *operational definition*).

A. Conceptual Definition

Because the clinical evidence shows a continuous relationship between blood pressure level and cardiovascular risk, the definition of hypertension still remains largely arbitrary. About 30 years ago, Sir George Pickering viewed arterial hypertension as a quantitative disease and related blood pressure values to mortality (1). Although many have attempted to numerically define this quantitative threshold, the real threshold level for hypertension is flexible, depending in large part on the total cardiovascular risk profile of an individual subject. Rose (2) has probably provided the best definition of hypertension as "the level of blood pressure at which the benefits of action (i.e., therapeutic intervention) exceed those of inaction."

B. Operational Definition

Operationally, the time-honored blood pressure values that identify hypertensive individuals are a systolic blood pressure of ≥140 mmHg or a diastolic blood pressure of ≥90 mmHg—values that are associated with an approximate doubling of cardiovascular risk, as compared to the values that characterize the normotensive state. Except for very high blood pressure values or the presence of cardiovascular disease and organ damage, these systolic and diastolic values must be confirmed by sphygmomanometric (clinical) blood pressure measurements made over a period of several weeks.

C. Definition of Hypertension: 2003 Guidelines

Recently, several sets of guidelines have been proposed by different professional organizations for defining hypertension. One updated definition of hypertension is proposed in the 2003 Guidelines of the European Society of Hypertension/European Society of Cardiology (3) (see Table 2.1).

These guidelines consider a patient as hypertensive when either the systolic or the diastolic blood pressure value is ≥140/90 mmHg upon repeated sphygmomanometric measurements in the physician's office. The guidelines also identify different categories of risk on the basis of the magnitude of blood pressure elevation. A patient is placed in a higher category whenever the patient's systolic and diastolic blood pressure values fall within different ranges. Guidelines were also established for classifying patients within the normotensive range according to the relationship between observed "normotensive" blood pressure values and cardiovascular risk. In addition, a separate classification was established for isolated systolic hypertension, which is defined as the concomitant presence of a systolic blood pressure of ≥140 mmHg and a diastolic blood pressure of <90 mmHg (3). Then a separate definition of hypertension also was established for children, where high blood pressure is defined as values equal to or greater than the values that correspond to the 95th percentile for that age (4) and borderline high blood pressure is identified by values between the 90th and the 94th percentile for that age (Table 2.2).

Table 2.1 ESH/ESC Definition and Classification of Normotension and Hypertension

Category	Systolic blood pressure (mmHg)	Diastolic blood pressure (mmHg)
Optimal	<120	<80
Normal	120–129	80–84
High normal	130–139	85–89
Grade 1 hypertension (mild)	140–159	90–99
Grade 2 hypertension (moderate)	160–179	100–109
Grade 3 hypertension (severe)	≥180	≥110
Isolated systolic hypertension	≥140	<90

Note: ESH/ESC, European Society of Hypertension/European Society of Cardiology.

Table 2.2 Definition of Hypertension in Children and Adolescents

Age	Normotension (systolic/ diastolic pressure in mmHg)	Borderline hypertension (systolic/ diastolic pressure in mmHg)	Defined hypertension (systolic/ diastolic pressure in mmHg)
<2 years	<104/70	<111/73	>112/74
3–5 years	<108/70	<115/75	>116/76
6–9 years	<114/74	<121/77	>122/78
10–12 years	<122/78	<125/81	>126/82
13–15 years	<130/80	<135/85	>136/86
16–18 years	<136/84	<139/89	>140/90

A second definition of hypertension also has been addressed by guidelines issued in the 7th Report of the Joint National Committee (5), which consistently differs from earlier guidelines and also differs from the 2003 Guidelines of the European Society of Hypertension/ European Society of Cardiology (3). One of the differences is the creation of a single category that encompasses blood pressure values that were previously defined as "normal" or "high normal". This category is called "prehypertension" and has a specific indication for nonpharmacological treatment. This new category has been criticized because defining an individual as prehypertensive may cause anxiety in that individual, thus favoring a further blood pressure rise. In addition, nonpharmacological interventions, such as those suggested in the case of the "prehypertensive state," have a relevant economic impact; engaging in physical training programs, adopting hypocaloric diets, and eating low-salt food have associated economic costs just as drug treatments do.

The definitions of hypertension proposed by the 2003 European Guidelines (3) and the 7th Report of the Joint National Committee (5) incorporate aspects of disease characterization that are not previously defined. One is the classification of patients into different categories at blood pressure values <140/90 mmHg, which is based on the continuous relationship to cardiovascular risk in the normotensive range, in addition to the classification of patients with blood pressures of 120–139 mmHg systolic or 80–89 mmHg diastolic (1), who upon reaching middle age, have a high risk of becoming hypertensive in their remaining lifetimes.

The second is the reference to a particular form of hypertension that is characterized by measured blood pressure elevations of ≥140/90 mmHg in the doctor's office and measured normal blood pressure values at home over 24 h (the so-called "white coat" hypertension) (6). Although the significance of this phenomenon is still controversial, it is likely that white-coat hypertension is

not entirely without pathological significance because of the evidence of its association with an increased prevalence of left ventricular hypertrophy, renal and vascular damage, and metabolic abnormalities (3,6). Thus, in the population of patients identified with this phenomenon, the recommendations are that once diagnosed, these patients be monitored closely. This way, treatment can be initiated when a patient's blood pressure values also reach hypertensive levels outside the physician's office. However, if there is evidence of organ damage or other cardiovascular risk factors, drug treatment should be implemented right away.

Other guidelines for the definition, diagnosis, and treatment of hypertension include those issued by the International Society of Hypertension in Blacks (7), the International Forum for Hypertension Control and Prevention in Africa (8), and the World Health Organization (WHO)/International Society of Hypertension (ISH) (9). These WHO/ISH guidelines appear to be more similar to the European than to the American guidelines, at least from the perspective of blood pressure targets, the definition of hypertension, and the assessment of global risk. Other issues that are related to specific sections of the various guidelines are discussed in detail in the relevant chapters of this book.

III. CLASSIFICATION

Classification of hypertension makes it possible to more precisely characterize blood pressure elevation in the individual patient from a clinical standpoint. Several factors are taken into account in classifying an hypertensive condition: the evolution of the disease, the magnitude of the increase in blood pressure values, the etiology of the hypertensive state, and the absolute level of the total cardiovascular risk profile. The total risk profile appears to be the most comprehensive because, as suggested by the European Guidelines (3), it encompasses not only the risk that is associated with blood pressure elevation, but also the risk associated with the negative interactions between hypertension and other factors (e.g., hyperlipidemia, cigarette smoking, obesity).

A. Classification of Hypertension According to Disease Evolution

The evolution of the hypertensive state allows classification of blood pressure elevation as two forms: malignant hypertension and benign hypertension.

1. Malignant Hypertension

Malignant hypertension, which was first described as a separate disease entity about 90 years ago by Volhard and Fahr, is characterized by a very high blood pressure

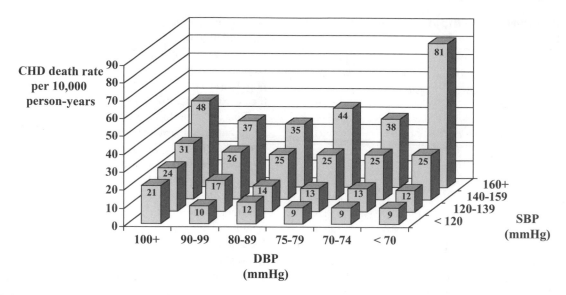

Figure 2.1   Relationship between high blood pressure values and coronary heart disease (CHD) mortality. For systolic blood pressure (SBP), the relationship is closer than for diastolic blood pressure (DBP). [Modified with permission from Kannell et al. (11).]

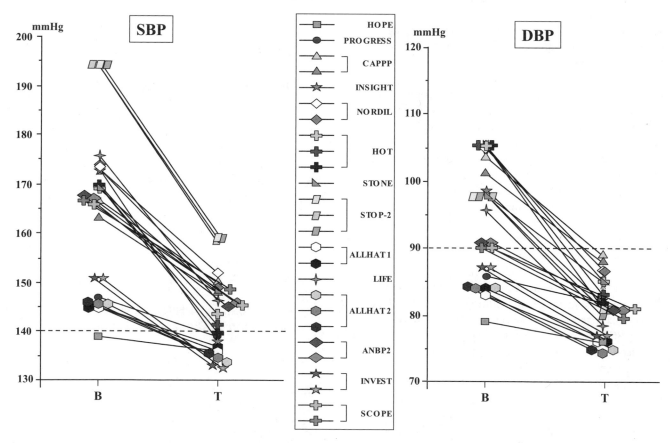

Figure 2.2   Effects of antihypertensive drug treatment on systolic blood pressure and diastolic blood pressure (SBP and DBP, respectively) in clinical trials with essential-hypertensive patients. Blood pressure values at the beginning of the clinical trials (B) and values achieved during treatment (T) are shown for each trial. [Modified with permission from Mancia and Grassi (12).]

elevation (usually $>200/120$ mmHg) that is most often associated with an increase in plasma creatinine levels, renal dysfunction and failure, left ventricular hypertrophy, microangiopathic hemolytic anemia, and neurological manifestations of hypertensive encephalopathy (10). The incidence of new cases of accelerated hypertension has decreased drastically in the past few years, primarily because earlier diagnosis and treatment of the disease prevents blood pressure increases in the vast majority of cases, as well as preventing the clinical manifestations and complications of such an elevation in pressure. The prognosis of malignant hypertension also has improved in the past few years because of the availability of new and effective antihypertensive compounds and the availability of renal dialysis and kidney transplantation.

2. Benign Hypertension

Benign hypertension is a frequently encountered clinical condition that includes hypertensive states in which the magnitude of the blood pressure increase is less marked than the increases that characterize malignant hypertension. Benign hypertension also includes hypertensive states in which there is no evidence of cardiac, renal, or cardiovascular organ damage and no symptoms that are related to an elevation in blood pressure values. The clinical evolution of the latter type of hypertension is usually slower than the evolution of accelerated hypertension, and the long-term prognosis is more benign.

B. Classification of Hypertension According to Blood Pressure Levels

In a comprehensive classification of the hypertensive state that is based on the magnitude of the blood pressure increase, such as that provided in the 2003 Guidelines of the European Society of Hypertension/European Society of Cardiology, one point should be stressed, namely that classification of hypertension according to blood pressure values is no longer based solely on the diastolic component, but also on the systolic blood component. This is in response to clinical evidence that systolic blood pressure values appear to predict the incidence of cardiovascular disease in several conditions more readily than those of diastolic blood pressure (11) (see Fig. 2.1).

Despite the predictive value of these systolic values, control of systolic blood pressure is achieved much less frequently in clinical practice than control of diastolic blood pressure. In a large number of antihypertensive drug trials, systolic blood pressure values remain higher than 140 mmHg in a consistent fraction (75%) of treated hypertensives, even though diastolic blood pressure is reduced by treatment well below 90 mmHg in most instances (12) (see Fig. 2.2). This means that systolic

blood pressure control is difficult to achieve in a hypertensive population and that this population remains at higher risk for cardiovascular events.

The classification of hypertension according to blood pressure levels is based on sphygmomanometric assessment of a patient's blood pressure values. However, despite its time-honored usefulness in clinical practice, the traditional Riva–Rocci–Korotkoff technique has a number of problems, the more clinical relevant being the so-called white coat effect, that is, the "alarm reaction" on the part of the patient, which produces an elevation in blood pressure that results in an overestimation of the patient's actual blood pressure levels (13). This phenomenon has been largely overcome by two approaches that have been adopted successfully in clinical practice, namely, home measurement of blood pressure and monitoring of 24 h ambulatory blood pressure (14,15).

1. Normality of 24 h Ambulatory Blood Pressure Values

Cross-sectional population studies have shown that 24 h ambulatory blood pressure values are usually less than blood pressure values measured in the physician's office. The discrepancy increases with an increase in office-measured

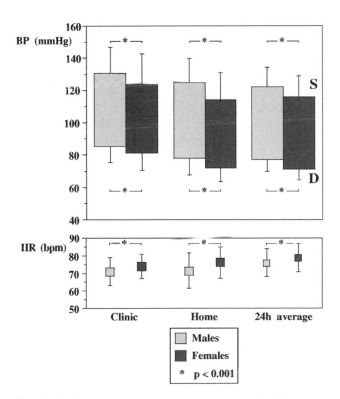

Figure 2.3 Clinic, home, and 24 h ambulatory blood pressure (BP) values in the PAMELA study in males and females. The corresponding heart rate (HR) values are shown in the lower panel. [Modified with permission from Mancia et al. (16).]

Table 2.3 Classification of Secondary Hypertension According to Its Etiology

---

Causes of Secondary Hypertension

Exogenous substance
- Oral contraceptive pills
- Glucocorticoids
- Glycyrrhizinic acid
- Erythropoietin
- Cyclosporine
- Non-steroidal anti-inflammatory drugs
- Acute alcohol

Renal disease
- Renovascular hypertension
- Rrenal parenchimal hypertension

Endocrine disease
- Corticoadrenal hypertension
- Hyperthyroidism and hypothyroidism
- Pheochromocytoma
- Acromegaly

Aortic coarctation

Pregnancy
- Pregnancy-induced hypertension

Neurological disease
- Acute cerebrovascular ischaemia
- Sleep-apnea syndrome
- Guillain-Barré syndrome
- Quadriplegia
- Familial disautonomia

---

values and are a magnitude of several mmHg difference relative to an office measurement of 140/90 mmHg. Although the upper limits of normality have not yet been defined conclusively, an agreement among results of most studies exists, which identifies threshold values of

normality as 125 mmHg for systolic blood pressure and 80 mmHg for diastolic blood pressure, as shown in Fig. 2.3 for the Pressioni Arteriose Monitorate E Loro Associazioni (PAMELA) study (16) and as indicated by the recent European Society of Hypertension/European Society of Cardiology Guidelines for the management of hypertension (3).

2. Normality of Home Blood Pressure Values

The 2003 Guidelines (3) identify the threshold values for definition of hypertension on the basis of blood pressure values as measured by the patient at home. The threshold values are 135/85 mmHg, which correspond to 140/90 mmHg measured in the office or clinic. These numbers are based on data provided by, among others, the PAMELA study (17) (see Fig. 2.3).

C. Classification According to Etiology of Hypertension

In ~90–95% of hypertension cases, the etiological factors that are responsible for the blood pressure increase remain unknown. Secondary forms of hypertension are relatively rare diseases; their prevalence amounts to 5–10% of all cases of hypertension (Table 2.3). A detailed description of the secondary forms of hypertension, including their diagnostic and therapeutic approach, is provided in Part E of this book.

D. Classification According to Global Cardiovascular Risk Profile

Hypertension often is associated with metabolic risk factors. Studies performed in several populations have shown that

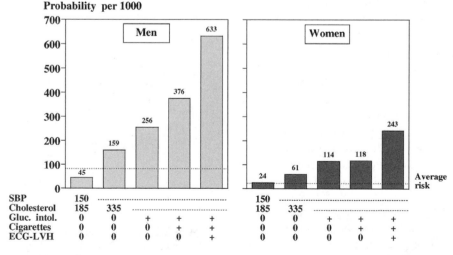

Figure 2.4 Additive (+) effects in males and females of hypertension (SBP), hypercholesterolemia (high cholesterol levels), hyperglycemia (glucose intolerance), cigarette smoking, and left ventricular hypertrophy (ECG-LVH) on cardiovascular risk in the Framingham Study. [Modified with permission from Kannel (18).]

Table 2.4 Blood Pressure Associated with Risk Factors and Disease History

Other risk factors and disease history	Blood pressure (mmHg)				
	Normal	High normal	Grade 1	Grade 2	Grade 3
No other risk factors	Average risk	Average risk	Low added risk	Moderate added risk	High added risk
1–2 risk factors	Low added risk	Low added risk	Moderate added risk	Moderate added risk	Very high added risk
≥3 risk factors, target organ damage, or diabetes	Moderate added risk	High added risk	High added risk	High added risk	Very high added risk
Associated clinical conditions	Very high added risk	Very high added risk	Very high added risk	Very high added risk	Very high added risk

individuals with high blood pressure have a greater prevalence of dyslipidemia, insulin resistance, and diabetes than normotensive individuals (17). This also is the case in individuals who have a high-normal blood pressure as compared to individuals who have normal or optimal blood pressure levels. The association of hypertension with other risk factors markedly increases the absolute risk of a cardiovascular event because individual risk factors interact additively, so that when two or three of these risk factors are present, the total risk is much greater than the sum of the individual contribution (18) (see Fig. 2.4).

This association of hypertension with other risk factors had led to the emphasis in the European Guidelines on the importance of total cardiovascular risk stratification through the approach illustrated in Table 2.4 (3).

It is clear that an individual can be at high risk for a cardiovascular event (≥20% within 10 years) if this individual has a marked elevation in blood pressure. But the patient also may belong to this high-risk category or to the very-high-risk category even when he or she has only a modest elevation in blood pressure, if there also is evidence of three or more other risk factors, diabetes, or subclinical damage and organ damage. A similar classification model exists for subjects in the high-normal blood pressure range. This stratification of risk factors for both groups of patients has a practical value because, as demonstrated by clinical trials, individuals in high-risk or very-high-risk categories do not require only lifestyle changes, but also prompt blood pressure lowering intervention through drug administration (3). They also may require nonhypertension-related intervention, such as the administration of antiplatelet drugs and statins (3).

REFERENCES

1. Pickering G. Hypertension. Definitions, natural histories and consequences. Am J Med 1972; 52:570–583.
2. Evans JG, Rose GA. Hypertension. Brit Med Bull 1971; 27:37–42.
3. Guidelines Committee. 2003 European Society of Hypertension/European Society of Cardiology guidelines for the management of arterial hypertension. J Hypertens 2003; 21:1011–1053.
4. Task Force on Blood Pressure Control in Children. Report of the School Task Force on Blood Pressure Control in Children. Paediatrics 1987; 79:1–25.
5. Chobanian AV, Bakris GL, Black HR, Cushman WC, Green LA, Izzo JL Jr, Jones DW, Materson BJ, Oparil S, Wright JT Jr, Roccella EJ. National Heart, Lung and Blood Institute Joint National Committee on Prevention, Detection, Evaluation and Treatment of High Blood Pressure. National High Blood Pressure Education Program Coordinating Committee, 7th Report. J Am Med Assoc 2003; 289:2560–2571.
6. Pickering TG, Coats A, Mallion JM, Mancia G, Verdecchia P. Task force V. White coat hypertension. Blood Press Monit 1999; 4:333–341.
7. Consensus statement of the hypertension in African Americans Working Group of the International Society of Hypertension in Blacks. Arch Intern Med 2003; 163:525–541.
8. World Health Organization/International Society of Hypertension Writing Group. 2003 World Health Organization (WHO)/International Society of Hypertension (ISH) statement on management of hypertension. J Hypertens 2003; 21:1983–1992.
9. International Forum for Hypertension Control and Prevention in Africa. Recommendations for prevention, diagnosis and management of hypertension and cardiovascular risk factors in sub-saharan Africa. J Hypertens 2003; 21:1993–2000.
10. Seedat YK. Malignant-accelerated hypertension. In: Mancia G, Chalmers J, Julius S, Saruta T, Weber M, Ferrari A, Wilkinson I, eds. Manual of Hypertension. London: Churchill Livingston, 2002: 623–634.
11. Kannell WB, Gordon T, Schwartz MJ. Systolic versus diastolic blood pressure and risk of coronary heart disease. Am J Cardiol 1971; 27:335–346.
12. Mancia G, Grassi G. Systolic and diastolic blood pressure control in antihypertensive drug trials. J Hypertens 2002; 20:1461–1464.
13. Mancia G, Bertinieri G, Grassi G, Parati G, Pomidossi G, Ferrari A, Gregorini L, Zanchetti A. Effects of blood pressure measurement by the doctor on patients' blood pressure and heart rate. Lancet 1983; ii:695–698.

14. Mancia G, Parati G, Omboni S, Ulian L, Zanchetti A. Ambulatory blood pressure monitoring. Clin Exp Hypertens 1999; 21:703–715.

15. Mancia G, Sega R, Grassi G, Cesana G, Zanchetti A. Defining ambulatory and home blood pressure normality. J Hypertens 2001; 19:995–999.

16. Mancia G, Sega R, Bravi C, De Vito G, Valagussa F, Cesana G, Zanchetti A. Ambulatory blood pressure normality: results from the PAMELA Study. J Hypertens 1995; 13:1377–1390.

17. Reaven GM, Lithell H, Landsberg L. Hypertension and associated metabolic abnormalities. New Engl J Med 1996; 334:374–381.

18. Kannel WB. Blood pressure as a cardiovascular risk factor. J Am Med Assoc 1996; 275:1571–1576.

3

Epidemiology of Hypertension

GILBERT R. KAUFMANN
University Hospital Basel, Basel, Switzerland

KEYPOINTS

- Hypertension is a serious health problem that results in major cardiovascular mortality and morbidity. It affects 25–30% of the entire adult population—up to 60–70% of individuals beyond the seventh decade.
- The prevalence of hypertension has declined in the Western world, but it has increased in many developing countries. The reason appears to be a change in life style as well as environmental factors.
- In the last 30 years, the awareness and control of hypertension has improved dramatically in developed countries, reducing cardiovascular complications. In developing countries, the awareness and control of hypertension still remains low.
- Hypertension has not been observed in a few isolated societies. Common to all these populations is the lack of acculturation.
- The prevalence of hypertension is higher in African-Americans and lower in Mexican-Americans when compared with United States residents of Caucasian origin.
- Mean blood pressure and the prevalence of hypertension are higher in men than in women.
- There is a direct relationship between elevations in blood pressure and increasing age of individuals in the population and increases in body weight.

- The influence of menopause, contraceptives, and hormone replacement therapy on blood pressure level remains controversial.
- Dietary factors, such as the intake of salt and unsaturated fats, may increase blood pressure in susceptible individuals.
- Genetic, socioeconomic, and environmental factors may affect blood pressure. For example, blood pressure tends to be higher in low-income earners, in migrants, and in individuals working in stressful environments.
- Hypertension causes end-organ damage, including left ventricular hypertrophy, congestive heart disease, coronary heart failure, stroke, renal failure, and peripheral arterial disease.
- The improved recognition and therapy of hypertension has led to a decline in cardiovascular mortality and morbidity. However, end-stage renal disease has increased in recent years.

SUMMARY

Hypertension is a serious health problem that results in major mortality and morbidity. It accounts for 6% of adult deaths worldwide. The current definition of hypertension is based on the increased risk of cardiovascular events above a certain threshold of blood pressure, but the dividing line between normal blood pressure and hypertension cannot be determined exactly and remains arbitrary. In developed countries, the prevalence of hypertension increases with age and affects 25–30% of the entire adult population—up to 60–70% of individuals beyond the seventh decade. The prevalence is higher in Europe than in North America, and, although it declined continuously between 1974 and 1991, it appears to have risen slightly since 1991. In developing countries, the prevalence of hypertension is lower, but is increasing parallel to environmental and social changes during the process of industrialization. Environmental factors appear to be more important in the development of hypertension than genetic factors. Nevertheless, certain populations, such as African-Americans, show a particularly high prevalence of hypertension. In addition, a higher prevalence of hypertension is generally found in men, in the elderly, and in obese individuals. Uncontrolled hypertension is closely associated with end-organ diseases, including coronary heart disease, congestive heart disease, left ventricular hypertrophy, stroke, renal failure, and peripheral arterial disease. Elevated systolic blood pressure and diastolic blood pressure, as well as pulse pressure, are predictors of end-organ disease. The improved recognition of hypertension has led to major reductions in cardiovascular disease. The incidence of coronary heart disease and stroke has declined with improved awareness, therapy, and control of hypertension, whereas the rate of end-stage renal disease has increased.

I. INTRODUCTION

Hypertension accounts for 6% of adult deaths worldwide and is found in all human populations, except for a minority of individuals living in isolated societies. In developed countries, the prevalence of hypertension rises with age and affects 25–30% of the entire adult population, reaching up to 60–70% of individuals beyond the seventh decade. The cardiovascular risk increases according to the level of hypertension; however, there is no clear-cut threshold above which the risk of cardiovascular disease suddenly increases (1,2). The dividing line between normal blood pressure and hypertension is therefore arbitrary, particularly because the majority of complications occur in persons with moderately elevated blood pressure (3). The current definition of hypertension adopts a blood pressure threshold of 140/90 mmHg. In patients with diabetes mellitus and chronic renal disease, a blood pressure below the threshold of 130/80 mmHg is the preferred goal (4). The improved recognition of hypertension has led to major reductions in cardiovascular disease (5). But despite this, hypertension remains a serious problem, resulting in major mortality and morbidity in developed countries, and it appears to be emerging as a major health threat in the developing world (6).

II. HYPERTENSION IN WESTERNIZED SOCIETIES

The incidence of hypertension is typically <1–2% in the first three decades of life and increases to 4–8% during the sixth and seventh decade (7–11). The prevalence of hypertension is difficult to determine in a standardized manner in population surveys. Accuracy depends on the measurement device that is used, the extent of training of survey personnel, and a variety of other factors that may potentially lead to random or even systematic errors. Nevertheless, the prevalence of hypertension has been studied in a large number of countries and in different geographic and regional areas (Table 3.1).

In the USA, a valuable source of epidemiological data originates from the National Health and Nutrition Examination Survey (NHANES) surveys that evaluate the prevalence of hypertension in regular time intervals. Another important source of data is the Framingham Heart Study that enrolled 4962 individuals between 1990 and 1995 (12,13). Other large epidemiologic studies that have provided important information include the Hypertension

Table 3.1 Prevalence of Hypertension in Persons 35–64 Years in Age, Stratified According to Country and Gender

Country	Prevalence in general population (%)	Prevalence in men (%)	Prevalence in women (%)	Hypertensive persons taking medication (%)	Body mass index
USA	27.8	29.8	25.8	52.5	27.4
Canada	27.4	31.0	23.8	36.3	26.8
Italy	37.7	44.8	30.6	32.0	26.4
Sweden	38.4	44.8	32.0	26.2	26.5
England	41.7	46.9	36.5	24.8	27.1
Spain	46.8	49.0	44.6	26.8	27.4
Finland	48.7	55.7	41.6	25.0	27.1
Germany	55.3	60.2	50.3	26.0	27.3

Source: Adapted from Wolf-Maier et al. (18).

Detection and Follow-up Program (HDFP), the Multiple Risk Factor Intervention Trial (MRFIT), the World Health Organization MONItoring CArdiovascular disease (WHO MONICA) study, and others (14–16).

In the Framingham study, data on Framingham residents 28–68 years in age was prospectively collected every 2 years, and in the case of the Framingham Offspring study, every 4 years. Blood pressure was optimal or normal (<130/85 mmHg) in 43.7% of the subjects and high normal (131–139/86–89 mmHg) in 13.4% of the subjects. Stage 1 hypertension (140–159/90–99 mmHg) was found in 12.9% of the subjects, and stage 2 hypertension or greater (≥160/100 mmHg) was found in 30% of the subjects (17).

A sample survey of six European countries in the 1990s evaluated the prevalence of hypertension and observed moderate heterogeneity of systolic blood pressure (Table 3.1). The highest age- and gender-adjusted prevalence of hypertension in Europe was found in Germany (55%), Finland (49%), Spain (47%), and England (42%) (18). Sweden and Italy both showed a lower prevalence (38%). The rank order of hypertension rates in European countries was similar for men and women. For all age groups, mean systolic blood pressure and diastolic blood pressure were higher in European countries (136/83 mmHg) than in the USA and Canada (127/77 mmHg). Consequently, a higher prevalence of hypertension was noted in Europe (28%) than in the USA and Canada, reaching particularly high levels of 78% in individuals aged 65–74 years in Europe, as compared to 53% in the USA in this age range. The higher mean blood pressure in Europe resulted in a mortality rate from stroke of 41.2/100,000 person-years in comparison to a rate of 27.6/100,000 person-years in the USA.

In the USA, the mean blood pressure and the prevalence of hypertension in adults (>140/90 mmHg) have declined from 29.7% in 1960 to 20.4% in 1991, affecting a slightly greater proportion of men than women (22.8% vs. 18.0%) (12,19). Interestingly, the most recent NHANES survey, which evaluated data from 1999 to 2000, reported a 3.7% average rise of the prevalence of hypertension since 1988 (2.2% for men and 5.6% for women) (20). The reason for this reverse trend remains unclear, but it may be attributed to the continuously increasing body mass index (BMI) in recent years.

A. Awareness, Treatment, and Control of Hypertension

In the most recent NHANES survey in the USA, one-third of all hypertensive individuals were unaware of elevated blood pressure. The level of awareness increased continuously from 51% in 1976–1980 to 70% in 1999–2000 (Table 3.2). The proportion of treated hypertension increased from 31% to 59% and the proportion of controlled hypertension increased from 10% to 34% (4).

Uncontrolled hypertension was more frequently found in women, older patients, and Mexican-Americans (Table 3.3). Of concern was the observation that only 25% of individuals with diabetes reached the preferred blood pressure of 130/85 mmHg.

In Canada, the situation is similar. In a population-based, cross-sectional survey in nine Canadian provinces, 26,293 men and women 18–74 years in age were selected from the health insurance registers from 1986 to 1990 (21). Most individuals had blood pressure measured at least twice. Sixteen percent of men and 13% of women showed a diastolic blood pressure of 90 mmHg or greater. About 26% of these subjects were unaware of their hypertension. Forty-two percent were treated and their condition was controlled; 16% were treated, but the hypertension remained uncontrolled; and 16% were neither treated nor their hypertension controlled. Only 2% had never measured their blood pressure (3% men and 1% women). Young men 18–34 years in age showed the lowest rate (6%) of measurement. In 51% of those who had their blood pressure measured, the last

Table 3.2 Hypertension Awareness, Treatment, and Control in Adults in the United States, 1976–1994

Patient treatment condition	1976–1980 NHANES II (%)	1988–1991 NHANES III (%)	1991–1994 NHANES III (%)	1999–2000 (%)
Hypertension awareness	51	73	68	70
Hypertension treated	31	55	54	59
Hypertension controlled	10	29	27	34

Note: NHANES, National Health and Nutrition Examination Survey; Hypertension controlled, Systolic blood pressure <140 mmHg; diastolic blood pressure <90 mmHg.
Source: Adapted from Chobanian et al. (4).

Table 3.3 Awareness, Treatment, and Control of Hypertension in the United States Population, 1988–2000

Patient characteristics	1988–1991 (% (SE))	1991–1994 (% (SE))	1999–2000 (% (SE))	Change 1988–2000 (% (95% CI))
	Awareness			
Age (years)				
18–39	61.5 (4.5)	49.1 (6.9)	51.8 (5.8)	−9.7 (−24.1–4.7)
40–59	73.2 (2.4)	72.7 (3.3)	73.3 (2.8)	0.1 (−7.1–7.3)
≥60	68.3 (1.3)	69.1 (1.6)	69.8 (1.9)	1.5 (−3.0–6.0)
Gender				
Male	63.2 (2.2)	60.1 (2.9)	66.3 (2.4)	3.1 (−3.3–9.5)
Female	75.1 (1.4)	73.6 (1.5)	71.2 (2.2)	−3.9 (−9.0–1.2)
Race or ethnicity				
Non-Hispanic white	70.6 (1.4)	67.5 (1.8)	69.5 (2.0)	−1.1 (−5.9–3.7)
Non-Hispanic black	73.3 (1.6)	72.6 (1.6)	73.9 (2.7)	0.6 (−5.6–6.8)
Mexican-American	54.4 (2.3)	62.0 (4.0)	57.8 (3.6)	3.4 (−5.0–11.8)
	Treatment			
Age (years)				
18–39	34.1 (5.4)	24.8 (3.5)	27.7 (5.3)	−6.4 (−21.2–8.4)
40–59	53.9 (2.7)	54.2 (2.4)	62.9 (3.1)	9.0 (0.9–17.1)
≥60	55.1 (1.2)	56.7 (1.6)	62.7 (2.0)	7.6 (−4.5–10.3)
Gender				
Male	44.5 (1.9)	42.6 (1.8)	54.3 (2.5)	9.8 (7.2–23.4)
Female	60.1 (1.5)	60.0 (1.5)	62.0 (2.3)	1.9 (−3.5–7.3)
Race or ethnicity				
Non-Hispanic white	53.9 (1.6)	51.9 (1.4)	60.1 (2.1)	6.2 (1.0–11.4)
Non-Hispanic black	55.8 (1.7)	56.4 (2.4)	63.0 (2.9)	7.2 (0.6–13.8)
Mexican-American	34.1 (1.5)	43.5 (0.2)	40.3 (3.4)	6.2 (−1.1–13.5)
	Control			
Age (years)				
18–39	61.5 (7.2)	70.2 (7.4)	51.9 (11.5)	−9.6 (−36.2–17.0)
40–59	53.7 (3.4)	54.2 (3.6)	66.4 (3.7)	12.7 (2.9–22.5)
≥60	40.8 (2.8)	35.2 (2.2)	43.7 (2.5)	2.9 (−4.5–10.3)
Gender				
Male	44.6 (2.6)	40.2 (3.7)	59.9 (3.2)	15.3 (7.2–23.4)
Female	48.5 (3.3)	45.7 (2.8)	47.8 (3.0)	−0.7 (−9.4–8.0)
Race or ethnicity				
Non-Hispanic white	47.4 (2.5)	43.8 (2.3)	55.6 (2.7)	8.2 (1.0–15.4)
Non-Hispanic black	43.7 (3.0)	41.2 (2.4)	44.6 (3.6)	0.9 (−8.3–10.1)
Mexican-American	40.2 (4.4)	37.5 (1.9)	44.0 (4.7)	3.8 (−8.8–16.4)

Note: SE, Standard error; CI, confidence interval.
Source: Adapted from Hajjar and Kotchen (20).

measurement was performed within the previous six months (45% men and 57% women).

Hypertension treatment and control in Europe is on the average poorer than in North America (18). In the age group of 35–64 years, 8% of European hypertensive individuals had their condition treated and controlled compared with 23% in the USA.

In developing countries, the awareness, treatment, and control of hypertension is usually lower than in industrialized countries. In China, Tao et al. found a 13.6% prevalence of hypertension in the population aged 15 years and older, but they noted a low level of awareness (25%) and control (3%) (22). In the Egyptian National Hypertension Project (NHP), Ibrahim et al. (23) found among a population aged 25 and over a hypertension prevalence of 26.3%, with a low level of awareness (38%), treatment (24%), and control (8%). In a survey of 21,242 Koreans 30 years in age or older, the prevalence of hypertension reached 20%, with a low level of awareness (25%), treatment (16%), and control (5%) (24).

B.   Geographic Patterns of Hypertension

According to previous national surveys, the prevalence of hypertension in China has increased dramatically during the past decades (25,26). In 1960, the estimated number of individuals with hypertension among adult Chinese was 30 million, and this number rose to 59 million in 1980 and 94 million in 1990 (27). From 1982 to 1994, the prevalence of hypertension in Chinese persons aged 35–59 years has increased from 17.8% to 25.5% in men and from 17.7% to 24.0% in women. A recent cross-sectional survey that included 15,540 individuals found an even larger prevalence of 34% in Northern China and 23% in Southern China (28). In another study, the age-adjusted prevalence of stage 1, stage 2, and stage 3 hypertension was 19.9%, 7.4%, and 3.8%, respectively, in the North, and 14.2%, 4.6%, and 2.1%, respectively, in the South. There was no significant difference between urban and rural areas (29.0% vs. 28.1%). Geographic variations in hypertension prevalence may have changed over the past decades due to dramatic economic development, urbanization, and associated lifestyle changes.

In a cross-sectional survey, Smith (29) studied hypertension in Sherpa men living in urban and rural regions of Nepal. Sherpas comprise a population of Tibeto-Burmese origin, and are world-renowned as high-altitude mountain guides. Individuals enrolled in this study were either living at lower altitude Kathmandu (1330 m) or at higher altitude in the Khumbu region (3400–3900 m). The results of this investigation suggested that the modernization of the last few years may have had a negative impact on blood pressure among the Sherpa population. This has been attributed primarily to lifestyle changes.

The highest prevalence of elevated blood pressure was found among Sherpa men who were living in the most acculturated areas, whose blood pressures reached a mean systolic blood pressure and diastolic blood pressure similar to levels found in the USA. The prevalence of elevated blood pressure has risen from none in the 1960s (30) to 24.8% of the higher altitude Sherpa men and 21.7% of the lower altitude Sherpa men in 1995. Individuals in the urban lower altitude showed the greatest prevalence of hypertension of 32.4%. Mean systolic blood pressure has increased from 113.5 mmHg in 1971–122.9 mmHg in 1995, and mean diastolic blood pressure has increased from 70.6–79.7 mmHg. During the past 30 years, the lives of Sherpas have changed dramatically with regard to lifestyle, activities performed, and acquisition of material wealth. Transitions in lifestyle for Sherpa men, including reduced physical activity and increased consumption of alcoholic drinks, appear to have contributed to a higher prevalence of obesity, a known risk factor for hypertension.

Sayeed et al. (31) studied the prevalence of hypertension and related risks in 2361 native Bangladeshis. Overall, the prevalence of systolic and diastolic hypertension was low, amounting to 14.4% and 9.1%, respectively, being almost comparable to that of other Asian populations and South Asian migrants. The prevalence of systolic hypertension was significantly higher in rural than in urban areas. A higher social class was associated with a significantly more elevated prevalence of systolic and diastolic hypertension.

The prevalence of hypertension and its associated risk factors also has been studied in an urban South Indian population at Chennai. The definition of hypertension was based on a systolic blood pressure ≥ 140 mmHg, a diastolic blood pressure ≥ 90 mmHg, treatment with antihypertensive drugs, or a combination of these factors. In 1262 subjects who were enrolled in this study, the crude prevalence of hypertension was 21.1%; the age-adjusted prevalence reached 17.0% (32). The prevalence of hypertension is lower in rural areas of India than it is in urban regions, but it is steadily increasing in rural areas as well (33). In 1994–1995, Malhotra et al. (34) carried out a population-based survey in seven rural, nonindustrialized villages around Raipur Rani in the state of Haryana in India to determine the prevalence of hypertension. A sample of 2559 individuals, 16–70 years old, was studied by using three blood pressure readings and a pretested, structured questionnaire to evaluate the relationship between hypertension and lifestyle characteristics. One hundred and fourteen individuals (4.5%) were found to be hypertensive according to the Fifth Joint National Committee on the Detection, Evaluation, and Treatment of High Blood Pressure (JNC V) criteria (4). In men, mean systolic blood pressure and diastolic blood pressure were 116.9 and 71.7 mmHg, respectively, and in women, 119.1 and 72.7 mmHg, respectively. Of note was the significantly higher prevalence of hypertension in women than in men (5.8% vs. 3.0%). Other risk factors of hypertension were higher body weight, higher body mass index, alcohol consumption, higher economic status, and smoking.

In Japan, the average prevalence of hypertension is 37% in men and 33% in women, reaching 53% in persons over 60 years of age (35). More than one-third have isolated systolic hypertension. Lee et al. (36) studied the effect of long-term body weight changes on the prevalence and incidence of hypertension in a large sample of community-residing Japanese persons from 30 to 69 years in age. Out of 3431 men and 2409 women, 11.7% of males and 8.9% of females developed hypertension over a 5-year observation period. Those individuals who developed hypertension were significantly older, had a higher body mass index, and had a higher systolic blood pressure and diastolic blood pressure at baseline. After adjustment for confounding factors, the slope of body mass index was positively associated with the incidence of hypertension in females as well as in males.

Current evidence suggests that African-Americans have higher blood pressures than black Africans (37,38). This has been attributed primarily to the lifestyle in westernized countries. Similarly, blood pressure in black Brazilians is higher than in black Africans, supporting the significance of environmental factors (38).

In some societies, blood pressure shows only a small age-related increase, or completely lacks the typical increase in blood pressure at older ages (39,40). Consequently, the incidence of cardiovascular disease in these places remains extraordinary low (41). In addition to the absence of hypertension, a lower serum cholesterol, lower blood glucose, and lower body mass index have been reported (45,46). These societies are located in Africa, South America, China, Australia, and Indonesia (42–44), and have in common a lack of acculturation (the process of adopting western social and cultural lifestyles). In addition, they are characterized by a low level of formal education, a more rural lifestyle, a lower consumption of food, and cultural isolation (47). As early as 1929, Donnison failed to find any cases of hypertension among 1000 individuals in a Kenyan tribe in eastern Africa. He concluded that a "civilized lifestyle" may contribute to the development of high blood pressure.

The survival of 175 indigenous groups in the Amazon basin in Brazil offers an excellent opportunity to study the impact of acculturation (48). The Yanomano are South American people with aboriginal traditions. Their contact with western society dates back to the early 20th century, and there are important differences between tribes with regard to the degree of acculturation (49).

Many Yanomano subjects who today are able to understand Portuguese also have higher blood pressures than native subjects who have not been acculturated. In the Rondonia state at the Bolivian border of northwest Brazil in the Amazon region, about 20 indigenous groups still exist. Many of these groups are still completely segregated. One study examined the Amondava people living in the Uru-Eu-Uau-Uau area. In contrast to other Brazilian Indians, their first official contact with the Brazilian National Indian Foundation came only in 1987. The cardiovascular risk profile of the Amondava is characterized by lower blood pressure levels, lower body mass index, lower total cholesterol, and lower glycemia than those found in control groups of more industrialized countries. The Amondava diet is characterized by low salt intake, low animal fat content, and high fiber content. Physical activity in this population is high; but social stress is very low. Similar observations have been made for the Xavante people in Mato Grosso (41). Shortly, after indigenous populations come into contact with western culture, cardiovascular risk patterns begin to change dramatically (50). This has been observed in the Chimbu in New Guinea, in individuals from the Cook Islands in Melanesia (51), in the Tarahumara in Mexico, and in the Pima Indians in Arizona (52). These observations suggest that environmental factors, not a particular genetic predisposition, seem to determine the blood pressure among these isolated populations.

C. Hypertension in Different Ethnic Groups

In the USA, the age-adjusted prevalence of hypertension is higher in nonHispanic blacks than in non Hispanic Caucasians and Mexican-Americans (33.5%, 28.9%, and 20.7%, respectively; Table 3.4). In the Caucasian population, hypertension develops on average 10 years later. The high rates of hypertension in African-Americans are greatest at younger ages, particularly in African-American women. By the age of 55, the majority of African-American men and women in the USA are hypertensive. Interestingly, hypertension is more prevalent in the African-American population in the USA than in Afro-Caribbeans and in native black African populations (43,44). Hence, the influence of ethnicity remains unclear.

A recent study also highlighted the relevance of lifestyle factors. Because hypertension is related to a higher body mass index, the difference in the prevalence of hypertension in African-Americans and Caucasians may be partly explained by the larger proportion of black individuals with obesity and the lack of adequate physical activity (54). Other factors that could potentially contribute to a higher prevalence of hypertension in this population are a lower intake of potassium and calcium and a greater salt sensitivity (55).

Table 3.4 Age Adjusted Prevalence of Hypertension in the United States Population, 1988–2000, Stratified by Race or Ethnicity

Patient characteristics	Prevalence 1988–1991 (% (SE))	1991–1994 (% (SE))	1999–2000 (% (SE))	Change 1988–2000 (%, (95% CI))
Age (years)				
18–39	5.1 (0.6)	6.1 (0.6)	7.2 (1.1)	2.1 (−0.3–4.5)
40–59	27.0 (1.4)	24.3 (2.2)	30.1 (1.8)	3.1 (−1.4–7.6)
≥60	57.9 (2.0)	60.1 (1.1)	65.4 (1.6)	7.5 (2.4–12.5)
Overall	25.0 (1.5)	25.0 (1.7)	28.7 (1.8)	3.7 (0–8.3)
Gender				
Male	24.9 (2.1)	23.9 (2.6)	27.1 (2.7)	2.2 (−4.5–8.9)
Female	24.5 (1.7)	26.0 (1.8)	30.1 (2.4)	5.6 (0–11.4)
Race or ethnicity				
Non-Hispanic white	25.9 (1.8)	25.6 (2.1)	28.9 (2.3)	3.1 (−2.7–8.7)
Non-Hispanic black	28.9 (2.2)	32.5 (2.1)	33.5 (3.2)	4.6 (−3–12.2)
Mexican-American	17.2 (1.6)	17.8 (2.0)	20.7 (2.7)	3.5 (−2.7–9.7)
Gender and race or ethnicity				
Male				
Non-Hispanic white	26.7 (2.7)	24.4 (2.4)	27.7 (3.4)	1.0 (−7.5–9.6)
Non-Hispanic black	29.1 (3.3)	29.5 (2.9)	30.9 (4.9)	1.8 (−9.8–13.4)
Mexican-American	17.9 (2.6)	17.8 (1.8)	20.6 (3.9)	2.7 (−6.5–11.9)
Female				
Non-Hispanic white	25.1 (2.1)	26.8 (2.3)	30.2 (3.1)	5.1 (−2.2–12.4)
Non-Hispanic black	28.6 (2.7)	35.0 (2.7)	35.8 (4.2)	7.2 (−2.6–17.0)
Mexican-American	16.5 (2.2)	17.9 (2.1)	20.7 (3.4)	4.2 (−3.8–12.2)

Note: SE, standard error; CI, confidence interval.
Source: Adapted from Hajjar and Kotchen (20).

In Hispanics, the prevalence of hypertension is slightly lower than in Caucasian Americans, despite a greater prevalence of obesity and diabetes (53,56,57). It has to take into account that Hispanics represent a heterogeneous population.

D. Age-Related Changes of Blood Pressure

In a Danish study, 24 h blood pressure profiles were assessed in normotensive healthy adults by using ambulatory blood pressure monitoring (58). The mean systolic blood pressure and diastolic blood pressure showed a progressive, age-dependent increase without significant differences between men and women (Fig. 3.1).

In the population-based cohort of 2036 patients in the original Framingham study, age-related changes in blood pressure of normotensive and untreated hypertensive individuals were evaluated (59). These investigators found a linear rise in systolic blood pressure from age 30 to 84, with a concomitant increase in diastolic blood pressure and mean arterial blood pressure. After the age of 50–60 years, diastolic blood pressure began to decline, which resulted in a steep increase in pulse pressure. The annual increase in blood pressure depended on the baseline value; patients with a high-normal diastolic blood pressure

(85–89 mmHg) had a two to three times higher risk of progressing to hypertension than individuals with normal diastolic blood pressure (<85 mmHg) (60). The late decline of diastolic blood pressure after the age of 60 years and the continuous rise in systolic blood pressure reflects the increased large artery stiffness in older age. Higher systolic blood pressure, if left untreated, may further accelerate large artery stiffness, perpetuating a vicious circle.

E. Body Weight and Hypertension

Obesity is a significant risk factor of hypertension. The odds of progression to hypertension increases by 20–30%/5% gain in body weight. Positive associations also have been documented between body mass index (weight/height^2) and blood pressure in both cross-sectional and prospective studies (61). In addition, body mass index is positively and independently associated with the morbidity and mortality resulting from hypertension, cardiovascular disease, type 2 diabetes mellitus, and other chronic diseases. In Caucasian populations, the association between body mass index and cardiovascular mortality is "J-shaped." The nadir of the curve occurs at a body mass index of 18.5–25 (63). On the basis of this

(A)

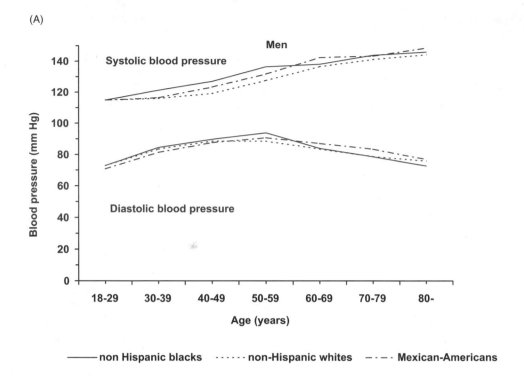

(B)

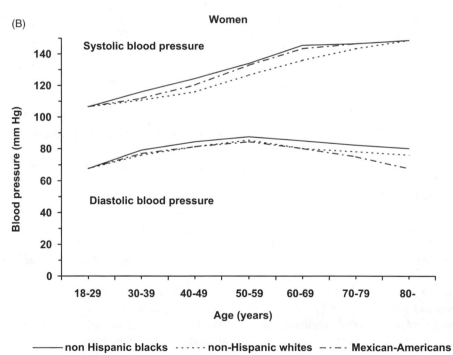

Figure 3.1 Diastolic and systolic blood pressure in men (A) and women (B) according to age. [Adapted from Wiinberg et al. (58).]

association, the World Health Organization has defined four categories. Persons with body mass indexes <18.5–24.9 are considered underweight; those above this range are considered overweight or "at risk"; and those with a body mass index ≥30 are considered obese. One way that body fat is thought to influence hypertension is through increased insulin resistance. Body fat, particularly abdominal fat, may lead to an increase in fatty acids in the portal blood vessels, enhancing insulin resistance and resulting in the development of hypertension and other metabolic complications (64).

Cross-sectional studies also have documented an association between body mass index and hypertension in East Asians, Chinese, and Filipinos (27,57,65,66). Deurenberg et al. (67) has noted discrepant body mass indexes in different ethnic groups despite similar percentages of body fat. Ko et al. (65) found that the body mass index cutoff that is associated with hypertension in Hong Kong Chinese persons is lower than in Caucasians (23.8 vs. 25 kg m^{-2}). The East Asian population is known to have a greater proportion of total body fat. In particular, the abdominal fat is increased despite a lower body mass index when compared with Caucasians. In Chinese, Indonesian, and Thai populations, body mass index values are on average 1.9, 3.2, and 2.9 units, respectively, lower than in Caucasians despite similar percentages of body fat. To explain the distinct strength of relationship between body mass index and hypertension in Asians and Caucasians, genetically determined differences in body composition and metabolic response need to be considered in conjunction with social and environmental factors. It is also possible that Asians are more insulin-resistant than Caucasians for reasons other than increased central adiposity (68).

F. Gender-Specific Issues of Hypertension

The mean blood pressure is usually higher in men than in women of similar age (Fig. 3.1). In addition, women appear to better tolerate elevated blood pressure, resulting in lower mortality from coronary heart disease (69,70).

In a cross-sectional study that enrolled 278 premenopausal and 184 postmenopausal women, hypertension was found in 10% of premenopausal women and in 40% of postmenopausal women (71). After adjusting for age and body mass index, postmenopausal women had 2.2 odds ratio of developing hypertension when compared with premenopausal women. Possible explanations for these findings include weight gain or estrogen withdrawal after menopause, which results in an overproduction of pituitary hormones and other neurohormones. However, the longitudinal Framingham study failed to identify a significant relationship between menopause and blood pressure elevation (72).

In the Baltimore Longitudinal Study of Aging, 226 healthy normotensive postmenopausal women with a mean age of 64 years were enrolled (73). The women were randomized to receive hormone replacement therapy in the form of oral or transdermal estrogen and progestin or a placebo. The treated group showed during the 10 year observation period a smaller increase in systolic blood pressure of only 7.6 mmHg compared with an increase of 18.7 mmHg in the untreated group. The diastolic blood pressure was not affected by hormone replacement therapy. Conversely, the postmenopausal Estrogen/Progestin Intervention trial reported no effect of hormone replacement therapy on blood pressure (74). In this study, 875 healthy postmenopausal women aged 45–64 years were randomized to receive conjugated equine estrogen or conjugated equine estrogen plus cyclic medroxyprogesterone acetate or a placebo. During a mean follow up of 3 years, no change in systolic and diastolic blood pressure was found in those women on hormone replacement therapy. However, the Women's Health Initiative (WHI) study reported a 25% higher rate of hypertension in women treated with an estrogen and progestin combination (75).

The Nurses' Health Study found that women who received contraceptives had an age-adjusted relative risk of 1.5 (95% CI 1.2–1.8) to develop hypertension (76). The absolute risk was modest, amounting to 41.5 cases/10,000 person-years. The negative effect of contraceptives on the development of hypertension rapidly declined after cessation of this therapy. Although the exact mechanism of the altered risk of hypertension by contraceptives remains unclear, it may rather be related to the progestogenic than the estrogenic component of the contraceptive preparation.

G. Hypertension in Children

Just 25 years ago, pediatricians started to pay attention to hypertension in childhood and adolescence. The introduction of blood pressure measurements during routine physical examinations of children revealed new cases of previously undetected asymptomatic secondary hypertension (77). However, hypertension and reference values cannot be defined in the same way they are defined in adults. The definition of hypertension in adults is based on epidemiological data. The cutoff point for hypertensive blood pressure in adults has been determined according to the risk for developing cardiovascular complications, but in children and adolescents, the definition of hypertension is based exclusively on statistical calculations (78). In 1977, the National Heart, Lung, and Blood Institute published a definition of hypertension that was based on a meta-analysis of three American studies that enrolled 5789 children. This definition was updated in 1987 and encompasses data from more than 70,000 children of all races. In 1993, demographic data of blood pressure in children was published that allowed a definition of hypertension according to the percentiles and categories of age, height, and gender (79,80). The Riva-Rocci method of blood pressure measurement that is used in adults cannot always be applied to children reliably because of the variability of Korotkoff sounds in adolescents. In some children, the sounds are even heard down to 0 mmHg. The 1996 update of the diagnosis of hypertension recommended using the fifth Korotkoff sound to determine the diastolic blood pressure (80).

Blood pressure is considerably lower in children than in adults, but it steadily increases during the first two decades of life. The height of the person is an independent predictor of blood pressure at all ages, but blood pressure is not gender specific. In addition, no significant differences between Caucasian, African-American, and Hispanic children in the USA have been noted (81).

The prevalence of hypertension in children and adolescents varies widely, ranging from 1% to 13% (82). Such variation may reflect the differences in the methodologies that were used. Children of families with known hypertension tend to have higher blood pressure than children of normotensive families. Several longitudinal studies also demonstrated that blood pressure in children, even if it is in the normal range, predicts the risk of hypertension in adulthood (83,84). A low birth weight seems to be a further independent prognostic factor of elevated blood pressure in adulthood (85,86). A decrease of 1 kg in birth weight increases diastolic pressure by 1.0 mmHg, and a decrease of 1 cm in chest circumference increases diastolic blood pressure by 0.3 mmHg. Barker et al. (87) demonstrated that men born with low birth weight and smaller chest circumferences had increased death rates due to cardiovascular events. Interestingly, placental weight was directly associated with the blood pressure at 8 years of age. Diastolic blood pressure increased by 0.7 mmHg/100 g increase in placental weight.

H. Effect of Dietary Factors

It is very likely that some diets negatively influence blood pressure. Energy intake (88), salt (89), and more recently, saturated fats (90–92) have been shown to affect either directly (93) or indirectly (94), the prevalence of hypertension in various populations (91,92). Members of lean populations typically living in developing countries have lower blood pressures than do persons of overweight populations in affluent countries (27,95).

There is a well-documented association between sodium intake and hypertension. Over 30 years ago, Dahl and Heine (96) demonstrated in a rat model that increased sodium intake results in a rapid rise of blood pressure. Similarly, an almost linear relationship between mean blood pressure and daily salt consumption was found in humans (97). Populations with sodium intake of <50 mmol/day are known to have lower blood pressures. Restricting sodium intake can significantly reduce blood pressure in hypertensive patients, usually by >10 mmHg (98). With greater sodium intake, hypertension develops even in regions where the prevalence of obesity is low.

A large multicenter study conducted by the INTERSALT Co-operative Research Group confirmed the relationship between increased sodium intake and hypertension after adjusting for confounding variables such as age, gender, body mass index, potassium intake, and alcohol intake (99). In this study, 10,079 persons 20–59 years in age were enrolled, 8344 of whom were normotensive.

Cutler and Stamler (100) conducted a meta-analysis, including 32 randomized clinical studies and 2635 individuals. With sodium intake was reduced, they found a decline of 4.8 and 2.5 mmHg in systolic and diastolic blood pressure, respectively, in hypertensive participants. In normotensive individuals, the reduction of blood pressure was less marked, ranging from 1.1 to 1.9 mmHg. However, there was a linear dose–response relationship between the reduction of salt intake and the decline of blood pressure. Falker and Michel (101) investigated the effect of dietary salt on blood pressure in children and adolescents. They demonstrated that a dietary salt restriction was more effective in persons with a positive family history of hypertension and in obese patients. The phenomenon is known as *sodium sensitivity* and is higher in patients with severe hypertension (102), in black individuals, in patients with a family history of hypertension, in the elderly, and in patients with hyperaldosteronism (103). However, not all individuals who consume larger amounts of dietary sodium develop hypertension.

Cross-sectional studies have shown a higher blood pressure and a higher prevalence of hypertension in individuals with increased alcohol intake (62,104). A consumption of more than three standard alcoholic drinks per day approximately doubles the risk of hypertension. Blood pressure declines again within days after alcohol intake has been discontinued. The exact mechanisms by which alcohol affects blood pressure remain unclear. It has been suggested that the increase in blood pressure may occur via the activation of the sympathetic nervous system or by affecting the cellular transport of electrolytes. The most recent evaluation of NHANES data suggested that there might be a causal relationship between dietary intake and blood pressure among regional populations within the USA (105). However, different dietary conditions or alcohol intake do not entirely explain regional differences of the prevalence of hypertension or the difference between European countries and the USA (99).

A high-fat diet also has been postulated to be one of the causes for the high prevalence of hypertension in Russia and Finland. In geographical areas where the consumption of saturated fat is higher, the prevalence of hypertension is usually elevated (106,107). Several studies have demonstrated that an "inverted" diet with a high unsaturated-to-saturated fat ratio tends to reduce the blood pressure (90,92,108,109). This may explain why members of religious groups that adhere to a diet that is low in meat show a lower blood pressure in general than persons who eat an omnivorous diet.

I. Socioeconomic Factors

Several other factors may be responsible for the geographic and regional patterns of hypertension, comprising genetic, socioeconomic, environmental, and psychosocial factors. It is conceivable that genetic polymorphisms may affect electrolyte transport, sympathetic, or endocrine control mechanisms. The occurrence of one genetic alteration or a combination of mutations may result ultimately in clinically manifested hypertension. Hereditary factors may confer 20–50% of the variation in blood pressure (110).

According to the United States Department of Health and Human Services, the prevalence of hypertension is lower in high-income earners in comparison to the poor, near poor, and middle-income populations (22% vs. 26–27%). Similarly, the British Regional Heart Study and the Nine Towns Study found that the mean systolic blood pressure is lower in individuals with skilled nonmanual occupations than in persons with unskilled manual occupations (111,112). Although there is now in industrialized countries a fairly consistent inverse association between socioeconomic status and blood pressure (113), this relationship is thought to have emerged only 40–60 years ago. Previous studies in the USA and UK found that a high socioeconomic status was associated with a higher risk of hypertension and more frequent cardiovascular complications (113). Interestingly, in a study from Jamaica, low-income as well as high-income earners showed a higher prevalence of hypertension than middle-income earners, resulting in a J-shaped curve (114).

The background for the inconsistent association between socioeconomic status and blood pressure remains unclear. The mechanisms by which socioeconomic factors influence blood pressure and hypertension are unknown (115,116). The dynamics of social and cultural transitions during the process of economic development are thought to change the pace at which hypertension and other risk factors of cardiovascular disease are emerging in developing countries (117). Hence, one explanation for the inconsistent association between socioeconomic status and blood pressure may be the heterogeneity of stages of modernization and economic development. In the least-developed countries, high socioeconomic status groups may adopt atherogenic and hypertensive lifestyles that are characterized by smoking, sedentary activities, and diets that are high in energy and fats (114), whereas in more industrialized countries persons with high socioeconomic status may be more prepared to adopt lifestyles that lower the risk of coronary vascular disease. In contrast, individuals with low socioeconomic status may adhere stronger to lifestyles that are adverse for their health. Assuming this hypothesis, one would expect a direct relationship between socioeconomic status and blood pressure in low-income countries, and an inverse relationship in industrialized countries. In developing countries, the relationship between socioeconomic status and blood pressure also may be influenced by other risk factors of hypertension and coronary vascular disease, such as fetal malnutrition and psychosocial stress (118).

Mass migration in the past century provided convincing evidence that environmental factors play an important role for the development of hypertension (119). Reports of people with similar ethnic backgrounds but distinctly different types of contact with modern societies indicate a strong relationship between westernized lifestyle and increased cardiovascular risk (120). An increase in blood pressure also was observed in individuals who moved from rural to urban areas (120). It remains to be determined whether migrating from urban to rural areas has the opposite effect and reduces blood pressure.

In an interesting study, Timio et al. studied blood pressure trends and cardiovascular events in 144 nuns in a secluded order in Umbria, Italy, over a period of 30 years. They compared the results with data from 138 laywomen who lived in the same region. Both groups were comparable with regard to baseline characteristics, including age, blood pressure, body mass index, race, ethnic background, menarche, family history of hypertension, and 24 h urinary sodium excretion. Smokers and individuals who used contraceptive agents or estrogen replacement therapy were excluded. Among nuns, blood pressure remained remarkably stable. None showed an increase in diastolic blood pressure to levels >90 mmHg. Conversely, laywomen showed the typical age-related increase in blood pressure that resulted in systolic and diastolic differences of blood pressure between both groups of >30 and 15 mmHg, respectively. In addition, there was a significantly larger number of fatal and nonfatal cardiovascular events in laywomen over the 30 year period. Hence, the study suggests that environmental stress and, in particular, psychosocial stress may be an important factor in the development of hypertension (121).

Stress in form of racial discrimination and migration also has been associated with an increased risk of hypertension (122). In addition, unfavorable working conditions, for example, noise and shift-work, are thought to result in an increase in blood pressure (123).

III. BURDEN AND DISEASE FROM HYPERTENSION

Hypertension is associated with an increased risk of atherosclerotic vascular disease outcomes. In 1925, the Society of Actuaries conducted a study that enrolled 560,000 insured men. The results of this investigation indicated that even mild hypertension may reduce life expectancy (124). It has been shown that high-normal blood pressure already increases the risk of cardiovascular complications (125). The contribution of hypertension to the risk of atherosclerotic vascular disease has been determined from large-scale epidemiologic studies and meta-analyses (126,127). The number of persons with cardiovascular disease has declined substantially in western countries over the past decades, but cardiovascular complications remain a serious problem. Even in developing countries, cardiovascular disease represents a heavy burden. For example, in the People's Republic of China, in Japan, and in other east Asian countries, stroke is the principal cause of death. In 1994, cardiovascular disease mortality had reached 544 of 100,000 Chinese men and 559 of 100,000 Chinese women age 35 years or older. Nearly 40% of all deaths (37.0% in men and 41.8% in women) were the direct result of cardiovascular disease. More than half of all cardiovascular disease deaths were the result of stroke (56.2% in men and 52.5% in women). The emergence of cardiovascular disease as a leading cause of death in China is believed to be the result of the dramatic and rapid economic transition, urbanization, industrialization, and globalization that has occurred over the past few decades. Even more worrying, the morbidity and mortality rate resulting from cardiovascular

disease in China has been projected to further increase over the next 20 years (128).

A. Cardiovascular Risk

Cardiovascular disease is the leading cause of death in adults in most industrialized countries. It affects males more frequently than females by a 4:1 ratio. Disability from cardiovascular disease steadily increases as individuals grow older. The incidence doubles approximately each decade after the age of 45 and accounts for nearly 50% of all deaths after the age of 65. The relationship between diastolic blood pressure and the risk of coronary heart disease follows a log–linear curve (127). However, a clear-cut threshold level of blood pressure where the risk of cardiovascular morbidity commences to increase cannot be determined. It has been estimated that a persistent elevation of diastolic blood pressure of 5 mmHg increases the risk of coronary heart disease by at least 21%, whereas an elevation of 10 mmHg changes the risk by +37% (Fig. 3.2) (127).

The risk of cardiovascular events appears also to be higher in persons with isolated systolic hypertension (13,125). Moreover, several studies found a significant association between pulse pressure, cardiovascular disease morbidity, and mortality (129–131). In an analysis of 2231 patients of the Survival and Ventricular Enlargement (SAVE) study and 6781 patients randomly assigned

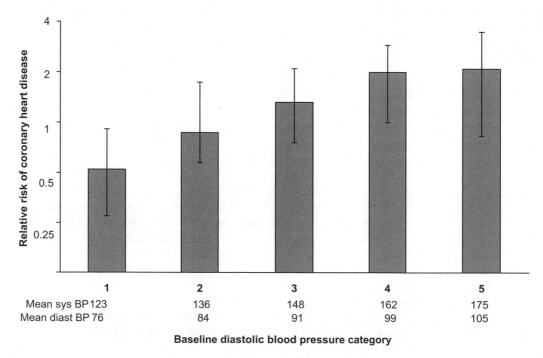

Figure 3.2 Relative risk of coronary heart disease in the Framingham Heart Study according to different strata of systolic and diastolic blood pressures. [Adapted from MacMahon et al. (127).]

to the Studies of Left Ventricular Dysfunction (SOLVD), pulse pressure predicted the risk of death after myocardial infarction and recurrent myocardial infarction (132,133). Similarly, pulse pressure predicted all-cause, cardiovascular, and coronary mortality in 19,083 middle-aged and elderly but otherwise healthy French men enrolled in a screening program (131). Madhavan et al. (134) found that pulse pressure, not systolic or diastolic blood pressure, was an independent predictor of cardiovascular outcomes in 2207 untreated hypertensive patients who were followed for almost 5 years. In the East Boston Senior Health Project (135), pulse pressure was found to be a dominant predictor of coronary artery disease. The risk of coronary heart disease is also influenced by other factors such as higher age, elevated blood lipids, cigarette smoking, and diabetes. However, hypertension and dyslipidemia are those atherosclerotic risk factors that can be modified most easily.

B. Stroke

Stroke is a heterogeneous condition, responsible for 20% of all cardiovascular deaths in the elderly. Most (72%) strokes occur after the age of 65 years, but almost 20% of strokes occur in persons 60 or younger. The risk of stroke doubles each successive decade after the age of 55. Approximately 85% of strokes are cerebral infarctions. Intracerebral or subarachnoid hemorrhages account for 15% of strokes.

The risk of stroke increases with increasing age, cigarette smoking, diabetes, and atrial fibrillation. Hypertension has been recognized as an independent risk factor of stroke. In the Seven Countries Study, the age-adjusted stroke rates varied substantially in different areas: North America and Northern Europe, 35–50/1000 person-years; Southern Europe, 44–70/1000 person-years; rural Serbia, Croatia, and Japan, 83–107/1000 person-years (136). MacMahon et al. (127) estimated that an elevation of diastolic blood pressure by >5 mmHg results in a 34% increase in stroke risk (Fig. 3.3), whereas a 10 mmHg elevation results in a 57% increase in stroke risk. Stage 2 or stage 3 hypertension increases the risk of stroke by ~50% and 100%, respectively, compared with individuals with stage 1 hypertension.

A 10 year period of permanent elevation of blood pressure by one standard deviation is associated with a relative risk of stroke of 1.68 (95% CI: 1.25–2.25) in men and of 1.92 (95% CI: 1.39–2.66) in women (137). In middle-aged Japanese adults enrolled in the ABCC-JNIH Adult Health Study examinations in Hiroshima-Nagasaki, Prentice et al. (138) found that the systolic blood pressure 2–4 years before the initiation of antihypertensive therapy already predicted the risk of future ischemic strokes. Similarly, elevated blood pressure measured at a single visit already predicted an increased risk of stroke (139). However, in the Zutphen Study, Kelli et al. (140) noted that a single determination of the

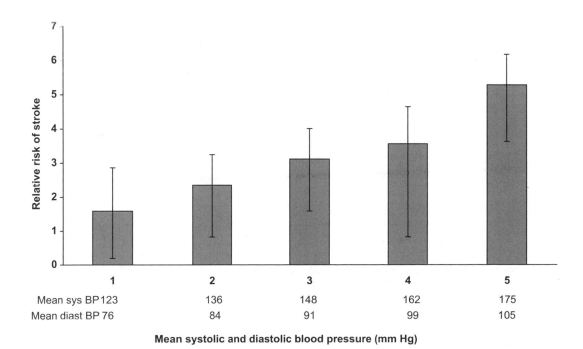

Figure 3.3 Relative risk of stroke in the Framingham Heart Study according to different strata of systolic and diastolic blood pressures. [Adapted from MacMahon et al. (127).]

systolic blood pressure underestimated the strength of the association between hypertension and the 15 year stroke incidence by 55% when compared with the average systolic blood pressure during the previous 11 years.

Although it was initially believed that diastolic blood pressure has a greater impact on the risk of stroke than systolic blood pressure, this concept was not supported by the Framingham study (141). It has been shown that the risk of stroke increases continuously after the age of 50 despite a declining diastolic blood pressure. The ideal blood pressure for reducing the risk of stroke has not been defined yet. However, a systolic blood pressure <125 mmHg and a diastolic blood pressure <85 mmHg appear to be reasonable thresholds.

C. Left Ventricular Hypertrophy and Congestive Heart Failure

Left ventricular hypertrophy is frequently the result of long-standing uncontrolled hypertension and volume overload. The first studies providing evidence of a close relationship between hypertension and left ventricular hypertrophy were based on ECG diagnosis. More recently, this relationship was confirmed with echocardiography.

Left ventricular hypertrophy is a prominent feature of evolving or manifest congestive heart failure. Approximately 20% of congestive heart failure cases had antecedent signs of left ventricular hypertrophy in the ECG and 60–70% according to the more sensitive echocardiography. After adjustment for age and other risk factors, left ventricular hypertrophy indicates a twofold to threefold higher risk of developing congestive heart failure (142). In one study, 140 men with uncomplicated hypertension were followed for a mean time period of 4.8 years (147). During this time, 14 cardiovascular events were recorded. The event rate was 4.6/100 patient-years in men with left ventricular hypertrophy and 1.4/100 patient-years in those without hypertrophy. In a multivariate model that takes into account age, systolic and diastolic blood pressure, and left ventricular fractional shortening, the left ventricular mass index was the most powerful predictor of cardiovascular morbidity.

According to the Framingham study, a 40% rise in the risk of major cardiovascular events can be expected for each 39 g/m^2 or standard deviation increase of left ventricular mass (145,146). A blood pressure of >160/95 mmHg was associated with a sixfold higher incidence of congestive heart failure. It was estimated that a 10 mmHg increase in diastolic blood pressure increased the incidence of congestive heart failure by 25%. In 1621 elderly men and women of the East Boston Senior Health Project, an association between increased pulse pressure and congestive heart failure was reported after adjustment for age, gender, mean blood pressure, history

of coronary artery disease, diabetes mellitus, atrial fibrillation, and treatment for hypertension (135). Pulse pressure increases steeply with age, especially after the fifth to sixth decade of life, a time when diastolic pressure tends to decline (59). If left untreated, hypertension may further accelerate the development of large-artery stiffness and further increase systolic blood pressure (129). These changes subsequently cause a deterioration of asymptomatic left ventricular dysfunction that results in overt congestive heart failure (143). Similarly, among 2152 participants of the Established Populations for Epidemiologic Studies of the Elderly program who were free of coronary disease and congestive heart failure at the baseline examination, pulse pressure showed a strong linear relationship with the risk of developing congestive heart failure after adjustment for demographic variables, co-morbidity, and risk factors. A 10 mmHg increment in pulse pressure was associated with a 14% increase in risk of congestive heart failure (144).

D. End-Stage Renal Disease

Long-term data of more than 10,000 men of the Veterans Administration study indicated a significant relationship between systolic blood pressure and renal disease (148). Conversely, end-stage renal disease may lead to hypertensive blood pressure. In an analysis of 26 geographic areas in the state of Maryland, the incidence of end-stage renal disease was closely related to the prevalence of hypertension (149). One of the highest rates of end-stage renal disease has been recorded in the Southeast of the USA, where the prevalence of hypertension is very high. The African-American population in the USA shows a very high prevalence of hypertension, but it also has a sixfold higher incidence of end-stage renal disease than the Caucasian population (150). Even individuals with high-normal blood pressure have a twofold increased risk of end-stage renal disease in comparison to subjects with optimum blood pressure (<120/80 mmHg). The relative risk of end-stage renal disease among individuals with hypertension stages 1–4 amounted to 3.1, 6.0, 11.2, and 22.1, respectively (Table 3.5).

Treating elevated blood pressure reduces the risk of end-stage renal disease. The Reduction of Endpoints in NIDDM with the Angiotensin II Antagonist Losartan (RENAAL) study indicated that a reduction of elevated blood pressure with an angiotensin II receptor blocker in patients with diabetes mellitus type 2 significantly reduced the time to end-stage renal disease (151,152). Further analysis of this study showed that baseline systolic blood pressure represents an independent risk factor for end-stage renal disease or death. During a 15-year follow up of 11,912 male hypertensive veterans, the pretreatment systolic blood pressure was more strongly

Table 3.5 Blood Pressure and All-Cause End-Stage Renal Disease

Blood pressure category	Age-adjusted rate/100,000 person-years	Adjusted relative risk (95% CI)
Optimal blood pressure (<120 mmHg systolic, <80 mmHg diastolic)	5.3	1.0
Normal but not optimal blood pressure (120–129/80–84 mmHg)	6.6	1.2 (0.8–1.7)
High normal blood pressure (130–139/85–89 mmHg)	11.1	1.9 (1.4–2.7)
Hypertension		
Stage 1	21.0	3.1 (2.3–4.3)
Stage 2	43.6	6.0 (4.3–8.4)
Stage 3	96.1	11.2 (7.7–16.2)
Stage 4	187.1	22.1 (14.2–34.3)
Overall	15.6	—

Note: CI, confidence interval.
Source: Adapted from Klag et al. (169).

Table 3.6 Risk of Intermittent Claudication by Systolic and Diastolic Blood Pressures in Subjects 35–84 Years of Age

Blood pressure (mmHg)	Men Biennial age-adjusted rate per 1000 (%)	Women Biennial age-adjusted rate per 1000 (%)
Systolic		
≤119	5.2	1.8
120–139	4.5	2.3
140–159	9.5	3.4
160–179	9.6	5.1
≥180	13.9	9.4
Diastolic		
≤75	6.2	2.9
76–80	6.8	2.8
81–86	6.8	2.8
87–94	5.5	4
≥95	10.6	5.8

Source: Adapted from Kannel and McGee (157).

associated with end-stage renal disease than the diastolic blood pressure (153). Any systolic blood pressure values >140 mmHg significantly increased the risk of end-stage renal disease compared with values <130 mmHg. Systolic blood pressure and pulse pressure appear to have similar predictive values for end-stage renal disease. A baseline pulse pressure >70 mmHg increases the risk of progression to end-stage renal disease (151). In contrast, baseline diastolic blood pressure in this study failed to predict poor renal outcomes in this population with type 2 diabetes and nephropathy. However, diastolic blood pressure was a useful predictor of renal outcomes in younger people with nondiabetic renal disease and type 1 diabetes in other studies (154–156).

The prognosis of end-stage renal disease is usually poor. After 5 years, only 38% of persons with the disease are still alive, the most common cause of death being coronary heart disease.

E. Peripheral Arterial Disease

The incidence and prevalence of peripheral arterial disease increase substantially with age in men and women (157,158). Both symptomatic and asymptomatic peripheral arterial disease are associated with significantly increased risks of coronary and cardiovascular mortality (158,159).

There is a steep, nonlinear relationship between baseline levels of systolic blood pressure and the risk of intermittent claudication (Table 3.6).

In an examination of peripheral arterial disease and its risk factors in the Framingham Offspring Study, patients

40 years or older were evaluated. The prevalence of intermittent claudication was 1.9% in men and 0.8% in women. In a multivariate adjusted analysis, age, hypertension, current smoking, pack-years of smoking, fibrinogen, HDL cholesterol, and coronary heart disease were associated with peripheral arterial disease. Each 10 year increment in age carried a 2.6-fold increase in the odds of peripheral arterial disease. Hypertension and coronary heart disease were associated with a more than twofold increase in the odds of peripheral arterial disease. Smokers showed twice the risk of developing peripheral arterial disease. An increase of 10-pack-years of smoking resulted in a 1.3-fold increase in the odds of peripheral arterial disease. Each 50 mg/dL increment in fibrinogen was associated with a 1.2-fold increase in the odds of peripheral arterial disease. HDL cholesterol was inversely associated with peripheral arterial disease; for each 5 mg/dL increase in HDL cholesterol, there was a 10% decrease in the odds of peripheral arterial disease (160). For baseline diastolic blood pressure, data suggests that the threshold where the risk of peripheral arterial disease increases commences at 87–94 mmHg in women and at 95 mmHg in men.

F. Predictive Value of Systolic and Diastolic Blood Pressure

Since the mid-1920s, a relationship has been known to exist between diastolic and systolic blood pressures and life expectancy. Highly elevated blood pressure was called malignant hypertension because 79% of affected individuals died within 1 year of this diagnosis (161). From the 1920s until the 1980s, the risks of coronary heart disease and stroke have been attributed predominantly to elevated diastolic blood pressure (162). In fact, it was a misconception that diastolic blood pressure would be a better predictor of cardiovascular risk. In 1971, the Framingham study indicated that isolated elevated systolic blood pressure is associated with an increased risk of cardiovascular disease (163). A large number of diverse prospective studies followed and confirmed that systolic blood pressure is in fact a superior predictor of cardiovascular risk. More recently, *pulse pressure* (the difference between diastolic and systolic blood pressure) has been recognized as a further significant predictor of cardiovascular events (145,164). Systolic blood pressure and diastolic blood pressure show distinct trends with progressing age. Diastolic blood pressure reaches a plateau at the age of 50 and subsequently commences to decline, whereas systolic blood pressure continues to increase after the age of 50. As a consequence, pulse pressure increases after the age of 50. Diastolic blood pressure rises with peripheral arterial resistance and falls with increased central artery stiffness. The contributions of these opposing forces determine diastolic blood pressure and, ultimately, the pulse pressure (165).

In the Framingham study, increments in pulse pressure at particular systolic pressures were associated with a greater risk of coronary heart diseases than were increments of systolic blood pressure at a fixed pulse pressure (145). Of note, the prediction of cardiac hypertrophy has been reported to be associated with high pulse pressure and low diastolic pressure (166). Hence, with increasing age the prognostic value of diastolic, systolic, and pulse pressure for coronary heart disease may change (167). From the age of 60 years onward, diastolic pressure is negatively correlated with coronary heart disease. At this age, pulse pressure may become a better predictor of coronary heart disease than systolic or diastolic blood pressure (167). However, the strong relationship between systolic blood pressure and pulse pressure makes a separation of the effects of each predictor extremely problematic, no matter what statistical method is used (168). This may explain why studies fail to agree on the prognostic importance of diastolic blood pressure, systolic blood pressure, and pulse pressure (165).

G. Trends in Hypertension Morbidity and Mortality

The early detection and treatment of hypertension is essential in order to prevent secondary complications such as stroke, heart failure, and coronary heart disease. Since 1972, the rates of coronary heart disease have declined by 46%, parallel to the decline in the prevalence of hypertension. The decline in cardiovascular mortality is independent of gender and race but is more pronounced in older persons. Stroke is the third leading cause of death in the USA and accounts for more than 160,000 deaths/annum. After 1972, a sharp decline in stroke mortality of 58% was observed, decreasing annually by 6%. The rate of decline was similar for all age groups and did not depend on race and gender. In contrast, the incidence of end-stage renal disease has increased since 1973, despite a decline in the prevalence of hypertension.

IV. CONCLUSIONS

In developed countries, hypertension affects 25–30% of the entire adult population, reaching 60–70% of individuals beyond the seventh decade. Hypertension is associated with older age, increased body mass index and other less defined psychosocial, environmental and nutritional factors. Preventive measures have led to a substantial decline in hypertension prevalence in the United States, particularly between 1974 and 1991. In addition, the incidence of coronary heart disease and the rate of cerebrovascular events have declined as a result of improved awareness, more potent therapy and better control of blood pressure. In contrast, the prevalence of hypertension is still increasing in developing countries, paralleling industrialization and the adoption of a Westernized lifestyle. Overall, the prevalence of hypertension remains high and represents a serious health problem, causing endorgan damage such as left-ventricular hypertrophy, congestive heart disease, coronary heart failure, stroke, renal failure, and periperal arterial disease. It requires large efforts to further reduce cardiovascular morbidity and mortality.

REFERENCES

1. Vasan RS, Larson MG, Leip EP, Evans JC, O'Donnell CJ, Kannel WB, Levy D. Impact of high-normal blood pressure on the risk of cardiovascular disease. N Engl J Med 2001; 345:1291–1297.
2. Thomas F, Bean K, Guize L, Quentzel S, Argyriadis P, Benetos A. Combined effects of systolic blood pressure and serum cholesterol on cardiovascular mortality in young (<55 years) men and women. Eur Heart J 2002; 23:528–535.
3. Stamler J, Stamler R, Neaton JD. Blood pressure, systolic and diastolic, and cardiovascular risks. US population data. Arch Intern Med 1993; 153:598–615.
4. Chobanian AV, Bakris GL, Black HR, Cushman WC, Green LA, Izzo JL Jr, Jones DW, Materson BJ, Oparil S, Wright JT Jr, Roccella EJ. National heart, lung, and blood institute joint national committee on prevention, detection, evaluation, and treatment of high blood pressure; national high blood pressure education program coordinating committee. The seventh report of the joint national committee on prevention, detection, evaluation, and treatment of high blood pressure: the JNC 7 report. JAMA 2003; 289:2560–2572.

5. Hunink MG, Goldman L, Tosteson AN, Mittleman MA, Goldman PA, Williams LW, Tsevat J, Weinstein MC. The recent decline in mortality from coronary heart disease, 1980–1990. The effect of secular trends in risk factors and treatment. JAMA 1997; 277:535–542.

6. Boersma E, Keil U, De Bacquer D, De Backer G, Pyorala K, Poldermans D, Leprotti C, Pilotto L, de Swart E, Deckers JW, Heidrich J, Sans S, Kotseva K, Wood D, Ambrosio GB, EUROASPIRE I and II Study Groups. Blood pressure is insufficiently controlled in European patients with established coronary heart disease. J Hypertens 2003; 21:1831–1840.

7. Andre JL, Monneau JP, Gueguen R, Deschamps JP. Five-year incidence of hypertension and its concomitants in a population of 11 355 adults unselected as to disease. Eur Heart J 1982; 3(suppl C):53–58.

8. Kahn HA, Medalie JH, Neufeld HN, Riss E, Goldbourt U. The incidence of hypertension and associated factors: the Israel ischemic heart disease study. Am Heart J 1972; 84:171–182.

9. Dischinger PC, Apostolides AY, Entwisle G, Hebel JR. Hypertension incidence in an inner-city black population. J Chronic Dis 1981; 34:405–413.

10. Paffenbarger RS Jr, Wing AL, Hyde RT, Jung DL. Physical activity and incidence of hypertension in college alumni. Am J Epidemiol 1983; 117:245–257.

11. Folsom AR, Prineas RJ, Kaye SA, Munger RG. Incidence of hypertension and stroke in relation to body fat distribution and other risk factors in older women. Stroke 1990; 21:701–706.

12. Burt VL, Cutler JA, Higgins M, Horan MJ, Labarthe D, Whelton P, Brown C, Roccella EJ. Trends in the prevalence, awareness, treatment, and control of hypertension in the adult US population. Data from the health examination surveys, 1960–1991. Hypertension 1995; 26:60–69.

13. Kannel WB, Wolf PA, Verter J, McNamara PM. Epidemiologic assessment of the role of blood pressure in stroke: the Framingham Study, 1970. JAMA 1996; 276:1269–1278.

14. Stamler J, Wentworth D, Neaton JD. Is relationship between serum cholesterol and risk of premature death from coronary heart disease continuous and graded? Findings in 356,222 primary screenees of the Multiple Risk Factor Intervention Trial (MRFIT). JAMA 1986; 256:2823–2828.

15. Geographical variation in the major risk factors of coronary heart disease in men and women aged 35–64 years. The WHO MONICA Project. World Health Stat Q 1988; 41:115–140.

16. Taylor J. The hypertension detection and follow-up program: a progress report. Circ Res 1977; 40(5 suppl 1):I106–I109.

17. Lloyd-Jones DM, Evans JC, Larson MG, O'Donnell CJ, Wilson PW, Levy D. Cross-classification of JNC VI blood pressure stages and risk groups in the Framingham Heart Study. Arch Intern Med 1999; 159:2206–2212.

18. Wolf-Maier K, Cooper RS, Banegas JR, Giampaoli S, Hense HW, Joffres M, Kastarinen M, Poulter N, Primatesta P, Rodriguez-Artalejo F, Stegmayr B, Thamm M, Tuomilehto J, Vanuzzo D, Vescio F. Hypertension prevalence and blood pressure levels in 6 European countries, Canada, and the United States. JAMA 2003; 289:2363–2369.

19. Goff DC, Howard G, Russell GB, Labarthe DR. Birth cohort evidence of population influences on blood pressure in the United States, 1887–1994. Ann Epidemiol 2001; 11:271–279.

20. Hajjar I, Kotchen TA. Trends in prevalence, awareness, treatment, and control of hypertension in the United States, 1988–2000. JAMA 2003; 290:199–206.

21. Joffres MR, Hamet P, Rabkin SW, Gelskey D, Hogan K, Fodor G. Prevalence, control and awareness of high blood pressure among Canadian adults. Canadian Heart Health Surveys Research Group. CMAJ 1992; 146:1997–2005.

22. Tao S, Wu X, Duan X, Fang W, Hao J, Fan D, Wang W, Li Y. Hypertension prevalence and status of awareness, treatment and control in China. Chin Med J (Engl) 1995; 108:483–489.

23. Ibrahim MM, Rizk H, Appel LJ, el Aroussy W, Helmy S, Sharaf Y, Ashour Z, Kandil H, Roccella E, Whelton PK. Hypertension prevalence, awareness, treatment, and control in Egypt. Results from the Egyptian National Hypertension Project (NHP). NHP Investigative Team. Hypertension 1995; 26:886–890.

24. Kim JS, Jones DW, Kim SJ, Hong YP. Hypertension in Korea: a national survey. Am J Prev Med 1994; 10:200–204.

25. Wu YK, Lu CQ, Gao RC, Yu JS, Liu GC. Nation-wide hypertension screening in China during 1979–1980. Chin Med J (Engl) 1982; 95:101–108.

26. Wu X, Duan X, Gu D, Hao J, Tao S, Fan D. Prevalence of hypertension and its trends in Chinese populations. Int J Cardiol 1995; 52:39–44.

27. He J, Klag MJ, Whelton PK, Chen JY, Qian MC, He GQ. Body mass and blood pressure in a lean population in southwestern China. Am J Epidemiol 1994; 139:380–389.

28. Reynolds K, Gu D, Muntner P, Wu X, Chen J, Huang G, Duan X, Whelton PK, He J, InterASIA Collaborative Group. Geographic variations in the prevalence, awareness, treatment and control of hypertension in China. J Hypertens 2003; 21:1273–1281.

29. Smith C. Blood pressures of Sherpa men in modernizing Nepal. Am J Human Biol 1999; 11:469–479.

30. Lang SD, Lang A. The Kunde hospital and a demographic survey of the upper Khumbu, Nepal. N Z Med J 1971; 74:1–8.

31. Sayeed MA, Banu A, Haq JA, Khanam PA, Mahtab H, Azad Khan AK. Prevalence of hypertension in Bangladesh: effect of socioeconomic risk factor on difference between rural and urban community. Bangladesh Med Res Counc Bull 2002; 28:7–18.

32. Shanthirani CS, Pradeepa R, Deepa R, Premalatha G, Saroja R, Mohan V. Prevalence and risk factors of hypertension in a selected South Indian population—the Chennai Urban Population Study. J Assoc Physicians India 2003; 51:20–27.

33. Gupta R, al-Odat NA, Gupta VP. Hypertension epidemiology in India: meta-analysis of 50 year prevalence rates and blood pressure trends. J Hum Hypertens 1996; 10:465–472.

34. Malhotra P, Kumari S, Kumar R, Jain S, Sharma BK. Prevalence and determinants of hypertension in an un-industrialised rural population of North India. J Hum Hypertens 1999; 13:467–472.

35. Ueshima H, Zhang XH, Choudhury SR. Epidemiology of hypertension in China and Japan. J Hum Hypertens 2000; 14:765–769.

36. Lee JS, Kawakubo K, Kashihara H, Mori K. Effect of long-term body weight change on the incidence of hypertension in Japanese men and women. Int J Obes Relat Metab Disord 2004; 28:391–395.

37. Gillum RF, Grant CT. Coronary heart disease in black populations. II. Risk factors. Am Heart J 1982; 104:852–864.

38. Wilson TW, Hollifield LR, Grim CE. Systolic blood pressure levels in black populations in sub-Sahara Africa, the West Indies, and the United States: a meta-analysis. Hypertension 1991; 18:I87–I91.

39. Carvalho JJ, Baruzzi RG, Howard PF, Poulter N, Alpers MP, Franco LJ, Marcopito LF, Spooner VJ, Dyer AR, Elliott P. Blood pressure in four remote populations in the INTERSALT Study. Hypertension 1989; 14:238–246.

40. Lengani A, Laville M, Serme D, Fauvel JP, Ouandaogo BJ, Zech P. Renal insufficiency in arterial hypertension in black Africa. Presse Med 1994; 23:788–792.

41. Carneiro O, Jardim PC. Blood pressure in a Xavante tribe. Comparison after 15 years. Arq Bras Cardiol 1993; 61:279–282.

42. Pavan L, Casiglia E, Braga LM, Winnicki M, Puato M, Pauletto P, Pessina AC. Effects of a traditional lifestyle on the cardiovascular risk profile: the Amondava population of the Brazilian Amazon. Comparison with matched African, Italian and Polish populations. J Hypertens 1999; 17:749–756.

43. Kaminer B, Lutz WP. Blood pressure in Bushmen of the Kalahari Desert. Circulation 1960; 22:289–295.

44. Truswell AS, Kennelly BM, Hansen JD, Lee RB. Blood pressures of Kung bushmen in Northern Botswana. Am Heart J 1972; 84:5–12.

45. Swai AB, McLarty DG, Kitange HM, Kilima PM, Tatalla S, Keen N, Chuwa LM, Alberti KG. Low prevalence of risk factors for coronary heart disease in rural Tanzania. Int J Epidemiol 1993; 22:651–659.

46. Knuiman JT, West CE, Burema J. Serum total and high density lipoprotein cholesterol concentrations and body mass index in adult men from 13 countries. Am J Epidemiol 1982; 116:631–642.

47. Poulter NR, Khaw KT, Hopwood BE, Mugambi M, Peart WS, Rose G, Sever PS. The Kenyan Luo migration study: observations on the initiation of a rise in blood pressure. BMJ 1990; 300:967–972.

48. Fleming-Moran M, Coimbra Junior CE. Blood pressure studies among Amazonian native populations: a review from an epidemiological perspective. Soc Sci Med 1990; 31:593–601.

49. Mancilha-Carvalho JJ, Carvalho JV, Lima JA, Sousa e Silva NA. The absence of risk factors for coronary disease in Yanomami Indians and the influence of acculturation on arterial pressure. Arq Bras Cardiol 1992; 59:275–283.

50. Patrick RC, Prior IA, Smith JC, Smith AH. Relationship between blood pressure and modernity among Ponapeans. Int J Epidemiol 1983; 12:36–44.

51. Hodge AM, Dowse GK, Erasmus RT, Spark RA, Nathaniel K, Zimmet PZ, Alpers MP. Serum lipids and modernization in coastal and highland Papua New Guinea. Am J Epidemiol 1996; 144:1129–1142.

52. Knowler WC, Pettitt DJ, Saad MF, Bennett PH. Diabetes mellitus in the Pima Indians: incidence, risk factors and pathogenesis. Diabetes Metab Rev 1990; 6:1–27.

53. Hajjar IM, Grim CE, Kotchen TA. Dietary calcium lowers the age-related rise in blood pressure in the United States: the NHANES III survey. J Clin Hypertens (Greenwich) 2003; 5:122–126.

54. Harris MM, Stevens J, Thomas N, Schreiner P, Folsom AR. Associations of fat distribution and obesity with hypertension in a bi-ethnic population: the ARIC study. Atherosclerosis Risk in Communities Study. Obes Res 2000; 8:516–524.

55. Gerber AM, James SA, Ammerman AS, Keenan NL, Garrett JM, Strogatz DS, Haines PS. Socioeconomic status and electrolyte intake in black adults: the Pitt County Study. Am J Public Health 1991; 81:1608–1612.

56. Lorenzo C, Serrano-Rios M, Martinez-Larrad MT, Gabriel R, Williams K, Gonzalez-Villalpando C, Stern MP, Hazuda HP, Haffner S. Prevalence of hypertension in Hispanic and non-Hispanic white populations. Hypertension 2002; 39:203–208.

57. Colin Bell A, Adair LS, Popkin BM. Ethnic differences in the association between body mass index and hypertension. Am J Epidemiol 2002; 155:346–353.

58. Wiinberg N, Hoegholm A, Christensen HR, Bang LE, Mikkelsen KL, Nielsen PE, Svendsen TL, Kampmann JP, Madsen NH, Bentzon MW. 24-h ambulatory blood pressure in 352 normal Danish subjects, related to age and gender. Am J Hypertens 1995; 8:978–986.

59. Franklin SS, Gustin W IV, Wong ND, Larson MG, Weber MA, Kannel WB, Levy D. Hemodynamic patterns of age-related changes in blood pressure. The Framingham Heart Study. Circulation 1997; 96:308–315.

60. Leitschuh M, Cupples LA, Kannel W, Gagnon D, Chobanian A. High-normal blood pressure progression to hypertension in the Framingham Heart Study. Hypertension 1991; 17:22–27.

61. Stamler R, Stamler J, Riedlinger WF, Algera G, Roberts RH. Weight and blood pressure. Findings in hypertension screening of 1 million Americans. JAMA 1978; 240:1607–1610.

62. MacMahon S. Alcohol consumption and hypertension. Hypertension 1987; 9:111–121.

63. Hoffmans MD, Kromhout D, de Lezenne Coulander C. The impact of body mass index of 78,612 18-year old

Dutch men on 32-year mortality from all causes. J Clin Epidemiol 1988; 41:749–756.

64. Lamarche B. Abdominal obesity and its metabolic complications: implications for the risk of ischaemic heart disease. Coron Artery Dis 1998; 9:473–481.

65. Ko GT, Chan JC, Cockram CS. Age, body mass index and 2-hour plasma glucose are the major determinants of blood pressure in Chinese women newly diagnosed to have glucose intolerance. Int J Cardiol 1999; 69:33–39.

66. Hu FB, Wang B, Chen C, Jin Y, Yang J, Stampfer MJ, Xu X. Body mass index and cardiovascular risk factors in a rural Chinese population. Am J Epidemiol 2000; 151:88–97.

67. Deurenberg P, Yap M, van Staveren WA. Body mass index and percent body fat: a meta analysis among different ethnic groups. Int J Obes Relat Metab Disord 1998; 22:1164–1171.

68. Chandalia M, Abate N, Garg A, Stray-Gundersen J, Grundy SM. Relationship between generalized and upper body obesity to insulin resistance in Asian Indian men. J Clin Endocrinol Metab 1999; 84:2329–2335.

69. Barrett-Connor E. Sex differences in coronary heart disease. Why are women so superior? The 1995 Ancel Keys Lecture. Circulation 1997; 95:252–264.

70. Isles C. Blood pressure in males and females. J Hypertens 1995; 13:285–290.

71. Staessen J, Bulpitt CJ, Fagard R, Lijnen P, Amery A. The influence of menopause on blood pressure. J Hum Hypertens 1989; 3:427–433.

72. Staessen JA, Celis H, Fagard R. The epidemiology of the association between hypertension and menopause. J Hum Hypertens 1998; 12:587–592.

73. Scuteri A, Bos AJ, Brant LJ, Talbot L, Lakatta EG, Fleg JL. Hormone replacement therapy and longitudinal changes in blood pressure in postmenopausal women. Ann Intern Med 2001; 135:229–238.

74. Effects of estrogen or estrogen/progestin regimens on heart disease risk factors in postmenopausal women. The Postmenopausal Estrogen/Progestin Interventions (PEPI) Trial. The Writing Group for the PEPI Trial. JAMA 1995; 273:199–208.

75. Wassertheil-Smoller S, Anderson G, Psaty BM, Black HR, Manson J, Wong N, Francis J, Grimm R, Kotchen T, Langer R, Lasser N. Hypertension and its treatment in postmenopausal women: baseline data from the Women's Health Initiative. Hypertension 2000; 36:780–789.

76. Chasan-Taber L, Willett WC, Manson JE, Spiegelman D, Hunter DJ, Curhan G, Colditz GA, Stampfer MJ. Prospective study of oral contraceptives and hypertension among women in the United States. Circulation 1996; 94:483–489.

77. Bartosh SM, Aronson AJ. Childhood hypertension. An update on etiology, diagnosis, and treatment. Pediatr Clin North Am 1999; 46:235–252.

78. Morgenstern B. Blood pressure, hypertension, and ambulatory blood pressure monitoring in children and adolescents. Am J Hypertens 2002; 15(2 Pt 2):64S–66S.

79. Rosner B, Prineas RJ, Loggie JM, Daniels SR. Blood pressure nomograms for children and adolescents, by height, sex, and age, in the United States. J Pediatr 1993; 123:871–886.

80. Update on the 1987 Task Force Report on High Blood Pressure in Children and Adolescents: a working group report from the National High Blood Pressure Education Program. National High Blood Pressure Education Program Working Group on Hypertension Control in Children and Adolescents. Pediatrics 1996; 98(4 Pt 1):649–658.

81. Muntner P, He J, Cutler JA, Wildman RP, Whelton PK. Trends in blood pressure among children and adolescents. JAMA 2004; 291:2107–2113.

82. Kay JD, Sinaiko AR, Daniels SR. Pediatric hypertension. Am Heart J 2001; 142:422–432.

83. Lauer RM, Clarke WR. Childhood risk factors for high adult blood pressure: the Muscatine Study. Pediatrics 1989; 84:633–641.

84. Burke GL, Voors AW, Shear CL, Webber LS, Smoak CG, Cresanta JL, Berenson GS. Cardiovascular risk factors from birth to 7 years of age: the Bogalusa Heart Study. Blood pressure. Pediatrics 1987; 80(5 Pt 2):784–788.

85. Barker DJ, Osmond C, Golding J, Kuh D, Wadsworth ME. Growth in utero, blood pressure in childhood and adult life, and mortality from cardiovascular disease. BMJ 1989; 298:564–567.

86. Moore VM, Miller AG, Boulton TJ, Cockington RA, Craig IH, Magarey AM, Robinson JS. Placental weight, birth measurements, and blood pressure at age 8 years. Arch Dis Child 1996; 74:538–541.

87. Barker DJ, Forsen T, Eriksson JG, Osmond C. Growth and living conditions in childhood and hypertension in adult life: a longitudinal study. J Hypertens 2002; 20:1951–1956.

88. Yamori Y. Preliminary report of cardiac study: cross-sectional multicenter study on dietary factors of cardiovascular diseases. CARDIAC Study Group. Clin Exp Hypertens A 1989; 11:957–972.

89. Staessen J, Fagard R, Lijnen P, Amery A. Body weight, sodium intake and blood pressure. J Hypertens Suppl 1989; 7:S19–S23.

90. Morck TA, Lynch SR, Cook JD. Inhibition of food iron absorption by coffee. Am J Clin Nutr 1983; 37:416–420.

91. Smith-Barbaro PA, Pucak GJ. Dietary fat and blood pressure. Ann Intern Med 1983; 98(5 Pt 2):828–831.

92. Puska P, Iacono JM, Nissinen A, Korhonen HJ, Vartianinen E, Pietinen P, Dougherty R, Leino U, Mutanen M, Moisio S, Huttunen J. Controlled, randomised trial of the effect of dietary fat on blood pressure. Lancet 1983; 1:1–5.

93. Myers JB. Reduced sodium chloride intake normalises blood pressure distribution. J Hum Hypertens 1989; 3:97–104.

94. Stehbens WE. Diet and atherogenesis. Nutr Rev 1989; 47:1–12.

95. Jones DW, Kim JS, Andrew ME, Kim SJ, Hong YP. Body mass index and blood pressure in Korean men and women: the Korean National Blood Pressure Survey. J Hypertens 1994; 12:1433–1437.

96. Dahl LK, Heine M. Primary role of renal homografts in setting chronic blood pressure levels in rats. Circ Res 1975; 36:692–696.

97. Schmieder RE, Messerli FH, Garavaglia GE, Nunez BD. Cardiovascular effects of verapamil in

patients with essential hypertension. Circulation 1987; 75:1030–1036.

98. MacGregor GA, Markandu ND, Sagnella GA, Singer DR, Cappuccio FP. Double-blind study of three sodium intakes and long-term effects of sodium restriction in essential hypertension. Lancet 1989; 2:1244–1247.

99. Intersalt: an international study of electrolyte excretion and blood pressure. Results for 24 hour urinary sodium and potassium excretion. Intersalt Cooperative Research Group. BMJ 1988; 297:319–328.

100. Cutler JA, Stamler J. Introduction and summary of the dietary and nutritional methods and findings in the Multiple Risk Factor Intervention Trial. Am J Clin Nutr 1997; 65(suppl 1):184S–190S.

101. Falkner B, Michel S. Blood pressure response to sodium in children and adolescents. Am J Clin Nutr 1997; 65(suppl 2):618S–621S.

102. Salgado CM, Carvalhaes JT. Arterial hypertension in childhood. J Pediatr (Rio J) 2003; 79(suppl 1):S115–S124.

103. Midgley JP, Matthew AG, Greenwood CM, Logan AG. Effect of reduced dietary sodium on blood pressure: a meta-analysis of randomized controlled trials. JAMA 1996; 275:1590–1597.

104. Marmot MG, Elliott P, Shipley MJ, Dyer AR, Ueshima H, Beevers DG, Stamler R, Kesteloot H, Rose G, Stamler J. Alcohol and blood pressure: the INTERSALT study. BMJ 1994; 308:1263–1267.

105. Hajjar I, Kotchen T. Regional variations of blood pressure in the United States are associated with regional variations in dietary intakes: the NHANES-III data. J Nutr 2003; 133:211–214.

106. Wright A, Burstyn PG, Gibney MJ. Dietary fibre and blood pressure. Br Med J 1979; 2:1541–1543.

107. Sacks FM, Rosner B, Kass EH. Blood pressure in vegetarians. Am J Epidemiol 1974; 100:390–398.

108. Beilin LJ. Diet and lifestyle in hypertension: changing perspectives. J Cardiovasc Pharmacol 1990; 7(suppl 16): S62–S66.

109. Srikumar TS, Kallgard B, Ockerman PA, Akesson B. The effects of a 2-year switch from a mixed to a lactovegetarian diet on trace element status in hypertensive subjects. Eur J Clin Nutr 1992; 46:661–669.

110. Pratt RE, Dzau VJ. Genomics and hypertension: concepts, potentials, and opportunities. Hypertension 1999; 33:238–247.

111. Shaper AG, Pocock SJ, Walker M, Cohen NM, Wale CJ, Thomson AG. British Regional Heart Study: cardiovascular risk factors in middle-aged men in 24 towns. Br Med J (Clin Res Ed) 1981; 283:179–186.

112. Bruce NG, Wannamethee G, Shaper AG. Lifestyle factors associated with geographic blood pressure variations among men and women in the UK. J Hum Hypertens 1993; 7:229–238.

113. Kaufman JS, Tracy JA, Durazo-Arvizu RA, Cooper RS. Lifestyle, education, and prevalence of hypertension in populations of African origin. Results from the International Collaborative Study on Hypertension in Blacks. Ann Epidemiol 1997; 7:22–27.

114. Mendez MA, Cooper R, Wilks R, Luke A, Forrester T. Income, education, and blood pressure in adults in Jamaica, a middle-income developing country. Int J Epidemiol 2003; 32:400–408.

115. Chang CL, Shipley MJ, Marmot MG, Poulter NR. Can cardiovascular risk factors explain the association between education and cardiovascular disease in young women? J Clin Epidemiol 2002; 55:749–755.

116. Cooper R, Rotimi C. Hypertension in blacks. Am J Hypertens 1997; 10:804–812.

117. Mackenbach JP. The epidemiologic transition theory. J Epidemiol Community Health 1994; 48:329–331.

118. Forrester TE, Wilks RJ, Bennett FI, Simeon D, Osmond C, Allen M, Chung AP, Scott P. Fetal growth and cardiovascular risk factors in Jamaican schoolchildren. BMJ 1996; 312:156–160.

119. Bursztyn M, Raz I. Blood pressure, glucose, insulin and lipids of young Ethiopian recent immigrants to Israel and in those resident for 2 years. J Hypertens 1993; 11:455–459.

120. He J, Klag MJ, Whelton PK, Chen JY, Mo JP, Qian MC, Mo PS, He GQ. Migration, blood pressure pattern, and hypertension: the Yi Migrant Study. Am J Epidemiol 1991; 134:1085–1101.

121. Timio M, Lippi G, Venanzi S, Gentili S, Quintaliani G, Verdura C, Monarca C, Saronio P, Timio F. Blood pressure trend and cardiovascular events in nuns in a secluded order: a 30-year follow-up study. Blood Press 1997; 6:81–87.

122. Krieger N, Sidney S. Racial discrimination and blood pressure: the CARDIA Study of young black and white adults. Am J Public Health 1996; 86:1370–1378.

123. Lang T, Pariente P, Salem G, Tap D. Social, professional conditions and arterial hypertension: an epidemiological study in Dakar, Senegal. J Hypertens 1988; 6:271–276.

124. Actuaries Society. Blood Pressure Study. New York: Society of Actuaries and Association of Life Insurance Medical Directors, 1940.

125. Kannel WB. Elevated systolic blood pressure as a cardiovascular risk factor. Am J Cardiol 2000; 85:251–255.

126. MacMahon S. Antihypertensive drug treatment: the potential, expected and observed effects on vascular disease. J Hypertens Suppl 1990; 8:S239–S244.

127. MacMahon S, Peto R, Cutler J, Collins R, Sorlie P, Neaton J, Abbott R, Godwin J, Dyer A, Stamler J. Blood pressure, stroke, and coronary heart disease. Part 1, Prolonged differences in blood pressure: prospective observational studies corrected for the regression dilution bias. Lancet 1990; 335:765–774.

128. Murray CJ, Lopez AD. Mortality by cause for eight regions of the world: Global Burden of Disease Study. Lancet 1997; 349:1269–1276.

129. Franklin SS, Weber MA. Measuring hypertensive cardiovascular risk: the vascular overload concept. Am Heart J 1994; 128:793–803.

130. Darne B, Girerd X, Safar M, Cambien F, Guize L. Pulsatile versus steady component of blood pressure: a cross-sectional analysis and a prospective analysis on cardiovascular mortality. Hypertension 1989; 13:392–400.

131. Benetos A, Safar M, Rudnichi A et al. Pulse pressure: a predictor of long-term cardiovascular mortality in a French male population. Hypertension 1997; 30:1410–1415.

132. Mitchell GF, Moye LA, Braunwald E, Rouleau JL, Bernstein V, Geltman EM, Flaker GC, Pfeffer MA. Sphygmomanometrically determined pulse pressure is a powerful independent predictor of recurrent events after myocardial infarction in patients with impaired left ventricular function. SAVE investigators. Survival and Ventricular Enlargement. Circulation 1997; 96:4254–4260.

133. Domanski MJ, Davis BR, Pfeffer MA, Kastantin M, Mitchell GF. Isolated systolic hypertension: prognostic information provided by pulse pressure. Hypertension 1999; 34:375–380.

134. Madhavan S, Ooi WL, Cohen H, Alderman MH. Relation of pulse pressure and blood pressure reduction to the incidence of myocardial infarction. Hypertension 1994; 23:395–401.

135. Chae CU, Pfeffer MA, Glynn RJ, Mitchell GF, Taylor JO, Hennekens CH. Increased pulse pressure and risk of heart failure in the elderly. JAMA 1999; 281:634–639.

136. Menotti A, Jacobs DR Jr, Blackburn H, Kromhout D, Nissinen A, Nedeljkovic S, Buzina R, Mohacek I, Seccareccia F, Giampaoli S, Dontas A, Aravanis C, Toshima H. Twenty-five-year prediction of stroke deaths in the seven countries study: the role of blood pressure and its changes. Stroke 1996; 27:381–387.

137. Seshadri S, Wolf PA, Beiser A, Vasan RS, Wilson PW, Kase CS, Kelly-Hayes M, Kannel WB, D'Agostino RB. Elevated midlife blood pressure increases stroke risk in elderly persons: the Framingham Study. Arch Intern Med 2001; 161:2343–2350.

138. Prentice RL, Shimizu Y, Lin CH, Peterson AV, Kato H, Mason MW, Szatrowski TP. Serial blood pressure measurements and cardiovascular disease in a Japanese cohort. Am J Epidemiol 1982; 116:1–28.

139. Marang-van de Mheen PJ, Gunning-Schepers LJ. Variation between studies in reported relative risks associated with hypertension: time trends and other explanatory variables. Am J Public Health 1998; 88:618–622.

140. Keli S, Bloemberg B, Kromhout D. Predictive value of repeated systolic blood pressure measurements for stroke risk. The Zutphen Study. Stroke 1992; 23:347–351.

141. Kannel WB, Wolf PA, Verter J, McNamara PM. Epidemiologic assessment of the role of blood pressure in stroke. The Framingham study. JAMA 1970; 214:301–310.

142. Kannel WB. Vital epidemiologic clues in heart failure. J Clin Epidemiol 2000; 53:229–235.

143. Vasan RS, Benjamin EJ, Levy D. Congestive heart failure with normal left ventricular systolic function. Clinical approaches to the diagnosis and treatment of diastolic heart failure. Arch Intern Med 1996; 156:146–157.

144. Vaccarino V, Holford TR, Krumholz HM. Pulse pressure and risk for myocardial infarction and heart failure in the elderly. J Am Coll Cardiol 2000; 36:130–138.

145. Franklin SS, Khan SA, Wong ND, Larson MG, Levy D. Is pulse pressure useful in predicting risk for coronary heart Disease? The Framingham heart study. Circulation 1999; 100:354–360.

146. Verdecchia P, Schillaci G, Reboldi G, Ambrosio G, Pede S, Porcellati C. Prognostic value of midwall shortening fraction and its relation with left ventricular mass in systemic hypertension. Am J Cardiol 2001; 87:479–482, A7.

147. Casale PN, Devereux RB, Milner M, Zullo G, Harshfield GA, Pickering TG, Laragh JH. Value of echocardiographic measurement of left ventricular mass in predicting cardiovascular morbid events in hypertensive men. Ann Intern Med 1986; 105:173–178.

148. Perry HM Jr, Miller JP, Fornoff JR, Baty JD, Sambhi MP, Rutan G, Moskowitz DW, Carmody SE. Early predictors of 15-year end-stage renal disease in hypertensive patients. Hypertension 1995; 25:587–594.

149. Brancati FL, Whelton PK, Whittle JC, Klag MJ. Epidemiologic analysis of existing data to investigate hypertensive renal disease: an example from the Maryland End-Stage Renal Disease Registry. Am J Kidney Dis 1993; 21(4 suppl 1):15–24.

150. Perneger TV, Whelton PK, Klag MJ, Rossiter KA. Diagnosis of hypertensive end-stage renal disease: effect of patient's race. Am J Epidemiol 1995; 141:10–15.

151. Bakris GL, Weir MR, Shanifar S, Zhang Z, Douglas J, van Dijk DJ, Brenner BM. RENAAL Study Group. Effects of blood pressure level on progression of diabetic nephropathy: results from the RENAAL study. Arch Intern Med 2003; 163:1555–1565.

152. Brenner BM, Cooper ME, de Zeeuw D, Keane WF, Mitch WE, Parving HH, Remuzzi G, Snapinn SM, Zhang Z, Shahinfar S. RENAAL Study Investigators. Effects of losartan on renal and cardiovascular outcomes in patients with type 2 diabetes and nephropathy. N Engl J Med 2001; 345:861–869.

153. Perry HM Jr, Miller JP, Baty JD, Carmody SE, Sambhi MP. Pretreatment blood pressure as a predictor of 21-year mortality. Am J Hypertens 2000; 13:724–733.

154. Jafar TH, Schmid CH, Landa M, Giatras I, Toto R, Remuzzi G, Maschio G, Brenner BM, Kamper A, Zucchelli P, Becker G, Himmelmann A, Bannister K, Landais P, Shahinfar S, de Jong PE, de Zeeuw D, Lau J, Levey AS. Angiotensin-converting enzyme inhibitors and progression of nondiabetic renal disease. A meta-analysis of patient-level data. Ann Intern Med 2001; 135:73–87.

155. Peterson JC, Adler S, Burkart JM, Greene T, Hebert LA, Hunsicker LG, King AJ, Klahr S, Massry SG, Seifter JL. Blood pressure control, proteinuria, and the progression of renal disease. The Modification of Diet in Renal Disease Study. Ann Intern Med 1995; 123:754–762.

156. Lewis JB, Berl T, Bain RP, Rohde RD, Lewis EJ. Effect of intensive blood pressure control on the course of type 1 diabetic nephropathy. Collaborative Study Group. Am J Kidney Dis 1999; 34:809–817.

157. Kannel WB, McGee DL. Update on some epidemiologic features of intermittent claudication: the Framingham Study. J Am Geriatr Soc 1985; 33:13–18.

158. Smith GD, Shipley MJ, Rose G. Intermittent claudication, heart disease risk factors, and mortality. The Whitehall Study. Circulation 1990; 82:1925–1931.

159. Criqui MH, Langer RD, Fronek A, Feigelson HS, Klauber MR, McCann TJ, Browner D. Mortality over a period of 10 years in patients with peripheral arterial disease. N Engl J Med 1992; 326:381–386.

160. Murabito JM, Evans JC, Nieto K, Larson MG, Levy D, Wilson PW. Prevalence and clinical correlates of peripheral arterial disease in the Framingham Offspring Study. Am Heart J 2002; 143:961–965.

161. Keith N, Wagener H, Kernohan J. The syndrome of malignant hypertension. Arch Intern Med 1928; 41:44.

162. Ramsay LE, Waller PC. Strokes in mild hypertension: diastolic rules. Lancet 1986; 2:854–856.

163. Kannel WB, Gordon T, Schwartz MJ. Systolic versus diastolic blood pressure and risk of coronary heart disease. The Framingham study. Am J Cardiol 1971; 27:335–346.

164. Khattar RS, Swales JD, Dore C, Senior R, Lahiri A. Effect of aging on the prognostic significance of ambulatory systolic, diastolic, and pulse pressure in essential hypertension. Circulation 2001; 104:783–789.

165. Kannel WB. Cardiovascular hazards of components of blood pressure. J Hypertens 2002; 20:395–397.

166. Pannier B, Brunel P, el Aroussy W, Lacolley P, Safar ME. Pulse pressure and echocardiographic findings in essential hypertension. J Hypertens 1989; 7:127–132.

167. Franklin SS, Larson MG, Khan SA, Wong ND, Leip EP, Kannel WB, Levy D. Does the relation of blood pressure to coronary heart disease risk change with aging? The Framingham Heart Study. Circulation 2001; 103:1245–1249.

168. Celentano A, Palmieri V, Di Palma Esposito N, Pietropaolo I, Arezzi E, Mureddu GF, de Simone G. Relations of pulse pressure and other components of blood pressure to preclinical echocardiographic abnormalities. J Hypertens 2002; 20:531–537.

169. Klag MJ, Whelton PK, Randall BL, Neaton JD, Brancati FL, Ford CE, Shulman NB, Stamler J. Blood pressure and end-stage renal disease in men. N Engl J Med 1996; 334:13–18.

Part B: Etiology, Physiology, and Pathophysiology

4

Genetics of Hypertension

STEPHEN J. NEWHOUSE, SABIH M. HUQ, GANESH ARUNACHALAM,
MARK J. CAULFIELD, PATRICIA B. MUNROE

*Clinical Pharmacology and Barts and the London Genome Centre, William Harvey Research Institute,
St. Bartholomew's Hospital, London, UK*

KEYPOINTS

- About 30–50% of blood pressure variance within a population is of genetic origin.
- Genetic and environmental factors interact to produce the final hypertensive phenotype.
- Single-gene disorders that have hypertension as a primary phenotype are rare.
- Genetic studies of essential and secondary hypertension suggest a common final pathway for the pathogenesis of hypertension via the kidney renin–angiotensin–aldosterone system (RAAS) and changes in renal sodium handling.
- Pharmacogenetics uses the patients' genetic profile to predict their response to a particular drug.

SUMMARY

Estimates are that 30–50% of the blood pressure variance within a population is of genetic origin. Essential hypertension is a complex, multifactorial, polygenic trait, where both genetic and environmental factors interact to produce the final phenotype. Thus, inherited genes may not cause hypertension directly, but confer susceptibility to develop hypertension given appropriate environmental cues. Single-gene disorders that have hypertension as a primary phenotype exist, and the genetic variants underlying the mechanism of hypertension have been demonstrated. These disorders provide insight into new pathways and genes involved in blood pressure regulation and the pathogenesis of hypertension. Over 60 candidate genes for essential hypertension have been studied in different populations, and genetic variants have been identified for all of these genes. To date, not one gene has been conclusively linked or associated with essential hypertension. Studies of essential and secondary hypertension suggest a common final pathway for the pathogenesis of hypertension via the kidney renin–angiotensin–aldosterone system and changes in renal sodium handling. Genome-wide screens for blood pressure loci have implicated numerous regions in different populations on all chromosomes except 13 and 20. The results confirm the polygenic and heterogeneous nature of the disorder and suggest that hypertension may result from the interaction of many genes with modest effect. Pharmacogenetics has demonstrated the potential of using a patient's genetic profile to predict their response to a particular drug.

I. INTRODUCTION

Hypertension is a major public health problem that affects >20% of the adult population worldwide. It is a major risk factor for cardiovascular disease, contributing greatly to morbidity and mortality from stroke, myocardial infarction, end-stage renal disease, and congestive heart failure (1). Considering the impact of hypertension on human health, substantial effort has been put into the study of the disorder. In ~5% of hypertensive patients, an underlying renal or adrenal disease or a single gene mutation is responsible for the disorder; these patients have what is called *secondary hypertension*. The remaining 95% of hypertensive patients have *essential hypertension*, in which there is no single, clearly identifiable cause for the elevated blood pressure (1). Family and epidemiological studies suggest that essential hypertension results from a complex interaction between genetic and environmental factors, including high salt intake, alcohol, and obesity. Although the environmental influences on blood pressure have been well established, we still have a limited understanding of the genetic factors that contribute to essential hypertension and the interactions that produce the disorder.

With the advent of modern genomics and its application to the discovery of disease genes, the genetic mechanisms that contribute to hypertension are beginning to reveal themselves. This chapter will outline the evidence that hypertension is a genetic disease, describe the nature of the disorder, and discuss some of the approaches that are used to study the genetics of hypertension. This discussion will be followed by an overview of some of the major findings from studies of both secondary and essential hypertension and the application of pharmacogenetics in hypertension research.

II. EVIDENCE FOR A GENETIC COMPONENT

It has been estimated that 30–50% of the blood pressure variance within a population is inherited, which suggests that hypertension is, in part, a genetically determined disease (2). The evidence comes primarily from studies of families, twins, and adopted children. Each type of study examines the proportion of genetic and environmental factors that contribute to blood pressure variation. If there is a genetic component to hypertension, it is expected that blood pressure levels and the incidence of hypertension would be similar between biological relatives.

Family studies do show that hypertension occurs more frequently in individuals who have a family history of hypertension (3). In addition, these studies show that these individuals are ~1.6 times more likely to develop high blood pressure if they have a first-degree relative with the condition (3,4). This trend has been termed "familial aggregation." The similarity of blood pressure levels within families is not restricted to individuals in the family who are hypertensive because familial aggregation of blood pressure can be seen for all blood pressure levels across all age groups (3). Familial aggregation, however, does not prove conclusively that there is a genetic component to hypertension. Families share both their genes and their environment; therefore, similarity also could be attributed to a shared environment.

Studies of twins and families with adopted children allow researchers to separate, to some extent, the relative effects of genes and environment on blood pressure levels. Studies of twins take advantage of the fact that monozygotic (identical) twins share 100% of their genes and dizygotic (nonidentical) twins share only 50% of their genetic make-up. This difference allows researchers to examine the "heritability" of a trait. Heritability refers to the proportion of phenotypic variation that can be explained by genetic factors. A higher correlation or similarity in blood pressure levels between monozygotic twins than between dizygotic twins indicates a genetic influence (5,6). For blood pressure levels, it has been demonstrated that monozygotic twins have a higher correlation coefficient than dizygotic twins, and that the incidence of hypertension is higher among monozygotic twins than among dizygotic twins. Overall, studies of twins have estimated the heritability of blood pressure levels to be in the range of 50–70% (7–9).

Studies of families with adopted children have the advantage of comparing different genetic influences in the same family environment. This type of study involves the comparison of genetically related relatives (i.e., biological relatives) and people who are relatives by adoption (i.e., genetically unrelated individuals who live in the same family). A greater similarity or concordance of a particular trait between biological relatives than between adopted relatives suggests a genetic influence. Alternatively, if adopted relatives show more similarity for a trait, this suggests a greater contribution from environmental factors. The similarity of blood pressure levels among biological relatives but not in adopted relatives lends further support for a role of genetic factors in hypertension. Studies of families with adopted children show that the incidence of hypertension is greater among biological siblings than between adopted siblings. There is also a greater concordance of blood pressure levels in general among biological siblings than among adopted siblings living in the same household, which demonstrates that familial aggregation of blood pressure cannot be attributed only to shared environmental factors (10–12).

Rare Mendelian disorders that have high blood pressure or a low blood pressure as the primary phenotype also have been identified (13). Although the mutations in the genes responsible for these disorders are rare and, therefore, unlikely to contribute to the overall prevalence of hypertension in the general population, these forms of hypertension have emphasized the importance of genetic factors in blood pressure control and in the development of hypertension.

III. THE NATURE OF THE GENETIC COMPONENT

The inheritance pattern of hypertension has been debated for many years. During the 1950s, studies to determine the genetic influences on hypertension sparked a debate between Sir George Pickering and Sir Robert Platt over whether hypertension is a monogenic or a polygenic disorder. Pickering argued that because blood pressure has a continuous distribution in the general population, there are multiple genes and environmental factors that determine the level of an individual's blood pressure and that hypertension is merely the upper end of this distribution (14). The Pickering school of thought put forward the theory that an individual with essential hypertension is

one who happens to have inherited an aggregate of genes and is exposed to environmental factors that favor hypertension (14). The Platt school of thought held that hypertension was a discrete genetic entity that displays Mendelian autosomal dominant inheritance (15).

Both theories proved to be correct. A small number of hypertensives within a population will have a high blood pressure level that is caused by a single gene disorder. (See Section V in this chapter.) However, in the vast majority of individuals in the hypertensive population, there is no clear pattern of Mendelian inheritance. This supports the notion that hypertension is influenced by a number of different genes in combination with environmental influences.

It is now generally accepted that essential hypertension is a *polygenic* disorder. This means that several genes, either a few "major" genes that exert moderate effects or many "minor" genes that exert smaller individual effects on blood pressure level, cause raised blood pressure.

However, there are probably more layers of complexity. First, multiple variants (*alleles*) of these genes are likely to exist, with each variant having a different effect on blood pressure level. Secondly, different combinations of genes can influence blood pressure in a unique manner, with certain combinations of genes more readily elevating blood pressure. Thirdly, environmental factors (e.g., salt intake) also will interact with genetic factors to influence blood pressure levels. Finally, genetic variability might predispose an individual to hypertension, but it may not be enough to cause hypertension outright. It will cause hypertension, however, when combined with the effects from genetic variants at other loci and environmental factors.

IV. STRATEGIES FOR IDENTIFYING BLOOD PRESSURE GENES

The two approaches commonly used for identifying the genetic determinants of human disease are linkage and association studies (16). These tools were developed initially for mapping simple Mendelian traits, but with advances in statistical genetics and technologies, they are now being applied to complex disease gene mapping (17). In genetic *linkage analysis*, the co-inheritance of blood pressure and a genetic marker (usually microsatellites) is tested between affected individuals within a family (e.g., sibling pairs). Chromosomal regions that harbor blood pressure genes are defined as those regions in which identical marker alleles are shared more often than would be expected by chance. Basically, if the location on a chromosome of a marker locus and a disease-causing gene locus are physically close, and the probability of recombination between the two loci is low, the genetic marker will *co-segregate*, or travel, with the disease-causing locus. The loci are then said to be in tight "linkage." Thus, it is possible to infer the chromosomal location of a disease locus from the location of the marker locus.

Linkage studies can either focus on genetic loci that have previously been implicated in hypertension or be carried out on a genome-wide scale. The genome-wide screen approach has become a standard tool for studying complex diseases like hypertension because it allows the identification of new genes that have been missed previously. The relative odds or the likelihood that the co-segregation of the marker and disease is due to linkage as opposed to chance is measured by the logarithm of odds (LOD) score. An LOD score of >3 is generally considered to be strong evidence for linkage (18).

When a candidate gene has been identified, either through linkage mapping studies or on the basis of its known function, *association studies* are designed to detect the association between the disease and specific alleles of the gene. Association studies are crucial for identifying the genes implicated in a disease. One of the most popular designs for studying allelic association between a disease and a marker is the *case–control design*. In this type of study, investigators search for the differences in the allele frequencies at a marker locus in unrelated groups of individuals with hypertension ("cases," i.e., patients) and groups of individuals without the disease (the *controls*). Significant differences in allelic frequencies at this marker locus between the two groups will implicate specific alleles at that locus in the etiology of the disease. If an allele is found more frequently in individuals with the disease than it is in individuals without the disease, the allele is said to be associated with the disease. The marker may be the causal mutation, or it may be in linkage disequilibrium with the true disease-causing allele.

In the hunt for blood pressure genes, a number of strategies have been employed to identify hypertension susceptibility loci. These have included the study of rare Mendelian forms of hypertension, the investigation of candidate genes, and genome-wide screens. Candidate gene analysis has been the primary strategy in determining and testing for genes that may be involved in essential hypertension. This approach assumes that either a single gene or a number of genes associated with specific physiological or cellular functions contribute to blood pressure variation. Candidate genes have been chosen on the basis of their recognized effects on cardiovascular and renal function and on the known pathophysiology of hypertension. Candidacy can also be based on linkage data. For example, if a gene maps to a region that has been linked to hypertension in a chromosomal or genome-wide mapping study, this gene can be considered

as a *positional candidate*. Although hypertension is considered a complex disease, candidate genes also can be selected on the basis of studies of the Mendelian forms of hypertension. Because the Mendelian disorders are extremely rare, they do not contribute greatly to the overall hypertensive burden (although they are probably under-diagnosed). However, the genes responsible for these rare disorders are providing insight into the pathogenesis of hypertension and, thus, highlight potential new genes and pathways for further study. The hypothesis is that subtle variations in these genes may contribute to the development of essential hypertension.

V. MONOGENIC HYPERTENSION

The most striking advances in blood pressure genetics have been made in the field of monogenic hypertension. Nine single-gene disorders are now known, seven of which have been characterized at the functional level (Table 4.1). An interesting feature is that despite the numerous physiological systems that are involved in the regulation of blood pressure, the abnormal gene product, in all of these disorders affects the same one system: renal salt handling.

A. Normal Physiology of the Kidney

The kidneys filter 188 L of plasma every day. This filtered load contains about 25 moles of salt, equivalent to nearly 25 kg, of which $<1\%$ is excreted. The whole process is highly energy intensive. The kidneys receive 7% of the total oxygen intake for the body, despite the fact that they comprise only 0.5% of the total body weight. Ninety-nine percent of this energy cost is attributable to active sodium transport. The mechanism by which salt is reabsorbed and modulated is complex. Knowledge of several elements of this system has come directly from research into the Mendelian forms of hypertension.

Sixty-seven percent of filtered sodium is reabsorbed in the proximal convoluted tubule, 24% of filtered sodium is reabsorbed in the thick, ascending loop of Henle via the sodium–potassium chloride co-transporter, and 7% of filtered sodium is reabsorbed in the distal convoluted tubule via the sodium chloride co-transporter. The remaining 2% of filtered sodium is reabsorbed in the cortical collecting tubule via the epithelial sodium channel. The last stage of sodium reabsorption is the most highly regulated in the system. Fine control is provided by modulating the activity of the epithelial sodium channel via aldosterone, which in turn is under the influence of the RAAS (19).

Given the huge volume of filtrate, even a small percentage of change in salt handling will result in a large change

Table 4.1 Monogenic Forms of Hypertension

Syndrome	Mode of inheritance	Chromosome	Gene product	Phenotype
Pseudohypoaldosteronism type 2	Autosomal dominant	12p, 17q, and 1q	WNK1, WNK4[a]	Hypertension, $\uparrow K^+$, metabolic acidosis
Glucocorticoid remediable aldosteronism	Autosomal dominant	8q	Chimeric protein: aldosterone synthase and 11-β-hydroxylase	Hypertension with other variable features
Apparent mineralocorticoid excess	Autosomal recessive	16q	$\downarrow$11-β-hydroxysteroid dehydrogenase	Hypertension, $\downarrow K^+$, metabolic alkalosis, $\downarrow$renin, $\downarrow\downarrow$aldosterone
Congenital adrenal hyperplasia	Autosomal recessive	8q	$\downarrow$11-β-hydroxylase	Hypertension with other variable features
		10q	$\downarrow$17-α-hydroxylase	Hypertension, absent sexual maturation, $\downarrow K^+$
Hypertension exacerbated by pregnancy	Autosomal dominant	4q	Abnormal MR[b]	Early hypertension exacerbated by pregnancy
Liddle's syndrome	Autosomal dominant	16q	Abnormal ENaC[c]: reduced receptor clearance	Hypertension, $\downarrow K^+$, metabolic alkalosis, $\downarrow$renin, $\downarrow$aldosterone
PPARγ mutations[d]	Autosomal dominant	3p	Malfunctioning nuclear receptor PPARγ	Hypertension, insulin resistance, type 2 diabetes
Hypertension and brachydactyly	Autosomal dominant	12p	Unknown	Hypertension, brachydactyly

[a]Specific enzymes in the WNK (with no lysine K) family of kinases.
[b]Mineralocorticoid receptor.
[c]Epithelial sodium channel.
[d]Peroxisome proliferator-activated receptor.

in the net sodium balance. Therefore, modifying any one of the steps in the pathway can lead to significant (and clinically relevant) changes. Mutations that increase sodium reabsorption and lead to hypertension have been identified at various points in the control pathway, and we will now look at these, working our way along the nephron (Fig. 4.1).

B. Pseudohypoaldosteronism Type 2

Also known as familial hyperkalemic hypertension (Gordon's syndrome), this is a genetically heterogeneous disease. The key feature is overactivity of the sodium chloride co-transporter in the distal convoluted tubule and the cortical collecting duct. This causes an increase in net sodium reabsorption, which, in turn, increases the plasma volume (because plasma osmolality is held constant) and, thus, cardiac output and blood pressure. Decreased delivery of sodium to the distal tubule decreases the electrical gradient that is generated by the epithelial sodium channel (lumen-negative gradient) and, thus, impairs hydrogen and potassium secretion. This explains the classical phenotypic features of hypertension, hyperkalemia, hyperchloremic metabolic acidosis,

suppressed renin activity, and normal or elevated aldosterone (inappropriately low for the level of hyperkalemia). All these abnormalities can be corrected by the administration of thiazide diuretics, which are specific sodium chloride co-transporter inhibitors (20).

How is increased sodium chloride co-transporter function mediated? Genetic studies have found mutations in specific enzymes, WNK (with no lysine K) kinases—a family of serine–threonine kinases that are involved in several signal transduction pathways. The WNK4 kinase inhibits the sodium chloride co-transporter naturally by decreasing its cell surface expression, and mutant WNK4 has been found to increase sodium chloride co-transporter activity *in vitro*. Various missense mutations that co-segregate with the disease in the WNK4 gene on chromosome 17 have been found (21).

This is not the only genetic abnormality that causes the pseudohypoaldosteronism 2 (PHA2) phenotype. Other regions on chromosomes 1q and 12p also have been linked in different families (21,22). Chromosome 12p contains the WNK1 kinase gene, and intronic deletions within this gene have been found to co-segregate precisely with the PHA2 phenotype. These intronic deletions lead to an increase in WNK1 expression. *In vitro* studies

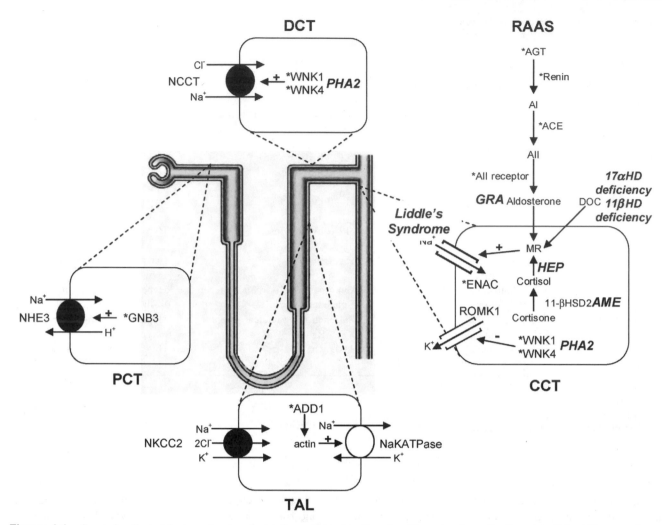

Figure 4.1 Genes implicated in hypertension that influence renal sodium handling. A schematic diagram of the kidney nephron, showing the major sites of sodium (Na$^+$) reabsorption. The major apical sodium transporters in the individual renal cells are the type 3 Na$^+$/H$^+$ exchanger (NHE3) in the proximal convoluted tubule (PCT), the bumetamide-sensitive type 2 Na-K-2Cl co-transporter (NKCC2) in the thick ascending limb (TAL), the thiazide-sensitive sodium chloride co-transporter (NCCT) in the distal convoluted tubule (DCT), and the amiloride-sensitive epithelial sodium channel (ENaC) in the cortical collecting tubule (CCT) and connecting ducts. In all cell types sodium is reabsorbed into the blood across the basolateral membrane by the Na-K ATPase (NaKATPase). (For the sake of clarity, only NaKATPase is shown in the TAL.) Also shown is the RAAS, which is involved in tightly regulating sodium reabsorption via the action of aldosterone. Genetic variants of these sodium transporters and their regulators have been shown to cause hypertension. The monogenic forms of hypertension (designated by bold, italicized font) and the gene responsible for each disorder are indicated. Candidate genes that are implicated in essential hypertension and that may influence renal sodium handling are designated by asterisks. Abbreviations used are as follows: 11βHD, 11-beta-hydroxylase; 11-βHSD2, 11-beta-hydroxysteroid dehydrogenase 2; 17αHD, 17-alpha-hydroxylase; ACE, Angiotensin-converting enzyme; ADD1, α-adducin; AGT, Angiotensinogen; AI, Angiotensin I; AII, Angiotensin II; AME, Apparent mineralocorticoid excess; DOC, Deoxycorticosterone; GNB3, G-protein beta3 subunit gene; GRA, Glucocorticoid-remediable aldosteronism; HEP, Hypertension exacerbated by pregnancy; MR, Mineralocorticoid receptor; PHA2, Pseudohypoaldosteronism type 2; ROMK1, Renal outer medullary potassium channel; WNK, Family of protein WNK kinases. From Lifton et al. (13) © 2001 Cell Press; adapted with permission from Elsevier.

have suggested that WNK1 does not inhibit sodium chloride co-transporter directly but does prevent WNK4-mediated inhibition of sodium chloride co-transporter (23). It should be noted that understanding of WNK protein function with respect to renal salt handling is still in a preliminary stage and that specific targets for the kinases and the complete signalling pathway have yet to be discovered.

C. Glucocorticoid-Remediable Aldosteronism

Glucocorticoid-remediable aldosteronism is an autosomal dominant disorder whereby ectopic aldosterone production causes increased sodium reabsorption at the epithelial sodium channel, which thus leads to hypertension. The last two steps in the biosynthesis of aldosterone from cholesterol are catalyzed by 11-β-hydroxylase and aldosterone synthase. These two enzymes are >90% identical, and the genes that code them are adjacent to each other on chromosome 8q. The genetic defect in glucocorticoid-remediable aldosteronism has been found to be due to unequal crossover during meiosis. This leads to the 5′ regulatory end of the 11-β-hydroxylase gene fusing to the catalytic 3′ end of aldosterone synthase gene, creating a chimeric gene. The resulting protein has the enzymatic activity of aldosterone synthase, but is under the regulatory control of adrenocorticotropic hormone. Therefore, it is expressed ectopically in adrenal fasiculata and does not respond to the usual signals (from angiotensin II and plasma potassium) for aldosterone release, but to adrenocorticotropic hormone. (Hence, it can be suppressed by therapy with an exogenous steroid.) Various crossover points have been identified in patients with glucocorticoid-remediable aldosteronism, all of which are proximal to exon 5 of aldosterone synthase, which suggest that this region is essential in maintaining catalytic aldosterone synthase activity (24).

The phenotype for glucocorticoid-remediable aldosteronism is variable. Hypokalemia is not present in many cases, and although individuals in some families have very high blood pressure with early death from stroke, this is not always the case. The hypertension may be mild (25). The hypertension and biochemical abnormalities can be reversed through dexamethasone therapy.

D. Non-Aldosterone Steroid Disorders

There are three autosomal recessive disorders in which steroids other than aldosterone activate a normal mineralocorticoid receptor—apparent mineralocorticoid excess and two types of congenital adrenal hyperplasia.

1. Apparent Mineralocorticoid Excess

In vitro, cortisol is a potent activator of the mineralocorticoid receptor. In the body, however, despite its high plasma concentrations, cortisol has little effect on the mineralocorticoid receptor. This is because 11-β-hydroxysteroid dehydrogenase type 2 converts cortisol to cortisone, a far less potent agonist. In apparent mineralocorticoid excess, homozygous mutations cause a loss of function of 11-β-hydroxysteroid dehydrogenase type 2, which leads to increased levels of cortisol in the distal nephron of the kidney, subsequent activation of the mineralocorticoid receptor, and increased epithelial sodium channel activity and, therefore, to hypertension (26). Phenotypic features of apparent mineralocorticoid excess are early onset hypertension with hypokalemia, metabolic alkalosis, suppressed renin levels, and very low aldosterone levels.

2. Congenital Adrenal Hyperplasia

Congenital adrenal hyperplasia encompasses several inherited disorders in which adrenal steroid synthesis is abnormal and the result is a deficiency of cortisol. Two of the rarer forms of congenital adrenal hyperplasia produce hypertension at an early age: 11-β-hydroxylase deficiency and 17-α-hydroxylase deficiency. This is the result of increased concentrations of steroids (metabolites of deoxycorticosterone) proximal to the defective step in the synthetic pathway. These steroids can activate the mineralocorticoid receptor, but they are not usually present in high enough concentrations to do so. More than 20 mutations in the 11-β-hydroxylase gene on chromosome 8q (27) and at least 18 mutations in the 17-α-hydroxylase gene on chromosome 10 have been identified that cause deficiencies in hydroxylase. The more severe forms of congenital adrenal hyperplasia completely destroy enzymatic activity; in milder forms of congenital adrenal hyperplasia, partial activity is retained. Phenotypically, both 11-β-hydroxylase deficiency and 17-α-hydroxylase deficiency often (but not always) cause early onset hypertension and hypokalemic metabolic alkalosis. 11-β-hydroxylase-deficient patients display various other phenotypic features, including signs of excess virilization. Features of 17-α-hydroxylase deficiency include ambiguous genitalia and primary amenorrhea (28).

E. Hypertension Exacerbated by Pregnancy

One rare type of Mendelian hypertension is caused not by excess ligand stimulating a normal mineralocorticoid receptor, but by a genetically abnormal receptor. The abnormal receptor is activated by molecules that usually do not activate this receptor. An autosomal dominant condition recently was identified, in which a leucine-to-serine mutation at position 810 in the mineralocorticoid receptor eliminates the need for agonists to have a 21-hydroxyl group. This allows steroids such as progesterone and spironolactone, which do not have a hydroxyl group at this position, to activate the receptor. All the affected members of the family in the study had hypertension before the age of 20, which became markedly worse during pregnancy as a result of the sharp increase in levels of progesterone (29).

F. Liddle's Syndrome

The final control point in renal salt balance is the epithelial sodium channel. The functioning of this channel is controlled by aldosterone, but mutations in the genes that encode the channel itself can cause an increase in sodium transport activity and, therefore, excessive salt reabsorption and hypertension. The channel is a heterotrimer (α, β, and γ subunits) (30), which is removed from the cell surface by endocytosis. The process of removing this heterotrimer depends on a conserved sequence (PPPXY) on both the β and γ subunits. Mutations in the β subunit and in the γ subunit have been found to reduce receptor complex clearance and thus increase the sodium flow, producing the disorder (31–33) (Fig. 4.1). Patients with these mutations have early onset hypertension, hypokalemic alkalosis, and decreased renin and aldosterone levels. The abnormalities respond to treatment with amiloride which blocks the epithelial sodium channel.

G. Other Monogenic Forms of Hypertension

Two other monogenic forms of hypertension are known. One form is an autosomal dominant hypertension with brachydactyly, in which affected individuals have severe hypertension that shortens life expectancy. RAAS responses are normal. This condition has been mapped to a 3.15 Mb area on chromosome 12p. A complex chromosomal rearrangement that involves a deletion, re-insertion, and inversion has been identified recently in one Turkish family (34). Although several candidate genes in the identified region of chromosome 12p have been studied, none seems to be the cause of the syndrome. Further research with more families is required.

Another monogenic form of hypertension comprises mutations in the peroxisome proliferator-activated receptor gamma (PPARγ) receptor. Three patients from two unrelated families were found to have autosomal dominant, loss-of-function mutations that involved the binding domain of the PPARγ receptor. The clinical syndrome consisted of severe insulin resistance, early onset diabetes, and hypertension (35). The PPARγ receptor is a key regulator of adipocyte differentiation, glucose regulation, and angiogenesis. It is also expressed in endothelial and vascular smooth muscle cells. The PPARγ receptor may play a part in blood pressure regulation by modulating vascular tone, but its exact role is unknown. Drugs that stimulate the receptor also lower blood pressure.

VI. ESSENTIAL HYPERTENSION

Essential hypertension accounts for $\sim$95% of all cases of hypertension, and in contrast to the rare Mendelian forms of hypertension, the genetic mechanisms that contribute to the disorder are less well understood. Various components of blood pressure regulatory systems have been found to exhibit genetic variability, and each of these is a potential cause of essential hypertension. In theory, mutations in a gene or genes that encode components from any of the blood pressure regulatory systems can contribute to or cause hypertension, producing an overwhelming number of potential candidate genes for hypertension.

Numerous genes have been studied ($>$60) and genetic variants that are associated with hypertension in various ethnic groups have been identified. These include genes from the RAAS (36–39), the epithelial sodium channel (40), the adrenergic receptor system (41), the renal kallikrein–kinin system (42), α-adducin (43), other systems that involve lipoprotein metabolism (44), and growth factors (45). Some of the genes implicated in the pathogenesis of hypertension that have either demonstrated familial aggregation and linkage or an association to human essential hypertension are given in (Table 4.2).

Of particular interest is the observation that many of these genes encode proteins that are either directly or indirectly involved with renal ion transport. These include genes that encode angiotensinogen, angiotensin-converting enzyme, α-adducin, the G-protein β3 subunit gene (GNB3), the sodium epithelial channel, and the WNK kinases (Fig. 4.1).

A. Angiotensinogen

The angiotensinogen gene was one of the first genes found to be associated with human essential hypertension.

Table 4.2 Genes Implicated in Essential Hypertension

Candidate gene	Reference
Aldosterone synthase	Davies et al. (39)
Angiotensin II type 1 receptor	Bonnardeaux et al. (38)
Angiotensin-converting enzyme	O'Donnell et al. (37)
Angiotensinogen	Jeunemaitre et al. (36)
Epithelial sodium channel	Persu et al. (40)
Glucocorticoid receptor	Lin et al. (46)
G-protein β3 subunit	Siffert et al. (47)
Kallikrein	Berge et al. (42)
α-2 adrenergic receptor	Lockette et al. (48)
α-Adducin	Cusi et al. (43)
β-2 adrenergic receptor	Timmermann et al. (49)
WNK4	Elrich et al. (50)

Because of the known role of the RAAS in the regulation of blood pressure, the angiotensinogen gene has been one of the most intensely studied candidate genes. It was first reported to be linked to hypertension by Jeunemaitre and colleagues (36) in 1992. Subsequent screening of the gene identified the M235T polymorphism (methionine → threonine at amino acid position 235) of the angiotensinogen gene. This polymorphism was found to be associated with hypertension and elevated plasma levels of angiotensinogen, with the 235T allele observed more frequently in hypertensives than in normotensives.

Since the original publication by Jeunemaitre and colleagues, a large number of studies have been performed, which confirm their results in some populations, but not in other populations (51). Despite inconsistencies among many of the angiotensinogen studies, the results of three large meta-analyses have concluded that the 235T allele is associated, although weakly, with an increased risk of hypertension (51–53).

The angiotensinogen gene has now been screened extensively for polymorphisms in several populations, and many new mutations have been described. Of particular interest is the M235T polymorphism, which has been found to be in tight linkage disequilibrium with a mutation in the promoter of the gene (54). This mutation is characterized by a single base change from adenine to guanine (A–6G) and lies six base pairs upstream of the transcription initiation start site. Studies have demonstrated that A–6G polymorphism can increase the rate of angiotensinogen transcription, which accounts for the variation in plasma angiotensinogen levels.

Exactly how angiotensinogen gene mutations might contribute to the pathogenesis of hypertension remains unclear. One view is that increased angiotensinogen levels might result in an increase in the production of angiotensin II (AII), which could lead to increased sodium retention and vasoconstriction and, therefore, contribute to an elevated blood pressure. It is important to note, however, that angiotensinogen levels can increase without any effect on blood pressure, as long as renin secretion is regulated normally. Renin cleaves angiotensinogen to angiotensin I, which is then cleaved by the angiotensin-I-converting enzyme to produce angiotensin II, a peptide hormone that stimulates the secretion of aldosterone, and through its effects on the heart, kidneys, and blood vessels, elevates blood pressure. Angiotensin II mediates all the effects of the RAAS. Therefore, it is likely that defects in the control of renin secretion, angiotensin-I-converting enzyme activity, and other components of the RAAS will interact with angiotensinogen gene polymorphisms to elevate blood pressure.

B. The Angiotensin-I-Converting Enzyme

The angiotensin-I-converting enzyme not only cleaves angiotensin I to produce angiotensin II, it also breaks down bradykinin, a potent vasodilator. The success of angiotensin-I-converting enzyme inhibitors in the treatment of hypertension has highlighted the importance of the angiotensin-I-converting enzyme and the RAAS in the development of hypertension and related cardiovascular disease (55).

An insertion–deletion polymorphism in intron 16 of the angiotensin-I-converting enzyme locus has been linked and associated with plasma angiotensin-I-converting enzyme levels and activity in humans (56). It has been shown that angiotensin-I-converting enzyme activity in individuals homozygous for the deletion–mutation genotype is about twice the angiotensin-I-converting enzyme activity in individuals homozygous for the insertion genotype (56). People who are heterozygous for the insertion–deletion genotype have intermediate levels of angiotensin-I-converting enzyme activity. It was thought that higher angiotensin-I-converting enzyme activity could result in increased levels of angiotensin II. Considering the action of angiotensin II on the cardiovascular and renal systems, it is not surprising that many researchers focused their attention on the angiotensin-I-converting enzyme, trying to find an association between hypertension and the angiotensin-I-converting enzyme gene insertion–deletion polymorphism. But this polymorphism has not been proven conclusively to be important in human essential hypertension. Most studies report a significant association with cardiovascular disease endpoints, but not with hypertension (57,58).

The angiotensin-I-converting enzyme insertion/deletion polymorphism is thought to be in linkage disequilibrium with the functional mutations that determine angiotensin-I-converting enzyme activity. Indeed, re-sequencing of the angiotensin-I-converting enzyme gene has identified many single-nucleotide polymorphisms that are in tight linkage disequilibrium and has allowed researchers to identify distinct variants of the angiotensin-I-converting enzyme gene that are associated with varying levels of angiotensin-I-converting enzyme activity (59–61). In 1998, two independent studies reported evidence of a link between the angiotensin-I-converting enzyme gene locus and hypertension (37,62). O'Donnell et al. (37) analyzed >3000 participants from the Framingham heart study and found evidence for association and linkage of the D allele with hypertension and diastolic blood pressure in men, but not in women. In a large sibling pair study, Fornage et al. (62) similarly demonstrated linkage in men to a region on chromosome 17 that encompasses the angiotensin-I-converting enzyme gene locus.

These studies were the first large, prospective studies to investigate the role of the angiotensin-I-converting enzyme gene in hypertension, and the results have generated some renewed interest in the angiotensin-I-converting enzyme gene locus. Although it is possible that genes near the angiotensin-I-converting enzyme gene locus may explain the observed results in these studies, the role of the angiotensin-I-converting enzyme in blood pressure regulation further supports the notion that the angiotensin-I-converting enzyme gene itself contributes to blood pressure variability in men. The mechanism by which angiotensin-I-converting enzyme gene influences blood pressure in a sex-specific manner remains to be more fully investigated.

C. Adducin

Adducin is an $\alpha-\beta$ heterodimeric membrane skeletal protein that is involved in the regulation of membrane ion transport and cellular signal transduction through changes in the actin cytoskeleton (63). The role of adducin in the etiology of essential hypertension was implicated originally in studies of the Milan-hypertensive and normotensive strains of rats. In the hypertensive strain of rats, a defect in renal sodium handling causes hypertension and also an increase in the level of ouabain-like factor. The renal alteration that leads to hypertension is produced by an increase in expression and activity of the renal sodium–potassium ATPase (NaKATPase) as the result of mutations in the adducin genes (64,65).

Two missense point mutations in the adducin α subunit (F316Y) and β subunit (Q529R) are associated with the blood pressure variation in Milan-hypertensive rats. They account for up to 50% of the blood pressure variation between the Milan-hypertensive and normotensive strains of rats (66). The precise mechanisms that link adducin polymorphisms to the increased NaKATPase activity enhanced renal sodium reabsorption, and hypertension have not yet been fully elucidated.

Human essential hypertension and salt sensitivity have been linked to the α-adducin locus on chromosome 4p. An association between the α-adducin gene and a functional polymorphism (Gly460Trp) also has been demonstrated in a number of independent studies (43). However, as has been the case for most candidate genes, both positive and negative associations have been found for the Gly460Trp polymorphism when it has been studied in different populations (65). When hypertensive patients who carry at least one 460Trp allele are compared with patients who are homozygous for the wild-type Gly460 allele, they have a demonstrable lower plasma renin activity, a larger increase in blood pressure after sodium infusion, enhanced proximal tubular reabsorption, a more pronounced fall in blood pressure after chronic diuretic (hydrochlorothiazide) treatment or acute sodium depletion, and a higher blood pressure (67–70). These observations suggest an important role for α-adducin in salt-sensitive hypertension. For example, the selective effect of diuretics on patients who carry the 460Trp allele suggests that screening hypertensive patients for this polymorphism could be used to identify individuals who might benefit from diuretic treatment and a sodium-restricted diet. Further work is required in other populations to confirm the role of α-adducin in human essential hypertension and to test whether genetic variants of this gene affect the outcome of diuretic therapy in hypertensive patients.

D. G-Protein Beta3 Subunit

A recent candidate gene for essential hypertension is the GNB3 gene. The G-proteins are a family of heterotrimeric proteins that consist of α, β, and γ subunits linked to a variety of secondary messenger systems.

A polymorphism in exon 10 of the GNB3 gene (C825T, cytosine-to-thymine at postion 825) creates an alternative splice site that results in an in-frame deletion of 41 amino acids and that is associated with an increased sodium–hydrogen exchange (47). In a small number of case–control studies, the 825T allele was found to be associated with hypertension; carriers of the T allele have been reported to have a 50% increased chance of having hypertension when compared with non-carriers of the allele (47,71). Exactly why and how this allele confers an increased susceptibility to the development of hypertension is not clear at present. Fifty percent of hypertensive patients also have been reported to have enhanced sodium–hydrogen exchange activity as a result of an altered signal transduction that is associated with mutations in the GNB3 gene. Whether this abnormality plays a role in the pathogenesis of hypertension remains unclear (72).

The GNB3 825T polymorphism also has been associated with increased renal perfusion (73). Because renal hemodynamic changes play a critical role in the pathogenesis of essential hypertension and because increased renal perfusion has been reported in early hypertension, the association of the GNB3 825T polymorphism with increased renal perfusion lends further support for the probability of increased G-protein activation in the pathogenesis of hypertension. In addition, a recent study of 461 patients enrolled in the Hypertension and Ambulatory Recording Venetia Study (HARVEST) showed that the 825T allele was associated with an increased risk of progression to more severe hypertension in young patients with grade I hypertension (CI = 1.108–1.843; $p = 0.006$) (74). At this time, the GNB3 825T allele should be considered a potential genetic marker for predisposition to hypertension. However, both negative and positive associations have been reported for GNB3.

E. Epithelial Sodium Channel

The epithelial sodium channel is involved in the control and fine tuning of sodium reabsorption in the distal nephron of the kidney. Studies of the Mendelian form of hypertension, Liddle's syndrome, have found mutations in the β and γ subunits of the epithelial sodium channel that cause hypertension, which suggests that the epithelial sodium channel might play a role in blood pressure regulation. It has been proposed that subtle variants of this gene might be important in the development in essential hypertension.

Several studies have been conducted to identify variants in the epithelial sodium channel subunits that may confer susceptibility to essential hypertension. Numerous mutations that result in a change in an amino acid have been identified; however, the majority are rare missense mutations and do not affect the carboxy terminus of the epithelial sodium channel β and γ subunits that are mutated or deleted in Liddle's syndrome (75,76).

Of particular interest, however, is a threonine 594 methionine (T594M) mutation in the epithelial sodium channel β subunit (77). This mutation is located in the last exon of the carboxy terminus of the epithelial sodium channel β subunit. It results in a change from threonine to methionine at amino acid position 594 and is found almost exclusively in populations of African descent. This variant is associated with increased epithelial sodium channel activity in lymphocytes from hypertensive patients, which suggests that the mutation could contribute to elevated blood pressure by increasing renal tubular sodium reabsorption in patients with essential hypertension. A case–control study that involved 206 black hypertensive patients and 142 normotensive black individuals living in London found the T594M variant to be associated with hypertension (odds ratio = 4.17, CI = 1.12–18.25, $p = 0.029$) (78). Individuals with the mutation also had lower plasma renin activity, lending further support to the idea of increased sodium reabsorption. In a larger cross-sectional study of 458 subjects of African origin from the same area of London, the frequency of the 594M allele increased with increasing blood pressure, and the T594M variant was found to be associated with hypertension ($p = 0.05$) (79). Although the T594M variant has been associated with hypertension in some populations of African descent, studies have failed to demonstrate an association in populations of white ancestry (80).

Evidence from linkage and association studies has suggested a role for the epithelial sodium channel in human essential hypertension in various populations. However, the susceptibility alleles have yet to be identified and the role of the epithelial sodium channel has yet to be assessed in large family-based studies. It is still an open question whether the genes that encode the epithelial sodium channel subunits are involved in the pathogenesis of essential hypertension.

F. The WNK Kinases

All the data accumulated about the genetic basis of pseudohypoaldosteronism type 2 (PHA2) suggests that WNK1 and WNK4 may be part of a previously unrecognized pathway that is involved in regulating sodium homeostasis and blood pressure control. The WNK1 and WNK4 kinases have been shown to regulate sodium reabsorption and potassium secretion in the distal nephron of the kidney (81). The WNK kinases, therefore, are also excellent candidate genes for essential hypertension. Indeed, individuals with essential hypertension often respond well to thiazide diuretics and have low renin activity, just as PHA2 patients do. This fact raises the possibility that variants in the WNK kinases might contribute to essential hypertension in the general population (82).

Genome-wide screens for blood pressure loci have implicated the region on chromosome 17q21 that contains the WNK4 gene (83,84). Re-sequencing of the WNK4 gene also has identified a genetic variant in intron 10 that is associated with essential hypertension in Caucasian subjects (165 hypertensives; 91 normotensives, $p < 0.05$), but not in subjects of African origin from the United States (50). Analysis of an additional WNK4 variant (a variable nucleotide tandem repeat in intron 11) in 155 hypertensive and 245 normotensive Anglo-Celtic white Australian subjects failed to find an association between WNK4 and hypertension (85).

Analysis of WNK1 variants in human essential hypertension has yet to be performed. However, it has been observed in some individuals with the PHA2 WNK1 deletion mutations that blood pressure increases over time in a way that mimics essential hypertension. In this subset of patients with mutations, the hypertension was less severe and did not develop until late in their fourth decade (86). Analysis of the patients revealed that urinary calcium excretion was normal, an observation that is not consistent with increased sodium chloride co-transporter activity. Therefore, it has been postulated that WNK1 also may play a role in the development of hypertension that is independent of renal sodium excretion. WNK1 is expressed in many different tissues; therefore, the abnormal regulation of WNK1 expression in vascular smooth muscle cells could alter vascular remodelling and lead to alterations in peripheral vascular resistance over time, thereby contributing to hypertension (86,87). Consistent with studies in humans, analyses of

WNK1-deficient mice have revealed a corresponding role for WNK1 in blood pressure regulation in mice. WNK1 heterozygous knockout mice have a significantly reduced blood pressure when compared with wild-type mice, and this reduced blood pressure is associated with decreased levels of WNK1 expression (88). Homozygous knockout mice die during embryonic development. These studies demonstrate the importance of the WNK1 gene not only in blood pressure control, but also in development.

It is early in the research of WNK kinases. Their roles in blood pressure regulation and hypertension are only just beginning to be elucidated. Further work is required to identify other WNK1 and WNK4 polymorphisms. Additional studies in larger human populations will be required to assess the role of the WNK kinases in essential hypertension.

VII. INCONSISTENCY AMONG CANDIDATE GENE STUDIES

Since the earliest publications of the association between a single gene (the angiotensinogen gene) and essential hypertension and the discovery of the genetic basis for the rare Mendelian diseases that affect blood pressure, a lot of excitement has been generated over the possibility of elucidating the genetic basis of human essential hypertension (36,89). There are now numerous studies covering a diverse range of candidate genes. However, for every positive study, there is at least one negative study; and the role of many of the genes studied remains, thus far, ambiguous. The inconsistencies among studies demonstrate the challenges of studying complex, multifactorial traits. Inconsistencies can arise from small sample sizes, the underlying population substructure, the varying effects of disease-susceptibility variants, gene-environment interactions, or poor study design. Each of these factors can hinder the detection of the modest contribution of an individual locus to a trait such as hypertension (90). The contribution of many of these factors to observed inconsistencies among studies has been reviewed by Corvol et al. (91). They discuss the contribution of the two genes (the angiotensinogen gene and the epithelial sodium channel gene) to essential hypertension and the lessons that can be learned from them and applied to other candidate gene studies in hypertension.

VIII. GENOME-WIDE SCREENS FOR BLOOD PRESSURE GENES IN HUMANS

The list of potential candidate genes is enormous, and it is unlikely that the genes studied to date represent all of the genes involved in the pathogenesis of hypertension.

Successive examination of each of these candidate genes is not the most efficient approach for identifying the major genetic factors involved in human essential hypertension. Therefore, researchers have been turning to a genome-wide screen approach to narrow the list of potential candidate genes and, more importantly, to identify new genes that may not have been considered previously.

In the genome-wide screen approach, family members with a trait in which researchers are interested are genotyped for highly polymorphic markers that are spaced at regular intervals (10–30 cM) across the entire genome. Each marker is then tested for links to the trait in which they are interested to identify genomic regions that might contain the trait-influencing loci.

There have been more than 30 studies that focus on genome-wide screens for human essential hypertension. The results of many of these studies are reviewed in Samani (2003) (92) and Garcia et al. (2003) (93). The studies that have been published to date are diverse with respect to phenotype, ethnic origin, selection criteria, and numbers and structures of families. They range from the analysis of single, large pedigrees to large sibling-pair resources of up to 1599 families.

The largest and most ambitious genome-wide screens for blood pressure loci have been those of the Medical Research Council-funded BRItish Genetics of HyperTension (BRIGHT) Study (94) and the National Heart Lung and Blood Institute's Family Blood Pressure Program (FBPP) (95–98). The BRIGHT study represents the largest study of a single ethnic group; it consists of 1599 sibling-pairs of white, British ancestry. The FBPP study comprised four multicenter networks [HyperGEN (95), GENOA (96), GenNet (97), and SAPPHIRe (98)], each designed to target multiple ethnic groups from the US population. The total number of people in the FBPP study was more than 6000 hypertensive individuals.

Both the BRIGHT study and the FBPP studies identified multiple chromosomal regions that are linked to hypertension. The BRIGHT study identified a locus on chromosome 6q with genome-wide significance (LOD score of 3.21) and three other loci on chromosomes 2q, 5q, and 9q (94). In contrast, the results of the FBPP studies found no loci with genome-wide significance. The GenNet study reported the highest LOD score (2.96); this was for a region on chromosome 1 that is linked to diastolic blood pressure in Caucasians (97). The HyperGen study found evidence for linkage to a region on chromosome 2p in African-Americans (LOD score of 2.0) (95). The SAPPHIRe study reported evidence for linkage to chromosome 10p, with an LOD score of 2.5 (98). In the GENOA study, no evidence of linkage to hypertension was found for any chromosomal locus (96). Furthermore, meta-analysis of the pooled FBPP data failed to provide evidence of linkage to any loci.

However, the loci on chromosomes 1q and 2p that were identified in the GenNet and HyperGen studies, respectively, replicate the results from other studies (99,100), highlighting these regions for further investigation.

From the many genome-wide screens for blood pressure loci, only six studies have identified regions that achieved genome-wide significance. The linked regions are located on chromosomes 2p (100), 4p, 6q (94), 14q (101), 17q (84), and 18q (102). Other studies have identified numerous regions that have nominal links or that suggest possible linkage to hypertension. Interestingly, a number of loci overlap with the results from other studies, strengthening the likelihood that these regions may contain "susceptibility" genes for hypertension.

Overall, the results of the genome-wide studies support the idea that blood pressure is governed by multiple genetic loci, each with relatively weak effects on blood pressure in the population at large. The fact that multiple chromosomal regions have been identified and that different regions have been implicated in different populations lends further evidence to the polygenic and heterogeneous nature of the disorder. A number of promising regions that might contain blood pressure loci have been identified. It is encouraging that the regions that demonstrate significant linkage to hypertension contain a number of potential gene candidates, which suggests that new genes or pathways might be discovered from studies in the near future.

IX. PHARMACOGENETICS IN HYPERTENSION

One of the driving forces behind the study of the genetics of essential hypertension is the potential for developing new therapeutics and diagnostic tests that are capable of predicting an individual's response to antihypertensive therapy. *Pharmacogenetics* can be defined as the study of the role of genetics in drug response. Less than 40% of hypertensive patients have their blood pressure adequately controlled. Patients often vary in their response to a particular antihypertensive drug, and this response cannot be easily predicted. The same class of drugs are not effective for everyone and might cause some patients to suffer adverse side-effects or even death. Some of the differences can be attributed to personal characteristics such as age, weight, and gender, to the particular nature of the disease, or to other medications they may be taking. Despite this fact, it also is thought that inter-individual variation in drug response may be influenced by genetic factors (103).

Pharmacogenetics in hypertension is still at an early stage. Only a limited number of studies have been performed, the results of which have been summarized in a recent review by Koopmans et al. (2003) (104).

In pharmacogenetic studies of hypertension, blood pressure reduction has been used as a surrogate marker for predicting drug response on the basis of genetic polymorphisms. Blood pressure reduction and its correlation to a particular genotype have been reported for polymorphisms of angiotensinogen, angiotensin-I-converting enzyme, α-adducin, GNB3, and the epithelial sodium channel. The $-6A$ allele and the 235T allele of the angiotensinogen gene have been associated with an increased response to atenolol and irbesartan. Carriers of the 235T allele also have been reported to have a greater response to angiotensin-I-converting enzyme inhibitors. The angiotensin-I-converting enzyme insertion/deletion polymorphism has been associated with an increased response to angiotensin-I-converting enzyme inhibitors, hydrochlorothiazide, β-blockers, and angiotensin II type 1 receptor blockers. Carriers of the α-adducin 460Trp polymorphism have demonstrated a greater response to acute or chronic treatment with furosemide or hydrochlorothiazide. Carriers of the GNB3 825T polymorphism have been reported to have greater response to clonidine and hydrochlorothiazide. The T594M polymorphism of the epithelial sodium channel gene has been associated with greater response to amiloride treatment (104).

DNA microarrays also have been introduced to study the pharmacogenetics of hypertension. In a pilot study to demonstrate the feasibility of this system, a panel of 74 single-nucleotide polymorphisms from 25 blood pressure-regulating genes were selected and genotyped in 97 hypertensive patients (105). The genes that were selected for analysis were chosen on the basis of their known function in the RAAS, in adrenergic and endothelial systems, and in lipid metabolism. The single-nucleotide polymorphisms that were chosen were polymorphisms thought to play a role in blood pressure regulation on the basis of evidence from the published literature. A microarray-based genotyping system that is capable of analyzing multiple single-nucleotide polymorphisms at the same time (microarray minisequencing) was used.

In this study, a subgroup of hypertensive patients from the Swedish Irbesartan Left Ventricular Hypertrophy Investigation vs. Atenolol (SILVHIA) trial were randomly chosen for treatment with either atenolol (an α 1 adrenergic receptor blocker) or irbesartan (an angiotensin II type 1 receptor blocker) and then tested for blood pressure reduction induced by the drug treatment. The results indicated that variants of the α-2 aderenergic receptor and β-2 aderenergic receptor could be used to predict the response to atenolol and that angiotensinogen, angiotensin-I-converting enzyme, and aldosterone synthase gene variants were associated with a greater response to irbesartan.

In 2004, another study by the same group applied DNA microarray technology to assess whether RAAS gene variants were related to the blood pressure-lowering effects of antihypertensive treatment. Once again, 97 patients were randomly chosen for treatment with either atenolol or irbesartan for 12 weeks. They were then genotyped at 30 single-nucleotide polymorphisms in seven RAAS genes and then tested for association of blood pressure-lowering response to specific antihypertensive therapy (106). The results demonstrated that specific angiotensinogen gene variants (−6A and 235T) were associated with a greater blood pressure reduction in response to treatment with atenolol than to treatment with irbesartan (105,106).

The pharmacogenetics studies performed thus far are encouraging, but they should be viewed as preliminary. There are conflicting results for many of the polymorphisms studied (104). For example, in the initial pilot study described earlier, angiotensinogen gene polymorphisms were found to be associated with response to irbesartan, but in the second study, the same polymorphisms were associated with a response to atenolol. Both studies involved a small sample of patients from a single population. Pharmacogenetic studies still suffer from the same inconsistencies as do genetic association studies (90,91,104). They are limited by small sample size and generally have focused on testing for association by using a small number of single-nucleotide polymorphisms in a few genes. Therefore, these studies should be followed up with larger prospective studies to confirm their results. Despite these limitations, however, the results of the initial studies illustrate the potential of using single-nucleotide polymorphism genotyping as a pharmacogenetic tool in antihypertensive treatment. They also demonstrate the potential of microarray-based technology, which makes it possible for a large number of genetic markers to be typed per patient.

X. GENERAL CONCLUSIONS AND FUTURE PERSPECTIVES

The prevention of hypertension and appropriate management of the disorder continue to pose a challenge for health care professionals all over the world. With the recognition of a genetic component to hypertension and the advances in molecular techniques, numerous studies have now been conducted to try to unravel the genetics of hypertension. Genetic research in relation to blood pressure will provide new insights into the underlying mechanisms behind inter-individual variation in blood pressure levels and control. Implementing the results of genetic research will have a substantial impact on public health. It is anticipated that this research will lead to the development of pre-clinical diagnostic tests that can identify individuals who are at risk of developing hypertension

and to the development of novel and more effective antihypertensive treatments.

The greatest advances in our understanding of the genetic influences, blood pressure control, and the pathogenesis of hypertension have come from the study of the rare monogenic forms of hypertension. The structure and function of the genes that are responsible for these disorders have been elucidated, and a direct link between a genetic variant and the underlying molecular mechanism that causes hypertension has been shown. The discovery of these single-gene disorders has provided insight into new pathways and other genes that regulate blood pressure, and has provided tools for clinical diagnosis and targeted therapy of these conditions.

The data obtained from genetic research into essential hypertension suggests that hypertension is likely to be the result of a complex interaction among environmental factors and many genes, each contributing a small percentage to blood pressure variation in the population at large. Despite the complex nature of the disorder, some progress has been made in our understanding of the genetics of essential hypertension and the genes that might contribute to the disorder. Although candidate gene studies have failed to identify any genes that have major genetic effects on essential hypertension, allelic variants in many of the genes that regulate blood pressure have been found to be associated with hypertension or blood pressure variation. However, many of these associations are weak, with each gene accounting only for a fraction ($\sim$1–2%) of the inter-individual variation in blood pressure levels. In addition, most reported associations are not robust, and many subsequent studies have failed to replicate the initial positive findings.

Until recently, the candidate gene approach has dominated the genetic research of essential hypertension. Now, technology permits whole-genome scanning for hypertension susceptibility loci. This method has the advantage of allowing researchers to identify new genes that may have not been previously recognized as candidates for essential hypertension. Numerous genome-wide screens in diverse populations have been performed, and a number of potential loci have presented themselves. One of the most striking observations from these studies, however, is the degree of heterogeneity between populations. Very few of the identified regions in one population overlap with the identified regions from other studies in other populations. Nevertheless, the genome-wide screens that have been published to date represent a major step toward identifying the genes for hypertension. The challenge facing us now is to determine the function of the newly discovered genes, to identify their genetic variants, and to assess their role in the pathogenesis of hypertension.

As yet, there are no genetic diagnostic tests for essential hypertension. Pharmacogenetic studies in hypertension are at early stage of development and should be considered only as generating hypotheses. However, applying the results of pharmacogenetic research has the potential of revolutionizing the treatment of hypertension. Genetic tests could eventually allow clinicians to identify which hypertensive patients are more likely to respond to specific drugs and less likely to be at risk for adverse reactions to the drugs.

The complete sequencing of the human genome initiatives such as the International HapMap project (107), the DNA microarray chip technologies (108), and programs such as UK Biobank, deCODE, the BRIGHT study, and the FBPP will allow larger and more sophisticated genetic studies of hypertension in the future.

The human genome project (http://www.ensembl.org, http://genome.ucsc.edu, and http://www.ncbi.nlm.nih.gov) has identified the location and DNA sequence of all genes in the genome. In addition, the HapMap project (http://www.hapmap.org) has made substantial progress in identifying all common patterns of genetic variation in the human genome from multiple ethnic populations. This should provide tools that will allow the association mapping to be applied to any functional candidate gene in the genome, to any region suggested by family-based linkage analysis, or, ultimately, for whole genome-wide scans for disease susceptibility loci (107). The implementation of new chip technologies will allow the rapid identification of single-nucleotide polymorphisms and the simultaneous analysis of multiple genes in whole populations.

The UK Biobank (http://www.ukbiobank.ac.uk), deCODE (http://www.decode.com), BRIGHT (http://www.brightstudy.ac.uk), and FBPP (http://www.sph.uth.tmc.edu/hgc/fbpp) programs will provide researchers with powerful resources for the study of complex diseases, increased statistical power to detect small effects, and the capability to analyze various subsets of patients, which will help in the detection of effects that are confounded by non-genetic factors.

ACKNOWLEDGMENTS

We are extremely grateful to the Medical Research Council, The British Heart Foundation, the Research Advisory Board of Barts and the London, and the Special Trustees of St. Bartholomew's Hospital for funding our research.

REFERENCES

1. Swales JD, Sever PS, Peart WS. Clinical Atlas of Hypertension. London, New York, Philadelphia: Gower Medical Pub., 1991. Distributed in the USA and Canada by J.B. Lippincott Co.

2. Ward R. Familial aggregation and genetic epidemiology of blood pressure. In: Laragh JH, Brenner, BM, eds. Hypertension: Pathophysiology, Diagnosis, and Management. New York: Raven Press, 1995.

3. Biron P, Mongeau JG. Familial aggregation of blood pressure and its components. Pediatr Clin North Am 1978; 25:29–33.

4. Katzmarzyk PT, Rankinen T, Perusse L, Rao DC, Bouchard C. Familial risk of high blood pressure in the Canadian population. Am J Human Biol 2001; 13:620–625.

5. Luft FC. Twins in cardiovascular genetic research. Hypertension 2001; 37:350–356.

6. Loos RJ, Beunen G, Fagard R, Derom C, Vlietinck R, Phillips DI. Twin studies and estimates of heritability. Lancet 2001; 357:1445.

7. Fagard R, Brguljan J, Staessen J, Thijs L, Derom C, Thomis M, Vlietinck R. Heritability of conventional and ambulatory blood pressures. A study in twins. Hypertension 1995; 26:919–924.

8. Hunt SC, Hasstedt SJ, Kuida H, Stults BM, Hopkins PN, Williams RR. Genetic heritability and common environmental components of resting and stressed blood pressures, lipids, and body mass index in Utah pedigrees and twins. Am J Epidemiol 1989; 129:625–638.

9. Slattery ML, Bishop DT, French TK, Hunt SC, Meikle AW, Williams RR. Lifestyle and blood pressure levels in male twins in Utah. Genet Epidemiol 1988; 5:277–287.

10. Biron P, Mongeau JG, Bertrand D. Familial aggregation of blood pressure in 558 adopted children. Can Med Assoc J 1976; 115:773–774.

11. Mongeau JG, Biron P, Sing CF. The influence of genetics and household environment upon the variability of normal blood pressure: the Montreal Adoption Survey. Clin Exp Hypertens A 1986; 8:653–660.

12. Rice T, Vogler GP, Perusse L, Bouchard C, Rao DC. Cardiovascular risk factors in a French Canadian population: resolution of genetic and familial environmental effects on blood pressure using twins, adoptees, and extensive information on environmental correlates. Genet Epidemiol 1989; 6:571–588.

13. Lifton RP, Gharavi AG, Geller DS. Molecular mechanisms of human hypertension. Cell 2001; 104(4):545–556.

14. Pickering GW. The nature of essential hypertension. Lancet 1959(ii):1027–1028.

15. Platt R. The nature of essential hypertension. Lancet 1959; 2:55–57.

16. Strachan T, Read AP. Human Molecular Genetics. 2nd ed. New York: Wiley, 1999.

17. Lander ES, Schork NJ. Genetic dissection of complex traits. Science 1994; 265:2037–2048.

18. Lander E, Kruglyak L. Genetic dissection of complex traits: guidelines for interpreting and reporting linkage results. Nat Genet 1995; 11:241–247.

19. Goodman LS, Hardman JG, Limbird LE, Gilman AG. Goodman & Gilman's The Pharmacological Basis of Therapeutics. 10th ed. New York: McGraw-Hill, 2001.

20. Mayan H, Vered I, Mouallem M, Tzadok-Witkon M, Pauzner R, Farfel Z. Pseudohypoaldosteronism type II: marked sensitivity to thiazides, hypercalciuria,

normomagnesemia, and low bone mineral density. J Clin Endocrinol Metab 2002; 87:3248–3254.

21. Wilson FH, Disse-Nicodeme S, Choate KA, Ishikawa K, Nelson-Williams C, Desitter I, Gunel M, Milford DV, Lipkin GW, Achard JM, Feely MP, Dussol B, Berland Y, Unwin RJ, Mayan H, Simon DB, Farfel Z, Jeunemaitre X, Lifton RP. Human hypertension caused by mutations in WNK kinases. Science 2001; 293:1107–1112.

22. Mansfield TA, Simon DB, Farfel Z, Bia M, Tucci JR, Lebel M, Gutkin M, Vialettes B, Christofilis MA, Kauppinen-Makelin R, Mayan H, Risch N, Lifton RP. Multilocus linkage of familial hyperkalaemia and hypertension, pseudohypoaldosteronism type II, to chromosomes 1q31-42 and 17p11-q21. Nat Genet 1997; 16:202–205.

23. Yang CL, Angell J, Mitchell R, Ellison DH. WNK kinases regulate thiazide-sensitive Na–Cl cotransport. J Clin Invest 2003; 111:1039–1045.

24. Lifton RP, Dluhy RG, Powers M, Ulick S, Lalouel JM. The molecular basis of glucocorticoid-remediable aldosteronism, a Mendelian cause of human hypertension. Trans Assoc Am Physicians 1992; 105:64–71.

25. Gates LJ, MacConnachie AA, Lifton RP, Haites NE, Benjamin N. Variation of phenotype in patients with glucocorticoid remediable aldosteronism. J Med Genet 1996; 33:25–28.

26. Stewart PM, Krozowski ZS, Gupta A, Milford DV, Howie AJ, Sheppard MC, Whorwood CB. Hypertension in the syndrome of apparent mineralocorticoid excess due to mutation of the 11 β-hydroxysteroid dehydrogenase type 2 gene. Lancet 1996; 347:88–91.

27. Geley S, Kapelari K, Johrer K, Peter M, Glatzl J, Vierhapper H, Schwarz S, Helmberg A, Sippell WG, White PC, Kofler R. CYP11B1 mutations causing congenital adrenal hyperplasia due to 11 β-hydroxylase deficiency. J Clin Endocrinol Metab 1996; 81:2896–2901.

28. Warrell DA. Oxford Textbook of Medicine. 4th ed. Oxford, New York: Oxford University Press, 2003.

29. Geller DS, Farhi A, Pinkerton N, Fradley M, Moritz M, Spitzer A, Meinke G, Tsai FT, Sigler PB, Lifton RP. Activating mineralocorticoid receptor mutation in hypertension exacerbated by pregnancy. Science 2000; 289:119–123.

30. Canessa CM, Schild L, Buell G, Thorens B, Gautschi I, Horisberger JD, Rossier BC. Amiloride-sensitive epithelial Na$^+$ channel is made of three homologous subunits. Nature 1994; 367:463–467.

31. Shimkets RA, Warnock DG, Bositis CM, Nelson-Williams C, Hansson JH, Schambelan M, Gill JR Jr, Ulick S, Milora RV, Findling JW. Liddle's syndrome: heritable human hypertension caused by mutations in the β subunit of the epithelial sodium channel. Cell 1994; 79(3):407–414.

32. Hansson JH, Nelson-Williams C, Suzuki H, Schild L, Shimkets R, Lu Y, Canessa C, Iwasaki T, Rossier B, Lifton RP. Hypertension caused by a truncated epithelial sodium channel γ subunit: genetic heterogeneity of Liddle's syndrome. Nat Genet 1995; 11(1):76–82.

33. Snyder PM, Price MP, McDonald FJ, Adams CM, Volk KA, Zeiher BG, Stokes JB, Welsh MJ. Mechanism by which Liddle's syndrome mutations increase activity of a human epithelial Na$^+$ channel. Cell 1995; 83(6):969–978.

34. Bahring S, Rauch A, Toka O, Schroeder C, Hesse C, Siedler H, Fesus G, Haefeli WE, Busjahn A, Aydin A, Neuenfeld Y, Muhl A, Toka HR, Gollasch M, Jordan J, Luft FC. Autosomal-dominant hypertension with type E brachydactyly is caused by rearrangement on the short arm of chromosome 12. Hypertension 2004; 43:471–476.

35. Barroso I, Gurnell M, Crowley VE, Agostini M, Schwabe JW, Soos MA, Maslen GL, Williams TD, Lewis H, Schafer AJ, Chatterjee VK, O'Rahilly S. Dominant negative mutations in human PPARγ associated with severe insulin resistance, diabetes mellitus and hypertension. Nature 1999; 402:880–883.

36. Jeunemaitre X, Soubrier F, Kotelevtsev YV, Lifton RP, Williams CS, Charru A, Hunt SC, Hopkins PN, Williams RR, Lalouel JM. Molecular basis of human hypertension: role of angiotensinogen. Cell 1992; 71(1):169–180.

37. O'Donnell CJ, Lindpaintner K, Larson MG, Rao VS, Ordovas JM, Schaefer EJ, Myers RH, Levy D. Evidence for association and genetic linkage of the angiotensin-converting enzyme locus with hypertension and blood pressure in men but not women in the Framingham heart study. Circulation 1998; 97:1766–1772.

38. Bonnardeaux A, Davies E, Jeunemaitre X, Fery I, Charru A, Clauser E, Tiret L, Cambien F, Corvol P, Soubrier F. Angiotensin II type 1 receptor gene polymorphisms in human essential hypertension. Hypertension 1994; 24:63–69.

39. Davies E, Holloway CD, Ingram MC, Inglis GC, Friel EC, Morrison C, Anderson NH, Fraser R, Connell JM. Aldosterone excretion rate and blood pressure in essential hypertension are related to polymorphic differences in the aldosterone synthase gene CYP11B2. Hypertension 1999; 33:703–707.

40. Persu A, Barbry P, Bassilana F, Houot AM, Mengual R, Lazdunski M, Corvol P, Jeunemaitre X. Genetic analysis of the β subunit of the epithelial Na$^+$ channel in essential hypertension. Hypertension 1998; 32:129–137.

41. Krushkal J, Xiong M, Ferrell R, Sing CF, Turner ST, Boerwinkle E. Linkage and association of adrenergic and dopamine receptor genes in the distal portion of the long arm of chromosome 5 with systolic blood pressure variation. Hum Mol Genet 1998; 7:1379–1383.

42. Berge KE, Bakken A, Bohn M, Erikssen J, Berg K. Analyses of mutations in the human renal kallikrein (hKLK1) gene and their possible relevance to blood pressure regulation and risk of myocardial infarction. Clin Genet 1997; 52:86–95.

43. Cusi D, Barlassina C, Azzani T, Casari G, Citterio L, Devoto M, Glorioso N, Lanzani C, Manunta P, Righetti M, Rivera R, Stella P, Troffa C, Zagato L, Bianchi G. Polymorphisms of α-adducin and salt sensitivity in patients with essential hypertension. Lancet 1997; 349:1353–1357.

44. Wu DA, Bu X, Warden CH, Shen DD, Jeng CY, Sheu WH, Fuh MM, Katsuya T, Dzau VJ, Reaven GM, Lusis AJ, Rotter JI, Chen YD. Quantitative trait locus mapping of human blood pressure to a genetic region at or near the lipoprotein lipase gene locus on chromosome 8p22. J Clin Invest 1996; 97:2111–2118.

45. Brand E, Bankir L, Plouin PF, Soubrier F. Glucagon receptor gene mutation (Gly40Ser) in human essential hypertension: the PEGASE study. Hypertension 1999; 34:15–17.

46. Lin RC, Wang WY, Morris BJ. Association and linkage analyses of glucocorticoid receptor gene markers in essential hypertension. Hypertension 1999; 34:1186–1192.

47. Siffert W, Rosskopf D, Siffert G, Busch S, Moritz A, Erbel R, Sharma AM, Ritz E, Wichmann HE, Jakobs KH, Horsthemke B. Association of a human G-protein $\beta3$ subunit variant with hypertension. Nat Genet 1998; 18:45–48.

48. Lockette W, Ghosh S, Farrow S, MacKenzie S, Baker S, Miles P, Schork A, Cadaret L. α 2-adrenergic receptor gene polymorphism and hypertension in blacks. Am J Hypertens 1995; 8:390–394.

49. Timmermann B, Mo R, Luft FC, Gerdts E, Busjahn A, Omvik P, Li GH, Schuster H, Wienker TF, Hoehe MR, Lund-Johansen P. β-2 adrenoceptor genetic variation is associated with genetic predisposition to essential hypertension: the Bergen blood pressure study. Kidney Int 1998; 53:1455–1460.

50. Erlich PM, Cui J, Chazaro I, Farrer LA, Baldwin CT, Gavras H, DeStefano AL. Genetic variants of WNK4 in whites and African Americans with hypertension. Hypertension 2003; 41:1191–1195.

51. Kunz R, Kreutz R, Beige J, Distler A, Sharma AM. Association between the angiotensinogen 235T-variant and essential hypertension in whites: a systematic review and methodological appraisal. Hypertension 1997; 30:1331–1337.

52. Kato N, Sugiyama T, Morita H, Kurihara H, Yamori Y, Yazaki Y. Angiotensinogen gene and essential hypertension in the Japanese: extensive association study and meta-analysis on six reported studies. J Hypertens 1999; 17:757–763.

53. Sethi AA, Nordestgaard BG, Tybjaerg-Hansen A. Angiotensinogen gene polymorphism, plasma angiotensinogen, and risk of hypertension and ischemic heart disease: a meta-analysis. Arterioscler Thromb Vasc Biol 2003; 23:1269–1275.

54. Inoue I, Nakajima T, Williams CS, Quackenbush J, Puryear R, Powers M, Cheng T, Ludwig EH, Sharma AM, Hata A, Jeunemaitre X, Lalouel JM. A nucleotide substitution in the promoter of human angiotensinogen is associated with essential hypertension and affects basal transcription in vitro. J Clin Invest 1997; 99:1786–1797.

55. Johnston CI. Biochemistry and pharmacology of the renin-angiotensin system. Drugs 1990; 39(suppl 1):21–31.

56. Rigat B, Hubert C, Alhenc-Gelas F, Cambien F, Corvol P, Soubrier F. An insertion/deletion polymorphism in the angiotensin I-converting enzyme gene accounting for

57. Harrap SB, Davidson HR, Connor JM, Soubrier F, Corvol P, Fraser R, Foy CJ, Watt GC. The angiotensin I converting enzyme gene and predisposition to high blood pressure. Hypertension 1993; 21:455–460.

58. Kuznetsova T, Staessen JA, Wang JG, Gasowski J, Nikitin Y, Ryabikov A, Fagard R. Antihypertensive treatment modulates the association between the D/I ACE gene polymorphism and left ventricular hypertrophy: a meta-analysis. J Hum Hypertens 2000; 14:447–454.

59. Keavney B, McKenzie CA, Connell JM, Julier C, Ratcliffe PJ, Sobel E, Lathrop M, Farrall M. Measured haplotype analysis of the angiotensin-I converting enzyme gene. Hum Mol Genet 1998; 7:1745–1751.

60. Rieder MJ, Taylor SL, Clark AG, Nickerson DA. Sequence variation in the human angiotensin converting enzyme. Nat Genet 1999; 22:59–62.

61. Cox R, Bouzekri N, Martin S, Southam L, Hugill A, Golamaully M, Cooper R, Adeyemo A, Soubrier F, Ward R, Lathrop GM, Matsuda F, Farrall M. Angiotensin-1-converting enzyme (ACE) plasma concentration is influenced by multiple ACE-linked quantitative trait nucleotides. Hum Mol Genet 2002; 11:2969–2977.

62. Fornage M, Amos CI, Kardia S, Sing CF, Turner ST, Boerwinkle E. Variation in the region of the angiotensin-converting enzyme gene influences interindividual differences in blood pressure levels in young white males. Circulation 1998; 97:1773–1779.

63. Barlassina C, Citterio L, Bernardi L, Buzzi L, D'Amico M, Sciarrone T, Bianchi G. Genetics of renal mechanisms of primary hypertension: the role of adducin. J Hypertens 1997; 15:1567–1571.

64. Manunta P, Barlassina C, Bianchi G. Adducin in essential hypertension. FEBS Lett 1998; 430:41–44.

65. Bianchi G, Tripodi G. Genetics of hypertension: the adducin paradigm. Ann NY Acad Sci 2003; 986:660–668.

66. Bianchi G, Tripodi G, Casari G, Salardi S, Barber BR, Garcia R, Leoni P, Torielli L, Cusi D, Ferrandi M. Two point mutations within the adducin genes are involved in blood pressure variation. Proc Natl Acad Sci USA 1994; 91(9):3999–4003.

67. Manunta P, Burnier M, D'Amico M, Buzzi L, Maillard M, Barlassina C, Lanella G, Cusi D, Bianchi G. Adducin polymorphism affects renal proximal tubule reabsorption in hypertension. Hypertension 1999; 33:694–697.

68. Morrison AC, Bray MS, Folsom AR, Boerwinkle E. ADD1 460W allele associated with cardiovascular disease in hypertensive individuals. Hypertension 2002; 39:1053–1057.

69. Psaty BM, Smith NL, Heckbert SR, Vos HL, Lemaitre RN, Reiner AP, Siscovick DS, Bis J, Lumley T, Longstreth WT Jr, Rosendaal FR. Diuretic therapy, the α-adducin gene variant, and the risk of myocardial infarction or stroke in persons with treated hypertension. J Am Med Assoc 2002; 287:1680–1689.

70. Sciarrone MT, Stella P, Barlassina C, Manunta P, Lanzani C, Bianchi G, Cusi D. ACE and α-adducin

half the variance of serum enzyme levels. J Clin Invest 1990; 86:1343–1346.

polymorphism as markers of individual response to diuretic therapy. Hypertension 2003; 41:398–403.

71. Beige J, Hohenbleicher H, Distler A, Sharma AM. G-Protein $\beta3$ subunit C825T variant and ambulatory blood pressure in essential hypertension. Hypertension 1999; 33:1049–1051.

72. Siffert W, Dusing R. Sodium-proton exchange and primary hypertension. An update. Hypertension 1995; 26:649–655.

73. Zeltner R, Delles C, Schneider M, Siffert W, Schmieder RE. G-protein $\beta(3)$ subunit gene (GNB3) 825T allele is associated with enhanced renal perfusion in early hypertension. Hypertension 2001; 37:882–886.

74. Sartori M, Semplicini A, Siffert W, Mormino P, Mazzer A, Pegoraro F, Mos L, Winnicki M, Palatini P. G-protein $\beta3$-subunit gene 825T allele and hypertension: a longitudinal study in young grade I hypertensives. Hypertension 2003; 42:909–914.

75. Persu A, Coscoy S, Houot AM, Corvol P, Barbry P, Jeunemaitre X. Polymorphisms of the γ subunit of the epithelial Na^+ channel in essential hypertension. J Hypertens 1999; 17:639–645.

76. Melander O, Orho M, Fagerudd J, Bengtsson K, Groop PH, Mattiasson I, Groop L, Hulthen UL. Mutations and variants of the epithelial sodium channel gene in Liddle's syndrome and primary hypertension. Hypertension 1998; 31:1118–1124.

77. Su YR, Rutkowski MP, Klanke CA, Wu X, Cui Y, Pun RY, Carter V, Reif M, Menon AG. A novel variant of the β-subunit of the amiloride-sensitive sodium channel in African Americans. J Am Soc Nephrol 1996; 7:2543–2549.

78. Baker EH, Dong YB, Sagnella GA, Rothwell M, Onipinla AK, Markandu ND, Cappuccio FP, Cook DG, Persu A, Corvol P, Jeunemaitre X, Carter ND, MacGregor GA. Association of hypertension with T594M mutation in β subunit of epithelial sodium channels in black people resident in London. Lancet 1998; 351:1388–1392.

79. Dong YB, Zhu HD, Baker EH, Sagnella GA, MacGregor GA, Carter ND, Wicks PD, Cook DG, Cappuccio FP. T594M and G442V polymorphisms of the sodium channel β subunit and hypertension in a black population. J Hum Hypertens 2001; 15:425–430.

80. Brand E, Herrmann SM, Nicaud V, Ruidavets JB, Evans A, Arveiler D, Luc G, Plouin PF, Tiret L, Cambien F. The 825C/T polymorphism of the G-protein subunit $\beta3$ is not related to hypertension. Hypertension 1999; 33:1175–1178.

81. Kahle KT, Wilson FH, Leng Q, Lalioti MD, O'Connell AD, Dong K, Rapson AK, MacGregor GG, Giebisch G, Hebert SC, Lifton RP. WNK4 regulates the balance between renal NaCl reabsorption and K^+ secretion. Nat Genet 2003; 35:372–376.

82. Reyes AJ. Diuretics in the therapy of hypertension. J Hum Hypertens 2002; 16(suppl 1):S78–S83.

83. Baima J, Nicolaou M, Schwartz F, DeStefano AL, Manolis A, Gavras I, Laffer C, Elijovich F, Farrer L, Baldwin CT, Gavras H. Evidence for linkage between essential hypertension and a putative locus on human chromosome 17. Hypertension 1999; 34:4–7.

84. Levy D, DeStefano AL, Larson MG, O'Donnell CJ, Lifton RP, Gavras H, Cupples LA, Myers RH. Evidence for a gene influencing blood pressure on chromosome 17. Genome scan linkage results for longitudinal blood pressure phenotypes in subjects from the Framingham heart study. Hypertension 2000; 36:477–483.

85. Benjafield AV, Katyk K, Morris BJ. Association of EDNRA, but not WNK4 or FKBP1B, polymorphisms with essential hypertension. Clin Genet 2003; 64:433–438.

86. Achard JM, Warnock DG, Disse-Nicodeme S, Fiquet-Kempf B, Corvol P, Fournier A, Jeunemaitre X. Familial hyperkalemic hypertension: phenotypic analysis in a large family with the WNK1 deletion mutation. Am J Med 2003; 114:495–498.

87. Choate KA, Kahle KT, Wilson FH, Nelson-Williams C, Lifton RP. WNK1, a kinase mutated in inherited hypertension with hyperkalemia, localizes to diverse Cl^--transporting epithelia. Proc Natl Acad Sci USA 2003; 100:663–668.

88. Zambrowicz BP, Abuin A, Ramirez-Solis R, Richter LJ, Piggott J, BeltrandelRio H, Buxton EC, Edwards J, Finch RA, Friddle CJ, Gupta A, Hansen G, Hu Y, Huang W, Jaing C, Key BW Jr, Kipp P, Kohlhauff B, Ma ZQ, Markesich D, Payne R, Potter DG, Qian N, Shaw J, Schrick J, Shi ZZ, Sparks MJ, Van Sligtenhorst I, Vogel P, Walke W, Xu N, Zhu Q, Person C, Sands AT. Wnk1 kinase deficiency lowers blood pressure in mice: a gene-trap screen to identify potential targets for therapeutic intervention. Proc Natl Acad Sci USA 2003; 100:14109–14114.

89. Lifton RP. Genetic determinants of human hypertension. Proc Natl Acad Sci USA 1995; 92:8545–8551.

90. Hirschhorn JN, Lohmueller K, Byrne E, Hirschhorn K. A comprehensive review of genetic association studies. Genet Med 2002; 4:45–61.

91. Corvol P, Persu A, Gimenez-Roqueplo AP, Jeunemaitre X. Seven lessons from two candidate genes in human essential hypertension: angiotensinogen and epithelial sodium channel. Hypertension 1999; 33:1324–1331.

92. Samani NJ. Genome scans for hypertension and blood pressure regulation. Am J Hypertens 2003; 16:167–171.

93. Garcia EA, Newhouse S, Caulfield MJ, Munroe PB. Genes and hypertension. Curr Pharm Des 2003; 9:1679–1689.

94. Caulfield M, Munroe P, Pembroke J, Samani N, Dominiczak A, Brown M, Benjamin N, Webster J, Ratcliffe P, O'Shea S, Papp J, Taylor E, Dobson R, Knight J, Newhouse S, Hooper J, Lee W, Brain N, Clayton D, Lathrop GM, Farrall M, Connell J. Genome-wide mapping of human loci for essential hypertension. Lancet 2003; 361:2118–2123.

95. Rao DC, Province MA, Leppert MF, Oberman A, Heiss G, Ellison RC, Arnett DK, Eckfeldt JH, Schwander K, Mockrin SC, Hunt SC. A genome-wide affected sibpair linkage analysis of hypertension: the HyperGEN network. Am J Hypertens 2003; 16:148–150.

96. Kardia SL, Rozek LS, Krushkal J, Ferrell RE, Turner ST, Hutchinson R, Brown A, Sing CF, Boerwinkle E. Genome-wide linkage analyses for hypertension genes in two ethnically and geographically diverse populations. Am J Hypertens 2003; 16:154–157.

97. Thiel BA, Chakravarti A, Cooper RS, Luke A, Lewis S, Lynn A, Tiwari H, Schork NJ, Weder AB. A genome-wide linkage analysis investigating the determinants of blood pressure in whites and African Americans. Am J Hypertens 2003; 16:151–153.

98. Ranade K, Hinds D, Hsiung CA, Chuang LM, Chang MS, Chen YT, Pesich R, Hebert J, Chen YD, Dzau V, Olshen R, Curb D, Botstein D, Cox DR, Risch N. A genome scan for hypertension susceptibility loci in populations of Chinese and Japanese origins. Am J Hypertens 2003; 16:158–162.

99. Allayee H, de Bruin TW, Michelle Dominguez K, Cheng LS, Ipp E, Cantor RM, Krass KL, Keulen ET, Aouizerat BE, Lusis AJ, Rotter JI. Genome scan for blood pressure in Dutch dyslipidemic families reveals linkage to a locus on chromosome 4p. Hypertension 2001; 38:773–778.

100. Angius A, Petretto E, Maestrale GB, Forabosco P, Casu G, Piras D, Fanciulli M, Falchi M, Melis PM, Palermo M, Pirastu M. A new essential hypertension susceptibility locus on chromosome 2p24-p25, detected by genomewide search. Am J Hum Genet 2002; 71:893–905.

101. von Wowern F, Bengtsson K, Lindgren CM, Orho-Melander M, Fyhrquist F, Lindblad U, Rastam L, Forsblom C, Kanninen T, Almgren P, Burri P, Katzman P, Groop L, Hulthen UL, Melander O. A genome wide scan for early onset primary hypertension in Scandinavians. Hum Mol Genet 2003; 12:2077–2081.

102. Kristjansson K, Manolescu A, Kristinsson A, Hardarson T, Knudsen H, Ingason S, Thorleifsson G, Frigge ML, Kong A, Gulcher JR, Stefansson K. Linkage of essential hypertension to chromosome 18q. Hypertension 2002; 39:1044–1049.

103. Evans WE, Johnson JA. Pharmacogenomics: the inherited basis for interindividual differences in drug response. Annu Rev Genomics Hum Genet 2001; 2:9–39.

104. Koopmans RP, Insel PA, Michel MC. Pharmacogenetics of hypertension treatment: a structured review. Pharmacogenetics 2003; 13:705–713.

105. Liljedahl U, Karlsson J, Melhus H, Kurland L, Lindersson M, Kahan T, Nystrom F, Lind L, Syvanen AC. A microarray minisequencing system for pharmacogenetic profiling of antihypertensive drug response. Pharmacogenetics 2003; 13:7–17.

106. Kurland L, Liljedahl U, Karlsson J, Kahan T, Malmqvist K, Melhus H, Syvanen AC, Lind L. Angiotensinogen gene polymorphisms: relationship to blood pressure response to antihypertensive treatment. Results from the Swedish Irbesartan Left Ventricular Hypertrophy Investigation vs Atenolol (SILVHIA) trial. Am J Hypertens 2004; 17(1):8–13.

107. Gibbs RA, Belmont JW, Hardenbol P, Willis TD, Yu F, Yang H, Chang LY, Huang W, Liu B, Shen Y, Tam PK, Tsui LC, Waye MM, Wong JT, Zeng C, Zhang Q, Chee MS, Galver LM, Kruglyak S, Murray SS, Oliphant AR, Montpetit A, Hudson TJ, Chagnon F, Ferretti V, Leboeuf M, Phillips MS, Verner A, Kwok PY, Duan S, Lind DL, Miller RD, Rice JP, Saccone NL, Taillon-Miller P, Xiao M, Nakamura Y, Sekine A, Sorimachi K, Tanaka T, Tanaka Y, Tsunoda T, Yoshino E, Bentley DR, Deloukas P, Hunt S, Powell D, Altshuler D, Gabriel SB, Zhang H, Matsuda I, Fukushima Y, Macer DR, Suda E, Rotimi CN, Adebamowo CA, Aniagwu T, Marshall PA, Matthew O, Nkwodimmah C, Royal CD, Leppert MF, Dixon M, Stein LD, Cunningham F, Kanani A, Thorisson GA, Chakravarti A, Chen PE, Cutler DJ, Kashuk CS, Donnelly P, Marchini J, McVean GA, Myers SR, Cardon LR, Abecasis GR, Morris A, Weir BS, Mullikin JC, Sherry ST, Feolo M, Daly MJ, Schaffner SF, Qiu R, Kent A, Dunston GM, Kato K, Niikawa N, Knoppers BM, Foster MW, Clayton EW, Wang VO, Watkin J, Sodergren E, Weinstock GM, Wilson RK, Fulton LL, Rogers J, Birren BW, Han H, Wang H, Godbout M, Wallenburg JC, L'Archeveque P, Bellemare G, Todani K, Fujita T, Tanaka S, Holden AL, Lai EH, Collins FS, Brooks LD, McEwen JE, Guyer MS, Jordan E, Peterson JL, Spiegel J, Sung LM, Zacharia LF, Kennedy K, Dunn MG, Seabrook R, Shillito M, Skene B, Stewart JG, Valle DL, Jorde LB, Cho MK, Duster T, Jasperse M, Licinio J, Long JC, Ossorio PN, Spallone P, Terry SF, Lander ES, Nickerson DA, Boehnke M, Douglas JA, Hudson RR, Kruglyak L, Nussbaum RL. The International HapMap Project. Nature 2003; 426:789–796.

108. Napoli C, Lerman LO, Sica V, Lerman A, Tajana G, de Nigris F. Microarray analysis: a novel research tool for cardiovascular scientists and physicians. Heart 2003; 89:597–604.

5

Hemodynamics, Circulation, and the Vascular Tree in Hypertension

MICHEL E. SAFAR

Hôpital Hôtel-Dieu, Paris, France

KEYPOINTS

- The blood pressure curve can be described by two essential parameters; mean blood pressure and pulse pressure.
- Ejection of blood into the aorta generates a forward-traveling pressure wave (incident pressure wave) that is propagated at a given velocity to other arteries throughout the body (pulse wave velocity).

- The incident pressure wave is reflected at any point of structural or functional discontinuity in the arterial tree (reflected "echo" wave).
- Pulse pressure and pulse pressure wave velocities increase with age due to increased arterial stiffness and vascular remodeling. Therefore, systolic blood pressure increases with age, while diastolic blood pressure tends to decrease after about 55 years of age.
- Hypertension exacerbates these changes due to further vascular remodeling

SUMMARY

Hypertension involves two different components of the blood pressure curve; mean and pulse pressure. The former relates to vascular resistance and microcirculation and the latter to arterial stiffness, wave reflections, and macrocirculation. This discription constitutes now a days a necessary approach for the understanding of the goals of antihypertensive drug therapy.

I. INTRODUCTION

Until the second half of the 20th century, systemic hypertension was considered as a cardiovascular and renal disease, and the principal research objective was to find its possible causes such as kidney and adrenal alterations, coarctation of the aorta, and renal artery stenosis. Although the definition of high blood pressure was based on two specific and arbitrary points on a curve of blood pressure values (peak systolic and end-diastolic blood pressures), in practice, pressure and flow were thought to be steady-state phenomena, that is, they were constant over time. The hemodynamics of human hypertension were limited to the determinations of mean blood pressure and cardiac output, and the calculation of total vascular resistance (MBP/CO where MBP represents mean blood pressure and CO, cardiac output) (1,2). The latter calculation is based on Poiseuille's law, which describes a fluid of viscosity μ in a straight pipe of length l, and diameter d. The pressure gradient across the pipe is proportional to μ, l, and Q, but inversely related to d^4. Thus, in subjects with hypertension, vascular resistance was considered the only opposition to flow, and it was thought that this vascular resistance would affect only the smaller arteries and the microvascular network. In addition, because cardiac output was observed to be normal despite the elevated blood pressure, hemodynamic studies focused on the nature of the observed homeostatic ("autoregulatory") mechanisms.

As a result of developments in cardiovascular epidemiology and, in particular, the development of antihypertensive drug therapy, hypertension came to be recognized increasingly as a risk factor for cardiovascular diseases. As a consequence, the mechanisms of hypertension were no longer studied from the perspective of a simple, stable, homeostatic system, but from the perspective of patient survival and cardiovascular morbidity and mortality. This "Darwinian" approach led to the understanding that the blood pressure curve should be investigated as a cyclic rather than as a steady-state phenomenon (3–5), thus elevating the potential role of blood pressure pulsatility in the mechanisms of cardiovascular death (Fig. 5.1). Hence, high blood pressure was no longer studied solely on the basis of a simple linear model of the circulation. In addition to microcirculation, the large arteries, pulse pressure, and arterial stiffness were shown to be extensively involved in the hemodynamics of hypertension (5).

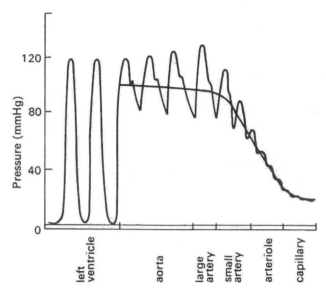

Figure 5.1 Pulsatile hemodynamic profile of blood pressure along the heart and the vascular tree. Note that from the aorta to the capillaries, mean aterial pressure (denoted as a straight line) is indicated in addition to pulsatile pressure. If only the mean pressure (and mean flow) are considered, the hemodynamics of hypertension are derived exclusively from Poiseuille's law by using a simple linear model of the circulation (1,2). If, more realistically, pulsatile pressure is considered as well, then more complex nonlinear models that include the status of the large arteries should be taken into account (3–5).

The primary purpose of this chapter is to describe in detail the characteristics of the blood pressure curve in normotensive and hypertensive populations. But the associated changes in cardiac structure and function also are examined, along with the vascular factors in hypertensive subjects, which involve successively the roles of the macrocirculation and microcirculation.

II. BLOOD PRESSURE CURVE IN HYPERTENSIVE SUBJECTS

The topics in this section include the functional components of the blood pressure curve, the propagation of a pressure wave, the relationship between blood pressure and arterial remodeling, and the role of age in the hemodynamics of hypertension.

A. Components of the Blood Pressure Curve (3–5)

The arterial system functions in two distinct ways: as a conduit, whereby an adequate supply of blood and oxygen is delivered from the heart to the peripheral organs and as a buffer (cushion), whereby the pulsations that result from intermittent ventricular ejection are dampened. These two functions are strongly interrelated, but can interact independently with the classical pathophysiological mechanisms of hypertension.

The role of the arteries is to maintain the continuous, steady, and constant flow of blood that is required for metabolic activity. To maintain this flow, there must be a steady pressure that will overcome the energy losses that result from the viscosity of the blood and friction, that is, overcome vascular resistance as defined by the relationship between a steady mean blood pressure and a steady blood flow. The mean blood pressure, calculated by measuring the area under the blood pressure curve and then dividing this measurement by the time interval involved, is equal to cardiac output multiplied by vascular resistance (1,2). In accordance with Poiseuille's law, the efficiency of the arterial conduit function depends on the number and diameter of the small arteries and of the constancy of mean blood pressure, with an almost imperceptible mean blood pressure gradient between the ascending aorta and the peripheral arteries. Because cardiac output is normal in subjects with hypertension, it is vascular resistance that clearly is increased.

The role of arteries as a cushion is to smooth out the pressure oscillations that are a result of intermittent ventricular ejection. Hemodynamically, the resulting pulsatile flow and pulsatile pressure characterize the cushioning function. Large arteries can accommodate the volume of blood ejected from the ventricles instantaneously, storing part of the stroke volume during systole and draining this volume during diastole, which permits continuous

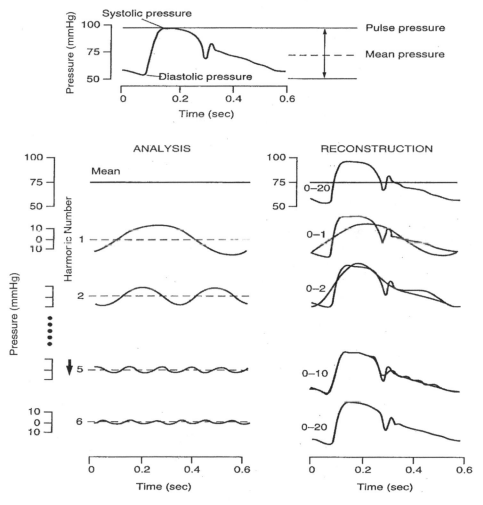

Figure 5.2 The two components of the blood pressure curve (upper panel) and Fourier analysis of the blood pressure curve. The technique for deriving a series of sine waves from a given pressure is mathematically simple, but the calculation, which is cumbersome, has been improved considerably during the last few years by the use of digital computers. An example of Fourier analysis of aortic pressure wave is provided in the lower panel (4). The harmonic zero reflects the mean value, which represents a sine wave with an infinite period. The first harmonic reflects the heart rate f; higher harmonics have a frequencies of $2f$, $3f$, and so forth. When all of the sine waves are known, adding them together leads to the mathematical reconstruction of the signal. In the cardiovascular system, about 20 harmonics are sufficient for an adequate reconstruction of the complete blood pressure curve, as shown by using digital computers. According to that methodology, a correct description of the curve (in the upper panel) takes into account not only peak-systolic and end-diastolic blood pressures, but also the mean blood pressure and the oscillation around the mean blood pressure, simplified as pulse pressure (3,4).

perfusion of peripheral organs and tissues. The cushioning function is the consequence of the viscoelastic properties of the arterial wall and can be evaluated from two perspectives: the "Windkessel" or air-chamber effect (time domain) and wave propagation (frequency domain) (3,4).

Because of the dual function of arteries, and in accordance with Fourier analysis of the blood pressure curve (3,4), blood pressure has two different components: mean blood pressure and pulse pressure (Fig. 5.2, upper section).

Both mean blood pressure and pulse pressure are elevated in subjects with hypertension. However, although mean blood pressure is determined by cardiac output and vascular resistance, pulse pressure, which represents the oscillation around the mean blood pressure, is determined by the pattern of left ventricular ejection, the viscoelastic and propagative properties of the large arteries, and the amplitude and timing of reflected waves. Both blood pressure components strongly affect the viscoelastic and propagative properties of the arterial system. But the relative contribution of each component varies widely according to the age of the patient, resulting in several varieties of hypertension.

B. Propagation of the Pressure Wave and Pulse Pressure Amplification

Ejection of blood into the aorta generates a pressure wave that is propagated at a given velocity (the so-called *pulse wave velocity*) to other arteries throughout the body (3–5) (Fig. 5.3).

This forward-traveling pressure wave (*incident pressure wave*) is reflected at any point of structural or functional discontinuity in the arterial tree, thereby generating a reflected ("echo") wave that travels backward toward the ascending aorta. Incident and reflected pressure waves interact constantly, and their sum is the aortic *measured wave* that indicates the level of blood pressure and the degree of hypertension (Fig. 5.2). The final amplitude and shape of this measured wave are determined by the phase relationship (timing) of the component waves. The timing of incident and reflected pressure waves depends on the pulse wave velocity, the distance the pressure waves must travel (i.e., arterial length, as determined by body height), and the duration of left ventricular ejection. The shape and amplitude of measured pulse pressure waves also depend on where in the arterial system the pressure is being recorded (Fig. 5.2). Peripheral arteries are close to sites where waves are reflected. The incident and reflected waves in these peripheral arteries are in phase and, thus, produce an additive effect. The ascending aorta and central arteries are located away from the sites where waves are reflected. In these arteries, depending on the pulse wave velocity, the return of the reflected wave is delayed in proportion to the arterial distance; thus, the incident and reflected waves are not in phase. The delay of reflected waves is influenced largely by the age of the patient, but this delay has identical consequences in both normotensive and hypertensive subjects (Fig. 5.4).

In young humans (≤50 years) with distensible arteries and low pulse wave velocity, the reflected waves affect the central arteries during diastole, after left ventricular ejection has ceased. This timing is desirable because the reflected waves cause an increase in ascending aortic pressure during early diastole, not during systole; this produces an aortic systolic blood pressure and pulse pressure that are lower than in the peripheral arteries (only the mean blood pressure remains almost constant throughout the arterial system). (Fig. 5.4, left panel.) This hemodynamic aspect, which involves pulse pressure amplification between the central and the peripheral arteries (Fig. 5.3), is advantageous physiologically because the increase of early diastolic blood pressure has a boosting effect on coronary perfusion without increasing the left ventricular afterload. This desired timing in younger subjects is disrupted in older subjects (>50 years) by an increase in pulse wave velocity as a result of arterial stiffening. (Fig. 5.4, right panel.) With an increase in pulse wave velocity, the sites where pressure waves are reflected appear to be closer to the ascending aorta, and these reflected waves occur earlier because they are more closely in phase with the incident waves in this region. The earlier return of reflected waves means that these waves affect the central arteries during systole rather than during diastole, thus amplifying aortic and left ventricular pressures during systole and reducing aortic pressure during diastole (3–6). (Fig. 5.4, right panel.) The pulse pressure and systolic blood pressure gradients along the arterial tree tend to disappear, resulting in temporal equalization of peripheral and aortic pressures and a loss of pulse pressure amplification.

Hypertension in middle-aged individuals involves increases in both mean blood pressure and pulse pressure, but it also is characterized by significant pulse pressure amplification. In older patients, pulse pressure amplification disappears as a result of the more pronounced effect of aging on the central arteries than on the peripheral arteries.

C. Blood Pressure and Arterial Remodeling

The arterial wall is a complex tissue that consists of different cell populations that are subject to structural and functional changes in response to direct injury and atherogenic factors or in response to modifications of long-term hemodynamic conditions. The principal geometric modifications that are induced by these alterations are changes of the arterial lumen or arterial wall thickness as a result of the activation, proliferation, and migration of smooth muscle cells and the rearrangements of cellular elements and extracellular matrix of the vessel wall.

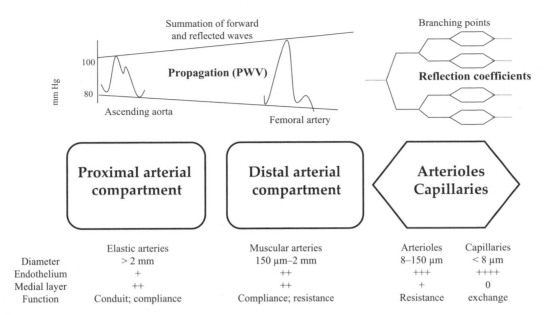

Figure 5.3 Schematic representation of the architecture of the arterial and arteriolar systems, and the propagation of blood pressure waves (personal view). In the middle and lower panels are indicated the proximal (central elastic arteries) and distal (peripheral muscular arteries) compartments of the arterial tree and finally the microvascular network, composed of arterioles and capillaries. The propagation of pressure waves at a given velocity (pulse wave velocity) along the proximal and distal arteries are shown in the upper panel, along with the bifurcations (branching points) of the microvascular network, which are the major sites of wave reflection. Each site has its own reflection coefficient. Note that the sum of the forward and backward pressure waves at each point of the arterial tree means that at the same mean blood pressure, pulse pressure is higher in the central arteries than it is in the peripheral arteries.

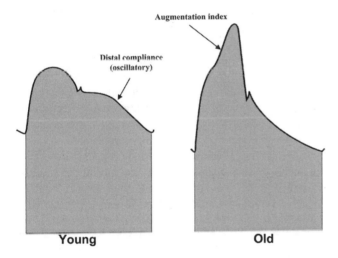

Figure 5.4 Invasive thoracic aorta blood pressure curves in younger and older subjects. Note that, for the same mean blood pressure (the same cross-sectional area beneath the blood pressure curve) in younger and older subjects, pulse pressure is higher in older subjects than it is in younger subjects. This is owing to both a higher systolic blood pressure and a lower diastolic blood pressure. This change in blood pressure curve with age is the result of increased arterial stiffness and pulse wave velocity and a change in the timing of wave reflections, which return to the heart during diastole in younger subjects. (this alteration is often evaluated as reduction in distal oscillatory compliance) (6) and during systole in older subjects (this alteration is often called: increase of augmentation index) (3,4).

The mechanical signals for arterial remodeling that are associated with hemodynamic overload are cyclic tensile stress or shear stress (7–10). Blood pressure is the principal determinant of arterial wall stretch and tensile stress; it creates radial and tangential forces that counteract the effect of intraluminal pressure. Blood flow alterations result in changes in *shear stress*, which is the dragging frictional force created by blood flow. Although acute changes in tensile stress or shear stress induce transient adjustments in vasomotor tone and arterial diameter, chronic alterations of mechanical forces lead to modifications of the geometry and composition of the vessel walls that can be considered adaptive responses to long-lasting changes in blood flow or blood pressure (8).

According to Laplace's law, tensile stress (σ) is directly proportional to arterial transmural pressure (P) and radius (r), and inversely proportional to arterial wall thickness (h), according to the formula $\sigma = Pr/h$ (3–7). In response to an increase in blood pressure or arterial radius, tensile stress is maintained within the physiological range by a thickening of the heart and vessel walls, a process that is consistently observed in the heart and in the small and large arteries of hypertensive subjects (2–9).

Shear stress is a function of the blood-flow pattern. In linear segments of the vasculature, blood is displaced in layers that are moving at different velocities. The middle of the stream moves more rapidly than the side layers, which generates a parabolic velocity profile. The slope of the velocity profile, that is, the change of blood velocity per unit distance across the vessel radius, defines the shear rate. Shear stress (τ) is directly proportional to blood flow (Q) and blood viscosity (η), and inversely proportional to the radius (r) of the vessel, according to the formula $\tau = Q\eta/\pi r^3$ (7–9). Because cardiac output is normal in hypertensive subjects, it is often thought that shear stress is of secondary importance in the mechanisms of hypertension. However, cardiac output decreases with age and is even significantly elevated during the early phase of hypertension (1,2). Furthermore, changes in shear stress and tensile stress are interrelated because any modification of the arterial radius that is caused by alterations in blood flow and shear stress induces changes in tensile stress as well (unless blood pressure varies in the opposite direction).

The characteristics of arterial remodeling depend primarily on the nature of hemodynamic stimuli that are applied to the arteries. To maintain tensile stress within physiological limits, arteries respond by thickening their walls (Laplace's law), but the increased tensile stress is a direct result of both high blood pressure and pressure-dependent passive distension of the arterial lumen. Studies in animals and humans have shown that this pressure-related distension of the arterial diameter is limited to central (elastic-type) arteries [i.e., it is not present in peripheral (muscular-type) arteries], and it causes an increase of the wall-to-lumen ratio that is proportional to the pressure (3,5,7). This ability to adjust the wall-to-lumen ratio efficiently maintains tensile stress within normal limits. The nature of the mechanism that prevents the passive dilation effect of pressure is unknown, but prevention of passive dilation does require the presence of an intact endothelium (7). It is worthwhile noting here that endothelial function is altered in subjects with hypertension (7,8,11).

Experimental and clinical data indicates that acute and chronic augmentations of arterial blood flow induce proportional increases in the vessel lumen, whereas decreasing flow reduces the arterial inner diameter (7,8). An example of flow-mediated remodeling associates arterial dilation and sustained high blood flow after the creation of an arteriovenous fistula (12). An increase in arterial inner diameter usually is accompanied by arterial wall hypertrophy and increased intima–media cross-sectional area (following increases in the radius of the arterial vessel and in arterial wall tension). As noted earlier, the presence of the endothelium is a prerequisite for normal vascular adaptation to chronic changes of blood flow; experimental data indicates that flow-mediated arterial remodeling can be limited through inhibition of nitric oxide synthase (11). Although the alterations of tensile stress and shear stress are interrelated, changes in tensile stress primarily induce alterations and hypertrophy of the arterial media. Changes in shear stress principally modify the dimensions

and the structure of the intima. It is noteworthy that alterations and hypertrophy of the arterial media predominate in subjects with hypertension (3,7,8,11).

D. Age and Hemodynamic Patterns of Hypertension

It is widely accepted that blood pressure increases with age, but this is true primarily for systolic blood pressure (Fig. 5.5) (13). Diastolic blood pressure increases progressively until 55 years of age but, thereafter, remains stable or even tends to decline spontaneously. From the observed age-related changes in systolic blood pressure and diastolic blood pressure, it can be concluded that, with age, mean blood pressure is modified only a little, whereas pulse pressure increases exponentially. All of these hemodynamic changes are more pronounced in hypertensive subjects than in normotensive subjects (Fig. 5.5).

From most classical longitudinal studies reported in the literature (Fig. 5.5), it appears that in young subjects (≤ 50 years), systolic blood pressure, diastolic blood pressure, mean blood pressure, and pulse pressure increase to the same extent with age. This indicates a predominant influence of an increase in mean blood pressure and vascular resistance that corresponds to the hemodynamic pattern of sustained essential hypertension in middle age. In older subjects (>50 years), systolic blood pressure and pulse pressure increase markedly with age, whereas mean blood pressure and diastolic blood pressure remain relatively stable—diastolic blood pressure even tends to decline. This pattern reflects a predominance of increased arterial stiffness and altered pressure wave reflections in the mechanisms of hypertension, which corresponds to the traditional picture of systolic hypertension.

It seems logical to divide the hemodynamic aspects of human hypertensive subjects into those that affect vascular resistance and the microcirculation, particularly as observed in young subjects, and those that affect the stiffness of arteries, wave reflection, and macrocirculation that are observed primarily in older subjects (5).

III. CARDIAC STRUCTURE AND FUNCTION IN HYPERTENSION

It is important to summarize the characteristics of the cardiac pump, which are common to both vascular aspects of hypertension. It should be noted that, in this review, these descriptions are limited to subjects with chronic, sustained, essential, uncomplicated hypertension. *Chronic* indicates that the disease is >3 years in duration, with a mean subject age of between 20 and 70 years. *Sustained* implies that the diastolic blood pressure is consistently >90 mmHg or that the systolic blood pressure is

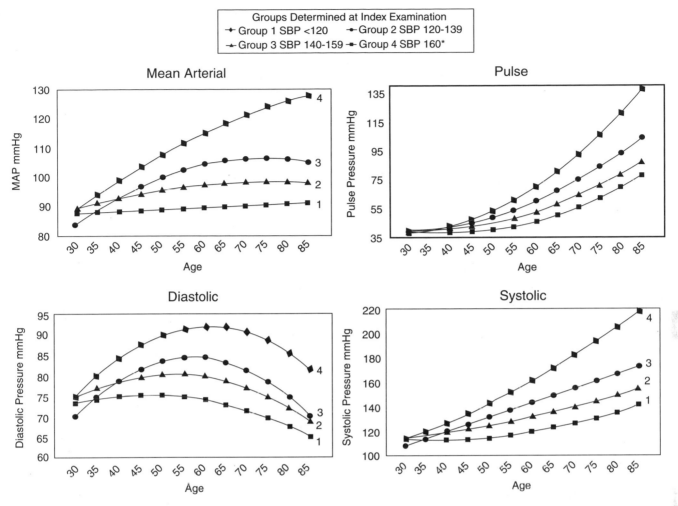

Figure 5.5 Relationship between blood pressure and age in normotensive and hypertensive subjects classified from 1 to 4 (13). Note that although systolic blood pressure ("systolic") (SBP) and pulse pressure ("Pulse") increase markcdly with age, diastolic blood pressure ("diastolic") increases up to 55 years of age and, thereafter, tends to decrease substantially. The mean blood pressure ("mean arterial") is little modified by age. In this study, no subject was treated with antihypertensive drugs *mmHg.

>140 mmHg (the standard definition of hypertension). *Essential* means that plasma and urinary electrolytes, urinary catecholamines, and renal arteries investigated by using echo-Doppler techniques are always within the normal range. *Uncomplicated* is defined as no history of stroke, congestive heart failure, or any vascular complication, and that plasma creatinine is <1.4 mg%. In the literature, data are frequently restricted to men who are compared with controls of the same age and sex, with both populations having a balanced sodium intake and urinary output. Sodium intake in the range of 80–150 mEq/day is considered to be the steady state.

A. Normal Cardiac Output and Cardiac Hypertrophy

In comparison to controls of the same age and sex, cardiac output (expressed as ml/min per m² body surface area) is normal in patients with uncomplicated, sustained, essential hypertension (14–19). Although some elevated values for cardiac output have been reported for patients with secondary forms of hypertension (14), the normal value for subjects with essential hypertension is observed in both supine and upright positions. Oxygen consumption is normal or slightly increased (15,17,18). The arteriovenous oxygen difference is elevated because of the reduction in oxygen venous content of red blood cells (15). Heart rate is slightly increased, but the stroke volume is normal. Blood flow in the liver and lower limbs remains within the normal range, but renal blood flow is reduced (16).

When subjects with essential hypertension are excercising, cardiac output remains adapted to the metabolic needs of the tissues. However, the slope of the curve plotting cardiac output (or stroke volume) against oxygen consumption is lower than it is for control subjects (15,17). In the past, this finding had been attributed to an early phase of heart failure, but the alterations of ventricular geometry that are associated with cardiac hypertrophy play a more important role (15). Investigations that are based on echocardiography have shown that symmetric cardiac hypertrophy is frequent in sustained, uncompli-cated, essential hypertension and parallels the blood pressure level, primarily the systolic blood pressure and the pulse pressure (19–22). In accordance with Laplace's law, cardiac hypertrophy helps to maintain a normal value for myocardial wall stress through an increase in ventricu-lar wall thickness. The change of ventricular geometry is associated with an increase of left ventricular wall stiff-ness, frequently in combination with a change of the dias-tolic function of the heart (21). Hence, a normal stroke volume is maintained through increases of systolic and diastolic intraventricular pressure.

Left ventricular function, as assessed by invasive studies (3,19) and noninvasive evaluation of ejection frac-tion, the mean velocity of circumferential fiber shortening, the mean normalized systolic ejection rate, and iso-volumetric indexes, is normal or enhanced in patients with hypertensive hypertrophy, even in patients with greater increases of muscle mass and with the presence of concomitant coronary artery disease (19–22). Impair-ment in left ventricular function is observed only when regional contraction abnormalities or ventricular dilatation above or both occur (22). The changes of cardiac function are then a reflection of cardiac size, systolic wall stress, and, hence, left ventricular oxygen consumption (21).

B. Cardiac Output and Filling Pressure of the Heart (23–25)

In human studies, the pressure that is considered to be most representative of circulatory filling is the right atrial pressure (central venous pressure). For patients with sus-tained essential hypertension, all reports in the literature have shown that right atrial pressure is slightly, but signifi-cantly increased, even in the absence of congestive heart failure (23–25). Parallel to the rise of atrial pressure, there is also an increase of pulmonary arterial and wedge pressures. The pressure gradient across the pulmonary cir-culation is identical to the pulmonary gradient in normal subjects, and the total resistance of the pulmonary circula-tion also is similar to the total resistance in normotensive controls. In addition, all circulatory pressures (arterial, right atrial, pulmonary, and pulmonary wedge) are posi-tively correlated with each other (25). Right atrial pressure is influenced by parameters that regulate both venous return and the pumping ability of the right ventricle. Theoretically, elevated central venous pressure in hyper-tension could result from three possibilities: decreased or modified pumping function of the heart, decreased vascu-lar compliance, or increased blood volume (1,2).

The basic mechanism for adjusting stroke volume to blood inflow is described as the Frank–Starling law of the heart, and it is expressed in terms of cardiac function curves by plotting stroke volume or cardiac output against right atrial pressure, for example, during volume expansion (1–3). In patients with essential hypertension when compared with controls right cardiac function curves exhibit a rightward shift of otherwise normally shaped blood pressure curves. The pump operates nor-mally but at a higher basic pressure level (23,24). This increase in basic pressure level theoretically might be a passive consequence of heart hypertrophy and the result of a backward effect of elevated arterial pressure. However, such a passive mechanism cannot be the princi-pal factor that accounts for an elevated central venous pressure in subjects with hypertension. Cardiopulmonary and low pressure systems are compliant and, as such, increase their volume when they are subjected to increased pressure. Nevertheless, elevated central venous pressure is observed in patients with essential hypertension, whereas cardiopulmonary blood volume and total blood volume are normal and decreased, respectively (25). Taking into account all these particularities, it appears that in subjects with hypertension, only a reduction in venous compliance could explain satisfactorily the right atrial pressure changes. Acute and rapid volume expansion has been induced in normal and hypertensive subjects by using iso-oncotic-dextran infusion (23–25). Central venous pressures increased significantly more in hypertensive sub-jects than it did in normotensive subjects for equivalent increases in intravascular blood volume (23,24). This finding indicates clearly that in the presence of normal cardiac function curves, effective venous capacity is reduced in hypertensive subjects. This interpretation is supported by the negative correlation that is observed in normal and hypertensive populations between central venous pressure and blood volume, and between central venous pressure and total effective vascular compliance (25). In other words, in subjects with essential hyperten-sion, the slight increase of central venous pressure that is observed under resting conditions is a result of concomi-tant lowering of total effective vascular compliance, not a result of the reduction in blood volume.

In patients with essential hypertension, the contribution of vascular capacitance to the regulation of cardiac output is especially important in view of the three hemodynamic features of the heart and vessels in hypertension: normal cardiac output, decreased intravascular blood volume, and cardiac hypertrophy without congestive heart failure. It is widely accepted that the normal cardiac output in the presence of increased afterload is achieved through cardiac hypertrophy, which causes a decrease of left ven-tricular compliance. In this situation, the presence of estab-lished cardiac hypertrophy would lead to a reduction of the stroke volume without adequate compensation (2). Such compensation could be found in the form of increased cardiac filling pressures in the left and right ventricles. In patients with essential hypertension, capillary wedge pressure is increased, indirectly reflecting an elevation in left atrial pressure (23–25). Right atrial pressure is also elevated, which could, in turn, lead to decreased venous compliance to obtain an adequate driving pressure for the hypertrophied heart. During isotonic saline intravenous volume loading, Ulrych et al. (26) showed that the cardiac output increase was enhanced in hypertensives and suggested that a reduction of peripheral vascular capacity was responsible. More direct evidence is provided by the observation of a negative correlation between cardiac output or stroke volume and effective vascular compliance in patients with essential hypertension: the more reduced the compliance, the higher the cardiac output (26). Thus, despite cardiac hypertrophy and decreased intravascular volume, normal cardiac output is achieved in sustained essential hypertension through a reduction of venous compliance.

C. Age-Related Changes in Cardiac Output in Subjects with Hypertension

Cardiac output decreases physiologically with age, but many investigators have shown that this decline is more pronounced in hypertensive than in normotensive subjects (15,18,27,28). Indeed, cardiac output that is measured in young patients with a mildly elevated blood pressure (systolic blood pressure and diastolic blood pressure ranges between 140 and 160 mmHg and between 90 and 95 mmHg, respectively) while they are at rest in the supine position is frequently elevated (15,27–30). This increased cardiac output is associated with an increase in stroke volume or heart rate, or both (15,18,27,28). Regional hemodynamics studies of this population of young subjects have shown that the elevated cardiac output was due to an increase in muscle blood flow; renal and hepatic blood flows remained within the normal range (16). The cardiac output is elevated in the supine position but not in the sitting position or tilted position, for which most authors found normal values (15,18,27). It is noteworthy that in these young subjects, cardiac output, as judged in relationship to oxygen consumption, is consistently normal, both at rest and during exercise. Cross-sectional studies also indicate that cardiac output is not particularly affected by intravascular volume, but it is affected significantly and directly by heart rate (18,27,28,30,31). A higher ratio between cardiopulmonary and total blood volumes is also observed, suggesting, as with the elevated heart rate, that sympathetic overactivity is present in this population of young patients (2,18,27,29–31).

On the basis of epidemiological studies, it is widely accepted that until 50–60 years of age, systolic blood pressure and diastolic blood pressure increase progressively as a person ages, while cardiac output decreases. This hemodynamic change also is observed when repeat hemodynamic measurements are made in young subjects with mildly elevated blood pressure (15,18,27,28,30,31). However, the younger population exhibits two peculiarities: first, the cardiac output decrease occurs more rapidly in hypertensive than in normotensive subjects; and second, in ~10–20% of these subjects with borderline hypertension, the hemodynamic pattern of sustained, essential hypertension occurs later, over the long-term. However, repeat investigations for this group are difficult to perform for two reasons. On the one hand, these hypertensive subjects frequently either are not re-examined or are upon follow-up found to have been treated with antihypertensive drug therapy. On the other hand, these subjects are matched with normotensive controls who are difficult to recruit in the first place and are subsequently difficult to follow-up. Nevertheless, when hypertensive subjects are followed up in later investigations, they all show the same pattern of changes in cardiac output control. First, the slope of the curve plotting cardiac output against oxygen consumption during exercise tends to be less steep with age (15,17). Secondly, in repeat, cross-sectional studies of large populations, the correlation between cardiac output and intravascular volume becomes more and more pronounced, although the significance of the correlation between heart rate and cardiac output tends to disappear during the follow-up (30–32).

Mathematical and statistical procedures have been developed to examine cross-sectional or longitudinal hemodynamic data from human subjects by using Guyton's cardiovascular model (1). In this model (Fig. 5.6), the kidney is considered to be a filter, and for each given value of sodium intake (which in steady-state and normal conditions is equal to urinary sodium output), a given, steady mean blood pressure is achieved.

As hypertension develops, the renal filter is altered and a higher mean blood pressure is required to maintain a normal sodium balance. Within the organism, this pressure–diuresis mechanism functions through a negative feedback loop, which in animal models, is defined by equations and blocks (with their corresponding specific coefficients) that characterize the resulting changes of fluid volumes, cardiac output, vascular resistance, and compliance.

In 1979, Chau et al. (31) used original statistical procedures that made it possible to determine what conditions could be applied to investigating human hemodynamic data by using Guyton's model. The goal was to evaluate which parts of the model (Fig. 5.6) would have to be modified to maintain the same cardiac output level in

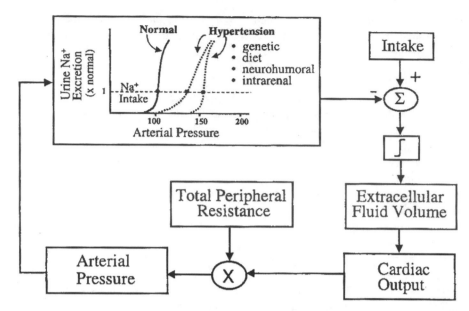

Figure 5.6 Pressure–diuresis mechanism and negative feedback loop of Guyton's model. In the Guyton's model, hypertension is characterized by a shift of pressure–diuresis mechanisms toward higher blood pressure values. In both normotensive and hypertensive populations, each time the blood pressure increases, there is a reduction in extracellular and intravascular volume, cardiac output, and vascular resistance, which making that finally, blood pressure returns back toward normal values. Each block of the negative feedback loop is characterized by its own regulation equation and, therefore, its own regulation coefficients. In animal models of hypertension, this mechanism is operating under the same conditions as normotensive models, that is, with the same regulation coefficients; but it requires a re-setting of the pressure–diuresis curve. Chau et al. (31,32) showed that in hypertensive humans, the regulation coefficients of the equations of the negative feedback loop also should be modified in parallel.

normotensive and hypertensive subjects (31). The response of the model showed that two primary modifications would be required to achieve a normal cardiac output in subjects with essential hypertension: changes of the arteriolar system and reduced vascular compliance. Reduced vascular compliance involves both the large arteries and the veins (32).

Further studies showed that under these conditions, control of cardiac output in hypertensive subjects always differs from that of normotensive subjects and that control of cardiac output involved predominantly neurogenic influences in the normotensive subjects and predominantly vascular structural changes in hypertensive subjects (31,32).

IV. MEAN ARTERIAL BLOOD PRESSURE, MICROCIRCULATION, AND SYSTOLIC–DIASTOLIC HYPERTENSION IN MIDDLE AGE

The principal functions of microcirculation are to optimize nutrient and oxygen supply within the tissues in response to variations in demand and to minimize large fluctuations of hydrostatic pressure in the capillaries that would cause disturbances to capillary exchange (33,34). For

microcirculation in the context of hypertension, the primary questions were to determine under which conditions a large drop in hydrostatic pressure might be achieved without substantial change of capillary pressure (33) and how the reflectance properties of the arterial tree could be optimized (5).

A. Location of Peripheral Vascular Resistances in Chronic Hypertension

The profile of the hydrostatic-pressure decline along the various vascular elements between the heart and the capillaries has been determined in the past in numerous animal studies (1–3). It is generally agreed that relatively little pressure is lost within the larger arteries and that although the pressure profile varies somewhat between studies and for different vascular beds, the pressure drop occurs predominantly in the precapillary vessels that range from 10 to 300 μm in diameter (33–35). In most forms of experimental and clinical hypertension, the cardiac output is close to normal and the peripheral vascular resistance is increased in proportion to blood pressure elevation. Several studies of skeletal muscle in spontaneously hypertensive rats have concluded that blood pressure is elevated approximately proportionally throughout the precapillary vasculature (33–35). For example, De Lano et al. (36) found that if the measured pressures are normalized by the systemic arterial pressure, pressures are virtually identical in normotensive rats and in spontaneously hypertensive rats at all of the locations studied in the system. These results suggest that because the major pressure drop occurs in the smallest arteries and arterioles, these vessels represent the principal sites of increased vascular resistance in hypertension, at least in spontaneously hypertensive rats.

The *in vivo* hemodynamic status represents the combined effects of a complex network of thousands of small arteries and arterioles that make up the resistance vasculature. Because small arteries constitute the most substantial proportion of peripheral resistance, alterations of resistance in these arteries in experimental and human hypertension have attracted considerable attention. In experimental models of hypertension, during its established phase, high blood pressure is associated with increased peripheral resistance and is attributed primarily to a modified vascular structure (33,34). The most striking evidence for this alteration is the marked increase in resistance that occurs when the vasculature is in a state of maximum relaxation. The classic experiments by Folkow (2) showed that minimum vascular resistance was increased by 37% in established hypertension (mean blood pressure increased by 55%), a finding that suggests two important conclusions:

1. According to Poiseuille's law, altered minimum vascular resistance could be the result of a diminution of the lumen diameter of individual vessels, of vessels being longer, or of their rarefaction (a decreased number of vessels connected in parallel) (33,34).
2. Another important paradigm is that increased vascular resistance is a result of modifications to the structure or the function of the microvascular network, or a combination of both.

B. Mechanisms of Increased Vascular Resistance in Hypertension

Most investigations of the mechanisms of hypertension have been performed by using animal models (1–3,33,34). The two models that have been used most often are the Goldblatt renal hypertensive model and the spontaneously hypertensive rats model. In hypertension, the structure and function of the microcirculation may be altered in at least three ways:

1. The mechanisms regulating vasomotor tone may be abnormal, leading to enhanced vasoconstriction, reduced vasodilating responses, or altered autoregulatory processes.

2. There may be anatomical alterations of the structure of individual precapillary resistance vessels, such as increases in their wall-to-lumen ratios.
3. There may be changes at the microvascular network level, perhaps involving a reduction in the density (rarefaction) of arterioles or capillaries within a given vascular bed. It is likely that the relative contributions of these factors may be different in the various vascular beds and among the different forms and models of hypertension.

1. Changes in Vasomotor Tone and Autoregulation

The most obvious mechanism in increased resistance to blood flow in arterioles is vasoconstriction. This is a very powerful mechanism for continuously controlling blood pressure and flow throughout the circulatory system. Because resistance through a vessel is inversely proportional to the fourth power of the vessel radius (Poiseuille's law), only small changes in lumen size are required to make large adjustments to flow and pressure. Functionally, arterioles are highly sensitive to active changes of diameter (1–3,33,34). These changes may range from complete closure to a threefold increase in diameter in the smallest arterioles and up to 50% variation in diameter in larger arterioles. Vasomotor tone in resistance arteries is controlled by both local or metabolic regulation and by the sympathetic nervous system. In addition, paracrine substances, which are released primarily by the endothelial cells, play a key role in the control of local vasomotor tone (37). For example, the altered vascular resistance in genetically hypertensive rats is reflected in their increased pressure response to infused agonists (35). This increase in pressure could be the result not only of alterations in the resistance vessels but also of different levels of intrinsic tone.

The tone of the microcirculation and, consequently, the levels of tissue perfusion are tightly coupled to the status of tissue oxygen consumption. When oxygen requirements increase, blood inflow increases accordingly. The ability of a vascular bed to constrict and dilate in order to maintain flow during changes of perfusion pressure, independently of any systemic neurohumoral regulation, is termed *autoregulation*. In coronary circulation, autoregulation is most effective between pressures of 40–160 mmHg (38). It is important to note that chronic hypertension shifts the range of pressures over which autoregulation occurs in the myocardium, so that flow begins to decline at greater pressure. A similar hemodynamic pattern has been observed within the renal and the cerebral circulations (1–3). The nature of the signaling molecules that link flow to demand and participate in the local autoregulation process has been studied for >40 years, but it still remains poorly elucidated. Adenosine, arachidonic acid derivatives, nitric oxide, oxygen, carbon dioxide, hydrogen, and potassium have all been considered candidates.

In experimental hypertension, vasoconstriction seems to be particularly enhanced at the initial stages, when arterial pressure increases rapidly and structural changes have not yet taken place. For instance, Meininger et al. (39) showed that small arterioles in the rat cremaster muscle constrict significantly during the onset of renal hypertension; protection of the hindquarters from the pressure increases reduces the amount of vasoconstriction, which indicates that autoregulatory mechanisms mediate part of the vascular tone increase. On the other hand, a loss of vasodilating properties, particularly of endothelial origin has been reported in various animal models (34,37). It is in human hypertensive subjects that the autoregulatory process is the most difficult to define. In the classical Guyton's model (1), enhanced cardiac output is an important initiating factor in the mechanism of elevated blood pressure. In models of hypertension that are secondary to volume expansion, cardiac output increases in an early phase of hypertension "beyond the oxygen needs of the tissues" and thereafter returns toward normal values through an autoregulatory process that involves arteriole changes and increases in vascular resistance (1). By using Guyton's model and changing its coefficients to obtain the same cardiac output level in normotensive and hypertensive subjects, Chau et al. (31,32) clearly established that structural changes in the arterioles were a necessary prerequisite to achieve normal cardiac output in the hypertensive population.

2. *Increased Wall-to-Lumen Ratio*

Hypertrophy of the vascular wall, which results in decreased lumen size, and medial hypertrophy, which results in heightened vasodilated vascular resistance, are concepts that are currently receiving considerable attention with respect to hypertension (2,35).

It has been known for many years that small resistance arteries can alter their diameters and their structures in response to blood pressure changes. Increases in the media/lumen ratio of small arteries have been widely documented in several forms of hypertension (34,35). The media/lumen ratio of small mesenteric arteries increases with increasing blood pressure in renal hypertensive rats. These changes are consistent with the view that vessels maintain constant wall stress in the face of changing pressure. However, it is not clear that arterioles undergo similar changes in primary hypertension. Arterioles of spontaneously hypertensive rats have not been reported to show consistently either reduced luminal diameter or wall thickening (40). Reduced arteriole lumen diameters are difficult to demonstrate in hypertensive humans (40–42) because only in vitro and not physiological conditions are available (Table 5.1).

It should be emphasized that the expression "altered structure of the arterial wall" is ambiguous. It is necessary to define precisely what parameter (media thickness, lumen diameter, or wall cross-sectional area) is being studied and under what experimental conditions (whether vessels are maximally dilated or not) the resistance vessels are being studied. As discussed extensively by Mulvany et al. (42), a narrowed lumen and the resulting increased media/lumen ratio can occur without any change in the amount of material in the vessel wall. Conversely, an increased media/lumen ratio need not result in a narrowed lumen, nor is an increased amount of wall material (demonstrated by an increase of the wall cross-sectional area) necessarily accompanied by a smaller lumen or elevated media/lumen ratio. The use of antihypertensive agents in animal models has clearly shown the absence of a parallel between blood pressure changes and wall/lumen ratio changes (35). Nevertheless, the changes in wall/lumen ratio may explain why the loss of vasodilating properties that are a result of structural changes in hypertensive subjects could favor the occurrence of cardiovascular events (34,35,38,42).

Table 5.1 Morphometry of Small Arteries Investigated on a Wire Myograph

Parameter	Normotensive ($n = 10$)	Untreated hypertensives ($n = 7$)	Treated hypertensives with atenolol ($n = 10$)	Treated hypertensives with nifedipine ($n = 10$)
Lumen (μm)	277 $\pm$ 10	223 $\pm$ 13	235 $\pm$ 11	258 $\pm$ 13
Media width (μm)	14.9 $\pm$ 0.61	14.6 $\pm$ 1.9	15.6 $\pm$ 0.65	14.1 $\pm$ 0.85
Media/lumen ratio (%)	5.37 $\pm$ 0.08	7.08 $\pm$ 0.12*	6.81 $\pm$ 0.18*	5.38 $\pm$ 0.18
Media cross-sectional area (μm^2)	13400 $\pm$ 1245	11326 $\pm$ 2897	13243 $\pm$ 1081	12284 $\pm$ 1207

*$P < 0.001$, vs. normotensive or hypertensive patients treated by nifedipine.

Note: Values are expressed as mean $\pm$ SEM. Note that lumen diameter does not differ in the four groups. Determinations of lumen diameter are performed *in vitro* and may differ markedly, depending on whether the diameters are measured at the same pressure or are measured at the same wall tension. In the latter case, because the media/lumen ratios are significantly different in the four groups, the distensibility also should differ significantly in the various groups.

Source: From Schiffrin and Deng (41).

3. Microvascular Rarefaction

Hutchins et al. (43) first described up to 50% rarefaction of the microvasculature in the cremaster muscles of spontaneously hypertensive rats, and Prewitt et al. (44) subsequently found rarefaction of capillaries and arterioles in gracilis muscle of spontaneously hypertensive rats. There is now much evidence that the development of hypertension is accompanied by the rarefaction of arterioles and capillaries in both animal and human models (45–48).

Rarefaction (34) can be functional, which is when it is the result of vasoconstriction that is strong enough to close the vascular lumen and prevent the perfusion of a capillary bed, or it can be structural, in which case the vessels are absent or the number of vessels is decreased in perfused tissues. Functional rarefaction of the capillary beds in skeletal muscles of normotensive animals has been recognized since many years (33,34). Some capillaries are not perfused under resting conditions but are perfused during hyperemia after muscles have had to work during exercise. Because the capillaries themselves cannot constrict, the terminal portion of the arteriole, by adapting its smooth-muscle tone, controls this functional capillary density. Functional rarefaction of arterioles in normotensive animals has been observed in vessels as large as third-order arterioles, which suggests that all of the smaller arterioles and most of the capillaries that are fed by a closed third-order arteriole would not be sufficiently perfused.

It has been suggested that rarefaction might occur in two phases (44), the first phase (functional rarefaction) leading to a second phase (structural or anatomical rarefaction) that cannot be reversed by maximal vasodilatation (34,44). In light of that interpretation, it is important to understand under what conditions the various forms of microvascular alteration might affect the resistance properties of a microvascular network (5,33,34,49). The resistance of tree-like, branched networks can be described by relatively simple extensions of Poiseuille's law, according to which the length of a vessel and its radius (to the fourth power) are the most important geometric features that determine the resistance of a vessel. For a tree-like network, the number of blood vessels that is coupled in parallel also is an important factor. Computer simulation studies have shown that the elimination of a number of small arterioles from such a vascular bed (rarefaction) causes an increase in total resistance (46).

The situation is considerably more complex for arcade-like networks because these networks contain both in-series and in-parallel coupled arteriole branches. In arcade-like networks, the lengths and diameters of individual arterioles, the branching angles of the arterioles, the location of each branching point, and the number of branches all are factors in resistance (49). This implies that in analyzing the role of microvascular densities controlling in resistance, the nature of the change to the network should be defined, as well as the absolute number of blood vessels in the network. This conclusion is in line with the findings of Greene et al. (46) in computer simulations of mammalian microvascular networks. In their model, removal of arteriole segments caused an increase in resistance. On the basis of microvascular rarefaction, the amount of the increase in resistance was sufficient to explain the enhanced vascular resistance that has been observed in some experimental forms of hypertension. However, whether some sites (such as the kidney) are specifically involved in the mechanism of hypertensive microvascular rarefaction remains to be investigated.

V. MACROCIRCULATION AND THE HEMODYNAMIC PATTERN OF SYSTOLIC HYPERTENSION IN THE ELDERLY

Two associated mechanisms might be responsible for systolic hypertension in older subjects: increased arterial stiffness and alterations in the amplitude and timing of wave reflections (3–5,50–53). Both of these mechanisms affect the walls of large arteries and, therefore, are closely interrelated. However, these mechanisms also might act independently as pathophysiological mechanisms in hypertensive disease. In older subjects with isolated systolic hypertension, vascular resistance is poorly modified when compared with normotensive controls of the same age and gender. But in older subjects with a high diastolic blood pressure and a disproportionate increase of systolic blood pressure over diastolic blood pressure, vascular resistance is increased (53).

A. Increased Arterial Stiffness

The ability of arteries to accommodate the volume ejected instantaneously by the left ventricle (Windkessel effect) can be described quantitatively in terms of "compliance," "distensibility", or stiffness of the aorta or an individual artery. These terms express the volume of blood that is contained in the vasculature (total or in a segment of the system) as a function of a given transmural pressure over a given physiological range (3,53). For a particular artery, *compliance* describes the absolute amount of strain change that follows a stress change. In physiology, compliance (C) is defined as the change in volume (ΔV) due to a change in pressure (ΔP); that is, $C = \Delta V/\Delta P$.

If an artery is represented as a long, cylindrical tube, compliance is the instantaneous slope of the pressure–volume relationship at a given point of the tube. The vessel's physical properties are determined primarily by the arterial media. Because the vessel wall comprises smooth-muscle cells and also connective tissue that contains elastin and collagen fibers, the pressure–volume relationship is nonlinear. Compliance, therefore, should be defined only at a given pressure. At a low distending pressure, the tension is borne by the elastin fibers. At a high distending pressure, the tension is borne predominantly by the less extensible collagen fibers, and the arterial wall becomes stiffer (less compliant). This structural arrangement is advantageous because it both prevents arterial blood from pooling at high pressures and protects arteries from high-pressure-induced rupture. To facilitate comparisons of the viscoelastic properties of structures whose dimensions are different, compliance can be expressed relative to the initial volume of the arterial vessels as a coefficient of distensibility Di, defined as $Di = \Delta V/\Delta PV$, where $\Delta V/\Delta P$ is compliance and V is the initial "unstressed" volume (3).

In all subjects, the mean blood pressure is almost the same throughout the large arteries in the system (5). However, there is a progressive increase in vessel stiffness from the proximal (central) to the distal (peripheral) segments of the arterial tree. This is a result of a combination of factors: the continuous decrease in vessel cross-sectional area along the branching points of the vascular tree (Fig. 5.2); the progressive increase in the rigidity of vessel wall fibers (primarily due to modification of the elastin/collagen ratio); and the physiological increase in pulse pressure from central to peripheral arteries as a result of wave reflections (Fig. 5.2) (3,5). Because compliance and distensibility are much higher in the proximal segments of the arterial tree than in the distal segments, it is possible to observe the distensibility gradient between these segments. For example, in humans, the decline in the distensibility gradient between the carotid artery and the radial artery is ~25% in normal, middle-aged subjects (53). With increasing age, this physiological gradient is reduced significantly because of lower compliance and distensibility (increased stiffness) in the central arteries, but not in the peripheral arteries (50–53). This age-related reduction of distensibility of central arteries requires no mean blood pressure change and reflects the intrinsic alterations of the central arterial walls with increasing age. It involves progressively: an enlargement of the mean diameter with a reduction of pulsatile diameter, a massive development of the extracellular matrix of the vessel wall, a lowering of the systolic blood pressure, and a loss of pulse pressure amplification (3,50–53). The latter reflects the more rapid increase with age of aortic systolic blood pressure and pulse pressure than of peripheral systolic blood pressure and pulse pressure as a result of both increased stiffness and altered reflectance properties of the arterial wall (3,50–53). A consequence of the age-dependent enlargement of

aortic diameter is that proximal compliance decreases less with age than does the proximal distensibility (51).

In hypertensive subjects, the mechanical factor represented by high blood pressure contributes necessarily to increasing stiffness in the central arteries and is the major factor that explains the reduced compliance and distensibility of central arteries that are observed in younger hypertensive subjects (3,5,53) (Table 5.2).

Systolic blood pressure, diastolic blood pressure, and pulse pressure are increased to the same extent in this population. In older subjects, alterations of the vascular wall that are independent of changes in mean blood pressure (i.e., isobaric reduction of compliance and distensibility) play a more important or even unique role in the mechanism of increased stiffness in the central arteries, which leads to the hemodynamic pattern of systolic hypertension. Increases in systolic blood pressure and pulse pressure in these subjects are much higher than increases in diastolic blood pressure (which, in many cases, is even lowered). Therefore, for this population, reduced isobaric compliance and distensibility are associated with a "sclerotic" remodeling of the arterial wall that involves increased collagen content and major modifications of the extracellular matrix (3,53). This structural change, called *arteriosclerosis*, is manifested primarily as medial degeneration that is generalized throughout the thoracic aorta and central arteries and causes dilatation, diffuse hypertrophy, and stiffening of the arteries.

Arteriosclerosis is sometimes considered to be a physiological aging phenomenon that results in diffuse, fibroelastic intima thickening, increased medial ground

Table 5.2 Untreated Hypertensive Subjects: Mechanical Properties of Conduit Arteries

	Hypertensive subjects	
	Young	Old
Compliance and distensibility		
Central (aorta; carotid artery)		
Operational	↘	↘
Isobaric	Normal	↘
Peripheral (radial; femoral)		
Operational	Normal	Normal
Isobaric	Normal	Normal
Pulse pressure (PP)		
Central (carotid; aortic) PP	↗	
Peripheral (brachial; radial) PP	↗	↗
PP amplification	Normal	Reduced according to age
(aorto-brachial; radial)		

Note: "Operational," the steady state mean arterial pressure of each group of subjects; Isobaric, the same mean arterial pressure as normotensive controls; PP, pulse pressure. Arrow means increased (↗) or reduced (↘)

substance and collagen, and fragmentation of the elastic lamellae with secondary fibrosis and calcification of the media. Age-related arterial alterations that lead to stiffening of arteries are heterogeneous, being more pronounced in the aorta and central, elastic-type, capacitive arteries than in the peripheral, muscular-type limb arteries (50–52). Changes that are similar to the ones noticed for the aging process also can be observed in systolic hypertension in older patients. However, some differences characterize the two conditions. In subjects with systolic hypertension, arterial dilation is limited or absent and collagen content is enhanced; aging is typified by alterations in the elastin of the arterial wall. In older subjects with cardiovascular diseases, diabetes, end-stage renal failure, or multiple atherosclerotic lesions, systolic hypertension also is a classical feature. Arteriosclerosis often is associated with the particular changes that are attributed to the primary disease (53–56).

B. Altered Wave Reflections

With the increased arterial stiffness and consequent higher pulse wave velocity observed in hypertensive older subjects, wave reflections return to the heart earlier, which means that reflected waves affect the central arteries during systole and not during diastole (Fig. 5.4). This produces an augmentation of aortic pressure during systole and a reduction of aortic pressure during diastole. Thus, the altered mechanical properties of the aortic wall are influencing the level of aortic systolic blood pressure and diastolic blood pressure. However, wave reflections not only alter systolic blood pressure and diastolic blood pressure through increased arterial stiffness and changed timing but also through modification of the reflectance properties that are associated primarily with the microvascular network of the arterial tree and, therefore, are influenced by the geometry, number, structure, and function of the smaller muscular arteries and arterioles (5). Taylor (57) was the first to report that an increase of arterial cross-section area at peripheral bifurcations causes a delay of wave reflections with subsequent selective reductions of systolic blood pressure and pulse pressure through changes in peripheral reflection patterns. Inversely, it is expected that a decrease of arterial cross-section area at peripheral bifurcations contributes to earlier wave reflection and to an increase in systolic blood pressure and pulse pressure through changes in peripheral reflection patterns. These alterations are influenced by distal structural and functional factors—primarily reduced distensibility and hypertrophy or remodeling of arterial and arteriolar vessels, but also by the following: a change in the number and branching angles of arterioles; modifications of the microenvironment (in particular the levels of sodium and other cations), reduction of endothelium-mediated vasodilation, changes in the extracellular matrix composition of small arteries and arterioles, and genetically mediated alterations of vasomotor tone that are a result of changes to smooth muscle or endothelial cells.

Thus, the architecture of the microvascular network plays a pivotal role as the principal site of wave reflection. Early mathematical studies of wave reflection suggested that a majority of reflection sites are in the microvascular area of the network (5). However, recent, careful measurements by Christensen and Mulvany (58) imply that pulse pressure is transmitted much deeper into the microcirculation than was previously thought. These observations have important implications for drug treatment of hypertension, which could possibly reverse specific alterations in microvascular architecture and, through these changes, selectively lower systemic systolic blood pressure and pulse pressure (5,33).

It is noteworthy that several other reflection sites primarily those located in larger arteries, also play a role in the mechanism of disturbed wave reflection and the resulting systolic hypertension. Under normal physiological conditions, these other sites probably have a minimal impact. However, they may become important in some pathological situations, such as those created by aortic coarctation, trauma that necessitates the amputation of the lower limbs, or atherosclerotic alterations that involve multiples sites in the lower limbs (5,53). For instance, changes in aorta geometry, particularly an accelerated age-induced and pressure-induced increase of aortic cross-sectional area (abdominal aneurysm) and the age-induced increase of aorta length (and, hence, tortuosities) (5), may modify the amplitude and timing of wave reflection. Intriguingly, these changes can differ markedly in men and women. In women, changes are largely influenced by their shorter arterial trees (59) but are also influenced by hormonal factors, such as the loss of estrogen. For both men and women, the presence of calcified plaques, particularly at aortic, carotid, and femoral bifurcations and at the origin of the renal arteries, also may serve as *de novo* reflection sites closer to the heart, thereby modifying wave reflection and raising systolic blood pressure and pulse pressure (53).

It is important to note that, in older people, increased arterial stiffness and disturbed wave reflection may be deleterious to the cardiovascular system. By favoring early wave reflections, arterial stiffening increases peak-systolic and end-systolic pressures in the ascending aorta, thereby increasing the systolic tension-time index (STTI) and myocardial oxygen consumption, decreasing the diastolic blood pressure and diastolic tension-time index (DTTI), and decreasing the DTTI/STTI ratio, a determinant of sub-endocardial blood-flow distribution (3,38). Canine studies have shown that aortic stiffening directly diminishes sub-endocardial blood flow, despite an increased mean coronary flow, and that chronic aortic stiffening reduces cardiac transmural perfusion and aggravates sub-endocardial ischemia (3,55). On the other hand, an increase in systolic blood pressure induces myocardial hypertrophy and impairs diastolic myocardial function and left ventricular ejection. Elevated systolic blood pressure and pulse pressure accelerate arterial damage, which in turn, enhances the fatigue of biomaterials, causing degenerative changes and further arterial stiffening. This initiates a process that perpetuates a vicious circle (5).

This review of the hemodynamics of hypertension emphasizes, by using nonlinear models of the circulation, that both macrocirculation and microcirculation are disturbed in human subjects with hypertension. The use of pulsatile hemodynamics helps in understanding to what extent high blood pressure is an important cardiovascular risk factor. In particular, the use of pulsatile hemodynamics makes it possible to better analyze the subtle links between mechanical factors and newly discovered aspects of hypertension that involve molecular biology and genetics.

REFERENCES

1. Guyton AC, Coleman TG, Granger HJ. Circulation: overall regulation. Annu Rev Physiol 1972; 34:13–46.
2. Folkow B. Physiological aspects of primary hypertension. Physiol Rev 1982; 62:347–504.
3. Nichols WW, O'Rourke M. McDonald's blood flow in arteries. In: Arnold E, ed. Theoretical, Experimental and Clinical Principles. 4th ed. London: Sydney, Auckland, 1998:54–113, 201–222, 284–292, 347–401.
4. Westerhof N, Huisman RM. Arterial haemodynamics of hypertension. Clin Sci 1987; 72:391–398.
5. Safar ME, Levy BI, Struijker-Boudier H. Current perspectives on arterial stiffness and pulse pressure in hypertension and cardiovascular diseases. Circulation 2003; 107(22):2864–2869.
6. Cohn JN, Finkelstein S, McVeigh G. Non invasive pulse wave analysis for the early detection of vascular disease. Hypertension 1995; 26:503–508.
7. Langille BL. Remodeling of developing and mature arteries: endothelium, smooth muscles, and matrix. J Cardiovasc Pharmacol 1993; 21(suppl I):S11–S17.
8. Kamiya A, Togawa T. Adaptative regulation of wall shear stress to flow change in the carotid artery. Am J Physiol 1980; 239:H14–H21.
9. Gibbons GH, Dzau VJ. The emerging concept of vascular remodeling. N Eng J Med 1994; 330:1431–1438.
10. Williams B. Mechanical influences on vascular smooth muscle cell function. J Hypertens 1998; 16:1921–1929.
11. Pohl U, Holtz J, Busse R, Bassenge E. Crucial role of endothelium in the vasodilator response to the increased flow in vivo. Hypertension 1986; 8:37–44.
12. Girerd X, London G, Boutouyrie P, Mourad JJ, Safar M, Laurent S. Remodeling of radial artery in response to a chronic increase in shear stress. Hypertension 1996; 27(part 2):799–803.
13. Franklin SS, Gustin W IV, Wong ND, Larson MG, Weber MA, Kannel WB, Levy D. Hemodynamic patterns of age-related changes in blood pressure. The Framingham Heart Study. Circulation 1997; 96:308–315.
14. Frohlich ED, Tarazi ED, Dustan HP. Re-examination of the hemodynamics of hypertension. Am J Med Sci 1969; 257:9–23.
15. Lund-Johansen P. Haemodynamics in essential hypertension. Clin Sci 1980; 59(Suppl 6):343s–354s.
16. Temmar MM, Safar ME, Levenson JA, Totomouko JJ, Simon AC. Regional blood flow in borderline and sustained essential hypertension. Clin Sci 1981; 60(6):653–658.
17. Amery A, Julius S, Whitlock S, Conway J. Influence of hypertension response to exercise. Circulation 1967; 36:231–237.
18. Birkenhager WH, De Leeuw PW, Schalekamp MADH. Control Mechanisms in Essential Hypertension. Amsterdam: Elsevier Biomedical Press, 1982:73–102, 118–127, 196–200.
19. Merillon JP, Fontenier GJ, Lerallut JF, Jaffrin MY, Motte GA, Genain CP, Gourgon RR. Aortic input impedance in normal man and arterial hypertension: its modification during changes in aortic pressure. Cardiovasc Res 1982; 16:646–656.
20. Savage DD, Drayer JIM, Henry WL, Mathiews EC Jr, Ware JH, Gardin JM, Cohen ER, Epstein SE, Laragh JH. Echocardiographic assessment of cardiac anatomy and function in hypertensive subjects. Circulation 1979; 59(4):623–632.
21. Frohlich ED, Apstein C, Chobanian AV, Devereux RB, Dunstan HP, Dzau V, Fouad Tarazi F, Horan MJ, Marcus M, Massieb, Pfeffer MA, Re RN, Rocella EJ, Savage D, Shub C. The heart in hypertension. N Engl J Med 1992; 327:998–1008.
22. Strauer BE. Ventricular function and coronary hemodynamics in hypertensive heart disease. Am J Cardiol 1979; 44(5):999–1006.
23. London GM, Safar ME, Simon AC, Alexandre JM, Levenson JA, Weiss YA. Total effective compliance, cardiac output and fluid volumes in essential hypertension. Circulation 1978; 57:995–1000.
24. Safar ME, London GM, Levenson JA, Simon AC, Chau NP. Rapid dextran infusion in essential hypertension. Hypertension 1979; 1:615–623.
25. Safar M, Plante G, London G. Vascular compliance and blood volume in essential hypertension. In: Laragh JH, Brenner BM, eds. Hypertension. New York: Raven Press Ltd., 1995:377–388.
26. Ulrych M, Hofman J, Heijl Z. Cardiac and renal hyperresponsiveness to acute plasma volume expansion in hypertension. Am Heart J 1964; 68:193–199.
27. Julius S, Schork MA. Borderline hypertension—a critical review. J Chronic Dis 1971; 23:723–754.
28. Weiss YA, Safar ME, London GM, Simon AC, Levenson JA, Milliez PM. Repeat hemodynamic determinations in borderline hypertension. Am J Med 1978; 64:382–387.

29. Safar ME, London GM, Weiss YA. Systemic hemodynamics in sustained essential and renovascular hypertension. In: Safar ME, Tarazi F, eds. The Heart in Hypertension. Dordrecht: Kluwer Academic, 1989:67–78.

30. Safar ME, Weiss YA, Levenson JA, London GM, Milliez PL. Hemodynamic study of 85 patients with borderline hypertension. Am J Cardiol 1973; 31:315–319.

31. Chau NP, Safar ME, London GM, Weiss YA, Levenson JA, Milliez PM. Essential hypertension: an approach to clinical data by the use of models. Hypertension 1979; 1:86–98.

32. Chau NP, Coleman TG, London GM, Safar ME. Meaning of the cardiac output–blood volume relationship in essential hypertension. Am J Physiol 1982; 243:R318–R328.

33. Levy BI, Ambrosio G, Pries AR, Struijker-Boudier HAJ. Microcirculation in hypertension. A new target for treatment? Circulation 2001; 104:735–740.

34. Struijker Boudier HA, Ambrosio G. Microcirculation and Cardiovascular Disease. London: Lippincott Williams & Wilkins, 2000:47–56, 77–88.

35. Mulvany MJ, Aalkjaer C. Structure and function of small arteries. Physiol Rev 1990; 70:921–961.

36. DeLano FA, Schmid-Schonbein GW, Skalak TC, Zweifach BW. Penetration of the systemic blood pressure into the microvasculature of rat skeletal muscle. Microvasc Res 1991; 41:92–110.

37. Küng CF, Lüscher TF. Different mechanisms of endothelial dysfunction with aging and hypertension in rat aorta. Hypertension 1995; 25:194–200.

38. Hoffman JIE. A critical view of coronary reserve. Circulation 1987; 75(suppl I):6–11.

39. Meininger GA, Lubrano VM, Granger HJ. Hemodynamic and microvascular responses in the hindquarters during the development of renal hypertension in rats. Evidence for the involvement of an autoregulatory component. Circ Res 1984; 55:609–622.

40. Struijker-Boudier HAJ, Le Noble JLML, Messing MWJ, Huijberts MSP, Le Noble FAC, Ven Essen H. The microcirculation and hypertension. J Hypertens 1992; 10(suppl 7): S147–S156.

41. Schiffrin EL, Deng LY. Structure and function of resistance arteries of hypertensive patients treated with a β-blocker or a calcium channel antagonist J Hypertens 1996; 14:1247–1255.

42. Mulvany MJ, Hansen PK, Aalkjaer C. Direct evidence that the greater contractility of resistance vessels in spontaneously hypertensive rats is associated with a narrowed lumen, a thickened media, and an increased number of smooth muscle cell layers. Circ Res 1978; 43:845–864.

43. Hutchins PM, Bond RF, Green HD. Participation of oxygen in the local control of skeletal muscle microvasculature. Circ Res 1974; 40(4):85–93.

44. Prewitt RL, Chen II, Dowell R. Development of microvascular rarefaction in the spontaneously hypertensive rat. Am J Physiol 1982; 243(2):H243–H251.

45. Greene AS, Lombard JH J, Cowley AW, Hansen-Smith FM. Microvessel changes in hypertension measured by Griffonia simplicifolia I lectin. Hypertension 1990. 15(6 Pt 2):779–783.

46. Greene AS, Tonellato PJ, Lui J, Lombard JH, Cowley AW Jr. Microvascular rarefaction and tissue vascular resistance in hypertension. Am J Physiol 1989; 256:H126–H131.

47. Antonios TF, Singer DRJ, Markandu ND. Rarefaction of skin capillaries in borderline essential hypertension suggests an early structural abnormality. Hypertension 1999; 34:655–658.

48. Sullivan JM, Prewitt RL, Joseph JA. Attenuation of the microcirculation in young patients with high-output borderline hypertension. Hypertension 1983; 5:844–851.

49. Le Noble FAC, Stassen FRM, Hacking WJG, Struijker Boudier HAJ. Angiogenesis and hypertension. J Hypertens 1998; 16:1563–1572.

50. Learoyd BM, Taylor MG. Alterations with age in the viscoelastic properties of human arterial walls. Circ Res 1966; 18:278–292.

51. Benetos A, Laurent S, Hoeks AP, Boutouyrie P, Safar ME. Arterial alterations with aging and high blood presure. A noninvasive study of carotid and femoral artery. Arterioscler Thromb 1993; 13:90–97.

52. Boutouyrie P, Laurent S, Benetos A, Girerd X, Hoek APG, Safar ME. Opposing effects of aging on distal and proximal large arteries in hypertensives. J Hypertens 1992; 10(suppl 6):S87–S92.

53. Safar ME, London GM. The arterial system in human hypertension In: Swales JD, ed. Textbook of hypertension. London: Blackwell Scientific, 1994:85–102.

54. Benetos A, Waeber B, Izzo JL, Mitchell GF, Resnik L, Asmar R, Safar M. Influence of age, risk factors, and cardiovascular and renal disease on arterial stiffness: clinical applications. Am J Hypertens 2002; 15:1101–1108.

55. Kass DA, Kelly RP. Ventriculo-arterial coupling: concepts, assumption and applications. Ann Biomed Engineering 1992; 20:41–62.

56. Mitchell GF, Tardif JC, Arnold JM, Marchiori G, O'Brien TX, Dunlap ME, Pfeffer MA. Pulsatile hemodynamics in congestive heart failure. Hypertension 2001; 38:1433–1439.

57. Taylor MG. Wave travel in arteries and the design of the cardiovascular system. In: Attinger EO, ed. Pulsatile Blood Flow. New York: Mc Graw Hill, 1964:343–347.

58. Christensen KL, Mulvany MJ. Location of resistance arteries. J Vasc Res 2001; 38:1–12.

59. London GM, Guerin AP, Pannier B, Marchais SJ, Benetos A, Safar ME. Influence of sex on arterial hemodynamics and blood pressure. Role of body height. Hypertension 1995; 26:514–519.

6

Vascular Remodeling in Hypertension

ROK HUMAR, THERESE RESINK, EDOUARD J. BATTEGAY

University Hospital Basel, Basel, Switzerland

KEYPOINTS

- Blood vessels undergo structural changes, for example, vascular remodeling and microvascular rarefaction.
- Structural changes are adaptive responses to changes in blood pressure and pulse.

- Small-resistance-vessel remodeling contributes to hypertension by a decrease in luminal diameter through eutrophic or hypertrophic inward remodeling.
- Reduction of microvessel density by microvascular rarefaction contributes to hypertension by a decrease in total arteriolar and capillary cross-sectional area.

SUMMARY

Changes in blood vessel morphology and function, including vascular remodeling, microvascular rarefaction, and endothelial dysfunction, accompany the increase in peripheral vascular resistance and blood pressure that are characteristics of hypertension. Blood vessels are capable of structural alteration. Remodeling of large and small arteries in hypertension contributes to an elevation in blood pressure and also may participate in the complications of hypertension. Large arteries exhibit increased lumen size and thickened media, which contribute to an elevated systolic blood pressure and pulse pressure. In small-resistance arteries, smooth muscle cells are restructured around a smaller lumen, with eutrophic inward remodeling, particularly in milder forms of hypertension; in severe forms of hypertension and in secondary hypertension (renovascular hypertension), hypertrophic inward remodeling has been reported. Finally, reduction of microvessel density, that is, capillary rarefaction which decreases total arteriolar and capillary cross-sectional area, and small artery remodeling which increases peripheral resistance in the basal state, together increase diastolic blood pressure and decrease vascular reserve.

I. INTRODUCTION

Vascular remodeling and angiogenesis represent two aspects of a series of events that determine the structure and arrangement of vascular beds. Both are complex processes involving cell growth, cell migration, cell rearrangement, or programmed cell death, as well as production, degradation, and reorganization of the extracellular matrix. Both restructuring processes are initiated by humoral factors generated by mechanisms that sense a change in hemodynamic conditions. The angiogenic process gives rise to new vessels; the remodeling process leads to structural changes in the vessel wall or to the loss of microvasculature (1).

Vascular remodeling can be viewed as a physiological protective response, but it can also contribute to certain circulatory disorders such as hypertensive vascular disease, atherosclerosis, restenosis, and aneurysm formation. These vascular changes are likely to enhance vasoconstriction and further reduce blood flow and reserve, which are major contributing factors to the clinical complications of hypertension such as myocardial ischemia and stroke (2,3).

Structural alterations of blood vessels have distinct features: in response to increased arterial pressure, the vessel structure is altered such that the ratio of the width of the wall to the width of the lumen is elevated by either increase in muscle mass or rearrangements of cellular and noncellular elements. These changes heighten vascular reactivity, which potentiates the increase in peripheral resistance, that is characteristic of hypertension (4). Another form of vascular remodeling involves changes in luminal dimensions. Here, active restructuring of the cellular and noncellular components of the vessel wall results in apparent changes in luminal dimensions, with relatively small changes in wall thickness. Vascular dilatation associated with sustained high blood flow or cell loss and matrix proteolysis that result in aneurysm formation can cause this form of remodeling (2). Conversely, a reduction of the vascular mass and caliber results from a long-term reduction in blood flow. Rarefaction of the microcirculation (a loss of capillary area) is another form of vascular remodeling that promotes hypertension and tissue ischemia (5). The architecture of the vessel wall is also markedly altered in response to vascular injury. A neointima forms as part of a reparative response to injury that involves thrombosis, migration and proliferation of vascular cells, matrix production, and inflammatory-cell infiltration (2).

II. REMODELING IN HYPERTENSION

A. Resistance Vessels

Small arteries classically consist of three layers: intima, media, and adventitia. The longitudinally arranged endothelial cells of the intima are separated from the circumferentially arranged smooth muscle cells and connective tissue of the media by an internal elastic lamina. The adventitia contains many components including sympathetic nerves, collagen, and fibroblasts. The primary functional characteristic of the vessels is the lumen diameter, which determines their resistance (to the fourth power according to the Poiseuille relation); this characteristic is determined by the active and structural properties of the vessel. Peripheral resistance is mainly determined by the distal part of the arterial vasculature (the resistance vessels), consisting of the small arteries (arteries with diameter <300 μm) and the arterioles (the arteries leading into the capillaries), and also in part by the microvasculature (diameter <100 μm). The active properties of a vessel are determined by the state of contraction of the individual smooth muscle cells, their number, and their arrangement. The structural properties of a vessel (lumen diameter, media thickness, and wall thickness) are determined with the smooth muscle cells relaxed and usually with the vessels exposed to a given intravascular pressure (6).

B. Definition of Remodeling

The ability of resistance vessels to undergo changes in their structure without changing their volume is called remodeling (7). This term, however, is also used to describe structural changes of the heart after myocardial infarction or structural changes of coronary arteries after angioplasty. Remodeling in these different organs and pathological conditions is caused by different processes. Mulvany and coworkers (3,7–9) proposed to use the term "remodeling" exclusively for changes in the lumen diameter of a relaxed vessel measured under standard intravascular pressure. The same authors have introduced a classification of the different forms of vascular remodeling and provided a nomenclature accordingly [Fig. 6.1(A)]. Remodeling is termed "inward remodeling" or "outward remodeling," depending on whether the remodeling process resulted in a decrease or an increase, respectively, in vessel diameter. Furthermore, an increase,

no change, or a decrease in the amount of the vessel material subclassify remodeling into hypertrophic, eutrophic, and hypotrophic, respectively [Fig. 6.1(A)]. Hypertrophic remodeling is a growth-related process that may involve an increased cell number (hyperplasia), increased cell size (hypertrophy), and increased deposition of fibrillar or nonfibrillar intercellular matrix or various combinations of these. Hypotrophic remodeling involves a reduction in the amount of vessel material. Eutrophic remodeling is characterized by no change in the amount of the material of the vessel wall and may result through rearrangement or restructuring of cellular and noncellular vessels components or a combination of growth and apoptosis in the vessel wall.

The terms "remodeling index" and "growth index" are used for the quantification of the remodeling process [Fig. 6.1(B)]. Knowledge of wall cross-sectional area indicates the amount of material within the vascular wall and thus provides information about the process of growth or regression. Another parameter for the study of vessel remodeling is the wall thickness/lumen diameter (or media thickness/lumen diameter) ratio. The calculation of the media thickness/lumen diameter ratio, according to the Laplace relation, provides information about the ability of the vessels to contract against intravascular pressure. This is a highly stable and reproducible parameter and is also of major hemodynamic significance because it correlates closely with minimal vascular resistance at maximal vasodilation in small arteries (10).

The term remodeling *per se* does not imply a pathological change, but rather a difference between the vessels of hypertensive patients and those of similarly aged normotensive subjects. Furthermore, arteries of the same branching order should be studied, if comparisons between them are to be valid (10).

C. Remodeling of Resistance Vessel Structure During Hypertension

Resistance vessels experience inward eutrophic remodeling during essential hypertension: increased media/lumen ratios in the resistance vasculature of essential hypertensive patients have been demonstrated in numerous studies (11). Other studies have shown that these increased media/lumen ratios were not associated with an increase in the cross-sectional area of the tunica media (12). The size of the individual smooth muscle cell within the media is also normal (13), leaving functional responses unaffected. Altered hemodynamic characteristics of resistance vessels during essential hypertension are therefore mainly due to a eutrophic rearrangement of normal cells around a smaller diameter (14) [Fig. 6.1(A), vessel c]. Different modes of remodeling have been noted for other situations. In human renal hypertension,

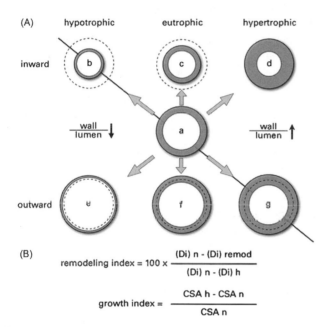

$$\text{remodeling index} = 100 \times \frac{(Di)\,n - (Di)\,remod}{(Di)\,n - (Di)\,h}$$

$$\text{growth index} = \frac{CSA\,h - CSA\,n}{CSA\,n}$$

Figure 6.1 (A) The starting point is the vessel at the center (vessel a). Dotted circles indicate the outer cross-sectional area of the starting vessel. Remodeling can be hypertrophic, that is, increase of cross-sectional area (vessels d and g), eutrophic, that is, no change in cross-sectional area (vessels c and f), or hypotrophic, that is, decrease of cross-sectional area (vessels b and e). These forms of remodeling can be inward, that is, reduction of luminal diameter (vessels b–d) or outward, that is, increase in luminal diameter (vessels e–g). The diagonal axis (from top left to bottom right) denotes vessels with the same wall-to-lumen ratio compared to the starting point vessel at the center. To the right of this line, the wall-to-lumen ratio increases; to the left of the line, the wall-to-lumen ratio decreases. [Adapted from Mulvany et al. (3,8).] (B) Calculation of remodeling and growth index. (Di) n and (Di) h are the internal diameters of normotensive and hypertensive vessels, respectively; CSAn, is the cross-sectional area of a normotensive vessel; and CSAh is the cross-sectional area of a hypertensive vessel. [Adapted from Zervoudaki and Toutouzas (10).]

that is, secondary hypertension and in a manner similar to that found in animal models, a pronounced activation of the renin–angiotensin–aldosterone system is associated with vascular smooth muscle cell hypertrophy (15). Here, reduction in resistance vessel lumen diameter is accompanied by an increase in media cross-sectional area, which is an inward hypertrophic response [Fig. 6.1(A), vessel d]. Inward hypotrophic remodeling [Fig. 6.1(A), vessel b] is found in kidney afferent arterioles in spontaneously hypertensive rats (SHRs) (3,16) and in rat mesenteric small arteries after reduced blood flow (17). In humans, antihypertensive treatment (18), specifically angiotensin-converting enzyme (ACE)-inhibition (19) results in an outward hypertrophic and eutrophic remodeling of resistance vessels [Fig. 6.1(A), vessels f and g]. Finally, outward hypotrophic remodeling [Fig. 6.1(A), vessel e] has been demonstrated with ACE-inhibitor treatment of SHRs (20).

All forms of remodeling denoted in Fig. 6.1 have been demonstrated in human hypertension or in animal models of hypertension. The clinically most relevant forms of resistance vessel remodeling in humans may be eutrophic inward remodeling during essential hypertension and inward hypertrophic remodeling during secondary hypertension.

D. Remodeling of Large Arteries

Remodeling in the resistance vessels of hypertensive individuals differs from that seen in large arteries. Patients with newly diagnosed and untreated hypertension have isobaric internal radial artery diameters similar to those of matched normotensive subjects (9). This probably reflects the different functional requirements of large arteries, their function being primarily to transport blood and their flow-rate being largely unchanged in hypertension (3). Thus, an increase in the wall-to-lumen ratio of a large artery will—with a normal lumen—involve an increase in the amount of material (9) and result in hypertrophic outward remodeling (9).

E. Microcirculation and Angiogenesis

The microcirculation is involved in the genesis and maintenance of hypertension and plays a major role in many of the functional changes that take place (21–23). A primary function of the microcirculation is to optimize nutrient and oxygen supply within the tissue in response to variations in demand. A second important function is to avoid large fluctuations in hydrostatic pressure at the level of the capillaries causing disturbances in capillary exchange. Finally, it is at the level of the microcirculation that a substantial proportion of the drop in hydrostatic pressure occurs.

Therefore, the microcirculation is extremely important in determining the overall peripheral resistance (24,25).

In mature (nongrowing) capillaries, the vessel wall is composed of an endothelial cell lining, a basement membrane, and a layer of cells called pericytes which partially surround the endothelium (26). The pericytes are contained within the same basement membrane as the endothelial cells, occasionally making direct contact with them. The microcirculation is generated by a morphogenic process called angiogenesis, that is, the formation of new microvessels from pre-existing ones (26,27). Angiogenic factors bind to endothelial cell receptors and initiate the sequence of angiogenesis. When endothelial cells are stimulated to grow, they secrete proteases that digest the base membrane surrounding the vessel. The junctions between endothelial cells are altered, cell projections pass through the space created, and the newly formed sprout grows towards the source of the stimulus. Continued capillary sprout growth is dependent upon several processes: the stimulus for growth (angiogenic factors, hypoxia, etc.) must be maintained; the endothelial cells must secrete the proteases required to break down the adjacent tissue; the endothelial cells must be capable of movement or migration; and the endothelial cell division must take place to provide the necessary number of cells (this takes place at a site behind the growth front of the sprout). Neighboring blind-ended sprouts then join together to form a capillary loop that later matures into a vessel similar to the one from which it derived. Increased shear forces in the microcirculation appear to be vasodilatatory and angiogenic. In normal situations, neoformation of capillaries promotes a restoration of normal shear forces.

In hypertension, a reduction in the number of parallel-connected arterioles, a process known as rarefaction (i.e., negative angiogenesis), is a further cause of increased peripheral resistance. Small differences in vessel number, length, diameter, and branching characteristics may be sufficient to shift pressure and flow distribution in particular tissues. In fact, the pressure drops gradually from the level of the small arteries to the capillaries without a specific, single site of resistance control along this segment of the vascular tree (Fig. 6.2). Despite their thin walls, capillaries are relatively nondistensible and their endothelial cell nuclei encroach on the lumen to reduce luminal cross-sectional area by 50%. These deformations are accompanied by a slowing or diversion of the blood stream to other vessels. Capillary endothelial cells in mammals also have been shown to contain actin filaments and heavy meromyosin, which may indicate some form of contractility (21,22).

The capillary network thus can contribute to the resistance control by virtue of their narrow caliber, by the reduction in their number (rarefaction or negative angiogenesis), or possibly by their deformation (21,22).

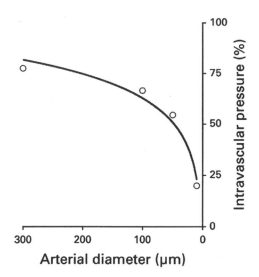

Figure 6.2 Fractional blood pressure at different lumen diameters. The pressure drops gradually from the levels in the small arteries to the levels in the capillaries.

III. MECHANISMS OF REMODELING

Although the morphological characteristics of resistance artery remodeling in hypertension are relatively well defined, the cellular mechanisms remain unclear. A dynamic interaction among humoral factors (e.g., angiotensin II), hemodynamic stimuli, (e.g., increased blood pressure or shear-stress) (i.e., signals) and their transduction within the cell and to adjacent cells (i.e., transducers, may lead to changes in cell growth, cell death or apoptosis, cell migration, and production or degradation of extracellular matrix and differential expression of adhesion molecules (i.e., mediators) (2,10).

Although all vascular cells may participate in the remodeling process, the endothelium is particularly suited to play a prominent part. The endothelial apical surface is constantly exposed to humoral factors and physical forces. The endothelium is strategically located to serve not only as a sensor and transducer of signals but also as an effector that elicits biologic responses through activation and release of substances involved in vascular remodeling (2,10). Furthermore, endothelial morphogenic changes in response to angiogenic stimuli are the basis of angiogenesis and control pericyte attachment and regulation of extracellular matrix components (26,27).

A. Signals in Remodeling

1. Humoral Factors

Endothelial cells can participate directly in vascular remodeling by releasing factors that influence the growth, death, and migration of cellular elements or influence the composition of the extracellular matrix (2). The factors

that regulate the growth of vascular cells involved in remodeling are listed in Table 6.1.

These factors can modulate one another's actions, and they may have multiple functions. For example, platelet-derived growth factor (PDGF) also has vasoactive properties, and transforming growth factor (TGF)-1 may have either growth-stimulating or growth-inhibiting properties, depending on the type of cell involved and the local cellular milieu (28,29). Vasoactive factors that have acute effects on vessel tone also might influence the growth and migration of vascular cells and matrix production. Angiotensin II facilitates vascular smooth-muscle cell growth by inducing the autocrine growth factors, PDGF-AA, basic fibroblast growth factor (bFGF), and TGF-1 (28,30). Hence, vasoactive factors may play an important part in determining vascular structure. In humans with a kallikrein gene polymorphism that lowers kallikrein activity (Bradykinin and lys-Bradykinin), the brachial artery undergoes eutrophic inward remodeling in the absence of hypertension or other hemodynamic changes (31). Alterations of the kallikrein-kinin system are also associated with formation of aortic aneurysms (32). Conversely, after vascular injury, kinins mediate the beneficial effect of angiotensin-converting enzyme inhibitors that prevent neointima formation. Thus, decreased kallikrein-kinin system activity may play an important role in the pathogenesis of vascular remodeling and disease, while increased activity may have

Table 6.1 Factors that Modulate the Growth of Vascular Smooth Muscle Cells

Growth promoters	Growth inhibitors
Acidic and basic fibroblast growth factor	Heparan sulfate
Platelet-derived growth factors AA, AB, and BB	Fibronectin
Transforming growth factors $\beta1$ and $\beta2$	Transforming growth factors $\beta1$ and $\beta2$
Heparin-binding growth factor	Interferon gamma
Epidermal growth factor	
Insulin-like growth factor	
Interleukin-1	
Interleukin-6	
Thrombin	Nitric oxide
Serotonin	Prostaglandins
Angiotensin II	Atrial natriuretic peptide
Endothelin	Type C natriuretic peptide
Norepinephrine	
Vasopressin	
Substance P and K	
Leukotrienes	
Thromboxane	
Stretch or wall tension	Shear stress

Source: Adapted from Gibbons and Dzau (2).

a beneficial effect (32). Despite the apparent complexity of these interactions, an elaborate set of checks and balances results in a co-ordinated local response to various stimuli.

2. Hemodynamic Stimuli

The capacity of the endothelium to sense shear-stress is not only an important determinant of luminal diameter and overall vessel structure, but also of shear-stress regulated of arterial tone, vascular remodeling, and atherogenesis (33). Thus, chronic, experimentally induced, or aging-induced or disease-induced alterations in blood pressure or flow which, respectively, perturb the circumferential wall and fluid shear-stress, may act as stimuli for arterial structural changes that alter vascular geometry in an attempt to reduce or normalize the stress. Therefore, altered endothelial function might be a key factor in the development of vascular changes characteristic of hypertension.

Electrophysiological studies have suggested that shear-stress activates a flow-sensitive potassium channel that induces hyperpolarization and promotes calcium influx, whereas pressure or tension stimulates a stretch-responsive cationic channel (34–37). *In vitro* increases in shear-stress alter the balance of endothelial-cell-derived mediators (Table 6.1) involved in the regulation of vascular tone, hemostasis, vascular-cell growth, and matrix production. Flow-mediated vasorelaxation *in vivo* is largely mediated by shear-stress-induced generation of the vasodilators prostacyclin and nitric oxide and decreased production of the vasoconstrictor endothelin-1 by the endothelium (38–41). Shear-stress activates a genetic program that alters the balance of the mediators of remodeling by activating the transcription of genes for factors such as nitric oxide synthase, PDGF, and TGF-1 (41–43) (Table 6.1). Various endothelial growth factor receptor activities appear to be significantly modulated by shear-stress: recent research suggests that shear-stress rapidly activates vascular endothelial growth factor receptor 2 (VEGFR2) in a ligand-independent manner and leads to endothelial nitric oxide synthase activation in cultured endothelial cells (33). Inhibiting VEGFR2 kinase significantly reduces flow-mediated nitric-oxide-dependent arteriolar dilation *in vivo*. VEGFR2 may act as a key mechano-transducer that activates endothelial nitric oxide synthase in response to blood flow (33,44). Importantly, vascular endothelial growth factor (VEGF) and nitric oxide are also key players in the regulation of angiogenesis. Other tyrosine kinase receptors involved in endothelial restructuring and angiogenesis are also modulated: rapid down-regulation of vascular endothelial receptor tyrosine kinase (*Tie1*) by shear-stress changes, and its rapid binding to angiopoietin-2 receptor tyrosine kinase (*Tie2*) may be required for destabilization of endothelial cells in order to initiate the process of vascular restructuring (44). Genetic

profiling also identified *Tie2* and VEGFR2-up-regulation after exposure of endothelial cell to shear-stress (45).

Investigations on the effects of shear-stress have demonstrated that, besides their contribution to control of cell adhesion and migration, integrins play significant roles in the shear-elicited signaling in endothelial cells and are involved in mechano-transduction. Both integrins and the small GTPase Rho are implicated in endothelial cell responses to shear (46–50). Shear-stress rapidly stimulates conformational activation of integrin $\alpha_v\beta_3$ in bovine aortic endothelial cells, followed by an increase in its binding to extracellular cell-matrix protein. This conformational change induces a transient inhibition of Rho kinase necessary for cytoskeletal alignment in the direction of flow (47). The shear-stress regulation of Rho is linked functionally to endothelial cell migration, mitogen-activated protein kinase signaling, and organization of the actin-based cytoskeleton. Many shear-stress-activated signaling events depend on the actin-based cytoskeleton. However, the detailed molecule interplay among integrins, Rho, and actin in mechano-transduction remains elusive (50).

B. Effectors of Remodeling

1. Apoptosis

Maintenance of media volume may involve a combination of growth and apoptotic processes. Programmed cell death localized to the outer periphery of the vessel may result in a reduction of the outer diameter of the vessel, whereas inward cell growth decreases lumen diameter. In contrast to cell necrosis, apoptosis is a selective process of cell loss that occurs without evoking an inflammatory response. Experimental studies propose reactive oxygen species, nitric oxide, endothelin system and angiotensin type 2 (AT2) receptors as possible apoptosis modulators (51,52). Some of the factors listed in Table 6.1, such as bFGF and interferon γ (IF-γ), may also be involved in regulation of apoptosis.

2. Matrix Modulation

Rearrangement of extracellular matrix components and their corresponding adhesion receptors might shift interactions between smooth muscle cells and extracellular matrix proteins quantitatively, topographically or both, thereby resulting in a rearrangement of smooth muscle cells and a restructured vascular wall. In experimental models of hypertension, expression of adhesion molecules in resistance vessels, specifically integrins, is abnormal. Integrins act as physical attachment points between extracellular matrix and cytoskeletal components and as signal-transducing receptors. Vascular remodeling may involve changes in these anchorage sites. Mesenteric arteries from SHRs exhibit an increase in the expression of $\alpha_v\beta_3$ and $\alpha_5\beta_1$ integrins and the volume density of collagen. In humans with essential hypertension, collagen also has been reported to increase in mesenteric small arteries (53). Such changes, representing an increase in cell-matrix attachment sites and their topographic localization, may modulate arterial structure (54). Augmented deposition of extracellular matrix proteins in the vessel wall seems to be, in part, a humorally determined event. Angiotensin II stimulates human vascular smooth muscle cell production of collagen I, via AT1 and possibly angiotensin type 2 receptors (51,55).

3. Smooth Muscle Cell Phenotype

Expression of extracellular matrix proteins and their cellular receptors is closely related to smooth muscle cell phenotype. Normally, vessel smooth muscle cells express a contractile, differentiated phenotype but upon injury they modulate to a synthetic phenotype. The synthetic smooth muscle cell phenotype is characterized by enhanced expression of extracellular matrix and by high motility and proliferation (56). Growth factor receptors, such as PDGF, and extracellular matrix receptors, such as integrins, can regulate phenotypic modulation of smooth muscle cell from a differentiated to synthetic state. Growth factor and extracellular matrix receptors interact with each other to coordinate activation of signaling cascades (57).

4. Smooth Muscle Cell Hypertrophy

Increased levels of angiotensin II account, in part, for vascular smooth muscle cell hypertrophy: angiotensin II-induced hypertrophy of vascular smooth muscle cells might involve two parallel pathways. Activation of mitogen-activated protein kinase (MAPK) is involved in growth mechanisms and thus may be related to hypertrophic remodeling (58). However, recent reports clearly favor activation of another signaling pathway that involves PI3-kinase-target of rapamycin (mTOR) phosphorylation (59). It was shown that angiotensin II induces phosphorylation of the mTOR downstream target 4E-BP1 through the mTOR pathway but not via MAPK (59). These results are important in the context of smooth muscle cell hypertrophy because mammalian cell size is regulated by mTOR (60). Inhibition of mTOR by rapamycin was also shown to regress established cardiac hypertrophy and improve cardiac function in an experimental mouse model of ascending aortic constriction (61).

C. Mechanisms of Rarefaction

In most forms of clinical and experimental hypertension, reduction in the number or density of microvessels has been reported. Several theories have been proposed to explain microvascular rarefaction in hypertension. Rarefaction may be either primary (i.e., antedates the onset of hypertension) or secondary (i.e., occurring as a consequence of prolonged elevation of blood pressure). Primary rarefaction may be the result of impaired angiogenesis, whereas secondary rarefaction may be associated with impaired recruitment of nonperfused capillaries or destruction of capillaries (25).

It has been suggested that rarefaction may occur in two phases. The first phase—functional rarefaction—involves microvessel constriction to the point of nonperfusion, possibly as a result of increased sensitivity to vasoconstrictor stimuli. Disappearance of the nonperfused vessels by necrosis or apoptosis may lead to the second phase—structural or anatomic rarefaction—which cannot be reversed by maximal vasodilation. In patients with primary hypertension, the reduction in density of capillaries in the skin of the dorsum of the fingers recently has been shown to be primarily a result of anatomic rather than functional rarefaction. It is therefore possible to view microvessel abnormality and rarefaction as responses to increased vascular pressure.

However, microvascular changes similar to those observed in hypertension can be found under conditions where elevation in arterial blood pressure is insignificant (62). An increase in the media-to-lumen ratio in mesenteric small-resistance arteries has been observed in SHRs at a prehypertensive stage (4 weeks of age) (63). Norrelund et al. (64) found that renal afferent arterioles are narrowed at a very young age in SHRs, with no correlation between renal afferent arteriolar diameter and blood pressure. Significant structural rarefaction of the skin capillaries also occurs in the early stages of human essential hypertension, with only mild intermittent elevation of blood pressure. Here, capillary density is inversely related to the cardiac index but not to blood pressure. For example, patients with mild borderline primary hypertension show as much dermal capillary rarefaction as those with established hypertension. Moreover, impaired microvascular vasodilation and capillary rarefaction are associated with a familial predisposition to essential hypertension. Offspring of parents with high blood pressure had fewer capillaries on the dorsum of fingers before the onset of significant hypertension (65). Thus, capillary rarefaction may be a primary or very early structural abnormality rather than a consequence of sustained hypertension (66). Primary rarefaction of capillaries supports theories of reduced angiogenesis and diminished microvascular growth in primary hypertension or inadequate upkeep and development of a vascularized connective tissue in target organs. Impaired angiogenesis in patients who are prone to hypertension may evolve because of a genetic disposition-deficient placental and embryonic vascular development and thus low birth weight and because of impaired

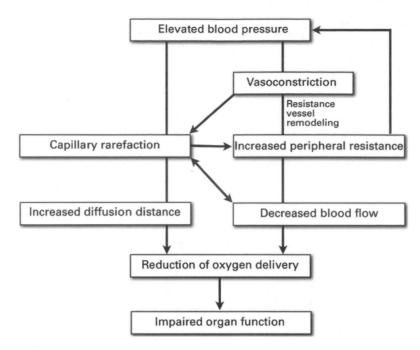

Figure 6.3 Relationship between capillary rarefaction, high blood pressure, and their impact on organ function.

postembryonic vascular growth. The potential genetic mechanisms are still unknown, although recently the SHR genetic abnormality has been localized in a chromosomal domain that also contains growth-related hormones and elements of the renin–angiotensin system. Inadequate formation of new blood vessels, that is, impaired angiogenesis, may thus be associated with hypertension and development of hypertension-dependent target-organ damage (21,22,25,65–67) (Fig. 6.3).

Mechanistically, interactions of angiogenesis and hypertension may involve inter alia, blood pressure itself, nitric oxide, angiogenic molecules, and the renin–angiotensin–aldosterone system. In the Dahl salt-sensitive rat experimental model of hypertension, blood pressure itself did not seem to affect the extent of angiogenesis, whereas decreased nitric oxide biosynthesis reduced angiogenesis. Thus, rather than resulting from elevated blood pressure itself, impaired angiogenesis in hypertension may be the consequence of metabolic changes associated with hypertension such as impaired nitric oxide biosynthesis, activation of the renin–angiotensin–aldosterone system, and other factors (68).

IV. PATHOPHYSIOLOGY

A. Remodeling

Although the pathogenic role of resistance vessels in causing high blood pressure is unclear, hypertension damage of arterioles and small arteries seems to contribute

to complications of hypertension, such as strokes (9) and nephroangiosclerosis (69) and possibly to myocardial ischemia (79).

1. Cardiac Failure

Significant reduction in coronary reserve is found in hypertensive patients with left ventricular hypertrophy. Substantial thickening of the coronary resistance vessels (medial hypertrophy) is considered sufficient to explain the impairment of coronary flow. This small-vessel abnormality correlates well with clinical findings in hypertensive heart disease (angina and electrocardiographic changes despite a normal coronary arteriogram). Structural adaptation of the small vessels may carry the inherent risk of an impaired oxygen supply to the hypertrophied myocardium. Thus, late cardiac failure of the hypertrophied heart in hypertension may be attributed in part to this microcirculation disorder (71,72).

2. Renovascular Hypertension

Structural changes in the preglomerular vasculature, which leads to increased wall thickness and lumen narrowing by hypertrophic inward remodeling (73), may cause hypertension by mimicking the hemodynamic effects of main renal artery stenosis. There is evidence compatible with this hypothesis in SHRs, and preliminary evidence indicates that experimentally increased intrarenal Ang II levels can cause structural changes in the walls of the preglomerular resistance vessels and hypertension. In human hypertension, the hypothesis remains conjectural because the necessary measurements of renal vessel structure (resistance vessel wall dimensions, lumen dimensions) are not possible; however, renal hemodynamic changes in early and borderline human hypertension are compatible with early structural changes (74).

B. Capillary Rarefaction

In addition to its contribution to increased peripheral vascular resistance, capillary rarefaction also contributes to complications that are associated with hypertension.

1. Target-Organ Blood Flow

Capillary rarefaction may display pathological complications similar to that after narrowing of small arteries and arterioles by inward remodeling. Indeed, rarefaction of intramyocardial vessels is one of the most relevant structural alterations in hypertension-induced left ventricular dysfunction, hypertrophy, and ischemia (21,65). Vessel rarefaction significantly influences tissue blood flow resistance to a degree comparable with vessel constriction; however, unlike constriction, microvascular rarefaction markedly alters blood flow distribution (5) (Fig. 6.3).

2. Renal Failure/Uremia

Cardiac capillary length density in patients with renal failure was noted to be reduced when compared with patients with essential hypertension and normotensive control patients. This finding implies that in left ventricular hypertrophy of uremic patients, capillary growth does not keep pace with cardiomyocyte growth, apparently because of some selective inhibition, or lack of stimulation, of capillary angiogenesis.

3. Pre-Eclampsia Syndrome

A low capillary density may account in part for the failure of blood pressure to fall in pre-eclamptic pregnancies and may reflect the maladaptive cardiovascular response that is part of the pre-eclampsia syndrome.

4. Insulin Resistance/Hyperinsulinemia

Metabolic abnormalities can influence capillary density. Capillary rarefaction is observed in patient with insulin resistance. In contrast, physiological hyperinsulinemia induces, in parallel with the increase in total leg blood flow, an increase in total skin microcirculatory blood flow and augments nitric-oxide-mediated vasodilatation in skin microcirculation.

5. Rheological Profile

Subjects with skin capillary density below the group median are younger, have higher diastolic pressure, higher blood viscosity at low shear, higher P-selection levels, higher erythrocyte and leukocyte filterability rates, and higher erythrocyte aggregation indexes. In contrast, patients with greater skin capillary density have a greater plasma viscosity. Thus, in untreated hypertensive men, capillary rarefaction and hyperviscosity are associated with an increased diastolic blood pressure and an adverse hemorheological profile (75).

C. Hypertension Treatment

1. Antihypertension Treatment and Reversal of Resistance Vessels Remodeling

Possible regression and reversal of structural and mechanical changes of resistance vessels under antihypertension treatment and ongoing normalization of the structure and function may improve clinical outcomes of hypertensive patients. Some classes of antihypertensive drugs can lead to normalization of resistance vessels structure in hypertensive patients. Normalization of the abnormalities in the structure of resistance vessels is obtained by facilitation of remodeling, that is, a rearrangement of the wall material around a larger lumen (76), rather than by inhibition of growth. The reversal of these changes concern all vascular beds and may also occur in coronary microcirculation (77,78).

However, different classes of antihypertensive drugs have differential effects on vessel structure normalization: beta-blocker treatment by atenolol did not cause normalization of resistance vessels structure and function, even when administered for up to 2 years (77). Isradipine, a potent calcium channel antagonist, showed no effect on structure normalization (79). Losartan, an AT1 receptor antagonist, improves structural abnormalities and normalize the endothelial function of small arteries in hypertensive patients (80). There is conflicting data in the literature regarding the effect of diuretic treatment on normalization of resistance vessels structure (10). Differential effects of various antihypertension therapies are possibly related to the different pharmacological action of these drugs.

Reduction in blood pressure without normalization of resistance vessels structure would reduce the vascular reserve and consequently aggravate the decreased coronary vascular reserve (10,76). Altered resistance vessels structure is a major characteristic of hypertensive disease and may be one of the fundamental causes of the observed reduced vascular reserve. Therefore, normalization of the structural, functional, and mechanical properties of resistance vessels should be considered an important goal of antihypertension therapy (10,76).

Further investigation is required to determine whether reversal of resistance vessel remodeling with antihypertension treatment also will improve clinical outcomes of essential hypertension, reducing morbidity (cardiac events, strokes, progression of hypertensive nephropathy), and mortality.

2. Treatment of Hypertension and Improvement of Angiogenesis

Setting the goal to reverse microvascular rarefaction by antihypertension therapy is based on the relationship of target-organ damage in hypertension to the microcirculation (68). Amongst the widely used classes of antihypertensive agents, ACE inhibitors and potentially AT1 receptor blockers are the most promising in reversion of microvascular rarefaction.

ACE inhibition leads to accumulation of bradykinin which has a strong angiogenic potential mediated via both its receptors. Accumulation of bradykinin leads to endothelium-dependent vasodilation and lowering of blood pressure (81). The beneficial effect of ACE inhibition on the microvasculature is probably due to angiogenesis via bradykinin and other molecules such as FGF, VEGF, endothelial nitric oxide synthase, and PKC (82,83). More clinically oriented *in vivo* models show that the ACE inhibitor perindopril increases vessel density and capillary number in ischemic hind limbs of mice (84). The BK2 receptor, together with an increase in endothelial nitric oxide synthase protein level, mediates this increase of vessel density (84,85). Spirapril, another ACE inhibitor, substantially increases myocardial capillary microvascular density in SHRs (86,87). Spirapril also improves left ventricular function by reducing its thickness and hypertrophic weight (86,87). It is not known whether improved function of the left ventricle is also due to enhanced angiogenesis. Another ACE inhibitor, quinaprilat, promotes angiogenesis in a rabbit model of hind limb ischemia *in vivo* (86).

Other classical antihypertensive agents, such as calcium antagonists, alpha- and beta-blockers, and diuretics, have not yet been extensively studied in the context of angiogenesis. AT1 receptor blockers and calcium antagonists may reduce microvascular rarefaction, that is, possibly improve angiogenesis (22). Initial studies have examined the effects of combination of different antihypertensive agents on angiogenesis. Promising results were obtained by combination of ACE inhibitors with diuretics (22). Thus, combination antihypertension therapies may be a promising modality to improve target-organ damage that is a result of hypertension and microvascular rarefaction.

V. PITFALLS AND DANGERS

A. Criteria for Resistance Vessels

A large amount of *in vivo* and *in vitro* research has been conducted on small 100–300 μm arteries in order to understand their function in the distribution of blood. However, although vessels of this size are frequently referred to as resistance arteries, the evidence for this is limited. There is evidence from conscious rats that 100–300 μm mesenteric arteries fulfill the criteria for resistance arteries. Less evidence is available for vessels from other vascular beds or in other species, particularly in humans. Most data were obtained under conditions of anesthesia and may not be representative of the physiological situation when a patient is conscious. Another crucial point is that experiments in larger animals, including humans, are rare. Thus, an unambiguous picture of the location of resistance arteries has yet to emerge (88,6).

B. Angiogenic Therapy

In adults, induction of angiogenesis may be beneficial in decreasing capillary resistance and increasing blood supply to insufficiently oxygenized organs in myocardial and peripheral ischemic disease. However, the "angiogenic" switch in tumors is a hallmark of the development of a fast-growing and metastasizing phenotype (89,90). Research in clinical trials now strongly focuses on anti-angiogenic therapy to treat tumor angiogenesis and cancer (91). Induction of angiogenesis as a therapy to reverse microvascular rarefaction in hypertension could awake dormant, nonvascularized tumors. Furthermore, potent angiogenic molecules, such as VEGF, also can cause a hemorrhage as a result of an increase in vascular permeability or the inappropriate formation of new microvessels. Therefore, a proangiogenic approach to increase capillary density by potent angiogenic molecules currently is not recommended. Rather, combination therapies using locally acting antihypertension drugs with proangiogenic properties are safer.

VI. CONCLUSIONS

In hypertension, vascular remodeling contributes to increased peripheral resistance, which affects both development and complications of hypertension. Although smooth muscle cell growth is the mechanism classically associated with vascular remodeling, it has increasingly been appreciated that apoptosis, low-grade inflammation, and vascular fibrosis are dynamic processes that also influence the degree of remodeling. Inward growth may be associated with peripheral apoptosis, contributing to eutrophic remodeling. Low-grade inflammation, perhaps angiotensin-dependent or endothelin-dependent and triggered in part by increased oxidative stress in the vascular wall, may elicit growth-factor-mediated, extracellular matrix remodeling. Changes in the anchorage of cells to extracellular fibrillar components may alter cell attachment, modifying vessel wall architecture. They also may promote abnormal intracellular transduction of extracellular input to the cytoskeleton of smooth muscle cells, contributing to smooth muscle cell restructuring. Chronic vasoconstriction may result in an inwardly remodeled blood vessel, as the contracted vessel structure becomes embedded in a remodeled extracellular matrix, further promoting rearrangement of smooth muscle cells around a smaller lumen. Growth, apoptosis, inflammation, and fibrosis of blood vessels thus may all contribute to vascular remodeling. Arterial remodeling may be adaptive initially but eventually become maladaptive and compromise organ function, contributing to cardiovascular complications of hypertension.

There is little doubt about the existence of abnormal angiogenesis in cardiovascular disease, and increasing evidence points towards some role in the pathogenesis of hypertension. Many of the currently available antihypertensive agents also may exert proangiogenic effects that have therapeutic potential for improvement of microvascular rarefaction and the corresponding target-organ damage and function.

REFERENCES

1. Scheirer J. Angiogenesis and vascular remodeling in the microvasculature. NIH guide 1995; 24.
2. Gibbons GH, Dzau VJ. The emerging concept of vascular remodeling. N Engl J Med 1994; 330:1431–1438.
3. Mulvany MJ. Vascular remodelling of resistance vessels: can we define this? Cardiovasc Res 1999; 41:9–13.
4. Owens GK. Control of hypertrophic versus hyperplastic growth of vascular smooth muscle cells. Am J Physiol 1989; 257:H1755–H1765.
5. Greene AS, Tonellato PJ, Lui J, Lombard JH, Cowley AW, Jr. Microvascular rarefaction and tissue vascular resistance in hypertension. Am J Physiol 1989; 256:H126–H131.
6. Mulvany M. Resistance vessels in hypertension. Textbook of Hypertension. Oxford: Blackwell Science 1994.
7. Baumbach GL, Heistad DD. Remodeling of cerebral arterioles in chronic hypertension. Hypertension 1989; 13:968–972.
8. Mulvany MJ, Baumbach GL, Aalkjaer C et al. Vascular remodeling. Hypertension 1996; 28:505–506.
9. Schiffrin EL, Hayoz D. How to assess vascular remodelling in small and medium-sized muscular arteries in humans. J Hypertens 1997; 15:571–584.
10. Zervoudaki A, Toutouzas P. Remodeling of resistance vessels in essential hypertension. Hellenic J Cardiol 2003; 44:116–124.
11. Nordborg C, Ivarsson H, Johansson BB, Stage L. Morphometric study of mesenteric and renal arteries in spontaneously hypertensive rats. J Hypertens 1983; 1:333–338.
12. Short D. The vascular fault in chronic hypertension with particular reference to the role of medial hypertrophy. Lancet 1966; 1:1302–1304.
13. Korsgaard N, Aalkjaer C, Heagerty AM, Izzard AS, Mulvany MJ. Histology of subcutaneous small arteries from patients with essential hypertension. Hypertension 1993; 22:523–526.
14. Rosei EA, Rizzoni D, Castellano M et al. Media/lumen ratio in human small resistance arteries is related to forearm minimal vascular resistance. J Hypertens 1995; 13:341–347.
15. Rizzoni D, Porteri E, Castellano M et al. Vascular hypertrophy and remodeling in secondary hypertension. Hypertension 1996; 28:785–790.
16. Skov K, Mulvany MJ, Korsgaard N. Morphology of renal afferent arterioles in spontaneously hypertensive rats. Hypertension 1992; 20:821–827.
17. Pourageaud F, De Mey JG. Structural properties of rat mesenteric small arteries after 4-wk exposure to elevated or reduced blood flow. Am J Physiol 1997; 273:H1699–H1706.
18. Thybo NK, Stephens N, Cooper A, Aalkjaer C, Heagerty AM, Mulvany MJ. Effect of antihypertensive treatment on small arteries of patients with previously untreated essential hypertension. Hypertension 1995; 25:474–481.
19. Skov K, Fenger-Gron J, Mulvany MJ. Effects of an angiotensin-converting enzyme inhibitor, a calcium antagonist, and an endothelin receptor antagonist on renal afferent arteriolar structure. Hypertension 1996; 28:464–471.
20. Thybo NK, Korsgaard N, Eriksen S, Christensen KL, Mulvany MJ. Dose-dependent effects of perindopril on blood pressure and small-artery structure. Hypertension 1994; 23:659–666.
21. le Noble FA, Stassen FR, Hacking WJ, Struijker Boudier HA. Angiogenesis and hypertension. J Hypertens 1998; 16:1563–1572.
22. Kiefer FN, Neysari S, Humar R, Li W, Munk VC, Battegay EJ. Hypertension and angiogenesis. Curr Pharm Des 2003; 9:1733–1744.
23. Tomanek RJ, Schalk KA, Marcus ML, Harrison DG. Coronary angiogenesis during long-term hypertension and left ventricular hypertrophy in dogs. Circ Res 1989; 65:352–359.
24. Vicaut E. Hypertension and the microcirculation: a brief overvierw of experimental studies. J Hypertens 1992; 10:S59–S68.
25. Levy BI, Ambrosio G, Pries AR, Struijker-Boudier HA. Microcirculation in hypertension: a new target for treatment? Circulation 2001; 104:735–740.
26. Risau W. Mechanisms of angiogenesis. Nature 1997; 386:671–674.
27. Flamme I, Frolich T, Risau W. Molecular mechanisms of vasculogenesis and embryonic angiogenesis. J Cell Physiol 1997; 173:206–210.

28. Gibbons GH, Pratt RE, Dzau VJ. Vascular smooth muscle cell hypertrophy vs. hyperplasia. Autocrine transforming growth factor-beta 1 expression determines growth response to angiotensin II. J Clin Invest 1992; 90:456–461.

29. Battegay EJ, Raines EW, Seifert RA, Bowen-Pope DF, Ross R. TGF-beta induces bimodal proliferation of connective tissue cells via complex control of an autocrine PDGF loop. Cell 1990; 63:515–524.

30. Itoh H, Mukoyama M, Pratt RE, Gibbons GH, Dzau VJ. Multiple autocrine growth factors modulate vascular smooth muscle cell growth response to angiotensin II. J Clin Invest 1993; 91:2268–2274.

31. Azizi M, Boutouyrie P, Bissery A, Agharazii M, Verbeke F, Stern N, Bura-Riviere A, Laurent S, Alhenc-Gelas F, Jeunemaitre X. Arterial and renal consequences of partial genetic deficiency in tissue kallikrein activity in humans. J Clin Invest 2005; 115(3):780–787.

32. Carretero OA. Vascular remodeling and the kallikrein-kinin system. J Clin Invest 2005; 115(3):588-591.

33. Jin ZG, Ueba H, Tanimoto T, Lungu AO, Frame MD, Berk BC. Ligand-independent activation of vascular endothelial growth factor receptor 2 by fluid shear stress regulates activation of endothelial nitric oxide synthase. Circ Res 2003; 93:354–363.

34. Davies PF, Tripathi SC. Mechanical stress mechanisms and the cell. An endothelial paradigm. Circ Res 1993; 72:239–245.

35. Olesen SP, Clapham DE, Davies PF. Haemodynamic shear stress activates a K+ current in vascular endothelial cells. Nature 1988; 331:168–170.

36. Nakache M, Gaub HE. Hydrodynamic hyperpolarization of endothelial cells. Proc Natl Acad Sci USA 1988; 85:1841–1843.

37. Shen J, Luscinskas FW, Connolly A, Dewey CF Jr, Gimbrone MA Jr. Fluid shear stress modulates cytosolic free calcium in vascular endothelial cells. Am J Physiol 1992; 262:C384–C390.

38. Cooke JP, Rossitch E Jr, Andon NA, Loscalzo J, Dzau VJ. Flow activates an endothelial potassium channel to release an endogenous nitrovasodilator. J Clin Invest 1991; 88:1663–1671.

39. Frangos JA, Eskin SG, McIntire LV, Ives CL. Flow effects on prostacyclin production by cultured human endothelial cells. Science 1985; 227:1477–1479.

40. Kuchan MJ, Frangos JA. Shear stress regulates endothelin-1 release via protein kinase C and cGMP in cultured endothelial cells. Am J Physiol 1993; 264:H150–H156.

41. Nishida K, Harrison DG, Navas JP et al. Molecular cloning and characterization of the constitutive bovine aortic endothelial cell nitric oxide synthase. J Clin Invest 1992; 90:2092–2096.

42. Resnick N, Collins T, Atkinson W, Bonthron DT, Dewey CF Jr, Gimbrone MA Jr. Platelet-derived growth factor B chain promoter contains a cis-acting fluid shear-stress-responsive element. Proc Natl Acad Sci USA 1993; 90:4591–4595.

43. Ohno M, Cooke JP, Dzau VJ, Gibbons GH. Fluid shear stress induces endothelial transforming growth factor beta-1 transcription and production. Modulation by potassium channel blockade. J Clin Invest 1995; 95:1363–1369.

44. Chen-Konak L, Guetta-Shubin Y, Yahav H et al. Transcriptional and post-translation regulation of the Tie1 receptor by fluid shear stress changes in vascular endothelial cells. FASEB J 2003; 17:2121–2123.

45. Chen BP, Li YS, Zhao Y et al. DNA microarray analysis of gene expression in endothelial cells in response to 24-h shear stress. Physiol Genomics 2001; 7:55–63.

46. Loirand G, Rolli-Derkinderen M, Pacaud P. RhoA and resistance artery remodeling. Am J Physiol Heart Circ Physiol 2005; 288(3):H1051–H1056.

47. Tzima E, del Pozo MA, Shattil SJ, Chien S, Schwartz MA. Activation of integrins in endothelial cells by fluid shear stress mediates Rho-dependent cytoskeletal alignment. EMBO J 2001; 20:4639–4647.

48. Li S, Chen BP, Azuma N et al. Distinct roles for the small GTPases Cdc42 and Rho in endothelial responses to shear stress. J Clin Invest 1999; 103:1141–1150.

49. Wojciak-Stothard B, Ridley AJ. Shear stress-induced endothelial cell polarization is mediated by Rho and Rac but not Cdc42 or PI 3-kinases. J Cell Biol 2003; 161:429–439.

50. Shyy JY, Chien S. Role of integrins in endothelial mechanosensing of shear stress. Circ Res 2002; 91:769–775.

51. Intengan HD, Schiffrin EL. Vascular remodeling in hypertension: roles of apoptosis, inflammation, and fibrosis. Hypertension 2001; 38:581–587.

52. Ueno H, Kanellakis P, Agrotis A, Bobik A. Blood flow regulates the development of vascular hypertrophy, smooth muscle cell proliferation, and endothelial cell nitric oxide synthase in hypertension. Hypertension 2000; 36:89–96.

53. Intengan HD, Deng LY, Li JS, Schiffrin EL. Mechanics and composition of human subcutaneous resistance arteries in essential hypertension. Hypertension 1999; 33:569–574.

54. Intengan HD, Thibault G, Li JS, Schiffrin EL. Resistance artery mechanics, structure, and extracellular components in spontaneously hypertensive rats: effects of angiotensin receptor antagonism and converting enzyme inhibition. Circulation 1999; 100:2267–2275.

55. Hu WY, Fukuda N, Ikeda Y et al. Human-derived vascular smooth muscle cells produce angiotensin II by changing to the synthetic phenotype. J Cell Physiol 2003; 196:284–292.

56. Thyberg J. Phenotypic modulation of smooth muscle cells during formation of neointimal thickenings following vascular injury. Histol Histopathol 1998; 13:871–891.

57. Turley EA. Extracellular matrix remodeling: multiple paradigms in vascular disease. Circ Res 2001; 88:2–4.

58. Eguchi S, Dempsey PJ, Frank GD, Motley ED, Inagami T. Activation of MAPKs by angiotensin II in vascular smooth muscle cells. Metalloprotease-dependent EGF receptor activation is required for activation of ERK and p38 MAPK but not for JNK. J Biol Chem 2001; 276:7957–7962.

59. Yamakawa T, Tanaka S, Kamei J, Kadonosono K, Okuda K. Phosphatidylinositol 3-kinase in angiotensin II-induced hypertrophy of vascular smooth muscle cells. Eur J Pharmacol 2003; 478:39–46.

60. Fingar DC, Salama S, Tsou C, Harlow E, Blenis J. Mammalian cell size is controlled by mTOR and its downstream targets S6K1 and 4EBP1/eIF4E. Genes Dev 2002; 16:1472–1487.

61. McMullen JR, Sherwood MC, Tarnavski O, Zhang L, Dorfman AL, Shioi T, Izumo S. Inhibition of mTOR signaling with rapamycin regresses established cardiac hypertrophy induced by pressure overload. Circulation 2004.

62. Le Noble JLML, Tangelder GJ, Slaaf DW, van Essen H, Reneman RS, Struyker-Boudier HA. A functional morphometric study of the cremaster muscle microcirculation in young spontaneously hypertensive rats. J Hypertens 1990; 8:741–748.

63. Rizzoni D, Castellano M, Porteri E, Bettoni G, Muiesan ML, Agabiti-Rosei E. Vascular structural and functional alterations before and after the development of hypertension in SHR. Am J Hypertens 1994; 7:193–200.

64. Norrelund H, Christensen KL, Samani NJ, Kimber P, Mulvany MJ, Korsgaard N. Early narrowed afferent arteriole is a contributor to the development of hypertension. Hypertension 1994; 24:301–308.

65. Noon JP, Walker BR, Webb DJ et al. Impaired microvascular dilatation and capillary rarefaction in young adults with a predisposition to high blood pressure. J Clin Invest 1997; 99:1873–1879.

66. Antonios TF, Rattray FM, Singer DR, Markandu ND, Mortimer PS, MacGregor GA. Rarefaction of skin capillaries in normotensive offspring of individuals with essential hypertension. Heart 2003; 89:175–178.

67. Kiefer FN, Misteli H, Kalak N et al. Inhibition of nitric oxide biosynthesis, but not elevated blood pressure, reduces angiogenesis in rat models of secondary hypertension. Blood Press 2002; 11:116–124.

68. Levy BI, Duriez M, Samuel JL. Coronary microvasculature alteration in hypertensive rats. Effect of treatment with a diuretic and an ACE inhibitor. Am J Hypertens 2001; 14:7–13.

69. Ruilope LM, Alcazar JM, Rodicio JL. Renal consequences of arterial hypertension. J Hypertens Suppl 1992; 10:S85–S90.

70. Strauer BE. Significance of coronary circulation in hypertensive heart disease for development and prevention of heart failure. Am J Cardiol 1990; 65:34G–41G.

71. Motz W, Vogt M, Strauer BE. Coronary microcirculation in hypertensive heart disease: functional significance and therapeutic implications. Clin Invest 1993; 71:S42–S45.

72. Strauer BE. Left ventricular hypertrophy, myocardial blood flow and coronary flow reserve. Cardiology 1992; 81:274–282.

73. Rizzoni D, Porteri E, Guefi D et al. Cellular hypertrophy in subcutaneous small arteries of patients with renovascular hypertension. Hypertension 2000; 35:931–935.

74. Anderson WP, Kett MM, Stevenson KM, Edgley AJ, Denton KM, Fitzgerald SM. Renovascular hypertension: structural changes in the renal vasculature. Hypertension 2000; 36:648–652.

75. Ciuffetti G, Pasqualini L, Pirro M et al. Blood rheology in men with essential hypertension and capillary rarefaction. J Hum Hypertens 2002; 16:533–537.

76. Schiffrin EL. Remodeling of resistance arteries in essential hypertension and effects of antihypertensive treatment. Am J Hypertens 2004; 17(12 Pt 1):1192–1200.

77. Schiffrin EL. Vascular protection with newer antihypertensive agents. J Hypertens Suppl 1998; 16:S25–S29.

78. Schwartzkopff B, Brehm M, Mundhenke M, Strauer BE. Repair of coronary arterioles after treatment with perindopril in hypertensive heart disease. Hypertension 2000; 36:220–225.

79. Thurmann PA, Stephens N, Heagerty AM, Kenedi P, Weidinger G, Rietbrock N. Influence of isradipine and spirapril on left ventricular hypertrophy and resistance arteries. Hypertension 1996; 28:450–456.

80. Schiffrin EL, Park JB, Intengan HD, Touyz RM. Correction of arterial structure and endothelial dysfunction in human essential hypertension by the angiotensin receptor antagonist losartan. Circulation 2000; 101:1653–1659.

81. Busse R, Fleming I, Hecker M. Signal transduction in endothelium-dependent vasodilatation. Eur Heart J 1993; 14(suppl I):2–9.

82. Hayashi I, Amano H, Yoshida S et al. Suppressed angiogenesis in kininogen-deficiencies. Lab Invest 2002; 82:871–880.

83. Miura S, Matsuo Y, Saku K. Transactivation of KDR/Flk-1 by the B2 receptor induces tube formation in human coronary endothelial cells. Hypertension 2003; 41:1118–1123.

84. Silvestre JS, Bergaya S, Tamarat R, Duriez M, Boulanger CM, Levy BI. Proangiogenic effect of angiotensin-converting enzyme inhibition is mediated by the bradykinin B(2) receptor pathway. Circ Res 2001; 89:678–683.

85. Thuringer D, Maulon L, Frelin C. Rapid transactivation of the vascular endothelial growth factor receptor KDR/Flk-1 by the bradykinin B2 receptor contributes to endothelial nitric-oxide synthase activation in cardiac capillary endothelial cells. J Biol Chem 2002; 277:2028–2032.

86. Fabre JE, Rivard A, Magner M, Silver M, Isner JM. Tissue inhibition of angiotensin-converting enzyme activity stimulates angiogenesis in vivo. Circulation 1999; 99:3043–3049.

87. Olivetti G, Cigola E, Lagrasta C et al. Spirapril prevents left ventricular hypertrophy, decreases myocardial damage and promotes angiogenesis in spontaneously hypertensive rats. J Cardiovasc Pharmacol 1993; 21:362–370.

88. Mulvany MJ, Aalkjaer C. Structure and function of small arteries. Physiol Rev 1990; 70:921–961.

89. Folkman J, Hanahan D. Switch to the angiogenic phenotype during tumorigenesis. Princess Takamatsu Symp 1991; 22:339–347.

90. Bergers G, Benjamin LE. Tumorigenesis and the angiogenic switch. Nat Rev Cancer 2003; 3:401–410.

91. Sato Y. Molecular diagnosis of tumor angiogenesis and anti-angiogenic cancer therapy. Int J Clin Oncol 2003; 8:200–206.

7

Vascular Function in Hypertension: Role of Endothelium-Derived Factors

LUKAS E. SPIEKER, THOMAS F. LÜSCHER
University Hospital, Zürich, Switzerland

KEYPOINTS

- The vascular endothelium actively synthesizes and releases vasoactive substances such as nitric oxide.
- Nitric oxide, released from endothelial cells in response to shear stress and to activation of a variety of receptors, exerts vasodilating and antiproliferative effects on smooth muscle cells, inhibits thrombocyte-aggregation and leukocyte-adhesion.
- Endothelin-1 (ET-1) exerts its major vascular effects—vasoconstriction and cell proliferation—through activation of specific ETA receptors on vascular smooth muscle cells. ET-1 acts as a natural counterpart to nitric oxide.
- Endothelial dysfunction in experimental hypertension depends on the model studied. In spontaneous hypertension, nitric oxide synthase is upregulated and nitric oxide is inactivated by superoxide anions. In salt-related hypertension, nitric oxide production is reduced and the endothelin system is upregulated.
- The superoxide anion, generated by angiotensin II-activated NAD(P)H oxidase, by dysfunctional nitric oxide synthase, or by cyclooxygenase, can scavenge the vasodilator nitric oxide to form the highly peroxynitrite which can damage cell membranes and oxidize lipids.
- Atherogenic risk factors in addition to hypertension such as increased cholesterol or diabetes impair endothelial function.

SUMMARY

The vascular endothelium synthesizes and releases a spectrum of vasoactive substances and, therefore, plays a fundamental role in the basal and dynamic regulation of the circulation. Nitric oxide—originally described as endothelium-derived relaxing factor—is released from endothelial cells in response to shear stress produced by blood flow and in response to activation of a variety of receptors. After diffusion from endothelial to vascular smooth muscle cells, nitric oxide increases intracellular cyclic guanosine monophosphate concentrations by activating the enzyme guanylate cyclase, which leads to a relaxation of the smooth muscle cells.

Nitric oxide also has antithrombogenic, antiproliferative, leukocyte-adhesion inhibiting effects, and it influences myocardial contractility. Endothelium-derived nitric oxide-mediated vascular relaxation is impaired in spontaneously hypertensive animals. Nitric oxide decomposition by free oxygen radicals is a major mechanism of impaired nitric oxide bioavailability. The resulting imbalance of endothelium-derived relaxing and contracting substances disturbs the normal function of the vascular endothelium. Endothelin acts as the natural counterpart to endothelium-derived nitric oxide. In addition to its arterial blood pressure-elevation effect in humans, endothelin-1 induces vascular and myocardial hypertrophies, which are independent risk factors for cardiovascular morbidity and mortality. Indeed, in patients with essential hypertension, carotid wall thickening and left ventricular mass correlate with reduced endothelium-dependent vasodilation.

In hypertensive animals, most classes of antihypertensive drugs [e.g., calcium channel blockers, angiotensin-converting enzyme (ACE) inhibitors, AT_1 receptor antagonists] improve endothelium-dependent vasodilation. Surprisingly, in patients with arterial hypertension, antihypertensive therapy does not consistently restore impaired endothelium-dependent vasodilation. However, depending on the antihypertensive drug used and its pharmacological profile, the delicate balance of endothelium-derived factors, which is disturbed in hypertension, can be restored by specific antihypertensive and antioxidant treatment.

I. INTRODUCTION

The endothelium—probably the largest and most extensive tissue in the body—forms a highly selective permeability barrier and is a continuous, uninterrupted, smooth, and nonthrombogenic surface. The endothelium synthesizes and releases a broad spectrum of vasoactive substances. Functional impairment of the vascular endothelium in response to injury occurs long before the development of visible atherosclerotic changes of the artery. Because of its strategic anatomical position, the endothelium is constantly exposed to the different physiopathological conditions that lead to atherosclerosis.

The evolving concept of endothelial dysfunction in arterial hypertension has its roots more than a decade ago. The discovery of an endothelium-derived relaxing substance—later identified as nitric oxide—and later of its natural antagonist, endothelin, led to a paradigm shift away from the endothelium as just a mechanical barrier to a role as an active regulator of cardiovascular homeostasis. The concept of an imbalance of vasodilator and vasoconstrictor substances in arterial hypertension evolved. Experimental studies characterized the role of endothelial mediators in different models of arterial hypertension. In humans, many investigators demonstrated that the altered balance of endothelium-derived vasoactive factors can be restored by specific pharmacological treatment.

II. PHYSIOLOGY OF ENDOTHELIUM-DERIVED NITRIC OXIDE

Nitric oxide—originally described as endothelium-derived relaxing factor—is released from endothelial cells in response to the shear stress produced by blood flow and in response to the activation of a variety of receptors (Fig. 7.1) (1). Nitric oxide is synthesized by nitric oxide synthase from L-arginine in the presence of the cofactors oxygen, tetrahydrobiopterin, and reduced nicotinamide adenine dinucleotide phosphate (NADPH) (2). L-Citrulline is a by-product. The conversion from L-arginine to nitric oxide can be inhibited by false substrates for the nitric oxide synthase (e.g., by NG-monomethyl-arginine). Nitric oxide is a free radical gas with an *in vivo* half-life of a few seconds, and it is readily able to cross biological membranes. After diffusion from endothelial to vascular smooth muscle cells, nitric oxide increases intracellular cyclic guanosine monophosphate concentrations, which leads to a relaxation of the smooth muscle cells (Fig. 7.1).

A. Role of Nitric Oxide in Circulation

As there is a continuous basal release of nitric oxide that determines the tone of peripheral blood vessels, systemic inhibition of nitric oxide synthesis causes an increase in arterial blood pressure. There are two types of nitric oxide synthases:

1. A constitutive isoform, which is present in endothelial cells and is therefore called endothelial nitric oxide synthase.

2. An inducible isoform, which is an important inflammatory mediator that is released by macrophages in response to immunological stimuli.

Nitric oxide also has antithrombogenic, antiproliferative, leukocyte-adhesion inhibiting effects, and it influences myocardial contractility. The hemodynamic effects of pharmacologic nitric oxide inhibition include an increase in systemic and pulmonary arterial blood pressure and a decrease in cardiac output (Table 7.1).

B. Endothelial Cell Membranes and Signal Transduction

Ionic channels in vascular endothelium play significant roles in controlling resting potential and in signal transduction to smooth muscle cells. Therefore, they are major determinants for blood flow. Channel activity is influenced by vasoactive factors and mechanical forces that are related to blood flow, as well as being influenced by metabolic conditions.

The resting potential of endothelial cells in intact arteries is between −40 and −60 mV. Lower potentials are found in intact veins and cultured endothelial cells. Endothelial cells do not generate action potentials and, thus, are classified as nonexcitable cells.

Gap and tight junctions maintain the electrical coupling of endothelial cells. These junctions also mediate

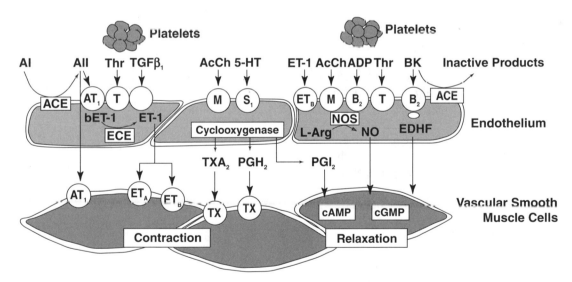

Figure 7.1 Endothelium-derived vasoactive substances. Nitric oxide is released from endothelial cells in response to shear stress and to activation of a variety of receptors. Nitric oxide exerts vasodilating and antiproliferative effects on smooth muscle cells and inhibits thrombocyte-aggregation and leukocyte-adhesion. ET-1 exerts its major vascular effects—vasoconstriction and cell proliferation—through activation of specific ET_A receptors on vascular smooth muscle cells. In contrast, endothelial ET_B receptors mediate vasodilation via release of nitric oxide and prostacyclin. In addition, ET_B receptors in the lung were shown to be a major pathway for the clearance of ET-1 from plasma. ACE, angiotensin-converting enzyme; Ach, acetylcholine; ADP, adenosine diphosphate; AII, angiotensin II; AT_1, angiotensin-1 receptor; BK, bradykinin; B_2, bradykinin receptor; COX, cyclooxygenase; ECE, endothelin-converting enzyme; EDHF, endothelium-derived hyperpolarizing factor; ET_A and ET_B, endothelin A and endothelin B receptors; ET-1, endothelin-1; L-Arg, L-arginine; M, muscarinergic receptor; PGH_2, prostaglandin H_2; PGI_2, prostacyclin; S, serotoninergic receptor; Thr, thrombine; T, thromboxane receptor; TXA_2, thromboxane; 5-HT, 5-hydroxytryptamine (serotonine). [Adapted from Lüscher and Noll (44).]

Table 7.1 Hemodynamic Effects of Nitric Oxide Synthase Inhibition in Healthy Volunteers

X	Baseline	L-NMMA (mg/kg per min)	
		0.3	1.0
SBP	134 ± 7	152 ± 5	150 ± 3[a]
DBP	73 ± 4	87 ± 5	85 ± 5[b]
SVR	1114 ± 124	1413 ± 145[a]	1973 ± 203[c]
HR	67 ± 4	70 ± 6	63 ± 6
CI	3.5 ± 0.3	3.1 ± 0.2[a]	2.3 ± 0.2[d]
SVI	53 ± 6	48 ± 6	38 ± 5 [b].
CVP	4 ± 0.7	3.6 ± 0.4	4.3 ± 0.05
B/min	23.1 ± 3.5	14 ± 4.5	18.6 ± 5.5

[a] $p < 0.05$ for each data point compared with baseline values.
[b] $p < 0.01$ for each data point compared with baseline values.
[c] $p < 0.001$ for each data point compared with baseline values.
[d] $p < 0.0001$, for each data point compared with baseline values.
Note: L-NMMA, NG-monomethyl-arginine; SBP, systolic blood pressure (mmHg); DBP, diastolic blood pressure (mmHg); SVR, systemic vascular resistance (dynes/s per cm^5); HR, heart rate (beats/min); CI, cardiac index (L/min m^2); SVI, stroke volume index (mL/min m^2); CVP, central venous pressure (mmHg); B/min, sympathetic bursts per minute.
Source: Adapted from Spieker et al. (30).

intercellular permeability to metabolites. Significant ion transport in endothelial cells occurs paracellularly rather than transcellularly. Gap junctions between endothelial cells and the underlying myocytes represent an important pathway for signal transduction.

Alterations in vascular tone translate into activation of mechanosensitive ion channels. Depending on species and the vascular bed, inward depolarization currents occur. Likewise, shear stress produced by flow activate inwardly-rectifying, calcium-activated potassium current. The flow-mediated activation of these channels results in hyperpolarization and the release of vasodilating nitric oxide.

Similarly, vasoactive agents such as acetylcholine, bradykinin, substance P, adenosine triphosphate, adenosine, and histamine produce outward currents and hyperpolarization in endothelial cells. The two principal classes of calcium-activated potassium channels are large-conductance bradykinin channels and small conductance (SK) channels.

Metabolic factors, such as hypoxia, influence endothelial cell membrane potential because of their adenosine triphosphate-sensitive potassium channels. These channels are blocked by sulfonylurea compounds such as glibenclamid.

III. ALTERATIONS IN VASCULAR FUNCTION IN EXPERIMENTAL HYPERTENSION

Endothelium-derived nitric oxide-mediated vascular relaxation is impaired in spontaneously hypertensive

animals (3). Thus, the bioavailability of nitric oxide is reduced. Surprisingly, the nitric oxide pathway is paradoxically upregulated in the resistance circulation and the heart of spontaneously hypertensive rats (SHRs) (4). Adult SHRs possess a higher activity of endothelial nitric oxide synthase than their normotensive counterparts (5). Very young prehypertensive SHRs have, in contrast, lower endothelial nitric oxide synthase activity than young normotensive rats without a genetic background for hypertension, which indicates that the increased activity of endothelial nitric oxide synthase in adult SHRs is indeed related to hypertension (Fig. 7.2). Moreover, the plasma concentrations of the oxidative product of nitric oxide metabolism, nitrate, are higher in hypertensive rats than in normotensive controls (4). These results indicate that the basal release of nitric oxide is increased in hypertensive rats.

Thus, in SHRs, there must be a factor blunting the hemodynamic effect of nitric oxide. Indeed, nitric oxide production is increased in stroke-prone SHRs, but bioavailability is reduced (6). Direct *in situ* measurement of nitric oxide release by a porphyrinic microsensor in stroke-prone SHRs confirmed that hypertension is associated with increased nitric oxide decomposition by superoxide anions, that is, free oxygen radicals (Fig. 7.3) (7).

In other models of hypertension—that is, in Dahl salt-sensitive rats, in two-kidney, one clip experimental hypertension, and in DOCA-salt hypertensive rats—endothelium-dependent relaxation also is impaired. However, nitric oxide production by endothelial nitric oxide synthase is rather reduced than upregulated in Dahl salt-sensitive rats (Fig. 7.3). L-arginine, the substrate of nitric oxide production by endothelial nitric oxide synthase, normalizes blood pressure and simultaneously increases urinary excretion of nitrate, the degradation product of nitric oxide, in Dahl salt-sensitive rats. Further mechanisms contribute to the pathogenesis of salt sensitive hypertension, for example, decreased expression of endothelial endothelin β receptors, which mediate nitric oxide release, and altered expression of the constitutive brain nitric oxide synthase and the inducible nitric oxide synthase isoform, possibly leading to alterations in renal sympathetic nervous activity and sodium handling.

IV. THE ENDOTHELIUM IN HUMAN HYPERTENSION

A. Measuring Endothelial Function

The measurement of endothelium-dependent vasodilation to various stimuli can serve as a clinical marker of global endothelial function. The magnitude of endothelium-dependent vasodilation is determined primarily

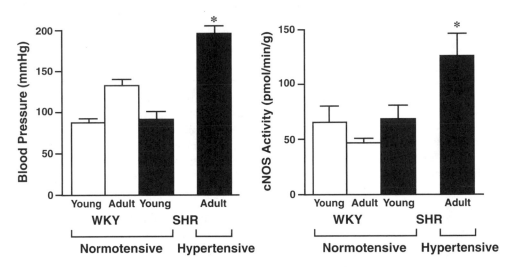

Figure 7.2 Increased activity of constitutive nitric oxide synthase in cardiac endothelium of spontaneously hypertensive rats (denoted by black bars). Adult spontaneously hypertensive rats possess a higher activity of constitutive nitric oxide synthase than their normotensive counterparts, Wystar Kyoto rats (denoted by open bars). Very young prehypertensive spontaneously hypertensive rats have, in contrast, lower constitutive nitric oxide synthase activity than the normotensive rats, which indicates that the increased activity of nitric oxide synthase in adult spontaneously hypertensive rats is indeed related to hypertension. NOS, nitric oxide synthase; SHRs, spontaneously hypertensive rats; WKY, Wystar Kyoto rats. [Adapted from Nava et al. (5).]

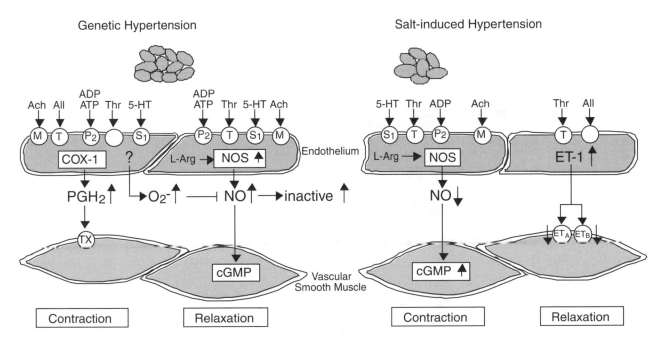

Figure 7.3 Heterogeneity of endothelial dysfunction in experimental hypertension. In spontaneous hypertension (left panel), nitric oxide synthase is upregulated and nitric oxide is inactivated by superoxide anions. In addition, the production of thromboxane and prostaglandin H$_2$ is increased. In salt-related hypertension (right panel), nitric oxide production is reduced and the endothelin system is upregulated. ACE, angiotensin-converting enzyme; ACh, acetylcholine; AII, angiotensin II; AT$_1$, angiotensin-1 receptor; cGMP, cyclic guanosine monophosphate; COX, cyclooxygenase; ET, endothelin; ET$_A$ and ET$_B$, endothelin A and endothelin B receptors; ET-1, endothelin-1; L-Arg, L-arginine; M, muscarinergic receptor; NO, nitric oxide; NOS, nitric oxide synthase; O$_2^-$, superoxide anion; PGI$_2$, prostacyclin; PGH$_2$, prostaglandin H$_2$; S, serotoninergic receptor; T, thrombine receptor; Thr, thrombine; TX, thromboxane receptor; TXA$_2$, thromboxane; 5-HT, 5-hydroxytryptamine (serotonine).

by endothelium-derived nitric oxide. There are several techniques for the assessment of nitric oxide bioavailability in man.

1. Flow-Mediated Vasodilation

Most often, flow-mediated vasodilation of the brachial artery—a noninvasive marker of endothelial function—is assessed by high-resolution ultrasonography (Fig. 7.4). Very elegantly, a physiological stimulus, that is, postischemic reactive hyperemia is used to increase blood flow. A cuff is placed around the wrist and after measurement of the basal radial or brachial artery diameter proximal to the cuff, it is inflated to suprasystolic pressure for several minutes. After release of the cuff, reactive hyperemia of the hand leads to an increased blood flow through the brachial artery (Fig. 7.4). The associated vasodilation of the brachial artery is assessed using high-resolution ultrasonography. Because of the tiny amount of vasodilation—the change in diameter reaches 10% in healthy volunteers—special sonographic equipment and analysis software is needed.

2. Intima-Media Thickness

The measurement of flow-mediated vasodilation of a large conduit artery as a functional measurement is sometimes combined with assessment of arterial intima-media thickness as a morphological parameter. Carotid intima-media

thickness correlates strongly with the cardiovascular risk. Indeed, asymptomatic subjects with cardiovascular risk factors such as hypertension or dyslipidemia show increased intima-media thickness. Therefore, measurement of intima-media thickness is often used as a surrogate endpoint in clinical trials, as is flow-mediated vasodilation itself. Not quite surprisingly, carotid intima-media thickness correlates strongly with flow-mediated vasodilation of the brachial artery, linking structural and functional abnormalities of the arteries.

3. Venous Occlusion Plethysmography

Alternatively, endothelium-dependent and endothelium-independent vasomotion in reaction to intra-arterially infused vasoactive substances are assessed by using venous occlusion plethysmography (Fig. 7.5). Among the most often used endothelium-dependent vasodilators are acetylcholine and serotonin. Sodium nitroprusside or nitroglycerine serve as endothelium-independent vasodilators. The technique of venous occlusion plethysmography experienced a renaissance in endothelial function research. A strain gage placed around the forearm changes its impedance in relation to the circumference. Therefore, an increase in arterial blood flow to the forearm changes the electrical signal, which is continuously recorded. Intra-arterial infusion of pharmacological substances is used to alter arterial blood flow for testing of vasomotion (Fig. 7.5).

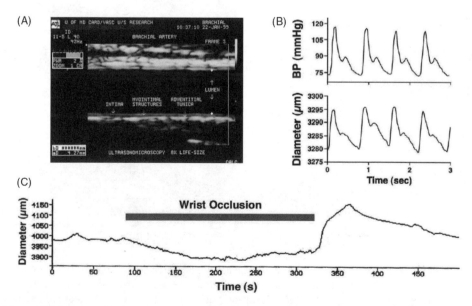

Figure 7.4   (A) Flow-mediated vasodilation of the brachial artery is measured by high-resolution ultrasonography. (B) With the use of echo-tracking, arterial diameter can be measured on a beat-to-beat base. (C) After establishing stable baseline conditions, flow-mediated vasodilation is measured after the release of a blood pressure cuff that was placed around the wrist and inflated to suprasystolic pressure for 5 min. The resulting hyperemic blood flow to the hand after release of the wrist cuff leads to a more-or-less pronounced vasodilation of the brachial artery, which is mediated by endothelium-derived nitric oxide.

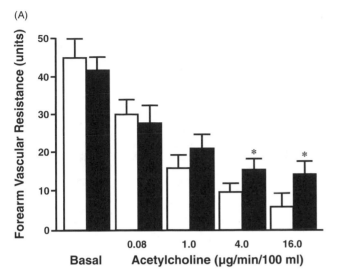

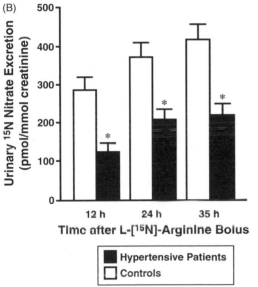

Figure 7.5 Endothelial dysfunction in arterial hypertension. (A) Decreased endothelium-dependent vasodilation in patients with hypertension in response to acetylcholine compared with normotensive controls. (B) Cumulative urinary excretion of [15N]nitrate after administration of 15N-labeled arginine, that is, the substrate for enzymatic production of nitric oxide. Urinary excretion of the metabolic oxidation product of nitric oxide (nitrate) is reduced in hypertensive patients compared with normotensive controls. This data show that whole-body nitric oxide production in patients with essential hypertension is diminished under basal conditions. [Adapted Linder et al. (8) and Forte et al. (13).]

4. Quantitative Coronary Angiography

The same pharmacological principle is commonly used for the assessment of endothelial function in coronary arteries. Quantitative coronary angiography allows detection of changes in diameter during intracoronary infusion of vasoactive substances or physiological stimuli to increase

coronary blood flow, (e.g., exercise). Atherosclerotic coronary arteries react to these stimuli with vasoconstriction, whereas the normal observation is vasodilation. Most commonly, endothelium-dependent vasodilators such as acetylcholine and serotonin are used. Sodium nitroprusside or nitroglycerine serve as endothelium-independent vasodilators.

B. Endothelial Dysfunction in Patients with Hypertension

Endothelium-dependent vasodilation in response to acetylcholine is impaired in patients with arterial hypertension, both in the forearm circulation (Fig. 7.5) (8,9) and in the coronary vascular bed (10). Endothelium-dependent vasodilation in the human forearm and coronary vascular beds are strongly correlated (11).

Basal nitric oxide activity is decreased in hypertensive patients (12). Furthermore, urinary excretion of the metabolic oxidation product of nitric oxide, [15N]nitrate, after administration of 15N-labeled arginine (i.e., the substrate for the generation of nitric oxide) is reduced in hypertensive patients compared with normotensive controls (Fig. 7.5) (13). Thus, whole-body nitric oxide production in patients with essential hypertension is diminished under basal conditions. In line with these findings, the vasoconstrictor response to NG-monomethyl-arginine, an inhibitor of nitric oxide synthesis, was significantly less in hypertensive patients compared with normotensive patients, whereas there was no difference in the response to norepinephrine, an endothelium-independent vasoconstrictor, between hypertensive patients and normotensive individuals (12).

Normotensive offspring of hypertensive parents exhibit impaired endothelium-dependent vasodilation to acetylcholine (14). In parallel to manifest hypertension in normotensive offspring, vasoconstriction which is a result of the inhibition of nitric oxide synthesis is decreased (15). Thus, derangement of endothelial function in hypertension is likely to be caused in part by genetic factors and not to be just a consequence of elevated blood pressure (although the hemodynamic factor is an important contributing factor to elevated pressure).

C. Interactions with Other Cardiovascular Risk Factors

Cardiovascular risk factors, such as hypercholesterolemia, smoking, diabetes mellitus, and hyperhomocysteinemia, impair endothelial function even in young asymptomatic individuals. The number of cardiovascular risk factors present relates to the degree of endothelial dysfunction. For example, long-term smoking potentiates endothelial dysfunction in hypercholesterolemic patients by enhancing the oxidation of low-density lipoprotein (LDL) cholesterol. Passive smoking is also associated with endothelial dysfunction.

Impressively, even a positive family history for premature coronary artery disease is sufficient to cause decreased endothelium-dependent coronary vasodilation to acetylcholine. In offspring of patients who had a myocardial infarction before the age of 60, flow-mediated vasodilation of the brachial artery is reduced and correlates with carotid intima-media thickness.

Aging is a primary determinant for the development of cardiovascular disease. Aging *per se* is associated with decreased endothelium-dependent vasodilation, even in the absence of other risk factors. In arteries exposed to high blood pressure, aging is associated with reduced nitric oxide production. Because nitric oxide synthase expression is actually increased, as is the production of free-oxygen-derived free radicals, aging seems to primarily affect the breakdown of nitric oxide by the superoxide anion, an oxygen radical. Also, endothelin-1 expression increases with age.

Male gender is associated with increased susceptibility to the noxious effects on endothelial function of cardiovascular risk factors such as elevated cholesterol levels. Estrogens mediate their protective actions partly over the nitric oxide pathway. In healthy postmenopausal women, short-term estrogen replacement therapy improves endothelium-dependent vasodilation in the coronary and brachial artery circulation. These beneficial effects are a result of improved endothelial function with increased nitric oxide bioavailability.

D. Endothelial Function in Patients with Atherosclerotic Vascular Disease

In patients with atherosclerotic vascular disease, endothelial nitric oxide synthase protein expression and nitric oxide release are markedly reduced (16). In contrast, circulating endothelin-1 levels are increased in patients with atherosclerotic vascular lesions and correlate with the severity of the disease (17). The amount of endothelin-1 in the vascular wall corresponds to blood pressure, total serum cholesterol, and number of atherosclerotic sites (18).

Indeed, endothelial dysfunction of the coronary arteries, which is paralleled by generalized endothelial dysfunction of the peripheral arteries, has both symptomatic and prognostic implications. In fact, impaired endothelium-dependent vasomotion is associated with myocardial ischemia and increased cardiac events. Exercise normally increases coronary artery diameter; however, in patients with coronary artery disease, the major physiological stimulus for endothelial nitric oxide release, increased blood flow, leads to coronary vasoconstriction. Exercise-induced vasoconstriction associated with endothelial dysfunction may be mediated by

unopposed α-adrenergic mechanisms. Similarly, acetylcholine, a receptor-dependent stimulator of nitric oxide release, evokes a paradoxical vasoconstriction in atherosclerotic coronary arteries; and epicardial atherosclerosis is associated with an impairment in endothelium-dependent dilation of the coronary microvasculature.

V. OXIDATIVE STRESS IN ARTERIAL HYPERTENSION

Oxidative stress plays an important role in the pathogenesis of hypertension (Fig. 7.6). Superoxide anions can scavenge nitric oxide to form peroxynitrite effectively reducing the bioavailability of endothelium-derived nitric oxide (Fig. 7.7) (19). In addition, the superoxide anion$^-$ can act as a vasoconstrictor (20). Reduced nicotinamide adenine dinucleotide (NADH) dehydrogenase, a mitochondrial enzyme of the respiratory chain, seems to be a major source of the superoxide anion. Expression of NAD(P)H oxidase in human coronary artery smooth muscle cells is upregulated by pulsatile stretch, generating increased oxidative stress. Another source of superoxide anions is cyclooxygenase. In contrast, xanthine oxidase, another generator of superoxide anions, does not appear to play a significant role in essential hypertension.

Paradoxically, nitric oxide synthase (i.e., the nitric oxide generating enzyme) can also produce superoxide anions. Production of superoxide anions in stroke-prone SHRs, an experimental model of genetic hypertension, can be prevented by nitric oxide synthase inhibition. Administration of exogenous tetrahydrobiopterin, an essential cofactor for nitric oxide synthase, can reduce excess superoxide anions in the aorta of stroke-prone SHRs (Fig. 7.6). In prehypertensive SHRs, the calcium ionophore A23187-stimulated (i.e., a receptor-independent activator of nitric oxide synthase) production of superoxide anions was significantly higher than in control rats. Nitric oxide release was reduced in SHR aortas, with opposite results in the presence of exogenous tetrahydrobiopterin. Thus, dysfunctional endothelial nitric oxide synthase may be a source of superoxide anions in prehypertensive SHRs and contribute to the development of hypertension and its vascular complications.

Superoxide anions are finally detoxified by superoxide dismutase forming hydrogen peroxide, which is further metabolized by catalase (Fig. 7.7). However, the reaction between the two radicals (superoxide anions) and nitric oxide is three times faster than the detoxification of superoxide anions by superoxide dismutase. Depending on the relative concentrations of nitric oxide and superoxide dismutase, there may be a propensity for superoxide to preferentially react with nitric oxide, resulting in decreased bioavailability of nitric oxide.

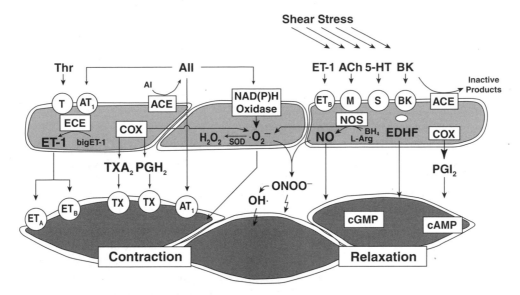

Figure 7.6 Role of oxidative stress in the pathogenesis of endothelial dysfunction in hypertension. The superoxide anion, generated by angiotensin II-activated NAD(P)H oxidase, by dysfunctional nitric oxide synthase, or by cyclooxygenase, can scavenge the vasodilator nitric oxide to form the highly reactive peroxynitrite. Peroxynitrite can damage cell membranes and oxidize lipids. In addition, the superoxide anion can act as a vasoconstrictor. ACE, angiotensin-converting enzyme; Ach, acetylcholine; AII, angiotensin II; AT_1, angiotensin-1 receptor; BH_4, tetrahydrobiopterine; BK, bradykinin; COX, cyclooxygenase; ECE, endothelin-converting enzyme; EDHF, endothelium-derived hyperpolarizing factor; ET_A and ET_B, endothelin A and endothelin B receptors; endothelin-1, ET-1; H_2O_2, hydrogen peroxide; L-Arg, L-arginine; NAD(P)H oxidase, nicotinamide adenine dinucleotide oxidase; O_2^-, superoxide anion; OH^-, hydroxyl radical; $ONOO^-$, peroxynitrite; PGH_2, prostaglandin H_2; PGI_2, prostacyclin; S, serotoninergic receptor; SOD, superoxide dismutase; Thr, thrombine; TXA, thromboxane receptor; TXA_2, thromboxane; 5-HT, 5-hydroxytryptamine (serotonine). [Adapted from Spieker et al. (43).]

The gene for cytosolic superoxide dismutase (i.e., superoxide dismutase 1) is located on the 21q22.1 region of chromosome 21. Therefore, patients with Down syndrome (trisomy 21) have an extra copy of the superoxide dismutase gene. Because of gene dosage excess, their superoxide dismutase activity is 50% greater than in the diploid population, which leads to reduced superoxide anion levels. Indeed, patients with Down syndrome have

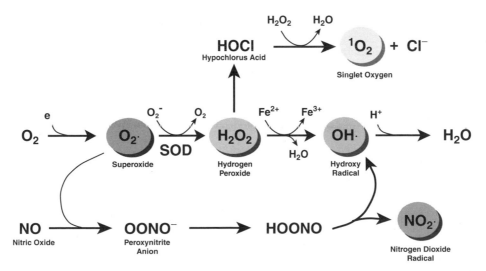

Figure 7.7 The superoxide anion, an oxygen radical, is detoxified by superoxide dismutase, forming hydrogen peroxide, which is further metabolized by catalase. However, the reaction between the two superoxide anions and nitric oxide is three times faster than the detoxification of the superoxide anion by superoxide dismutase. Depending on the relative concentrations of nitric oxide and superoxide dismutase, there may be a propensity for superoxide to preferentially react with nitric oxide. The superoxide anion can scavenge nitric oxide to form peroxynitrite, effectively reducing the bioavailability of endothelium-derived nitric oxide. H_2O_2, hydrogen peroxide; O_2^-, superoxide anion; $ONOO^-$, peroxynitrite; SOD, superoxide dismutase.

lower blood pressure levels, indicating a major role for superoxide anions in the regulation of arterial blood pressure. In addition, the normal age-associated increase of blood pressure is absent in patients with Down syndrome (21).

The renin–angiotensin–aldosterone system plays a major role in hypertension (Fig. 7.1). Apart from direct vasoconstrictor effects of angiotensin II, there are important interactions among angiotensin II, oxygen radicals, and nitric oxide.

Angiotensin II stimulates generation of superoxide anions by increasing the expression of the NAD(P)H oxidase gene (p22phox) and increasing the activity of NAD(P)H oxidase. The vasoconstrictor effect of angiotensin II is enhanced in the absence of nitric oxide and diminished during coinfusion of antioxidant vitamin C. Thus, the vasoconstrictive effect of angiotensin II is modulated by reactive oxygen species, primarily superoxide anions, and their interaction with endothelium-derived nitric oxide (Fig. 7.6). Furthermore, angiotensin II increases the production of endothelin in the blood vessel wall, which exerts vasoconstriction and induces proliferation of the vascular smooth muscle cells (22).

VI. PROSTAGLANDINS

Prostacyclin is a further endothelium-derived relaxing factor, which is released in response to shear stress (Fig. 7.1). Prostacyclin is synthesized by cyclooxygenase from arachidonic acid (23). Prostacyclin increases intracellular cyclic adenosine monophosphate in smooth muscle cells and platelets. In contrast to nitric oxide, prostacyclin does not contribute to the maintenance of basal vascular tone of large conduit arteries (24). Instead, its platelet inhibitory effects are most important. The synergistic effect of both prostacyclin and nitric oxide enhances the antiplatelet activity.

Depending on the animal model of hypertension and the vascular bed, endothelium-dependent contractions to acetylcholine, a muscarinic receptor-dependent stimulator of nitric oxide synthesis, have been documented (Fig. 7.3). As this response is inhibited by cyclooxygenase inhibitors and thromboxane receptor antagonists, the most likely contractile factors are thromboxane A_2 and prostaglandin H_2.

Interactions between cyclooxygenase products and nitric oxide have been demonstrated. In hypertensive patients, indomethacin, a cyclooxygenase inhibitor, significantly increased the response to acetylcholine, an effect that could be blocked by coinfusion of NG-monomethylarginine, an inhibitor of nitric oxide synthesis. Therefore, cyclooxygenase inhibition restores nitric oxide-mediated vasodilation in essential hypertension, which suggests

that cyclooxygenase-dependent substances can impair nitric oxide bioavailability. Cyclooxygenase is, indeed, a source of the nitric oxide-scavenger superoxide anions. A novel interesting concept in atherosclerosis is selective inhibition of cyclooxygenase-2, which lowers C-reactive protein (CRP) levels and improves endothelial function.

VII. ENDOTHELIUM-DERIVED HYPERPOLARIZING FACTOR

Inhibitors of the L-arginine pathway do not prevent all endothelium-dependent relaxations. As vascular smooth muscle cells become hyperpolarized under endothelium-dependent relaxation, an endothelium-dependent hyperpolarizing factor of unknown chemical structure has been proposed (Fig. 7.1). There is evidence that a calcium-dependent potassium channel on endothelial or smooth muscle cells is important in mediating endothelium-dependent hyperpolarization, a mechanism that is impaired in arterial hypertension. Endothelium-dependent hyperpolarization may also be involved in the compensation for the impaired nitric oxide-system in patients with essential hypertension.

VIII. ENDOTHELIN

Over a decade ago, a novel vasoconstrictor peptide synthesized by vascular endothelial cells has been identified (25,26). The family of endothelins consists of three closely related peptides—endothelin-1, endothelin-2, and endothelin-3—which are converted by endothelin-converting enzymes from "big endothelins" that originate from large preproendothelin peptides cleaved by endopeptidases. The endothelin peptides are not only synthesized in vascular endothelial and smooth muscle cells, but also in neural, renal, pulmonal, and some circulatory cells holding the genes for endothelins. The chemical structure of the endothelins is closely related to neurotoxins (sarafotoxins) produced by scorpions and snakes. Factors modulating the expression of endothelin-1 are shear-stress, epinephrine, angiotensin II, thrombin, inflammatory cytokines (tumor necrosis factor α, interleukin-1, and interleukin-2), transforming growth factor β, and hypoxia. Endothelin-1 is metabolized by a neutral endopeptidase, which also cleaves natriuretic peptides.

Imbalance of endothelium-derived relaxing and contracting substances disturbs the normal function of the vascular endothelium. Endothelin acts as the natural counterpart to endothelium-derived nitric oxide, which exerts vasodilating, antithrombotic, and antiproliferative effects, and inhibits leukocyte-adhesion to the vascular wall (Fig. 7.8). In addition to its effect on arterial blood

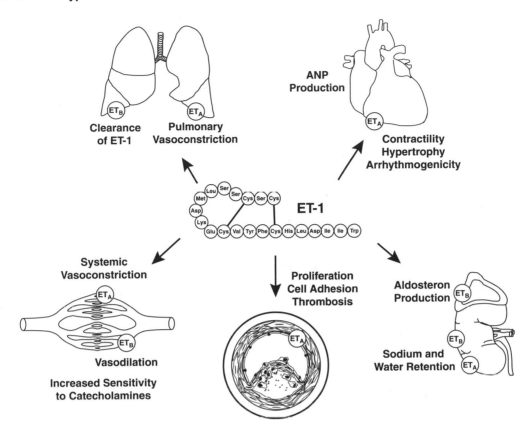

Figure 7.8 Pathophysiological role of ET-1. In the heart, endothelin-1 contributes to contractility. In addition to its vasoconstrictive effects in the systemic and pulmonary circulation, ET-1 leads to hypertrophy of myocardial and smooth muscle cells. The pulmonary circulation is an important source of ET-1, but it is also involved in the clearance of ET-1. In the kidney, endothelin-1 regulates sodium and water excretion. ET-1, endothelin-1. [Adapted from Spieker et al. (45).]

pressure in humans (27), endothelin-1 induces vascular and myocardial hypertrophies (28), which are independent risk factors for cardiovascular morbidity and mortality. Indeed, in patients with essential hypertension, carotid wall thickening and left ventricular mass correlate with reduced endothelium-dependent vasodilation.

Endothelin-1 rather acts in a paracrine than an endocrine mode of action, which is reflected by plasma levels of endothelin-1 in the picomolar range. Infusion of an endothelin receptor antagonist into the brachial artery or systemically in healthy humans leads to vasodilation, indicating a role of endothelin-1 in the maintenance of basal vascular tone. When endothelin-1 itself is infused, vasoconstriction follows a brief phase of vasodilation, which may be explained by relaxation of smooth muscle cells caused by ET$_B$ receptor-mediated release of the vasodilators nitric oxide and prostacyclin (Fig. 7.1). In addition, endothelin-1 may also exert effects on the central and autonomic nervous system and alter baroreflex function. In the kidney, sodium reabsorption is modulated.

The endothelin system is activated in several but not in all animal models of arterial hypertension. Correspondingly,

endothelin plasma levels have been reported to be elevated in certain patients with essential hypertension (29), but this is a subject to controversy. The causal role of endothelin-1 in the pathogenesis of hypertension thus remains unclear.

However, it might attain a higher concentration in the vessel wall than in the plasma because most endothelin-1 synthesized in endothelial cells is secreted abluminally. In fact, significant correlations between the amount of immunoreactive endothelin-1 in the tunica media and blood pressure, total serum cholesterol, and number of atherosclerotic sites were found (18). In blood vessels of healthy controls, endothelin-1 was detectable almost exclusively in endothelial cells, whereas in patients with coronary artery disease or arterial hypertension, sizable amounts of endothelin-1 were detectable in the tunica media of different types of arteries (18). In addition, there is evidence that certain gene polymorphisms of endothelin-1 and endothelin receptors could be associated with blood pressure levels. Moreover, in hypertensive patients, infusion of an ET$_{A/B}$ receptor antagonist causes significantly greater vasodilation than in normotensive subjects (Fig. 7.9).

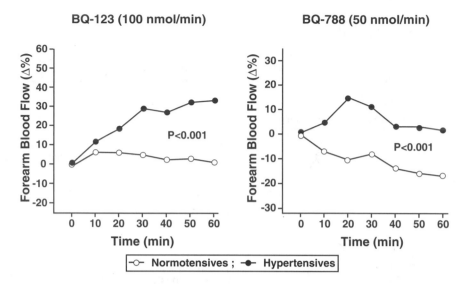

Figure 7.9 Forearm blood flow responses to intra-arterial infusion of the selective endothelin A receptor antagonist BQ-123 (100 nmol/min) and the endothelin B receptor antagonist BQ-788 (50 nmol/min) in hypertensive patients and normotensive controls. The vasodilator response to endothelin antagonism is significantly enhanced in hypertensives. ET_A, endothelin A receptor; ET_B, endothelin B receptor. [Adapted from Cardillo et al. (46).]

Because plasma levels of endothelin-1 were similar in normotensive and hypertensive patients in this study, increased sensitivity to endogenous endothelin-1 has to be postulated. As in some patients with arterial hypertension, endogenous catecholamine production is increased, and catecholamines potentiate endothelin-1 induced vasoconstriction (Fig. 7.10), these interactions with the endothelin-1 pathway is likely to be involved in the

pathogenesis of hypertension. Decreased bioavailability of nitric oxide is also involved in this phenomenon because nitric oxide antagonizes some of the effects of endothelin-1.

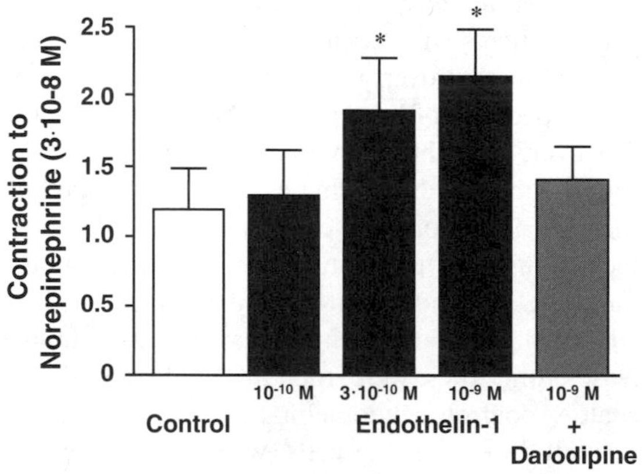

IX. INTERACTIONS BETWEEN THE ENDOTHELIUM AND THE SYMPATHETIC NERVOUS SYSTEM

The sympathetic nervous system is an important regulator of cardiovascular homeostasis. Although it is essential to be able to stand erect, sympathetic overactivity may be deleterious and turn "a beauty into a beast." Activation of the renin–angiotensin–aldosterone system is closely coupled to that of the sympathetic nervous system as the two neurohormonal regulators stimulate each other.

Sympathetic activity is regulated primarily by baroreceptors located in the cardiopulmonary and carotid vessel walls, which centrally inhibit sympathetic outflow. These stretch-activated mechanoreceptors not only regulate short-term changes of blood pressure, but they also react to a chronic elevation in blood pressure by resetting sensitivity to a lower level. In hypertension, altered baroreflex-mediated regulation of sympathetic nerve activity has been described. Similarly, in congestive heart failure, an abnormal baroreflex contributes to sympathetic activation, which is a negative prognostic factor.

Abnormal endothelial function with an imbalance of endothelium-derived relaxing and contracting factors affects baroreceptor function because the baroreceptor

Figure 7.10 Threshold concentrations of ET-1 that potentiate contractions to norepinephrine and serotonin in human arteries. In mammary artery rings, the contractions to norepinephrine were potentiated by threshold concentrations and low concentrations of ET-1. The calcium antagonist darodipine prevented the potentiation of the response to norepinephrine that is evoked by ET-1. Similarly, contractions to serotonin were amplified by ET-1 in the mammary artery rings and in the coronary arteries. [Adapted from Yang et al. (47).]

nerve endings and the endothelium are located very near each other (30). Various endothelial substances (e.g., nitric oxide, PGI$_2$, and endothelin-1) influence baroreceptor function in an experimental setting.

Interactions between the sympathetic nervous system and the vascular endothelium become major clinical importance in presence of a dysfunctional endothelium. Exercise normally increases coronary artery diameter; however, in patients with endothelial dysfunction, the major physiological stimulus for endothelial nitric oxide release, increased blood flow, leads to coronary vasoconstriction (Fig. 7.11). Phentolamine, an α-adrenoceptor blocker, prevents exercise-induced coronary vasoconstriction in patients with endothelial dysfuntion. Thus, unopposed α-adrenergic vasoconstriction in presence of impaired endothelial nitric oxide release results in paradoxical coronary vasoconstriction. Similar mechanisms also may be involved in the pathogenesis of coronary vasospasm.

Catecholamine release is increased in certain patients with arterial hypertension. Particularly in younger patients with hypertension, circulating catecholamine levels are increased. In hypertension, there are abnormalities on various levels of the catecholamine system, for example, increased neuronal as well as cerebral norepinephrine release, impaired neuronal norepinephrine re-uptake, and increased adrenal epinephrine release. Interestingly, the cardiovascular response to mental stress is exaggerated in patients with hypertension. Abnormalities in the response to mental stress are likely a result of genetic factors because normotensive offspring of hypertensive parents exhibit an exaggerated sympathetic activation in response to mental stress.

Particularly, wide-ranging are the effects of sympathetic activation on hemostasis. Platelets are activated by epinephrine via the α-adrenergic receptor pathway. Sympathetic overactivity in arterial hypertension thus has the potential to provoke a prothrombotic state.

X. ENDOTHELIUM AND THROMBOSIS IN HYPERTENSION

Maintaining the balance of blood flow and thrombus formation in case of vascular injury is one major task of the vascular endothelium. On the other hand, some of the most feared clinical sequelae of longstanding arterial hypertension, that is, stroke and myocardial infarction, are commonly mediated by thrombosis of the respective arterial vessel. Indeed, the long-term consequences of high blood pressure are generally ischemic rather than hemorrhagic.

A. Platelet Activation and Adhesion

The adhesion of platelets to basement membrane components exposed to blood after disruption of endothelial integrity is mediated by von Willebrand factor and its glycoprotein Ibα receptor, as well as platelet membrane GPIa–IIa (integrin-$\alpha_2\beta_1$) and GPVI interacting directly with collagen (Fig. 7.12). Activation of platelets by thrombin, adenosine diphosphate, thromboxane A$_2$, and epinephrine is under negative control by nitric oxide and prostacyclin. Thrombin directly stimulates platelets to release thromboxane A$_2$, inducing potent vasoconstriction, which is prevented by the simultaneous thrombin-induced release of prostacyclin and nitric oxide from endothelial cells (31). The feedback regulation of endothelial nitric oxide and prostacyclin release majorly contributes to the antithrombotic properties of the vascular endothelium.

B. Platelet Aggregation

Platelet aggregation leads to hemostasis via linking of accumulating platelets by fibrinogen (mediated by GPIIb–IIIa), von Willebrand factor, and fibronectin. The activation of the coagulation cascade resulting in the conversion of fibrinogen to fibrin by thrombin is triggered by tissue factor, which is present in blood and abundantly in atherosclerotic plaques. P-selectin and CD40L (also termed CD154), among other agonists, stabilize the plug (Fig. 7.12). In addition, CD40L mediates the cross-talk between platelets, endothelium, and inflammatory blood cells, which is an important step in the pathogenesis of atherosclerosis (32).

C. Hypertension and Atherothrombosis

Arterial hypertension is a risk factor for the development of stroke and myocardial infarction. These catastrophic

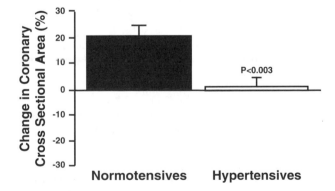

Figure 7.11 Coronary luminal area change during exercise in hypertensive patients and normotensive control subjects. Although exercise leads to coronary vasodilation in normotensive control subjects, exercise-induced coronary vasodilation is impaired in hypertensive patients and is sometimes even leads to vasoconstriction. [Adapted from Frielingsdorf et al. (48).]

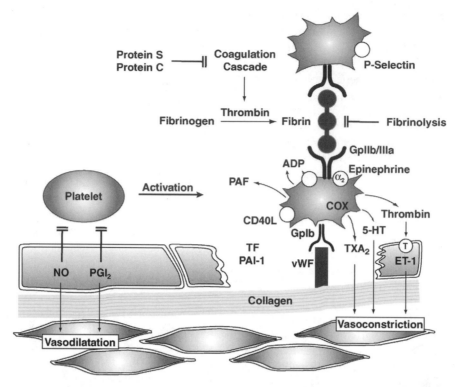

Figure 7.12 Interactions between the vascular endothelium and platelets in the pathogenesis of arterial thrombosis. ADP, adenosine diphosphate; GP, glycoprotein; NO, nitric oxide; PGI_2, prostacyclin; T, thrombin; TXA_2, thromboxane A_2; TF, tissue factor; vWF, von Willebrand factor.

events are most often mediated by thrombosis and subsequent occlusion of the nurturing arteries. Damage to vessel walls may develop after years of exposure to cardiovascular risk factors. Virchow's classical triad of blood flow, hemostatic blood factors, and vessel wall damage determines the susceptibility for thrombosis.

Platelets as major hemostatic blood constituents play a crucial role in the pathogenesis of acute coronary and cerebral ischemia. However, platelets also essentially contribute to the development and progression of chronic atherosclerotic lesions (33). Interaction with the arterial vessel wall, the endothelium in particular, determines the propensity of platelets to adhere and aggregate (Fig. 7.12). Therefore, endothelial dysfunction in patients with arterial hypertension contributes to a chronic prothrombotic state. Impaired bioavailability of endothelium-derived nitric oxide weakens the antithrombotic features of the vascular endothelium. Further morphologic, biochemical, and functional alterations in platelets contribute to atherothrombosis in hypertension (34).

1. Morphologic Platelet Alterations

Arterial hypertension is associated with certain morphologic platelet alterations. Patients with hypertension show increased platelet volume, as well as changes in shape, and an increased platelet turnover. The latter may partly be due to generation of platelets microparticles. These microparticles are released after activation, have procoagulant effects and promote thrombin generation. Increased shear stress in arterial hypertension is a likely underlying factor for microparticle generation. Over the long-term, increasing numbers of platelet microparticles may promote atherothrombosis in hypertension through particle deposition in the vessel wall, which propagates atherothrombosis. In turn, shear stress is further increased locally at sites of atherosclerotic lesions, thus promoting platelet stimulation.

2. Changes in Platelet Function

In addition to the morphologic alterations, there is increased platelet activation in patients with arterial hypertension. P-selectin expression, a platelet surface protein that implying increased platelet activation, is enhanced in patients with hypertension. Also, patients with arterial hypertension show increased plasma β-thromboglobulin release. β-thromboglobulin is a multimeric glycoprotein that is synthesized in megakaryocytes and is released upon activation of the platelets. Intraplatelet calcium is increased in hypertensive patients. An increase in intracellular platelet calcium concentration is the primary event that signals platelet activation. Platelet intracellular free-calcium correlates with systolic and diastolic blood pressure in patients with hypertension (35), and antihypertensive therapy normalizes intraplatelet calcium. The altered intracellular free-calcium homeostasis may likely be a result of increased sensitivity to catecholamines because epinephrine provokes an exaggerated intraplatelet free-calcium increase in patients with essential hypertension. Indeed, expression of platelet α-2-adrenergic receptors is enhanced in hypertensive patients. Activation of the renin–angiotensin–aldosterone system in hypertension contributes to platelet function alteration because angiotensin II also stimulates platelets. Moreover, in some patients with arterial hypertension, endogenous catecholamine production is increased, and genetic polymorphisms of the α-2-adrenoreceptor may further contribute to altered platelet function in arterial hypertension.

In addition to enhanced platelet activation, platelets from hypertensive patients have an increased tendency to aggregate, both spontaneously and in response to agonists such as collagen and adenosine diphosphate.

3. Impaired Fibrinolysis in Hypertension

On the other hand, the counter-regulatory mechanism of fibrinolysis is also functionally altered in patients with arterial hypertension. The activity of the fibrinolytic system is determined primarily by activators of fibrinolysis such as tissue-type plasminogen activators and inhibiting modulators such as a plasminogen activator inhibitor. The presence of atherothrombosis is associated with a marked disturbance in the relation of tissue-type plasminogen activator to plasminogen activator inhibitor, with a dominating presence of plasminogen activator inhibitor. Also in arterial hypertension, the plasminogen activator inhibitor to tissue-type plasminogen activator ratio is increased and correlates with increases in blood pressure. The impairment of fibrinolysis thus complements the chronic prothrombotic state in arterial hypertension.

D. Prothrombotic State and Hypertensive Target-Organ Damage

Target-organ damage in hypertension mainly manifests in the heart, brain, kidney, peripheral arteries, and eye. Patients with hypertensive target-organ damage are at particularly high risk for the development of cardiovascular and cerebrovascular events.

The presence of target-organ damage such as left ventricular hypertrophy or hypertensive kidney disease is associated with a prothrombotic state in hypertension (36). For example, microalbuminuria is related to increased plasma levels of von Willebrand factor, which mediates platelet adhesion to the vessel wall basement

membrane components that are exposed to blood after a disruption of endothelial integrity. Also, fibrinogen plasma levels correlate with the presence of hypertensive target-organ damage. Circulating fibrinogen levels are independently linked to increased cardiovascular risk in hypertensive patients.

Hypertension is a common cause of atrial fibrillation, which itself is associated with a prothrombotic state. The risk of stroke increases in presence of hypertensive heart disease with atrial fibrillation. Heart failure, which develops late after long-standing arterial hypertension, also confers an increased risk for thromboembolic events.

E. Hypertension, Dyslipidemia, and Diabetes

Arterial hypertension often is associated with dyslipidemia and diabetes because overweight is a common predisposing factor. The prevalence of arterial hypertension is as high as 50% in diabetic patients. The combination of arterial hypertension with diabetes has a particularly negative impact on endothelial function. These patients often have low levels of high-density lipoprotein (HDL) cholesterol. HDL levels determine thrombus formation because the anticoagulant activities of protein S and activated protein C are enhanced. Furthermore, HDL cholesterol has pro-fibrinolytic properties. The characteristic metabolic alterations associated with hypertension and diabetes thus confer a prothrombotic state.

XI. IMPACT OF ANTIHYPERTENSIVE THERAPY ON VASCULAR FUNCTION

In hypertensive animals, most classes of antihypertensive drugs (e.g., calcium channel blockers, ACE inhibitors, and AT_1 receptor antagonists) improve endothelium-dependent vasodilation (Fig. 7.13).

Surprisingly, and in contrast to animal experiments, antihypertensive therapy cannot restore impaired endothelium-dependent vasodilation consistently in patients with arterial hypertension. However, depending on the antihypertensive drug used and its pharmacological profile, improvements in endothelium-dependent vasodilation can be achieved (Table 7.2). The multi-factorial etiology of essential hypertension, as well as the duration of blood pressure elevation, may explain some of the inconsistent results from different investigators.

Antihypertensive therapy also has an impact on altered platelet function in patients with arterial hypertension. Antihypertensive therapy positively influences the prothrombotic state associated with hypertension. Although there might be differences between classes of antihypertensive drugs, their blood-pressure-lowering effect may

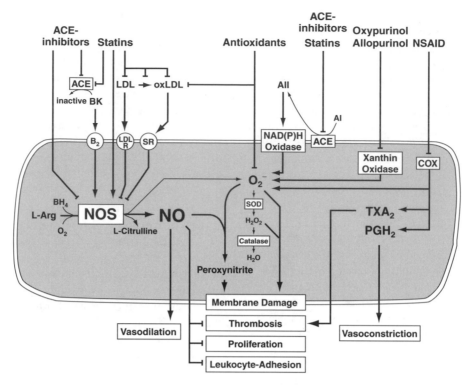

Figure 7.13 Potential mechanisms of action of cardiovascular drugs on the endothelial L-arginine nitric oxide pathway. Statins as well as ACE inhibitors increase endothelial nitric oxide synthase expression. In addition, ACE inhibitors inhibit the breakdown of bradykinin, which in turn increases the release of nitric oxide via B_2-bradykinergic receptors. Furthermore, they inhibit the formation of angiotensin II, which activates NAD(P)H oxidase to synthesize superoxide anions. Antioxidants, such as vitamin C or certain calcium channel antagonists, prevent scavenging of nitric oxide by superoxide anions. Exogenous supply of L-arginine and tetrahydrobiopterin increases their bioavailability in endothelial cells, which may be diminished in certain disease states. Nebivolol, a β_1-adrenoceptor blocker, directly activates nitric oxide release by an unknown mechanism. ACE, angiotensin-converting enzyme; AII, angiotensin II; B_2, bradykinin receptor; BK, bradykinin; COX, cyclooxygenase; eNOS, endothelial nitric oxide synthase; LDL-R, low-density lipoprotein receptor; NO, nitric oxide; O_2^-, superoxide anions; oxLDL, oxidatively modified LDL; PGH_2, prostaglandin H_2; PGI_2, prostacyclin; SR, scavenger receptor; BH_4, tetrahydrobiopterin.

be most important in mediating the attenuation of the prothrombotic state (36).

A. β-Blockers

It is interesting that the infusion of nebivolol, but not other β-blockers, intra-arterially in the forearm of healthy subjects is associated with an increase in forearm blood flow (Fig. 7.14). The increase in forearm blood flow achieved by nebivolol can be prevented by co-infusion of the nitric oxide synthesis inhibitor NG-monomethyl-arginine. Similar results have been obtained in the human venous circulation. This strongly suggests that nebivolol stimulates the formation of nitric oxide in the vasculature and may therefore have an interesting hemodynamic profile that leads—unlike other β-blockers—to peripheral vasodilation, in addition to the classical β-blocking effects on the sympathetic nervous system, heart rate, and cardiac contractility. Nebivolol also

causes nitric-oxide-dependent vasodilation in hypertensive patients. However, this favorable effect did not last during chronic treatment (6 months) with this new type of β_1-blocker. Nebivolol also inhibits platelet aggregation by its nitric-oxide-dependent mechanism. Traditional β-blockers have little effect on platelet aggregation.

B. ACE Inhibitors

In the Trial on Reversing ENdothelial Dysfunction (TREND) study, ACE inhibition with quinapril improved endothelial dysfunction in patients who were normotensive and who did not have severe hyperlipidemia or evidence of heart failure (37). However, the specific pharmacological features of an ACE inhibitor may be important for its effects on endothelial function, for example, high tissue permeability. ACE inhibitors inhibit the breakdown of bradykinin, a stimulator of nitric

Table 7.2 Effect of Antihypertensive Therapy on Endothelial Function in Patients with Arterial Hypertension

Author	Antihypertensive therapy by drug class	Duration of treatment	Nitric oxide-release agonist/antagonist	Improvement in endothelium-dependent vasomotion
	ACE inhibitors			
Hirooka et al.	Captopril	Acute	ACh	Yes
Creager et al.	Captopril	7–8 weeks	MCh	No
	Enalapril	7–8 weeks	MCh	No
Taddei et al.	Lisinopril	Acute	ACh	No
			Bk	Yes
		1 and 12 months	ACh	No
			Bk	Yes
Lyons et al.	Enalapril	6 weeks	L-NMMA	Yes
Millgard et al.	Captopril	Acute	MCh	Yes
		3 months	MCh	Yes
Schiffrin et al.	Cilazapril	1 and 2 years	ACh	Yes
Yavuz et al.	Enalapril	6 months	FMD	Yes
Ghiadoni et al.	Perindopril	6 months	FMD	Yes
	AII antagonists			
Ghiadoni et al.	Candesartan	2 months	ACh	No
		12 months	ACh	Yes[a]
Bragulat et al.	Irbesartan	6 months	ACh	Yes[a]
Yavuz et al.	Losartan	6 months	FMD	No
Ghiadoni et al.	Telmisartan	6 months	FMD	No
	β-blockers			
Schiffrin et al.	Atenolol	2 years	ACh	No
Dawes et al.	Nebivolol	Acute	L-NMMA	Yes
Ghiadoni et al.	Nebivolol	6 months	FMD	No
Ghiadoni et al.	Atenolol	6 months	FMD	No
	Calcium antagonists			
Hirooka et al.	Nifedipine	Acute	ACh	No
Millgard et al.	Nifedipine	Acute	MCh	No
Sudano et al.	Nifedipine	6 months	ACh	Yes
Schiffrin et al.	Nifedipine	Chronic	ACh	Yes
Ghiadoni et al.	Nifedipine	6 months	FMD	No
Taddei et al.	Lacidipine	2 and 8 months	ACh and Bk	Yes
Lyons et al.	Amlodipine	6 weeks	L-NMMA	Yes
Perticone et al.	Isradipine	2 and 6 months	ACh	Yes
Ghiadoni et al.	Amlodipine	6 months	FMD	No
	Other			
Panza et al.	Various (diuretics, verapamil, β-blockers, clonidine, α-methyldopa)	Chronic vs. two-week withdrawal	ACh ACh	No No
Taddei et al.	Potassium	Acute	ACh	Yes

[a]Effect was paralleled by an enhanced endothelium-independent vasodilation to sodium nitroprusside.
Note: ACE, angiotensin-converting enzyme; AII, angiotensin II; Ach, acetylcholine; Bk, bradykinin; FMD, flow-mediated dilation; L-NMMA, NG-monomethyl-L-arginine; MCh, methacholine; NO, nitric oxide.
Source: Adapted from Spieker et al. (43).

oxide release, and antioxidant properties further improve nitric oxide bioavailability. They inhibit the endothelial production of angiotensin II and endothelin-1. Indeed, only quinapril, not enalapril, was associated with a significant improvement in flow-mediated dilation of the brachial artery (38). Improved nitric oxide bioavailability also affects platelet function. Inhibitors of the renin–angiotensin–aldosterone system inhibit platelet

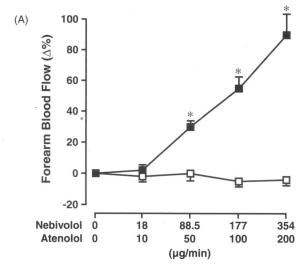

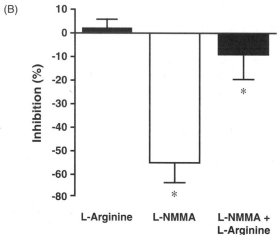

Figure 7.14 (A) Effects of nebivolol on forearm blood flow. In healthy human subjects, the effects of Nebivolol, but not the β-blocker atenolol, increases forearm blood flow, (B) an effect which is prevented by co-infusion of the inhibitor of nitric oxide, L-NMMA. L-NMMA, NG-monomethyl-L-arginine. [Adapted from Cockcroft et al. (49).]

aggregation *in vitro*. The favorable effects of ACE inhibitors on endothelial function with antithrombotic, antiproliferative, and antimigratory actions may explain how they can prevent cardiovascular events in patients with atherosclerosis, even in the absence of hypertension.

C. Angiotensin II Receptor Antagonists

Treatment with candesartan, an AT_1 receptor antagonist, reduced the vasodilator response to the mixed $ET_{A/B}$ receptor antagonist TAK-044 that was initially more pronounced in hypertensive patients than in normotensive controls (39). This was paralleled by a reduction in circulating plasma endothelin-1 levels. Furthermore, the impaired

vasoconstrictor response to NG-monomethyl-arginine, an inhibitor of nitric oxide synthesis, was augmented by antihypertensive treatment in patients with hypertension. Thus, the angiotensin II receptor blocker candesartan improves tonic nitric oxide release and reduces vasoconstriction to endogenous endothelin-1 in the forearm of hypertensive patients. Irbesartan, another AT_1 receptor antagonist, also has been investigated in hypertensive patients. Long-term irbesartan treatment enhanced both endothelium-dependent and endothelium-independent vascular vasodilation responses. In addition, irbesartan restored the vasoconstrictor capacity of the nitric oxide synthase inhibitor NG-monomethyl-arginine, which suggests a direct effect on tonic nitric oxide release and decreased endothelin-1 production. Other AT_1 receptor antagonists, such as telmisartan and losartan, did not improve endothelium-dependent vasodilation in hypertensive patients. The potency of angiotensin II receptor blockers to increase nitric oxide bioavailability may be even greater in platelets than in endothelial cells. Indeed, angiotensin II receptor antagonists show antiaggregatory effects on platelets.

D. Calcium Channel Blockers

In addition to particular ACE inhibitors, several calcium channel blocking agents were successful in improving endothelial function in human hypertension (Fig. 7.15 and Table 7.2).

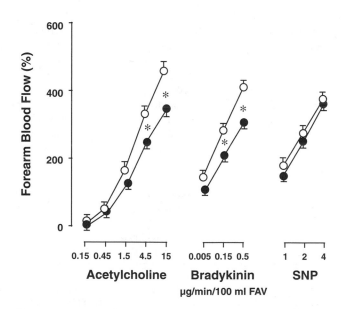

Figure 7.15 Effect of lacidipine, a calcium channel blocker, on endothelial function in hypertensive patients. After chronic treatment with lacidipine, vasodilation response to the endothelium-dependent vasodilators acetylcholine and bradykinin (but not to the endothelium-independent vasodilator sodium nitroprusside) was significantly increased. FAV, forearm volume; SNP, sodium nitroprusside. [Adapted from Taddei et al. (50).]

The antioxidant properties of an antihypertensive drug are important because oxidative stress plays a central role in the pathophysiology of human hypertension. The endothelial function of patients with hypertension is improved by ascorbic acid, an antioxidant vitamin that restores the imbalance of increased nitric oxide decomposition by superoxide anions. Scavenging reactive oxygen species by antioxidants may become an important therapeutic strategy because chronic treatment with vitamin C does, in fact, lower blood pressure in patients with hypertension (40). The beneficial effects of calcium antagonists on endothelial function may not be confined to hypertension. Nifedipine, a dihydropyridine calcium channel blocker, also improves endothelium-dependent vasodilation to acetylcholine in hypercholesterolemics (41). Also, in coronary circulation, calcium antagonists reverse abnormal vasomotion in hypercholesterolemia. In the International Nifedipine Trial on Antiatherosclerotic Therapy (INTACT), angiographic progression of coronary artery disease was retarded by nifedipine (42). However, in patients with coronary artery disease, the calcium antagonist amlodipine did not improve endothelial function.

An increase in intracellular platelet calcium concentration mediated by calcium channels is the primary signal event in platelet activation. Therefore, it is not surprising that calcium channel blockers have been shown to inhibit platelet activation.

E. Endothelin Antagonists and Vasopeptidase Inhibitors

In rats with angiotensin II-induced and chronic nitric-oxide-deficient hypertension, endothelial dysfunction is ameliorated by treatment with an endothelin receptor antagonist. Furthermore, endothelin receptor antagonism prevents vascular hypertrophy in a variety of other experimental models of hypertension. Similarly, treatment with a selective ET_A receptor antagonist attenuates the development of left ventricular hypertrophy in renovascular hypertensive rats. In hypertension and hypercholesterolemia, endothelin antagonism may be superior to endothelin-converting enzyme inhibition because vascular endothelin-converting enzyme activity is inversely correlated to serum LDL levels and blood pressure.

In hypertensive patients, bosentan, a mixed $ET_{A/B}$ receptor antagonist, effectively decreases arterial blood pressure in patients with essential hypertension. This effect is not accompanied by neurohormonal activation, as reflected by a lack of increase in heart rate, plasma catecholamines, plasma renin activity, and plasma angiotensin II levels. Further trials are needed to clarify whether endothelin receptor antagonists offer additional benefits over conventional antihypertensive drugs.

F. Aspirin

There are important interactions between nitric oxide and cyclooxygenase products. Cyclooxygenase-dependent substances (e.g., thromboxane A_2 and prostaglandin H_2) impair nitric oxide bioavailability. Cyclooxygenase is a source of the nitric oxide-scavenger superoxide anions. Aspirin improves the abnormal vasomotion in the forearm of hypertensive and hypercholesterolemic patients. It is most likely that aspirin restores the altered balance between vasoconstrictor and dilator prostanoids that favored vasoconstriction and thrombosis. These findings may explain in part the favorable effects of aspirin in patients with cardiovascular disease.

G. Antioxidant Vitamins

Antioxidants scavenge reactive oxygen species and thereby reduce nitric oxide breakdown. In patients with familial hypercholesterolemia, 5-methyltetrahydrofolate, the active form of folic acid, improves endothelial function both when given acutely and when given chronically. The effects of folic acid supplementation on morbidity and mortality in patients with coronary artery disease are currently tested in large clinical studies.

Vitamin C (ascorbic acid), an antioxidant vitamin, restores endothelial function in patients with hypercholesterolemia or diabetes mellitus and in patients who smoke. In addition, in patients with hypertension, endothelial dysfunction is improved by ascorbic acid, both in the coronary circulation and in the peripheral circulation. Scavenging of reactive oxygen species by antioxidants may become an interesting therapeutic strategy because chronic treatment with vitamin C in fact lowers blood pressure in patients with hypertension. In patients with coronary artery disease, long-term ascorbic acid supplementation also improves endothelial function.

The effects of vitamin E supplementation on endothelial function in patients at risk from or with established atherosclerotic vascular disease are less consistent. The beneficial effects of vitamin E may be confined to subjects with increased exposure to oxidized LDL cholesterol, as is the case for hypercholesterolemics who smoke. Combined vitamin E and simvastatin therapy leads to an improvement in flow-mediated vasodilation of the brachial artery of hypercholesterolemic men that is more pronounced than the improvement with lipid-lowering therapy alone. The results of clinical trials studying the clinical outcome of patients with coronary artery disease administered vitamin E supplementation have been disappointing. Indeed, vitamin E supplementation had no effect on cardiovascular endpoints in the Heart Outcomes Prevention Evaluation (HOPE) study.

H. Tetrahydrobiopterin and L-Arginine

Tetrahydrobiopterin, a cofactor for nitric oxide synthesis by endothelial nitric oxide synthase, ameliorates endothelial dysfunction in hypercholesterolemic patients and smokers. In patients with coronary artery disease, tetrahydrobiopterin restores endothelium-dependent vasodilation to acetylcholine. Experimentally, tetrahydrobiopterin also improves endothelial function in arterial hypertension. In human studies, tetrahydrobiopterin improves endothelium-dependent vasodilation to acetylcholine in patients with arterial hypertension.

L-arginine, the substrate for nitric oxide synthesis, improves endothelium-dependent vasodilation in both the coronary circulation and in the peripheral circulation of patients with hypercholesterolemia. However, L-arginine does not improve endothelial function in diabetic subjects, which indicates that the underlying pathophysiology in subjects with different risk factors calls for differential treatment strategies.

XII. CONCLUSIONS

The vascular endothelium, which synthesizes and releases vasoactive substances, plays a crucial role in the pathogenesis of hypertension. Because of its position between blood pressure level and the smooth muscle cells that are responsible for peripheral resistance, the endothelium is thought to be both victim and offender in arterial hypertension. A clinically important consequence of endothelial dysfunction in patients with arterial hypertension is the generation of a prothrombotic situation. The delicate balance of endothelium-derived factors that is disturbed in hypertension can be restored by specific antihypertensive and antioxidant treatment.

REFERENCES

1. Furchgott RF, Zawadzki JV. The obligatory role of endothelial cells in the relaxation of arterial smooth muscle by acetylcholine. Nature 1980; 288:373–376.
2. Palmer RM, Ashton DS, Moncada S. Vascular endothelial cells synthesize nitric oxide from L-arginine. Nature 1988; 333:664–666.
3. Lüscher TF, Vanhoutte PM. Endothelium-dependent contractions to acetylcholine in the aorta of the spontaneously hypertensive rat. Hypertension 1986; 8:344–348.
4. Nava E, Farre AL, Moreno C, Casado S, Moreau P, Cosentino F, Luscher TF. Alterations to the nitric oxide pathway in the spontaneously hypertensive rat. J Hypertens 1998; 16:609–615.
5. Nava E, Noll G, Lüscher TF. Increased activity of constitutive nitric oxide synthase in cardiac endothelium in spontaneous hypertension. Circulation 1995; 91:2310–2313.
6. McIntyre M, Hamilton CA, Rees DD, Reid JL, Dominiczak AF. Sex differences in the abundance of endothelial nitric oxide in a model of genetic hypertension. Hypertension 1997; 30:1517–1524.
7. Tschudi MR, Mesaros S, Luscher TF, Malinski T. Direct in situ measurement of nitric oxide in mesenteric resistance arteries. Increased decomposition by superoxide in hypertension. Hypertension 1996; 27:32–35.
8. Linder L, Kiowski W, Bühler FR, Lüscher TF. Indirect evidence for release of endothelium-derived relaxing factor in human forearm circulation in vivo. Blunted response in essential hypertension. Circulation 1990; 81:1762–1767.
9. Panza JA, Quyyumi AA, Brush JJ, Epstein SE. Abnormal endothelium-dependent vascular relaxation in patients with essential hypertension. N Engl J Med 1990; 323:22–27.
10. Treasure CB, Klein JL, Vita JA, Manoukian SV, Renwick GH, Selwyn AP, Ganz P, Alexander RW. Hypertension and left ventricular hypertrophy are associated with impaired endothelium-mediated relaxation in human coronary resistance vessels. Circulation 1993; 87:86–93.
11. Anderson TJ, Uehata A, Gerhard MD, Meredith IT, Knab S, Delagrage D, Lieberman EH, Ganz P, Creager MA, Yeung AC, Selwyn AP. Close relation of endothelial function in the human coronary and peripheral circulation. J Am Coll Cardiol 1995; 26:1235–1241.
12. Calver A, Collier J, Moncada S, Vallance P. Effect of local intra-arterial NG-monomethyl-L-arginine in patients with hypertension: the nitric oxide dilator mechanism appears abnormal. J Hypertens 1992; 10:1025–1031.
13. Forte P, Copland M, Smith LM, Milne E, Sutherland J, Benjamin N. Basal nitric oxide synthesis in essential hypertension. Lancet 1997; 349:837–842.
14. Taddei S, Virdis A, Mattei P, Arzilli F, Salvetti A. Endothelium-dependent forearm vasodilation is reduced in normotensive subjects with familial history of hypertension. J Cardiovasc Pharmacol 1992; 20:S193–S195.
15. McAllister AS, Atkinson AB, Johnston GD, Hadden DR, Bell PM, McCance DR. Basal nitric oxide production is impaired in offspring of patients with essential hypertension. Clin Sci (Colch) 1999; 97:141–147.
16. Oemar BS, Tschudi MR, Godoy N, Brovkovich V, Malinski T, Luscher TF. Reduced endothelial nitric oxide synthase expression and production in human atherosclerosis. Circulation 1998; 97:2494–2498.
17. Lerman A, Edwards BS, Hallett JW, Heublein DM, Sandberg SM, Burnett JJ. Circulating and tissue endothelin immunoreactivity in advanced atherosclerosis. N Engl J Med 1991; 325:997–1001.
18. Rossi GP, Colonna S, Pavan E, Albertin G, Della Rocca F, Gerosa G, Casarotto D, Sartore S, Pauletto P, Pessina AC. Endothelin-1 and its mRNA in the wall layers of human arteries ex vivo. Circulation 1999; 99:1147–1155.
19. Rubanyi GM, Vanhoutte PM. Superoxide anions and hyperoxia inactivate endothelium-derived relaxing factor. Am J Physiol 1986; 250:H822–H827.
20. Katusic ZS, Vanhoutte PM. Superoxide anion is an endothelium-derived contracting factor. Am J Physiol 1989; 257:H33–H37.

21. Morrison RA, McGrath A, Davidson G, Brown JJ, Murray GD, Lever AF. Low blood pressure in Down's syndrome, a link with Alzheimer's disease? Hypertension 1996; 28:569–575.

22. Moreau P, d'Uscio LV, Shaw S, Takase H, Barton M, Luscher TF. Angiotensin II increases tissue endothelin and induces vascular hypertrophy: reversal by ET(A)-receptor antagonist. Circulation 1997; 96:1593–1597.

23. Moncada S, Gryglewski R, Bunting S, Vane JR. An enzyme isolated from arteries transforms prostaglandin endoperoxides to an unstable substance that inhibits platelet aggregation. Nature 1976; 263:663–635.

24. Joannides R, Haefeli WE, Linder L, Richard V, Bakkali EH, Thuillez C, Lüscher TF. Nitric oxide is responsible for flow-dependent dilatation of human peripheral conduit arteries in vivo. Circulation 1995; 91:1314–1319.

25. Yanagisawa M, Kurihara H, Kimura S, Tomobe Y, Kobayashi M, Mitsui Y, Yazaki Y, Goto K, Masaki T. A novel potent vasoconstrictor peptide produced by vascular endothelial cells. Nature 1988; 332:411–415.

26. Hickey KA, Rubanyi G, Paul RJ, Highsmith RF. Characterization of a coronary vasoconstrictor produced by cultured endothelial cells. Am J Physiol 1985; 248:C550–C556.

27. Vierhapper H, Wagner O, Nowotny P, Waldhausl W. Effect of endothelin-1 in man. Circulation 1990; 81:1415–1418.

28. Ito H, Hirata Y, Hiroe M, Tsujino M, Adachi S, Takamoto T, Nitta M, Taniguchi K, Marumo F. Endothelin-1 induces hypertrophy with enhanced expression of muscle specific genes in cultured neonatal rat cardiomyocytes. Circ Res 1991; 69:209–215.

29. Saito Y, Nakao K, Mukoyama M, Imura H. Increased plasma endothelin level in patients with essential hypertension [letter]. N Engl J Med 1990; 322:205.

30. Spieker LE, Corti R, Binggeli C, Luscher TF, Noll G. Baroreceptor dysfunction induced by nitric oxide synthase inhibition in humans. J Am Coll Cardiol 2000; 36:213–218.

31. Yang Z, Arnet U, Bauer E, von Segesser L, Siebenmann R, Turina M, Lüscher TF. Thrombin-induced endothelium-dependent inhibition and direct activation of platelet-vessel wall interaction. Role of prostacyclin, nitric oxide, and thromboxane A2. Circulation 1994; 89:2266–2272.

32. Henn V, Slupsky JR, Grafe M, Anagnostopoulos I, Forster R, Muller-Berghaus G, Kroczek RA. CD40 ligand on activated platelets triggers an inflammatory reaction of endothelial cells. Nature 1998; 391:591–594.

33. Ruggeri ZM. Platelets in atherothrombosis. Nat Med 2002; 8:1227–1234.

34. Lip GY, Blann AD. Does hypertension confer a prothrombotic state? Virchow's triad revisited. Circulation 2000; 101:218–220.

35. Erne P, Bolli P, Burgisser E, Buhler FR. Correlation of platelet calcium with blood pressure. Effect of antihypertensive therapy. N Engl J Med 1984; 310:1084–1088.

36. Lip GY. Target organ damage and the prothrombotic state in hypertension. Hypertension 2000; 36:975–977.

37. Mancini GB, Henry GC, Macaya C, O'Neill BJ, Pucillo AL, Carere RG, Wargovich TJ, Mudra H, Luscher TF, Klibaner MI, Haber HE, Uprichard AC, Pepine CJ, Pitt B. Angiotensin-converting enzyme inhibition with quinapril improves endothelial vasomotor dysfunction in patients with coronary artery disease. The TREND (Trial on Reversing ENdothelial Dysfunction) Study [published erratum appears in Circulation 1996; 94:1490]. Circulation 1996; 94:258–265.

38. Anderson TJ, Elstein E, Haber H, Charbonneau F. Comparative study of ACE-inhibition, angiotensin II antagonism, and calcium channel blockade on flow-mediated vasodilation in patients with coronary disease (BANFF study). J Am Coll Cardiol 2000; 35:60–66.

39. Ghiadoni L, Virdis A, Magagna A, Taddei S, Salvetti A. Effect of the angiotensin II type 1 receptor blocker candesartan on endothelial function in patients with essential hypertension. Hypertension 2000; 35:501–506.

40. Duffy SJ, Gokce N, Holbrook M, Huang A, Frei B, Keaney JFJ, Vita JA. Treatment of hypertension with ascorbic acid. Lancet 1999; 354.

41. Verhaar MC, Honing ML, van Dam T, Zwart M, Koomans HA, Kastelein JJ, Rabelink TJ. Nifedipine improves endothelial function in hypercholesterolemia, independently of an effect on blood pressure or plasma lipids. Cardiovasc Res 1999; 42:752–760.

42. Lichtlen PR, Hugenholtz PG, Rafflenbeul W, Hecker H, Jost S, Deckers JW. Retardation of angiographic progression of coronary artery disease by nifedipine. Results of the International Nifedipine Trial on Antiatherosclerotic Therapy (INTACT). INTACT Group Investigators. Lancet 1990; 335:1109–1113.

43. Spieker LE, Noll G, Ruschitzka FT, Maier W, Luscher TF. Working under pressure: the vascular endothelium in arterial hypertension. J Hum Hypertens 2000; 14:617–630.

44. Lüscher TF, Noll G. Endothelium-derived vasoactive substances. In: Braunwald E, ed. Heart Disease. 5th ed. Philadelphia: W.B. Saunders Company, 1997:1165.

45. Spieker LE, Noll G, Ruschitzka FT, Luscher TF. Endothelin receptor antagonists in congestive heart failure: a new therapeutic principle for the future? J Am Coll Cardiol 2001; 37:1493–1505.

46. Cardillo C, Kilcoyne CM, Waclawiw M, Cannon RO 3III, Panza JA. Role of endothelin in the increased vascular tone of patients with essential hypertension. Hypertension 1999; 33:753–758.

47. Yang ZH, Richard V, von Segesser L, Bauer E, Stulz P, Turina M, Luscher TF. Threshold concentrations of endothelin-1 potentiate contractions to norepinephrine and serotonin in human arteries. A new mechanism of vasospasm? Circulation 1990; 82:188–195.

48. Frielingsdorf J, Seiler C, Kaufmann P, Vassalli G, Suter T, Hess OM. Normalization of abnormal coronary vasomotion by calcium antagonists in patients with hypertension. Circulation 1996; 93:1380–1387.

49. Cockcroft JR, Chowienczyk PJ, Brett SE, Chen CP, Dupont AG, Van Nueten L, Wooding SJ, Ritter JM. Nebivolol vasodilates human forearm vasculature: evidence for an L-arginine/NO-dependent mechanism. J Pharmacol Exp Ther 1995; 274:1067–1071.

50. Taddei S, Virdis A, Ghiadoni L, Uleri S, Magagna A, Salvetti A. Lacidipine restores endothelium-dependent vasodilation in essential hypertensive patients. Hypertension 1997; 30:1606–1612.

8

Regulation of Fluid and Electrolyte Balance in Hypertension: Role of Hormones and Peptides

JOHN E. HALL, JOEY P. GRANGER

University of Mississippi Medical Center, Jackson, Mississippi, USA

KEYPOINTS

- A complex array of natriuretic and antinatriuretic hormones interacts with intrarenal mechanisms to control body fluid, electrolyte balance and arterial pressure.

- Long-term control of arterial pressure by hormones is closely linked to their effects on excretion of water, electrolytes and renal pressure natriuresis.

- In all forms of chronic hypertension, renal pressure natriuresis is reset to higher blood pressures, and sodium excretion matches sodium intake despite increased arterial pressure.

- Although the causes of impaired pressure natriuresis in essential hypertension is not completely understood, abnormal hormonal control of renal hemodynamics and tubular reabsorption play an important role in many cases.

SUMMARY

Long-term blood pressure control is closely intertwined with body fluid and electrolyte balances which, in turn, are regulated by a complex array of neurohumoral and intrarenal mechanisms. A common pathway for long-term hormonal blood pressure control is by altering renal-pressure natriuresis. In all forms of chronic hypertension, including human essential hypertension, renal-pressure natriuresis is reset to higher blood pressures so that sodium excretion is the same as in normotension despite increased blood pressure. Considerable evidence indicates that resetting of pressure natriuresis plays a key role in causing hypertension, rather than merely occurring as an adaptation to increased blood pressure. In this chapter, we discuss the multiple hormones that influence long-term blood pressure regulation through their effects on renal-pressure natriuresis and regulation of body fluid volumes.

I. INTRODUCTION

The maintenance of a stable volume and electrolyte composition of the extracellular fluid is absolutely essential for normal cell function and overall homeostasis. Although body fluid volume is determined by the balance between intakes and outputs of salt and water, intakes are highly variable and governed largely by dietary habits in most people. Therefore, the burden of regulating the volume and composition of the extracellular fluid usually falls on the kidneys which must rapidly adapt their excretion to precisely match intake and output of salt and water under steady-state conditions. This remarkable feat is achieved with a complex array of intrarenal mechanisms as well as systemic hemodynamic and neurohumoral changes that influence glomerular filtration and tubular reabsorption of salt and water.

A key principle in understanding long-term control of body fluid volumes and blood pressure is that there must always be a precise balance between the intake and output of fluid and electrolytes under steady-state conditions regardless of whether a person has normal or elevated blood pressure. This balance can sometimes be achieved mainly by intrarenal and hormonal changes that alter renal excretion, with minimal changes in extracellular fluid volume or systemic hemodynamics. When kidney function is markedly impaired or when the various neurohumoral mechanisms malfunction, systemic hemodynamic adjustments, such as changes in blood pressure, often must be invoked to help re-establish salt and water balance.

In this chapter, we discuss the renal-body fluid feedback, one of the most powerful systems for controlling arterial pressure and maintaining fluid balance, and its interactions with multiple hormonal and intrarenal factors.

II. LONG-TERM CONTROL OF ARTERIAL PRESSURE BY RENAL-BODY FLUID FEEDBACK SYSTEM

Because arterial pressure is the product of cardiac output and total peripheral resistance, it is easy to overlook the role of renal excretory function in regulating arterial pressure and to focus on factors that directly affect vascular and cardiac function in considering mechanisms of hypertension. However, hypertension is a disturbance of long-term blood pressure control and is closely intertwined with regulation of extracellular fluid volume, which is determined by the balance between fluid intake and renal excretion. Even temporary imbalances between fluid intake and output can alter extracellular fluid volume, cardiac output, and eventually peripheral vascular resistance via autoregulatory mechanisms (1–3).

To maintain life, there must be a precise balance between fluid intake and output in the steady-state, a task that is performed by multiple systems that regulate renal excretion in response to changes in intake. In fact, it is more critical for the body to maintain fluid balance than a normal level of arterial pressure. Therefore, chronic increase in blood pressure often serves as a compensatory mechanism to increase renal excretion and re-establish electrolyte and fluid balance in the face of impaired kidney function.

A. Pressure Natriuresis as a Key Component of the Renal-Body Fluid Feedback

The term *pressure natriuresis* refers to the effect of the increased arterial pressure to raise renal sodium excretion. This effect is especially potent with chronic changes in arterial pressure so that sustained increases in arterial pressure of only a few mmHg can evoke large increases in sodium excretion, as long as kidney function is not impaired (1,2,4,5). One of the main reasons that the chronic pressure natriuresis mechanism is so potent is that it is modulated by the various hormonal systems.

Renal-pressure natriuresis is a key component of a feedback system that normally stabilizes arterial pressure and body fluid volumes (Fig. 8.1). For example, a disturbance that tends to elevate arterial pressure, such as an

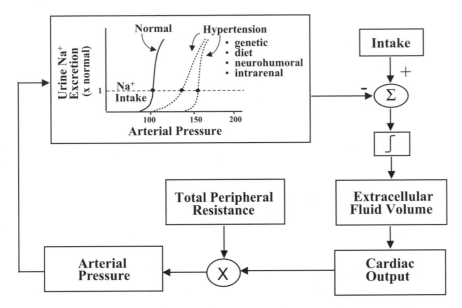

Figure 8.1 Renal-body fluid feedback mechanism for long-term regulation of arterial pressure and body fluid volumes.

increase in peripheral vascular resistance, will provoke an increase in sodium and water excretion via pressure natriuresis, if kidney function is not impaired. As long as renal excretion exceeds fluid intake, extracellular fluid volume will continue to decrease, reducing venous return and cardiac output until blood pressure returns to normal and fluid intake and output are balanced once again. The opposite occurs when blood pressure decreases.

B. Resetting of Renal-Pressure Natriuresis in Hypertension

A key feature of the renal-pressure natriuresis mechanism is that it has an infinite feedback gain, which means that it continues to operate until arterial pressure returns to the initial set-point (1). Therefore, as long as pressure natriuresis is unaltered, any disturbance that tends to increase arterial pressure, such as an increase in total peripheral vascular resistance, will be counteracted by increased sodium excretion and decreased extracellular fluid volume. For sodium balance to be maintained in the face of sustained hypertension, there must be a concomitant shift of pressure natriuresis to higher blood pressures.

Although renal-pressure natriuresis is clearly reset in all forms of hypertension, the precise causes of impaired kidney function have remained elusive, especially for human essential hypertension. Measurements of many indices of kidney function, such as serum creatinine, glomerular filtration rate, or renal blood flow, after hypertension is established, or even during the slow insidious development of hypertension, often do not reveal major abnormalities. The reason for this is that these

measurements represent a summation of the pathophysiological processes that cause hypertension and compensatory mechanisms that alter renal function and usually restore fluid balance to nearly normal. In some patients with essential hypertension, certain indices of kidney function, such as renal plasma flow and glomerular filtration rate, are actually increased, suggesting that the impairment of pressure natriuresis may be due primarily to increased renal tubular reabsorption rather than renal vasoconstriction. In other patients, glomerular filtration rate and renal plasma flow may be normal or reduced. It therefore seems likely that multiple aberrations of renal function may contribute to impaired pressure natriuresis in different patients with essential hypertension. The one measure of renal function, however, that is impaired in all patients with hypertension is renal-pressure natriuresis.

An important characteristic of renal-pressure natriuresis in normotensive and hypertensive subjects is that it is modulated by multiple neurohumoral systems that control renal hemodynamics and tubular reabsorption. It is through these effects that the various hormone systems have their most important effects on long-term blood pressure regulation. The rest of this chapter will, therefore, be devoted to some of the hormone systems that have a major influence on renal-pressure natriuresis and long-term blood pressure regulation.

III. RENIN–ANGIOTENSIN SYSTEM

The renin–angiotensin system is perhaps the body's most powerful hormone system for regulating body fluid volumes and arterial pressure. Angiotensin II, the major active component of this system, is a potent vasoconstrictor but its long-term effects on arterial pressure are closely related to its direct and indirect effects on the kidneys (6–9).

Figure 8.2 shows the powerful influence of angiotensin II on long-term renal-pressure natriuresis. When the renin–angiotensin system is fully functional, the chronic relationship between arterial pressure and sodium excretion is extremely steep, so that minimal changes in arterial pressure are needed to maintain sodium balance over a wide range of sodium intakes (10). A major reason for the steepness of the normal pressure natriuresis curve is that angiotensin II levels are suppressed when sodium intake is raised and, conversely, angiotensin II levels are increased when sodium intake is restricted. These changes in angiotensin II, in turn, alter renal hemodynamics and tubular sodium reabsorption, helping to adjust renal sodium excretion appropriately during changes in sodium intake without the need to invoke large changes in arterial pressure to maintain sodium balance. In other words, when the renin–angiotensin system is functioning normally, blood pressure is relatively salt-insensitive in most cases.

If the renin–angiotensin system cannot respond effectively to changes in salt intake, either because of a very low, fixed angiotensin II or because of a high, fixed angiotensin II, blood pressure becomes very salt-sensitive. For example, if angiotensin II is infused at a low rate, which initially has no major blood pressure effect, but it prevents angiotensin II levels from being suppressed, this impairs pressure natriuresis, thereby necessitating greater

increases in arterial pressure to maintain sodium balance when salt intake is raised (10). Blockade of angiotensin II formation, with angiotensin II receptor antagonists or angiotensin-converting enzyme (ACE) inhibitors also makes blood pressure very salt-sensitive, although it increases renal excretory capability so that sodium balance can be maintained at lower blood pressures (9,10).

Thus, the inability to suppress angiotensin II formation greatly attenuates the effectiveness of pressure natriuresis and causes blood pressure level to be very salt-sensitive. This is true whether angiotensin II levels are inappropriately elevated or whether they are inappropriately reduced; in either case, the inability to decrease angiotensin II formation as salt intake is increased causes blood pressure to increase as salt intake is raised and to decrease as salt intake is reduced below normal. However, inappropriately high levels of angiotensin II obviously cause blood pressure to be regulated at an elevated level.

The extreme importance of the interrelationships between arterial pressure, sodium excretion, and angiotensin II can be illustrated if renal perfusion pressure is servo-controlled to prevent pressure natriuresis during chronic angiotensin II hypertension. Infusion of angiotensin II normally usually causes a transient decrease in sodium excretion lasting for 1–2 days, followed by a rapid return of sodium excretion to normal (11). This is similar to the "escape" from sodium retention associated with mineralocorticoid excess (12). However, when renal perfusion pressure was servo-controlled at the normal pressure

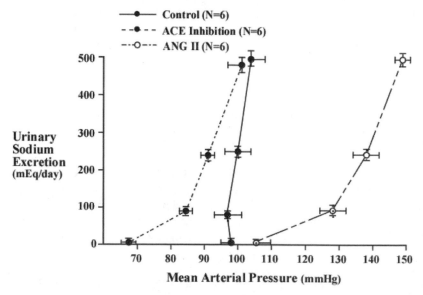

Figure 8.2 Steady-state relationships between arterial pressure and sodium intake and excretion. Sodium intake and excretion is shown under normal conditions with a functional renin–angiotensin system, after blockade of angiotensin II formation with an ACE inhibitor, and after angiotensin II infusion at a low dose to prevent angiotensin II levels from being suppressed when sodium intake is increased. The numbers in parentheses are estimated angiotensin II levels expressed as times normal. [Adapted from Hall et al. (10).]

during angiotensin II hypertension, escape from sodium retention did not occur and cumulative sodium balance continued to increase until symptoms of pulmonary edema developed after only a few days (Fig. 8.3) (11).

We also found similar results in other models of hypertension caused by chronic infusion of antinatriuretic or antidiuretic hormones, such as aldosterone, vasopressin, norepinephrine, and adrenocorticotrophic hormones (ACTH) (2,13). In each case, pressure natriuresis played a dominant role in maintaining sodium and water balance when excretory function of the kidneys was impaired by excessive levels of antinatriuretic hormones.

A. Renal Hemodynamic Actions of Angiotensin II

The sodium-retaining effect of angiotensin II and its modulation of pressure natriuresis could occur as a result of decreased glomerular filtration rate or increased tubular reabsorption. However, considerable evidence indicates that physiologic levels of angiotensin II, such as those that occur when the renin–angiotensin system is

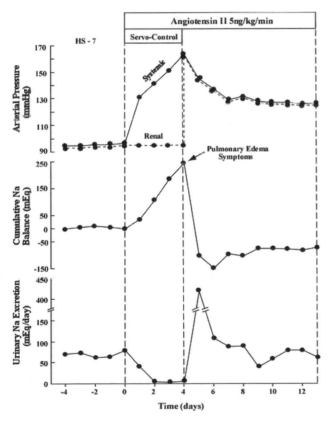

Figure 8.3 Effects of angiotensin II infusion. Effects of infusion in a dog in which renal perfusion pressure was servo-controlled at a normal level. After 4 days, severe sodium and water retention resulted in pulmonary edema. [Adapted from Hall et al. (11).]

activated by sodium depletion or renal artery stenosis, do not usually reduce glomerular filtration rate, but rather increase tubular reabsorption and help to prevent decreases in glomerular filtration rate (8,9).

1. Angiotensin II-Mediated Constriction of Efferent Arterioles

Activation of the renin–angiotensin system usually occurs as a *compensation* for conditions associated with decreased arterial pressure and underperfusion of the kidney, such as severe sodium depletion, renal artery stenosis, or congestive heart failure. In these instances, blockade of intrarenal or circulating angiotensin II, by infusion of angiotensin II antagonists or ACE inhibitors, may reduce glomerular filtration rate even though renal blood flow is preserved (6,9). The impairment of glomerular filtration rate (glomerular filtration rate) caused by angiotensin II blockade in these situations appears to be related to inhibition of the constrictor effects of angiotensin II on efferent arterioles as well as the reduced blood pressure.

The renin–angiotensin system usually works cooperatively with other autoregulatory mechanisms, such as tubuloglomerular feedback and myogenic activity, to maintain a relatively constant glomerular filtration rate during reduced perfusion of the kidney. The effect of angiotensin II appears to be the most important when renal perfusion pressure is reduced to very low levels, near the limits of autoregulation, or when other disturbances such as sodium depletion are superimposed on low renal perfusion pressure (6,9). The importance of the angiotensin II constrictor effect on efferent arterioles becomes especially important in patients with bilateral renal artery stenosis or stenosis of a solitary kidney; in these cases, ACE inhibition or angiotensin II blockade may cause severe decreases in glomerular filtration rate (14,15). The vasoconstrictor effect of angiotensin II on efferent arterioles also helps to prevent decreases in glomerular filtration rate during congestive heart failure, Bartter's syndrome, severe sodium depletion, or when high plasma protein concentration is reduced because of cirrhosis or hypoalbuminemia [see Refs. (6,9) for review].

By stabilizing glomerular filtration rate, the constrictor effect of angiotensin II on efferent arterioles helps to maintain normal excretion of metabolic waste products that depend primarily upon glomerular filtration rate for their renal clearance. At the same time, angiotensin II causes sodium and water retention through multiple mechanisms that increase renal tubular reabsorption.

2. Increased Angiotensin II Exacerbates Glomerular Injury in Overperfused Kidneys

Although blockade of the constrictor action of angiotensin II on efferent arterioles can cause a further decline in glomerular filtration rate in underperfused nephrons, renin–

angiotensin system blockade is beneficial when the kidneys are overperfused and angiotensin II formation is not appropriately suppressed, as occurs in diabetes mellitus and in certain forms of hypertension that lead to progressive glomerulosclerosis. In these instances, renin–angiotensin system blockade reduces efferent arteriolar resistance as well as arterial pressure, and therefore lowers glomerular hydrostatic pressure and wall stress in the overperfused and overstretched glomerular capillaries. Experimental and clinical studies suggest that renin–angiotensin system blockers may be more effective than other antihypertensive agents in preventing glomerular injury and in slowing the progression of renal disease probably due, at least in part, to greater reductions in glomerular hydrostatic pressure (16,18).

3. Does Angiotensin II Cause Renal Injury via Nonhemodynamic Effects?

There is little doubt that renin–angiotensin system blockade, with ACE inhibitors or angiotensin II receptor antagonists, can slow progression of renal disease in patients with diabetes and hypertension. What has been less clear is whether the deleterious renal effects of excessive renin–angiotensin system activation are mainly due to direct tissue specific actions of angiotensin II or to hemodynamic effects of angiotensin II, including increased blood pressure and efferent arteriolar constriction, which both raise glomerular hydrostatic pressure.

Physiological studies do not support the concept that moderate increases in angiotensin II, in the absence of increased arterial pressure, promote renal injury. For example, activation of the renin–angiotensin system by sodium depletion does not cause renal injury. Also, there does not appear to be any evidence of glomerular injury in the clipped kidney of the 2-kidney, 1-clip model of Goldblatt hypertension, which is chronically exposed to very high levels of angiotensin II but protected from increased arterial pressure by the clip on the renal artery (19). In contrast, the unclipped kidney which is exposed to high blood pressure and only moderate increases in angiotensin II has severe renal injury (19).

The belief that angiotensin II contributes to target organ damage by directly promoting tissue fibrosis is largely based on two main lines of evidence: (1) In vitro studies have shown that angiotensin II can directly cause vascular hypertrophy and increase collagen formation in various tissues, including mesangial cells; (2) Some experimental studies suggest that renin–angiotensin system blockade may reduce renal injury and proteinuria through mechanisms that are independent of reductions in blood pressure (20). Most in vitro studies, however, are limited because of the high concentrations of angiotensin II (often 10^{-6} moles/L or higher) needed to produce tissue fibrosis.

Many of the in vivo experimental studies are complicated by the fact that blood pressure has usually been measured intermittently with indirect methods. Studies in rats in which blood pressure was measured directly by radio-telemetry, 24 h/day, suggest that reductions in blood pressure may be primarily responsible for the renal protection associated with renin–angiotensin system blockade (21).

Clinical trials in both diabetic and nondiabetic nephropathy have shown some benefit of renin–angiotensin system blockade, compared with other antihypertensive therapies, in slowing progression of renal disease. However, most of these studies have not assessed blood pressure throughout the day to determine accurately the hemodynamic load on the kidneys. Results from two major clinical trials, the Reduction of Endpoints in NIDDM with the Angiotensin II Antagonist Losartan (RENAAL) and Irbesartan Diabetic Nephropathy (IDNT), illustrate the limitations of the usual approach in assessing the role of blood pressure in renal disease (17,22). Patients with diabetic nephropathy who were treated with angiotensin receptor antagonists had a decline in glomerular filtration rate of ∼5 mL/min per year, whereas diabetic patients treated with other antihypertensive drugs had a decline in glomerular filtration of ∼6 mL/min per year. Because the usual rate of decline in glomerular filtration rate in patients with diabetic nephropathy and untreated hypertension is ∼12 mL/min per year, all antihypertensive therapies that effectively lowered blood pressure appear to protect the kidneys (23). The further glomerular filtration rate protection of 1 mL/min per year observed with angiotensin II receptor blockade, compared to other therapies, was modest and might be explained by the slightly greater reductions in blood pressure observed in this group (23). Therefore, results from clinical trials and from animal studies in which very accurate measurements of arterial pressure have been made, 24 h/day, suggest that reductions in systemic arterial pressure and glomerular hydrostatic pressure may explain most, if not all, of the beneficial renal effects of renin–angiotensin system blockade.

4. Effects of Inability to Suppress Angiotensin II Formation in Overperfused Kidneys

We have already noted that the lack of an appropriate reduction in angiotensin II formation may cause salt-sensitive hypertension as well as increased glomerular pressure which itself tends to cause renal injury. The glomerulus initially responds to increased pressure and wall stress with mesangial cell proliferation and increased collagen which helps to prevent the glomerular capillaries from being overstretched. Over the long-term, however, the continued structural fortification impinges on the lumen of the capillary and, along with increased thickening of basement membranes, eventually causes loss of glomerular capillary function if the increased capillary wall stress is not relieved by reduction of glomerular pressure.

The loss of glomerular capillary function tends to cause sodium and water retention and further impairment of pressure natriuresis, causing additional increase in blood pressure. Although higher blood pressure serves the immediate need of restoring sodium balance, it also causes further glomerular injury. Thus, glomerular over-perfusion, especially in the presence of increased levels of angiotensin II and systemic hypertension, may initiate a slow insidious cycle that causes more and more nephron loss, a greater shift of pressure natriuresis, and higher and higher blood pressures that are needed to maintain sodium and water balance (8) (Fig. 8.4). Blockade of the renin–angiotensin system can break this cycle not only by lowering arterial pressure, but also by reducing efferent arteriolar resistance that lowers glomerular capillary hydrostatic pressure and wall stress.

B. Angiotensin II Promotion of Sodium Reabsorption

The antinatriuretic actions of angiotensin II are mediated mainly by increased renal tubular reabsorption, except in pathophysiological conditions in which angiotensin II contributes to progressive glomerulosclerosis and loss of nephron function.

Angiotensin II increases tubular sodium reabsorption by intrarenal as well as extrarenal effects, such as stimulation of aldosterone (8,9). The direct intrarenal actions

of angiotensin II occur at very low concentrations, considerably below those needed for extrarenal effects such as peripheral vasoconstriction. For example, angiotensin II constricts isolated efferent arterioles at concentrations as low as 10^{-12} M, whereas peripheral arterioles are much less sensitive to angiotensin II (6,9). angiotensin II also directly increases tubular transport at concentrations as low as 10^{-13} M (24,25). Thus, two intrarenal effects of angiotensin II that occur at very low concentrations and that contribute to sodium and water retention include constriction of efferent arterioles and direct stimulation of tubular sodium transport.

1. Altered Peritubular Capillary Dynamics and Medullary Blood Flow

Angiotensin II-mediated constriction of efferent arterioles reduces renal blood flow and peritubular capillary hydrostatic pressure, while raising peritubular colloid osmotic pressure as a result of increased filtration fraction (8,9). These changes reduce renal interstitial fluid hydrostatic pressure (RIHP) and raise interstitial fluid colloid osmotic pressure, thereby increasing the driving force for fluid reabsorption across the tubular epithelium and by diminishing backleak of sodium actively transported into the intercellular spaces (8,9).

Angiotensin II-mediated reductions in renal medullary blood flow, either as a result of efferent arteriolar constriction or direct effects on the vasa recta contractile elements, may also contribute to increased reabsorption in the loop of Henle and collecting ducts (8,9). Thus, there are several potential mechanisms by which subtle changes in renal hemodynamics, with little or no change in glomerular filtration rate and filtered sodium load, could enhance sodium reabsorption.

2. Increased Proximal Tubular Sodium Reabsorption

Multiple studies indicate that angiotensin II, at very low, physiologic concentrations of angiotensin II (10^{-13}– 10^{-10} M), directly increases proximal tubular reabsorption (8,24,25). On the luminal membrane of the proximal tubule, angiotensin II stimulates hydrogen ion secretion and sodium bicarbonate reabsorption via activation of the sodium–hydrogen antiporter (26) (Fig. 8.5). On the basolateral membrane, angiotensin II stimulates sodium–potassium ATPase activity as well as sodium bicarbonate co-transport (27,28). At least part of the stimulatory effect of angiotensin II on proximal sodium transport appears to be coupled to inhibition of the adenylyl cyclase and increased phospholipase C activity (26,29). Thus, angiotensin II, at physiologic concentrations, increases proximal reabsorption by multiple mechanisms that enhance sodium entry into the epithelial cells as well as sodium extrusion

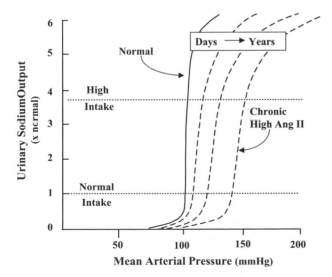

Figure 8.4 Postulated effect of inappropriately increased angiotensin II. Figure illustrates possible chronic effects of greater increases in angiotensin II on pressure natriuresis, shifting it to higher and higher arterial pressures.

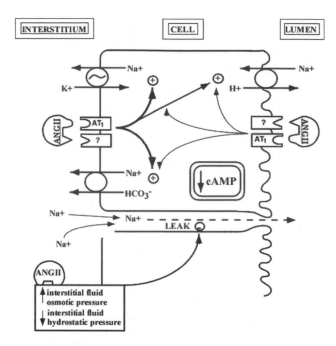

Figure 8.5 Increased proximal tubular reabsorption through action by angiotensin II. Angiotensin II binds to receptors in the luminal and basolateral membranes and stimulates the Na^+/H^+ antiporter, Na^+/HCO_3^- co-transport, and Na^+/K^+ ATPase activity. Angiotensin II also increases reabsorption by increasing interstitial fluid colloid osmotic pressure and by decreasing interstitial fluid hydrostatic pressure.

into the interstitial fluid and then into the peritubular capillaries.

3. Increased Sodium Reabsorption in Distal Parts of the Nephron

Specific binding of angiotensin II has been demonstrated at almost all sites along the distal nephron, including the thick ascending loop of Henle, distal convoluted tubule, and cortical and medullary collecting tubules (30,31). Autoradiographic studies also indicate a high level of angiotensin II binding in the renal medulla.

Whole kidney studies, using the lithium clearance technique suggest that physiological concentrations of angiotensin II increase reabsorption in the distal nephron, although this method does not allow assessment of specific sites at which angiotensin II may increase reabsorption (8,9). *In vivo* microperfusion studies indicate that angiotensin II, at physiological concentrations, increases bicarbonate reabsorption in the loop of Henle (32). Also, angiotensin II stimulates sodium–potassium-2 chloride transport in the medullary thick ascending loop of Henle (33). Angiotensin II also stimulates amiloride-sensitive sodium channels in the initial part of the collecting tubule (34). In sodium chloride-restricted rats administration of

an angiotensin receptor antagonist markedly decreased the abundance of the alpha-subunit of the epithelial sodium channel, which suggests that angiotensin II regulates epithelial sodium channel abundance and collecting duct function (35).

One of the strongest pieces of evidence suggesting that angiotensin II has powerful effects on distal sodium reabsorption is the fact that angiotensin II is capable of reducing sodium excretion to virtually zero without decreases in glomerular filtration rate. Thus, angiotensin II increases sodium reabsorption at multiple sites, including the distal parts of the nephron, where final processing of the urine takes place.

4. Increased Macula Densa Feedback Sensitivity

One distal tubular site that is particularly important in determining the final urinary excretion of sodium chloride is the macula densa. The macula densa is a crucial component of tubuloglomerular feedback that operates as follows: when there is an increase in sodium chloride delivery to the macula densa, this causes (through mechanisms that have not been fully elucidated) constriction of afferent arterioles, which reduces glomerular hydrostatic pressure and glomerular filtration rate, thereby helping to return macula densa sodium chloride delivery toward normal (36). The signal sensed by the macula densa appears to be closely related to sodium chloride transport by these cells rather than tubular fluid sodium chloride delivery or concentration *per se* because inhibition of sodium chloride reabsorption in the loop of Henle dissociates distal tubular sodium chloride concentration and tubuloglomerular feedback (36,37).

There are angiotensin II AT_1 binding receptors on macula densa cells and multiple studies have demonstrated that angiotensin II increases tubuloglomerular feedback sensitivity (31,36,37). It is unlikely that angiotensin II influences tubuloglomerular feedback by directly increasing afferent arteriolar tone because other vasoconstrictors, such as norepinephrine, which have even greater effects on afferent arterioles, do not markedly enhance tubuloglomerular feedback sensitivity. On the basis of experimental studies and results of mathematical modeling of renal hemodynamics and the renin–angiotensin system, we suggested almost 20 years ago that angiotensin II increases tubuloglomerular feedback sensitivity by stimulating macula densa sodium chloride transport (9,38) (Fig. 8.6). Bell and co-workers (39,40), using isolated, perfused macula densa preparations, have more recently shown that angiotensin II directly stimulates Na^+—H^+ exchange as well as Na^+—$2Cl^-$—K^+ co-transport in the apical membrane of macula densa cells. Thus, angiotensin II stimulated sodium chloride transport by the macula densa shifts the relationship between the distal sodium

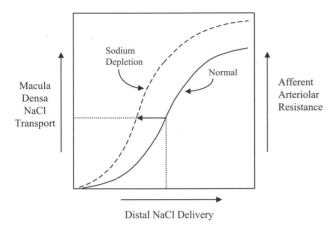

Figure 8.6 Postulated relationships among macula densa sodium chloride delivery, macula densa sodium chloride transport, and afferent arteriolar resistance. Relationships illustrated for normal conditions and for conditions when angiotensin II levels are increased by sodium depletion.

chloride delivery and the macula densa transport, thereby increasing tubuloglomerular feedback sensitivity; for any given level of sodium delivery, a greater rate of transport and a greater degree of afferent arteriolar constriction would occur in the presence of increased angiotensin II (8,9).

From a physiological point of view, a stimulatory effect of angiotensin II on macula densa sodium chloride transport and increased tubuloglomerular feedback sensitivity are highly beneficial because this permits decreased distal sodium chloride delivery to be maintained without a compensatory increase in glomerular filtration rate. A maintained reduction in distal sodium chloride delivery, due to increased proximal tubule and loop of Henle reabsorption and the resetting of the macula densa feedback, can then combine with a stimulatory effect of angiotensin II on reabsorption in more distal sites to provide a very powerful mechanism for conserving sodium. However, excessive formation of angiotensin II could impair renal-pressure natriuresis and cause hypertension by stimulating sodium reabsorption at the macula densa as well as other sites in the renal tubule.

IV. ALDOSTERONE AND PRESSURE NATRIURESIS

Aldosterone is a powerful sodium-retaining hormone, exerting multiple effects on the collecting ducts to stimulate sodium reabsorption and potassium secretion (1,7). These effects are due, in large part, to binding of aldosterone with intracellular mineralocorticoid receptors (MR) and activation of transcription of target genes which, in turn, increase synthesis or activation of the Na^+—K^+ ATPase pump and activate amiloride-sensitive Na^+ channels on the luminal side of the epithelial membrane. These effects are termed "genomic" because they are mediated by activation of gene transcription and require 30–60 min to occur after administration of aldosterone.

Recent studies suggest that aldosterone may also elicit more rapid nongenomic effects (42). For example, in principal cells of the cortical collecting tubule, aldosterone has been reported to increase the sodium current through the amiloride-sensitive channel in <2 min after application (43). Aldosterone also rapidly stimulates Na^+—H^+ exchange in kidney epithelial cells (42,43). The putative membrane receptor responsible for these rapid nongenomic actions of aldosterone has not yet been cloned and the cell signaling mechanisms involved have not been fully elucidated. Therefore, the importance of the nongenomic effects of aldosterone in long-term regulation of renal-pressure natriuresis and blood pressure are still unclear.

The overall effects of aldosterone on renal-pressure natriuresis are similar to those observed for angiotensin II, except they are somewhat less potent. Excess aldosterone secretion decreases the slope of pressure natriuresis so that blood pressure becomes very salt-sensitive. Although raising plasma aldosterone 6–10-fold may cause marked hypertension when sodium intake is normal or elevated, very little effect on blood pressure occurs when sodium intake is low (1).

Because angiotensin II is a major physiological regulator of aldosterone secretion, some of the effects of angiotensin II on tubular reabsorption are mediated by aldosterone. However, several other factors besides angiotensin II also regulate aldosterone secretion and it is increasingly recognized that blockade of MR may provide additional reductions in blood pressure even after blockade of the renin–angiotensin system. For example, the combination of a renin–angiotensin system blocker (e.g., ACE inhibitor) and a MR blocker is more effective than either alone in lowering arterial pressure in hypertensive patients (43).

The role of excess aldosterone in human hypertension has been a topic of renewed interest in recent years, with some investigators suggesting that hyperaldosteronism may be more common than previously believed, especially in patients with resistant hypertension. For example, the prevalence of primary hyperaldosteronism was reported to be almost 20% among patients referred to a hypertension specialty clinic for resistant hypertension (44). The resistant subjects in that cohort were generally obese (53), as is true for many patients with primary (essential) hypertension (45).

Studies in experimental animals and in humans have provided evidence that antagonism of aldosterone may provide an important therapeutic tool for attenuating target organ injury as well as for lowering blood pressure in experimental and human hypertension (46). We have shown, for example, that antagonism of aldosterone markedly attenuated sodium retention, hypertension, and glomerular hyperfiltration in obese dogs fed with a high fat diet (47) (Fig. 8.7). This finding was somewhat surprising in view of the fact that obesity causes only small increases in plasma aldosterone concentration (45,47). However, even modest increases in plasma aldosterone

concentration may contribute to increases in arterial pressure when accompanied by marked sodium retention and volume expansion as occurs in obesity hypertension. The attenuation of sodium reabsorption and hypertension by aldosterone antagonism was especially impressive considering the fact that PRA, and presumably angiotensin II formation, was several fold higher after aldosterone antagonism. This suggests that combined blockade of aldosterone and angiotensin II might be even more effective in preventing obesity-induced sodium retention and hypertension.

The fact that aldosterone antagonism markedly attenuated glomerular hyperfiltration associated with obesity may have important implications for renal protection. Although there are no studies, to our knowledge, which have tested this concept directly in hypertensive subjects, previous studies in various experimental models of hypertension have provided evidence that aldosterone antagonism attenuates hypertension induced renal injury as well injury in other organs (46). These observations suggest that aldosterone antagonism may be an important therapeutic tool for treatment or preventing target organ injury in hypertension, although the precise mechanisms by which aldosterone antagonism protects against renal and cardiovascular disease have not been fully elucidated.

V. ATRIAL NATRIURETIC PEPTIDE

Atrial natriuretic peptide is a 28 amino acid peptide synthesized and released from atrial cardiocytes in response to stretch. After atrial natriuretic peptide is released from the atria, it enhances sodium excretion through extrarenal and intrarenal mechanisms (48,49) (Fig. 8.8). Atrial natriuretic peptide increases glomerular filtration rate, while having no effect on renal blood in flow. However, an increase glomerular filtration rate is not a prerequisite for atrial natriuretic peptide to enhance sodium excretion. Atrial natriuretic peptide may alter tubular sodium reabsorption either directly by inhibiting the active tubular transport of sodium or indirectly via alterations in medullary blood flow, physical factors, and intrarenal hormones (49).

Whole-kidney clearance and micropuncture studies have provided evidence for an effect of atrial natriuretic peptide in the proximal tubule (48). However, this effect of atrial natriuretic peptide in the proximal tubule is caused mainly by antagonizing angiotensin II-stimulated sodium transport (48). Biochemical and physiological data indicate that the collecting tubules and ducts are also important nephron sites for direct actions of atrial natriuretic peptide. Results from microcatheterization studies suggest that atrial natriuretic peptide lowers fractional sodium reabsorption in the medullary collecting ducts (48). Administering atrial natriuretic peptide to

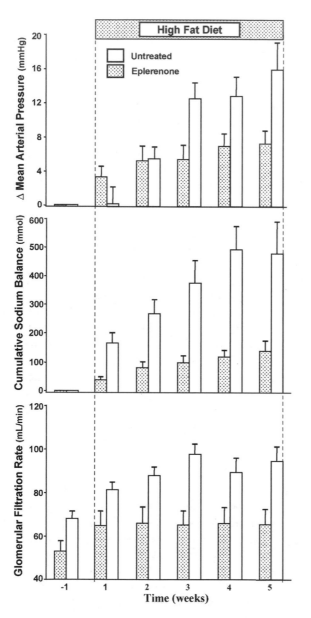

Figure 8.7 Changes (Δ) in mean arterial pressure (mmHg), cumulative sodium balance (mmol), and glomerular filtration rate (mL/min). Changes shown in control, untreated dogs and in eplerenone-treated (10 mg/kg, twice daily) dogs that were fed a high-fat diet for 5 weeks to develop obesity. [Adapted from de Paula, da Silva, and Hall (47).]

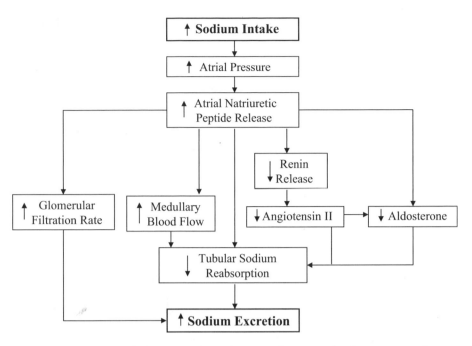

Figure 8.8 Mechanisms whereby atrial natriuretic peptide enhances sodium excretion in response to increases in sodium intake.

inner medullary collecting duct cells decreased oxygen consumption, which mainly reflects active sodium transport in these cells. Atrial natriuretic peptide has also been reported directly to inhibit sodium and water absorption in the cortical collecting duct (48). Thus, it appears that atrial natriuretic peptide directly inhibits sodium transport in the outer and inner medullary collecting ducts.

Atrial natriuretic peptide also has important actions at several sites of the renin–angiotensin system cascade (48). Intrarenal or intravenous infusion of atrial natriuretic peptide reduces renin secretion rate, presumably by a macula densa mechanism because atrial natriuretic peptide failed to reduce renin secretion in nonfiltering kidneys. The reduction in renin secretion would decrease intrarenal levels of angiotensin II, which could contribute to atrial natriuretic peptide-induced natriuresis. When intrarenal levels of angiotensin II were prevented from decreasing, the natriuretic effects of atrial natriuretic peptide were blunted (48).

Atrial natriuretic peptide also decreases aldosterone release from the adrenal zona glomerulosa cells (48,49). Two mechanisms for atrial natriuretic peptide-induced suppression of aldosterone release have been suggested: a direct action on adrenal glomerulosa cells and reduced circulating levels of angiotensin II that are a result of suppressed renin secretion under *in vivo* conditions (48). Although the suppression of aldosterone release would not play a role in mediating the acute natriuretic responses to atrial natriuretic peptide, decreases in circulating levels of aldosterone could contribute to the long-term actions of

atrial natriuretic peptide on sodium balance and arterial pressure regulation.

Plasma levels of atrial natriuretic peptide are elevated in numerous physiological conditions associated with enhanced sodium excretion (48,49). Acute saline of blood volume expansion consistently elevates circulating levels of atrial natriuretic peptide. Some, but not all, investigators have reported that chronic increases in dietary sodium intake raise circulating levels of atrial natriuretic peptide. Several studies have reported that infusions of exogenous atrial natriuretic peptide at rates that result in physiologically relevant plasma concentrations, comparable to those observed during volume expansion, have significant renal and cardiovascular effects (48,50). Infusion of atrial natriuretic peptide at a rate that causes a twofold increase in plasma atrial natriuretic peptide elicits significant natriuresis, especially in the presence of other natriuretic stimuli, such as high renal perfusion pressure (48). Long-term physiological elevations in plasma atrial natriuretic peptide also shift the renal-pressure natriuresis relationship and reduce arterial pressure (50).

The development of genetic mouse models that exhibit chronic alterations in expression of the genes for atrial natriuretic peptide or its receptors (NPR-A, NPR-C) have also provided compelling evidence for a role of atrial natriuretic peptide in chronic regulation of renal-pressure natriuresis and blood pressure (51). Transgenic mice overexpressing atrial natriuretic peptide gene are hypotensive relative to the nontransgenic littermates, whereas mice harboring functional disruptions of the atrial natriuretic peptide or *NPR-A* genes are hypertensive. The atrial natriuretic peptide gene knockout mice develop a salt-sensitive form of hypertension associated with failure to adequately suppress the renin–angiotensin system. These findings suggest that genetic deficiencies in atrial natriuretic peptide or natriuretic receptor activity could play a role in the pathogenesis of salt-sensitive hypertension.

VI. RENAL PROSTAGLANDINS

Renal prostaglandins are thought to be important mediators of vascular function, sodium and water homeostasis, and renin release (48,52). Cyclooxygenase metabolizes arachidonic acid into prostaglandin G_2 and subsequently to PGH_2, which is then further metabolized by tissue-specific isomerases to prostaglandins and thromboxane.

Although the kidney produces many types of prostaglandins with multiple functions, the major renal prostaglandin controlling sodium excretion is probably PGE_2 (48,52). However, production of other arachidonate acid metabolites, such as prostacyclin, thromboxane, and 20-HETE, may also influence renal-pressure natriuresis and blood pressure regulation. The largest production of PGE_2 occurs in the medulla with decreasing synthesis in the cortex. PGE_2 is synthesized and rapidly inactivated and, after it has been synthesized, is released and not stored. After being released, PGE_2 could influence sodium transport by several intrarenal mechanisms (48).

Support for a possible role for renal prostaglandins in regulating sodium excretion initially came from studies that demonstrated a potent natriuresis and diuresis during intrarenal infusion of PGE2 (48,52). Intrarenal infusion of PGE_2 produces a natriuresis that is associated with increased renal hemodynamics. Thus, prostaglandins may reduce sodium reabsorption by a hemodynamic mechanism and/or through a direct action on tubular sodium chloride transport. Evidence for a role of endogenous renal prostaglandins in regulating sodium excretion derives from investigations of the renal effects of nonspecific prostaglandin synthesis inhibitors such as indomethacin and meclofenamate. Administration of indomethacin and meclofenamate in anaesthetized animals undergoing saline volume expansion significantly attenuates sodium excretion (52). Furthermore, prostaglandin synthesis inhibitors significantly blunt the acute pressure natriuretic response.

Despite numerous reports that prostaglandins may contribute to the natriuresis of acute physiological perturbations, the importance of endogenous renal prostaglandins in the long-term regulation of sodium balance remains

unclear (48). Increases in dietary sodium intake have little or no effect on urinary prostaglandin excretion. In addition, nonspecific cyclooxygenase inhibitors do not affect the sodium excretory or blood pressure responses to chronic alterations in dietary sodium intake. Thus, it appears that endogenous renal prostaglandins may not play a major role in regulating sodium excretion during chronic changes in sodium intake (48).

Although long-term administration of prostaglandin synthesis inhibitors has very little effect on volume and/ or arterial pressure regulation under normal physiological conditions, renal prostaglandins may be important in pathophysiological states associated with enhanced activity or the renin–angiotensin system (48). *In vitro* and *in vivo* studies indicate that renal prostaglandins protect the preglomerular vessels form excessive angiotensin II-induced vasoconstriction (48). In the absence of this protective mechanism in pathophysiological states, the renal vasculature could be exposed to the potent vasoconstrictor actions of angiotensin II. This could lead to significant impairment of renal hemodynamics, reduced excretory function and hypertension.

It is now known that there are at least two distinct cyclooxygenases, COX-1 and COX-2 (52). COX-1 is called the constitutive enzyme because of its wide tissue distribution; COX-2 has been termed as inducible because of its more restricted basal expression and its upregulation by inflammatory or proliferative stimuli (52). On the basis of the concept that COX-1 performs cellular housekeeping functions for normal physiological activity and that COX-2 acts at inflammatory sites, it was initially hypothesized that the renal effects of nonsteriodal anti-inflammatory drugs (NSAIDS) might be linked to COX-1 inhibition (52). However, increasing experimental and clinical evidence has indicated that COX-2 metabolites may play a role in the regulation of renal function under various physiological and pathophysiological conditions (52). COX-2 inhibition has been shown to decrease urine sodium excretion and induce mild to moderate increases in arterial pressure. Moreover, blockade of COX-2 activity can have deleterious effects on renal blood flow and glomerular filtration rate. In addition to physiological regulation of COX-2 expression in the kidney, increased renal cortical COX-2 expression is seen in experimental models associated with altered renal hemodynamics and progressive renal injury. Long-term treatment with selective COX-2 inhibitors ameliorates functional and structural renal damage in these conditions (52).

In addition to renal prostaglandins generated via the COX pathway, other eicosanoids that inhibit tubular sodium transport are produced by cytochrome P450 (CYP) monooxygenase metabolism of arachidonic acid (53). CYP enzymes metabolize arachidonic acid primarily to 20-HETE and EETs. 20-HETE is a potent constrictor of renal arterioles that may have an important role in auto-regulation of renal blood flow and tubuloglomerular feedback (53). 20-HETE and EETs also inhibit sodium reabsorption in the proximal tubule and TALH. Compelling evidence suggests that the renal production of CYP metabolites of arachidonic acid is altered in genetic and experimental models of hypertension and that this system contributes to the resetting of pressure natriuresis and the development of hypertension. In the SHR, the renal production of 20-HETE is increased and inhibitors of the formation of 20-HETE decrease arterial pressure (53). Blockade of 20-HETE synthesis also reduces blood pressure or improves renal function in deoxycorticosterone acetate (DOCA)-salt, angiotensin II-infused, and Lyon hypertensive rats (53). In contrast, 20-HETE formation is reduced in the thick ascending limb of Dahl S rats and this contributes to elevated sodium reabsorption (53). Enhanced 20-HETE synthesis improves pressure natriuresis and lowers blood pressure in Dahl S rats, whereas inhibitors of 20-HETE production promote the development of hypertension in Lewis rats (53).

Studies in humans also suggest that CYP metabolites may play a role in sodium homeostasis. Urinary 20-HETE excretion is regulated by salt intake and is differentially regulated in salt-sensitive vs. salt-resistant subjects (54). Moreover, there appears to be a strong negative relationship between the excretion of 20-HETE and body mass index, which suggests that some factor related to obesity may be responsible for decreased synthesis or excretion of this eicosanoid in hypertension (55). These observations support the possibility that impaired renal production of 20-HETE could contribute to impaired renal-pressure natriuresis in human hypertension, especially when associated with obesity. However, further mechanistic studies are needed to test the importance of 20-HETE in human hypertension.

VII. ENDOTHELIN

In 1988, Yanagsawa and co-workers characterized an endothelial-derived vasoconstrictor, a 21 amino acid peptide subsequently called endothelin (56–58). Endothelin-1 is derived from a 203 amino acid peptide precursor, preproendothelin, which is cleaved after translation to form proendothelin. In the presence of a converting enzyme located within the endothelial cells, proendothelin or big endothelin is cleaved to produce the 21 amino acid peptide, endothelin. Increased synthesis of endothelin has been reported in various diseases associated with cardio-vascular abnormalities such as hypertension, diabetes, and chronic renal failure (56–58).

Endothelin receptor binding sites have been identified throughout the body with the greatest number of receptors in the kidneys and lungs (56,58). Although the biochemical and molecular nature of endothelin has been well characterized, the physiological importance of endothelin in the regulation of renal and cardiovascular function in disease processes is still unclear. ET_A receptors are primarily located on vascular smooth muscle cells. These receptors are thought to be involved in mediating endothelin-1 vasoconstriction and cellular proliferation in various cardiovascular disease states (56–58). Endothelin-1, via ET_A-mediated vasoconstriction, has been shown to play a role in various rat models of hypertension including the DOCA-salt, Dahl salt-sensitive, stroke-prone spontaneously hypertensive, and angiotensin-infused models (56–60).

More recent studies have focused on the potential physiological and pathophysiological roles of ET_B receptor activation (61,62). ET_B receptors are located on multiple cell types in the brain, on vascular endothelial cells, and renal epithelial cells. Although the location and the signal transduction pathways for ET_B receptors have been well characterized, the physiological role of these receptors has not been fully elucidated. ET_B receptors appear to play a role as clearance receptors, removing endothelin from the circulation and interstitial spaces (57,61). A significant role for ET_B receptors in the development of enteric neurons and melanocytes has been established. Loss of ET_B receptors result in failure of melanocytes and enteric neurons to develop resulting in abnormal development of the gastrointestinal tract and megacolon (58). Activation of vascular ET_B receptors by endothelin-1 or other ligands results in vasodilation, however, the physiological importance of ET_B-mediated vasodilatation is still unclear.

Experimental evidence suggests that endothelin-1, acting through the ET_B receptors, is involved in the regulation of sodium balance (57,61,62). The kidneys are important sites of endothelin-1 production and ET_B receptors are expressed at important renal sites of endothelin synthesis, particularly in the renal medulla. Some of the first studies using synthetic endothelin-1 demonstrated that nonpressor doses of endothelin-1 produced significant natriuresis and diuresis, effects that may be mediated by activation of ET_B receptors (57). It is now known that ET_B receptors are located in various parts of the nephron including the proximal tubule, medullary thick ascending limb, collecting tubule and the inner medullary collecting duct. The highest concentration of ET_B receptors appears to be on the inner medullary collecting duct in the renal medulla (57). Activation of ET_B receptors has been reported to inhibit sodium and water reabsorption along various parts of the nephron. Taken together, these data indicate that endothelin-1, via ET_B receptors, may influence the renal handling of sodium and water.

In order for the renal endothelin system to be an important control system for the regulation of sodium balance, the production of renal endothelin must change in response to variations in sodium intake. Although there are ample data showing that endothelin-1 can influence sodium reabsorption, there is a paucity of data in the literature examining the relationship between sodium intake and renal production of endothelin-1 (57,61). The most compelling evidence that the endothelin system may play a significant role in regulating sodium balance and arterial pressure is the report that transgenic rat deficient in ET_B receptors develop a severe form of salt-sensitive hypertension (62) (Fig. 8.9). In addition, long-term infusions of endothelin-1 in rats produce significant chronic hypertension, which was extremely salt-sensitive. Additional evidence comes from studies indicating that pharmacological antagonism of ET_B receptors produces significant hypertension in rats (61). The fact that ET_B receptor blockade produces greater elevations in blood pressure in rats maintained on a high sodium intake than those on a normal sodium intake indicates that ET_B receptor blockade produces a salt-sensitive form of hypertension.

Although endothelin-1 clearly plays a significant role in the pathogenesis some forms of experimental hypertension, especially salt-sensitive models, its role in human primary hypertension is unclear. Bosentan, a combined ET_A/ET_B receptor antagonist, significantly lowered blood pressure in a large, double-blind clinical trial, which indicates that endothelin system plays a role in maintaining blood pressure in human hypertension (63). However, the magnitude of the blood pressure reduction by bosentan was almost the same as that observed in normotensive humans. This observation suggests that endothelin probably does not play a major role in contributing to increased blood pressure in most patients with essential hypertension. Nevertheless endothelin-1 could be more important in severe, salt-sensitive hypertension, a possibility that deserves further investigation.

VIII. NITRIC OXIDE

In 1980, Furchgott and Zawadzki reported that the vascular endothelium releases a short acting substance which induces local relaxation of preconstricted arterial rings. Palmer and co-workers and Ignarro et al. independently demonstrated that this endothelial-derived relaxing factor was nitric oxide. Intravenous infusion of competitive inhibitors of the enzyme responsible for nitric oxide production (nitric oxide synthase) induced rapid increases in blood pressure in various species of animals (64–71). These effects were rapidly reversed with intravenous infusion of L-arginine, the substrate for nitric oxide synthase. These studies suggested that tonic release of nitric oxide by vascular endothelium may be important for regulation of vascular function. To investigate this concept further, the long-term effects of nitric oxide synthase inhibition were examined in normal dogs and rats (64–68). Continuous administration of a competitive inhibitor of nitric oxide production caused sustained hypertension associated with reductions in renal hemodynamic function. In the dog, the magnitude of the increase in blood pressure was dependent on the dietary sodium intake. The increase in blood pressure was prevented by simultaneous administration of L-arginine despite maintenance of a high sodium intake. These studies suggest that nitric oxide is an important factor for the long-term regulation of blood pressure in normotensive animals and is in some way related to renal sodium handling.

The renal effector mechanisms whereby reduced nitric oxide synthesis alters pressure natriuresis can be divided into hemodynamic and tubular components each of which may be modulated by processes which are intrinsic and extrinsic to the kidney (Fig. 8.10). For example, reductions in nitric oxide synthesis could lead to a decrease in renal sodium excretory function by directly increasing basal renal vascular resistance or tubular reabsorption or indirectly by activating the renin–angiotensin

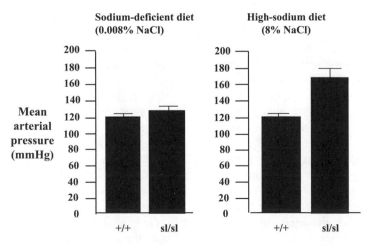

Figure 8.9   Salt-sensitive hypertension in endothelin-B receptor-deficient rats. [Adapted from Gariepy et al. (62).]

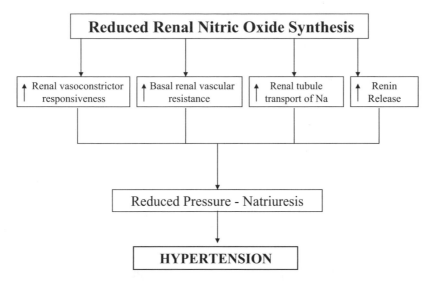

Figure 8.10 Mechanisms whereby a decrease in renal nitric oxide synthesis reduces renal-pressure natriuresis and causes hypertension.

system or by enhancing the renal vascular responsiveness to vasoconstrictors.

Significant increases in renal vascular resistance, reductions in renal plasma flow, and reductions in glomerular filtration rate were the earliest changes recognized in kidneys during inhibition of nitric oxide synthesis (64–68). Acute intravenous administration of nitric oxide synthesis inhibitor to normal rats also reduced glomerular plasma flow, single nephron glomerular filtration rate, and glomerular ultrafiltration coefficient, while increasing afferent and efferent renal arteriolar resistances and glomerular capillary pressure (64). In the conscious dog, inhibition of nitric oxide synthesis caused a reduction in renal plasma flow, while having no effect on glomerular filtration rate (72). Thus, the effect of nitric oxide synthesis inhibitors on renal hemodynamics may be species dependent or dependent upon the physiological status of the animal.

Direct effects of nitric oxide synthesis inhibition on the renal afferent arteriole have been confirmed *in vitro* (64). The effects of nitric oxide synthesis inhibition on renal hemodynamics may also involve potentiation of endogenous vasoconstrictors such as angiotensin II and norepinehrine (64,71). Inhibition of nitric oxide synthase potentiates the action of angiotensin II on the afferent arteriole in microperfused isolated glomeruli. Inhibition of nitric oxide synthesis potentiates the renal hemodynamic effects of exogenously administered angiotensin II in rats and dogs. Under normal conditions, a low intrarenal dose of angiotensin II or norepinephrine had no effect on glomerular filtration rate in dogs. In sharp contrast, the same dose of angiotensin II or norepinephrine decreased glomerular filtration rate by 30–40% in dogs pretreated with a nitric oxide synthesis inhibitor (64,71). Thus, it

appears that nitric oxide can oppose the preglomerular actions of angiotensin II and norepinephrine. Loss of this protective mechanism in diseases associated with endothelial dysfunction could lead to reductions in glomerular filtration rate, impaired pressure natriuresis and hypertension.

There is also evidence for an interaction between nitric oxide and the sympathetic nervous system (64,73). Several studies have shown that renal sympathetic nerve activity is suppressed following stimulation of nitric oxide production and increased after systemic administration of nitric oxide synthesis inhibitors (64). As changes in sympathetic nervous system activity are known to alter both renal hemodynamics and renal sodium reabsorption, changes in renal sympathetic nerve activity might also contribute to the blunted pressure natriuresis observed in conditions of abnormal nitric oxide production. In favor of this concept, the development of hypertension following nitric oxide synthesis inhibition has been shown to be both delayed and attenuated in renal denervated rats (64). In contrast, we have found that bilateral renal denervation in dogs does not alter the renal or hypertensive effects of chronic systemic nitric oxide synthesis inhibition (73). Thus, the importance of the interaction between nitric oxide and the sympathetic nervous system in long-term blood pressure control is unclear.

Another mechanism whereby nitric oxide synthesis inhibition may reduce pressure natriuresis is via activation of the renin–angiotensin system (64,70). Inhibition of nitric oxide production enhances renin release from rat cortical kidney slices. Inhibitors of nitric oxide synthesis also increase plasma renin activity *in vivo* when there are changes in renal perfusion pressure and adrenergic activity. We have shown that intrarenal inhibition of nitric oxide increased renin release in dogs, an effect that depends on the macula densa mechanism (71). These findings indicate that nitric oxide may have a direct effect in suppressing renin release. The effects of nitric oxide that is derived from various sources within the kidney, however, may be complex (64).

Reductions in nitric oxide synthesis may also reduce sodium excretory function either through direct effects on tubular transport or through changes in intrarenal physical factors such as renal interstitial hydrostatic pressure or medullary blood flow (64). Inhibition of nitric oxide synthesis leads to marked reductions in RIHP and urinary sodium excretion (68). Furthermore, normalization of the blunted pressure natriuretic response in Dahl S rats produced during stimulation of nitric oxide production results from improvement in the kidney's ability to generate RIHP in response to changes in renal perfusion pressure (64). Thus, changes in RIHP appear to be an important component of the effect of nitric oxide on sodium reabsorption *in vivo*.

Most investigators attribute the alterations in RIHP to changes in flow and pressure in the medullary circulation (64). Consistent with this hypothesis are observations that the acute infusion of a v synthase inhibitor directly into the renal medulla significantly reduces papillary blood flow, RIHP, and decreases urinary sodium and water excretion without affecting glomerular filtration rate or systemic pressure (66). Chronic medullary interstitial infusion of nitric oxide synthase inhibitors in conscious rats results in sustained reductions in medullary blood flow, sustained sodium and water retention, and hypertension which are reversed when the infusion is discontinued (66). These findings demonstrate that reductions in medullary blood flow may be another important mechanism whereby inhibition of nitric oxide in the kidney leads to a hypertensive shift in pressure natriuresis.

Inhibition of nitric oxide synthesis may have direct effects on renal tubule transport. Nitric oxide has direct effects on sodium uptake in cultured cortical collecting duct cells by altering apical sodium channels (66). Sodium transport in the cortical collecting duct *in vivo* is mediated through changes in cyclic guanosine monophosphate. Micropuncture studies have shown nitric oxide synthase inhibitors decrease proximal tubule reabsorption in anesthetized rats (65). This effect has been attributed to antagonism of angiotensin II-mediated sodium transport. An effect of nitric oxide on proximal reabsorption has also been inferred from changes in lithium clearance induced during inhibition of nitric oxide production. Thus, nitric oxide can affect sodium reabsorption via direct effects on tubular transport or indirectly via alteration in medullary blood flow or renal interstitial hydrostatic pressure.

Several lines of evidence suggest that nitric oxide may play an important role in the regulation of sodium balance and in pathogenesis of salt-sensitive hypertension (69). An increase in renal nitric oxide production or release, as evidenced by increased urinary excretion of nitric oxide metabolites or the nitric oxide second messenger, cyclic guanosine monophosphate, has been reported to be essential for the maintenance of normotension during a dietary salt challenge. Prevention of this increase in renal nitric oxide production resulted in salt-sensitive hypertension (64).

There is also *in vitro* evidence demonstrating that nitric oxide synthesis is impaired in some vascular beds in human essential hypertension. The extent to which these observations reflect effects of the hypertensive process or reflect important mechanisms for the pathogenesis of the hypertensive condition remains unclear.

IX. OXIDATIVE STRESS

Oxidative stress occurs when the total oxidant production exceeds the antioxidant capacity. Multiple studies suggest that reactive oxygen species may play a role in the initiation and progression of cardiovascular dysfunction associated with diseases such as hyperlipidemia, diabetes mellitus, and hypertension (74,75). In many forms of hypertension, the increased reactive oxygen species are derived from NADPH oxidases, which could serve as a triggering mechanism for uncoupling endothelial NOS by oxidants (74–78).

Reactive oxygen species produced by migrating inflammatory cells or vascular cells have distinct functional effects on each cell type (74). These effects include endothelial dysfunction, renal tubule sodium transport, cell growth, migration, inflammatory gene expression, and matrix regulation. Reactive oxygen species, by regulating vascular endothelial, smooth muscle, and renal tubule cell function, can play a role in altering renal-pressure natriuresis and blood pressure regulation (74–80).

Growing experimental evidence supports a role for reactive oxygen species in various animal models of sodium-sensitive hypertension (74–78). The Dahl salt-sensitive (S) rat has increased vascular and renal superoxide production and increased levels of hydrogen peroxide. The renal protein expression of superoxide dismutase is decreased in the kidney of Dahl S rats, and long-term administration of Tempol, a superoxide dismutase - mimetic, significantly decreases arterial pressure and renal damage. Another salt-sensitive model, the stroke-prone spontaneously hypertensive rats (SHRs), has elevated levels of superoxide and decreased total plasma antioxidant capacity. Superoxide production is also increased in the DOCA-salt hypertensive rat. Treatment of the DOCA-salt rats with apocynin, an NADPH oxidase inhibitor, decreases aortic superoxide production and arterial pressure.

The importance of oxidative stress in human hypertension is unclear. An imbalance between total oxidant production and the antioxidant capacity in human hypertension has been reported to occur in some but not all studies (74). The equivocal findings in human studies are most likely due to difficulty of assessing oxidative stress in humans. Moreover, most of recent human studies have found that vitamin E and vitamin C supplementation has little or no effect on blood pressure (74).

X. LEPTIN—AN ADIPOCYTE HORMONE

The discovery of leptin, an adipocyte hormone, led to a radical change in the view of adipose tissue which previously had been regarded mainly as a site for storing energy. White adipocytes are now recognized as serving endocrine and paracrine functions, secreting a large number of proteins, including angiotensinogen, adipsin, acylation-stimulating protein, adiponectin, retinol-binding protein, tumor neorosis factor α, interleukin 6, plasminogen activator inhibitor-1, fibrinogen-angiopoietin-related protein, metallothionein, and resistin (81,82). Some of these proteins play a role in lipid metabolism; others circulate in the blood and act as inflammatory cytokines, or they are involved in sympathetic nervous system regulation, vascular hemostasis, or the complement system.

One of the most widely studied hormones secreted from adipose tissue is leptin, a 167 amino acid protein produced by adipocytes in proportion to the degree of adiposity. Leptin circulates in the blood and crosses the blood–brain barrier via a saturable receptor-mediated transport system (81–83). Leptin binds to its long-form cytokine receptor in various regions of the hypothalamus and activates signaling pathways, especially in the arcuate nucleus, that regulate body weight by decreasing appetite and increasing energy expenditure (81–83). Evidence that leptin acts as a powerful controller of body weight comes from genetic studies of mice and humans demonstrating that missense mutations of the leptin gene cause extreme, early-onset obesity (84). Mutations of the leptin gene, however, are very rare in humans and the importance of abnormalities of leptin production or sensitivity of leptin receptors in contributing to obesity is still unclear.

Growing evidence suggests that leptin may be also an important link between obesity, sympathetic nervous system activation and hypertension (84) (Fig. 8.11). There is substantial evidence in rodents that high levels of leptin can activate sympathetic nervous system activity and increase arterial pressure (84–86). The rise in blood pressure with hyperleptinemia is slow in onset and occurs over a period of several days, despite decreased food intake that would otherwise tend to lower blood pressure (86). Moreover, the hypertensive effect of leptin

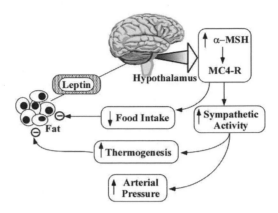

Figure 8.11 Possible links among leptin and its effects on the hypothalamus, sympathetic activation, and hypertension. Leptin may mediate much of its effects on appetite and sympathetic activity by stimulating other neurochemical pathways, including alpha-melanocyte-stimulating hormone, which activates melanocortin 4-receptors (MC4-R).

is enhanced when nitric oxide synthesis is inhibited (87), as often occurs in obese subjects with endothelial dysfunction. The chronic effects of leptin to raise arterial pressure are completely abolished by α-adrenergic and β-adrenergic blockade, which indicates that they are mediated by adrenergic activation (88).

An observation that favors leptin as a potential link between obesity and hypertension is the finding that mice with leptin deficiency and rats with mutations of the leptin receptor usually have little or no increase in arterial pressure despite severe obesity, when compared with their leaner weight controls (84,89). In contrast, animals with normal leptin production and normal leptin receptors have substantial increases in blood pressure during the development of dietary-induced obesity and this is associated with marked increases in circulating levels of leptin (84,90,91).

There have been few studies in which blood pressure has been measured in obese children with leptin gene mutations. In one study by Ozata et al. (92) four young patients with homozygous missense mutations of the leptin gene were found to have early-onset, morbid obesity but no indication of hypertension. Each of these children also had impaired sympathetic activity, postural hypotension, and attenuated renin–angiotensin–aldosterone system responses to upright posture (92). Moreover, the absence of hypertension occurred in spite of severe insulin resistance and hyperinsulinemia. These observations are consistent with those in leptin-deficient mice and suggest that hyperleptinemia may be an important factor in linking obesity with sympathetic nervous system activation and hypertension in humans as well as in rodents. However, these studies do not rule out the possibility that prolonged obesity may also activate other mechanisms that raise blood pressure, such as renal injury (91).

Leptin's stimulatory effect on sympathetic nervous system activity may be mediated, in part, by interaction with other hypothalamic factors, especially the pro-opiomelanocortin (POMC) pathway. Antagonism of the melanocortin 3/4 receptor (MC3/4-R) completely abolished leptin's acute effects on renal sympathetic nervous system activity (93). In addition, chronic blockade of the MC3/4-R in rats caused rapid weight gain but little or no increase in arterial pressure and a decrease in heart rate (94). Because weight gain usually increases blood pressure and heart rate, these findings are consistent with the possibility that a functional MC3/4-R is important in linking excess weight gain with increased sympathetic nervous system activity, impaired renal-pressure natriuresis and hypertension. However, the importance of the POMC pathway and MC3/4-R in controlling sympathetic nervous system activity and raising blood pressure in obese humans has not, to our knowledge, been investigated.

Although leptin appears to be a promising link between obesity sympathetic nervous system activation and hypertension, further studies are needed to understand the complex neurohumoral pathways by which the fat cells signal to the kidneys and cardiovascular system, and therefore influence blood pressure regulation. Because obesity may account for as much as 65–75% of the risk for primary (essential) hypertension (90,91), understanding the mechanisms of obesity-associated hypertension will like provide the key to understanding the pathogenesis of hypertension in most humans.

XI. CONCLUSIONS

A complex array of neurohumoral and intrarenal mechanisms interact to control body fluid and electrolyte balances and arterial pressure in hypertension as well as in normotension. In all forms of chronic hypertension, including human essential hypertension, renal-pressure natriuresis is reset to higher blood pressures so that sodium excretion is the same as in normotension despite increased blood pressure. The causes of this resetting in human essential hypertension are still uncertain, but many studies indicate that abnormal hormonal control of renal hemodynamics and tubular reabsorption play a key role.

ACKNOWLEDGMENTS

The authors' research was supported by a grant (P01 HL51971) from the National Heart, Lung and Blood Institute.

REFERENCES

1. Guyton AC. Arterial Pressure and Hypertension. Circulatory Physiology II. Philadelphia: W.B. Saunders, 1980.
2. Hall JE, Mizelle HL, Hildebrandt DA, Brands MW. Abnormal pressure natriuresis—a cause or a consequence of hypertension. Hypertension 1990; 15:547–559.
3. Cowley AW Jr. Long-term control of arterial blood pressure. Physiol Rev 1992; 72:231–300.
4. Hall JE, Guyton AC, Brands MW. Pressure–volume regulation in hypertension. Kidney Int 1996; 49(suppl 55):S35–S41.
5. Hall JE, Brands MW, Shek EW. Central role of the kidney and abnormal fluid volume control in hypertension. J Hum Hypertens 1996; 10:633–639.
6. Hall JE, Guyton AC, Brands MW. Control of sodium excretion and arterial pressure by intrarenal mechanisms and the renin–angiotensin system. In: Laragh JH, Brenner BM, eds. Hypertension: Pathophysiology, Diagnosis, and Management. 2nd ed. New York: Raven Press Ltd., 1995:1451–1475.
7. Laragh JH, Sealey JE. The renin–angiotensin–aldosterone hormonal system and regulation of sodium, potassium, and blood pressure homeostasis. In: Orloff J, Berliner RW, eds. Handbook of Physiology, Section 8, Renal Physiology. Washington, DC: The American Physiological Society, 1973:831–908.
8. Hall JE, Brands MW, Henegar JR. Angiotensin II and long-term arterial pressure control: the overriding dominance of the kidney. J Am Soc Nephrol 1999; 10:s258–s265.
9. Hall JE. Control of sodium excretion by angiotensin II: intrarenal mechanisms and blood pressure regulation. Am J Physiol 1986; 250:R960–R972.
10. Hall JE, Guyton AC, Smith MJ Jr, Coleman TG. Blood pressure and renal function during chronic changes in sodium intake: Role of angiotensin. Am J Physiol 1980; 239:F271–F280.
11. Hall JE, Granger JP, Hester RL, Coleman TG, Smith MJ Jr, Cross RB. Mechanisms of escape from sodium retention during angiotensin II hypertension. Am J Physiol 1984; 246:F627–F634.
12. Hall JE, Granger JP, Smith MJ Jr, Premen AJ. Role of renal hemodynamics and arterial pressure in aldosterone 'escape.' Hypertension 1984; 6(suppl I):I183–I192.
13. Hall, JE, Mizelle HL, Woods LL. The renin–angiotensin system and long-term regulation of arterial pressure. J Hypertens 1986; 4:387–397.
14. Hricik DE. Captopril-induced renal insufficiency and the role of sodium balance. Ann Intern Med 1985; 103:222–223.
15. Textor SC, Tarazi RC, Novick AC, Bravo EM, Fouad FM. Regulation of renal haemodynamics and glomerular filtration in patients with renovascular hypertension during converting enzyme inhibition with captopril. Am J Med 1984; 76:29–37.
16. Anderson S, Rennke HG, Brenner BM. Therapeutic advantage of converting enzyme inhibitors in arresting progressive renal disease associated with systemic hypertension in the rat. J Clin Invest 1986; 77:1993–2000.

17. Lewis EM, Hunsicker LG, Bain RP, Rohde ED. The effect of angiotensin-converting enzyme inhibition on diabetic nephropathy. N Engl J Med 1993; 329:1456–1462.

18. Matsuaka M, Hymes J, Ichikawa I. Angiotensin in progressive renal diseases: theory and practice. J Am Soc Nephrol 1996; 7:2025–2043.

19. Eng E, Veniants M, Floege J, Finerle J, Alpers CE, Menard J, Clozel J, Johnson RJ. Renal proliferative and phenotypic changes in rats with two-kidney, one-clip Goldblatt hypertension. Am J Hypertens 1994; 7:177–185.

20. Border WA, Noble NA. Interactions of transforming growth factor-beta and angiotensin II in renal fibrosis. Hypertension 1998; 3:181–188.

21. Griffin KA, Abu-Amarah I, Picken M, Bidani AK. Renoprotection by ACE inhibition or aldosterone blockade is blood pressure-dependent. Hypertension 2003; 41:201–206.

22. Brenner BM, Cooper ME, de Zeeuw D, Keane WF, Mitch WE, Parving HH, Remuzzi G, Snapinn SM, Zhang Z, Shahinfar S, RENAAL Study Investigators. Effects of losartan on renal and cardiovascular outcomes in patients with type 2 diabetes and nephropathy. N Engl J Med 2001; 345:861–869.

23. Kurtz TW. False claims of blood pressure-independent protection by blockade of the renin angiotensin aldosterone system? Hypertension 2003; 4:193–196.

24. Schuster VL. Effects of angiotensin on proximal tubular reabsorption. Fed Proc 1986; 45:1444–1447.

25. Harris PJ, Young JA. Dose-dependent stimulation and inhibition of proximal tubular sodium reabsorption by angiotensin II in the rat kidney. Pflugers Arch 1977; 367:295–297.

26. Liu FY, Cogan MG. Angiotensin II stimulates early proximal bicarbonate absorption in the rat by decreasing cyclic adenosine monophosphate. J Clin Invest 1989; 84:83–91.

27. Garvin J. Angiotensin stimulates glucose and fluid reabsorption by rat proximal straight tubules. J Am Soc Nephrol 1990; 1:272–277.

28. Geibel J, Giebisch G, Boron WF. Angiotensin II stimulates both Na^+-H^+ exchange and Na^+/HCO_3- cotransport in the rabbit proximal tubule. Proc Natl Acad Sci USA 1990; 87:7912–7920.

29. Schelling JR, Singh H, Marzec R, Linas S. Angiotensin II-dependent proximal tubular sodium transport is mediated by cAMP modulation of phospholipase C. Am J Physiol 1994; 267:C1239–C1245.

30. Navar LG, Harrison-Bernard LM, Nishiyama A, Kobori H. Regulation of intrarenal angiotensin II in hypertension. Hypertension 2002; 39:316–322.

31. Harrison-Bernard LM, Navar LG, Ho MM, Vinson GP, el-Dahr SS. Immunohistochemical localization of angiotensin II, AT1 receptor in adult rat kidney using a monoclonal antibody. Am J Physiol 1997; 273:F170–F177.

32. Capasso G, Unwin R, Ciani F, DeSanto NG, Detommaso G, Russo F, Giebisch G. Bicarbonate transport along the loop of Henle. II. Effects of acid-base, dietary and neurohumoral determinants. J Clin Invest 1994; 94:830–838.

33. Amlal H, LeGoff C, Vernimmen C, Soleimani M, Paillard M, Bichara M. ANG II controls Na^+—K^+(NH4+)–2Cl-cotransport via 20-HETE and PKC in

34. Peti-Peterdi J, Warnock DG, Bell PD. Angiotensin II directly stimulates ENaC activity in the cortical collecting duct via AT(1) receptors. J Am Soc Nephrol 2002; 13:1131–1135.

35. Beutler KT, Masilamani S, Turban S, Nielsen J, Brooks HL, Ageloff S, Fenton RA, Packer RK, Knepper MA. Long-term regulation of ENaC expression in kidney by angiotensin II. Hypertension 2003; 41:1143–1150.

36. Schnermann J, Levine DZ. Paracrine factors in tubulo-glomerular feedback: adenosine, ATP, and nitric oxide. Annu Rev Physiol 2003; 65:501–529.

37. Schnermann J. Juxtaglomerular cell complex in the regulation of renal salt excretion. Am J Physiol Regul Integr Comp Physiol 1998; 274:R263–R279.

38. Coleman TG, Hall JE. A Mathematical model of renal hemodynamics and excretory function. In: Iyengar SS, ed. Structuring Biological Systems—a Computer Modeling Approach. Boca Raton: CRC Press, 1992:89–124.

39. Kovacs G, Peti-Peterdi J, Rosivall L, Bell PD. Angiotensin II directly stimulates macula densa Na-2Cl-K cotransport via apical AT(1) receptors. Am J Physiol Renal Physiol 2002; 282:F301–F306.

40. Bell PD, Peti-Peterdi J. Angiotensin II stimulates macula densa basolateral sodium/hydrogen exchange via type 1 angiotensin II receptors. J Am Soc Nephrol 1999; 10(suppl 11):S225–S229.

41. Boldyreff B, Wehling M. Aldosterone: refreshing a slow hormone by swift action. News Physiol Sci 2004; 19:97–100.

42. Zhou ZH, Bubien JK. Nongenomic regulation of ENaC by aldosterone. Am J Physiol Cell Physiol 2001; 281:C1118–C1130.

43. Krum H, Nolly H, Workman D, He W, Roniker B, Krause S, Fakouhi K. Efficacy of eplerenone added to renin–angiotensin blockade in hypertensive patients. Hypertension 2002; 40:117–123.

44. Calhoun DA, Nishizaka MK, Zaman MA, Thakkar RB, Weissman P. Hyperaldosteronism among black and white subjects with resistant hypertension. Hypertension 2002; 40:892–896.

45. Hall JE. The kidney, hypertension, and obesity. Hypertension 2003; 41:625–633.

46. Rocha R, Stier CT Jr. Pathophysiological effects of aldosterone in cardiovascular tissues. Trends Endocrinol Metab 2001; 12:308–314.

47. de Paula RB, da Silva AA, Hall JE. Aldosterone antagonism attenuates obesity-induced hypertension and glomerular hyperfiltration. Hypertension 2004; 43:41–47.

48. Knox FG, Granger JP. Control of sodium excretion: An integrative approach. In: Windhager E, ed. Handbook of Renal Physiology. New York: Oxford University Press, 1992:927–967.

49. Vesely DL. Atrial natriuretic peptides in patho-physiological diseases. Cardiovasc Res 2001; 51(4):647–658.

50. Granger JP, Opgenorth TJ, Salazar J, Romero JC, Burnett JC Jr. Long-term hypotensive and renal effects of

chronic infusions of atrial natriuretic peptide in conscious dogs. Hypertension 1986; 8:II112–II116.

51. Melo LG, Steinhelper ME, Pang SC, Tse Y, Ackermann U. ANP in regulation of arterial pressure and fluid-electrolyte balance: lessons from genetic mouse models. Physiol Genomics 2000; 3(1):45–58.

52. Cheng HF, Harris RC. Cyclooxygenases, the kidney, and hypertension. Hypertension 2004; 43(3):525–530.

53. Hoagland KM, Flash AK, Roman RJ. Inhibitors of 20-HETE formation promote salt-sensitive hypertension in rats. Hypertension 2003; 42:669–673.

54. Laffer CL, Laniado-Schwartzman M, Wang MH, Nasjletti A, Elijovich F. Differential regulation of natriuresis by 20-hydroxyeicosatetraenoic acid in human salt-sensitive versus salt-resistant hypertension. Circulation 2003; 107:574–578.

55. Laffer CL, Laniado-Schwartzman M, Wang MH, Nasjletti A, Elijovich F. 20-HETE and furosemide-induced natriuresis in salt-sensitive essential hypertension. Hypertension 2003; 41:703–708.

56. Iglarz M, Schiffrin EL. Role of endothelin-1 in hypertension. Curr Hypertens Rep 2003; 5(2):144–148.

57. Granger JP. Endothelin. Am J Physiol Regul Integr Comp Physiol 2003; 285(2):R298–R301.

58. Schiffrin EL. Role of endothelin-1 in hypertension. Hypertension 1999; 34(4 Pt 2):876–881.

59. Kassab S, Miller MT, Novak J, Reckelhoff JF, Clower B, Granger JP. Endothelin-A receptor antagonism attenuates the hypertension and renal injury in Dahl salt-sensitive rats. Hypertension 1998; 30(1):397–402.

60. Alexander BT, Cockrell KL, Herrington JN, Granger JP. Enhanced renal expression of preproendothelin mRNA during chronic angiotensin II hypertension. Am J Physiol 2001; 280:R1388–R1392.

61. Pollock DM, Pollock JS. Evidence for endothelin involvement in the response to high salt. Am J Physiol Renal Physiol 2001; 281(1):F144–F150.

62. Gariepy CE, Ohuchi T, Williams SC, Richardson JA, Yanagisawa M. Salt-sensitive hypertension in endothelin-B receptor-deficient rats. J Clin Invest 2000; 105(7):925–933.

63. Krum H, Viskoper RJ, Lacourciere Y, Budde M, Charlon V. The effect of an endothelin-receptor antagonist, bosentan, on blood pressure inpatients with essential hypertension. Bosentan Hypertension Investigators. N Engl J Med 1998; 338:784–790.

64. Schnackenberg CG, Kirchner K, Patel A, Granger JP. Nitric oxide, the kidney, and hypertension. Clin Exp Pharmacol Physiol 1997; 24:600–606.

65. Ortiz PA, Garvin JL. Role of nitric oxide in the regulation of nephron transport. Am J Physiol Renal Physiol 2002; 282(5):F777–F784.

66. Cowley AW Jr, Mori T, Mattson D, Zou AP. Role of renal NO production in the regulation of medullary blood flow. Am J Physiol Regul Integr Comp Physiol 2003; 284(6):R1355–R1369.

67. Granger JP, Alexander BT. Abnormal pressure natriuresis in hypertension: Role of nitric oxide. Acta Physiol Scand 2000; 168(1):161–168.

68. Nakamura T, Alberola A, Granger JP. Role of renal interstitial pressure as a mediator of sodium retention during blockade of endothelium derived nitric oxide hypertension. Hypertension 1993; 21:956–960.

69. Sanders PW. Sodium intake, endothelial cell signaling, and progression of kidney disease. Hypertension 2004; 43(2):142–146.

70. Schnackenberg C, Tabor B, Strong M, Granger JP. Intrarenal NO blockade enhances renin secretion rate by a macula densa mechanism. Am J Physiol 1997; 272:R879–R886.

71. Schnackenberg C, Wilkins C, Granger JP. Role of nitric oxide in modulating the vasoconstrictor actions of angiotensin II in preglomerular and postglomerular vessels in dogs. Hypertension 1995; 26(2):1024–1029.

72. Granger JP, Alberola A, Salazer F, Nakamura T. Control of renal hemodynamics during intrarenal systemic EDNO synthesis blockade. J Cardiovasc Pharmacol 1992; 20:S160–S162.

73. Granger JP, Novak J, Schnackenberg C, Williams S, Reinhart G. Role of renal nerves in mediating the hypertensive effects of nitric oxide synthesis inhibition. Hypertension 1996; 27(2):613–618.

74. Taniyama Y, Griendling KK. Reactive oxygen species in the vasculature: molecular and cellular mechanisms. Hypertension 2003; 42(6):1075–1081.

75. Wilcox CS. Reactive oxygen species: roles in blood pressure and kidney function. Curr Hypertens Rep 2002; 4(2):160–166.

76. Manning RD Jr, Meng S, Tian N. Renal and vascular oxidative stress and salt-sensitivity of arterial pressure. Acta Physiol Scand 2003; 179(3):243–250.

77. Reckelhoff JF, Romero JC. Role of oxidative stress in angiotensin-induced hypertension. Am J Physiol Regul Integr Comp Physiol 2003; 284(4):R893–R912.

78. Romero JC, Reckelhoff JF. State-of-the-Art lecture. Role of angiotensin and oxidative stress in essential hypertension. Hypertension 1999; 34(4 Pt 2):943–949.

79. Sedeek M, Alexander BT, Abram SR, Granger JP. Role of oxidative stress in endothelin-induced hypertension in rats. Hypertension 2003; 42:806–810.

80. Garvin JL, Ortiz PA. The role of reactive oxygen species in the regulation of tubular function. Acta Physiol Scand 2003; 179(3):225–232.

81. Ahima RS, Flier JS. Adipose tissue as an endocrine organ. Trends Endocrinol Metab 2000; 11:327–332.

82. Trayhurn P, Beattie JH. Physiological role of adipose tissue: white adipose tissue as an endocrine and secretory organ. Proc Nutr Soc 2001; 60:329–339.

83. Jequier E. Leptin signaling, adiposity, and energy balance. Ann NY Acad Sci 2002; 967:379–388.

84. Hall JE, Hildebrandt DA, Kuo JJ. Obesity hypertension: role of leptin and sympathetic nervous system. Am J Hypertens 2001; 14:103s–115s.

85. Correia MLG, Morgan DA, Sivitz WI, Mark AL, Haynes WG. Leptin acts in the central nervous system to produce dose-dependent changes in arterial pressure. Hypertension 2001; 27:936–942.

86. Shek EW, Brands MW, Hall JE. Chronic leptin infusion increases arterial pressure. Hypertension 1998; 31:409–414.

87. Kuo J, Jones OB, Hall JE. Inhibition of NO synthesis enhances chronic cardiovascular and renal actions of leptin. Hypertension 2001; 37:670–676.

88. Carlyle M, Jones OB, Kuo JJ, Hall JE. Chronic cardio-vascular and renal actions of leptin-role of adrenergic activity. Hypertension 2002; 39:496–501.

89. Mark AL, Shaffer RA, Correia ML, Morgan DA, Sigmund CD, Haynes WG. Contrasting blood pressure effects of obesity in leptin-deficient ob/ob mice and agouti yellow mice. J Hypertens 1999; 17:1949–1953.

90. Hall JE, Jones DW, Kuo JJ, daSilva AA, Tallam LS, Liu J. Impact of the obesity epidemic on hypertension and renal disease. Curr Hypertens Rep 2003; 5:386–392.

91. Hall JE, Henegar JR, Dwyer TM, Liu J, daSilva AA, Kuo JJ, Tallam L. Is obesity a major cause of chronic kidney disease? Adv Ren Replace Ther 2004; 11:41–54.

92. Ozata M, Ozdemir IC, Licinio J. Human leptin deficiency caused by a missense mutation: multiple endo-crine defects, decreased sympathetic tone, and immune system dysfunction indicate new targets for leptin action, greater central than peripheral resistance to the effects of leptin, and spontaneous correction of leptin-mediated defects. J Clin Endocrinol Metab 1999; 10:3686–3695.

93. Haynes WG, Morgan DA, Djalali A, Sivitz WI, Mark AL. Interactions between the melanocortin system and leptin in control of sympathetic nerve traffic. Hypertension 1999; 33:542–547.

94. Kuo JJ, Silva AA, Hall JE. Hypothalamic melano-cortin receptors and chronic regulation of arterial pressure and renal function. Hypertension 2003; 41:768–774.

9

The Renin–Angiotensin–Aldosterone System

LUCIA MAZZOLAI, JÜRG NUSSBERGER

Centre Hospitalier Universitaire Vaudois (CHUV), Lausanne, Switzerland

KEYPOINTS

- The renin–angiotensin–aldosterone system plays a decisive role in regulating vessel diameter and sodium and water re-absorption. Thus, it controls blood pressure.
- The renin–angiotensin–aldosterone system contributes to cardiac and vascular hypertrophy, primarily via its AT1 receptor.
- Renin regulates both systemic and tissue angiotensin II concentrations; and both systemic and local angiotensin II affect blood pressure control and cardiac and vascular hypertrophy.

SUMMARY

Over 100 years after the discovery of renin, the first component of the renin–angiotensin–aldosterone system to be described, knowledge about this system continues to emerge. The renin–angiotensin–aldosterone system plays a major role in blood pressure and volume homeostasis. Most of the known biological actions of the renin–angiotensin–aldosterone system appear to be mediated by angiotensin II. Angiotensin II is generated through an enzymatic cascade, and it exerts its actions primarily through binding to the AT1 receptor. With respect to the latter, a major advance has been made in the last few years in understanding of the physiopathology of the renin–angiotensin–aldosterone system. Studies have shown that when angiotensin II binds to AT1 receptors, it stimulates the internalization and processing of the ligand–receptor complex by endocytosis. Internalization is important for controlling receptor function, because it regulates the number of available cell surface receptors. The renin–angiotensin–aldosterone system is a finely regulated system, and studies of the last decade support the idea that local plasma and tissue concentrations of angiotensin II appear to be determined primarily by circulating renal renin.

I. INTRODUCTION

Renin was first described by Tigerstedt and Bergmann (1) >100 years ago. Their simple observation of increased blood pressure in rabbits infused with rabbit kidney led them to propose the existence of an endocrine substance, which they named "renin". Since then, our knowledge of the renin–angiotensin–aldosterone system has not yet finished evolving. In fact, beyond its well-known effects on blood pressure and on sodium and fluid homeostasis, the renin–angiotensin–aldosterone system appears to play a role in a variety of other processes such as growth, atherosclerosis, thrombosis, hematopoiesis, and reproduction (2–6).

II. RENIN–ANGIOTENSIN–ALDOSTERONE–SYSTEM COMPONENTS

A. Renin and Angiotensins

Renin is a glycoprotein (aspartyl protease) of molecular weight of ~40,000 Da. It is expressed, stored, and released in a regulated manner by the juxtaglomerular cells of the kidneys. Renin secretion from the juxtaglomerular apparatus is calcium dependent. However, unlike other hormones, calcium plays an inhibitory action on renin release (7). Renin is synthesized initially as an inactive zymogen known as prorenin that contains an additional 29-amino acid amino-terminal fragment. Prorenin is expressed in a variety of tissues, but the only physiological maturation into active renin takes place exclusively in the kidneys, as demonstrated by the disappearence of angiotensin I and angiotensin II from plasma sampled and tested after a nephrectomy (8). Juxtaglomerular cells are modified smooth muscle cells located at the distal end of the afferent arteriole of the glomerulum. Renin has exquisite substrate specificity, and its only known substrate is angiotensinogen (Fig. 9.1). Angiotensinogen is an α-2 globulin of 55,000 Da and belongs to the family of the serine-protease inhibitors, the serpins. It is coded by a single gene and is mainly synthesized in the liver. Angiotensinogen is the only precursor of angiotensin peptides. Renin cleaves the amino-terminus of circulating angiotensinogen to form the Ang-(1–10)decapeptide or angiotensin I (Figs. 9.1 and 9.2). On the basis of the results

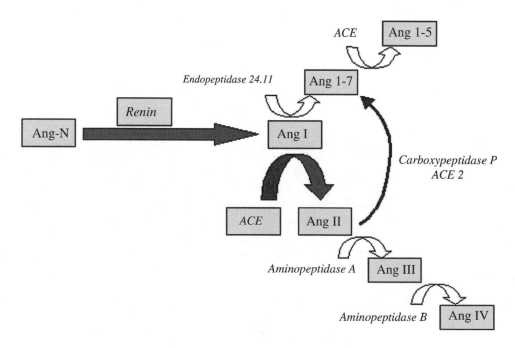

Figure 9.1 Renin and angiotensinogen system.

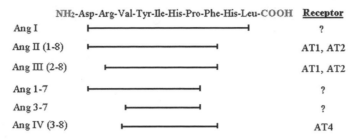

Figure 9.2 Angiotensins.

from *in vitro* experiments, it has been suggested that cathepsin D also may cleave angiotensinogen alternatively to renin. Cathepsin D is a lysosomal enzyme that would cleave angiotensinogen, contrary to renin, at an acidic pH (9,10). However, evidence that cathepsin D is of importance *in vivo* is currently lacking.

Angiotensin I is an inactive peptide, and no specific receptor for this Ang-(1–10)decapeptide has so far been established. Angiotensin I is cleaved by the endothelial cell-associated or soluble dipeptidyl carboxypeptidase angiotensin-converting enzyme (ACE) to form the biologically active Ang-(1–8)octapeptide or angiotensin II (Figs. 9.1 and 9.2). A minor portion of angiotensin I is alternatively cleaved by tissue-specific endopeptidases into the Ang-(1–7)heptapeptide, which is sequentially converted by ACE into Ang-(1–5)pentapeptide. From angiotensin II, aminopeptidase A or carboxypeptidase P cleave the amino- or carboxy-terminal amino acid to form either Ang-(2–8)heptapeptide, that is, angiotensin III or Ang-(1–7)heptapeptide, respectively; angiotensin III is further converted by aminopeptidase B into Ang-(3–8)hexapeptide, which is also called angiotensin IV. Aminopeptidases are enzymes of limited specificity and are widely present in human tissues.

Several studies have shown that alternative pathways exist for the production of angiotensin II. Enzymes other than ACE (tonin, trypsin, kallikrein, cathepsin G, chymotrypsin, chymase) have been demonstrated to be able to transform angiotensin I into angiotensin II (11–15). Among all the serine proteases, chymase has gained a major interest (16–18); it is mainly found in the heart and in the blood vessel wall and can be located in mastocytes. The pathophysiological relevance of these alternative pathways is still being debated.

B. Angiotensin-Converting Enzymes

The ACE, also known as kininase II, was first described by Erdos and co-workers (19). ACE is a type-I membrane-anchored dipeptidyl carboxypeptidase belonging to the zinc metallopeptidases family. It is synthesized as a 1306 amino acid polypeptide and processed to a mature form of 1277 residues which is heavily glycosylated

(30% by weight). ACE exists in two isoforms transcribed from the same gene in a tissue-specific manner. In somatic tissues, it exists as a glycoprotein that is composed of a single, large polypeptide chain of 1277 amino acids; in adult sperm cells, it is a lower molecular mass glycoform of 701 amino acids. ACE is found primarily on endothelial and epithelial cell surfaces. It can be released from endothelial cells by the action of an ACE secretase that cleaves the peptide near the transmembrane region. This soluble form of ACE accounts for barely 1% of all physiological ACE activities.

Recently, a homolog of ACE, ACE2, has been described (20). This is a carboxypeptidase found primarily in the heart, kidney, and testis. In contrast to ACE, ACE2 cleaves the carboxy-terminal leucine from angiotensin I, giving rise to the Ang-(1–9)nanopeptide, which may play a role in arachidonic acid production by bradykinin (21). In addition, ACE2 degrades angiotensin II to Ang-(1–7)heptapeptide with superior kinetics than carboxypeptidase P. Therefore, in tissues where ACE2 is present, the ACE2 is the preferred angiotensinase. Interestingly, ACE2 is not inhibited by many of the known ACE inhibitors.

ACE is an enzyme of little selectivity and it catalyses the hydrolytic cleavage of angiotensin I, bradykinin, and Ang-(1–7). Nevertheless, bradykinin is the preferred substrate of ACE with a K_m of 0.18 μM and with a k_{cat}/K_m ratio that is some 30 times higher than that of angiotensin I.

Bradykinin is a nonapeptide hormone generated from kininogen by kallikrein, either directly or via kallidin (Fig. 9.3). *In vivo* bradykinin has an extremely short half-life of some 2 min. It is rapidly degraded by kininases such as ACE, neutral endopeptidase (NEP), aminopeptidase P, and the carboxypeptidases M and N (22). Bradykinin is liberated from high or low molecular weight kininogen by the tissue or plasma kallikrein. Bradykinin exerts its actions via two G-protein coupled receptors: the B1 receptor and the B2 receptor. B1 receptors are weakly detectable under physiological conditions, but they are strongly induced by inflammatory mediators and tissue damage (23). B2 receptors are constitutively expressed in a variety of cells, including endothelial cells, vascular smooth muscle cells, and cardiomyocytes (24,25). Activation of

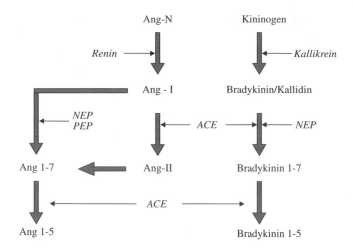

Figure 9.3 Generation of bradykinin from kininogen.

B2 receptors results in vasodilation in part mediated by stimulation of nitric oxide synthase and subsequent nitric oxide generation. Furthermore, bradykinin stimulates tissue plasminogen activator (tPA), which activates fibrinolysis (26–28).

C. Angiotensin Receptors

1. AT1 and AT2 Receptors

The two main angiotensin receptors are the angiotensin II receptor subtypes 1 (AT1) and 2 (AT2); both stem from single genes found on chromosome 3 and X, respectively. AT1 and AT2 are 7-transmembrane G-protein coupled receptors. The AT1 receptor comprises 359 amino acids, whereas the AT2 is 363 amino acids long sharing a 30% homology with AT1. Both receptors are expressed at very low levels, the AT1 is mainly expressed in blood vessels, adrenal cortex, liver, and brain; the AT2 are found primarily in fetal tissues, adrenal medulla, and uterus. Most of the known physiological functions of angiotensin II appear to be mediated by the AT1 receptor, whereas the AT2 receptor appears to mediate apoptosis and growth inhibition or fetal growth regulation (29–31).

Activation of the AT1 receptor by its ligand angiotensin II stimulates a variety of intracellular signal pathways, including those typically activated by G-protein coupled receptors, growth factor receptors, and cytokines, as well as events leading to the regulation of receptor function, such as phosphorylation and internalization of the receptor (32,33). Binding of angiotensin II to the AT1 receptor activates, via the $G_{q/11}$ family of G-proteins, inositol phosphate-induced Ca^{2+} signals, phospholipase C, and protein kinase C (34). AT1 receptor activation also regulates gene expression leading to a variety of growth-related responses, including activation of receptor and

nonreceptor protein tyrosine kinases (epidermal growth factor receptor, platelet-derived growth factor receptor, insulin-like growth factor-I receptor, Janus kinases, c-Src, focal adhesion kinase, and Ca^{2+}-dependent tyrosine kinases) (32,35,36). In addition, AT1 activation by angiotensin II stimulates signal transducers and activators of transcription pathway, small G-proteins, and expression of other important regulatory enzymes, such as phospholipase D, phospholipase A_2, and NAD(P)H oxidase (36–39).

Angiotensin II binding to AT1 receptors also stimulates the internalization and processing of the ligand–receptor complex (Fig. 9.4). Although other pathways have been implicated, internalization of the AT1 receptor occurs predominantly by endocytosis via clathrin-coated pits (40,41). At physiological angiotensin II concentrations, this process is dynamin-dependent and β-arrestins serve as adaptor proteins (42,43). Internalization is important for controlling receptor function by regulating the number of available cell surface receptors and facilitating resensitization of membrane receptors that have been desensitized by GPCR kinase (GRK)-mediated phosphorylation (44). Dephosphorylation probably occurs within the endosomes after receptor endocytosis; subsequent recycling of the resensitized receptor to the cell surface maintains signal generation. Recycling of internalized AT1 receptors to cell surface occurs via PI 3-kinase dependent and independent pathways (45).

Although the AT2 receptor belongs to the 7-transmembrane family, it did not reveal any functional features commonly attributed to this class of receptors, and the signaling of AT2 still remains largely unknown. Currently, AT2 signaling does not seem to modulate cytosolic calcium. Furthermore, agonist binding does not induce receptor internalization (46,47). AT2 signaling appears to activate phosphorylases-mediated inhibition of phosphorylation

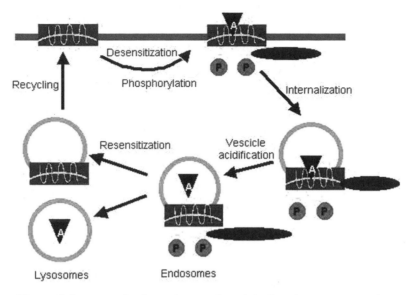

Figure 9.4 Internalization and processing of the ligand–receptor complex.

steps and to inactivate mitogen activated protein kinase via the serine/threonine phosphatase PP2A activation (48). Overall, diverse putative AT2 receptor signaling pathways have been hypothesized; however, intense research is still ongoing to further understand mechanisms underlying receptor activation and signaling.

2. AT4 Receptor

The AT4 receptor was recently described (49). This was the first receptor described in bovine adrenal membranes. It has been demonstrated that $[^{125}I]$AngIV does bind to the AT4 site reversibly, saturably, and with high affinity. This binding is insensitive to guanine nucleotides, which suggests that the AT4 receptor is not G-protein linked as the AT1 receptor is. In fact, AT4 is a type II integral-membrane protein that consists of 1025 amino acids and a large extracellular domain. Three isoforms of the AT4 receptor have been described, all of which are synthesized by a single gene on chromosome 5. AT4 is expressed primarily in the heart, placenta, kidney, small intestine, and skeletal muscle. A certain level of AT4 also is found throughout the brain and is concentrated particularly in regions involved in cognition (50). The AT4 receptor has been identified as the insulin-regulated amino-peptidase. Angiotensin IV binds to, but is not cleaved by this insulin-regulated aminopeptidase. Very little is known about the regulation of the AT4 receptor (49–55).

3. AT-(1–7) Receptor

The existence of a specific Ang-(1–7) receptor that is found primarily in the brain has been postulated (56–58). Studies conducted in cultured rat mesangial cells showed an Ang-(1–7) binding to the AT2 receptor with an affinity 40-fold higher than its affinity for the AT1 receptor. Conversely, other studies demonstrated that Ang-(1–7) binds poorly to both AT1 and AT2 receptors in human myometrium membranes. Final proof of the existence of an AT-(1–7) receptor remains to be sought.

4. Aldosterone and Aldosterone Receptor

Aldosterone is a mineralcorticoid hormone that is synthesized in the adrenal glomerulosa not only in response to angiotensin II but also in response to adrenocorticotropin hormone and potassium. Aldosterone exerts its action on epithelial cells of the distal renal tubules, colon, salivary, and sweat glands. Its renal effects are the best known and the most widely studied. In the kidney, aldosterone can either diffuse directly through the cell membrane or bind to an inactive form of mineralcorticoid receptor. Binding to mineralcorticoid receptor leads to the dissociation of the receptor from a multiprotein complex, which induces a translocation of the mineralcorticoid receptor through the nuclear pores to the chromatin. In the nucleus, the activated mineralcorticoid receptor acts as a positive transcription factor, modulating the expression of multiple proteins and triggering a cascade of events that lead to increased absorption of sodium ions and water through the epithelial sodium channel and that indirectly increase potassium ion excretion. The net result is expansion of intravascular volume and elevation in blood pressure. Recent studies have shown that mineralcorticoid receptors are present also in nonepithelial tissues such as the heart, brain, and blood vessels (59–61). A minute local production of aldosterone in these tissues also has been postulated, which suggests a possible local paracrine role (62–65). However, >99% of immunoreactive aldosterone disappears from rat cardiac tissue after an adrenalectomy (Nussberger, unpublished data). The adrenal glands are the main source of cardiac aldosterone (66). There is good evidence that aldosterone plays a key role in the pathogenesis of angiotensin II–induced end-organ damage. Both angiotensin II receptor antagonism (by losartan) and aldosterone synthase inhibition (by fadrazol) as well as adrenalectomy decrease circulating and tissue levels of aldosterone and provide anti-inflammatory effects and cardiac and renal protection which are at least partially independent of blood pressure lowering in hypertensive rats (66).

III. FUNCTION OF ANGIOTENSINS

Angiotensinogen and angiotensin I are inactive peptides for which no function has yet been described. Angiotensins other than angiotensin II are active peptides that are normally produced in small amounts. Their physiological relevance is still not completely understood, and their role may become more significant during angiotensin II inhibition.

A. Angiotensin II

Angiotensin II exerts most of the physiological functions of the renin–angiotensin–aldosterone system by activating membrane-bound receptors. Almost all the known pathophysiological effects of angiotensin II are mediated by the AT1 receptor (Table 9.1).

1. Cardiovascular Homeostasis

Adequate function of the cardiovascular system in vertebrates depends, according to Poiseuille's law, on

Table 9.1 Effects of Angiotensin II

AT1-mediated
Vasoconstriction
Sodium retention
Water retention
Activation of sympathetic nervous system
Myocyte and smooth muscle cell hypertrophy
Cardiac and vascular fibrosis
Stimulation of PAI-1
Induction of superoxide formation
Increased endothelin secretion
Atherosclerosis/inflammation
Renin suppression (negative feedback)
AT2-mediated
Antiproliferative
Apoptosis

physiological interplay between blood volume (and composition), vessel width (and quality), and blood pressure maintained by the pump function of the heart. As long as these three parameters remain within physiological limits, the cardiovascular system stays adequately balanced, homeostatic.

The renin–angiotensin–aldosterone system is intimately involved in the maintenance of cardiovascular homeostasis. Angiotensin II, the key hormone of the renin–angiotensin–aldosterone system, plays a pivotal role for both regulation of vessel width and sodium/water re-absorption and it therefore importantly contributes to blood pressure control.

First, angiotensin II constricts arterioles by direct stimulation of vascular smooth muscle cells. Indirectly, it facilitates norepinephrine-mediated vasoconstriction by central sympathetic stimulation and eventually by enhanced peripheral norepinephrine release. Furthermore, angiotensin II stimulates vascular endothelial cells to release the potent vasoconstrictor peptide endothelin-1. Angiotensin II also controls pituitary vasopressin release which, in extreme cases, raises blood pressure. In the kidneys, angiotensin II also causes vasoconstriction and decreases renal blood flow. Acting mainly at the level of efferent arterioles, angiotensin II prevents reductions in glomerular filtration rate by maintaining adequate filtration pressure even at low levels of perfusion pressure.

Secondly, angiotensin II increases re-absorption of sodium in the kidneys. In the proximal tubule, angiotensin II promotes sodium transport at the luminal and basolateral membranes of the epithelial cells. Indirectly, angiotensin II increases sodium re-absorption by stimulating adrenal release of aldosterone. Angiotensin II is the main stimulator of the aldosterone synthase in the adrenal cortical cells of the zona glomerulosa. Aldosterone mediates sodium re-absorption mainly in the late distal tubule including the beginning portion of the collecting tubule. All these sodium retaining effects of angiotensin II increase the total body volume and contribute to the maintenance of blood pressure. Angiotensin II participates in increasing body water by stimulating thirst and pituitary release of antidiuretic hormone.

Finally, angiotensin II exerts a negative feedback through the AT1 receptor on renin release from the juxtaglomerular cells: increased levels of angiotensin II inhibit renin secretion and thus limit further angiotensin production. This feedback mechanism is deficient in certain forms of hypertension with excessive generation of angiotensin II, and blood pressure can be reduced whenever the renin–angiotensin–aldosterone system is blocked by either ACE inhibitors or renin inhibitors or AT1 or aldosterone antagonists.

The primary goal of the renin–angiotensin system may well be an appropriate function of the nephrons. Healthy kidneys maintain this function at normal blood pressure levels. Local disturbance of nephron function may require locally increased angiotensin II concentrations and raised blood pressure. Enhanced renin secretion and generation of angiotensin II have their impact on extrarenal targets. However, an increase in systemic blood pressure is maintained only after a resetting of the renin–angiotensin system because a contralateral, well-functioning kidney and ipsilateral, undisturbed nephrons compensate by tuning down renin secretion and also by actually extracting renin from the circulation and by a pressure diuresis that reduces the circulating volume. Other neuronal mechanisms also are involved in maintaining cardiovascular homeostasis. However, there is no doubt that an insufficient shutting down of renin secretion at any given circulating volume will tend to cause hypertension. After more than two decades of clinical research hypothesizing that specific inhibition of renin should decrease blood pressure in hypertensive patients, we have recently entered a new era of successful cardiovascular treatment by orally active specific renin inhibitors (67,68).

2. Cardiac and Vascular Hypertrophy

It is well known that increased blood pressure is a potent stimulus for cardiovascular hypertrophy. However, for a long time it has been debated whether angiotensin II, in addition to its effect on blood pressure, could act directly on cardiomyocytes to trigger the hypertrophic response. Data from several in vitro and in vivo studies have demonstrated a relationship between angiotensin II and hypertrophy Angiotensin II AT1 receptors are widely distributed on cardiomyocytes, fibroblasts, and vascular smooth muscle cells. It has been demonstrated that genetically determined hypertension, and its subsequent cardiac hypertrophy, can be normalized by ACE inhibitor treatment (69). Furthermore, the administration of an ACE inhibitor completely prevented left ventricular hypertrophy that develops after coarctation of the abdominal aorta or in the "two kidney one clip" model of renovascular hypertension (70,71). Angiotensin II could act on the development of cardiac hypertrophy indirectly, via its effect on blood pressure and/or by inducing a direct cellular response in cardiomyocytes. The latter hypothesis is supported by several observations. For instance, the use of direct vasodilators has beneficial effects on blood pressure, but it does not cause regression of the cardiac hypertrophy. Angiotensin II triggers hypertrophic responses in pure cardiac cell cultures. Moreover, angiotensin II also is capable of inducing, in muscle cells, expression of cellular oncogenes involved in cell proliferation. Finally, cultured cardiomyocytes exposed to angiotensin II increase protein synthesis. Taken together, this data suggests that local angiotensin II accumulation, through its growth factor effect, could participate in the development of cardiac hypertrophy in vivo. It could be demonstrated in normotensive transgenic mice with increased cardiac angiotensin II production that locally increased angiotensin II concentrations can induce cardiac hypertrophy in the absence of blood pressure changes (72). Moreover, reversal or prevention of cardiac hypertrophy in this model was achieved by ACE inhibition or AT1 blockade (2).

Angiotensin II also has multiple effects on vascular smooth muscle cells. These depend on the cell phenotype, the density of receptors on cell surface, and the environment to which cells are exposed. Binding of angiotensin II to the AT1 receptor induces vessel contraction, hypertrophy, and hyperplasia; binding to the AT2 receptor has been suggested to mediate growth inhibition (73). These events are each mediated by unique signaling pathways. Angiotensin II-induced vessel contraction is mediated by rapid increase in intracellular calcium, which is released from intracellular stores. Calcium binds to calmodulin and associates with the myosin light-chain kinase, which is then converted to an active form and phosphorylates myosin light-chain, allowing the catalysis of adenosine triphosphate hydrolysis and generating tension. This process takes place in a cyclic manner for the duration of contraction. In addition to this pathway, angiotensin II stimulates calcium influx through calcium channels that are activated by free G-$\beta\gamma$ subunits, which seem to play a role in contraction of vessels that respond to angiotensin II tonically (74). Beyond contraction, angiotensin II stimulates growth of vascular smooth muscle cells. This hypertrophic response depends in part on gene transcription (75). Recent data have shown that angiotensin II-mediated vascular smooth muscle cell hypertrophy is mediated by intracellular production of superoxide that is partially derived from membrane-bound NADH/NADPH oxidase (37,38).

3. Atherosclerosis and Inflammation

The potential etiologic link between angiotensin II and atherosclerosis has been suggested by several clinical trials. The Cooperative North Scandinavian Enalapril Survival Study (CONSENSUS), Studies of Left Ventricular Dysfunction (SOLVD), and Survival and Ventricular Enlargement (SAVE) studies on heart failure demonstrated that treatment with an ACE inhibitor significantly reduced the incidence of acute coronary events in patients with heart failure when compared with conventional therapy suggesting that inhibition of the renin–angiotensin system may prevent atherosclerosis (76,77). Furthermore, results from the Heart Outcomes Prevention Evaluation (HOPE) study showed that chronic ACE inhibition reduces the rates of death, myocardial infarction, and stroke in patients with atherosclerosis (77).

Parallel with clinical trials, various experimental studies have shown that treatment with ACE inhibitors or angiotensin II receptor antagonists attenuates the development of atherosclerosis. Indeed, treatment with an ACE inhibitor inhibited atherosclerosis in the ApoE$^{-/-}$ mouse model and in the Watanabe rabbit model. Along the same line, losartan (an AT1 antagonist) reduced atherosclerosis in monkeys fed cholesterol (78,79).

Angiotensin II may play a role in the pathogenesis of atherosclerosis, not only through its hemodynamic effects but also through a direct cellular action on the vessel wall. Interestingly, many of the proposed mechanisms of atherogenesis show similar features with angiotensin II-mediated events. In recent years, the renin–angiotensin system has been shown to play a role in the inflammatory processes. Both macrophages and T-cells express the AT1 receptor on their surface (80). Angiotensin II may influence recruitment and activation of both macrophages and T-cells into the vessel wall, presumably by influencing expression of proinflammatory chemokines. Indeed, angiotensin II increases monocyte chemoattractant protein-1 expression in cultured vascular smooth muscle cells and in monocytes (81). In patients, treatment with an ACE inhibitor lowers plasma levels of monocyte chemoattractant protein-1 after myocardial infarction (82). Moreover, exposure of cultured vascular smooth muscle cells and macrophages to angiotensin II induce IL-6 expression (83). IL-6 is mainly expressed in atherosclerotic plaques by macrophages (84). IL-6 has multiple biological activities including T-cell activation and stimulation of matrix-degrading enzymes such as metalloproteinases. Therefore, angiotensin II has the capacity to induce an inflammatory response. However, the contribution of this pathway *in vivo* is still unknown.

Angiotensin II also induces cellular adhesion molecules (VCAM-1 and ICAM-1, in cultured endothelial cells and vascular smooth muscle cells), and it increases smooth muscle lipoxygenase activity, which itself can increase inflammation and low-density lipoprotein (LDL) oxidation (85,86). Angiotensin II has been shown to increase oxidative stress in the vasculature by increasing both hydrogen peroxide and free radical formation (87). Free radicals reduce the bioavailability of nitric oxide (a potent vasodilator) from the endothelium. Attenuation of endothelium-dependent vasodilatation is a characteristic of early stages of atherosclerosis. Angiotensin II has been shown to behave as a growth factor by directly inducing cardiomyocytes and vascular smooth muscle cell hypertrophy, as well as fibrosis, independent of its blood pressure effect (2,72). One of the characteristics of atherosclerotic lesions is arterial wall remodeling arising from hypertrophy, proliferation, migration of vascular smooth muscle cells, and matrix deposition. Rupture of atherosclerotic plaque and subsequent thrombus formation are important mechanisms

that underlie the acute manifestations of atherosclerosis. The thrombogenicity of the plaque is favored by a disturbance in the balance of coagulation and fibrinolysis. Angiotensin II is involved in both coagulation and fibrinolysis. Angiotensin II increases expression of tissue factor in cultured endothelial and vascular smooth muscle cells. Tissue factor is found in abundance in atherosclerotic plaques. It initiates blood coagulation, directly stimulates smooth muscle cell proliferation, and activates metalloproteinases. In the same cells, Ang II induces plasminogen activator inhibitor 1 expression, thus inhibiting also the fibrinolytic process (88). To study the contribution of Ang II in plaque vulnerability we generated hypertensive hypercholesterolemic ApoE$^{-/-}$ mice with either normal or endogenously increased Ang II production (renovascular hypertension models). Hypertensive high Ang II ApoE$^{-/-}$ mice developed unstable plaques while in hypertensive normal Ang II ApoE$^{-/-}$ mice plaques showed a stable phenotype (89). Moreover, in mice with high Ang II a skewed T helper type 1-like phenotype was observed. Splenocytes from high Ang II ApoE$^{-/-}$ mice produced significantly higher amounts of interferon-γ than those from ApoE$^{-/-}$ mice with normal Ang II. Secretion of IL4 and IL10 was not different. These findings suggest a new mechanism in plaque vulnerability demonstrating that Ang II, within the context of hypertension and hypercholesterolemia, independently form its hemodynamic effect behaves as a local modulator promoting the induction of vulnerable plaques probably via a T helper switch.

B. Angiotensin-(1–7)heptapeptide

The Ang-(1–7)heptapeptide is the most extensively studied among all the active angiotensin peptides besides angiotensin II. Its plasma levels in healthy humans are lower than those of angiotensin II. Most of the effects of Ang-(1–7)heptapeptide are opposite to those observed for angiotensin II, and they seem to be somehow co-mediated by the AT1 receptor because they can be prevented by AT1 blockade (90,91). In the central nervous system, Ang-(1–7)heptapeptide behaves as a neuromodulator by affecting tonic and reflex control of blood pressure. In fact, it induces release of vasopressin, modulates the baroreflex and heart rate, and it does not affect thirst (92,93). In the kidney, Ang-(1–7)heptapeptide has a potent natriuretic/diuretic action, probably via prostaglandin I_2 release and inhibition of tubular sodium and bicarbonate re-absorption (94). In the heart and blood vessels, Ang-(1–7)heptapeptide behaves as an angiotensin II antagonist. It generally promotes vasodilation either via bradykinin potentiation or directly by binding to a specific receptor other than AT1 or AT2. Ang-(1–7)heptapeptide has also been shown to stimulate DNA synthesis in human skin fibroblasts and to promote growth of cardiac fibroblasts, whereas it inhibits vascular smooth muscle cell growth with an overall antiangiogenic effect (95).

C. Angiotensin III

The heptapeptide angiotensin III derives from angiotensin II and it mainly exerts its effects on the central nervous system, leading to increased blood pressure by increasing vasopressin release and thirst (96). Vasopressin is released from the posterior pituitary into the blood after stimulation by neurons that originate from the supraoptic nucleus and the paraventricular nucleus. Because there is no AT1 or AT2 receptor mRNA in these brain areas, the stimulatory action of angiotensin III on supraoptic nucleus and paraventricular nucleus might be an indirect effect involving another neuromediator, or it might involve another Ang receptor subtype specific for angiotensin III. In the heart and vessels, the effects of angiotensin III are similar to those of angiotensin II, i.e. induction of vasoconstriction and sodium retention. Like angiotensin II, angiotensin III also induces aldosterone release by the adrenal gland (97–100). Angiotensin III displays other features similar to angiotensin II proinflammatory properties. In fact in mononuclear cells, angiotensin III regulates monocyte chemoattractant protein-1 chemokine production and activates the transcription factors NF-κB and AP-1 (101). In pathological situations, such as diabetes, hypertension, and nephritis, renal aminopeptidase A, the enzyme that degrades angiotensin II to angiotensin III is increased. Moreover, in mesangial cells, angiotensin III induces overexpression of growth-related, profibrotic, and proinflammatory genes. All these data suggest that angiotensin III could regulate cell growth, extra cellular matrix accumulation, and inflammatory cell responses and therefore contribute to the progression of kidney damage. Angiotensin III-mediated intracellular signaling pathways, such as calcium mobilization, induction of c-fos gene expression, and the activation of various transcription factors are similar to those of angiotensin II.

D. Angiotensin IV

Angiotensin IV is primarily produced by cleavage of angiotensin III. Its half-life is very short because it is converted rapidly to inactive fragments by various enzymes (aminopeptidases, endopeptidases, carboxypeptidases) that are widely distributed in the various tissues. Angiotensin IV is believed to exert its actions via a specific receptor the AT4, which is not affected by AT1 or AT2 blockers (102). Angiotensin IV has been postulated to be the link between the fibrinolytic system and the renin–angiotensin–aldosterone system. It is believed to induce plasminogen activator inhibitor 1 secretion, thus inhibiting fibrinolysis (Fig. 9.5) (103). In addition, angiotensin IV has been shown *in vivo* to reduce vascular resistance in renal and cerebral vascular beds, effects that are inhibited by AT4 antagonism (104,105). Moreover, angiotensin IV has been shown to mediate central nervous system effects. Indeed, binding of angiotensin IV to the AT4 receptor enhances learning and memory in normal rodents and reverses the memory deficits seen in animal models of amnesia (50). Angiotensin IV binds to the AT4 receptor with high affinity. Because the AT4 receptor is identical with the insulin-regulated aminopeptidase and because angiotensin IV is not cleaved by insulin-regulated aminopeptidase, this peptide could become a prototype inhibitor of insulin-regulated aminopeptidase. Such inhibitors are of interest for the treatment of memory loss like in Alzheimer's disease (106).

IV. SYSTEMIC vs. LOCAL RENIN– ANGIOTENSIN–ALDOSTERONE SYSTEM

The observation by Ganten et al. (107) of renin-like activity in the brain led to the concept of tissue renin–angiotensin–aldosterone system in various organs. These systems are hypothesized to produce angiotensins independently of renal renin. A landmark paper of Campbell (108) in 1987 proposed the cross-talk between circulating and vascular tissue components of the renin–angiotensin

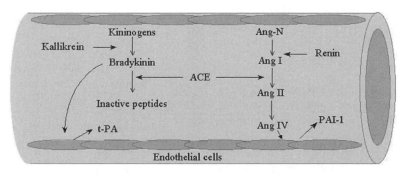

Figure 9.5 Angiotensin IV links fibrinolytic system and renin–angiotensin–aldosterone system.

system. Later, in addition to the well-established role of the circulating renin–angiotensin–aldosterone system in regulating pressure and fluid balance, it became clear that angiotensin II also exerts local effects in various organs that are independent of its hemodynamic effects. The degree to which individual tissue production of angiotensin II is in fact independent of renal renin remains controversial, but virtually all investigators agree that local Ang II concentrations are the key issue. Furthermore, several nonrenin enzymes (tonin, cathepsin, pepsin, etc.) have been shown to generate angiotensin peptides from angiotensinogen. Thus, angiotensinogen, but not necessarily renin, is required for the production of angiotensin I or angiotensin II. In addition, the conversion of angiotensin I to angiotensin II does not depend exclusively on the classic ACE (109); it also may be catalyzed in tissues, such as the heart, by chymostatin-sensitive chymases (110). Messenger RNA for angiotensinogen or renin has been found in many organs (111). Because the corresponding protein often localizes in tissues, the question of uptake from plasma or local protein synthesis had to be answered. It has been claimed that cultured rat cardiac myocytes released angiotensin II when they were stretched, but such results have never been confirmed. It would not be surprising, in this context, if distinct organs, such as the brain, ovary, and placenta, could generate angiotensin II independently of renal renin. However, theories about any angiotensin II-producing system in tissues should be based on reliable measurements of tissue concentrations of angiotensins and careful comparison with plasma concentrations and other components of the system. Studies of the last decade support the idea that local concentrations of angiotensin II appear to be determined largely by circulating renal renin, possibly by the tissue uptake of angiotensinogen (generated in the liver) from the circulation, and finally from the number of half-life prolonging-specific angiotensin II receptors. A recently discovered new renin receptor may or may not signal via angiotensin II (112,113). In healthy volunteers who were treated with an oral renin inhibitor, plasma levels of angiotensin II could be predicted precisely from measured plasma renin, angiotensinogen, and drug concentration (114). This predictability could not be expected, if a nonrenal tissue source of renin contributed to plasma angiotensin II in a nonsynchronized manner. Similar observations were made in human volunteers during a study of ACE inhibition (115).

In various animal experiments (rat, mouse, pig), a linear correlation exists between plasma and tissue concentrations of angiotensin II in various organs (116). In these animals, tissue concentrations of angiotensin II could not be explained by plasma contamination (values that are too high), and the slope of the correlation of tissue to plasma angiotensin II was quite different in various

organs (1–1000 fmol/g per fmol/mL), thus excluding simple plasma uptake. In a rodent model of renovascular hypertension (the two-kidneys, one-clip hypertension), circulating renin and angiotensin II levels are high. Interestingly, these animals show equally increased tissue levels of angiotensin II in the heart, adrenal glands, liver, and other organs, and thus this also suggests a major impact of the enhanced circulating renal renin. The same increased angiotensin II levels were found in the tissues of salt-depleted rats with very high circulating renal renin (116). One of the most convincing pieces of evidence for the predominant role of renal renin is the fact that angiotensin II virtually disappears from the plasma and tissues after a bilateral nephrectomy (116,117). Angiotensin II levels fell from the normal value of 4 to <2 fmol/mL within 2 days after a binephrectomy. Similar results have been obtained in binephrectomized rats and pigs; in these animals, angiotensin II and renin disappeared from the plasma and from the tissues. Of six anephric patients who were on dialysis treatment for months or years, we found no plasma angiotensin II in three of the patients (<0.1 fmol/mL) and ≤10% of normal plasma angiotensin II levels in the other three patients.

These observations emphasize the important role of renal renin in the regulation of both plasma and tissue angiotensin II concentrations.

V. CONCLUSIONS

The renin–angiotensin–aldosterone system (RAAS) plays a major role in regulating blood pressure and fluid homeostasis. In addition, more recent findings demonstrate that the RAAS is also a major contributor to processes such as cardiovascular remodelling, inflammation, and atherosclerosis. The RAAS can no longer be questioned as a pivotal player in physiology and pathophysiology.

REFERENCES

1. Tigerstedt R, Bergmann P. Niere und Kreislauf. Scand Arch Physiol 1898; 223–271.
2. Mazzolai L, Pedrazzini T, Nicoud F, Gabbiani G, Brunner HR, Nussberger J. Increased cardiac angiotensin II levels induce right and left ventricular hypertrophy in normotensive mice. Hypertension 2000; 35:985–991.
3. Mazzolai L, Duchosal MA, Korber M, Bouzourene K, Aubert JF, Hao H, Vallet V, Brunner H-R, Nussberger J, Gabbiani G, Hayoz D. Endogenous angiotensin II induces atherosclerotic plaque vulnerability and elicits a Th1 response in ApoE−/− mice. Hypertension 2004; 44:277–282.
4. Vaughan DE. The renin–angiotensin system and fibrinolysis. Am J Cardiol 1997; 79:12–16.

5. Haznedaroglu IC, Ozturk MA. Towards the understanding of the local hematopoietic bone marrow renin–angiotensin system. Int J Biochem Cell Biol 2003; 35:867–880.

6. Leung PS, Sernia C. The renin–angiotensin system and male reproduction: new functions for old hormones. J Mol Endocrinol 2003; 30:263–270.

7. Della BR, Pinet F, Corvol P, Kurtz A. Opposite regulation of renin gene expression by cyclic AMP and calcium in isolated mouse juxtaglomerular cells. Kidney Int 1995; 47:1266–1273.

8. Nussberger J, Fluckiger JP, Hui KY, Evequoz D, Waeber B, Brunner HR. Angiotensin I and II disappear completely from circulating blood within 48 hours after binephrectomy: improved measurement of angiotensins in rat plasma. J Hypertens 1991; 9(suppl):S230–S231.

9. Hackenthal E, Hackenthal R, Hilgenfeldt U. Isorenin, pseudorenin, cathepsin D and renin. A comparative enzymatic study of angiotensin-forming enzymes. Biochim Biophys Acta 1978; 522:574–588.

10. Morris BJ, Reid IA. A "renin-like" enzymatic action of cathepsin D and the similarity in subcellular distributions of "renin-like" activity and cathepsin D in the midbrain of dogs. Endocrinology 1978; 103:1289–1296.

11. Araujo RC, Lima MP, Lomez ES, Bader M, Pesquero JB, Sumitani M, Pesquero JL. Tonin expression in the rat brain and tonin-mediated central production of angiotensin II. Physiol Behav 2002; 76:327–333.

12. Ikeda M, Sasaguri M, Maruta H, Arakawa K. Formation of angiotensin II by tonin-inhibitor complex. Hypertension 1988; 11:63–70.

13. Nishimura II, Buikcma H, Baltatu O, Ganten D, Urata H. Functional evidence for alternative ANG II-forming pathways in hamster cardiovascular system. Am J Physiol 1998; 275:H1307–H1312.

14. Erdos EG, Deddish PA. The kinin system: suggestions to broaden some prevailing concepts. Int Immunopharmacol 2002; 2:1741–1746.

15. Liao Y, Husain A. The chymase-angiotensin system in humans: biochemistry, molecular biology and potential role in cardiovascular diseases. Can J Cardiol 1995; 11(suppl F):13F–19F.

16. Matsumoto T, Wada A, Tsutamoto T, Ohnishi M, Isono T, Kinoshita M. Chymase inhibition prevents cardiac fibrosis and improves diastolic dysfunction in the progression of heart failure. Circulation 2003; 107:2555–2558.

17. Takai S, Miyazaki M. The role of chymase in vascular proliferation. Drug News Perspect 2002; 15:278–282.

18. Urata H, Kinoshita A, Misono KS, Bumpus FM, Husain A. Identification of a highly specific chymase as the major angiotensin II-forming enzyme in the human heart. J Biol Chem 1990; 265:22348–22357.

19. Stewart TA, Weare JA, Erdos EG. Human peptidyl dipeptidase (converting enzyme, kininase II). Methods Enzymol 1981; 80(Pt C):450–460.

20. Harmer D, Gilbert M, Borman R, Clark KL. Quantitative mRNA expression profiling of ACE 2, a novel homologue of angiotensin-converting enzyme. FEBS Lett 2002; 532:107–110.

21. Donoghue M, Hsieh F, Baronas E, Godbout K, Gosselin M, Stagliano N, Donovan M, Woolf B, Robison K, Jeyaseelan R, Breitbart RE, Acton S. A novel angiotensin-converting enzyme-related carboxy-peptidase (ACE2) converts angiotensin I to angiotensin 1–9. Circ Res 2000; 87:E1–E9.

22. Skidgel RA. Bradykinin-degrading enzymes: structure, function, distribution, and potential roles in cardiovascular pharmacology. J Cardiovasc Pharmacol 1992; 20(suppl 9):S4–S9.

23. Burch RM, Kyle DJ. Recent developments in the understanding of bradykinin receptors. Life Sci 1992; 50:829–838.

24. Yayama K, Nagaoka M, Takano M, Okamoto H. Expression of kininogen, kallikrein and kinin receptor genes by rat cardiomyocytes. Biochim Biophys Acta 2000; 1495:69–77.

25. Ritchie RH, Marsh JD, Lancaster WD, Diglio CA, Schiebinger RJ. Bradykinin blocks angiotensin II-induced hypertrophy in the presence of endothelial cells. Hypertension 1998; 31:39–44.

26. Witherow FN, Dawson P, Ludlam CA, Webb DJ, Fox KA, Newby DE. Bradykinin receptor antagonism and endothelial tissue plasminogen activator release in humans. Arterioscler Thromb Vasc Biol 2003; 23:1667–1670.

27. Matsumoto T, Minai K, Horie H, Ohira N, Takashima H, Tarutani Y, Yasuda Y, Ozawa T, Matsuo S, Kinoshita M, Horie M. Angiotensin-converting enzyme inhibition but not angiotensin II type 1 receptor antagonism augments coronary release of tissue plasminogen activator in hypertensive patients. J Am Coll Cardiol 2003; 41:1373–1379.

28. Pretorius M, Rosenbaum D, Vaughan DE, Brown NJ. Angiotensin-converting enzyme inhibition increases human vascular tissue-type plasminogen activator release through endogenous bradykinin. Circulation 2003; 107:579–585.

29. Miura S, Saku K, Karnik SS. Molecular analysis of the structure and function of the angiotensin II type 1 receptor. Hypertens Res 2003; 26:937–943.

30. Schiffrin EL, Touyz RM. Multiple actions of angiotensin II in hypertension: benefits of AT1 receptor blockade. J Am Coll Cardiol 2003; 42:911–913.

31. Kaschina E, Unger T. Angiotensin AT1/AT2 receptors: regulation, signalling and function. Blood Press 2003; 12:70–88.

32. de Gasparo M, Catt KJ, Inagami T, Wright JW, Unger T. International Union of Pharmacology. XXIII. The angiotensin II receptors. Pharmacol Rev 2000; 52:415–472.

33. Hunyady L, Catt KJ, Clark AJ, Gaborik Z. Mechanisms and functions of AT(1) angiotensin receptor internalization. Regul Pept 2000; 91:29–44.

34. Spat A, Enyedi P, Hajnoczky G, Hunyady L. Generation and role of calcium signal in adrenal glomerulosa cells. Exp Physiol 1991; 76:859–885.

35. Berk BC, Corson MA. Angiotensin II signal transduction in vascular smooth muscle: role of tyrosine kinases. Circ Res 1997; 80:607–616.

36. Saito Y, Berk BC. Angiotensin II-mediated signal transduction pathways. Curr Hypertens Rep 2002; 4:167–171.

37. Ushio-Fukai M, Zafari AM, Fukui T, Ishizaka N, Griendling KK. p22phox is a critical component of the superoxide-generating NADH/NADPH oxidase system and regulates angiotensin II-induced hypertrophy in vascular smooth muscle cells. J Biol Chem 1996; 271:23317–23321.

38. Griendling KK, Minieri CA, Ollerenshaw JD, Alexander RW. Angiotensin II stimulates NADH and NADPH oxidase activity in cultured vascular smooth muscle cells. Circ Res 1994; 74:1141–1148.

39. Griendling KK, Ushio-Fukai M. Reactive oxygen species as mediators of angiotensin II signaling. Regul Pept 2000; 91:21–27.

40. Thomas WG. Regulation of angiotensin II type 1 (AT1) receptor function. Regul Pept 1999; 79:9–23.

41. Catt KJ, Olivares Reyes AJ, Zhang M, Smith RD, Hunyady L. Activation and phosphorylation of angiotensin AT1 and AT2 receptors. Endocr Res 2000; 26:559–560.

42. Werbonat Y, Kleutges N, Jakobs KH, van Koppen CJ. Essential role of dynamin in internalization of M2 muscarinic acetylcholine and angiotensin AT1A receptors. J Biol Chem 2000; 275:21969–21974.

43. Gaborik Z, Szaszak M, Szidonya L, Balla B, Paku S, Catt KJ, Clark AJ, Hunyady L. Beta-arrestin- and dynamin-dependent endocytosis of the AT1 angiotensin receptor. Mol Pharmacol 2001; 59:239–247.

44. Ferguson SS. Evolving concepts in G protein-coupled receptor endocytosis: the role in receptor desensitization and signaling. Pharmacol Rev 2001; 53:1–24.

45. Hunyady L, Baukal AJ, Gaborik Z, Olivares-Reyes JA, Bor M, Szaszak M, Lodge R, Catt KJ, Balla T. Differential PI 3-kinase dependence of early and late phases of recycling of the internalized AT1 angiotensin receptor. J Cell Biol 2002; 157:1211–1222.

46. Dudley DT, Hubbell SE, Summerfelt RM. Characterization of angiotensin II (AT2) binding sites in R3T3 cells. Mol Pharmacol 1991; 40:360–367.

47. Csikos T, Balmforth AJ, Grojec M, Gohlke P, Culman J, Unger T. Angiotensin AT2 receptor degradation is prevented by ligand occupation. Biochem Biophys Res Commun 1998; 243:142–147.

48. Bottari SP, King IN, Reichlin S, Dahlstroem I, Lydon N, de Gasparo M. The angiotensin AT2 receptor stimulates protein tyrosine phosphatase activity and mediates inhibition of particulate guanylate cyclase. Biochem Biophys Res Commun 1992; 183:206–211.

49. Zhuo J, Moeller I, Jenkins T, Chai SY, Allen AM, Ohishi M, Mendelsohn FA. Mapping tissue angiotensin-converting enzyme and angiotensin AT1, AT2 and AT4 receptors. J Hypertens 1998; 16:2027–2037.

50. Albiston AL, Mustafa T, McDowall SG, Mendelsohn FA, Lee J, Chai SY. AT4 receptor is insulin-regulated membrane aminopeptidase: potential mechanisms of memory enhancement. Trends Endocrinol Metab 2003; 14:72–77.

51. Mehta JL, Li DY, Yang H, Raizada MK. Angiotensin II and IV stimulate expression and release of plasminogen activator inhibitor-1 in cultured human coronary artery endothelial cells. J Cardiovasc Pharmacol 2002; 39:789–794.

52. Pawlikowski M, Gruszka A, Mucha S, Melen-Mucha G. Angiotensins II and IV stimulate the rat adrenocortical cell proliferation acting via different receptors. Endocr Regul 2001; 35:139–142.

53. Kramar EA, Armstrong DL, Ikeda S, Wayner MJ, Harding JW, Wright JW. The effects of angiotensin IV analogs on long-term potentiation within the CA1 region of the hippocampus in vitro. Brain Res 2001; 897:114–121.

54. Krishnan R, Hanesworth JM, Wright JW, Harding JW. Structure-binding studies of the adrenal AT4 receptor: analysis of position two- and three-modified angiotensin IV analogs. Peptides 1999; 20:915–920.

55. Patel JM, Martens JR, Li YD, Gelband CH, Raizada MK, Block ER. Angiotensin IV receptor-mediated activation of lung endothelial NOS is associated with vasorelaxation. Am J Physiol 1998; 275:L1061–L1068.

56. Diz DI, Ferrario CM. Angiotensin receptor heterogeneity in the dorsal medulla oblongata as defined by angiotensin-(1–7). Adv Exp Med Biol 1996; 396:225–235.

57. Santos RA, Campagnole-Santos MJ, Baracho NC, Fontes MA, Silva LC, Neves LA, Oliveira DR, Caligiorne SM, Rodrigues AR, Gropen JC. Characterization of a new angiotensin antagonist selective for angiotensin-(1–7): evidence that the actions of angiotensin-(1–7) are mediated by specific angiotensin receptors. Brain Res Bull 1994; 35:293–298.

58. Ferrario CM, Iyer SN. Angiotensin-(1–7): a bioactive fragment of the renin–angiotensin system. Regul Pept 1998; 78:13–18.

59. Lombes M, Farman N, Bonvalet JP, Zennaro MC. Identification and role of aldosterone receptors in the cardiovascular system. Ann Endocrinol (Paris) 2000; 61:41–46.

60. Gomez-Sanchez EP. Central hypertensive effects of aldosterone. Front Neuroendocrinol 1997; 18:440–462.

61. Takeda R, Hatakeyama H, Takeda Y, Iki K, Miyamori I, Sheng WP, Yamamoto H, Blair IA. Aldosterone biosynthesis and action in vascular cells. Steroids 1995; 60:120–124.

62. Weber KT, Sun Y, Wodi LA, Munir A, Jahangir E, Ahokas RA, Gerling IC, Postlethwaite AE, Warrington KJ. Toward a broader understanding of aldosterone in congestive heart failure. J Renin Angiotensin Aldosterone Syst 2003; 4:155–163.

63. Mill JG, Milanez MC, de Resende MM, Gomes MG, Leite CM. Spironolactone prevents cardiac collagen proliferation after myocardial infarction in rats. Clin Exp Pharmacol Physiol 2003; 30:739–744.

64. Funder J. Mineralocorticoids and cardiac fibrosis: the decade in review. Clin Exp Pharmacol Physiol 2001; 28:1002–1006.

65. Delcayre C, Silvestre JS, Garnier A, Oubenaissa A, Cailmail S, Tatara E, Swynghedauw B, Robert V. Cardiac aldosterone production and ventricular remodeling. Kidney Int 2000; 57:1346–1351.

66. Fiebeler A, Nussberger J, Shagdarsuren E, Rong S, Hilfenhaus G, Al-Saadi N, Dechend R, Wellner M, Meiners S, Maser-Gluth C, Jeng AY, Webb RL, Luft FC, Muller DN. An aldosterone synthase inhibitor ameliorates angiotensin II–induced end-organ damage. Circulation 2005; in press.

67. Zusman RM, Burton J, Nussberger J, Christensen D, Dodds A, Haber E. Hemodynamic effects of a competitive renin inhibitory peptide in humans: evidence for multiple mechanisms of action. Trans Assoc Am Physicians 1983; 96:365–374.

68. Gradman AH, Schmieder RE, Nussberger J, Lins RL, Chiang Y, Bedigian MP. Aliskiren, a novel orally active effective renin inhibitor, provides dose-dependent antihypertensive efficacy and placebo-like tolerability in hypertensive patients. Circulation 2005, 111:1012–1018.

69. Harrap SB, Van der Merwe WM, Griffin SA, Macpherson F, Lever AF. Brief angiotensin-converting enzyme inhibitor treatment in young spontaneously hypertensive rats reduces blood pressure long-term. Hypertension 1990; 16:603–614.

70. Makino N, Sugano M, Hata T, Taguchi S, Yanaga T. Chronic low-dose treatment with enalapril induced cardiac regression of left ventricular hypertrophy. Mol Cell Biochem 1996; 163–164:239–245.

71. Veniant M, Clozel JP, Heudes D, Banken L, Menard J. Effects of Ro 40–5967, a new calcium antagonist, and enalapril on cardiac remodeling in renal hypertensive rats. J Cardiovasc Pharmacol 1993; 21:544–551.

72. Mazzolai L, Nussberger J, Aubert JF, Brunner DB, Gabbiani G, Brunner HR, Pedrazzini T. Blood pressure-independent cardiac hypertrophy induced by locally activated renin–angiotensin system. Hypertension 1998; 31:1324–1330.

73. Itoh H, Mukoyama M, Pratt RE, Gibbons GH, Dzau VJ. Multiple autocrine growth factors modulate vascular smooth muscle cell growth response to angiotensin II. J Clin Invest 1993; 91:2268–2274.

74. Macrez N, Morel JL, Kalkbrenner F, Viard P, Schultz G, Mironneau J. A betagamma dimer derived from G13 transduces the angiotensin AT1 receptor signal to stimulation of Ca2+ channels in rat portal vein myocytes. J Biol Chem 1997; 272:23180–23185.

75. Berk BC, Vekshtein V, Gordon HM, Tsuda T. Angiotensin II-stimulated protein synthesis in cultured vascular smooth muscle cells. Hypertension 1989; 13:305–314.

76. Yusuf S, Pepine CJ, Garces C, Pouleur H, Salem D, Kostis J, Benedict C, Rousseau M, Bourassa M, Pitt B. Effect of enalapril on myocardial infarction and unstable angina in patients with low ejection fractions. Lancet 1992; 340:1173–1178.

77. Yusuf S, Sleight P, Pogue J, Bosch J, Davies R, Dagenais G. Effects of an angiotensin-converting-enzyme inhibitor, ramipril, on cardiovascular events in high-risk patients. The Heart Outcomes Prevention Evaluation Study Investigators. N Engl J Med 2000; 342:145–153.

78. Chobanian AV, Haudenschild CC, Nickerson C, Drago R. Antiatherogenic effect of captopril in the Watanabe heritable hyperlipidemic rabbit. Hypertension 1990; 15:327–331.

79. Strawn WB, Chappell MC, Dean RH, Kivlighn S, Ferrario CM. Inhibition of early atherogenesis by losartan in monkeys with diet-induced hypercholesterolemia. Circulation 2000; 101:1586–1593.

80. Thomas DW, Hoffman MD. Identification of macrophage receptors for angiotensin: a potential role in antigen uptake for T lymphocyte responses? J Immunol 1984; 132:2807–2812.

81. Chen XL, Tummala PE, Olbrych MT, Alexander RW, Medford RM. Angiotensin II induces monocyte chemoattractant protein-1 gene expression in rat vascular smooth muscle cells. Circ Res 1998; 83:952–959.

82. Soejima H, Ogawa H, Yasue H, Kaikita K, Takazoe K, Nishiyama K, Misumi K, Miyamoto S, Yoshimura M, Kugiyama K, Nakamura S, Tsuji I. Angiotensin-converting enzyme inhibition reduces monocyte chemoattractant protein-1 and tissue factor levels in patients with myocardial infarction. J Am Coll Cardiol 1999; 34:983–988.

83. Funakoshi Y, Ichiki T, Ito K, Takeshita A. Induction of interleukin-6 expression by angiotensin II in rat vascular smooth muscle cells. Hypertension 1999; 34:118–125.

84. Schieffer B, Schieffer E, Hilfiker-Kleiner D, Hilfiker A, Kovanen PT, Kaartinen M, Nussberger J, Harringer W, Drexler H. Expression of angiotensin II and interleukin 6 in human coronary atherosclerotic plaques: potential implications for inflammation and plaque instability. Circulation 2000; 101:1372–1378.

85. Pueyo ME, Gonzalez W, Nicoletti A, Savoie F, Arnal JF, Michel JB. Angiotensin II stimulates endothelial vascular cell adhesion molecule-1 via nuclear factor-kappaB activation induced by intracellular oxidative stress. Arterioscler Thromb Vasc Biol 2000; 20:645–651.

86. Tummala PE, Chen XL, Sundell CL, Laursen JB, Hammes CP, Alexander RW, Harrison DG, Medford RM. Angiotensin II induces vascular cell adhesion molecule-1 expression in rat vasculature: A potential link between the renin–angiotensin system and atherosclerosis. Circulation 1999; 100:1223–1229.

87. Rajagopalan S, Kurz S, Munzel T, Tarpey M, Freeman BA, Griendling KK, Harrison DG. Angiotensin II-mediated hypertension in the rat increases vascular superoxide production via membrane NADH/NADPH oxidase activation. Contribution to alterations of vasomotor tone. J Clin Invest 1996; 97:1916–1923.

88. Nishimura H, Tsuji H, Masuda H, Nakagawa K, Nakahara Y, Kitamura H, Kasahara T, Sugano T, Yoshizumi M, Sawada S, Nakagawa M. Angiotensin II increases plasminogen activator inhibitor-1 and tissue factor mRNA expression without changing that of tissue type plasminogen activator or tissue factor pathway inhibitor in cultured rat aortic endothelial cells. Thromb Haemost 1997; 77:1189–1195.

89. Mazzolai L, Duchosal M, Korber M, Bouzourene K, Aubert J-F, Vallet V, Hao H, Nussberger J, Gabbiani G, Hayoz D. Endogeneous angiotensin II induces atherosclerotic plaque vulnerability eliciting a Th1 response in ApoE$^{-/-}$ mice. Hypertension 2004; 44:277–282.

90. Ferrario CM, Iyer SN. Angiotensin-(1–7): a bioactive fragment of the renin–angiotensin system. Regul Pept 1998; 78:13–18.

91. Kucharewicz I, Pawlak R, Matys T, Chabielska E, Buczko W. Angiotensin-(1–7): an active member of the renin–angiotensin system. J Physiol Pharmacol 2002; 53:533–540.

92. Pawlak R, Napiorkowska-Pawlak D, Takada Y, Urano T, Nagai N, Ihara H, Takada A. The differential effect of angiotensin II and angiotensin 1–7 on norepinephrine, epinephrine, and dopamine concentrations in rat hypothalamus: the involvement of angiotensin receptors. Brain Res Bull 2001; 54:689–694.

93. Magaldi AJ, Cesar KR, de Araujo M, Simoes e Silva AC, Santos RA. Angiotensin-(1–7) stimulates water transport in rat inner medullary collecting duct: evidence for involvement of vasopressin V2 receptors. Pflugers Arch 2003; 447:223–230.

94. Burgelova M, Kramer HJ, Teplan V, Velickova G, Vitko S, Heller J, Maly J, Cervenka L. Intrarenal infusion of angiotensin-(1–7) modulates renal functional responses to exogenous angiotensin II in the rat. Kidney Blood Press Res 2002; 25:202–210.

95. Freeman EJ, Chisolm GM, Ferrario CM, Tallant EA. Angiotensin-(1–7) inhibits vascular smooth muscle cell growth. Hypertension 1996; 28:104–108.

96. Reaux A, Fournie-Zaluski MC, Llorens-Cortes C. Angiotensin III: a central regulator of vasopressin release and blood pressure. Trends Endocrinol Metab 2001; 12:157–162.

97. Blair-West JR, Coghlan JP, Denton DA, Fei DT, Hardy KJ, Scoggins BA, Wright RD. A dose-response comparison of the actions of angiotensin II and angiotensin III in sheep. J Endocrinol 1980; 87:409–417.

98. Campbell WB, Brooks SN, Pettinger WA. Angiotensin II- and angiotensin 3-induced aldosterone release vivo in the rat. Science 1974; 184:994–996.

99. Suzuki S, Doi Y, Aoi W, Kuramochi M, Hashiba K. Effect of angiotensin III on blood pressure, renin–angiotensin–aldosterone system in normal and hypertensive subjects. Jpn Heart J 1984; 25:75–85.

100. Zager PG, Luetscher JA. Effects of angiotensin III and ACTH on aldosterone secretion. Clin Exp Hypertens A 1982; 4:1481–1504.

101. Ruiz-Ortega M, Lorenzo O, Egido J. Angiotensin III increases MCP-1 and activates NF-kappaB and AP-1 in cultured mesangial and mononuclear cells. Kidney Int 2000; 57:2285–2298.

102. Wright JW, Krebs LT, Stobb JW, Harding JW. The angiotensin IV system: functional implications. Front Neuroendocrinol 1995; 16:23–52.

103. Kerins DM, Hao Q, Vaughan DE. Angiotensin induction of PAI-1 expression in endothelial cells is mediated by the hexapeptide angiotensin IV. J Clin Invest 1995; 96:2515–2520.

104. Loufrani L, Henrion D, Chansel D, Ardaillou R, Levy BI. Functional evidence for an angiotensin IV receptor in rat resistance arteries. J Pharmacol Exp Ther 1999; 291:583–588.

105. Kramar EA, Harding JW, Wright JW. Angiotensin II- and IV-induced changes in cerebral blood flow. Roles of AT1, AT2, and AT4 receptor subtypes. Regul Pept 1997; 68:131–138.

106. Albiston AL, Fernando R, Ye S, Peck GR, Chai SY. Alzheimer's, angiotensin IV and an aminopeptidase. Biol Pharm Bull 2004; 27:765–767.

107. Ganten D, Marquez-Julio A, Granger P, Hayduk K, Karsunky KP, Boucher R, Genest J. Renin in dog brain. Am J Physiol 1971; 221:1733–1737.

108. Campbell DJ. Circulating and tissue angiotensin systems. J Clin Invest 1987; 79:1–6.

109. Yang HY, Erdos EG, Levin Y. A dipeptidyl carboxypeptidase that converts angiotensin I and inactivates bradykinin. Biochim Biophys Acta 1970; 214:374–376.

110. Urata H, Kinoshita A, Misono KS, Bumpus FM, Husain A. Identification of a highly specific chymase as the major angiotensin II-forming enzyme in the human heart. J Biol Chem 1990; 265:22348–22357.

111. Dzau VJ, Ellison KE, Brody T, Ingelfinger J, Pratt RE. A comparative study of the distributions of renin and angiotensinogen messenger ribonucleic acids in rat and mouse tissues. Endocrinology 1987; 120:2334–2338.

112. Nguyen G, Burckle CA, Sraer JD. Renin/prorenin-receptor biochemistry and functional significance. Curr Hypertens Rep 2004; 6:129–132.

113. Nguyen G, Burckle C, Sraer JD. The renin receptor: the facts, the promise and the hope. Curr Opin Nephrol Hypertens 2003; 12:51–55.

114. Camenzind E, Nussberger J, Juillerat L, Munafo A, Fischli W, Coassolo P, van Brummelen P, Kleinbloesem CH, Waeber B, Brunner HR. Effect of the renin response during renin inhibition: oral Ro 42–5892 in normal humans. J Cardiovasc Pharmacol 1991; 18:299–307.

115. Juillerat L, Nussberger J, Menard J, Mooser V, Christen Y, Waeber B, Graf P, Brunner HR. Determinants of angiotensin II generation during converting enzyme inhibition. Hypertension 1990; 16:564–572.

116. Nussberger J. Circulating versus tissue angiotensin II. In: Epstein M, Brunner H, eds. Angiotensin II Receptor Antagonists. Philadelphia: Hanley & Belfus, 2000.

117. Campbell DJ, Kladis A, Skinner SL, Whitworth JA. Characterization of angiotensin peptides in plasma of anephric man. J Hypertens 1991; 9:265–274.

10

The Autonomic Nervous System in Hypertension

ALBERTO U. FERRARI, STEFANO PERLINI, MARCO CENTOLA
Università di Milano-Bicocca, Milano, Italy
Università di Pavia, Pavia, Italy
Centro Interuniversitario di Fisiologia Clinica e Ipertensione, Milano, Italy

KEYPOINTS

- Autonomic imbalance may play a causative factor in initiating hypertension.
- Sympathetic overactivity is a feature of the established hypertensive state.
- The autonomic nervous system and many molecules such as insulin, leptin, nitric oxide, reactive oxygen species, vasopressin, cytokines and many other substances that interact with neural mechanisms affect blood pressure, cardiovascular homeostasis, and hypertensive complications.

SUMMARY

Altered autonomic modulation of cardiac output, peripheral vascular resistance and renal water, and sodium handling may contribute to the genesis of high blood pressure. Derangements in neural cardiovascular control have been documented in human hypertension as well as in experimental hypertensive models. Gaining mechanistic insight into such derangements is challenging because along with the autonomic nervous system, numerous nonneural systems such as insulin, leptin, nitric oxide, reactive oxygen species, vasopressin, cytokines, and many others, powerfully affect cardiovascular homeostasis by acting either directly or by interacting with neural mechanisms. Finally, sympathetic influences are clearly involved in the genesis of hypertensive complications including myocardial hypertrophy and fibrosis, left ventricular dysfunction and failure, myocardial infarction, and atherogenesis.

I. INTRODUCTION

Arterial blood pressure and cardiovascular function at large are controlled by the autonomic nervous system whose parasympathetic and sympathetic divisions mediate inhibitory and excitatory influences, respectively. Even minute variations of the modulatory activity of either autonomic division may in the long run promote physiologically and clinically important cardiovascular alterations. In the frame of the multifactorial origin of high blood pressure, the hypothesis that hypertension may indeed represent one such alteration, that is at least in a sizeable proportion of the hypertensive population, the rise in blood pressure depends upon an abnormal autonomic cardiovascular regulation, has long been investigated, although its experimental confirmation has been far from complete. Because limitations in our methodological armamentarium have certainly represented one of the major difficulties encountered along this line of research, it is fortunate that recent technical advances allowed more and more cogent evidence in this direction to be collected.

At the same time, however, autonomic function was shown to be affected by complex interactions of diverse nonneural influences and in turn to exert a regulatory role on nonneural functions such as growth processes, cell metabolism, fluid and electrolyte balance, immune/inflammatory responses, the coagulatory cascade, and so on. Considering the strict dependence of blood pressure on autonomic neural activity, a contemporary picture about the autonomic origin of hypertension has to be outlined in the framework of the multifold earlier mentioned factors; each of them having the potential to play a causative role via modulation of autonomic influences.

In the present discussion, we will summarize the status of our knowledge about (i) the available methods to assess autonomic function, (ii) the physiological mechanisms of short-term and long-term autonomic regulation of blood pressure, (iii) the role of autonomic imbalance as a causative factor in initiating hypertension, (iv) sympathetic overactivity as a feature of the established hypertensive state, (v) the possible mechanisms underlying autonomic imbalance, and (vi) autonomic involvement in the genesis of hypertensive complications.

II. METHODS TO STUDY AUTONOMIC FUNCTION IN MAN

The time-honored measurement of plasma concentrations of norepinephrine and epinephrine provides a somewhat rough estimate of the extent of sympathetic activity (1); although still employed to this purpose, it has serious limitations especially because of low sensitivity and because of its inability to provide information on differential activation of the sympathetic system in different territories. Furthermore, plasma norepinephrine concentrations do not by definition directly reflect sympathetic firing and

neurotransmitter release but are also dependent on plasma clearance of this substance.

A much refined biochemical method to assess sympathetic activity is the measurement of tritiated norepinephrine spillover rate by which the appearance rate of the neurotransmitter (in mixed venous blood or in blood from single regional beds) can be accurately measured (2,3); this approach overcomes some of the most significant limitations of systemic venous plasma norepinephrine concentrations but obviously suffers from the inconveniences of being a time consuming, invasive (regional venous catheters have to be implanted), and costly procedure: in addition, only a few determinations can be performed in a given session.

A quite different approach has been represented by clinical microneurography. This now well-established technique provides direct measurement of efferent sympathetic nerve firing by means of thin tungsten electrodes inserted in neural trunks accessible through the skin, usually the peroneal or the median nerve (4,5). It has the advantage of being minimally invasive and of allowing prolonged recordings to be performed, so that neural responses to physiological stimuli can be evaluated; it has however the limitations of not permitting measurements in nonsuperficial nerves (splanchnic, renal, cardiac) and of involving almost complete patient's immobility.

Analysis of the variability of cardiovascular signals, heart rate, and, to a lesser extent, blood pressure and regional blood flows has been widely used to gain information on sympathetic and parasympathetic influences (6): time domain as well as frequency domain computer analysis allows overall variability or different frequency variability components in given spectral bands to be quantified. It is believed that the extent of parasympathetic or sympathetic outflows to the heart and to the blood vessels is quantitatively related to the magnitude of given variability parameters, namely, overall variability or its high-frequency spectral component reflecting the parasympathetic and the mid-frequency spectral component reflecting the sympathetic influences; although as for any indirect approach, the reliability of the various parameters as autonomic indices is far from being optimal (7,8). It is also to be mentioned, although it will not be reviewed in detail, that even more sophisticated mathematical processing of cardiovascular signals aimed at dissecting out autonomic modulation has been performed and is continuingly advanced.

Recent advances in nuclear techniques made it possible to visualize the release of norepinephrine from adrenergic nerve endings by administration of a radio-iodinated compound chemically homologous to catecholamines, metaiodo-benzylguanidine. This approach may be utilized at sites rich in adrenergic endings, mainly the heart (9,10).

III. AUTONOMIC REGULATION OF BLOOD PRESSURE

Arterial baroreceptors work to buffer any blood pressure fluctuations by sensing mechanical carotid sinus and aortic arch distension and reflexly promoting reciprocal variations of cardiovascular sympathetic outflows, as well as consensual variations of cardiac parasympathetic outflow. In contrast, the same autonomic effectors also work to generate marked blood pressure variations when their modulation is part of specific patterns associated with everyday life behavior such as exercise, emotion, sleep, and so on (11). Thus, a peculiar feature of autonomic influences is that they may either favor or oppose short-term blood pressure modifications, according to whether they are driven by reflex or by central influences (12).

Other reflex systems contributing to blood pressure control include the vagal cardiopulmonary reflex (13): mechanoreceptors sensing the distension of multiple central circulatory structures (atria, ventricles, pulmonary veins) reach the central nervous system via vagal afferent fibers and mediate in the short-term sympathetic inhibition (similar to the arterial baroreflex), but in the longer term also mediate neurohumoral changes majorly involved in water and sodium handling by the kidney.

Autonomic influences on blood pressure homeostasis are not confined to modulate vascular tone and cardiac function and rather extend to control a number of humoral systems, which may ultimately affect blood pressure via the control of vasomotor tone, sodium balance, cardiac performance, and cardiovascular trophic effects (14). These include the renin–angiotensin–aldosterone system, vasopressin, adrenomedullary epinephrine, insulin, cortisol, and others.

Renal handling of salt and water has long been known to be under neural control with both direct sympathetic modulation of renal blood flow and of proximal tubular sodium reabsortion and with effects mediated via the sympathetic control of renin secretion (15) and hence of angiotensin-mediated changes in systemic arterial pressure, intraglomerular pressure, aldosterone release, and distal tubular sodium reabsortion (16,17).

Autonomic cardiovascular influences are also significantly affected (via so far only partially understood mechanisms) by body's energy/nutritional balance. There is now substantial evidence that overeating and fat accumulation are associated with increased sympathetic activity, especially that directed to the kidney (18). As most obese subjects live a sedentary lifestyle—a feature also known to be associated with increased sympathetic activity (19), it remains to be clarified whether the two factors, overweight/obesity and physical inactivity, work in concert or independently in determining

sympathetic overactivity and its cardiovascular homeostatic consequences.

Among the behavioral factors associated with increased sympathetic activity, alcohol consumption and cigarette smoking are well known to be accompanied by sympathetic activation (20), again with only limited understanding of the exact underlying mechanisms. We have also limited knowledge of the importance and mode of contribution of autonomic effects to the adverse cardiovascular consequences of excess alcohol and tobacco use.

A number of heterogeneous nonneural mechanisms may at least partly act via autonomic cardiovascular influences and include leptin, insulin, endothelin, nitric oxide, reactive oxygen species, interleukins, tumor necrosis factors, complement fractions, and many others (21,22).

IV. AUTONOMIC IMBALANCE AND THE GENESIS OF HYPERTENSION

A. Animal Models

Extensive research efforts attempted to demonstrate, on one hand, that in various genetic hypertension models, sympathetic overactivity is the primary derangement underlying the blood pressure elevation, and on the other hand, to "produce" neurogenic forms of hypertension by altering neural cardiovascular control mechanisms via different experimental approaches. Clear-cut indications of neural overactivity have been obtained in the spontaneously hypertensive rat (SHR) model originally developed by Okamoto and Aoki (23): in this strain, which is unanimously viewed as the best rat model of human essential hypertension, there is an increased efferent sympathetic activity, especially that supplying the kidney; furthermore, the neurogenic vasoconstrictor responses to a variety of excitatory stimuli are exaggerated and the turnover of norepinephrine in pressor areas of the central nervous system is accelerated (24). This is of considerable interest inasmuch as similar alterations have been documented in human hypertension (discussed subsequently). Notably, in SHRs, the development of hypertension can be prevented or delayed by chemical sympathectomy or even by just denervating the kidneys (25).

The crucial hypertensinogenic role of neural mechanisms was also supported by Henry et al. (26), using a totally different approach, namely, by exposing mouse colonies to heavily stressful psycho-social stimuli (animals had to compete for space, access to food and water as well as for mating) for prolonged periods of time: besides demonstrating marked blood pressure elevations during the stressful stimulus application, this author could document the persistence of high blood pressure values in many of the stressed mice even long after stimulus removal, that is, when normal environmental conditions had been restored; furthermore, these animals also displayed the well-known features of the chronic hypertension syndrome such as myocardial fibrosis, coronary lesions, renal involvement, and so on.

The neural origin of high blood pressure was also supported by a furtherly different strategy, on the basis of experimental manipulations of cardiovascular reflexogenic areas or of neural pathways involved in cardiovascular homeostasis. In virtually all species tested, surgical denervation of sino-aortic baroreceptors or lesioning of the first central relay station of the baroreflex, that is, the nucleus tractus solitarii, was followed by immediate (and sometimes fulminating) blood pressure rises. Less univocal evidence was obtained as to the blood pressure levels prevailing in the later stages of sino-aortic denervation, with some groups reporting sustained, although less marked hypertension and some others reporting restoration of virtually normal average blood pressure levels in spite of larger than normal blood pressure fluctuations (27–30).

B. Human Hypertension

Addressing the primary role of autonomic mechanisms in human hypertension is an exceedingly difficult task considering that blood pressure elevation usually develops over years or decades; thus, preventing pathophysiological assessment to be performed in a truly prehypertensive stage. This would be essential in order for abnormalities responsible for initiation of the hypertensive process to be documented. A variety of alternative strategies have nonetheless been pursued. These include examination of normotensive offspring of hypertensive patients, in whom neurally mediated cardiovascular responses to excitatory stimuli were shown to be enhanced when compared with age-matched offspring of normotensive parents (31). In addition, studies conducted in the 70s by Julius et al. (32) could provide in young borderline hypertensive subjects evidence of reduced parasympathetic and enhanced sympathetic drive to the heart, whereas later studies using the tritiated norepinephrine method could document enhanced neurotransmitter release (especially to the heart and kidney) in younger hypertensive patients (33,34); the peculiar approach employed by these authors allowed them to show that on the other hand, the augmented circulating norepinephrine levels typical of older hypertensive subjects depends on a reduced clearance rather than by enhanced release (33).

Along a quite different conceptual line, other investigators addressed the blood pressure effects of null or very limited exposure to stressful stimuli as it may occur in secluded nuns: their unique observations showed lack of age-related increase in lifetime blood pressure, urinary norepinephrine excretion, and hypertension

incidence (35). Taken together, these albeit indirect observations concur to support the notion that autonomic mechanisms may play a primary role in the genesis of blood pressure elevation in at least a subset of the hypertensive population.

Since the initial documentation of insulin resistance in essential hypertension in 1987 (36), a new line of investigation on the etiology of hypertension was started. Because of the multifaceted properties of insulin, this may involve a number of possible mechanisms, including altered autonomic function: the sympathoexcitatory effect of insulin is well recognized (37) and may trigger vasoconstriction and enhanced peripheral vascular resistance. On the other hand, vasoconstriction may *per se* interfere with glucose uptake, especially in skeletal muscles, thus giving rise to a vicious circle (38). This is a still open and controversial area in which the primary vs. secondary nature of given alterations may not be easily demonstrated; whatever the exact sequence of pathophysiological events, derangements involving insulin action—the so-called metabolic syndrome—may be relevant hypertensinogenic factors in a significant subset of hypertensive patients such as those characterized by obesity or overweight, overt diabetes, and dyslipidemia.

V. SYMPATHETIC OVERACTIVITY IN ESTABLISHED HYPERTENSION

Both the neurochemical and the electrophysiological approaches mentioned earlier (2–6) applied to assess whether sympathetic overactivity is a feature of human hypertension have undisputably demonstrated this to be the case: renal and cardiac norepinephrine spillover have been found to be enhanced in most essential hypertensive patients (33), as clearly documented in Fig. 10.1; it is worth remarking that the extent of the sympathetic activation was inversely related to the subject's age, with the highest spillover values in the 20–40 year age range, more modest elevations between 40 and 60 years and no longer detectable enhancement in the >60 year age range.

Accordingly, microneurographic studies from different groups have all reported increased skeletal muscle sympathetic firing in subjects with established hypertension, borderline hypertension, and even in the normotensive offspring of hypertensive parents (39–41). An example of the findings obtained by the electrophysiological studies is provided in Fig. 10.2; it is notable that the authors could show a parallel increase of sympathetic activity and of blood pressure values, that is, a progressive increase in sympathetic discharge on going from normotensive to moderate and severe hypertensive subjects; they could also exclude that sympathetic overactivity was nonspecifically associated with high blood pressure values inasmuch

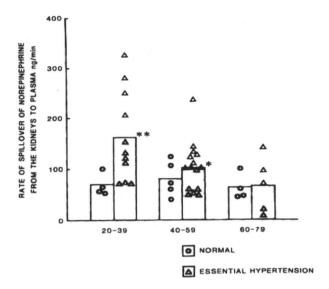

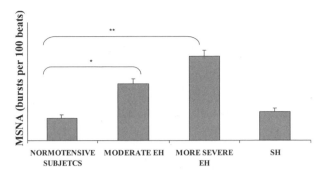

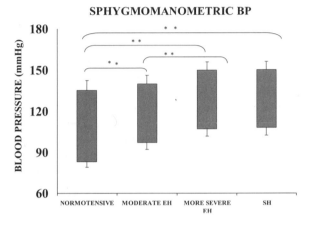

Figure 10.1 Renal norepinephrine spillover in normotensive and essential hypertensive subjects. Mean values (bars) and individual figures (circles, triangles) are separately shown in three age subgroups. Note the markedly enhanced renal norepinephrine spillover rate from the kidneys of young hypertensive patients, but not of healthy individuals or older hypertensives. Single ($p < 0.05$) and double ($p < 0.01$) asterisks indicate significant difference. [Reproduced from Esler et al. (3).]

Figure 10.2 Progressively increased sympathetic discharge (MSNA: muscle sympathetic nerve activity) on going from normotensive subjects to moderate and severe essential hypertensive patients, but not in secondary hypertensive patients (SH). Single ($p < 0.05$) and double ($p < 0.01$) asterisks indicate significant difference. [Data from Grassi et al. (41).]

as the study's protocol included the assessment of secondary hypertensive patients as well, in whom no evidence of sympathoexcitation could be detected.

Albeit limited to the cardiac territory, evidence of sympathetic activation in human hypertension has been further supported by studies based on ^{123}I-MIBG injection in which compared with normotensive subjects, the radionuclide washout rate from the heart was enhanced in early and even more so in established hypertensive patients (42).

VI. MECHANISMS UNDERLYING AUTONOMIC IMBALANCE IN HYPERTENSION

The contribution of cardiovascular reflex dysfunction and of exposure to psychological stress have been discussed earlier as possible primary etiologic factors in hypertension and will no longer be referred to. On the other hand, intensive investigation of the central neural mechanisms regulating autonomic outflows led to the demonstration of significant alterations in hypertensive humans as well as experimental animal models: neurochemically evaluated norepinephrine release from subcortical structures, including the hypothalamic paraventricular nucleus, was shown to be markedly enhanced in hypertensive vs normotensive subjects (43). In the brainstem of both

genetically and DOC-salt hypertensive rats, the adrenaline-forming enzyme, phenylethanolamine N-methyltransferase (PNMT) was abnormally elevated, the elevation being probably of etiologic importance because administration of a specific PNMT inhibitor normalized blood pressure values (44). Furthermore, in the same rat models, the number of catecholamine-containing brainstem neurons was found to be enhanced (45). This was also implicated as an important etiologic factor because the destruction of these neurons prevented the development of hypertension. Significant alterations identified in the SHR relate to metabolism of central peptides such as angiotensin, endothelin, and natriuretic peptides, as well as of excitatory amino acids such as GABA, glutamate, and aspartate (46). Compared to normotensive control Wistar-Kyoto (WKY) rats, the SHRs were also shown to carry augmented number and cell body volume in various hypothalamic nuclei. It was even reported that hypothalamic transplantation from SHR to WKY embryos was followed by sizeable increases in blood pressure postnatally (47) in the recipient rats.

It is important to emphasize that due to the multifactorial origin of hypertension, the range of "candidate" etiologic factors has been very wide. This helped investigators (including those interested in autonomic mechanisms) to recognize that alterations of different nature may importantly affect each other; thus, neural controllers may be significantly modulated by a variety of nonneural (hormonal, trophic/hemodynamic, metabolic, nutritional) influences. Because a thorough analysis of all possible interactions between neural and nonneural mechanisms is beyond the scope of this chapter, some among the most relevant examples will be discussed herein.

An important contribution on the role of structural factors in initiating or maintaining hypertension was given by the seminal work of Folkow (48) in the 70s. These authors observed that in the spontaneously hypertensive rat, the pressor and tachycardic responses to a stressful stimulus are exaggerated. The concept they developed and experimentally supported to explain this alteration is that the hemodynamic effect of sympathetically mediated vasoconstriction may be sizeably enhanced in the presence of vascular hypertrophy, especially in the case of inward remodeling of resistance vessels. Interestingly, they could document that the structural adaptive response may be triggered by short-lived, repeated blood pressure elevations such as those occurring in daily life in response to stressful stimuli. It is to be emphasized that at the time these investigations were conducted, the currently well established notion of the pro-hypertrophic effect of sympathetic (over)activity (49) was unknown, although it would fit well in the picture these authors envisaged. Indeed, based on their premise, progressive blood pressure elevation would in the long run almost invariably develop and one might somewhat provocatively wonder how normotension can be maintained in most individuals. The (far from exhaustive) answer is that genetically determined interindividual differences, on one hand, in autonomic responsiveness to stressful stimuli and, on the other hand, in the propensity to develop a cardiovascular hypertrophic response underlie the long-term setting of blood pressure levels in any given subject.

A further and well known "nonneural" factor involved in blood pressure homeostasis is sodium intake. A major contribution to the pro-hypertensinogenic effect exerted by dietary salt in a subset of the hypertensive population unquestionably depends on extracellular fluid and intravascular volume expansion. It is less often considered, however, that this is by no means the only mechanism in play and that dietary salt has multifold links with cardiovascular autonomic influences. In humans, the usual response to a high salt diet is characterized by a reduction in peripheral vascular resistance and in circulating catecholamines, whereas an opposite pattern is observed in

hypertensive patients (50,51). In the most commonly used animal model of sodium-dependent hypertension, the Dahl salt-sensitive rat, variations of salt intake have been associated with prominent changes in neural cardiovascular control mechanisms and impaired cardiovascular reflex function was also shown to be present in the prehypertensive stage before the animals are exposed to the high salt diet. In addition, even in the established phase of salt-dependent hypertension, acute removal of sympathetic cardiovascular drive by administration of a ganglion blocker abolishes the difference in blood pressure between the salt-sensitive and salt-resistant rat strain (52). Finally, it was also demonstrated that in the genetically salt-resistant strain, the increase in dietary salt not only fails to impair but also indeed potentiated baroreceptor function and cardiovascular reflexes responses from both the sino-aortic and cardiopulmonary reflexogenic areas (53–56) (Fig. 10.3).

If the earlier-mentioned observations clearly document the influences of salt intake on neural cardiovascular control mechanisms, there may be a reciprocal aspect of this relationship due to the sympathetic dependence of major components of renal function (discussed earlier) (15–17).

Moving from strictly nutritional to metabolic factors able to interact with autonomic function, obesity/overweight is undoubtedly of major pathophysiological relevance (and is nowadays of growing epidemiological relevance also). Obesity is associated with enhanced sympathetic activity, even in absence of hypertension, but there is evidence that the more marked degrees of sympathetic overactivity are observed when the two alterations coexist (57). Because it is also well established that obesity or overweight are more prevalent among hypertensive compared with normotensive individuals, the question arises whether an "upstream" alteration shared by the two conditions may contribute to the sympathetic activation observed in both; a hypothesis currently given strong consideration identifies insulin as such a common factor. One of the physiological actions of insulin (probably via its effects on thermogenesis) is to mediate the modulation of sympathetic nerve activity exerted by changes in caloric intake, namely, the sympathoexcitation associated with feeding and the sympathoinhibition associated with fasting. Thus, a disregulation of these mechanisms may play a causative role in hypertension, in particular, in the case of coexisting overweight/obesity/type II diabetes mellitus. According to this hypothesis, a genetically determined reduction in the tissue sensitivity to insulin action or an excessive caloric intake, or even more likely a combination of both, may trigger a sustained increase in insulin release, an attendant exaggeration of sympathetic activity, and eventually the development of high blood pressure (36,58).

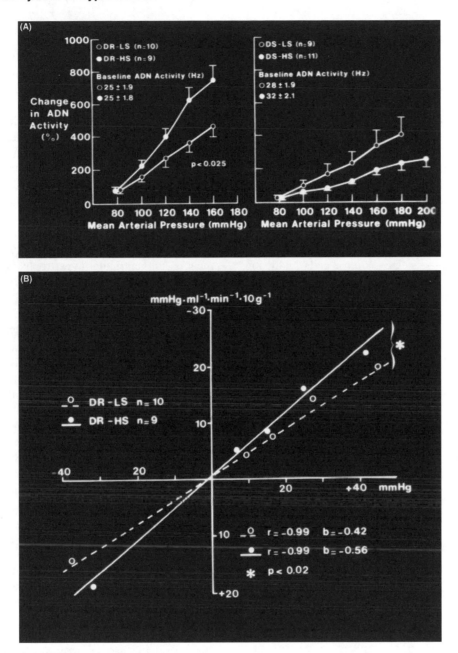

Figure 10.3 (A) Afferent arterial baroreceptor function evaluated from the aortic nerve (ADN) discharge/systemic pressure relationship in Dahl salt-resistant (DR) and Dahl salt-sensitive (DS) rats eating low-salt (LS, open symbols) or high-salt (HS, filled symbols) diets. Note the defective baroreceptor function in the salt-sensitive animals even before dietary salt loading and the opposite effect of high-salt diet in the resistant vs. sensitive animals. [Data from Ferrari and Mark (53).] (B) Baroreflex-mediated changes in vascularly isolated hind limb resistance (mmHg mL^{-1} min^{-1} 10 g^{-1}) elicited by arterial baroreceptor stimulation and deactivation via respectively phenylephrine and nitroprusside iv infusions in Dahl salt-resistant (DR) rats eating low-salt (LS, open symbols) or high-salt (HS, filled symbols) diets. Note the salt-induced potentiation of the reflex responses, quantified as slopes (b) of the stimulus–response relationship. [Data from Ferrari and Mark (54).]

Among the nonneural mechanisms implicated in sympathetic activation in hypertension, a final mention is to be devoted to inflammatory phenomena. Two among the major inflammatory cytokines, tumor necrosis factor-alpha (TNF-α) and interleukin 6 (IL-6) were found to be produced in excessive amounts in hypertensive animal models, as well as in human hypertension (59–61), although not all studies came to unanimous conclusions (62), and there is evidence that these substances can activate the central nervous system and enhance efferent sympathetic activity (63,64). Interestingly, epidemiological studies showed that enhanced inflammatory markers predict the development of diabetes and insulin resistance (65), and the recent IRAS study (66) suggests that subclinical, low grade inflammation is one of the features of the insulin-resistance syndrome. Moreover, both hypertensive and insulin-resistant individuals show enhanced acute-phase inflammatory responses (67,68). Although a mechanistic relationship between the earlier-mentioned observations and sympathetically mediated hypertension is far from being established, it is to be reminded that distinct similarities characterize IL-6 and leptin, a known sympatho-excitatory peptide which was lately very much studied as a possible etiologic factor in hypertension, especially in obese/overweight hypertensives. Both leptin and IL-6 are largely produced by adipose cells, and leptin was shown to exert part of its influences by modulating inflammatory phenomena and by binding to receptors that belong to the IL-6 receptor family (69–71). A schematic representation summarizing the interplay of metabolic, inflammatory, and neural mechanisms believed to contribute to the genesis of hypertension and atherosclerosis is illustrated in Fig. 10.4.

VII. AUTONOMIC INVOLVEMENT IN THE GENESIS OF COMPLICATIONS

Besides participating in the initiation and maintenance of the hypertensive state, autonomic imbalance significantly contributes to the genesis of major complications of hypertension, ranging from well-known acute cardiovascular events such as myocardial infarction, cardiac arrhythmias, and sudden death to more slowly developing entities such as left ventricular hypertrophy, congestive heart failure, and atherogenic/thrombotic processes.

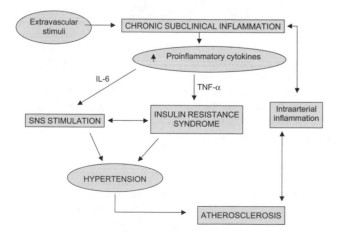

Figure 10.4 Interactions among heterogeneous mechanisms potentially acting as hypertensinogenic factors.

High blood pressure levels and sympathetic overactivity work in concert to enhance systolic wall stress, heart rate, and myocardial contractility, thus increasing myocardial oxygen demand; on the other hand, epicardial coronary artery disease and exaggerated small vessel constriction may curtail oxygen delivery to the heart. Such an imbalance may precipitate myocardial ischemia, causing further activation of sympathetic reflexes and establishing a vicious circle. Furthermore, sympathetic overactivity is clearly implicated as a crucial "trigger" of sudden cardiac death (72,73), mainly via its arrhythmogenic effects (74,75). Its influences on platelet function and on pro-coagulant/antifibrinolytic mechanisms (76,77) may further precipitate acute ischemic events (78).

Sustained sympathetic overactivity favors the development of left ventricular hypertrophy both directly through the well-known hypertrophic effect of cardiomyocyte adrenergic receptor stimulation (79) and indirectly through the facilitatory action of catecholamines on the local effects of angiotensin II (80). This has been convincingly documented by various reports that noradrenaline or isoproterenol chronically administered at subpressor doses induce cardiac hypertrophy in experimental animals (81), which implicates both alpha- and beta-adrenoceptors as the mediators of this effect. Needless to say, sympathetic overactivity may also directly promote left ventricular hypertrophy via its hemodynamic actions affecting both absolute blood pressure levels and blood pressure variability (82).

Sympathetic stimulation also profoundly influences arterial blood vessels with both structural and functional effects. Pressure-independent pro-hypertrophic actions of catecholamines are known to be exerted on the arterial wall (49,83), whereas arterial mechanical properties are also under direct sympathetic control as documented by the marked increase in arterial distensibility following removal of tonic sympathetic influences in both humans (84,85) and in experimental animals (86) (Fig. 10.5). A further albeit less direct way an autonomic imbalance may affect the arterial tree is via its ability to induce tachycardia, which was shown to *per se* exert an arterial stiffening effect (87). If one additionally considers the known ability of catecholamines to also unfavorably affect lipid metabolism and cholesterol synthesis (88), there is little question that sympathetic activation may exert significant proatherogenic effects; in conjunction with the adverse mechanical influence of high blood pressure, the overall impact of such effects may not be trivial, which makes it tempting to speculate that sympathetic overactivity may at least in part contribute to the facilitation of atherosclerosis notoriously associated with hypertension.

Although sympathetic activation was long believed to represent a compensatory response "helping" the heart to

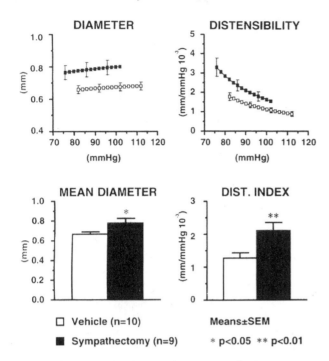

Figure 10.5 Effects of sympathectomy on diameter–pressure curves, distensibility–pressure curves, mean diameter and distensibility (dist.) index in the rat femoral artery. Note the arterial dilatation despite lower arterial distending pressure as well as the enhanced distensibility of the sympathectomized vs. intact animals. [Reproduced from Mangoni et al. (86).]

sustain an abnormally elevated mechanical load such as it occurs in chronic hypertension, growing experimental evidence challenges this notion and indicates that the overall effects of cardiac sympathetic drive are detrimental to the heart and facilitate rather than prevent cardiac decompensation. Along this line we could recently show that in a rat model of aortic banding-induced pressure overload cardiac hypertrophy, sympathectomy had beneficial effects on the course of the disease inasmuch as it markedly attenuated and delayed the transition to left ventricular dysfunction and failure; even more importantly, heart failure-related mortality was strikingly reduced (89). These observations demonstrate that sympathetic (over)activity favors the development and accelerates the progression of cardiac dysfunction in hypertensive heart disease; although the underlying mechanisms are not fully elucidated, they may include noxious effects to both the cardiomyocyte (necrosis/apoptosis) and the cardiac interstitium (fibrosis).

VIII. CONCLUSIONS

Having followed the above discussion, which touched upon some of the multifold factors relevant to the pathophysiology of hypertension, the reader should have realized that most if not all of them, including high salt intake, insulin-resistance, low-grade inflammation, overweight, dyslipidemia, physical inactivity are strongly interrelated in a sort of network in which activation of any element directly or indirectly calls in play the other ones. In the setting of our topic it may be important to recall that sympathetic overactivity makes no exception, although it may at present be difficult to tell whether it has to be viewed as just one of the elements in play or as the one ultimately giving rise to the hemodynamic landmark of most hypertensive conditions, that is the exaggerated peripheral vascular resistance, no matter which was (were) the primary derangement(s) that triggered the hypertensive process. It was additionally outlined that beside providing a significant contribution to the etiology of hypertension in at least a proportion of patients, autonomic mechanisms have a strong impact in the development and course of the major and often fatal complications of the hypertensive disease.

REFERENCES

1. Goldstein DS. Plasma catecholamines and essential hypertension: an analytical review. Hypertension 1983; 5:86–99.
2. Esler M, Lambert G, Jennings G. Increased regional sympathetic nervous activity in human hypertension: causes and consequences. J Hypertension 1990; 8(suppl 7):S53–S57.
3. Esler M, Jennings G, Korner P, Willet I, Lambert G et al. Assessment of human sympathetic nervous system activity from measurements of norepinephrine turnover. Hypertension 1988; 1:3–20.
4. Vallbo AB, Hagbarth KE, Torebjork HE et al. Somatosensory, proprioceptive and sympathetic activity in human peripheral nerves. Physiol Rev 1979; 59:919–957.
5. Grassi G, Cattaneo BM, Seravalle G, Lanfranchi A, Mancia G. Baroreflex control of sympathetic nerve activity in essential and secondary hypertension. Hypertension 1988; 31:68–72.
6. Mancia G, Parati G, Di Rienzo M, Zanchetti A. Bloood pressure variability. In: Zanchetti A, Mancia G, eds. Handbook of Hypertension. Vol. 17. Pathophysiology of Hypertension. Amsterdam: Elsevier Science, 1997: 117–169.
7. Daffonchio A, Franzelli C, Radaelli A, Castiglioni P, Di Rienzo M, Mancia G, Ferrari AU. Sympathectomy and cardiovascular spectral components in conscious normotensive rats. Hypertension 1995; 25:1287–1293.
8. Kingwell BA, Thompsom JM, Jennings G, Esler MD. Heart rate spectral analysis, cardiac norepinephrine spillover, and muscle sympathetic nerve activity during human sympathetic nervous activation and failure. Circulation 1994; 90: 234–240.
9. Sakata K, Shirotani M, Yoshida H, Kurata C. Comparison of effects of enalapril and nitrendipine on cardiac sympathetic nervous system in essential hypertension. J Am Coll Cardiol 1998; 32:438–443.

10. Sakata K, Shirotani M, Kurata C et al. Cardiac sympathetic nervous system in early essential hypertension assessed by ^{123}I-MIBG. J Nucl Med 1999; 40:6–11.

11. Mancia G, Ferrari A, Ludbrook J, Zanchetti A. Carotid baroreceptor influence on blood pressure in normotensive and hypertensive subjects. In: Sleight P, ed. Arterial Baroreceptors and Hypertension. Oxford University Press, Oxford: 1980:484–490.

12. Ferrari AU, Franzelli C, Daffonchio A, Perlini S, Di Rienzo M. Sympathovagal interplay in the control of overall blood pressure variability in unanesthetized rats. Am J Physiol 1996; 270:H2143–H2148.

13. Mancia G, Romero JC, Shepherd JT. Continuous inhibition of renin release in dogs by vagally innervated receptors in the cardiopulmonary region. Circ Res 1975; 36:529–535.

14. Mancia G. Bjorn Folkow Award Lecture. The sympathetic nervous system in hypertension. J Hypertens 1997; 15:1553–1565

15. Zanchetti A, Stella A. Neural control of renin release. Clin Sci 1975; 2:215–223.

16. Barrett CJ, Ramchendra R, Malpas SC et al. What sets the long-term level of renal sympathetic nerve activity. A role for angiotensin II and baroreflexes? Circ Res 2003; 92:1330–1336.

17. Lohmeier TE. The sympathetic nervous system and long-term blood pressure regulation. Am J Hypertens 2001; 14:147S–154S.

18. Landsberg L. Pathophysiology of obesity-related hypertension: role of insulin and the sympathetic nervous system. J Cardiovasc Pharmacol 1994; 23(suppl 1):s1–s8.

19. Jennings GL, Nelson L, Esler MD, Korner PI. Effects of changes in physical activity on blood pressure and sympathetic tone. J Hypertension Suppl 1984; 2: S139–S141.

20. Marano G, Ramirez A, Mori I, Ferrari AU. Sympathectomy inhibits the vasoactive effects of nicotine in conscious rats. Cardiovasc Res 1999; 42:201–205.

21. Brook RD, Julius S. Autonomic imbalance, hypertension, and cardiovascular risk. Am J Hypertens 2000; 13:112S–122S.

22. Fernandez-Real JM, Ricart W. Insulin resistance and chronic cardiovascular inflammatory syndrome. Endocr Rev 2003; 24:278–301.

23. Okamoto K, Aoki K. Development of strain of spontaneously hypertensive rats. Jnp Circ J 1963; 27:282–293.

24. Judy WJ, Watanabe AM, Murphy WR, Aprison BS, Yu PL. Sympathetic nerve activity and blood pressure in normotensive backcross rats genetically related to the spontaneously hypertensive rat. Hypertension 1979; 1:598–604.

25. Winternitz SR, Katholi RE, Oparil S. Role of the sympathetic nerves in the development and maintenance of hypertension in the spontaneously hypertensive rat. J Clin Invest 1980; 66:971–978.

26. Henry JP, Meehan JP, Stephens PM. The use of psychosocial stimuli to induce prolonged systolic hypertension in mice. Psychosom Med 1967; 29:408–432.

27. Koch E, Mies A. Chronische arterielle Hochdruck durch experimentelle Dauerausschaltung der Blutdruckzugler. Krankheitforschung 1929; 7:241–256.

28. Ferrario CM, Cubbin Mc JW, Page IH. Hemodynamic characteristics of chronic experimental neurogenic hypertension in unanesthetized dogs. Circ Res 1969; 24:911–922.

29. Laubie M, Schmitt H. Destruction of the nucleus tractus solitarii in the dog: comparison with sinoaortic denervation. Am J Physiol 1979; 236:H736–H743.

30. Cowley AW Jr, Liard JF, Guyton AC. Role of baroreceptor reflex in daily control of arterial blood pressure and other variables in dogs. Circ Res 1973; 32:564–576.

31. Falkner B, Onesti G, Langman G. Cardiovascular responses to mental stress in normal adolescents with hypertensive parents. Hypertension 1979; 1:23–30.

32. Julius S, Pasqual AV, London R. Role of parasympathetic inhibition in the hypercinetic type of bordeline hypertension. Circulation 1971; 44:413–418.

33. Esler M, Jennings G, Lambert G, Meredith I, Horn M, Elsenhofer G. Overflow of catecolamines neurotransmitter to the circulation: source, fate and functions. Physiol Rev 1990; 70:963–985.

34. Grassi G, Esler MD. How to assess sympathetic activity in humans. J. Hypertens 1999; 17:719–734.

35. Timio M, Lippi G, Venenzi S, Gentili S, Verdura C et al. Blood pressure trend and cardiovascular events in a secluded order: a 30-year follow up study. Blood Press 1997; 6:81–87.

36. Ferranini E, Buzzigoli G, Bonadonna R, Oleggini M, Graziadei L, Pedrinelli R, Brandi L, Bevilacqua S. Insulin resistance in essential hypertension. New Engl J Med 1987; 317:350–357.

37. Lembo G, Napoli R, Capaldo B, Rendina V, Triamarco B, Saccà L. Abnormal sympathetic overactivity evoked by insulin in the skeletal muscle of patients with essential hypertension. J Clin Invest 1992; 90:24–29.

38. Julius S, Gudbrandsson T, Jammerson KA. The hemodynamic link between insulin resistance and hypertension (hypothesis). J Hypertens 1991; 9:983–986.

39. Yamada Y, Mijajima E, Tochikubo O, Shionori H, Ishii M, Kaneko Y et al. Impaired baroreflex changes in muscle sympathetic nerve activity in adolescents who have a family history of essential hypertension. J Hypertens 1988; 6(suppl 4):s525–s528.

40. Anderson EA, Sinkey CA, Lawton WJ, Mark AL. Elevated sympathetic nerve activity in borderline hypertensive humans: evidence from direct intraneural recordings. Hypertension 1988; 14:177–183.

41. Grassi G, Cattaneo BM, Seravalle G, Lanfranchi A, Mancia G. Baroreflex control of sympathetic nerve activity in essential and secondary hypertension. Hypertension 1998; 31:68–72.

42. Sakata K, Shirotani M, Yoshida H, Kurata C. Cardiac sympathetic nervous system in early essential hypertension assessed by ^{123}I-MIBG. J Nucl Med 1999; 40:6–11.

43. Ferrier C, Jennings GL, Eisenhofer G. Evidence for increased noradrenaline release from subcortical brain regions in essential hypertension. J Hypertens 1993; 11:1217–1227.

44. Saavedra JM, Grobecker H, Axelrod J. Adrenaline-forming enzyme in brainstem: elevation in genetic and experimental hypertension. Science 1976; 191:483–484.

45. Chalmers JP, Howe PRC, Wallman Y, Tumuls I. Adrenaline neurons and PNMT activity in the brain and spinal cord of genetically hypertensive rats and rats with DOCA-salt hypertension. Clin Sci 1980; 61:219–221.

46. Ito S, Komatsu K, Sved AF. Excitatory amino acids in the rostral ventrolateral medulla support blood pressure in spontaneously hypertensive rats. Hypertension 2000; 35:413–417.

47. Eilam R, Malach R, Bergman F, Segal M. Hypertension induced by hypothalamic transplantation from genetically hypertensive to normotensive rats. J Neurosci 1991; 11:401–411.

48. Folkow B. The fourth Vohlard Lecture. Cardiovascular structural adaptation; its role in the inititation and maintenance of primary hypertension. Cli Sci Mol Med 1978; 4(suppl 3):3s–22s.

49. Dao HH, Lemay J, de Champlain J, de Blois D, Moreau P. Norepinephrine-induced aortic hyperplasia and extracellular matrix deposition are endothelin-dependent. J Hypertens 2001; 19:1965–1973.

50. Luft FC, Rankin LI, Henry DP. Plasma and urinary values at extremes of sodium intake in normal man. Hypertension 1979; 1:261–266.

51. Mark AL, Lawton WJ, Abboud FM, Fitz AE, Connor WE, Heistad DD. Effects of high and low sodium intake on arterial pressure and forearm vascular resistance in borderline hypertension. A preliminary report. Circ Res 1975; 36(suppl 1):s194–s198.

52. Takeshita A, Mark AL. Prevention of salt-induced hypertension in the Dahl strain by 6-hydroxydopamine. Am J Physiol 1979; 236:H48–H52.

53. Ferrari AU, Mark AL. Sensitization of aortic baroreceptors by high salt diet in Dahl salt-resistant rats. Hypertension 1987; 10:55–60.

54. Ferrari A, Mark AL. Salt-induced sensitization of the baroreflex control of vascular resistance in Dahl salt-resistant rats. Eur J Clin Invest 1984; 14:14.

55. Ferrari AU, Gordon FJ, Mark AL. Impairment of cardiopulmonary baroreflexes in Dahl-sensitive rats fed low salt. Am J Physiol 1984; 247:119–123.

56. Mark AL, Victor RG, Ferrari A, Morgan DA, Thoren P. Cardiac sensory receptors in Dahl salt-resistant and salt-sensitive rats. Circulation 1987; 75:I137–I140.

57. Grassi G, Seravalle G, Turri C, Dell'Oro R, Bolla GB, Mancia G. Adrenergic and reflex abnormalities in obesity-related hypertension. Hypertension 2000; 36:538–542.

58. Landsberg L. Diet, obesity and hypertension: a hypothesis involving insulin, the sympathetic nervous system, and adaptive thermogenesis. Q J Med 1986; 236:1081–1090.

59. Zinman B, Hanley AJG, Harris SB, Kwan J, Fantus IG. Circulating tumour necrosis factor-α concentrations in a native Canadian population with high rates of type 2 diabetes mellitus. J Clin Endocrinol Metab 1999; 84:272–278.

60. Pausova Z, Deslauries B, Gaudet D, Cowley AW, Hamet P. Role of tumor necrosis factor-α gene locus in obesity and obesity-associated hypertension in French Canadians. Hypertension 2000; 36:14–19.

61. Humphries SE, Luong LA, Ogg MS, Miller GJ. The interleukin-6-174 G/C promoter polymorphism is associated with risk of coronary heart disease and systolic blood pressure in healthy men. Eur Heart J 2001; 22:2243–2252.

62. Chae CU, Lee RT, Rifai N, Ridker PM. Blood pressure and inflammation in apparently healthy men. Hypertension 2001; 38:399–403.

63. Papanicolau DA, Petrides JS, Tsigos C, Bina S, Gold PW, Chrousos GP. Exercise stimulates interleukin-6 secretion: inhibition by glucocorticoids and correlation with catecholamines. Am J Physiol 1996; 271:E601–E605.

64. Besedovsky HO, Del Rey A. Immune-neuro-endocrine interactions: facts and hypotheses. Endocr Rev 1996; 17:64–102.

65. Pickup JC, Mattock MB, Chusney G, Burt D. NIDDM as a disease of innate immune system: association of the acute-phase reactants and interleukin-6 with metabolic syndrome X. Diabetologia 1997; 40:1286–1292.

66. Festa A, D'Agostino R Jr, Howard G, Mykkanen L, Tracy RP, Haffener SM et al. Chronic subclinical inflammation as a part of the insulin resistance syndrome: the Insulin Resistance Atherosclerosis study (IRAS). Circulation 2000; 102:42–47.

67. Schmidt MI, Duncan BB, Sharret AR, Lindberg G, Savage PJ, Offenbacher S, Tracy RP, Heiss G. Markers of inflammation and prediction of diabetes mellitus in adults (Atherosclerosis Risk in Communities study): a cohort study. Lancet 1999; 353:1649–1652.

68. Barzilay JI, Abraham L, Heckbert SR, Cushman M, Tracy RP. The relation of markers of inflammation to the development of glucose disorders in the elderly. The cardiovascular Health Study. Diabetes 2001; 50:2384–2389.

69. Haynes WG, Morgan DA, Walsh SA, Mark AL, Sivitz WI. Receptor-mediated regional sympathetic nerve activation by leptin. J Clin Invest 1997; 100:270–278.

70. Shek EW, Brands MW, Hall JE. Chronic leptin infusion increase arterial pressure. Hypertension 1998; 31:409–414.

71. Aizawa-Abe M, Ogawa Y, Masuzaky H, Ebihara K, Hayshi T, Hosoda K, Nakao K. Pathophysiological role of leptin in obesity-related hypertension. J Clin Invest 2000; 105:1243–1252.

72. Barron HV, Lesh MD. Autonomic nervous system and sudden cardiac death. J Am Coll Cardiol 1996; 27:1053–1060.

73. Schwartz PJ. QT proloungation, sudden death, and sympathetic imbalance: pendulum swings. J Cardiovasc Electrophysiol 2001; 12:1074–1077.

74. Pellizon OA, Beloscar JS, Mariani E. Adrenergic nervous system influences on the induction of ventricular tachycardia. Ann Noninvasive Electrocardiol 2002; 7:281–288.

75. Anderson KP. Sympathetic nervous system activity and ventricular tachyarrhythmias: recent advances. Ann Noninvasive Electrocardiol 2003; 8:75–89.

76. Anfossi G, Trovati M. Role of catecholamines in platelet function: pathophysiological and clinical significance. Eur J Clin Invest 1996; 26:353–370.

77. Bjorkman JA, Jern S, Jern C. Cardiac sympathetic stimulation triggers coronary t-PA release. Arterioscler Thromb Vasc Biol 2003; 23:1091–1097.

78. Muller JE. Circadian variation and triggering of acute coronary events. Am Heart J 1999; 137:S1–S8.

79. Schlaich MP, Kaye DM, Lambert E, Sommerville M et al. Relation between cardiac sympathetic activity and hypertensive left ventricular hypertrophy. Circulation 2003; 108:560–565.

80. Makino N, Sugano M, Otsuka S, Hata T. Molecular mechanism of angiotensin II type I and type II receptors in cardiac hypertrophy of spontaneously hypertensive rats. Hypertension 1997; 30:796–802.

81. Leenen FH, White R, Yuan B. Isoprotenerol-induced cardiac hypertrophy: role of circulatory versus cardiac renin-angiotensin system. Am J Physiol Heart Circ Physiol 2001; 281:H2410–H2416.

82. Greenwood JP, Scott EM, Stoker JB, Mary DA. Hypertensive left ventricular hypertrophy: relation to peripheral sympathetic drive. J Am Coll Cardiol 2001; 38:1711–1717.

83. Simon G, Csiky B. Effect of neonatal sympathectomy on the development of structural vascular changes in angiotensin II-treated rats. J Hypertension 1998; 16:77–84.

84. Grassi G, Giannattasio C, Failla M, Pesenti A, Peretti G, Marinoni E, Fraschini N, Vailati S, Mancia G. Sympathetic modulation of radial artery compliance in congestive heart failure. Hypertension 1995; 26:348–354.

85. Failla M, Grappiolo A, Emanuelli G, Vitale G, Fraschini N, Bigoni M, Grieco N, Denti M, Giannattasio C, Mancia G. Sympathetic tone restrains arterial distensibility of healthy and atherosclerotic subjects. J Hypertens 1999; 17:1117–1123.

86. Mangoni AA, Mircoli L, Giannattasio C, Mancia G, Ferrari AU. Effect of sympathectomy on mechanical properties of common carotid and femoral arteries. Hypertension 1997; 30:1085–1088.

87. Mangoni AA, Mircoli L, Giannattasio C, Ferrari AU, Mancia G. Heart rate-dependency of arterial distensibility in vivo. J Hypertension 1996; 14:897–901.

88. Jordan J, Furlan R, Tank J, Furlan S, Luft FC, Boschmann M. Adrenergic responsiveness of adipose tissue lipolysis in autonomic failure. Clin Auton Res 2004; 14:80–83.

89. Perlini S, Ferrero I, Fallarini S, Palladini G, Tozzi R, Radaelli A, Busca G, Fogari R, Ferrari AU. Chronic sympathectomy improves survival and attenuates cardiac dysfunction in experimental pressure overload hypertrophy. J Hypertension 2003; 21(suppl 4):s221–s222.

11

The Effects of Macronutrients and Dietary Patterns on Blood Pressure

BRETT ALYSON ANGE
Johns Hopkins Bloomberg School of Public Health, Baltimore, Maryland, USA

LAWRENCE J. APPEL
Johns Hopkins Medical Institutions, Baltimore, Maryland, USA

KEYPOINTS

- Multiple dietary factors affect blood pressure level.
- There is an expanding body of evidence suggesting that protein intake, specifically plant protein, may lower blood pressure.
- A high intake of omega-3 fatty acids can reduce blood pressure in individuals with hypertension.
- Consumption of an overall healthy diet pattern, such as the DASH Dietary Pattern or a vegetarian diet, has emerged as an effective means to lower blood pressure.

SUMMARY

High blood pressure is a significant public health problem, but one that is potentially controllable or preventable. One means of control and prevention is by dietary modification. A large body of evidence has shown that many dietary factors affect blood pressure. Current knowledge supports reducing salt intake, increasing potassium intake, controlling weight, moderating of alcohol intake (among those who drink) and consuming an overall healthy dietary pattern as appropriate modifications to help lower blood pressure. Additional emerging evidence has shown that increased protein intake, particularly plant protein, and high intake of omega-3 fatty acids can also reduce blood pressure. Whether increased fiber intake lowers blood pressure is remains unproven. For other macronutrients, as well as for cholesterol, evidence is currently limited or equivocal.

I. INTRODUCTION

Multiple dietary factors affect blood pressure. Reduced salt intake, increased potassium intake, weight loss, moderation of alcohol intake (among those who consume alcohol), and an overall healthy diet, termed the "Dietary Approaches to Stop Hypertension (DASH) diet," are effective dietary strategies that lower blood pressure. The DASH diet emphasizes fruits, vegetables, and low-fat dairy products and is reduced in saturated fat, total fat, and cholesterol. A very high intake of omega-3 fatty acid (fish oil) from pill supplements also lowers blood pressure in hypertensive individuals, but at doses that are commonly associated with side effects.

A variety of evidence suggests that other dietary factors affect blood pressure. This chapter reviews evidence with respect to the effects of macronutrients (fat, protein, and carbohydrate), fiber, cholesterol, and dietary patterns on blood pressure. Table 11.1 provides a summary of this evidence and Table 11.2 provides an overview of relevant findings from two major observational studies.

II. FAT

Cross-cultural (ecologic) studies, as well as migration studies, have documented that individuals who live in economically developed industrialized countries have higher blood pressure and a steeper age-related rise in blood pressure than those who live in nonindustrialized countries (1). Nonindustrialized societies are characterized by less meat and lower fat consumption. Within industrialized societies, vegetarians tend to have lower blood pressure than nonvegetarians. Although many components of the diet may differ between nonindustrialized and industrialized countries and between vegetarians and nonvegetarians, dietary fat, particularly saturated fat, has been associated with atherosclerosis and dyslipidemia. Therefore, it seemed plausible to explore the effects of fat intake on blood pressure.

Table 11.1 Summary of the Effects of Nutrients, Fiber, Cholesterol, and Dietary Patterns on Blood Pressure

Dietary component	Direction of effect	Evidence
Electrolytes		
Sodium chloride (salt)	Direct	++
Potassium	Inverse	++
Calcium	Inverse	+/−
Magnesium	Inverse	+/−
Weight	Direct	++
Alcohol	Direct	++
Fats[a]		
Saturated	Direct	+/−
Omega-3 polyunsaturated	Inverse	++
Omega-6 polyunsaturated	Inverse	+/−
Monounsaturated	Inverse	+/−
Proteins[a]		
Total	Inverse	+
Vegetable	Inverse	+
Animal	Uncertain	+/−
Carbohydrates[a]		
Total	Uncertain	+/−
Simple sugars	Direct	+/−
Starch	Uncertain	+/−
Fiber[a]	Inverse	+
Cholesterol[a]	Direct	+/−
Vitamin C	Inverse	+/−
Dietary patterns[a]		
Vegetarian	Inverse	++
Mediterranean-style	Inverse	+/−
DASH diet	Inverse	++

[a]Discussed in chapter.
Note: ++, convincing evidence, typically from clinical trial; +/−, limited or equivocal evidence; +, suggestive evidence, typically from observational studies and some clinical trials.

Different study designs have been used to investigate the relationship of fat intake with blood pressure. Cross-sectional studies have examined associations between tissue levels of fat and blood pressure, and cohort studies have assessed the effects of dietary fat intake on blood pressure change or incident hypertension. Clinical trials have tested the effects of different levels and/or types of fat intake on blood pressure. A review by Morris (1) has summarized this vast and complex literature.

A. Total Fat

Total fat includes saturated fat, monounsaturated fat, omega-3 polyunsaturated fat, and omega-6 polyunsaturated fat. It has been hypothesized that saturated fat increases blood pressure, polyunsaturated fat lowers blood pressure, a high polyunsaturated fat/saturated fat (P/S) ratio lowers blood pressure, and monounsaturated

Table 11.2 Overview of Major Findings from Two Observational Studies That Assessed the Effects of Macronutrients, Fiber, and Cholesterol on Blood Pressure[a]

Description	Multiple Risk Factor Intervention Trial	Chicago Western Electric Study
Type of dietary assessment	24 h dietary recalls (5 or 6 times)	Interviews (to assess eating patterns over previous 28 days)
Significant direct association	Starch	Cholesterol (SBP only)
	Saturated fat (DBP only)	Keys dietary lipid score (SBP only)
	Cholesterol (DBP only)	Alcohol use
	Keys dietary lipid score (DBP only)	
Significant inverse association	Fiber	Vegetable protein
	Protein (DBP only in usual care; SBP only in special intervention group)	
	Polyunsaturated fat (DBP only)	
	P/S ratio (DBP only)	
	Simple carbohydrates (DBP only)	
Adjustment factors	Age	Age (baseline)
	Race	Time
	Education	Height
	Serum cholesterol	Weight
	Smoking	Education
	Body mass index	Alcohol use
	Diet status (intervention or usual care)	Cigarette use
	Alcohol intake	

[a]See Stamler et al. (4), Slattery et al. (60), Yamori et al. (64), and Miura et al. (163) for further information regarding associations.
Note: DBP, diastolic blood pressure; SBP, systolic blood pressure; P/S, polyunsaturated fat/saturated fat.

fat lowers blood pressure. Hence, the net effect of fat intake on blood pressure may depend on the distribution of types of fat consumed. However, as documented by Morris (1), there is little evidence to support an effect of total fat intake on blood pressure.

B. Saturated Fat

Many observational studies and a few clinical trials have examined the effect of saturated fat on blood pressure. In most observational studies, saturated fat intake was not associated with elevations in blood pressure. For example, in the Nurses' Health Study and the Health Professionals Follow-Up Study (HPFS), there was no association among saturated, polyunsaturated, or total fat intake and incident hypertension during 4 years of follow-up in analyses that controlled for potential dietary and nondietary confounders (2,3). In these studies, food frequency questionnaires were used to assess fat intake, expressed as a percentage of total kilocalories (kcal). In contrast, in observational analyses of the Multiple Risk Factor Intervention Trial (MRFIT), there was a significant direct association between saturated fat intake, as measured by replicate 24 h dietary recalls, and diastolic blood pressure. The investigators also reported a significant inverse association between P/S ratio and diastolic blood pressure (4).

Clinical trials have documented that diets reduced in saturated or total fat intake have no effect on blood pressure. Some trials tested diets that were reduced in both total and saturated fat; other trials increased polyunsaturated fat intake and reduced saturated fat intake in order to hold total fat constant. Over a 1 year period, the National Diet Heart Study (5), with 1007 subjects, tested four diets, all with 30–37% of total calories from fat, but with varied P/S ratios (0.3, 1.5, 2.0, and 4.5). A Medical Research Council (MRC)-supported trial, with 393 subjects and five years of follow-up, tested two diets with different P/S ratios (0.2 and 2.0), but the same percent of kcal as fat (45%) (6). In these two large trials, as well as in several smaller trials, a reduction in saturated fat had no impact on blood pressure. The diets that were tested in these trials had increased levels of polyunsaturated fat; therefore, the lack of effect on blood pressure by these diets also suggests no beneficial effect from polyunsaturated fat.

Even well-controlled clinical trials have limitations, most of which would lead to false negative results. Potential limitations include enrollment of large numbers of nonhypertensive individuals and inadequate measurement of blood pressure. In addition, if the biological effects of saturated fat on blood pressure result from long-term exposure (for e.g., effects on arterial stiffness rather than vascular resistance), then a trial of even 5 years duration might not be long enough.

C. Monounsaturated Fat

Few studies have investigated the relationship between monounsaturated fat and blood pressure. Most cross-sectional studies did not detect any relationship (1). Likewise, two prospective studies did not find an effect of monounsaturated fat on incident hypertension (2,3). Early clinical trials did not support the hypothesis that monounsaturated fat had an effect on blood pressure. However, these trials were small and included nonhypertensives (1); hence, the trials may have been underpowered.

Two recent trials documented an inverse relationship between monounsaturated fat intake and blood pressure. In a trial of persons with type 2 diabetes, replacing carbohydrate with monounsaturated fat significantly lowered systolic blood pressure and ambulatory daytime diastolic blood pressure (7). In a cross-over trial, replacement of saturated fat with monounsaturated fat (as olive oil) significantly reduced blood pressure and the need for antihypertensive medication when compared with replacement with sunflower oil (polyunsaturated fat, mostly linoleic acid) (8). Overall, it is unclear whether an increased intake of monounsaturated fatty acids lowers blood pressure.

D. Omega-6 Polyunsaturated Fat

Omega-6 polyunsaturated fat is consumed mainly as linoleic acid in Western diets (9). In observational studies, there was no clear relationship between tissue or blood levels of omega-6 polyunsaturated fat and blood pressure (1). One small, randomized cross-over trial of elderly hypertensive subjects ($n = 44$) found that both fish oil (omega-3) and corn oil (omega-6) lowered systolic and diastolic blood pressure; however, these reductions were only significant during the first diet period (10).

E. Omega-3 Polyunsaturated Fat

Laboratory studies, observational epidemiologic studies, and clinical trials have documented that an increased intake of omega-3 polyunsaturated fat lowers blood pressure. In these studies, omega-3 polyunsaturated fat is usually consumed from fatty fish (e.g., mackerel, lake trout, herring, sardines, albacore tuna, and salmon) or from pill supplements, termed "fish oil."

There are many plausible mechanisms for an effect of omega-3 polyunsaturated fat on blood pressure. One mechanism is the inhibition of vasoconstrictor prostaglandins (e.g., thromboxane A2) (11). Another study found that in rats, supplementation with docosahexaenoic acid (DHA), one type of omega-3 fatty acid, altered the amount of adenosine triphosphate (ATP) released from the vascular endothelial cells (12). In a clinical trial that enrolled of 59 overweight, mildly hyperlipidemic men,

DHA—but not eicosapentaenoic acid (EPA)—enhanced vasodilator responses and attenuated constrictor responses in the forearm microcirculation (13). Other potential mechanisms include a decrease in vascular contractility and platelet aggregation (14), attenuation of vascular responses to sympatho-adrenal stimulation (15), an increase in systemic arterial compliance and reduction in pulse pressure (16), an increase in vasodilatory prostaglandins (e.g., prostacyclin) (9), and an increase in endothelial nitric oxide release. Various studies have shown that DHA may be the principal active component conferring cardiovascular protection rather than EPA (13,17).

1. Observational Studies

The low incidence of cardiac death in Greenland Eskimos, who consume a diet high in fat (mainly from seal and whale blubber), sparked interest in the health effects of omega-3 polyunsaturated fat (18). Several subsequent studies demonstrated an association among increased consumption of omega-3 fatty acid and decreased risk of coronary heart disease (19) and sudden death (20,21). Few observational studies examined the effects of omega-3 fatty acid intake on blood pressure.

2. Clinical Trials

Clinical trials have documented that high doses of omega-3 polyunsaturated fat can reduce blood pressure, at least in hypertensive individuals. In a trial of 156 Norwegian men and women with untreated mild hypertension, supplementation with 6 g/day of 85% EPA and DHA significantly lowered systolic blood pressure by 6.4 mmHg and diastolic blood pressure by 2.8 mmHg, net of control. A number of other clinical trials have shown similar benefit from supplementation with high dose fish oil supplements in hypertensive individuals (22–28). The effects of low dose fish oil have been disappointing. A recent trial tested a supplement containing a 4:1 ratio of EPA to gamma linoleic acid (GLA); GLA is an omega-6 polyunsaturated fatty acid that might act synergistically to lower blood pressure and allow for a reduced dose of EPA and hence, reduced side effects. However, this supplement had no significant effect on blood pressure (29). In other trials, consuming fish, which are rich in omega-3 polyunsaturated fat, reduced blood pressure (30). There was an additive effect of fish oil combined with weight loss (31), and DHA appeared to be a more effective omega-3 polyunsaturated fat than EPA (32).

Three meta-analyses of clinical trials confirmed that high doses of omega-3 polyunsaturated fat supplementation (typically at levels of ≥ 3 g/day) can reduce blood pressure, especially in hypertensive individuals (33–35). In each meta-analysis, fish oil supplementation was effective in untreated hypertensives. However, side effects were frequent, the most common being a fishy taste and belching. The most recent meta-analysis found that fish oil supplementation (median dose of 3.7 g/day) significantly reduced systolic blood pressure by 2.1 mmHg (95% CI: 1.0–3.2 mmHg) and diastolic blood pressure by 1.6 mmHg (95% CI: 1.0–2.2 mmHg) (34). Reductions in blood pressure tended to be larger in older subjects (>45 years of age) and in hypertensives (defined as individuals with a pretrial blood pressure >140/90 mmHg). The authors concluded that the effect seen in older subjects was only partly explained by their higher initial blood pressure levels. The effect appeared to be stronger in females, but there were not enough female subjects to make adequate statistical comparisons.

In summary, a very high intake of omega-3 fatty acid (fish oil) from pill supplements lowers blood pressure in hypertensive individuals, but at doses that are commonly associated with side effects.

III. PROTEIN

A paradigm shift has occurred regarding the effects of protein on blood pressure. The prevailing belief regarding protein's effect on blood pressure has been that there is either no association (36) between protein consumption and blood pressure, or that increased protein intake raises blood pressure (37–39). As discussed subsequently, the best available evidence is that increased protein intake, particularly from plant sources, can lower blood pressure.

Evidence for a direct association is based on several types of data. For example, individuals with protein malnutrition often have low blood pressure (40), and diets that are low in protein also appear to retard the progression of renal-insufficiency (41). The Kempner rice diet, which was a low-protein (20 g/day), low-sodium (150 mg/day), and high-carbohydrate (420–570 g/day) diet, successfully treated severe hypertension before the introduction of pharmacologic therapy (42,43). However, it is not known whether the blood pressure-lowering effect resulted from the low protein aspect of the diet. Vegetarians tend to have lower blood pressures when compared with nonvegetarians, although factors other than the intake of animal protein, such as lower body mass index in vegetarians (44), also differ between the two groups.

The contemporary view is that protein intake is inversely related to blood pressure (45–47). Recent studies, both observational and clinical trials, have shown that increasing protein intake, especially protein from nonmeat sources, may reduce blood pressure and prevent cardiovascular disease (48). New findings build upon observations from the 1970s and 1980s in Asian countries,

especially Japan and China, in which there was an inverse association between protein intake in certain parts of these countries and rates of hypertension and stroke (49,50). In addition, experimental data [e.g., the response to salt loading in salt-sensitive rats (50)] has shown that diets high in protein can slow the rise in blood pressure and reduce stroke rates in laboratory animals.

The mechanism by which protein may lower blood pressure is uncertain. One potential set of mechanisms is through the actions of constituent amino acids. Synthesis of catecholamines in the central nervous system is affected by the intake of tyrosine and phenylalanine (51). Tyrosine (52) and tryptophan (53) lower blood pressure when injected intraperitoneally in animals. Histidine (a precursor for the synthesis of histamine) contributes to regulatory activity on the sympathetic nervous system (54) and dilation of peripheral vessels (55). Arginine is the metabolic precursor of nitric oxide, a potent vasodilator that acts on the endothelium (56). Moncada and Higgs (56) have hypothesized that increased ingestion of arginine may reverse vascular reactivity changes and reduce intimal thickness in atherosclerosis, reduce the excessive proliferation of smooth-muscle cells in hypertension, and lower blood pressure. Taurine may exert a blood pressure lowering effect by natriuretic and diuretic effects in the kidney or inhibitory effects on the renin–angiotensin system (57). Alternatively, or in tandem, biologically active peptides (e.g., peptides with angiotensin-converting enzyme inhibitor activity) may lower blood pressure (58). There may be additional mechanisms by which soy protein operates.

A. Epidemiologic Studies

Both cross-sectional and longitudinal studies have been performed to assess the relationship between protein and blood pressure.

1. Cross-Sectional Studies

Of the available 18 cross-sectional studies, two found no association between protein intake and blood pressure (59,60), eight found a significant inverse association in at least one analysis (4,61–71), two found a direct association (72,73), and four found either an inverse association (74–77) or no association (78–80). One of the largest and most rigorous of these studies is the INTERSALT study, which documented a significant inverse association of systolic blood pressure and diastolic blood pressure with total nitrogen and urea nitrogen (measured by 24 h urine collections as a biomarker for total protein intake) in fully adjusted models; a direct association was seen when the model was adjusted only for age and sex (81). A study by Pellum and Madeiros (82) also found opposite associations depending on the adjustment procedures; the association of systolic blood pressure and pulse pressure with protein intake was inverse in multiple regression analyses, but in univariate analysis in males, a direct association for diastolic blood pressure and an inverse association for pulse pressure was found. A recent study conducted in Japan documented an inverse relationship between protein intake (estimated by the daily urinary excretion of urea nitrogen) and blood pressure in men (83). In women, a similar pattern was observed, but the relationship was not statistically significant.

An important concern in assessing the relationship between protein intake and blood pressure is the variation in reported energy intake (84). Blood pressure and excess body weight are positively associated, however, overweight individuals are more likely to underreport energy intake (85,86). Because of this underreporting of energy intake a spurious direct association between low protein intake and blood pressure may result. This phenomenon may be responsible for some of the discordant findings, including those from the first National Health and Nutrition Examination Survey (NHANES-I) (75,77), the Honolulu Heart Program (HHP) (61,63), and perhaps the Caerphilly Study (74). Other studies typically adjusted for energy intake or expressed protein intake as a percentage of kilocalories in statistical models.

2. Longitudinal Studies

Six reports of longitudinal analyses from five studies are available. Stamler et al. (4,87) reported on men in the MRFIT cohort. Among 11,000 men with 6 years of follow-up, a significant inverse association was observed between change in protein intake (as a percentage of kcal) and change in blood pressure. This association was seen in both the special intervention group (for systolic blood pressure) and the usual care group (for diastolic blood pressure). Twenty-four hour dietary recall information was collected from all men four to five times in the trial. In the Chicago Western Electric Study (88), there was an inverse association between intake of vegetable protein and change in systolic blood pressure and diastolic blood pressure, with up to 9 years of follow-up. There was also the suggestion of a direct association with animal protein. However, this study did not adjust for known determinants of blood pressure such as sodium and potassium intake. In a 10 year follow-up analysis of NHANES-I data (89), there was an inverse association between protein intake and incidence of hypertension in unadjusted analysis. Investigators of the Coronary Artery Risk Development in Young Adults (CARDIA) cohort, at 7 and 10 years of follow-up, found no association between protein intake and change in blood pressure (90,91). Similarly, a study by Morris et al. (92) found no

statistically significant association between protein and blood pressure in pregnant women.

In a study of children (93), there were small differences in blood pressure between groups that varied in protein, fat, and carbohydrate intake, but these differences were confounded by body size and maturity. A statistically significant association between diastolic blood pressure and protein intake was found among 9-year-olds (94), but the significance diminished once the authors adjusted for energy intake. A statistically significant inverse relationship between protein intake (measured with three 24 h dietary recalls) and blood pressure was found in one study with three years of follow-up in 7–10-year-olds. The relationship was no longer significant when many other dietary variables (including calcium, magnesium, potassium, carbohydrates, total fat, saturated fat, polyunsaturated fat, monounsaturated fat, dietary cholesterol, and total dietary fiber) were added to the model (95). The final study found no association between protein intake and blood pressure (96).

B. Clinical Trials

Results of early trials of protein supplementation, protein restriction, or substitution of meat for vegetarian products have been inconsistent, perhaps because of design limitations including small sample size (39,46). In a series of randomized trials, Sacks and colleagues (97–100) examined the short-term (2–6 weeks) effects on blood pressure of beef consumption, low vs. high protein intake, soy protein, and eggs. The only significant finding was that systolic blood pressure increased when beef was added to the diet (97).

Recent trials tested the effects of soy protein supplementation (101–107), and despite some variation, these trials tend to show a blood pressure-lowering effect. A 2 × 2 factorial study by Burke et al. (101) that tested the effects of high vs. low fiber and high vs. low protein on blood pressure, documented significant reductions in systolic and diastolic blood pressure of 5.9 and 2.6 mmHg, respectively, from a 66 g/day soy protein supplement. However, most of the benefit was seen in the high protein, high fiber arm of the study. He et al. (103) and Teede et al. (105) reported significant decreases in blood pressure with 40 g/day of soy supplementation.

Soy supplements also provide isoflavones; hence, there is the possibility that the observed reductions in blood pressure result from these bioactive compounds. However, two trials have shown that isolated isoflavones have no effect on blood pressure (108,109). A third trial by Jenkins et al. (110) varied the soy protein and isoflavone content in diets fed to hyperlipidemic men and postmenopausal women. Systolic blood pressure in men was significantly lower after administration of the diets high in soy protein, regardless of isoflavone status. No significant difference was seen in the women.

In spite of some inconsistencies, data from both epidemiological studies and clinical trials support the hypothesis that increased intake of protein, especially from vegetable sources, lowers blood pressure. However, this relationship has not been adequately tested in a clinical trial with size and rigor. Hence, available evidence is not yet sufficient to establish a relationship between protein consumption and blood pressure.

IV. CARBOHYDRATE

Carbohydrates include simple sugars, such as monosaccharides (glucose and fructose) and disaccharides (sucrose, maltose, and lactose) and complex carbohydrates, which are called polysaccharides (starch, cellulose, and glycogen). Starch is found in cereal grains, corn, legumes, and potatoes. Interest in the effects of carbohydrates results largely from their possible associations with insulin resistance, the metabolic syndrome, obesity, and, most recently, the glycemic index (111,112). A review by the National Research Council in 1989 (113) on diet and health (in relation to chronic diseases) made no mention of the possible effects of carbohydrates on blood pressure. A 1983 review (114) and more recent reviews (45,111) focused on simple sugars in relation to glucose tolerance and the well-known acute pressor effect of sucrose and fructose intake in animal models (115–118). Some of the mechanisms suggested for this acute direct effect on blood pressure include interactions with salt intake, promotion of salt retention (119,120), and increased catecholamine production or release with stimulation of the sympathetic nervous system (121–124). In contrast to the direct association found in animal studies, the Kempner rice diet that previously was used to treat severe hypertension was high in carbohydrate. A recent review by Hung et al. (125) concluded that diets high in carbohydrates, consumed as fruits and vegetables, together with dairy products, tend to lower blood pressure. However, fruits and vegetables are also high in fiber, potassium, and vitamin C (among other nutrients).

A. Epidemiologic Studies

Of 18 observational studies, eight studies found no significant association of carbohydrate intake with blood pressure. In other studies, the relationship was often inverse. However, direct associations also have been reported. Inverse associations were reported from NHANES-I (75,77) and the HHP (61,63), but these associations could be spurious because of inadequate adjustment for caloric intake and residual confounding. Other studies that adjusted for energy intake also found inverse associations. The Yi Migrant Study (67), NHANES-III (80), and the NHANES-I follow-up study (89) all found significant inverse associations between carbohydrate intake and blood pressure. In the MRFIT cohort, there was a direct association between carbohydrate intake and blood pressure at baseline, although there was an inverse association of 6 year change in total carbohydrate (and simple sugars) with change in diastolic blood pressure in the special intervention group (87). Direct associations of carbohydrate intake and blood pressure (or prevalent hypertension) were also seen in other studies (73,82). A cross-sectional analysis of NHANES-III data evaluated the relationship of carbohydrate intake and cardiovascular disease risk factors, one of which was systolic blood pressure (126). They found no significant relationship between carbohydrate intake and the systolic blood pressure in men or women.

In children, an inverse association between energy-adjusted carbohydrate intake and diastolic blood pressure >3 years of follow-up was seen in a study by Simons-Morton et al. (95). However, this association did not persist when other nutrients were added to the regression model.

B. Clinical Trials

Few trials have tested the effects of carbohydrates on blood pressure (45,111). A trial by Rebella et al. (120) assessed the effects of five solutions of simple sugars in 20 nonhypertensive men. Glucose and sucrose ingestion was associated with significant increases in blood pressure at 1 h (increase of 9–10 mmHg), as well as antinatriuresis. In a cross-over study of 24 subjects (men and women) who were classified as "carbohydrate-sensitive" due to their inflated insulin response upon sucrose loading, diastolic blood pressure significantly increased after a 6 week diet that contained one-third of the calories as sucrose (127). Another study found no association between blood pressure and sodium retention (secondary to glucose loading) (128). Sacks et al. (129) found no effect from replacement of saturated fat with carbohydrate.

In summary, data regarding the effects of carbohydrate on blood pressure are inconsistent. Further research is clearly warranted.

V. FIBER

There are various definitions of dietary fiber, and none is entirely adequate (130). The differences in definition and measurement of fiber intake have made the interpretation of study findings difficult (45). In 1972, Trowell (131) defined dietary fiber as the components of the plant cell wall that cannot be digested by the secretions of the human alimentary tract (cellulose, hemicelluloses, pectin, and lignin). A refined definition includes nondigestible plant materials that are not components of the cell wall, such as gums and mucilages (132). In the year 2000, the American Association of Cereal Chemists (AACC) (133) provided a definition of dietary fiber and criteria for analyzing the methodology used in fiber studies. The new definition does not greatly differ from Trowell's earlier definition.

Fiber can be classified as either water soluble or insoluble. Soluble fibers include pectins, gums, mucilages, and some hemicelluloses. Insoluble fibers include lignins and most hemicelluloses (113). Soluble fibers are of interest, as they affect gastrointestinal function by decreasing the rate at which digestion takes place, as well as the absorption of nutrients, and by indirectly affecting glucose and lipid metabolism (45). Animal studies have shown that increased intake of fiber can reduce the elevation in blood pressure that is associated with a sucrose load (134) or a fat-enriched diet (135).

There is an interest in the effect of high-fiber diets on insulin sensitivity and glucose metabolism, because a potential mechanism for fiber's effect on blood pressure is due to its association with insulin resistance (111,112). Another mechanism by which fiber could affect blood pressure is absorption of short-chain fatty acids in the large bowel by fermentable fiber components, which possibly has a beneficial effect on blood pressure (135).

A. Epidemiologic Studies

Many studies that have investigated macronutrient intake also have examined the association of fiber intake with blood pressure.

1. Cross-Sectional Analyses

The Caerphilly Study produced conflicting results; in two reports there was an inverse association between cereal fiber and systolic blood pressure (78,136), but a third study did not show the same relationship (74). The HHP (61), Yi Migrant Study (67), and a report from NHANES-III (80) all found an inverse association of dietary fiber with both systolic and diastolic blood pressure. In a sample of men free of clinical hypertension (137), systolic blood pressure was inversely associated with the intake of fruit fiber (adjusted for age, body habitus, and alcohol consumption). Diastolic blood pressure was also associated, but failed to reach statistical significance. Some cross-sectional studies indicate the potential for factors such as age, gender, race, and hypertension risk to affect the relationship between fiber intake and blood pressure (47).

2. Longitudinal Analyses

In the MRFIT cohort (4,87), investigators found an inverse association of change in fiber intake (g/1000 kcal) with change in blood pressure; inverse cross-sectional associations between reported dietary fiber intake and systolic and diastolic blood pressure were also found. The CARDIA study was a multicenter population-based cohort study that examined change in cardiovascular disease risk factors >10 years. It showed an inverse association of fiber intake at year seven (when diet history was assessed) and a 10 year change in blood pressure in white men and women (91). In the NHANES-I follow-up study, fiber was inversely associated with incident hypertension (89).

In predominantly white male health professionals in the United States, those with a fiber intake of <12 g/day were at greater risk for self-reported hypertension (4 year cumulative risk) compared with men with an intake of >24 g/day after adjustment for total energy intake. In addition, an association with systolic blood pressure change was found after adjustment for other dietary variables (2). In a prospective study that enrolled 58,000 predominantly white US female nurses, a 1989 (138) report documented an inverse association between fiber intake, adjusted for total energy consumption, and 4 year cumulative risk of self-reported hypertension. The increased risk was no longer significant when calcium and magnesium were included in the statistical model. However, another report from the Nurses' Health Study that had additional follow-up (3) adjusted for calcium, magnesium, and potassium reported an inverse association of dietary fiber with systolic and diastolic blood pressure. In the Baltimore Longitudinal Study of Aging, dietary records from 380 men (three to eight records over a period of 8 years) showed an inverse association between dietary fiber intake and both systolic and diastolic blood pressure (139).

Few studies have examined the association of blood pressure with dietary fiber in children. One study found an inverse association between energy-adjusted fiber intake and diastolic blood pressure in 9-year-old boys (94). Another study reported an inverse association with both systolic and diastolic blood pressure over up to 3 years of follow-up (95). After adjustment for other dietary variables, the relationship remained for diastolic blood pressure only.

B. Clinical Trials

Early, nonrandomized clinical trials showed a reduction in blood pressure after administration of dietary fiber supplementation (140,141); however, the trials were small. The study by Wright et al. (141) examined the effects of both reducing and increasing fiber intake on blood pressure. Two trials of increasing dietary fiber showed reductions in blood pressure. Over a 4 week period in 17 subjects, an increase from 16.2 to 24.5 g/day led to a decrease in systolic/diastolic blood pressure of 3.9/3.7 mmHg. The other trial ($n = 14$) showed decreases of 1.8/2.7 mmHg with an increase in fiber consumption from 16.8 to 28.6 g/day. A third trial, which reduced fiber intake from 30.8 to 14.8 g/day, showed an increase in blood pressure of 7.7/2.8 mmHg.

Subsequently, a large number of randomized controlled trials involving fiber supplementation have been carried out, several of which were well-controlled with sufficient sample size (142–144). However, most did not measure blood pressure as a primary outcome (47), and most did not detect a reduction in blood pressure with increased fiber intake.

A meta-analysis of the trials was carried out by He et al. (145). Twenty of 47 identified trials were included in the meta-analysis, with an average fiber intake of 14 g/day. Studies were excluded mainly because of simultaneous changes in dietary sodium, potassium, or fat intake in the active treatment arm. The average reductions in systolic and diastolic blood pressure were 1.6 mmHg (95% CI: 0.4–2.7 mmHg) and 2.0 mmHg (95% CI: 1.1–2.9 mmHg), respectively. Trials that used concentrated and purified fiber showed greater reductions in blood pressure than trials that tested fiber in foods. One potential reason for this difference is that compliance with fiber supplementation was higher than adherence to dietary changes; physical or chemical differences of the types of fiber also may have had a role.

After this meta-analysis, other studies were published. Burke et al. (101) examined the effects of both protein and fiber intake in a 2×2 factorial trial. They documented a significant decrease in 24 h systolic blood pressure (5.9 mmHg, 95% CI: 8.1–3.7) with addition of dietary fiber (15 g psyllium/day). The effect on diastolic blood pressure was not significant. The majority of the fiber (and protein) effect was seen in the higher fiber/high protein arm of the trial. A recent 12 week intervention study of oat consumption (soluble fiber) vs. wheat consumption (insoluble fiber) in men with hypertension ($n = 18$ in both groups) did not show a blood pressure-lowering effect of the oats (146).

In general, there appears to be an inverse association between dietary fiber and blood pressure (or incident hypertension), in both observational epidemiological studies and clinical trials. Interpretation of results from observational studies are complicated because of nonstandardized fiber definitions, suboptimal quantification of dietary fiber intake (e.g., with 24 h food recalls or with food diaries),

and potential confounding factors. Similarly, clinical trials have substantial problems including insufficient statistical power, inadequate measurement of blood pressure, and uncertain exposure (i.e., the type of fiber that was tested). Hence, evidence of an inverse association of dietary fiber with blood pressure, though suggestive, is not yet conclusive.

VI. CHOLESTEROL

Very few studies have addressed the effect of dietary cholesterol on blood pressure. In the MRFIT cohort, there was a direct positive relationship between increasing cholesterol intake (based on repeated 24 h dietary recalls measured in mg/1000 kcal per day) and both systolic and diastolic blood pressure (4,87). In addition, the Keys score was associated with diastolic blood pressure but not with systolic blood pressure in this cohort. In the Chicago Western Electric Study, there was a significant positive relationship between change in systolic blood pressure over 8 years of follow-up with both dietary cholesterol and Keys score (88). Both studies were able to adjust for possible demographic, dietary, and medical confounders. Yet, in view of the lack of available evidence, the relationship between dietary cholesterol intake and blood pressure is uncertain.

VII. DIETARY PATTERNS

The effects of dietary patterns on blood pressure and cardiovascular risk factors are of substantial interest.

A. Vegetarian Dietary Patterns

As reviewed by Beilin (147), vegetarians tend to have lower blood pressure than nonvegetarians, even after adjustment for age, gender, and body weight (44,100). In addition, vegetarians appear to have a lower age-related increase in blood pressure than nonvegetarians (Fig. 11.1) (37,100). Yet, it is difficult to isolate the effects of meat consumption from the effects of other dietary factors and lifestyle habits. Hence, some of the observed reductions in blood pressure that can be attributed to vegetarian diets may result from other dietary factors.

1. Observational Studies

Several cross-sectional studies have compared vegetarian with nonvegetarian populations, and some compared different types of vegetarians. In a study of 11,400 British adults, self-reported blood pressure of four groups were compared—meat eaters, fish eaters,

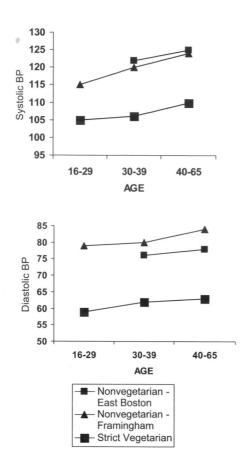

Figure 11.1 Blood pressure by age in a strict vegetarian population in Boston and in nonvegetarian populations in East Boston and Framingham, MA, USA. [From Sacks et al. (100), adapted with permission.]

vegetarians, and vegans (44). The lowest prevalence of hypertension occurred in the male vegan group, followed by the female vegan group. The highest prevalence of hypertension occurred in meat eaters. Vegetarians and fish eaters had a slightly higher prevalence of hypertension than the vegans. Mean systolic and diastolic blood pressures were also significantly different between the groups. Age-adjusted systolic blood pressure differences between meat eaters and vegans were 4.2 and 2.6 mmHg for men and women, respectively, corresponding diastolic blood pressure differences were 2.8 and 1.7 mmHg, respectively. Differences in body mass index (BMI) explained much of the differences between groups.

Another study obtained anthropometric measurements and recorded electrolyte excretion (including sodium and potassium) in matched pairs of vegetarians and nonvegetarians. The vegetarians were mainly Seventh-Day Adventists. Mean blood pressure was lower in vegetarians, and the authors concluded that these differences were not due to dietary sodium (37).

In a study of individuals who were vegetarian for at least 5 years, Melby et al. (148) compared vegetarians and nonvegetarians, stratified by race. Older black vegetarians had significantly lower blood pressure than black nonvegetarians, but they still had significantly higher blood pressure than white vegetarians and nonvegetarians. Such findings suggest that long-term adherence to a vegetarian diet lowers blood pressure in blacks, but that it does not eliminate differences in blood pressure that are attributable to racial differences.

2. Clinical Trials

Few trials have tested the effects of vegetarian diets on blood pressure. One trial was a randomized cross-over trial that evaluated the effect of an omnivorous diet vs. either of two lacto–ovo vegetarian diets for 6 week periods in 58 individuals with untreated hypertension (149). On the vegetarian diets, systolic blood pressure fell 5 mmHg, on average, and rose upon consumption of the omnivorous diet.

Another trial enrolled 59 nonhypertensive, nonvegetarian individuals, and randomized them either to a control group (omnivorous diet) or to one of two experimental diets (omnivorous diet for the first 2 weeks and a lacto–ovo vegetarian diet for one of two 6 week experimental periods) (150). Consumption of the lacto–ovo vegetarian diets led to significant reductions in systolic blood pressure (5–6 mmHg) and diastolic blood pressure (2–3 mmHg), when compared with consumption of the nonvegetarian diet. Blood pressure also significantly rose in the experimental group that reverted to the omnivorous diet. Yet, neither trial tightly controlled the dietary factors which might partially account for the observed benefit of the vegetarian diet and which might have differed across randomized groups.

Overall, available evidence indicates that vegetarian diets can lower blood pressure. However, it is possible that established dietary factors (salt intake, potassium intake, and weight) partially account for the effects of these diets on blood pressure.

B. Mediterranean-Style Diets

The *Mediterranean diet* is not a single dietary pattern. Rather, this term is used to describe a variety of diets consumed in this region of the world. Mediterranean diets typically emphasize fruits, vegetables, legumes, beans, nuts, seeds, cereals, and breads. Intake of olive oil is high, whereas intake of saturated fat is low. Fish consumption is often high, but the amount depends on proximity of the populace to the sea. The diets include dairy products, wine, and some meat and poultry (151,152). In view of the relatively lower coronary heart disease and total mortality that is characteristic of several Mediterranean regions (152), the effects of these diets on blood pressure and other cardiovascular disease risk factors are of considerable interest.

The seven countries study provides indirect evidence that a Mediterranean-style diet may have beneficial effects on blood pressure. In the part of Greece where traditional diets are eaten, the prevalence of hypertension was half that of Western Europe and the United States (153). Subsequently, a cross-sectional study of 1154 Greek women and 1128 Greek men who were free of cardiovascular disease documented that consumption of a Mediterranean-style diet was associated with a statistically significant (26%) decrease in prevalence of hypertension, even after controlling for potential confounding factors (154).

Yet, the few trials that have investigated the effect of a Mediterranean-style diet on blood pressure have been inconsistent. In one small study of 57 nonhypertensive rural dwellers in Southern Italy, replacement of usual diet with a diet increased in saturated fat and decreased in carbohydrates and monounsaturated fats led to a significant rise in systolic and diastolic blood pressure (155). However, in the Lyon Diet Heart Study, a Mediterranean-style diet had no effect on blood pressure (156,157). The Lyon Diet Heart Study was a randomized, single-blind secondary prevention trial that tested whether a Mediterranean-style diet can prevent a second myocardial infarction. Participants were randomized to a control or an experimental group. The experimental group consumed significantly less lipids, saturated fat, cholesterol, and linoleic acid, but more oleic and linolenic acid, confirmed by plasma measurements. After a mean follow-up at 27 months, there were fewer cardiac deaths and nonfatal myocardial infarction events in the experimental group (risk ratio = 0.27). However, blood pressure remained similar in both groups (157).

Overall, although consumption of traditional Mediterranean-style diets are associated with reduced coronary heart disease mortality and total mortality, there is little direct evidence that such diets lower blood pressure.

C. DASH Dietary Pattern

The DASH trial was designed to test whether modification of a whole dietary pattern as opposed to just one or two nutrients might affect blood pressure. The DASH trial tested two main hypotheses:

1. Increased intake of fruits and vegetables will lower blood pressure (the "fruits and vegetables" diet).
2. An overall healthy dietary pattern (the "combination diet," now referred to as the "DASH diet") will lower blood pressure.

The DASH trial was a controlled study; in which participants received all their food for a period of 11 weeks from the study. Average blood pressure at baseline was 131/85 mmHg, and 29% of the participants had stage 1 hypertension. Blacks compromised 65% of the study population; the reminder were predominantly white. Participants were randomized to one of three diets. The control diet was typical of what many people in the United States eat (Table 11.3 and Fig. 11.2).

The "fruits and vegetables" diet was higher in potassium, magnesium, and fiber, but otherwise similar to the control diet. The DASH diet emphasized fruits, vegetables, and low-fat dairy products, included whole grains, poultry, fish and nuts, and was reduced in fats, red meat, sweets, and sugar-containing beverages. Sodium intake levels averaged 3000 mg/day in all three diets. Energy intake was adjusted to maintain body weight. The maximum permissible alcohol intake was two or fewer drinks per day. By controlling weight, sodium intake, and alcohol intake, the study tested the effects of the diets independent of these established risk factors.

Among all the participants, the DASH diet significantly reduced blood pressure (Fig. 11.3). Systolic blood pressure decreased by 5.5 mmHg and diastolic blood pressure by 3.0 mmHg. Blood pressure reduction from the fruits and vegetables diet was about half of the DASH effect (158). The dietary effect was apparent after only 2 weeks on the two diets. In subgroup analyses, the DASH diet significantly lowered blood pressure in all major subgroups—men, women, blacks, nonblacks, hypertensives, and nonhypertensives (159). The effect of the DASH diet was significantly greater in blacks (with systolic and diastolic blood pressure reductions of 6.9 and 3.7 mmHg, respectively) than in whites (with systolic and diastolic

Table 11.3 Nutrient Profile of Diets Tested in the Dash Trial[a]

Nutrients	Control	Fruits and vegetables	Combination
Fat (% kcal)	37	37	27
Saturated fat	16	16	6
Monounsaturated fat	13	13	13
Polyunsaturated fat	8	8	8
Carbohydrates (% kcal)	48	48	55
Protein (% kcal)	15	15	18
Cholesterol (mg/day)	300	300	150
Fiber (g/day)	9	31	31
Potassium (mg/day)	1700	4700	4700
Magnesium (mg/day)	165	500	500
Calcium (mg/day)	450	450	1240
Sodium (mg/day)	3000	3000	3000

[a]For 2100 kcal energy level.
Source: From Appel et al. (158), adapted with permission.

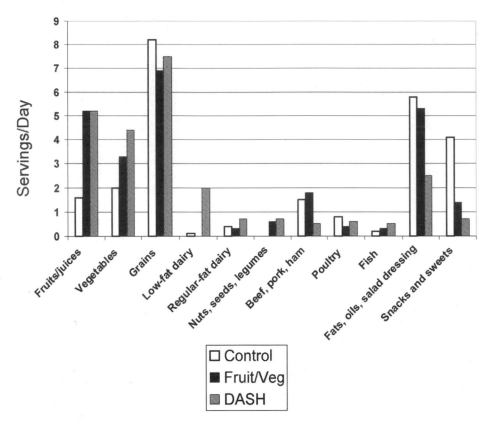

Figure 11.2 Servings per day of food groups by diet in the DASH clinical trial.

blood pressure reductions of 3.3 and 2.4 mmHg, respectively). Hypertensive subjects had an average reduction of 11.6 mmHg in systolic blood pressure and 5.3 mmHg in diastolic blood pressure; nonhypertensive subjects had net reductions in systolic and diastolic blood pressure of 3.5 and 2.2 mmHg, respectively.

A separate feeding study, the DASH-Sodium trial, tested the effects of the DASH diet by itself and the combined effects of the DASH diet and sodium reduction on blood pressure. In brief, the DASH diet lowered blood pressure in either case, but lowered it to a lesser extent when the sodium intake was ~1500 mg/day than when the sodium intake was 2300 mg/day (160). Finally, a behavioral intervention trial, the PREMIER study, documented that free-living individuals outside of the confines of a controlled diet studies such as DASH and DASH-sodium, can make dietary and other lifestyle changes including weight loss, exercise, and reduced salt intake (161).

There is considerable speculation about which components of the DASH diet lowered blood pressure. Fruits and vegetables are rich in potassium, magnesium, and fiber. Potassium has been shown to effectively lower blood pressure, particularly in individuals with a low intake of fruits and vegetables, in individuals with hypertension, and in blacks (162). Except for the "fruits and vegetables" food group, the DASH trial was not designed to test the effects of specific nutrients or food groups. Results from the DASH trial, as well as other studies, indicate that increased fruit and vegetable intake can lower blood pressure (163,164). Because the DASH diet also

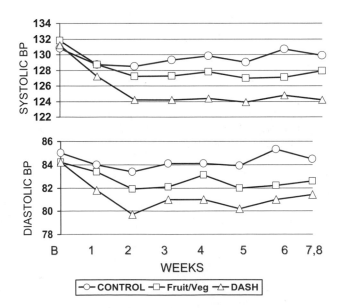

Figure 11.3 Blood pressure by week during the DASH trial, according to diet. [From Appel et al. (158), adapted with permission.]

lowered blood pressure when compared with the "fruits and vegetables" diet, some other aspect(s) of the DASH diet contributed to lowering blood pressure.

VIII. CONCLUSIONS

Available evidence is sufficiently strong to conclude that certain dietary patterns, specifically, following the DASH diet or vegetarian diets, can lower blood pressure. A very high intake of omega-3 polyunsaturated fat also can reduce blood pressure in hypertensive individuals.

Other factors also may influence blood pressure. Specifically, an expanding body of evidence suggests that increased protein intake, particularly protein intake from vegetable sources, may lower blood pressure. Whether increased fiber intake lowers blood pressure remains unproven. For other macronutrients and for cholesterol, corresponding evidence is either limited or equivocal.

Further research, especially well-designed trials with sufficient sample size, is required. In the meantime, a reduced salt intake, increased potassium intake, weight control, consumption of the DASH diet, and moderation of alcohol intake (among those who drink) remain prudent public health recommendations to lower blood pressure in hypertensive as well as nonhypertensive individuals.

REFERENCES

1. Morris MC. Dietary fats and blood pressure. J Cardiovasc Risk 1994; 1:21–30.
2. Ascherio A, Rimm EB, Giovannucci EL, Colditz GA, Rosner B, Willett WC, Sacks FM, Stampfer MJ. A prospective study of nutritional factors and hypertension among US men. Circulation 1992; 86:1475–1484.
3. Ascherio A, Hennekens CH, Willett WC, Sacks FM, Rosner B, Manson J, Witteman J, Stampfer MJ. A prospective study of nutritional factors, blood pressure, and hypertension among US women. Hypertension 1996; 27:1065–1072.
4. Stamler J, Caggiula A, Grandits GA, Kjelsberg M, Cutler JA. Relationship to blood pressure of combinations of dietary macronutrients. Findings of the Multiple Risk Factor Intervention Trial (MRFIT). Circulation 1996; 94:2417–2423.
5. National Diet Heart Study Research Group. The national diet and heart study final report. Circulation 1968; 37–38 (suppl 1):1228–1230.
6. Research Committee to the Medical Research Council. Controlled trial of soya-bean oil in myocardial infarction. Lancet 1968; 11:693–699.
7. Rasmussen OW, Thomsen C, Hansen KW, Vesterlund M, Winther E, Hermansen K. Effects on blood pressure, glucose, and lipid levels of a high-monounsaturated fat diet compared with a high-carbohydrate diet in NIDDM subjects. Diabetes Care 1993; 16:1565–1571.
8. Ferrara LA, Raimondi AS, d'Episcopo L, Guida L, Dello RA, Marotta T. Olive oil and reduced need for antihypertensive medications. Arch Intern Med 2000; 160:837–842.
9. Lorenz R, Spengler U, Fischer S, Duhm J, Weber PC. Platelet function, thromboxane formation and blood pressure control during supplementation of the Western diet with cod liver oil. Circulation 1983; 67:504–511.
10. Margolin G, Huster G, Glueck CJ, Speirs J, Vandegrift J, Illig E, Wu J, Streicher P, Tracy T. Blood pressure lowering in elderly subjects: a double-blind crossover study of omega-3 and omega-6 fatty acids. Am J Clin Nutr 1991; 53:562–572.
11. Yin K, Chu ZM, Beilin LJ. Blood pressure and vascular reactivity changes in spontaneously hypertensive rats fed fish oil. Br J Pharmacol 1991; 102:991–997.
12. Hashimoto M, Shinozuka K, Gamoh S, Tanabe Y, Hossain MS, Kwon YM, Hata N, Misawa Y, Kunitomo M, Masumura S. The hypotensive effect of docosahexaenoic acid is associated with the enhanced release of ATP from the caudal artery of aged rats. J Nutr 1999; 129:70–76.
13. Mori TA, Watts GF, Burke V, Hilme E, Puddey IB, Beilin LJ. Differential effects of eicosapentaenoic acid and docosahexaenoic acid on vascular reactivity of the forearm microcirculation in hyperlipidemic, overweight men. Circulation 2000; 102:1264–1269.
14. Yoshimura T, Matsui K, Ito M, Yunohara T, Kawasaki N, Nakamura T, Okamura H. Effects of highly purified eicosapentaenoic acid on plasma beta thromboglobulin level and vascular reactivity to angiotensin II Artery 1987; 14:295–303.
15. Chu ZM, Yin K, Beilin LJ. Fish oil feeding selectively attenuates contractile responses to noradrenaline and electrical stimulation in the perfused mesenteric resistance vessels of spontaneously hypertensive rats. Clin Exp Pharmacol Physiol 1992; 19:177–181.
16. Nestel PJ, Shige H, Pomeroy S, Cehun M, Abbey M, Raederstorff D. The n-3 fatty acids eicosapentaenoic acid and docosahexaenoic acid increase systemic arterial compliance in humans. Am J Clin Nutr 2002; 76:326–330.
17. McLennan P, Howe P, Abeywardena M, Muggli R, Raederstorff D, Mano M, Rayner T, Head R. The cardiovascular protective role of docosahexaenoic acid. Eur J Pharmacol 1996; 300:83–89.
18. Bang HO, Dyerberg J, Nielsen AB. Plasma lipid and lipoprotein pattern in Greenlandic West-coast Eskimos. Lancet 1971; 1:1143–1145.
19. Kromhout D, Bosschieter EB, de Lezenne CC. The inverse relation between fish consumption and 20-year mortality from coronary heart disease. N Engl J Med 1985; 312:1205–1209.
20. Albert CM, Hennekens CH, O'Donnell CJ, Ajani UA, Carey VJ, Willett WC, Ruskin JN, Manson JE. Fish consumption and risk of sudden cardiac death. JAMA 1998; 279:23–28.
21. Wang C, Chung M, Lichtenstein A, Balk E, DeVine D, Lawrence A et al. Effects of Omega-3 Fatty Acids on

Cardiovascular Disease. Evidence Report/Technology Assessment No. 94. 04-E009-2. Agency for Healthcare Research and Quality, Rockville, MD, 2004.

22. Knapp HR, FitzGerald GA. The antihypertensive effects of fish oil. A controlled study of polyunsaturated fatty acid supplements in essential hypertension. N Engl J Med 1989; 320:1037-1043.

23. Levinson PD, Iosiphidis AH, Saritelli AL, Herbert PN, Steiner M. Effects of n-3 fatty acids in essential hypertension. Am J Hypertens 1990; 3:754-760.

24. Norris PG, Jones CJ, Weston MJ. Effect of dietary supplementation with fish oil on systolic blood pressure in mild essential hypertension. Br Med J (Clin Res Ed) 1986; 293:104-105.

25. Prisco D, Paniccia R, Bandinelli B, Filippini M, Francalanci I, Giusti B, Giurlani L, Gensini GF, Abbate R, Neri Serneri GG. Effect of medium-term supplementation with a moderate dose of n-3 polyunsaturated fatty acids on blood pressure in mild hypertensive patients. Thromb Res 1998; 91:105-112.

26. Radack K, Deck C, Huster G. The effects of low doses of n-3 fatty acid supplementation on blood pressure in hypertensive subjects. A randomized controlled trial. Arch Intern Med 1991; 151:1173-1180.

27. Singer P, Berger I, Luck K, Taube C, Naumann E, Godicke W. Long-term effect of mackerel diet on blood pressure, serum lipids and thromboxane formation in patients with mild essential hypertension. Atherosclerosis 1986; 62:259-265.

28. Toft I, Bonaa KH, Ingebretsen OC, Nordoy A, Jenssen T. Effects of n-3 polyunsaturated fatty acids on glucose homeostasis and blood pressure in essential hypertension. A randomized, controlled trial. Ann Intern Med 1995; 123:911-918.

29. Dokholyan RS, Albert CM, Appel LJ, Cook NR, Whelton P, Hennekens CH. A trial of omega-3 fatty acids for prevention of hypertension. Am J Cardiol 2004; 93:1041-1043.

30. Pauletto P, Puato M, Caroli MG, Casiglia E, Munhambo AE, Cazzolato G, Bittolo BG, Angeli MT, Galli C, Pessina AC. Blood pressure and atherogenic lipoprotein profiles of fish-diet and vegetarian villagers in Tanzania: the Lugalawa study. Lancet 1996; 348:784-788.

31. Bao DQ, Mori TA, Burke V, Puddey IB, Beilin LJ. Effects of dietary fish and weight reduction on ambulatory blood pressure in overweight hypertensives. Hypertension 1998; 32:710-717.

32. Mori TA, Bao DQ, Burke V, Puddey IB, Beilin LJ. Docosahexaenoic acid but not eicosapentaenoic acid lowers ambulatory blood pressure and heart rate in humans. Hypertension 1999; 34:253-260.

33. Appel LJ, Miller ER, III, Seidler AJ, Whelton PK. Does supplementation of diet with 'fish oil' reduce blood pressure? A meta-analysis of controlled clinical trials. Arch Intern Med 1993; 153:1429-1438.

34. Geleijnse JM, Giltay EJ, Grobbee DE, Donders AR, Kok FJ. Blood pressure response to fish oil supplementation: metaregression analysis of randomized trials. J Hypertens 2002; 20:1493-1499.

35. Morris MC, Sacks F, Rosner B. Does fish oil lower blood pressure? A meta-analysis of controlled trials. Circulation 1993; 88:523-533.

36. Meyer TW, Anderson S, Brenner BM. Dietary protein intake and progressive glomerular sclerosis: the role of capillary hypertension and hyperperfusion in the progression of renal disease. Ann Int Med 1983; 98(Part 2):832-838.

37. Armstrong B, van Merwyk AJ, Coates H. Blood pressure in Seventh-Day Adventists. Am J Epidemiol 1977; 105:444-449.

38. McCarron DA, Henry HJ, Morris CD. Human nutrition and blood pressure regulation: an intergrated approach. Hypertension 1982; 4 (suppl III):III-2-III-13.

39. Sacks FM, Rosner B, Kass EH. Blood pressure in vegetarians. Am J Epidemiol 1974; 100:390-398.

40. Viart P. Hemodynamic findings in severe protein-calorie malnutrition. Am J Clin Nutr 1977; 30:334-348.

41. Ihle BU, Becker GJ, Whitworth JA, Charlwood RA, Kincaid-Smith PS. The effect of protein restriction on the progression of renal insufficiency. New Engl J Med 1989; 321:1773-1777.

42. Kempner W. Treatment of hypertensive vascular disease with rice diet. Am J Med 1948; 4:545-577.

43. Watkin DM, Froeb HF, Hatch FT, Gutman AB. Effect of diet in essential hypertension. II. Results with unmodified Kempner rice diet in fifty hopsitalized patients. Am J Med 1950; 9:441-493.

44. Appleby PN, Davey GK, Key TJ. Hypertension and blood pressure among meat eaters, fish eaters, vegetarians and vegans in EPIC-Oxford. Public Health Nutr 2002; 5:645-654.

45. Burke V, Beilin LJ, Sciarrone S. Vegetarian diets, protein and fibre. In: Swales JD, ed. Textbook of Hypertension. Oxford: Blackwell, 1994:619-632.

46. Obarzanek E, Velletri PA, Cutler JA. Dietary protein and blood pressure. JAMA 1996; 275:1598-1603.

47. He J, Whelton PK. Effect of dietary fiber and protein intake on blood pressure: a review of epidemiologic evidence. Clin Exp Hypertens 1999; 21:785-796.

48. Appel LJ. The effects of protein intake on blood pressure and cardiovascular disease. Curr Opin Lipidol 2003; 14:55-59.

49. Liu L. Hypertension studies in China. Clin Exper Hypertens 1989; 11:859-868.

50. Yamori Y, Horie R, Nara Y, Kihara M, Ikeda K, Mano M, Fujiwara K. Dietary prevention of hypertension in animal models and its applicability to humans. Ann Clin Res 1984; 16(suppl 43):28-31.

51. Anderson GH. Proteins and amino acids: effects on the sympathetic nervous system and blood pressure regulation. Can J Physiol Pharmacol 1986; 64:863-870.

52. Sved AF, Fernstrom JD, Wurtman RJ. Tyrosine administration reduces blood pressure and enhances brain norepinephrine release in spontaneously hypertensive rats. Proc Natl Acad Sci 1979; 76:3511-3514.

53. Sved AF, van Itallie CM, Fernstrom JD. Studies on the antihypertensive action of L-tryptophan. J Pharmacol Exp Ther 1982; 221:329-333.

54. Akins VF, Bealer SL. Central nervous system histamine regulates peripheral sympathetic activity. Am J Physiol 1991; 260:H218–H224.

55. Bender DA. Histidine. In: Bender DA, ed. Amino Acid Metabolism. 2nd ed. Chichester, UK: Wiley, 1985:188–200.

56. Moncada S, Higgs A. The L-arginine-nitric oxide pathway. N Engl J Med 1993; 329:2003–2012.

57. Martin DS. Dietary protein and hypertension: where do we stand? Nutrition 2003; 19:385.

58. FitzGerald RJ, Murray BA, Walsh DJ. Hypotensive peptides from milk proteins. J Nutr 2004; 134:980S–988S.

59. Dawber TR, Kannel WB, Kagan A, Donabedian RK, McNamara PM, Pearson G. Environmental factors in hypertension. In: Stamler J, Stamler R, Pullman TN, eds. The Epidemiology of Hypertension. New York: Grune & Stratton, 1967:255–288.

60. Slattery ML, Bishop DT, French TK, Hunt SC, Meikle AW, Williams RR. Lifestyle and blood pressure levels in twins in Utah. Genet Epidemiol 1988; 5:277–287.

61. Joffres MR, Reed DM, Yano K. Relationship of magnesium intake and other dietary factors to blood pressure: the Honolulu heart study. Am J Clin Nutr 1987; 45:469–475.

62. Kihara M, Fujikawa J, Ohtaka M, Mano M, Nara Y, Horie R, Tsunematsu T, Note S, Fukase M, Yamori Y. Hypertension. Hypertension 1984; 6:736–742.

63. Reed D, McGee D, Yano K, Hankin J. Diet, blood pressure, and multicollinearity. Hypertension 1985; 7:405–410.

64. Yamori Y, Kihara M, Nara Y, Ohtaka M, Horie R, Tsunematsu T, Note S. Hypertension and diet: multiple regression analysis in a Japanese farming community. Lancet 1981; 1:1204–1205.

65. Zhou BF, Wu XZ, Tao SQ, Yang J, Cao TX, Zheng RP, Tian XZ, Lu CQ, Maio HY, Ye FM et al. Dietary patterns in 10 groups and the relationship with blood pressure. Chin Med J 1989; 102:257–261.

66. Elliott P, Freeman J, Pryer J, Brunner E, Marmot M. Dietary protein and blood pressure: a report from the Dietary and Nutritional Survey of British Adults [abstr]. J Hypertens 1992; 109(suppl 1):S141.

67. He J, Klag MJ, Whelton PK, Chen J-Y, Qian M-C, He G-Q. Dietary macronutrients and blood pressure in southwestern China. J Hypertens 1995; 13:1267–1274.

68. Liu LJ, Ikeda K, Yamori Y. Twenty-four hour urinary sodium and 3-methylhistidine excretion in relation to blood pressure in Chinese: results from the China–Japan cooperative research for the WHO-CARDIAC Study. Hypertens Res 2000; 23:151–157.

69. Liu LJ, Liu LS, Ding Y, Huang Z, He B, Sun S, Zhao G, Zhang H, Miki T, Mizushima S, Ikeda K, Nara Y, Yamori Y. Ethnic and environmental differences in various markers of dietary intake and blood pressure among Chinese Han and three other minority peoples of China: results from the WHO Cardiovascular Diseases and Alimentary Comparison (CARDIAC) Study. Hypertens Res 2001; 24:315–322.

70. Liu LJ, Mizushima S, Ikeda K, Hattori H, Miura A, Gao M, Nara Y, Yamori Y. Comparative studies of diet-related factors and blood pressure among Chinese and Japanese: results from the China–Japan Cooperative Research of the WHO-CARDIAC Study. Cardiovascular disease and alimentary comparison. Hypertens Res 2000; 23:413–420.

71. Zhou BF, Zhang X, Zhu A, Zhao L, Zhu S, Ruan L, Zhu L, Liang S. The relationship of dietary animal protein and electrolytes to blood pressure: a study on three Chinese populations. Int J Epidemiol 1994; 23:716–722.

72. Havlik RJ, Fabsitz RR, Kalousdian S, Borhani NO, Christain JC. Dietary protein and blood pressure in mono-zygotic twins. Prev Med 1990; 19:31–39.

73. Rafie M, Boshtam M, Sarraf Zadegan N, Abdar N, Sedigheh K, Asgary S, Naderi G. The impact of macro and micronutrients daily intake on blood pressure [abstr]. Atherosclerosis 1998; 136(suppl 1):S62.

74. Elliott P, Fehily AM, Sweetnam PM, Yarnell JWG. Diet, alcohol, body mass, and social factors in relation to blood pressure: the Caerphilly Heart Study. J Epidemiol Comm Health 1987; 41:37–43.

75. Gruchow HW, Sobocinski KA, Barboriak JJ. Alcohol, nutrient intake, and hypertension in US adults. JAMA 1985; 253:1567–1570.

76. Hajjar IM, Grim CE, George V, Kotchen TA. Impact of diet on blood pressure and age related changes in blood pressure in the US population: analysis of NHANES III. Arch Intern Med 2001; 161:589–593.

77. McCarron DA, Morris CD, Henry HJ, Stanton JL. Blood pressure and nutrient intake in the United States. Science 1984; 224:1392–1398.

78. Fehily AM, Milbank JE, Yarnell JWG, Hayes TM, Kubiki AJ, Eastham RD. Dietary determinants of lipoproteins, total cholesterol, viscosity, fibrinogen, and blood pressure. Am J Clin Nutr 1982; 36:890–896.

79. Harlan WR, Hull AL, Schmouder RL, Landis JR, Thompson FE, Larkin FA. Blood pressure and nutrition in adults. The National Health and Nutrition Examination Survey. Am J Epidemiol 1984; 120:17–28.

80. He J, Loria C, Vupputuri S, Whelton PK. Dietary macro-nutrient intake and level of blood pressure: results from the Third National Health and Nutrition Examination Survey (NHANES-III) [abstr]. Circulation 1998; 98 (suppl 1):858.

81. Stamler J, Elliott P, Kesteloot H, Nichols R, Claeys G, Dyer AR, Stamler R. Inverse relation of dietary protein markers with blood pressure. Findings for 10,020 men and women in the INTERSALT Study. INTERSALT Cooperative Research Group. INTERnational study of SALT and blood pressure. Circulation 1996; 94:1629–1634.

82. Pellum LK, Madeiros DM. Blood pressure in young adult normotensives: effect of protein, fat, and cholesterol intakes. Nutr Rep Int 1983; 27:1277–1285.

83. Iseki K, Iseki C, Itoh K, Sanefuji M, Uezono K, Ikemiya Y, Fukiyama K, Kawasaki T. Estimated protein intake and blood pressure in a screened cohort in Okinawa, Japan. Hypertens Res 2003; 26:289–294.

84. Willet W, Stampfer M. Implications of total energy intake for epidemiologic analyses. In: Willet W, ed. Nutrtional Epidemiology. 2nd ed. Oxford: Oxford University Press, 1998:273–301.

85. Hill RJ, Davies PS. The validity of self-reported energy intake as determined using the doubly labelled water technique. Br J Nutr 2001; 85:415–430.

86. Pryer JA, Vrijheid M, Nichols R, Kiggins M, Elliott P. Who are the 'low energy reporters' in the dietary and nutritional survey of British adults? Int J Epidemiol 1997; 26:146–154.

87. Stamler J, Caggiula A, Grandits GA. Relation of body mass and alcohol, nutrient, fiber, and caffeine intakes to blood pressure in the special intervention and usual care groups in the Multiple Risk Factor Intervention Trial. Am J Clin Nutr 1997; 65(suppl):338S–365S.

88. Stamler J, Liu K, Ruth KJ, Pryer J, Greenland P. Eight-year blood pressure change in middle-aged men: relationship to multiple nutrients. Hypertension 2002; 39:1000–1006.

89. Vupputuri S, He J, Ogden LG, Loria C, Whelton PK. Dietary intake of macronutrients and risk of hypertension: a prospective study using the First National Health and Nutrition Examination Survey (NHANES) cohort. Circulation 1998; 98(suppl 1):859.

90. Liu K, Ruth KJ, Flack JM, Jones-Webb R, Burke G, Savage PJ, Hulley SB. Blood pressure in young blacks and whites: relevance of obesity and lifestyle factors in determining differences. The CARDIA Study. Coronary Artery Risk Development in Young Adults. Circulation 1996; 93:60–66.

91. Ludwig DS, Pereira MA, Kroenke CH, Hilner JE, van Horn L, Slattery ML, Jacobs DR. Dietary fiber, weight gain, and cardiovascular disease risk factors in young adults. JAMA 1999; 282:1539–1546.

92. Morris CD, Jacobson S-L, Anand R, Ewell MG, Hauth JC, Curet LB, Catalano PM, Sibai BM, Levine RJ. Nutrient intake and hypertensive disorders of pregnancy: evidence from a large prospective cohort. Am J Obstet Gynecol 2001; 184:643–651.

93. Boulton TJC. Nutrition in childhood and its relationships to early somatic growth, body fat, blood pressure and physical fitness. Acta Paediatr Scand 1981; 284 (suppl):68–79.

94. Jenner DA, English DR, Vandongen R, Beilin L, Armstrong BK, Miller MR, Dunbar D. Diet and blood pressure in 9-year-old Australian children. Am J Clin Nutr 1988; 47:1059.

95. Simons-Morton DG, Hunsberger SA, van Horn L, Barton BA, Robson AM, McMahon RP, Muhonen LE, Kwiterovich PO, Lasser NL, Kimm SYS, Greenlick MR. Nutrient intake and blood pressure in the Dietary Intervention Study in Children. Hypertension 1997; 29:930–936.

96. Frank GC, Berenson GS, Webber F. Dietary studies and the relationship of diet to cardiovascular disease risk factor variables in 10-year old children—the Bogalusa Heart Study. Am J Clin Nutr 1978; 31:328–340.

97. Sacks FM, Donner A, Castelli WP, Gronemeyer J, Pletka P, Margolius HS, Landsberg L, Kass EH. Effect of ingestion of meat on plasma cholesterol of vegetarians. JAMA 1981; 246:640–646.

98. Sacks FM, Marais GE, Handysides GH, Salazar J, Miller L, Foster JM, Rosner B, Kass EH. Lack of an effect of dietary saturated fat and cholesterol on blood pressure in normotensives. Hypertension 1984; 6:193–198.

99. Sacks FM, Wood PG, Kass EH. Stability of blood pressure in vegetarians receiving dietary protein supplements. Hypertension 1984; 6:199–201.

100. Sacks FM, Kass EH. Low blood pressure in vegetarians: effects of specific foods and nutrients. Am J Clin Nutr 1988; 48:795–800.

101. Burke V, Hodgson JM, Beilin LJ, Giangiulioi N, Rogers P, Puddey IB. Dietary protein and soluble fiber reduce ambulatory blood pressure in treated hypertensives. Hypertension 2001; 38:821–826.

102. Crouse JR III, Morgan T, Terry JG, Ellis J, Vitolins M, Burke GL. A randomized trial comparing the effect of casein with that of soy protein containing varying amounts of isoflavones on plasma concentrations of lipids and lipoproteins. Arch Intern Med 1999; 159:2070–2076.

103. He J, Wu XG, Gu DF, Duan XF, Whelton PK. Soybean protein supplementation and blood pressure: a randomized, controlled clinical trial [abstr]. Circulation 2000; 101:711.

104. Hermansen K, Sondergaard M, Hoie L, Carstensen M, Brock B. Beneficial effects of a soy-based dietary supplement on lipid levels and cardiovascular risk markers in type 2 diabetic subjects. Diabetes Care 2001; 24:228–233.

105. Teede HJ, Dalais FS, Kotsopoulos D, Liang YL, Davis S, McGrath BP. Dietary soy has both beneficial and potentially adverse cardiovascular effects: a placebo-controlled study in men and postmenopausal women. J Clin Endocrinol Metab 2001; 86:3053–3060.

106. Washburn S, Burke GL, Morgan T, Anthony M. Effect of soy protein supplementation on serum lipoproteins, blood pressure, and menopausal symptoms in perimenopausal women. Menopause 1999; 6:7–13.

107. Effects of a soy diet on blood pressure and vascular reactivity in hypertensive men and postmenopausal women. Third International Symposium on the Role of Soy in Preventing and Treating Chronic Disease, Washington, DC, 99 Nov, 1999.

108. Hodgson JM, Puddey IB, Beilin LJ, Mori TA, Burke V, Croft KD, Rogers PB. Effects of isoflavonoids on blood pressure in subjects with high-normal ambulatory blood pressure levels: a randomized controlled trial. Am J Hypertens 1999; 12(1 Pt 1):47–53.

109. Nestel PJ, Yamashita T, Sasahara T, Pomeroy S, Dart A, Komesaroff P, Owen A, Abbey M. Soy isoflavones improve systemic arterial compliance but not plasma lipids in menopausal and perimenopausal women. Arterioscler Thromb Vasc Biol 1997; 17:3392–3398.

110. Jenkins DJA, Kendall CWC, Jackson CC, Connelly PW, Parker T, Faulkner D, Vidgen E, Cunnane SC, Leiter LA, Josse RG. Effects of high- and low-isoflavone soyfoods on blood lipids, oxidized LDL, homocysteine,

and blood pressure in hyperlipidemicmen and women. Am J Clin Nutr 2002; 76:365–372.

111. Preuss HG, Gondal JA, Lieberman S. Association of macronutrients and energy intake with hypertension. J Am Coll Nutr 1996; 15:21–35.

112. Reaven GM, Hoffman BB. Hypertension as a disease of carbohydrate and lipoprotein metabolism. Am J Med 1989; 87(suppl 6A):6A-2S–6A-6S.

113. National Research Council. Diet and Health. Washington, DC: National Academy Press, 1989:291–309.

114. Hodges RE, Rebello T. Carbohydrates and blood pressure. Ann Int Med 1983; 98(Part 2):838–841.

115. Hwang I-S, Ho H, Hoffman BB, Reaven GM. Fructose-induced insulin resistance and hypertension in rats. Hypertension 1987; 10:512–516.

116. Martinez FJ, Rizza RA, Romero JC. High-fructose feeding elicits insulin resistance, hyperinsulinism, and hypertension in normal mongrel dogs. Hypertension 1994; 23:456–463.

117. Preuss HG, Knapka JJ, MacCarthy P, Yousufi AK, Sabnis SG, Antonovych TT. High sucrose diets increase blood pressure of both salt-sensitive and salt-resistant rats. Am J Hypertens 1992; 5:585–591.

118. Zein M, Areas JL, Knapka JJ, MacCarthy P, Yousufi AK, DiPette D, Holland B, Goel R, Preuss HG. Excess sucrose and glucose ingestion acutely elevate blood pressure in spontaneously hypertensive rats. Am J Hypertens 1990; 3:380–386.

119. Preuss HG. Interplay between sugar and salt on blood pressure in spontaneously hypertensive rats. Nephron 1994; 68:385–387.

120. Rebello T, Hodges RE, Smith JL. Short-term effects of various sugars on antinatriuresis and blood pressure changes in normotensive men. Am J Clin Nutr 1983; 38:84–94.

121. Bunag RD, Tomita T, Sasaki S. Chronic sucrose ingestion induces mild hypertension and tachycardia in rats. Hypertension 1983; 5:218–225.

122. Fournier RD, Chiueh CC, Kopin IJ, Knapka JJ, DiPette D, Preuss HG. Refined carbohydrate increases blood pressure and catecholamine excretion in SHR and WKY. Am J Physiol 1986; 250:E381–E385.

123. Gradin K, Nissbrand H, Ehrenstom F, Henning M, Persson B. Adrenergic mechanisms during hypertension induced by sucrose and/or salt in the spontaneously hypertensive rat. Arch Pharmacol 1988; 337:47–52.

124. Young JB, Landsberg L. Stimulation of the sympathetic nervous system during sucrose feeding. Nature 1977; 269:615–617.

125. Hung T, Sievenpiper JL, Marchie A, Kendall CW, Jenkins DJ. Fat versus carbohydrate in insulin resistance, obesity, diabetes and cardiovascular disease. Curr Opin Clin Nutr Metab Care 2003; 6:165–176.

126. Yang EJ, Chung HK, Kim WY, Kerver JM, Song WO. Carbohydrate intake is associated with diet quality and risk factors for cardiovascular disease in U.S. adults: NHANES III. J Am Coll Nutr 2003; 22:71–79.

127. Israel KD, Michaelis OE, Reiser S, Keeney M. Serum uric acid, inorganic phosphorus, and glutamic-oxalacetic transaminase and blood pressure in carbohydrate-sensitive adults consuming three different levels of sucrose. Ann Nutr Metab 1983; 27:425–435.

128. Kraikitpanitch S, Chrysant SG, Lindenmann RD. Natriuresis and carbohydrate induced antinatriuresis in fasted, hydrated, hypertensives. Proc Soc Exp Biol Med 1975; 149:319–324.

129. Sacks FM, Rouse IL, Stampfer MJ, Bishop LM, Lenherr CF, Walter RJ. Effect of dietary fats and carbohydrate on blood pressure of mildly hypertensive patients. Hypertension 1987; 10:452–460.

130. Trowell HC, Burkitt DP. The development of the concept of dietary fibre. Mol Aspects Med 1986; 9:7–15.

131. Trowell H. Crude fibre, dietary fibre and atherosclerosis. Atherosclerosis 1972; 16:138–140.

132. Trowell H, Southgate DAT, Wolever TMS, Leeds AR, Gassull MA, Jenkins DJA. Dietary fiber redefined. Lancet 1976; i:967.

133. De Vries JW. On defining dietary fibre. Proceedings of the Nutrition Society 2003; 62:37–43.

134. Gondal JA, MacArthy P, Myers AK, Preuss HG. Effects of dietary sucrose and fibers on blood pressure in hypertensive rats. Clin Nephrol 1996; 45:163–168.

135. MacIver DH, McNally PG, Ollerenshaw JD, Sheldon TA, Haegerty AM. The effect of short chain fatty acid supplementation on membrane elctrolyte transport and blood pressure. J Hum Hypertens 1990; 4:485–490.

136. Lichtenstein MJ, Burr ML, Fehilly AM, Yarnell JWG. Heart rate, employment status, and prevalent ischaemic heart disease confound the relation between cereal fibre and blood pressure. J Epidemiol Comm Health 1986; 40:330–333.

137. Ascherio A, Stampfer MJ, Colditz GA, Willett WC, McKinlay J. Nutrient intakes and blood pressure in normotensive males. Int J Epidemiol 1991; 20:886–891.

138. Witteman JCM, Willett WC, Stampfer MJ, Colditz GA, Sacks F, Speizer FE, Rosner B, Hennekens CH. A prospective study of nutritional factors and hypertension among US women. Circulation 1989; 80:1320–1327.

139. Hallfrisch J, Tobin JD, Muller DC, Andres R. Fiber intake, age, and other coronary risk factors in men of the Baltimore Longitudinal Study (1959–1975). J Gerontol 1988; 43:M64–M68.

140. Kelsay JL, Behall KM, Prather ES. Effect of fiber from fruits and vegetables on metabolic responses of human subjects I. Bowel transit time, number of defecations, fecal weight, urinary excretions of energy and nitrogen and apparent digestibilities of energy, nitrogen, and fat. Am J Clin Nutr 1978; 31:1149–1153.

141. Wright A, Burstyn PG, Gibney MJ. Dietary fibre and blood pressure. BMJ 1979; 2:1541–1543.

142. Brussaard JH, van Raaij JM, Stasse-Wolthuis M, Katan MB, Hautvast JG. Blood pressure and diet in normotensive volunteers: absence of an effect of dietary fiber, protein, or fat. Am J Clin Nutr 1981; 34:2023–2029.

143. Fehily AM, Burr ML, Butland BK, Eastham RD. A randomised controlled trial to investigate the effect of a high fibre diet on blood pressure and plasma fibrinogen. J Epidemiol Comm Health 1986; 40:334–337.

144. Margetts BM, Beilin LJ, Vandongen R, Armstrong BK. A randomized controlled trial of the effect of dietary fibre on blood pressure. Clin Sci (Lond) 1987; 72:343–350.

145. He J, Whelton PK, Klag MJ. Dietary fiber supplementation and blood pressure reduction: a meta-analysis of controlled clinical trials [abstr]. Am J Hypertens 1996; 9:74A.

146. Davy BM, Melby CL, Beske SD, Ho RC, Davrath LR, Davy KP. Oat consumption does not affect resting casual and ambulatory 24-h arterial blood pressure in men with high-normal blood pressure to stage I hypertension. J Nutr 2002; 132:394–398.

147. Beilin LJ. Vegetarian and other complex diets, fats, fiber, and hypertension. Am J Clin Nutr 1994; 59 (suppl):1130S–1135S.

148. Melby CL, Goldflies DG, Toohey ML. Blood pressure differences in older black and white long-term vegetarians and nonvegetarians. J Am Coll Nutr 1993; 12:262–269.

149. Margetts BM, Beilin LJ, Vandongen R, Armstrong BK. Vegetarian diet in mild hypertension: a randomised controlled trial. BMJ 1986; 293:1468–1471.

150. Rouse IL, Beilin LJ, Armstrong BK, Vandongen R. Blood pressure-lowering effect of a vegetarian diet: controlled trial in normotensive subjects. Lancet 1983; i:5–10.

151. Kris-Etherton P, Eckel RH, Howard BV, St Jeor S, Bazzarre TL. AHA Science Advisory: Lyon Diet Heart Study. Benefits of a Mediterranean-style, National Cholesterol Education Program/American Heart Association Step I Dietary Pattern on Cardiovascular Disease. Circulation 2001; 103:1823–1825.

152. Trichopoulou A, Costacou T, Bamia C, Trichopoulos D. Adherence to a Mediterranean diet and survival in a Greek population. N Engl J Med 2003; 348:2599–2608.

153. Keys A. Seven Countries Study. Cambridge, MA: Harvard University Press, 1980.

154. Panagiotakos DB, Pitsavos CH, Chrysohoou C, Skoumas J, Papadimitriou L, Stefanadis C, Toutouzas PK. Status and management of hypertension in Greece: role of the adoption of a Mediterranean diet: the Attica study. J Hypertens 2003; 21:1483–1489.

155. Strazzullo P, Ferro-Luzzi A, Siani A, Scaccini C, Sette S, Catasta G, Mancini M. Changing the Mediterranean diet: effects on blood pressure. J Hypertens 1986; 4:407–412.

156. De Lorgeril M, Renaud S, Mamelle N, Salen P, Martin JL, Monjaud I, Guidollet J, Touboul P, Delaye J. Mediterranean alpha-linolenic acid-rich diet in secondary prevention of coronary heart disease. Lancet 1994; 343:1454–1459.

157. De Lorgeril M, Salen P, Martin JL, Monjaud I, Delaye J, Mamelle N. Mediterranean diet, traditional risk factors, and the rate of cardiovascular complications after myocardial infarction: final report of the Lyon Diet Heart Study. Circulation 1999; 99:779–785.

158. Appel LJ, Moore TJ, Obarzanek E, Vollmer WM, Svetkey LP, Sacks FM, Bray GA, Vogt TM, Cutler JA, Windhauser MM, Lin PH, Karanja N. A clinical trial of the effects of dietary patterns on blood pressure. DASH Collaborative Research Group. N Engl J Med 1997; 336:1117–1124.

159. Svetkey LP, Simons-Morton D, Vollmer WM, Appel LJ, Conlin PR, Ryan DH, Ard J, Kennedy BM. Effects of dietary patterns on blood pressure: subgroup analysis of the Dietary Approaches to Stop Hypertension (DASH) randomized clinical trial. Arch Intern Med 1999; 159:285–293.

160. Sacks FM, Svetkey LP, Vollmer WM, Appel LJ, Bray GA, Harsha D, Obarzanek E, Conlin PR, Miller ER, III, Simons-Morton DG, Karanja N, Lin PH. Effects on blood pressure of reduced dietary sodium and the Dietary Approaches to Stop Hypertension (DASH) diet. DASH-Sodium Collaborative Research Group. N Engl J Med 2001; 344:3–10.

161. Appel LJ, Champagne CM, Harsha DW, Cooper LS, Obarzanek E, Elmer PJ, Stevens VJ, Vollmer WM, Lin PH, Svetkey LP, Stedman SW, Young DR. Effects of comprehensive lifestyle modification on blood pressure control: main results of the PREMIER clinical trial. JAMA 2003; 289:2083–2093.

162. Dietary Reference Intakes for Water, Potassium, Sodium, Chloride, and Sulfate. Washington, DC, Institute of Medicine, National Academy of Sciences, 2004.

163. Miura K, Greenland P, Stamler J, Liu K, Daviglus ML, Nakagawa H. Relation of vegetable, fruit, and meat intake to 7-year blood pressure change in middle-aged men: the Chicago Western Electric Study. Am J Epidemiol 2004; 159:572–580.

164. John JH, Ziebland S, Yudkin P, Roe LS, Neil HA. Effects of fruit and vegetable consumption on plasma antioxidant concentrations and blood pressure: a randomised controlled trial. Lancet 2002; 359:1969–1974.

12

Alcohol and Hypertension

D. GARETH BEEVERS

University Department of Medicine, Birmingham, UK

KEYPOINTS

- Population studies demonstrate a close relationship between alcohol intake and the height of the blood pressure.
- Acute alcohol loading studies demonstrate an acute pressor response, with no clear threshold.
- The mechanism of alcohol rotates hypertension is unknown.
- There is no clear relationship between alcohol intake and the cardiovascular consequence of hypertension.
- Alcohol moderation does lower blood pressure in hypertensive patients.

SUMMARY

A close relationship exists between alcohol consumption and the height of the blood pressure. These remain however several unanswered questions. As yet no clear mechanism has been demonstrated to explain how alcohol raises blood pressure. The other problem is there does not appear to be a close relationship between alcohol intake and the cardiovascular complications of hypertension, namely heart attack, stroke, peripheral vascular disease and renal damage.

Reliable short-term clinical trials have shown that reducing alcohol intake brings about a rapid fall in systolic and diastolic blood pressure. Thus moderation of intake is one component of the recommendations on the non-pharmacological management of hypertension. There does not appear to be any benefit from reducing alcohol intake from moderate levels to none at all hypertensive patients, along with the population at large, should be advised to limit their alcohol intake to no more than 3 drinks per day in men and 2 drinks per day in women.

I. INTRODUCTION

Of all of the lifestyle factors implicated as a cause of hypertension, alcohol has received the least attention and is possibly, therefore, the least well understood. Furthermore, the long-term consequences of the relationship between alcohol intake and blood pressure and its vascular sequelae, namely heart attack and stroke, remain controversial. Finally, there is a lack of a coherent or plausible mechanism whereby alcohol raises blood pressure, either acutely or over the long term.

II. HISTORY

It is generally held that the first scientific paper to report an association between high alcohol intake and hypertension was published in Paris in 1915 by Camile Lian in his study of French soldiers (1). He reported the prevalence of hypertension in "les tres grands buveurs, les grands buveurs, les moyens bouvers et les sobres." ("Les sobres" were those who drank <1 L of wine per day.) There was a direct linear relationship between alcohol intake and prevalence of hypertension. However, in 1877, Frederick Henry Horatio Akhbar Mahomed (2), who was working at Guy's Hospital in London, was measuring blood pressure with the aid of the sphygmograph. He noted high-tension pulses in patients whom he termed "alcoholists." In 1922, Batty Shaw (3) in his text book of hypertension (Hyperpiesia and Hyperpiesis) commented that the relationship between alcohol intake and high blood pressure was "well known." A total of 10 of the 47 patients he studied in detail were "addicted to alcohol." Be that as it may, there are almost no further references to alcohol and hypertension for another 50 years. Notably, alcohol received no mention in Sir George Pickering's great textbook of hypertension that was first published in 1955.

In 1959, Shah and Kunjannam (4) in India reported that the blood pressures of citizens listed on the Bombay Alcohol Register were higher than those in citizens who were not so labeled. At this time in the city of Bombay, a person had to register with the city before he or she was allowed to buy alcoholic drinks.

It was not until the 1970s that large-scale epidemiological studies appeared that showed a relationship between alcohol intake and height of the blood pressure. Since then, the association has been almost universally confirmed.

III. MODERN EPIDEMIOLOGICAL RESEARCH

One of the first of the modern studies of the relationship between alcohol intake and blood pressure was the Copenhagen Heart Study published in 1974 (5). This study of 5249 Danish men demonstrated a close association between alcohol intake (primarily beer) and height

of their blood pressure, which was independent of body mass index, physical exercise, or smoking habit.

The year 1977 was an important year; Klatsky et al. (6), who were examining the data file of the Kaiser Permanente multiphasic health examination survey, were able to demonstrate a close relationship between alcohol intake and blood pressure that held true in men, women, Caucasians, African-Americans, and Asian-Americans of Chinese origin. This effect also was found to be independent of age, salt intake, obesity, and educational level as an indicator of socioeconomic status.

Later that same year, Ramsay (7) and Beevers (8), working independently in Glasgow, reported an association between hypertension and abnormal liver function tests and concluded that the most likely mechanism was the differences in alcohol intake. Plasma alanine and aspartate aminotransferase levels were significantly higher in hypertensive men than in normotensive controls. In women, only aspartate aminotransferase levels were significantly higher in hypertensive patients compared with controls. In the hypertensive individuals, reported alcohol intake correlated with the reported levels of these blood tests. Since then, however, it has become clear that part of the association between hypertension and abnormal liver function tests also may be seen in nondrinkers as a result of nonalcoholic hepatic steatosis (fatty liver) or, occasionally, of nonalcoholic steatohepatitis (9). This syndrome is associated with central obesity, insulin resistance, type 2 diabetes mellitus, impaired glucose tolerance, hyperlipidaemia, and hypertension in the metabolic syndrome X.

IV. ALCOHOL DOSE RESPONSE CURVE

People who drink more than six standard units of alcohol per day (a unit corresponds to a glass of wine, a small measure of spirits, or a half-pint of beer) appear to have a two to three times higher prevalence of hypertension when compared with nondrinkers or people who consume very little alcohol (10). The question, however, remains whether the relationship between alcohol and blood pressure is linear. Several studies have suggested that people who drink fewer than two drinks per day may have slightly lower blood pressures than people who claim to drink nothing at all (11). This trend was seen in particular among women in the Kaiser Permanente multiphasic health examination survey, and in a study from London. This J-shaped relationship has been seen only occasionally and only in men, but even in men there appears to be no significant gradient between no drinks per day and fewer than two drinks per day (12). Therefore, this raises the possibility that there is a threshold above which alcohol raises blood pressure. An alternative explanation is a cynical one—that is, to question the validity of reports by people who claim that they consume no alcohol. Although many of these people may have been genuine teetotalers all of their lives, some of them also may have been ex-drinkers—some of whom may have stopped drinking by virtue of physical illness. Many people simply may have succeeded in deceiving their examiners. There also may be another threshold at the top end of the alcohol–blood pressure relationship. In the second Kaiser Permanent survey, published in 1986, there was a trend for examinees who consumed more than nine drinks per day to have lower blood pressure than those who consumed six to eight drinks per day (12).

V. EX-DRINKERS

Ex-drinkers may represent a diverse population, including some people who may now be too unwell to drink alcohol, but it is important to note that ex-drinkers appear to have the same blood pressure profile of people who have never drunk alcoholic beverages (12). This strongly suggests that the alcohol–blood pressure relationship is reversible. This is of some interest because with most other causes of high blood pressure, removing the underlying cause does lower blood pressure, but it does not usually lead to complete normalization. The remarkable reversibility of the blood pressure–alcohol relationship is addressed later in this chapter and raises the possibility that alcohol does not so much cause hypertension, but that it simply causes a reversible and harmless rise in blood pressure.

VI. TYPE OF ALCOHOLIC BEVERAGE

Epidemiological studies in different countries have all shown an alcohol–blood pressure relationship and also found that this relationship exists in people who drink predominantly beer (Copenhagen), in people who drink primarily wine (Paris), and in people who drink a mixture of alcoholic beverages (13). Therefore, there does not seem to be any major difference among alcoholic beverages. These findings are borne out by acute alcohol loading studies in normotensive volunteers and in patients in whom alcohol-free beer was found to have no effect on blood pressure, but in whom the same beer with alcohol added did raise blood pressure. Furthermore, the blood pressure rose and fell parallel to increases and decreases in blood alcohol levels (14). There has been speculation that the nonalcoholic constituents of some alcoholic beverages, particularly of red wine, might exert a protective effect, particularly against heart disease (15). The problem is that the people who drink primarily red wine are frequently from a higher socioeconomic group than those who drink alcohol mostly in the form of beer or

spirits. Thus, the apparent protection in drinkers of red wine may be a marker for other safe personal habits, including a low frequency of cigarette smoking (15).

VII. PATTERN OF ALCOHOL CONSUMPTION

It is possible that binge drinking of a specific amount of alcohol has a greater effect than consuming the same total amount of alcohol over several days each week. A comparison between people in Northern Ireland and France, where total weekly alcohol intake was the same, showed that drinkers in Belfast tended to drink more on the weekends, whereas drinkers in Paris tended to drink smaller quantities regularly everyday, with no "binge effect" (16). This raises the possibility that binge drinking itself has a harmful effect (17,18). The variation of blood pressure over a work-week has been investigated in several population studies. There was a tendency for blood pressures to be higher on Monday after a weekend of presumed drinking. It did not take long; however, for blood pressure to return to normal levels during the remainder of the week.

VIII. MECHANISMS

Perhaps, the least understood issue is the mechanisms by which alcohol might increase blood pressure. An early study from Birmingham that involved 132 alcoholic patients admitted to the hospital showed that during the early detoxification process, blood pressures were elevated (17). As the effects of the alcohol withdrawal wore off, the patients' blood pressures settled. Among alcoholics who, 6 weeks later, were still not drinking, blood pressures remained low, whereas alcoholics who had relapsed and gone back to their former drinking habits, blood pressures had risen again. This study also showed that there was a significant linear relationship between the severity of alcohol withdrawal symptoms and the height of the blood pressure. This raises the possibility that it was not the alcohol itself that increased blood pressure, but rather the withdrawal from alcohol. During withdrawal, some of the alcoholics were found to have very high levels of plasma catecholamines, levels comparable to those seen in patients with phaeochromocytoma (14). At this point, it was suggested that the alcohol withdrawal mechanism might be the explanation; but it was difficult to extrapolate this to large-scale population studies among more moderate drinkers. It was argued; however, that if an epidemiological survey were carried out during the morning hours, a pressor effect also might be observed in moderate drinkers because of the alcohol that had been consumed on the preceding evening—the examinee would be in a state of mild, subclinical alcohol withdrawal. This possibility was backed up by the Lipid Research Clinics project, where people who had consumed alcohol within 24 h of screening had a lower blood pressure than people who had consumed no alcohol during this same period (18).

In sharp contrast to the alcohol withdrawal syndrome hypothesis were the results of studies of acute alcohol loading and withdrawal. Potter and Beevers (19) conducted the first randomized, parallel group study of alcohol consumption in hypertensive patients in an in-patient, clinical environment in Birmingham. During three further days of moderate alcohol consumption in hospital, blood pressures remained elevated but then fell rapidly during three subsequent days with no alcohol consumption. Conversely, patients who were allowed no alcohol for 3 days and then started drinking again moderately on day 4, sustained an increase in blood pressure. Therefore, this finding was in sharp contrast to the suggestion that the alcohol pressor effect was owing to the withdrawal from alcohol. Similarly, alcohol loading studies conducted both among healthy volunteers and among hypertensive patients showed that an increase in blood pressure that occurs after drinking alcohol roughly parallels the increase in blood alcohol levels (14,20). This strongly suggested that alcohol must have a direct pressor effect or a rapid pressor effect that is mediated by other hormones. During these acute alcohol loading studies over a period of 3 h, no significant changes were found in plasma renin or angiotensin levels, in plasma cortisol levels, or in plasma adrenaline or noradrenaline levels (20). This also strongly suggests that none of these hormones was involved in the pressor response that was observed. At a later stage of these experiments, plasma renin levels rose. This effect was thought to be a result of mild, subclinical dehydration associated with an alcohol-induced diuresis. At this stage, the blood pressure had returned to baseline levels.

If the increase in blood pressure that is induced by alcohol in acute experiments is not mediated by activation of the synthetic nervous system or the renin–angiotensin system, the possibility is that alcohol has a direct effect on arterial vascular tone that is possibly mediated by an increase in the intracellular calcium and intracellular sodium that are associated with the inhibition of the sodium potassium pump (21–23).

It remains possible that alcohol has at least two mechanisms by which it raises blood pressure. First, blood pressure may be raised because of the stress of the alcohol withdrawal syndrome, and this elevation in pressure may well be mediated by an increase in plasma catecholamine levels. Secondly, alcohol may have direct pressor effect on the arteriolar wall tension, which causes an increase in systemic pressure that parallels the prevailing blood alcohol levels (24).

Given that alcohol does raise blood pressure both acutely and at the time of alcohol withdrawal, the question arises whether alcohol actually causes hypertension. The rapid reversibility of the alcohol effect and its acute onset are not consistent with the idea that alcohol causes chronic hypertension with its associated end-organ damage (25). A low-salt diet does not normalize blood pressure in hypertensive patients, it merely reduces it. Why is it, therefore, that the cessation of alcohol intake normalizes blood pressure so quickly? Does alcohol cause an innocent, transient increase in blood pressure that is not clinically important?

IX. ALCOHOL AND END-ORGAN DAMAGE

If alcohol causes hypertension, it also should cause the end-organ damage associated with hypertension, namely, left ventricular hypertrophy, heart attack, stroke, and renal damage. In addition, it also should probably cause peripheral vascular disease. There is very little information about renal damage or peripheral vascular disease in association with alcohol consumption, but there is absolutely no evidence to suggest that alcohol causes renal damage or that it worsens peripheral vascular disease. Indeed, alcohol may sometimes relieve the symptoms of peripheral vascular disease. When we look at the association of alcohol consumption with heart attacks and strokes, the topic becomes more complicated.

A. Alcohol and Coronary Heart Disease

There is no convincing evidence that alcohol causes coronary heart disease either directly or through an increase in blood pressure.

Long-term population studies and studies of survivors from myocardial infarction show that alcohol has a modest protective effect, at least in low doses, in preventing coronary heart disease (26,27). In high doses, any association to alcohol and coronary mortality may be explained by an arrhythmic effect rather than by the generation of coronary heart disease associated with atheroma deposition (28). There is no doubt that alcohol in high doses, both acutely and during the withdrawal phase, can cause tachyarrhythmias and atrial fibrillation (29). Atrial fibrillation, in turn, may be associated with increased mortality and morbidity from heart failure and thromboembolic stroke.

Could it be that the harmful effects of alcohol on the heart are offset by the beneficial effects on other risk factors? Even though alcohol increases blood pressure, it also increases lipid levels—but in a rather unusual manner (30). Alcohol in large quantities increases the total plasma cholesterol, but most of this increase is explained by an increase in plasma HDL cholesterol, which has a protective effect against heart disease.

Overall, one must conclude that although alcohol causes an increase in blood pressure and might even cause hypertension, it does not cause hypertensive end-organ damage in the form of coronary heart disease.

B. Alcohol and Stroke

The relationship between alcohol and strokes is slightly more consistent with a possible positive correlation. In the Yugoslavia Cardiovascular Diseases Study, alcohol intake and mortality were investigated (31). A possible protective effect against coronary heart disease was confirmed, but a close relationship was found between alcohol intake and stroke mortality. In the first West Birmingham case-controlled stroke study, a close relationship was found between alcohol and stroke; although there was a threshold effect, no association observed unless the patient had been consuming more than four drinks per day prior to the stroke onset (32). Below that level, there was some evidence of a protective effect in men, with a U-shape relationship between alcohol intake and stroke. Teetotalers, therefore, appear to have slightly higher risk of stroke than patients who drink very small quantities of alcohol. This study found no such effect in women, primarily because of the very small numbers of women who drank alcohol in sufficient quantities for the investigators to draw any conclusions. Although many other population studies have confirmed a relationship between alcohol intake and stroke, there are some important negative studies, in particular those that evaluate the association between alcohol and stroke mortality (33).

The relationship between stroke and alcohol may be complicated by the nature or by the manner of alcohol consumption. There are reports of binge drinking being associated with acute stroke, but binge drinkers usually are also heavy drinkers, so it is not certain whether it is the quantity of alcohol or the pattern of drinking that is causing strokes (34). In Robert Louis Stevenson's Treasure Island, the old sea captain who resided at the Admiral Benbow Inn consumed a very high level of alcohol in the form of rum. The captain was attacked by the villainous "Black Dog", and, soon after, he collapsed. It was thought that the captain was wounded. Dr. Livsey was called "'Wounded? A fiddlesticks end,' said the doctor, 'no more wounded than you or I. The man has had a stroke as I warned him'". The captain's rum consumption remained high, and soon after he was "struck dead by thundering apoplexy".

The relationship between high alcohol intake and stroke might be explained either by a dehydration effect of the alcohol-induced disease with a rise in hematocrit or by an increase in plasma catecholamine levels that is associated with the stress of the alcohol withdrawal in the ensuing 24 h after ceasing to drink.

If alcohol does cause strokes, it does so only when consumed in high quantities and does not demonstrate the close linear response curve that one would find if alcohol were a major actual cause of stroke in the population at large (34).

X. ALCOHOL AND CLINICAL HYPERTENSION

Despite all of the uncertainties described in the preceding sections, the fact remains that in clinical practice there is an observed association between alcohol intake and high blood pressure. Furthermore, among hypertensive patients, a reduction of alcohol intake or even total cessation is associated with a drop in blood pressure (19,35). This drop in pressure, therefore, should lead to a reduction in the number of antihypertensive drugs that are required for treatment. From an epidemiological perspective, it had been thought that alcohol might be the cause of hypertension in 5–11% of hypertensive patients, and alcohol has been reported to be associated with 24% of untreated hypertension in Australian men (36,37).

There are a few studies that assess the effects of a reduction or cessation of alcohol consumption on blood pressure in hypertensive patients. In an early study from Birmingham, hospitalized nonalcoholic hypertensive patients went through a period of moderate alcohol consumption, followed by cessation of drinking. Twenty-four hours after altering alcohol intake either upward or downward, blood pressure had increased or decreased (22).

Two other very reliable studies were conducted in Perth, Western Australia on a double-blind basis with either canned and specially labeled low-alcohol content beer or normal beer. These studies showed a close relationship between alcohol and blood pressure in both hypertensive patients and normotensive volunteers (37,38). Other studies that have included both hypertensive individuals and normotensive individuals have demonstrated that in both groups, reduction or cessation of drinking alcohol was associated with a decrease in blood pressure (39).

XI. ALCOHOL AND ANTIHYPERTENSIVE DRUGS

There is evidence that the antihypertensive response to drug therapy is reduced in people who consume a relatively large quantity of alcohol (40), although one study reported no interference of alcohol in the antihypertensive effect of the beta-blocker metoprolol (41). In general, there is very little consistent evidence that alcohol specifically interacts with any particular class of antihypertensive drugs, but this area has not been studied in detail.

XII. EXPERIMENTATION

Just has been the case in human research, experiments with animals have provided confusing results. Acute alcohol loading studies in rats have shown that blood pressures were lower with alcohol, but in dogs, intravenous (but not intragastric alcohol) did cause an increase in blood pressure (42). Very little work has been done in this area.

XIII. CONCLUSIONS

Both acute and chronic alcohol consumptions are important causes of high blood pressure. Reducing alcohol intake is beneficial in terms of reducing blood pressure and, presumably, also in reducing the need for antihypertensive medication. There is no convincing evidence that alcohol causes end-organ damage of hypertension in the heart. There is some evidence that alcohol does cause strokes, but possibly only when alcohol is consumed in large quantities (32). It would appear that the relationship between alcohol and blood pressure differs from other lifestyle factors in that there is a remarkable reversibility and also a possible threshold effect with no linear dose response curve. In practice, therefore, it is sensible to conclude that unlike tobacco smoking, which is always harmful at any level, alcohol intake in moderation is not harmful and may have some beneficial effects. The recommendations that the amount of alcohol intake in men should be limited to no more than three drinks per day and in women to no more than two drinks per day should be emphasized as part of good clinical practice.

REFERENCES

1. Lian C. L'alcoolism cause d'hypertension arterielle. Bull Acad Med (Paris) 1915; 74:525–528.
2. Mahomed FA. On the sphygmographic evidence of arteriocapilliary fibrosis. Trans Path Soc 1877; 28:394.
3. Shaw HB. Hyperpiesia and Hyperpiesis. A Clinical, Pathological and Experimental Study. London: Henry Frowde, 1922. Oxford Medical Publication.
4. Shah VV, Kunjannam PV. The incidence of hypertension in liquor permit holders and teetotallers. J Assoc Physicians India 1959; 7:243–267.
5. Glyntelberg F, Meyer J. Relationship between blood pressure and physical fitness, smoking and alcohol consumption in Copenhagen males age 40–59. Acta Med Scand 1974; 95:375–380.
6. Klatsky AL, Friedman GD, Siegelaub AB, Gerard MJ. Alcohol consumption and blood pressure: Kaiser Permanente multiphasic health examination data. N Engl J Med 1977; 296:1194–2000.
7. Ramsay LE. Liver dysfunction and hypertension. Lancet 1977; 2:111–114.
8. Beevers DG. Alcohol and hypertension. Lancet 1977; 2:114–115.
9. Yamada Y, Ishizaki M, Kido T, Honda R, Tsuritani I, Yamaya H. Relationship between serum gamma-glutamyl transpeptidase activity and blood pressure in middle aged male and female non-drinkers. J Hum Hypertens 1990; 4:609–614.
10. Klatsky AL, Friedman GD, Siegelaub AB. Alcohol and hypertension. Comp Ther 1978; 4:60–68.
11. Bulpitt CJ, Shipley MJ, Semmence A. The contribution of moderate intake of alcohol and the presence of hypertension. J Hypertens 1987; 5:85–91.
12. Klatsky AL, Friedman GP, Armstron MA. The relationship between alcohol beverage use and other traits on blood pressure: a new Kaiser Permanente Study. Circulation 1986; 73:628–636.
13. Milon H, Froment A, Gaspard P, Guidollet J, Ripole JF. Alcohol consumption and blood pressure in a French epidemiological study. Eur Heart J 1982; 3:59–64.
14. Potter JF, Watson RDS, Skan W, Beevers DG. The pressor and metabolic effects of alcohol in normotensive subjects. Hypertens 1986; 8:625–631.
15. Nuttall SL, Kendall MJ, Martin V. Antioxidants therapy for the prevention of cardiovascular disease. Quart J Med 1999; 92:239–244.
16. Marques-Vidal P, Arveiler D, Evans A, Amouyel P, Ferrieres B, Ducimetiere P. Different alcohol drinking and blood pressure relationships in France and Northern Ireland. The PRIME Study. Hypertension 2001; 38:1361–1366.
17. Saunders JB, Beevers DG, Paton A. Alcohol-induced hypertension. Lancet 1981; 2:653–656.
18. Criqui MH, Wallace RB, Mishkel M, Barrett-Connor E, Heiss G. Alcohol consumption and blood pressure: the Lipid Research Clinics prevalence study. Hypertension 1981; 3:557–565.
19. Potter JF, Beevers DG. Pressor effects of alcohol in hypertension. Lancet 1989; 1:119–122.
20. Potter JF, MacDonald IA, Beevers DG. Alcohol raised blood pressure in hypertensive patients. J Hypertens 1986; 4:435–441.
21. Awkwright PD, Beilin LJ, Rouse I, Armstrong BK, Vandongeh R. Effects of alcohol use and other aspects of lifestyle on blood pressure levels and hypertension in a working population. Circulation 1982; 66:60–66.
22. Stokes GS. Hypertension and alcohol: is there a link? J Chronic Dis 1982; 35: 759–762.
23. Knochel JP. Cardiovascular effects of alcohol. Ann Intern Med 1983; 98(part 2):849–859.
24. Potter JF, Beevers DG. Factors determining the acute pressor response to alcohol. Clin Exp Hypertens (A) 1991; A13:13–34.
25. Lip GYH, Beevers DG. Alcohol, hypertension, coronary disease and stroke. Clin Exp Pharmacol Physiol 1995; 22:189–194.
26. Moore RD, Pearson TA. Moderate alcohol consumption and coronary artery disease. Medicine 1986; 65:242–267.

27. Shaper AG, Philip AW, Pocock SJ, Walker M. Alcohol and ischaemic heart disease in middle-aged British men. Br Med J 1987; 294: 733–737.

28. Portal RW. Alcoholic heart disease. Br Med J 1981; 283:1202–1203.

29. Kupari M. Acute cardiovascular effects of ethanol. A controlled non-invasive study. Br Heart J 1983; 49:174–182.

30. Rimm EB, Williams P, Fosher K, Criqui M, Stampfer MJ. Moderate alcohol intake and lower risk of coronary heart disease: meta-analysis of effects on lipids and haemostatic factors. Br Med J 1999; 319:1523–1528.

31. Kozara DJ, Vojvodic N, Dawber T. Frequency of alcohol consumption and morbidity and mortality. The Yugoslavia Cardiovascular Disease study. Lancet 1989; 1:613–616.

32. Gill JS, Zezulka AV, Shipley MJ, Gill SK, Beevers DG. Stroke on alcohol consumption. N Engl J Med 1986; 315:1041–1046.

33. Hillbom M, Kaste M. Does alcohol intoxication promote brain infarction in young adults? Lancet 1982; 2:1181–1183.

34. Gill JS, Zezulka AV, Beevers DG. Binge drinking and stroke. Br Med J 1985; 291:1645.

35. Maheswaran R, Beevers M, Beevers DG. Alcohol and hypertension. Hypertension 1992; 19:79–84.

36. Cooke KM, Frost GW, Thornell R, Stokes GS. Alcohol consumption and blood pressure: Survey of the relationship in a health-screening clinic. Med J Aust 1982; 1:65.

37. Puddey IB, Beilin LJ, Vandongen R, Rouse IR, Rogers P. Evidence of a direct effect of alcohol consumption and blood pressure in normotensive men. A randomised controlled trial. Hypertension 1985; 7:707–713.

38. Puddey IB, Beilin LJ, Vandouge R. Regular alcohol use raises blood pressure in treated hypertensive subjects. Lancet 1987; 1:647–651.

39. Wallace P, Cutler S, Haines A. Randomised controlled trail of general practitioner intervention in patients with excessive alcohol consumption. Br Med J 1988; 297:663–668.

40. Beevers DG. Alcohol, blood pressure and antihypertensive drugs. J Clin Pharm Ther 1990; 15:395–397.

41. Maheswaran R, Beevers DG, Kendall MJ, Davies P. Prediction of the acute pressure response to oral alcohol. J Clin Pharm Ther 1990; 15:405–410.

42. Ganz V. The acute effect of alcohol and the circulation and on the oxygen metabolism of the heart. Am Heart J 1963; 66:494–497.

13

Physical Activity, Exercise, Fitness, and Blood Pressure

ROBERT H. FAGARD, VERONIQUE A. CORNELISSEN
University of K.U. Leuven, Leuven, Belgium

KEYPOINTS

- Exercise-induced increases in blood pressure and decreases in systemic vascular resistance are roughly parallel in hypertensive and normotensive subjects.
- Observational studies suggest that greater physical activity and fitness are associated with lower blood pressure and reduced incidence of hypertension.
- Dynamic aerobic endurance training decreases blood pressure through a reduction of systemic vascular resistance, in which the sympathetic nervous system and the renin angiotensin system appear to be involved. The blood pressure reduction is more pronounced in hypertensive than in normotensive subjects.

- Moderate "resistance" training, designed to increase muscular strength, power, and/or endurance, decreases blood pressure.

SUMMARY

Acute dynamic and static exercise increase blood pressure. The increase is roughly parallel in hypertensive and normotensive individuals. Many epidemiological studies have analyzed the relationship between engaging in regular physical activity or being physically fit and blood pressure, but the results are not quite consistent. Although several epidemiological studies did not observe significant independent relationships, others concluded that blood pressure or the incidence of hypertension is lower in individuals who are more fit or more active. Longitudinal intervention studies are more appropriate for assessing the effects of physical activity and training on blood pressure. A meta-analysis of 44 randomized controlled trials revealed that dynamic aerobic training reduces resting blood pressure on average by 2.6/1.8 mmHg in normotensive patients and by 7.4/5.8 mmHg in hypertensive patients ($P < 0.001$ for all), on the basis of a reduction in systemic vascular resistance. This type of training also lowered blood pressure measured during ambulatory monitoring or during exercise. It is likely that the sympathetic nervous system, the renin–angiotensin system, and endothelial function are involved in the training-induced blood pressure reduction. Static exercise (strength or resistance training) has been less well studied than dynamic aerobic training. A meta-analysis of nine randomized controlled trials revealed a reduction of blood pressure of 3.2 ($P = 0.10$)/3.5 ($P = 0.01$) mmHg associated with exercise. However, it should be noted that most exercise in these studies was dynamic in nature.

I. INTRODUCTION

Essential hypertension is undoubtedly a multifactorial disease, and it is very unlikely that only one causal factor is involved. Its pathogenesis is based on the interaction among genetic and environmental and lifestyle factors. The genetic variance has been shown in family and twins studies, but the exact nature of the postulated genetic defect remains largely unknown. Environmental and lifestyle factors that have been suggested as factors to explain an elevated blood pressure include sodium, alcohol, caloric intake, stress, and physical inactivity. In the present review, the impact of physical activity and fitness on blood pressure is evaluated from cross-sectional and longitudinal epidemiological data and from longitudinal intervention studies in humans. But, first, we will describe the effects of acute exercise on blood pressure. This review is restricted to studies in adults.

II. HEMODYNAMIC RESPONSE TO ACUTE EXERCISE

Dynamic (predominantly isotonic) and static (isometric) efforts are the two major forms of exercise. The former involves rhythmic contractions of flexor and extensor muscle groups and is performed against a relatively constant load. Exercise that is primarily static involves muscle contractions with limited or no movement and is, thus, performed at a relatively constant muscle length. Walking, running, cycling, and swimming are examples of dynamic activities. Blood pressure rises during such activities; and, in general, the blood pressure during exercise is proportional to the blood pressure at rest. As can be seen in Fig. 13.1, intra-arterial systolic pressure clearly rises with bicycle exercise in men with a normal blood

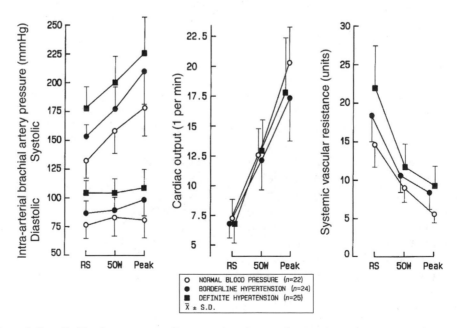

Figure 13.1 Systolic and diastolic blood pressure, cardiac output, and systemic vascular resistance at supine resting position (RS), 50 W exercise, and peak exercise (peak) in subjects with normal blood pressure, borderline hypertension, and definite hypertension, according to intra-arterial brachial artery pressure at supine rest and the 1978 WHO criteria.

pressure at rest. In patients with borderline or definite hypertension, the exercise-induced increases in systolic pressures are roughly parallel to the changes in the normotensive subjects (1).

In a previous study (2), the exercise-induced change in systolic pressure was similar in hypertensive individuals and normotensive individuals at a young age, but the systolic pressure showed a greater increase in older hypertensive patients. The changes in intra-arterial diastolic pressure are less pronounced, but the differences in blood pressure at rest persist during exercise. Cardiac output behaves similarly in these three groups, and the differences in blood pressure are clearly related to systemic vascular resistance—those individuals with the highest blood pressure at rest have the highest vascular resistance during exercise (Fig. 13.1). It is generally accepted that the increase in blood pressure is more pronounced during predominantly static effort, such as strength training, particularly when the intensity exceeds 40% of the maximal voluntary contraction. It is noteworthy, however, that the blood pressures achieved during maximal dynamic effort, such as cycling, also can be quite high in hypertensive patients. Therefore, when resting blood pressure is high, it seems logical to control blood pressure before embarking on a training program; furthermore, patients with uncontrolled blood pressure are dissuaded from intense static physical exercise. However, there is no convincing evidence that the exercise-induced increase in blood pressure is harmful, at least not in patients with no ischemic heart disease or other cardiovascular disease.

III. EPIDEMIOLOGICAL AND CROSS-SECTIONAL STUDIES

Many studies have analyzed the relationship between physical activity and blood pressure. In some studies, physical fitness was estimated from an exercise test; other studies used questionnaires and sometimes an interview relating to the subject's physical activity at work, at leisure, or both. It is accepted by most authors that the estimation of physical activity by questionnaire and interview is a poor but nevertheless useful, and possibly the best, available tool. Furthermore, the relationships between data of physical fitness tests and physical activity pattern by interview or questionnaire are of low order. In general, therefore, the methodology for estimating physical activity lacks accuracy. There are various confounding variables that might affect the relationship between physical activity and blood pressure. Some of these, such as age, weight, or indices of body fatness, can be accounted for in the analysis. Others, such as self-selection, are hardly controllable. Indeed, "fit" subjects may have lower blood pressures and choose a more active lifestyle,

whereas subjects with higher blood pressures may suffer from cardiovascular disease, which results in a lower degree of physical activity. Another problem is that the level of physical activity is low in most western societies, which may hamper the finding of an association with blood pressure. In the present review, only studies that had a reasonable sample size and that took into account at least age and anthropometric characteristics are considered.

A. Regular Ongoing Physical Activity and Blood Pressure

Miall and Oldham (3) classified 2832 South Wales males on the basis of the physical demands of their usual occupations and found that blood pressure was lower in the most physically active individuals, even after taking into account age and arm girth. Montoye et al. (4) also demonstrated a lower systolic and diastolic blood pressure in men with the most active occupations in a sample of 1696 men from Tecumseh, Michigan, but the relationship was stronger when both occupational and leisure time activities were considered; the results were adjusted for age and weight.

Criqui et al. (5) reported on the association of blood pressure with regular exercise in Caucasian adults (2482 men and 2298 women) in nine North American populations [the Lipid Research Clinics Prevalence Study (LRC)]. Exercise history was determined by a yes or no answer to the question: "Do you regularly engage in strenuous exercise or hard physical labor?" In men, diastolic blood pressure was inversely and independently related to exercise ($P < 0.01$), whereas the association was weak and nonsignificant for systolic pressure. Systolic pressure was inversely related to exercise in younger women ($P = 0.03$), but not in older women. The results were controlled for age, body mass index, and several other confounding variables.

Folsom et al. (6) measured energy expenditure in leisure time physical activity by using the Minnesota Leisure Time Physical Activity Questionnaire for residents 25–74 years old (738 men and 878 women) of the seven-county metropolitan area of Minneapolis-St. Paul, MN, USA. After controlling for age, systolic blood pressure was found to be inversely related to heavy intensity activity in women ($r = -0.09$; $P < 0.01$), but not in men. The relationship was no longer significant in multiple regression analysis, with inclusion of body mass index and other confounders. In addition, blood pressure was not related to total leisure time energy expenditure.

Reaven et al. (7) studied 641 older Caucasian women between the ages of 50 and 89 in a community-based study. The women were classified into categories of heavy physical activity (6%), moderate physical activity (24%), light physical activity (58%), or no physical activity (12%) by the estimated metabolic rate required for various leisure time activities in which they engaged during the 2 week period preceding their visit. Mean blood pressure differed significantly among the four groups. After adjustment for age and body mass index, systolic and diastolic blood pressure decreased stepwise with greater reported physical activity intensity and averaged 141/76, 136/75, 132/74, and 131/72 mmHg, respectively, from the least to the most active individuals.

Staessen et al. (8) investigated what lifestyle factors were correlated with the level and the variability of systolic and diastolic blood pressure in a random population sample in Flanders, Belgium. Ten blood pressure readings were obtained at home in 405 men and 379 women (20–84 years of age). Calories expended at work and in sports were assessed from a self-administered questionnaire. A P_{10} to P_{90} increase in the calories expended in sports was accompanied by a decrease in blood pressure, averaging 1.5 mmHg for diastolic blood pressure in men and 2.4 and 1.8 mmHg for systolic and diastolic blood pressure in women, after controlling for age, body mass index, and other significant covariates. After adjustment for age, the variability of diastolic blood pressure was inversely correlated with self-reported physical activity in men. Calories expended at work were not identified as a determinant of blood pressure.

Eaton et al. (9) studied the relationships between physical activity and coronary artery disease risk factors measured in a large community sample in the Health and Religion Project (HARP). Subjects included 381 men and 556 women, randomly selected from membership rolls ($n = 1367$ members) of 20 randomly selected Catholic, Baptist, and Episcopal churches in the state of Rhode Island. Physical activity was established during an interview by the following question: "In the past month, how often on the average do you do continuous vigorous exercise for 20 min or more?" The age-adjusted inverse correlations for physical activity levels and blood pressure were significant in women, but not in men. In women, the correlation coefficients amounted to -0.10 ($P < 0.05$) for systolic and -0.13 ($P < 0.01$) for diastolic pressure; adjusting for body mass index only moderately attenuated these correlations.

Liu et al. (10) analyzed the influence of various lifestyle factors on blood pressure in young African-Americans and Caucasians, aged 18–30 at baseline, in the Coronary Artery Risk Development in Young Adults (CARDIA) study, which included 1154 African-American women, 853 African-American men, 1126 Caucasian women, and 1013 Caucasian men. Baseline, self-reported regular, ongoing physical activity derived from the CARDIA Physical Activity History, a modified version of the Minnesota Leisure Time Physical Activity Questionnaire, was significantly and negatively related to average

diastolic blood pressure over four examinations in a period of 7 years in both African-American and Caucasian men, but not in women. Blood pressure was positively related with baseline age and body mass index. Systolic blood pressure was not independently related to physical activity.

Palatini et al. (11) studied 796 hypertensive patients, 18–55 years old (592 of whom were men), who had never been treated and took part in the Hypertension and Ambulatory Recording Venetia Study (HARVEST). They were classified as exercisers if they reported at least one session of aerobic sports per week ($n = 169$ exercisers) and as nonexercisers if they did not engage in regular sports activities ($n = 627$ nonexercisers). Physically active men exhibited a lower 24 h and daytime diastolic blood pressure than the inactive men, although there were no group differences in office blood pressure or in nighttime diastolic blood pressure and in ambulatory systolic blood pressure. The ambulatory diastolic blood pressure difference between groups remained statistically significant after adjustment for age, body mass index, alcohol intake, and smoking ($P < 0.001$). Adjusted 24 h pressure averaged 81.2 mmHg in nonexercisers and 78.8 mmHg in exercisers ($P = 0.001$); these values were 83.3 and 80.4 mmHg, respectively, for daytime diastolic blood pressure ($P < 0.001$).

The goal of Wareham et al. (12) was to assess the independent associations among energy expenditure and cardio-respiratory fitness and blood pressure. Volunteers were 775 participants of the Isle of Ely Study. A highly significant negative linear trend ($P < 0.001$) between increasing energy expenditure and decreasing blood pressure was found across quintiles of the physical activity level. The age- and treatment-adjusted difference in the mean systolic/diastolic blood pressure between the top and bottom quintile was 6.3/4.4 mmHg in men and 10.7/5.9 mmHg in women. These effects were independent of obesity and cardio-respiratory fitness.

Hu et al. (13) studied the relationship between both commuting and leisure time physical activity and a selection of cardiovascular risk factors in a cross-sectional population survey in urban Tianjin, China. Subjects were 15–69 years old. In this group, 2002 men and 1974 women completed the survey. A commuting physical activity or combined commuting and leisure time physical activity of >60 min was related to the highest systolic blood pressure in men and the highest diastolic blood pressure and systolic blood pressure in women ($P < 0.01$). Thirty-one to sixty minutes of commuting activity only or of commuting activity plus leisure time physical activity was associated with the lowest diastolic blood pressure and systolic blood pressure in women. Results were adjusted for age, body mass index, smoking, alcohol consumption, and education.

B. Physical Fitness and Blood Pressure

Gyntelberg and Meyer (14) determined physical fitness from a submaximal exercise test in 5249 employed men 40–59 years old in Copenhagen and found significant inverse relationships between physical fitness and systolic and diastolic blood pressure that were independent of age and weight. The regression coefficient indicated that a 10 mL/min per kg higher estimated maximal oxygen uptake was associated with a 2 mmHg lower blood pressure.

Sedgwick et al. (15) examined the relationships between predicted maximal oxygen uptake and risk factors for coronary heart disease in 1500 men and women 20–65 years in age. After controlling for the effects of age, physique, smoking, alcohol use, and stress, it was found that men and women who were more physically fit had lower blood pressure than their less fit counterparts. However, the relationships were seen as weak trends, probably of minor clinical importance. For men, fitness accounted independently for 3.6% and 2.4% of the variances of systolic and diastolic blood pressure, respectively; similar results were found for women (3.5% and 2.7%, respectively).

Siconolfi et al. (16) measured systolic and diastolic blood pressure and estimated maximal oxygen uptake in 184 men and 227 women, 18–65 years in age, who were randomly selected as part of a cardiovascular risk factor survey conducted in two New England cities in the United States. Initially, both measures of blood pressure were strongly and inversely correlated with estimated maximal oxygen uptake, expressed as mL/min per kg ($P < 0.001$). However, when the results were adjusted for age, the strength of the correlations decreased sharply. The proportion of the variance in systolic pressure that could be explained by differences in maximal oxygen uptake decreased from 9.6% to 0.8% (NS) for males and from 21.2% to 2.3% ($P < 0.05$) for females. Similar decreases were demonstrated for diastolic pressure in males [14.4–2.9% ($P < 0.05$)] and females [18.5–5.3% ($P < 0.01$)].

In the Framingham Offspring Study (17), 2606 young and middle-aged healthy adults (1232 men and 1374 women) participated in submaximal treadmill tests to determine the association between exercise endurance and cardiovascular risk factor profiles. For both men and women, exercise endurance was inversely related to the resting systolic blood pressure. After adjusting for age, body mass index, and resting heart rate, the relationship remained significant in men, but not in women.

Hartung et al. (18) categorized exercise tolerance, as determined by maximal treadmill testing, into six age-specific levels by gender. The participants (15,612 men and 3855 women) were self-referred Caucasian subjects, seen at the Cooper Clinic in Dallas, TX for preventive medical examinations. Both systolic and diastolic blood pressures were significantly and negatively related to exercise tolerance in both men and women ($r = -0.21$ in men and $r = -0.31$ in women for systolic pressure). These relations remained after covariance adjustment for among others age, and body mass index. For women, there was an adjusted mean difference of -6.8 mmHg in systolic blood pressure and -3.6 mmHg in diastolic blood pressure from the lowest exercise tolerance group to the highest; the corresponding differences for men were -4.7 and -4.1 mmHg, respectively.

In the Health and Religion Project (9), maximal oxygen uptake was estimated from a graded submaximal step test. With adjustment for age and body mass index, systolic blood pressure ($r = -0.14$ in men; $r = -0.25$ in women) and diastolic blood pressure ($r = -0.10$ in men; $r = -0.24$ in women) were significantly related to the physical fitness level, categorized as low, moderate, and high, according to age and gender.

IV. LONGITUDINAL OBSERVATIONAL STUDIES

A. Physical Activity, Fitness, and Future Blood Pressure

Paffenbarger et al. (19) assessed the incidence of hypertension in 14,998 Harvard University male alumni during a follow-up period of 6–10 years beginning 16–50 years after college entrance. Presence or absence of a background of collegiate sports did not influence the risk of hypertension in this study population, nor did stair-climbing, walking, or light sports activity by alumni, based on physical activity information obtained through questionnaires mailed in a postcollege health survey. However, alumni who did not engage in vigorous sports activity in postcollege years (59%) were at 35% greater risk of hypertension than the 41% who did participate in such activity ($P < 0.001$), and this relationship held for all ages between 35 and 74 years of age. Lack of strenuous exercise independently predicted increased risk of hypertension. Therefore, current vigorous exercise was inversely related to hypertension risk, but chiefly among alumni overweight-for-height. In a similar study of 5463 University of Pennsylvania alumni, Paffenbarger et al. (20) confirmed that vigorous sports activity reduced the incidence of hypertension and that this was not the case for collegiate sports activity and current walking, stair-climbing, or light sports activity. Folsom et al. (21) examined the 2 year incidence of hypertension in a cohort of 41,837 women 55–69 years of age. High levels of leisure physical activity were associated with a significant (30%) reduction in risk of hypertension, but physical activity no longer contributed to hypertension risk after adjustment for age, body mass index, waist-to-hip ratio, and smoking history in this short-term follow-up study. Haapanen et al. (22) studied the effect of the total amount and intensity of leisure time physical activity on the 10 year incidence of hypertension in a cohort of 1340 men and 1500 women 35–63 years of age. The men's total amount of activity and vigorous activity one or more times in a week were inversely associated with the age-adjusted risk of hypertension ($P = 0.02$). After further control for body mass index and diabetes, the associations were only statistically suggestively significant ($P = 0.08$). For women, neither of these leisure time physical activity measures was significantly associated with risk of hypertension. Hayashi et al. (23) investigated the association of the duration of the walk-to-work and leisure time physical activity with the 10 year risk of hypertension in 6017 Japanese men, 35–60 years of age. Both measures of activity were significantly associated with a reduction in the risk for incident hypertension. The multivariate adjusted risk for hypertension was significantly reduced by 12% when the duration of the walk-to-work was increased by 10 min and by 30% in men who engaged in regular physical activity at least once weekly. In the Atherosclerosis Risk in Communities Study (ARIC), Percira et al. (24) related leisure time physical activity with incident hypertension in 7459 African-American and Caucasian adults 45–65 years of age. After multivariate adjustment, Caucasian men in the highest quartile of leisure activity, primarily cycling and walking, had a 34% lower odds of developing hypertension >6 years compared with the least active men. Baseline activity was not significantly associated with incident hypertension in Caucasian women or in African-Americans.

During a 10 year follow-up period (1985–1995), Hernelahti et al. (25) investigated the incidence of hypertension in old age among males who were formerly elite athletes in endurance and mixed sports or in power sports and among healthy male controls. The men were athletes who represented Finland at least once in the Olympic Games, a world or European championship in sports, or other international sports competition between 1920 and 1965; the controls were selected from among Finnish men who at 20 years of age had been classified as completely healthy. The men included in the analysis were ≤65 years of age, had no history of hypertension in 1985, and had been healthy at the age of 20. To determine the level of physical activity in 1985, a leisure time activity index was calculated. The endurance sports and mixed sports group had a significantly lower cumulative incidence of hypertension than both the power sports group ($P = 0.014$) and the control group ($P = 0.013$). Compared with the controls, the endurance and mixed

sports athletes had a lower age-adjusted risk (odds ratio = 0.67; $P = 0.019$) for hypertension between 1986 and 1995. After further control for body mass index, alcohol intake, activity index, smoking, and occupational group, the odds ratio was 0.78 ($P = 0.21$). When a leisure activity index was used instead of data for the athlete groups in the analysis, the age-adjusted odds ratio for hypertension decreased by 14% per increasing quartile in activity index ($P = 0.02$). After additional adjustment for body mass index and other confounding covariates, the odds ratio decreased by 12% per increasing quartile, which was no longer statistically significant.

Hu et al. (26) prospectively followed 302 Finnish men and 9139 women 25–64 years in age without a history of antihypertensive drug use, coronary heart disease, stroke, or heart failure at baseline. Physical activity was measured at baseline by a self-administered questionnaire and included occupational, commuting, and leisure time physical activity. During a mean follow-up period of 11 years, 787 men and 813 women developed an incident of drug-treated hypertension. Hazard ratios of hypertension associated with light, moderate, and high physical activity; adjusted for age, body mass index, systolic blood pressure at baseline, and other confounding factors were 1.00, 0.60, 0.59 in men and 1.00, 0.80, 0.72 in women.

Blair et al. (27) related physical fitness, assessed by maximal treadmill testing in healthy normotensive men ($n = 4820$) and women ($n = 1219$) 20–65 years in age, to the incidence of hypertension. After a preventive medical examination at the Cooper Clinic in Texas, the subjects participated in a follow-up mail survey; the follow-up interval ranged from 1 to 12 years, with a median of 4 years. Subjects were divided into age-specific and gender-specific categories of physical fitness. The reference high-physical fitness category comprised those with excellent and superior fitness (28% of the participants), whereas the comparison group comprised the remaining participants (72%) in four physical fitness categories (very poor to good). After adjustment for age, gender, baseline body mass index, blood pressure, and follow-up interval, persons with low levels of physical fitness had a relative risk of 1.52 for the development of hypertension when compared with the highly fit persons ($P = 0.02$). Sawada et al. (28) investigated the relationship between physical fitness and incidence of hypertension through a prospective study in 3305 Japanese men whose blood pressure was normal when they received their first physical examination before the age of 50. The blood pressure of 425 subjects was diagnosed as hypertension in the fifth year. Fitness levels were divided into quintiles according to estimated maximal oxygen uptake levels. The relative risk of hypertension, after adjustment for age, initial blood pressure, body fat, and other confounders, was 1.9 times higher in the least fit individuals when compared with the group of most fit individuals ($P < 0.01$).

B. Changes in Physical Activity, Fitness, and Blood Pressure

A number of studies concentrated on the relationships between changes in physical activity or fitness and changes in blood pressure over time. Sallis et al. (29) studied representative samples of adults 20–35 years in age from four northern California cities in order to examine the relationships between a self-reported measure of habitual vigorous physical activity and risk factors. In the 1 year longitudinal follow-up, exercise groups were defined as sedentary, adopter, quitter, or maintainer. There were no significant differences in the change in systolic blood pressure between sedentary subjects and adopters or between quitters and maintainers of vigorous activity.

Hubert et al. (30) investigated the lifestyle and behavioral correlates of change in coronary heart disease risk factors measured 8 years apart in the young adult offspring of the Framingham Heart Study cohort, that is, in 397 men and 497 women who were 20–29 years old at the time of their entry in the study. Stepwise linear regression procedures were used to identify characteristics that were independently associated with risk factor changes during the study period. Changes in self-assessed physical activity were not related to the changes in blood pressure in either men or women.

Young et al. (31) assessed associations between a composite self-reported physical activity change score and risk factor change in the cohort sample of the Stanford (University) Five-City Project, which consisted of 380 men and 427 women between the ages of 18 and 74 years. In men and in postmenopausal women, there was no relationship between changes in physical activity and changes in blood pressure over the 5 years of observation. In contrast, in premenopausal women the change in systolic blood pressure was inversely related to the change in physical activity score ($P = 0.005$).

In the CARDIA study, Liu et al. (10) found that the changes in systolic and diastolic blood pressure over 7 years were significantly related to the change in body mass index, but not to the change in physical activity score. Sawada et al. (28) reported that subjects whose maximal oxygen uptake improved $\geq 15\%$ over a 5 year period, showed a smaller increase in systolic ($P < 0.05$) and diastolic ($P < 0.01$) blood pressure than the others.

Sedgwick et al. (32) aimed to assess relationships between increased aerobic fitness sustained >4 years and changes in blood pressure in middle-aged subjects who were entering a fitness program. The 342 selected men and women were either consistent fitness "gainers"

(predicted maximal oxygen uptake improved by >5%) or "nongainers" (improved by ≤5%). For men, comparison of these groups and multiple regression analyses failed to show significant relationships between changes in fitness over the 4 year period. For women, gainers improved more than nongainers in systolic blood pressure (-4 mmHg; $P < 0.03$); regression analyses resulted in a significant relationship between changes in fitness and blood pressure ($P < 0.05$).

V. DYNAMIC AEROBIC TRAINING AND BLOOD PRESSURE

It remains difficult to ascribe differences in blood pressure within a population to differences in levels of physical activity or fitness because of the potentially incomplete statistical correction for known confounders and because of the possible influence of confounding factors that were not considered or that cannot be taken into account, such as self-selection. Therefore, longitudinal intervention studies are more appropriate to assess the effect of physical activity and training on blood pressure. Most investigators assessed the effect of dynamic aerobic training on blood pressure; others assessed static exercises. Blood pressure was most often measured in resting conditions, but it also was measured by using ambulatory monitoring techniques or measured in response to stress, particularly during exercise testing.

A. Blood Pressure at Rest

Many longitudinal studies have assessed the effect of dynamic aerobic training on resting blood pressure, but essential scientific criteria have not always been observed. Inclusion of a control group or control phase is mandatory. To avoid selection bias, allocation to the active or control group or the order of the training and nontraining phases should be determined at random. Ideally, the subjects in the control group or in the control phase should be seen regularly, preferably as frequently as those in the training program; some authors even included low-level exercise as placebo treatment. We recently presented a meta-analysis of 44 randomized controlled trials on the effect of dynamic aerobic or endurance exercise on blood pressure at rest in otherwise healthy normotensive or hypertensive individuals (33).

1. Overall Results on Resting Blood Pressure

In the 44 trials included in the meta-analysis, which included a total of 2674 participants (65% of whom were men), 19 studies comprised only men, four studies comprised only women, and the other studies comprised both men and women. Some studies involved several groups of subjects or applied different training regimens in the same participants, so that a total of 68 training groups and programs were available for analysis. Average age in the groups ranged from 21 to 79 years (median = 44 years). Duration of training ranged from 4 to 52 weeks (median = 16 weeks) with a frequency of 1–7 weekly sessions (median = 3 sessions) of 15–70 min each (median = 50 min), including warm-up and cool-down activities. The exercises involved walking, jogging, and running in 69% of the studies, cycling in 50% of the studies, swimming in 3% of the studies, and other exercises in 23% of the training regimens. Average training intensity in the various groups varied between 30% and 85% of maximal exercise performance (median = 65%).

Control data were collected only at the beginning and at the end of the control period in 23 studies. Three control groups were subjected to light dynamic or recreational exercises; 10 groups were seen at least once in the research facilities; and another eight groups were contacted regularly by the investigators. Resting blood pressure was measured by an automatic device in five of the 44 studies. When pressure was measured by the use of a random zero device ($n = 15$ studies) or by conventional (or unspecified) methodology ($n = 24$ studies), the investigator was "blinded to the treatment" in only five and three studies, respectively. Table 13.1 summarizes the overall results.

In the 68 study groups, the changes of blood pressure in response to training, after adjustment for the control observations, ranged from +9 to −20 mmHg for systolic blood pressure and from +11 to −11 mmHg for diastolic pressure. The overall net changes averaged −3.4/−2.4 mmHg ($P < 0.001$), that is, after adjustment for control observations and after weighing for the number of trained participants that could be analyzed in each study group (the total number of participants was 1529). Peak oxygen uptake increased significantly, whereas heart rate and body mass index decreased (Table 13.1). When expressed as net percent change, peak oxygen uptake increased by 11.8% (95% CL: 10.3; 13.4), and heart rate and body mass index decreased by 6.8% (5.5; 8.2) and 1.2% (0.8; 1.7), respectively. In 16 of 68 study groups in which average baseline blood pressure was in the hypertensive

range (systolic blood pressure ≥ 140 mmHg or diastolic blood pressure ≥ 90 mmHg), the weighted net blood pressure decrease was significant and averaged 7.4/5.8 mmHg. The blood pressure reduction also was significant and averaged 2.6/1.8 mmHg in the 52 study groups in which baseline blood pressure was normal, regardless of the type of antihypertensive therapy. In addition, when normotensive and hypertensive subjects followed the same training program, the blood pressure decrease was greatest in the hypertensive subjects (34).

In other recent meta-analyses, which included 29 (35) and 54 (36) randomized controlled trials irrespective of baseline blood pressure of the participants, the training-mediated decreases of systolic/diastolic blood pressure averaged 4.7/3.1 (35) and 3.8/2.8 mmHg (36), respectively.

2. Influence of Other Characteristics

The conclusions of the meta-analyses were that there was no significant effect of age (37) or of baseline body mass index (36,37) on the exercise-induced changes in blood pressure. The blood pressure response also was not related to the changes in body mass index (36,37), which ranged from approximately −1.5 to +0.5 kg/m^2 among the various study groups. The influence of gender is more difficult to assess because many studies included both men and women. Kelley (38) reported a small but significant reduction of blood pressure in studies that only involved women, all of whom were normotensive at baseline. Among the three ethnic groups included in the study, African-American participants had significantly greater reductions in systolic blood pressure and Asian-American participants had significantly greater reductions in diastolic blood pressure when compared with white participants (36). However, there were only four studies of African-American women and six studies of Asian-American women. With respect to the characteristics of the training program, exercise frequency (33,35,36), type of exercise (36,39), intensity of exercise (33,35,36) (Fig. 13.2), and amount of time per session (33) did not appear to have an effect on the blood pressure response.

Table 13.1 Baseline Data and Net Change in Response to Dynamic Exercise Training

Type of data	n	Baseline data[a]	Net change in response[a]	P-value
Blood pressure (mmHg)				
Systolic	68	126.2 (123.3; 129.0)	−3.4 (−4.5; −2.3)	<0.001
Diastolic	68	79.9 (77.9; 82.0)	−2.4 (−3.2; −1.6)	<0.001
Peak oxygen uptake (mL/min per kg)	59	31.4 (29.6; 33.2)	+3.7 (+3.2; +4.3)	<0.001
Heart rate (beats/min)	48	71.1 (69.3; 72.9)	−4.9 (−5.9; −3.9)	<0.001
Body mass index (kg/m^2)	64	25.6 (25.0; 26.1)	−0.34 (−0.46; −0.22)	<0.001

[a]Weighted mean value and 95% confidence limits (CL).
Note: n, number of study groups.

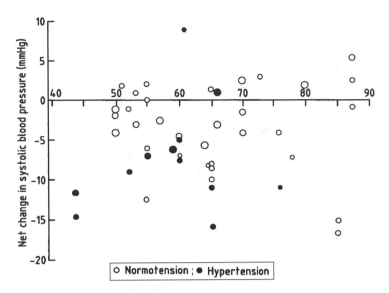

Figure 13.2 Changes in systolic blood pressure with training, adjusted for control data, vs. training intensity, in normotensive and hypertensive study groups. Training intensity is expressed as percent of maximal work load, heart rate reserve, or oxygen uptake reserve. The four sizes of the circles represent the number of analyzable trained subjects in each group, that is, less than 10, 10–19, 20–29, and greater than or equal to 30, respectively. The weighted meta-regression coefficient $r = 0.19$ ($P = 0.21$). [From Fagard (33).]

However, the change of blood pressure was somewhat smaller in studies of longer duration (33,36), most likely because participant adherence to the intervention program decreased over time.

B. Ambulatory Blood Pressure

Among randomized controlled trials, 12 used ambulatory blood pressure monitoring (40). Six trials reported the average 24 h blood pressure, nine trials the average daytime blood pressure from early morning to late evening, and four trials the nighttime pressure. Because an earlier analysis based on controlled and uncontrolled studies suggested that nighttime blood pressure is not influenced or is much less influenced by exercise training (34), the current analysis is based on daytime blood pressure in nine studies and on 24 h blood pressure in the three studies that did not report a separate full-day ambulatory pressure. Baseline blood pressures averaged 135/86 mmHg, and the exercise-induced, weighted net change in blood pressure averaged -3.0 (-4.8; -1.3)/-3.2 (-4.3; -2.2) mmHg.

C. Exercise Blood Pressure

The effect of endurance training on blood pressure during exercise can be analyzed, either by considering the data at a fixed workload or by considering the effect at a relative workload—that is, at a certain percentage of the pretraining maximal aerobic power and of the usually higher post-training maximal aerobic power. In the current overview,

only the more relevant first approach will be used. In eight randomized controlled trials (40), blood pressure was measured during bicycle exercise at a median work load of 100 W (range = 60–140 W). Blood pressure was measured during treadmill exercise at an energy expenditure of ~4 METS in two other studies. Baseline exercise systolic blood pressure averaged 180 mmHg and heart rate 124 beats per min (bpm). The weighted net training-induced change in systolic blood pressure amounted to -7 (-9.5; -4.5) mmHg, and heart rate decreased by 6.0 (2.7; 9.2) bpm.

D. Limitations

Several limitations of individual studies should be mentioned. Subjects in the control group or control phase seldom were examined as regularly as those in the training program, or they were not followed during control. In addition, it is difficult if not impossible to blind the participants to the treatment in training studies. Many studies did not mention that the investigator who measured blood pressure at rest or during exercise was not aware of the treatment group, and automated techniques were not often used. Participants were not always advised to keep their diet or lifestyle constant throughout the study periods. Other shortcomings include methodological issues, such as the methods of randomization, statistical analysis, handling of drop-outs from the study, keeping of log books, monitoring exercise intensity, and controlling the time interval between the last exercise session and the subsequent blood pressure measurement.

Table 13.2 Net Hemodynamic Change in Response to Dynamic Aerobic Endurance Training

Type of data	n	Net % change in response[a]	P-value
Mean blood pressure	17	−4.3 (−6.4; −2.1)	<0.001
Cardiac output	17	+3.3 (−3.1; +9.7)	NS
Stroke volume	17	+15.4 (+7.5; +23.5)	<0.01
Heart rate	17	−9.3 (−13; −6.0)	<0.001
Systemic vascular resistance	17	−7.1 (−14; −1.4)	<0.05

[a]Weighted mean value and 95% confidence limits (CL).
Note: n, number of study groups.

E. Mechanisms of the Training-Induced Changes of Blood Pressure

We identified 12 randomized controlled studies (17 study groups or programs) in which blood pressure, cardiac output, and heart rate were measured and stroke volume and systemic vascular resistance were calculated. Baseline mean blood pressure ranged from 85 to 121 mmHg and averaged 101.5 mmHg. Table 13.2 summarizes the weighted net percent changes of the hemodynamic variables. Training reduced mean blood pressure by 4.3% in these studies. On average, there was no significant effect of training on cardiac output, so the change in blood pressure could be attributed to a decrease in systemic vascular resistance. Heart rate decreased by 9% and stroke volume increased by 15%.

Possible mechanisms linking blood pressure, physical activity, and fitness have been reviewed elsewhere (1,40,41). It is likely that the sympathetic nervous system is involved. A meta-analysis of 13 study groups from nine randomized controlled training studies showed a highly significant weighted net reduction of plasma noradrenaline of 29% (95% CL: 15; 42) ($P < 0.001$). In addition, the lack of an effect on blood pressure during sleep, when sympathetic activity is low, indirectly supports the involvement of the sympathetic nervous system in the hypotensive effect of training. The renin–angiotensin–aldosterone system is also potentially important through its effect on blood volume and arterial pressure. A meta-analysis of 10

randomized controlled study groups revealed a significant reduction of plasma renin activity with −20% (95% CL: −35; −47) (1). More recently, it has been suggested that improvement of endothelial function contributes to the reduction of blood pressure after training (42–44). It is likely that the lowering of blood pressure by training is multifactorial, and further studies are needed to determine the mechanisms (40).

VI. STATIC STRENGTH AND RESISTANCE TRAINING AND BLOOD PRESSURE

Static strength and resistance training have been less well studied than dynamic aerobic training. We identified nine randomized controlled studies (12 study groups or programs) on the effect of training designed to develop strength (45). Most of the 341 participants were men. The average age of the groups ranged from 22 to 72 years, and the weighted mean age was 56 years. Baseline systolic blood pressure was between 110 and 152 mmHg, and baseline diastolic pressure was between 66 and 95 mmHg. Duration of the training ranged from 6 to 26 weeks (median = 14 weeks), with a frequency of three weekly sessions in all but two studies ($n = 2$). The results are shown in Table 13.3.

In the 12 study groups, the changes of blood pressure in response to training, after adjustment for the control observations, ranged from +2.0 to −16.8 mmHg for systolic pressure, and from +1.4 to −16.5 mmHg for diastolic

Table 13.3 Baseline Data and Net Change in Response to Resistance Exercise Training

Type of data	n	Baseline data[a]	n	Net change in response[a]	P
Blood pressure (mmHg)					
Systolic	12	131.0 (123.0; 138.8)	12	−3.2 (−7.1; +0.7)	=0.10
Diastolic	12	81.1 (74.5; 87.7)	12	−3.5 (−6.1; −0.9)	=0.01
VO$_2$ max (mL/min per kg)	9	24.7 (19.2; 30.2)	6	+2.6 (+0.3; +4.8)	<0.05
Heart rate (beats/min)	10	70.7 (66.9; 74.4)	8	+1.0 (−1.7; +3.7)	NS

[a]Weighted mean value and 95% confidence limits (CL). Results are weighted for the number of trained participants.
Note: n, number of study groups.

pressure. The overall weighted net change averaged -3.5 mmHg ($P = 0.01$) for diastolic pressure; however, the 3.2 mmHg decrease in systolic pressure did not reach statistical significance. It is important to consider the training regimens in these studies. The change in blood pressure cannot be attributed to pure static or isometric training. In all but one study, most exercises were dynamic and, therefore, involved movement of the arms, legs, and trunk. Furthermore, training intensity was not always high and ranged from 30% to 60% in half of the study groups and from 70% to 80% in the others. It is noteworthy that aerobic power increased by 11% in the six study groups in which it was measured, which would not be expected from static training. Finally, it should be mentioned that there is no evidence that strength training leads to an increase in blood pressure.

VII. CONCLUSIONS

Greater physical activity and fitness are associated with lower blood pressure and reduced incidence of hypertension. Therefore, exercise is a cornerstone therapy for the primary prevention, treatment, and control of hypertension. It is recommended to exercise at moderate intensity for at least 30 min per day on most, preferably all days of the week; the recommended exercise comprises primarily endurance physical activity supplemented by resistance exercise (40).

ACKNOWLEDGMENTS

The authors gratefully acknowledge the secretarial assistance of N. Ausseloos. R. Fagard is holder of the Prof. Amery Chair in Hypertension Research, founded by M.S.D. Belgium.

REFERENCES

1. Fagard R, Amery A. Physical exercise in hypertension. In: Laragh JH, Brenner BM, eds. Hypertension: Pathophysiology, Diagnosis and Management, 2nd ed. New York: Raven Press, 1995:2669–2681.
2. Amery A, Julius S, Whitlock LS, Conway J. Influence of hypertension on the hemodynamic response to exercise. Circulation 1967; 36:231–237.
3. Miall WE, Oldham OD. Factors influencing arterial blood pressure in the general population. Clin Sci 1958; 17:409–444.
4. Montoye HJ, Metzner HL, Keller JB, Johnson BC, Epstein FH. Habitual physical activity and blood pressure. Med Sci Sports 1972; 4:175–181.
5. Criqui MH, Mebane I, Wallace RB, Heiss G, Holdbrook MJ. Multivariate correlates of adult blood pressures in 9 North American populations: The Lipid Research Clinics Prevalence Study. Prev Med 1982; 11:391–402.
6. Folsom AR, Caspersen CJ, Taylor HL, Jacobs DR, Luepker RV, Gomez-Marin O, Gillum RF, Blackburn H. Leisure time physical activity and its relationship to coronary risk factors in a population based sample. The Minnesota Heart Survey. Am J Epidemiol 1985; 121:570–579.
7. Reaven PD, Barrett-Connor E, Edelstein S. Relation between leisure-time physical activity and blood pressure in older women. Circulation 1991; 83:559–565.
8. Staessen JA, Fagard R, Amery A. Lifestyle as a determinant of blood pressure in the general population. Am J Hypertens 1994; 7:685–694.
9. Eaton CB, Lapane KL, Garber CE, Assaf AR, Lasater TM, Carleton RA. Physical activity, physical fitness and coronary heart disease risk factors. Med Sci Sports Exerc 1995; 27:340–346.
10. Liu K, Ruth KJ, Flack JM, Jones-Webb R, Burke G, Savage PJ, Hulley SB. Blood pressure in young blacks and whites: relevance of obesity and lifestyle factors in determining differences. The CARDIA Study. Circulation 1996; 93:60–66.
11. Palatini P, Graniero GR, Mormino P, Nicolosi L, Mos L, Visentin P, Pessina A. Relation between physical training and ambulatory blood pressure in stage I hypertensive subjects. Results of the HARVEST Trial. Circulation 1994; 90:2870–2876.
12. Wareham NJ, Wong MY, Hennings S, Mitchell J, Kirsten R, Cruickshank K, Day NE. Quantifying the association between habitual energy expenditure and blood pressure. Int J Epidemiol 2000; 29:655–660.
13. Hu G, Pekkarinen H, Hänninen O, Yu Z, Guo Z, Tian H. Commuting, leisure-time physical activity, and cardiovascular risk factors in China. Med Sci Sports Exerc 2002; 34:234–238.
14. Gyntelberg F, Meyer J. Relationship between blood pressure and physical fitness, smoking and alcohol consumption in Copenhagen males aged 40–59. Acta Med Scand 1974; 195:375–380.
15. Sedgwick AW, Taplin RE, Davidson AH, Thomas DW. Relationships between physical fitness and risk factors for coronary heart disease in men and women. Aust NZ J Med 1984; 14:208–214.
16. Siconolfi SF, Lasater TM, McKinlay S, Boggia P, Carleton RA. Physical fitness and blood pressure: the role of age. Am J Epidemiol 1985; 122:452–457.
17. Abbott RD, Levy D, Kannel WB, Castelli WP, Wilson PWF, Garrison RJ, Stokes J. Cardiovascular risk factors and graded treadmill exercise endurance in healthy adults. The Framingham Offspring Study. Am J Cardiol 1989; 63:342–346.
18. Hartung GH, Kohl HW, Blair SN, Lawrence SJ, Harrist RB. Exercise tolerance and alcohol intake. Blood pressure relation. Hypertension 1990; 16:501–507.
19. Paffenbarger RS, Wing AL, Hyde RT, Jung DL. Physical activity and incidence of hypertension in college alumni. Am J Epidemiol 1983; 117:245–257.
20. Paffenbarger RS, Dexter L, Leung RW, Hyde RT. Physical activity and hypertension: an epidemiological view. Ann Med 1991; 3:319–327.

21. Folsom AR, Prineas RJ, Kaye SA, Munger RG. Incidence of hypertension and stroke in relation to body fat distribution and other risk factors in older women. Stroke 1990; 21:701–706.

22. Haapanen N, Miilunpalo S, Vuori I, Oja P, Pasanen M. Association of leisure time physical activity with the risk of coronary heart disease, hypertension and diabetes in middle-aged men and women. Int J Epidemiol 1997; 26:739–747.

23. Hayashi T, Tsumura K, Suematsu C, Okada K, Fujii S, Endo G. Walking to work and the risk for hypertension in men. The Osaka Health Survey. Ann Intern Med 1999; 130:21–26.

24. Pereira MA, Folsom AR, McGovern PG, Carpenter M, Arnett DK, Liao D, Szklo M, Hutchinson RG. Physical activity and incident hypertension in black and white adults: the Atherosclerosis Risk in Communities Study. Prev Med 1999; 28:304–312.

25. Hernelahti M, Kujala UM, Kaprio J, Sarna S. Long-term vigorous training in young adulthood and later physical activity as predictors of hypertension in middle-aged and older men. Int J Sports Med 2002; 23:178–182.

26. Hu G, Barengo NC, Tuomilehto J, Lakka TA, Nissinen A, Jousilahti P. Relationship of physical activity and body mass index to the risk of hypertension: a prospective study in Finland. Hypertension 2004; 43:25–30.

27. Blair SN, Goodyear NN, Gibbons LW, Cooper KH. Physical fitness and incidence of hypertension in healthy normotensive men and women. J Am Med Assoc 1984; 252:487–490.

28. Sawada S, Tanaka H, Funakoshi M, Shindo M, Kono S, Ishiko T. Five-year prospective study on blood pressure and maximal oxygen uptake. Clin Exp Pharmacol Physiol 1993; 20:483–487.

29. Sallis JF, Haskell WL, Wood PD, Fortmann SP, Vranizan KM. Vigorous physical activity and cardiovascular risk factors in young adults. J Chronic Dis 1986; 39:115–120.

30. Hubert HB, Eaker ED, Garrison RJ, Castelli WP. Lifestyle correlates of risk factor change in young adults: an eight-year study of coronary heart disease risk factors in the Framingham offspring. Am J Epidemiol 1987; 125:812–831.

31. Young DR, Haskell WL, Jatulis DE, Fortmann SP. Associations between changes in physical activity and risk factors for coronary heart disease in a community-based sample of men and women: the Stanford five-city project. Am J Epidemiol 1993; 138:205–216.

32. Sedgwick AW, Thomas DW, Davies M. Relationships between change in aerobic fitness and changes in blood pressure and plasma lipids in men and women: the "Adelaide 1000" 4-year follow-up. J Clin Epidemiol 1993; 46:141–151.

33. Fagard RH. Exercise characteristics and the blood pressure response to dynamic physical training. Med Sci Sports Exerc 2001; 33:S484–S492.

34. Fagard RH. Physical activity, fitness and blood pressure. In: Birkenhäger WH, Reid JL, Bulpitt CJ, eds. Handbook of hypertension, Vol. 20. Epidemiology of Hypertension. Amsterdam: Elsevier, 2000:191–211.

35. Halbert JA, Silagy CA, Finucane P, Withers RT, Hamdorf PA, Andrews GR. The effectiveness of exercise training in lowering blood pressure: a meta-analysis of randomized controlled trials of 4 weeks or longer. J Hum Hypertens 1997; 11:641–649.

36. Whelton SP, Chin A, Xin X, He J. Effect of aerobic exercise on blood pressure: a meta-analysis of randomized, controlled trials. Ann Intern Med 2002; 136:493–503.

37. Fagard RH. Physical activity in the prevention and treatment of hypertension in the obese. Med Sci Sports Exerc 1999; 31:S624–S630.

38. Kelley GA. Aerobic exercise and resting blood pressure among women: a meta-analysis. Prev Med 1999; 28:264–275.

39. Kelley G, Tran ZV. Aerobic exercise and normotensive adults: a meta-analysis. Med Sci Sports Exerc 1995; 27:1371–1377.

40. Pescatello LS, Franklin B, Fagard R, Farquhar WB, Kelley GA, Ray CA. American College of Sports Medicine Position Stand: Exercise and Hypertension. Med Sci Sports Exerc 2004; 36:533–553.

41. Arakawa K. Antihypertensive mechanisms of exercise. J Hypertens 1993; 11:223–229.

42. Kingwell BA, Sherrard D, Jennings GM, Dart AM. Four weeks of cycle training increases basal production of nitric oxide from the forearm. Am J Physiol 1997; 272:H1070–H1077.

43. Higashi Y, Sasaki S, Kurisu S, Yoshimizu A, Sasaki N, Matsuura H, Kajiyama G, Oshima T. Regular aerobic exercise augments endothelium-dependent vascular relaxation in normotensive as well as hypertensive subjects. Role of endothelium-derived nitric oxide. Circulation 1999; 100:1194–1202.

44. Higashi Y, Sasaki S, Sasaki N, Nakagawa K, Ueda T, Yoshimizu A, Kurisu S, Matsuura H, Kajiyama G, Oshima T. Daily aerobic exercise improves reactive hyperemia in patients with essential hypertension. Hypertension 1999; 33:591–597.

45. Cornelissen VA, Fagard RH. Effect of resistance training on resting blood pressure: a meta-analysis of randomized controlled trials. J Hypertens 2005; 23:251–259.

Part C: Diagnosis, Clinical Assessment, and Sequelae of Hypertension

14

Diagnosis and Clinical Assessment

WILLIAM J. ELLIOTT
Rush University Medical Center, Chicago, Illinois, USA

KEYPOINTS

- Hypertension is traditionally diagnosed by blood pressure measurements in the health care office using a mercury sphygmomanometer.
- Newer methods are increasingly being used, some for home use, including ambulatory blood pressure monitoring and devices that do not use liquid mercury.
- The initial assessment of a hypertensive patient should include a detailed history and physical examination, but with tests limited to: serum chemistries (including a lipid profile), urinalysis, electrocardiogram (ECG), and hematocrit. Other tests are warranted only when supported by an appropriate clinical suspicion.
- These measures help limit expensive and possibly dangerous drug therapy to those individuals who are most likely to benefit from it.
- The follow-up interval should be inversely proportional to both the patient's absolute cardiovascular risk and whether goal blood pressure has been attained. In worst cases, this should be 2–4 weeks; in best cases semiannually.

SUMMARY

Elevated blood pressure (or hypertension) is typically detected by the Korotkoff technique (appropriately-sized cuff, stethoscope, and mercury manometer), but home measurements (typically using oscillometric methods) and ambulatory blood pressure monitoring are becoming more common. Many types of technical problems can confound the proper estimation of blood pressure. Accurate measurements are important to assess the absolute risk for future cardiovascular events, and to guide the intensity of antihypertensive therapy. The initial assessment of the hypertensive patient includes a thorough history and physical examination, with special efforts made to detect hypertensive target-organ damage and clinical clues that would suggest secondary hypertension. This approach should limit expensive testing to those who are most likely to benefit from it.

I. INTRODUCTION

According to the Seventh Report of the Joint National Committee (JNC 7) on Prevention, Detection, Evaluation, and Treatment of High Blood Pressure (1), hypertension can be diagnosed if a person is taking antihypertensive medication or has two sets of appropriately measured pressures with either a systolic blood pressure ≥ 140 mmHg or a diastolic blood pressure ≥ 90 mmHg. Outside the United States, a higher threshold of 160/95 mmHg is sometimes used (2). Traditionally, these blood pressures are obtained in the medical office setting using the Korotkoff technique, but other methods (described in detail below) are being more commonly used.

II. DIAGNOSIS OF HYPERTENSION

Many methods have been proposed for estimating the pressure generated by the heart during its normal contractile cycle. The standard method using a mercury column and stethoscope has changed little in > 100 years. Over the last decade, this method has come under fire from regulatory authorities who have banned mercury, a recognized health hazard, from most worksites including healthcare environments. This led to the need for alternative methods for measuring blood pressure. Also, the worldwide trend favoring Système International units has led some to recommend adoption of the kiloPascal (kPa) as the standard, replacing the traditional "millimeter of mercury" (1 mmHg = 0.1333 kPa).

Until the late nineteenth century, it took extensive experience to learn to palpate the pulse and appreciate the contour and pressure within a peripheral artery. In 1906, Riva-Rocci, Janeway, and Korotkoff characterized the sounds heard by placing a stethoscope over the compressed artery, making objective measurements easier. Korotkoff's terminology is still used today. Systolic blood pressure is recorded when the first of at least two clear and repetitive tapping sounds are heard. Diastolic blood pressure is recorded when these sounds disappear. If Korotkoff sounds are continuously audible to 0 mmHg, in addition to the 0 mmHg (3), the clinician records the pressure at which "muffling" of the sounds occurs (Korotkoff phase IV). Since the early 1930s, insurance companies have recognized the value of blood pressure readings as a useful, if imprecise, predictor of mortality. This is ~ 25 years before healthcare epidemiologists reached the same conclusion.

III. MEASURING TECHNIQUES

The proper technique for accurate blood pressure measurement is typically taught very early during medical training, but rarely executed correctly thereafter. Many expert panels have made recommendations regarding the methodology of blood pressure measurement. These frequently do not agree in all details, but several general principles can be extracted (3):

- Match the size of the blood pressure cuff (newborn, infant, child, standard adult, large adult, or thigh) to the size of the subject's arm. A smaller than recommended cuff on a larger arm typically results in an overestimation of blood pressure. The large adult-size cuff is required for all those obese or muscular individuals with an arm circumference of > 38 cm at the mid-humerus.
- Deflate the cuff slowly. To be precise (within 2 mmHg), the observer should hear at least one Korotkoff sound at each 2 mmHg gradation of the mercury column. The heart rate of the subject therefore dictates the correct deflation rate, generally $2-3$ mmHg/s.
- Take several blood pressure readings on each occasion. It has been traditional to average the second and third in a series of measurements in a single position, whether supine, seated, or standing, and record this as the average blood pressure at a given visit. More recently, the standard practice is to record several individual readings in different positions, especially in the standing position. "Quality care auditors" use the lowest reading in any position as the "blood pressure at that visit," and taking several blood pressure measurements in different positions increases the likelihood of having at least one which is acceptable.
- Measure blood pressure on several occasions in the medical office before committing a person to

long-term therapy. Most long-term data on hypertension treatment has been derived from "casual" measurements made with a mercury sphygmomanometer and stethoscope in a healthcare provider's office, but in clinical trials, multiple visits are required before enrolling the patient. Physicians and patients often are more interested and impressed by blood pressure readings taken with out-of-office methods, such as home monitors or ambulatory blood pressure monitoring devices, both of which are discussed subsequently. However, nearly all data linking blood pressure measurements to adverse clinical sequelae (including myocardial infarction, stroke, and death) have been gathered in medical offices. Therefore, in all but a few special situations, office readings taken by a trained professional should be used for diagnosing and treating hypertension.

Blood pressure is subject to a large degree of intrinsic variability. Several steps can be taken to minimize this variability, including the following:

- Take multiple measurements, especially when the pulse is irregular (e.g., atrial fibrillation). This is necessary because ventricular filling pressures vary considerably as a result of fluctuations in diastolic filling time, especially in older persons with elevated systolic blood pressures.

- Center the bladder of the cuff over the brachial artery with its lower edge within 2.5 cm of the antecubital fossa. This leaves enough space to apply the stethoscope head beneath it, without touching the cuff and generating background noise.

- Ensure that the subject abstains from tobacco, caffeine, or alcohol for 30 min before a blood pressure measurement.

- Assure silent and comfortable rest of at least 5 min (with back support, if seated) before and during blood pressure measurement. Talking or listening, having legs crossed, sitting with an unsupported back, or standing with an unsupported arm all increase blood pressure. Both the muscular work of tensed muscles around the elbow and the hydrostatic pressure caused by a "dangling arm" increase the pressure necessary to obliterate the pulse and lead to overestimation of systolic blood pressure.

- Question the subject regarding the most recent meal or evacuation of bowels or bladder. Distended abdominal viscera can routinely cause elevated blood pressure, presumably because of anxiety or pain. In addition, older persons typically have a lower blood pressure postprandially.

- Listen over the brachial artery with the bell of the stethoscope, and minimize pressure exerted on the skin, leaving no lasting indentations. Too much pressure directly over the artery will likely cause overestimation of systolic blood pressure and underestimation of diastolic blood pressure.

- Determine the "peak inflation level" of the mercury column by palpating the radial pulse during cuff deflation before applying the stethoscope. Then typically inflate the cuff 20 mmHg higher than the pressure at which the palpable pulse at the radial artery disappeared. This will minimize potential loss of important prognostic information owing to not detecting the "auscultatory gap."

- Use a properly calibrated and clean sphygmomanometer. This is less of a concern with mercury columns, but environmental concerns about these are increasing. All sphygmomanometers used to measure blood pressure should be cleaned and calibrated frequently and routinely against a standard (usually mercury every 6 months). Also, check for proper cuff size and nonleaking tubing to ensure accuracy.

- Avoid "terminal digit preference." Traditionally, blood pressure measurements have been made to the nearest 2 mmHg, the typical markings on a mercury sphygmomanometer. Theoretically, in a large collection of systolic and diastolic blood pressure measurements, there should be an equal number of readings ending in 0, 2, 4, 6, or 8 mmHg. However, there is a marked statistical preference for terminal digits in inpatient medical services, decreasing reading accuracy to ±10 mmHg.

- Measure blood pressure in more than one extremity at the initial visit. If the difference is >10/5 mmHg, select the location with the higher blood pressure for all future measurements. This often raises concern about coarctation of the aorta, Takayasu's arteritis, or Moyamoya disease, but these are seldom seen on ultrasonography or other confirmatory testing. Blood pressure measurement in a leg should be commonplace in all young hypertensives at the first visit and may be useful in older people as a peripheral indicator of aortic insufficiency or "Hill's Sign."

A. Mercury Columns vs. Other Devices

Technology for obtaining accurate and reproducible blood pressure measurements outside the traditional medical environment has improved greatly in the last 25 years. Three major types of devices, oscillometric devices, hand-held aneroid ("dial") sphygmomanometers, and wrist monitors, are convenient, inexpensive, and relatively accurate (Table 14.1). Even persons with hearing difficulties, problems with hand-eye coordination, and other

Table 14.1   Advantages and Disadvantages of Methods of Blood Pressure Measurement Available to Patients in the Outpatient Setting

Attribute	Oscillometric with digital readout	Oscillometric with stethoscope	Anaeroid with stethoscope
Coordination necessary	Less so	Yes	Yes
Affected by presbyacusis	No	Yes	Yes
Affected by presbyopia	Less so	Less so	Yes
Widely available	Increasingly	Less so	Yes
Inexpensive	Increasingly	Less so	Yes
Quality results	Yes	Yes, with effort	Yes, with effort
Increases patients' interest in managing blood pressure	Yes	Yes	Yes
Battery powered	Yes	Yes	No
Affected by impaired grip strength	No	No	Yes
Independently validated by prospective studies	Little data	No	No

Source: Adapted from Elliott WJ, Black HR. Special situations in the management of hypertension. In: Hollenberg NK ed. Atlas of Hypertension. 4th ed. Philadelphia, PA: Current Medicine, Inc., 2003:257–281.

disabilities can operate semiautomatic devices with digital readouts and printers to estimate blood pressure. Some authorities believe that such devices should be provided to every person with elevated blood pressure. Others are concerned about possible misuse and over-interpretation of the data, as these methods have not been used in decision-making in clinical trials, and therefore should not be used routinely in practice to make diagnostic or therapeutic decisions (4). Very few "professional" blood pressure measurement devices have been as thoroughly tested (5) and proven as reliable, accurate, and long-lived as the mercury column. Most of the inexpensive devices currently on the market are meant for home use where they are activated perhaps once or twice daily. These are neither accurate nor durable enough to be recommended for a busy healthcare facility, at which blood pressure is measured hundreds to thousands of times each day.

Oscillometric devices are now the most widely used and probably the most accurate devices available. These rely on detection of small changes in volume by the blood pressure cuff during pulsation of the brachial artery and can be inaccurate even when properly executed. Several methods of improving this technology are now commercially available, including the use of "fuzzy logic" to improve the detection and identification of faint or irregular signals during a constant decrease in surrounding pressure, for example, in a blood pressure cuff (6).

The hand-held aneroid sphygmomanometer is being recommended to healthcare providers, particularly by those in purchasing departments in large medical centers, because it is small, portable, inexpensive, and widely available. These devices have a long history of declining accuracy with prolonged use, however, even if they pass visual inspection.

Monitors that measure blood pressure at the wrist are attractive for several reasons including convenience and the fact that circumference of the wrist is fairly constant across people of all sizes. Unfortunately, most of the tested devices that measure blood pressure at the wrist have not been as accurate as the more traditional arm measurement devices (7) and are therefore not recommended.

B. Home Measurements

Home blood pressure readings are typically lower (by ~5–12/5–7 mmHg) than measurements taken in the traditional medical environment, even in normotensive subjects. Home readings are more frequently correlated with both the extent of target organ damage (TOD) and the risk of future mortality than are readings taken in the physician's office (8). These readings can be helpful in evaluating symptoms suggestive of hypotension, especially if the symptoms are intermittent or infrequent. Reliable home readings can lower costs by allowing for less frequent visits to healthcare providers. Persons who routinely measure blood pressure at home probably have a better prognosis than do those who do not for two reasons: these individuals tend to be more interested in their blood pressure than are those who refuse to purchase and use a home blood pressure machine, and they often have better social support, having another person involved in blood pressure measurement and overseeing pill-taking and appointment-keeping behaviors.

However, there are several caveats about home blood pressure readings (4,5,9). Despite several reports of benefit in short-term blood pressure control (10–12) and at least two studies showing long-term prognosis to be better predicted by home readings than by one or two "casual" office measurements, there are no long-term clinical trials that based all treatment decisions solely on home readings. Unlike ambulatory blood pressure monitoring, home blood pressure readings have not yet become widely accepted for demonstrating the efficacy of

Table 14.2 Advantages and Disadvantages of Ambulatory Blood Pressure Monitoring

Advantages	Disadvantages
Identifies white coat hypertension (for which cost is now reimbursed by Medicare)	Cost
Many blood pressure and pulse measurements during 24 h period	Limited availability of equipment
Measures diurnal variation (including during sleep)	Potential disruption of daily activities due to noise or discomfort (e.g., sleep quality, flaccid arm during measurement)
Measures blood pressure and pulse during daily activities	Limited "normative" data
No "alerting response"	Limited guidelines (or consensus) for interpretation of data in individuals
No placebo effect	
Better correlation with target organ damage than with other methods of blood pressure measurement	Relatively few long-term prospective studies demonstrating utility compared with traditional (and much less expensive) blood pressure measurements
Adds to prognostic value of clinic measurements (in a few studies)	

Source: Adapted from Elliott WJ, Black HR. Special situations in the management of hypertension. In: Hollenberg NK, ed. Atlas of Hypertension. 4th ed. Philadelphia, PA: Current Medicine, Inc., 2003:257–281.

antihypertensive drugs (13). Many of the factors that contribute to blood pressure variability are more difficult to control in the home environment, including intrinsic circadian variation, food and alcohol ingestion, exercise, and stress. There is also concern that home blood pressure measurements will become an obsession. However, home readings can be a useful adjunct to information obtained in the physician's office, especially when the two are widely disparate (4); if they are to be taken, the instrument should be calibrated against a mercury sphygmomanometer using a Y-tube and the measuring technique checked.

Table 14.3 Threshold Values for Normal Blood Pressure

Source of data	Office measurements (mmHg)	Home measurements (mmHg)	ABPM measurements (mmHg)
JNC 7	140/90		
Ohasama	140/90	137/84	
ASH	140/90	135/85	135/85
Staessen et al.	140/90		133/82

Note: ABPM, ambulatory blood pressure monitoring. JNC 7: Chobanian AV, Bakris GL, Black HR et al. The seventh report of the Joint National Committee on Prevention, Detection, Evaluation, and Treatment of High Blood Pressure: The JNC 7 Report. JAMA 2003; 289:2560–2572; Ohasama: Tsuji I, Imai Y, Nagai K et al. Proposal of reference values for home blood pressure measurement: prognostic criteria based on a prospective observation of the general population in Ohasama, Japan. Am J Hypertens 1997; 10:409–418; American Society of Hypertension (ASH): Pickering TG. Chair for an American Society of Hypertension Ad Hoc Panel. Recommendations for the use of home (self) and ambulatory blood pressure monitoring. Am J Hypertens 1996; 9:1–11; Staessen et al.: Staessen JA, Bieniaszewski L, O'Brien ET, Fagard R. What is normal blood pressure in ambulatory monitoring? Nephrol Dial Transplant 1996; 11:241–245.
Source: Adapted from Elliott WJ, Black HR. Special situations in the management of hypertension. In: Hollenberg NK ed. Atlas of Hypertension. 4th ed. Philadelphia, PA: Current Medicine, Inc., 2003:257–281.

C. Ambulatory Blood Pressure Monitoring

Extensive research has led to a better definition of the role of automatic recorders that measure blood pressure frequently over a 24 h period during a person's usual daily activities including sleep (14). The use of these devices by practitioners in the United States was limited until April 1, 2002, when the Center for Medicare and Medicaid Services authorized reimbursement (of approximately $40–55 per session) for ambulatory blood pressure monitoring only for the evaluation of "white coat hypertension" (15). This decision removed a barrier to more widespread use of this important diagnostic modality. As a research tool, the advantages and disadvantages of ambulatory blood pressure monitoring have been well

Table 14.4 Situations in Which ABPM is Useful

Diagnosing office or "white-coat" hypertension, in patients with office hypertension, but no target organ damage[a,b]
Diagnosis of "high normal" blood pressure without target organ damage
Assessing refractory or resistant hypertension[a]
Evaluating episodic hypertension (at least once a day)
Evaluating symptoms consistent with hypotension[a]
Deciding whether drug treatment is warranted in older patients
Assuring efficacy of antihypertensive drug therapy over 24 h
Evaluating hypertension with autonomic dysfunction
Identifying nocturnal hypertension[a]
Managing hypertension during pregnancy
Evaluation of efficacy of antihypertensive drugs in clinical research

[a]Denotes situations for which a repeat ambulatory blood pressure monitoring session may be considered; some would include "after major changes in drug therapy" to this list.
[b]Denotes the situation for which ambulatory blood pressure monitoring is reimbursed by Medicare in the United States.
Source: O'Brien et al. (22).

documented (Table 14.2), normal values have been defined (Table 14.3), and publications correlating abnormal results of ambulatory blood pressure monitoring with adverse outcomes have appeared (16–21). Several expert panels have defined the special situations in which ambulatory blood pressure monitoring is particularly useful (Table 14.4) (22).

Several varieties of ambulatory blood pressure monitoring devices are currently available. In the United States, those that measure blood pressure indirectly (i.e., without arterial cannulation) employ either an auscultatory or an oscillometric technique. The auscultatory type uses a microphone placed over the artery to detect Korotkoff sounds in the traditional fashion. The oscillometric measures biophysical oscillations of the brachial artery. These use a standardized algorithm to compare the oscillometric measurements with those observed in previous calibrations using a mercury sphygmomanometer. Systolic blood pressure is determined directly from the threshold oscillation, mean arterial pressure is estimated, and diastolic blood pressure is calculated. Both types of monitors are small (<450 g), simple to use, accurate, relatively quiet, and powered by two to four small batteries. The monitors store data from 80 to 120 blood pressure and pulse measurements in a small microprocessor and then download it into a desktop computer, which edits the readings and prints the report.

All of the existing ambulatory blood pressure monitoring devices have drawbacks. Direct blood pressure measurement requires 24 h of arterial cannulation, which may be dangerous and is therefore rarely used even in research. Indirect blood pressure measurements using auscultatory techniques can be confused by ambient noise levels, despite R-wave gating, which requires electrocardiographic leads attached to the chest. Oscillometric techniques require that the subject keep the arm straight and flaccid during the measurement, and the data can be easily corrupted, if the subject has a tremor. A thorough diary of the subject's activities helps interpret the ambulatory blood pressure monitoring readings, but these diaries are not always completed.

Ambulatory blood pressure monitoring routinely measures blood pressure during sleep and has renewed interest in the circadian variation of heart rate and blood pressure. Most normotensives and perhaps 80% of hypertensives have a ≥10% drop in blood pressure during sleep when compared with the daytime average. Several prospective studies have shown an increased risk of cardiovascular events among those with a nocturnal "nondipping" blood pressure or pulse pattern such as with blacks and the elderly (16,23–27). Type 1 diabetics with a "nondipping" 24 h blood pressure pattern had a greater incidence of proteinuria during follow-up than those with the normal "dipping" profile (28). These data

support the idea that "24 h blood pressure load" is an important factor, as individuals with the "nondipping" pattern have a higher proportion of elevated blood pressures during the 24 h period. In several studies in Japan, elderly people with >20% drop in blood pressure during sleep ("excessive dippers") may suffer unrecognized ischemia in "watershed areas" (of the brain and other organs) during sleep, if their blood pressure declines below the autoregulatory threshold (18). They are also at higher risk for future stroke (20,29).

The clinical importance of the circadian blood pressure pattern determined by ambulatory blood pressure monitoring is complicated by several factors. The definitions of "dipper" and "nondipper" hypertension have not been consistent across the world's literature. Most studies attribute the increased prevalence of the "nondipping pattern" to advancing age. The reproducibility of the "nondipping pattern" has been poor in several studies that repeated ambulatory blood pressure monitoring during placebo treatment. Perhaps the most troublesome difficulty is that one class of antihypertensive drugs has converted individuals from a "nondipping pattern" to the more common "dipping pattern," even when the drug was not expected to affect nocturnal blood pressures on the basis of its pharmacodynamic parameters and time of administration.

Ambulatory blood pressure monitoring readings correlate quite accurately with the prevalence and extent of TOD in hypertensives. Compared with "casual" blood pressure measurements made in the healthcare office, ambulatory blood pressure monitoring measurements are a better predictor of left ventricular hypertrophy, cardiac function, and overall scores summing optic, carotid, cardiac, renal, and peripheral vascular damage resulting from elevated blood pressure.

Perhaps, the most important data demonstrating the value of ambulatory blood pressure monitoring has come from recent prospective studies that focused on cardiovascular events (death, myocardial infarction, and stroke) as the primary endpoint. In the first study on this from Italy, ambulatory blood pressure monitoring was the best predictor of future cardiovascular events. "Nondipper hypertensives'" risk was approximately three times that of hypertensives whose blood pressure dropped 10% lower at night ("dippers"). Continued follow-up and refinements in these analyses come to the same conclusions (25,26). A population-based study involving 1572 men and women comparing ambulatory blood pressure monitoring vs. casual and home blood pressures has been ongoing since 1987 in Ohasama, Japan. After almost 5 years of follow-up, cardiovascular mortality was much more strongly related to ambulatory blood pressure measurements than to a single office blood pressure reading (8). The value of ambulatory blood pressure monitoring in refractory hypertension was demonstrated in another study of 86 hypertensive people taking an average of three antihypertensive medications daily (30). Follow-up data collected ~4 years later showed that the patients having ambulatory blood pressure monitoring results in the lowest tertile to have significantly lower rates of cardiovascular complications per 100 patient-years: first tertile 2.2, second tertile 9.5, third tertile 13.5 events. These data suggest that ambulatory blood pressure monitoring may be helpful in sorting out which patients with elevated office blood pressure measurements who already are taking multiple antihypertensive medications ought to have intensified treatment. A sub-study of the Systolic Hypertension in Europe (Syst-Eur) trial involved 808 patients who had ambulatory blood pressure monitoring in addition to the usual clinic blood pressure measurements before being randomly assigned to placebo or active treatment (16). In the group placed on placebos, ambulatory blood pressure monitoring was clearly a better predictor of future cardiovascular events than was the office blood pressure measurement. In the other groups, active treatment reduced the difference in prognosis between ambulatory and office measurements. Furthermore, the risk of a cardiovascular event was much higher in patients who did not display a nocturnal decline in blood pressure. These data suggest (but do not prove) that the poor prognosis seen with nondipping hypertension can be mitigated by active antihypertensive drug treatment.

Perhaps, the most impressive study so far demonstrating the added value of ambulatory blood pressure monitoring was carried out in a study of 1963 hypertensive European patients (21). All had an ambulatory blood pressure monitoring, and then were followed for a median of 5 years, with treatment dictated by the office blood pressure as usual. New cardiovascular events occurred in 157 patients. After adjusting for all the traditional risk factors, ambulatory blood pressure (whether 24 h mean, daytime or nighttime; systolic or diastolic) was found to be a significant independent predictor of cardiovascular events.

D. White Coat Hypertension

Approximately 10–20% of American hypertensives have substantially lower blood pressure measurements outside the healthcare provider's office than in it (31). In Italy, this phenomenon is observed in 30% of pregnant women (32). The name white coat hypertension has been given to the situation in which blood pressure measurements outside the healthcare setting are considerably lower than those within it. Studies originally done in Italy, and later corroborated in other countries, show that blood pressure rises in response to an unknown physician approaching the subject. This does not happen if a nurse

approaches the subject, even when the nurse is wearing a white coat (33).

The clinical consequences and prognostic significance of white coat hypertension continue to be hotly debated in the medical literature. One school of thought suggests that if a person has an acute rise in blood pressure caused by stress related to an approaching physician, similar elevations in blood pressure are likely whenever a stressful stimulus is encountered. Thus, some literature supports the concept that the white coat response is merely a precursor to "more substantial and more sustained hypertension." This point of view is buttressed by several clinical and population-based studies in which people with "white coat hypertension" have a greater prevalence of sub-clinical risk factors for cardiovascular disease, including left ventricular hypertrophy, a family history of hypertension and heart disease, hypertriglyceridemia, elevated fasting insulin levels, and lower high-density lipoprotein (HDL) cholesterol levels (34–36).

A second school of thought, on the basis of careful and more conservative definitions of the white coat effect, proposes that some individuals consistently show a similar and marked elevation in blood pressure in response to the healthcare environment. Using more stringent criteria than the studies cited earlier, several long-term studies have shown a greatly reduced risk of either TOD or major cardiovascular sequelae among people with the white coat phenomenon (37,38). Whether the future risk of such individuals for cardiovascular events is similar (or even identical) to that of completely normotensive people is open to question. Another possibility is that white coat hypertension simply represents an unrepresentative sampling (biased toward the high end) of blood pressure levels in those with considerable blood pressure variability.

The best approach to the treatment of white coat hypertension is undetermined. Clearly, such individuals should benefit from lifestyle modifications, which could reduce the likelihood of progression to sustained hypertension. Withholding antihypertensive medication from white coat hypertensive patients appears unwise (39). The risk of future cardiovascular events did not appear to differ between white coat and sustained hypertensives when both were treated with antihypertensive medications (40). Whether intensive treatment with continuous antihypertensive medication is warranted for only temporary increases in blood pressure is debatable. The initial ambulatory blood pressure monitoring session is cost-saving because it limits expensive therapy in the 20% of patients with white-coat hypertension but frequent ambulatory blood pressure monitoring sessions would be required to monitor such therapy, which would be cost-prohibitive. One ambulatory blood pressure monitoring session annually is usually the upper limit (22). Because of the potential high cost, several authoritative groups have recommended that ambulatory blood pressure monitoring be used sparingly in the general hypertensive population. In managed care, veterans' hospitals, and other situations where minimal incremental direct costs are involved, ambulatory blood pressure monitoring could be performed more widely (22).

E. White Coat Normotension

A relatively small proportion of individuals (61 of 234 or 26% of the original series from New York City) have hypertension-related target-organ damage, despite office blood pressures that are consistently below the "normal" threshold. These individuals have been called white coat normotensives, and this diagnosis can really only be made with ambulatory blood pressure monitoring. These individuals would have not been given potentially useful antihypertensive therapy if they had not had carotid ultrasound examinations that showed carotid wall thickening similar to that usually seen in sustained hypertensives; echocardiograms that showed left ventricular hypertrophy; and ambulatory blood pressure monitoring sessions that disclosed the higher out-of-office blood pressures (41). It is unclear whether these individuals have greater stresses and resulting blood pressure elevations outside the medical office than in it. One would expect that if they were not diagnosed with white coat normotension then their prognosis should be similar to untreated hypertensives, but this has not yet been proven.

F. Isolated Systolic Hypertension

Prior to 1997, isolated systolic hypertension could be diagnosed when the systolic blood pressure was elevated, but the diastolic blood pressure was below threshold ($\geq 140/<90$ mmHg in the United States; often $\geq 160/<95$ mmHg in other countries). This pattern is seen in ~60–70% of older hypertensives and is thought to derive pathophysiologically from "stiff" arteries and reduced vascular compliance. Three large-scale clinical trials specifically enrolled patients with isolated systolic hypertension, defined as systolic blood pressure >160 mmHg with a normal diastolic blood pressure: Systolic Hypertension in the Elderly Program (SHEP) in the USA, Systolic Hypertension (Syst-Eur) in Europe, and Systolic Hypertension in China (Syst-China). Each independently showed that older individuals with blood pressure elevations only in the systolic have a reduced risk of cardiovascular events if given pharmacologic treatment. In a meta-analysis of 15,693 patients with isolated systolic hypertension enrolled in eight clinical trials, drug therapy reduced the initial blood pressure (174/83 mmHg) on average by only 10.4/4.1 mmHg.

However, large clinical benefits were observed: 30% reduction in fatal and nonfatal stroke, 23% reduction in fatal and nonfatal coronary heart disease, 26% reduction in cardiovascular events, and 13% reduction in all-cause mortality (42). As a result, there is no longer any debate about the wisdom of lowering blood pressure in patients with isolated systolic hypertension.

The high risk of untreated isolated systolic hypertension prompted investigations of pulse pressure, the numerical difference between systolic and diastolic blood pressure, as a cardiovascular risk factor, particularly in older individuals. Although many studies found that a widened pulse pressure was associated with lower survival rates, the Prospective Studies Collaborative Group gathered data from 61 prospective trials involving nearly 1 million people and found that pulse pressure was a much poorer predictor of future cardiovascular events than systolic blood pressure (43). In other words, a blood pressure of 180/130 mmHg does not have the same prognosis as 130/80 mmHg, even though both have a pulse pressure of 50 mmHg. This has led some to rely less on pulse pressure as an independent cardiovascular risk factor, although as a secondary factor, prognosis is generally poorer for a higher pulse pressure at any given systolic blood pressure. This may simply be a reflection of the decreased vascular compliance seen in individuals with a wide pulse pressure.

IV. ASSESSMENT OF THE HYPERTENSIVE PATIENT

During the initial office evaluation of a person with elevated blood pressure readings, six important issues must be addressed:

- Documenting an accurate diagnosis of hypertension (discussed earlier).
- Defining the presence or absence of TOD related to hypertension.
- Screening for other cardiovascular risk factors that often accompany hypertension.
- Assessing future risk for cardiovascular disease, which suggests the appropriate intensity of treatment.
- Assessing whether the person is likely to have an identifiable cause of hypertension (secondary hypertension) and should have further diagnostic testing to confirm or exclude the diagnosis.
- Obtaining data that may be helpful in the initial and subsequent choices of therapy.

There are many possibilities that might explain a single set of elevated blood pressure readings (Table 14.5). Elevated blood pressure does not necessarily correspond

Table 14.5 Causes of Hypertension

I. Systolic and diastolic hypertension
  A. Primary, essential or idiopathic
  B. Secondary
    1. Renal
      a) Renal parenchymal disease
        (1) Acute glomerulonephritis
        (2) Chronic nephritis
        (3) Polycystic disease
        (4) Diabetic nephropathy
        (5) Hydronephrosis
      b) Renovascular
        (1) Renal artery stenosis
        (2) Intrarenal vasculitis
      c) Renin-producing tumors
      d) Renoprival
      e) Primary sodium retention (Liddle's syndrome, Gordon's syndrome)
    2. Endocrine
      a) Acromegaly
      b) Hypothyroidism
      c) Hyperthyroidism
      d) Hypercalcemia (hyperparathyroidism)
      e) Adrenal
        (1) Cortical
          (a) Cushing's syndrome
          (b) Primary aldosteronism
          (c) Congenital adrenal hyperplasia
          (d) Apparent mineralocorticoid excess (licorice)
        (2) Medullary pheochromocytoma
      f) Extra-adrenal chromaffin tumors
      g) Carcinoid
      h) Exogenous hormones
        (1) Estrogen
        (2) Glucocorticoids
        (3) Mineralocorticoids
        (4) Sympathomimetics
        (5) Tyramine-containing foods and monoamine oxidase inhibitors
    3. Coarctation of the aorta
    4. Pregnancy-induced hypertension
    5. Sleep apnea
    6. Neurologic disorders
      a) Increased intracranial pressure
        (1) Brain tumor
        (2) Encephalitis
        (3) Respiratory acidosis
      b) Quadriplegia
      c) Acute porphyria
      d) Familial dysautonomia
      e) Lead poisoning
      f) Guillain–Barré syndrome
    7. Acute stress, including surgery
      a) Psychogenic hyperventilation
      b) Hypoglycemia

(continued)

Table 14.5 *Continued*

      c) Burns
      d) Pancreatitis
      e) Alcohol withdrawal
      f) Sickle cell crisis
      g) Postresuscitation
      h) Postoperative
    8. Increased intravascular volume
    9. Alcohol and drug use
II. Systolic hypertension
  A. Increased cardiac output
    1. Aortic valvular insufficiency
    2. Atrioventricular fistula, patent ductus arteriosus
    3. Thyrotoxicosis
    4. Paget's disease of bone
    5. Beriberi
    6. Hyperkinetic circulation
  B. Rigidity of aorta or small arteries
III. Iatrogenic hypertension

Source: Adapted from Kaplan NM. Systemic hypertension: mechanisms and diagnosis. In: Braunwald E ed. Heart Disease. 5th ed. Philadelphia, PA: W.B. Saunders Company 1997:807–839.

to hypertension. Except for people who take one of several types of drugs known to elevate blood pressure (Table 14.6), many individuals with only one elevated blood pressure reading will have their blood pressure return to the normal range over time. This is the reason for recommending at least two or three sets of blood pressure measurements before diagnosing hypertension.

A. Routine Assessment in Hypertensive Patients

The recommendations of JNC 7 (1) and other national and international expert panels (2) limit the number of and the expense related to initial tests for the routine evaluation of every hypertensive patient (Table 14.7). Tests that are used in assessing the presence or absence of TOD include physical examination, serum creatinine, urinalysis, and an ECG. Assessing the number of cardiovascular risk factors can be accomplished with the medical history, chemistry panel (glucose, lipid profile), and urinalysis. Although the EXPRESS version of JNC 7 no longer includes a formal risk stratification system, other expert panels have very elaborate systems for linking the assessment of cardiovascular risk and the intensity of antihypertensive treatment (44,45).

In general, direct the physical examination toward clues that might indicate an identifiable secondary cause of hypertension. These might include an abdominal or flank bruit, which is a sign of renal artery disease, or an abdominal or flank mass, which is consistent with either pheochromocytoma or polycystic kidney.

Table 14.6   Partial List of Drugs Known to Elevate Blood Pressure

Chemical elements and other industrial chemicals	*Venoms and toxins*
Lead	Spider bites (especially the brown recluse or "fiddleback" spider)
Mercury	Scorpion bites
Thallium and other heavy metals	Snake bites
Lithium salts, especially the chloride	*Prescription Drugs*
Chloromethane	Cortisone and other steroids (both corticosteroids and mineralocorticoids)[a]
Carbon disulfide	Estrogens (usually oral contraceptive agents with high estrogenic activity)[a]
Polychlorinated (and polybrominated) biphenyls	Nonsteroidal antiinflammatory drugs (including cyclooxygenase-2 inhibitors)[a]
Parathion and other insecticides	Phenylpropanolamines and analogs[a]
Food substances	Cyclosporine and tacrolimus[a]
Sodium chloride[a]	Erythropoietin
Licorice	Naloxone
Caffeine	Ketamine
Tyramine-containing foods (with MAO-I)	Desflurane
Ethanol	Carbamazepine
Street Drugs and other "Natural Products"	Bromocriptine
Anabolic steroids	Metoclopramide
Cocaine ("?") (and cocaine withdrawal)	Antidepressants (especially venlafaxine)
Heroin withdrawal	Buspirone
Methylphenidate	Disulfuram
Phencyclidine	Clonidine, β-blocker (and maybe calcium antagonist) withdrawal
γ-hydroxybutyric acid (and withdrawal from it)	Pheochromocytoma: β-blocker without α-blocker first; glucagon
Ma Huang, "herbal ecstasy," and other phenylpropanolamine analogs[a]	Pentagastrin
Nicotine ("?") (and nicotine withdrawal)	Digitalis
Ketamine	Thyrotropin-releasing hormone (Protirelin)
Ergotamine and other ergot-containing herbal preparations	Synthetic ACTH (Corticotropin)
St. John's Wort	Sibutramine
	Alkylating agents (typically used for cancer chemotherapy)
	Clozapine
	Orlistat?

[a]Substances of greatest current clinical importance.

Table 14.7   Tests Recommended by JNC 7 for the Initial Evaluation of a Hypertensive Patient

Serum chemistries (glucose, potassium, creatinine, calcium)
Urinalysis
Hematocrit
ECG
Lipid profile (including HDL-cholesterol, triglycerides, and calculated LDL-cholesterol, preferably obtained in the fasting state)
An estimate of urinary albumin excretion (24 h urine or urinary albumin/creatinine ratio); optional, but quite helpful in patients with diabetes or chronic kidney disease

Source: Chobanian et al. (1).

B. Ophthalmic Assessment

A thorough examination of the optic fundus is a valuable tool for evaluating hypertensive patients. Before effective antihypertensive drug therapy became available, the most important predictor of future cardiovascular events was not the blood pressure level, but the appearance of the optic fundi. The prognosis of hypertensive patients has improved greatly since that time, but the appreciation of hypertension-related changes in the optic fundus is still a valuable clue to both the severity and the duration of the elevated blood pressure. The optic fundus is the only site in the entire body where blood vessels can be examined directly. Patients with Keith–Wagener–Barker (KWB) grade III or IV fundi, characterized by hemorrhages or exudes, or papilledema, generally have long-term hypertension as opposed to a recent onset.

With prolonged hypertension, the normal yellowish-white color of the retinal arteries gradually changes to a reddish-brown tone ("copper wire"), and the ratio of artery/vein diameters is reduced from the normal 2:3 to less than 1:3. Gradually over months to years, the column of blood within the artery gradually diminishes, and the artery is reduced to a whitish thread ("silver wire") despite persistent blood flow. Atrioventricular nicking is perhaps the most easily recognized ocular abnormality in hypertensive retinopathy. When the thickened artery containing blood at elevated pressure compresses a low-pressure, thin-walled vein within the shared adventitial sheath, the vein disappears. Hypertension is therefore both epidemiologically and pathophysiologically a risk factor for retinal vein occlusion. When arterial blood flow is reduced sufficiently to cause infarction of underlying retinal tissue, this forms round or oval white patches with fluffy borders called cytoid bodies or cotton–wool spots. Intraretinal "flame-shaped" hemorrhages occur after breakdown in the blood-retinal barrier caused by a ruptured aneurysm, neovascularization (typically in diabetics), or "blowout" hemorrhages resulting from hypertension. A leakage of plasma into the macular space often precedes an acute reduction in visual acuity and is followed by the "macular star figure" which is visible for many years thereafter. Increased intraocular or intracranial pressure and diminished axoplasmic flow in the optic nerve fibers can cause ischemia in the optic nerve circulation. This can lead to papilledema from either a retinal vein occlusion or a hypertensive emergency. An alternative cause for papilledema should be sought if both the fundi are otherwise free of hypertensive retinopathy and there is no evidence of acute, ongoing damage to other target organs.

The importance of controlling hypertension to prevent ophthalmic endpoints such as vision loss, retinal hemorrhages, and laser photocoagulation procedures has not received much attention in recent medical literature. There are nonetheless several reports of improved blood pressure control reducing the risk of these problems in large prospective clinical trials, especially in diabetics.

C. Cardiac Assessment

Two major prognostic factors associated with the heart can be obtained in the initial physical examination in hypertensive patients. These include both left ventricular hypertrophy and aortic sclerosis. A murmur of aortic sclerosis can be auscultated in ~21–26% of adults >65 years of age. In the Cardiovascular Health Study, 29% of the 5621 subjects older than 65 years of age had this valvular abnormality detected on echocardiography; it was found much more commonly among hypertensives and those with left ventricular hypertrophy. Perhaps most important, its presence was associated with a highly significant 50% increase in cardiovascular events during 5 years of follow-up. Much of this increased risk was due to concomitant hypertension, however; after adjustment for baseline differences in risk factors (between those who had or did not have aortic sclerosis), only one of four studied endpoints remained statistically significant. An atrial (S_4) gallop is common in hypertensive patients, and may be the first sign of hypertensive heart disease, but has little prognostic importance (particularly in older people).

An ECG is recommended during the initial evaluation of all persons with hypertension. The ECG is used to document previously undetected myocardial infarction, myocardial ischemia, and cardiac rhythm disturbances, and it is possibly the most cost-effective way to screen for left ventricular hypertrophy. The ECG is not the most sensitive or specific method of detecting left ventricular hypertrophy, but it is less expensive than echocardiography, computed axial tomographic (CAT) scanning, or magnetic resonance imaging (MRI) of the heart. The "limited echocardiogram" that accurately calculates left ventricular size and assesses ventricular geometry at a very affordable price has been recommended and implemented in some centers in Canada, but not yet in the United States.

Left ventricular hypertrophy is perhaps the most important indicator of prognosis in hypertensive patients. It is often considered the "hemoglobin A_{1c} of blood pressure" because it objectively measures both the severity and the duration of elevated blood pressure. In the Framingham Heart Study, ECG evidence of left ventricular hypertrophy has been associated with an approximately three-fold increase in the incidence of cardiovascular events when compared with those without it. Echocardiographically detected left ventricular hypertrophy has proven an even better predictor of cardiovascular events.

The geometry of the enlarged ventricle also plays a role. Concentric hypertrophy of the left ventricle is most commonly seen in hypertension, perhaps as a result of concentric remodeling. In one series, concentric left ventricular hypertrophy carried a four-fold increased risk of cardiac morbidity and mortality when compared with individuals with nonhypertrophied hearts. Eccentric hypertrophy, most commonly seen in athletes, imparted only a two-fold increased risk of events in the same series. In a variety of reports, left ventricular hypertrophy has been the most influential of all traditional cardiovascular risk factors in predicting not only death or myocardial infarction, but also stroke, heart failure, and other cardiovascular end points (46). Echocardiographically determined left ventricular mass is an important predictor of prognosis; however, there is sufficient intrinsic variability in a single echocardiogram (perhaps 10–15%) that serial determinations are imprecise, which makes it an inefficient screening test. An exception might be a person with uncomplicated stage 1 hypertension and a normal ECG, where the presence of concentric left ventricular hypertrophy would usually require antihypertensive drug treatment.

Left ventricular hypertrophy is associated both epidemiologically and pathophysiologically with intimal hyperplasia of the epicardial coronary arteries, increased coronary vascular resistance, increased severity and frequency of ventricular dysrhythmias, decreased flow reserve, and reduced diastolic relaxation. Heart failure with preserved left ventricular function often manifests clinically as "flash pulmonary edema" and carries a poor prognosis even when carefully treated (47). Hypertension probably plays a major role in the pathogenesis of this syndrome, which has been identified in up to 40% of patients admitted to the hospital with heart failure (48). The new Cornell voltage-duration criteria show the status of left ventricular hypertrophy as a powerful risk factor for cardiovascular events, making it the major inclusion criterion for the recent Losartan Intervention For Endpoint reduction (LIFE) study. In this important clinical trial where nearly all of the benefit was in stroke reduction (49), an angiotensin receptor blocker with or without a diuretic was more effective at reducing both the degree of left ventricular hypertrophy and the overall cardiovascular risk than a β-blocker with or without a diuretic.

The most contentious aspect of left ventricular hypertrophy lies in its treatment and possible reversal. Short-term clinical studies that evaluated changes in left ventricular hypertrophy show different conclusions about which class of antihypertensive drug best regresses left ventricular hypertrophy. The LIFE study is currently the only outcome study to show a correlation between reduction in left ventricular hypertrophy and prevention of cardiovascular events. Because left ventricular hypertrophy is unlikely to regress without reducing blood pressure, most authorities recommend allocating resources to blood pressure control, rather than on serial echocardiograms, to see whether the left ventricular mass index is returning to normal during treatment.

D. Renal Assessment

JNC 7 recommends only a serum creatinine and a dipstick for proteinuria in the evaluation of renal function, although performing either a "spot" urine protein/creatinine ratio or a 24 h urine test is optional. The US National Kidney Foundation recommends screening for microalbuminuria, which is defined as an albumin excretion of 30–300 mg/d. This level is below the detection limit for the conventional dipstick. Because the traditional 24 h urine collection is cumbersome and potentially inaccurate in many patients, an early morning "spot" urine for protein/creatinine ratio is recommended. This methodology has been widely validated in several clinical studies (e.g., LIFE, AASK, IRMA-2, and RENAAL). Microalbuminuria has been strongly associated with the risk for future cardiovascular events, in both diabetics and nondiabetics. There is concern about whether it is simply a marker for increased cardiovascular risk or is an independent predictor of cardiovascular events, especially in younger individuals and those with earlier stages of hypertension (50). The prevalence of microalbuminuria ranges from 12% to 36% (averaging 20%) in type 2 diabetics and is slightly lower in nondiabetics (5–40%) and becomes more common after age 55. Important confounders include various types of dyslipidemia, duration of hypertension, degree of blood pressure control, and a "nondipping" circadian pattern of blood pressure. All monotherapies except dihydropyridine calcium antagonists and central or peripheral sympathetic blockers can reduce albuminuria. Both ACE-inhibitors and angiotensin II receptor blockers have been shown in prospective studies to retard the progression from microalbuminuria to proteinuria ($\geq$300 mg/day of protein in a 24 h collection) in type 2 diabetics.

E. Assessment of the Vasculature

One of the hallmarks of hypertensive circulation is decreased vascular compliance. When blood pressure is acutely elevated, the elastic behavior of both large and small arteries changes. The muscular layers of the arterial wall become unable to relax as quickly or transmit pressure waves as easily and reproducibly as they did when blood pressure was lower. This is a passive and reversible phenomenon that typically lasts minutes to hours. However, when the blood pressure is continually elevated, the internal elastic lamina of blood vessels becomes gradually infiltrated with thinned, split, and frayed elastic fibers, and a new intercellular matrix is created. In extreme cases, medial necrosis develops within the arterial wall. This process of arteriosclerosis is often attributed to aging, hypertension, or a combination of both and leads to chronic, irreversible stiffening of the arterial tree.

There are several methods of assessing arterial compliance (Table 14.8), but most are invasive, expensive, or not widely used in clinical medicine. Large clinical studies are now using new methods of calculating total arterial compliance that are based on pulse contour analysis (51,52).

Pseudohypertension is the name given to the rarely diagnosed circumstance in which blood pressure measurements

Table 14.8 Methods for Determining Arterial Compliance

Type of method	Measured in	Invasive	Drawbacks
Direct			
Angiography	Aorta	Yes	Expensive
Echocardiography	Aorta	No	Expensive
Intravascular ultrasound	Peripheral or coronary arteries	Yes	Expensive
Echo-tracking	Peripheral arteries	No	Not widely available
Venous occlusion plethysmography	Peripheral arteries	Not always	Time- and operator-intensive
Indirect			
Stroke volume/pulse pressure ratio	Total arterial compliance	No	Reproducibility questionable
Pulse wave velocity	Segmental arteries	No	Limited to large arteries
Fourier pulse analysis	Peripheral arteries	No	Reproducibility questionable
Total compliance	Total arterial compliance	No	Expensive
Pulse contour analysis	Total arterial compliance	No	Time- and operator-intensive

Source: Adapted from Elliott WJ, Black HR. Special situations in the management of hypertension. In: Hollenberg NK ed. Atlas of Hypertension. 4th ed. Philadelphia, PA: Current Medicine, Inc., 2003:257–281.

by indirect sphygmomanometry are much higher than direct intra-arterial measurement. These differences are usually attributed to very stiff and calcified arteries that are nearly impossible to compress with the bladder in the usual blood pressure cuff. Palpating the walls of the brachial artery when blood flow is stopped by inflating the cuff higher than systolic pressure, or the "Osler Maneuver," is a simple way to diagnose this condition. Note that this technique is less accurate than initially reported. Perhaps because repeated intra-arterial measurements would be required to document and then calibrate the difference between indirect and direct blood pressure measurements, few physicians diagnose pseudohypertension routinely.

F. Assessment of Other Organs

Generally, few other blood or urine tests are necessary. In specific circumstances, plasma renin activity, 24 h urine collections, and sometimes serum insulin levels can be useful during a specialized evaluation for a specific patient. Some newly appreciated markers of cardiovascular risk, such as C-reactive protein and homocyteine, have not yet been shown to be sensitive or specific enough to warrant routine testing, but interest in these markers is growing (53,54).

G. Assessment for Identifiable Causes of Hypertension

There are many identifiable causes of hypertension (secondary hypertension, Table 14.5). In some of these, the elevated blood pressure can be improved with specific treatment such as angioplasty or surgery or by removing the agent that caused the hypertension. By far, the most common

identifiable cause is chronic renal failure. Although chronic renal disease is mostly incurable, the hypertension associated with it can often be controlled with adequate volume regulation using diuresis or dialysis. In contrast, renal artery stenosis, pheochromocytoma, and some mineralocorticoid-excess states are potentially curable. These conditions are sufficiently common to warrant specialized tests to screen for and confirm the diagnosis. If a secondary cause of hypertension is suspected, a referral to a hypertension specialist may be appropriate (1,2).

1. Renovascular Hypertension

Patients with renovascular hypertension often have very elevated blood pressures despite multiple-drug therapy, considerable TOD, and are at high risk of losing renal function due to ischemic nephropathy (55). Atherosclerotic renal artery stenosis is found in ~90% of those with renovascular hypertension, and primarily affects older people who had easily controlled primary hypertension, but then developed refractory hypertension after age 55. Many have evidence of atherosclerotic disease in other vascular beds (carotids, coronaries, and peripheral arteries) and are or were heavy cigarette smokers. Most of the remainder is due to fibromuscular dysplasia, most common in 10- to 25-year-old Caucasian women with very high blood pressures, and is particularly well treated with angioplasty. Although more common in Caucasians, African Americans also develop renovascular hypertension. A simple and relatively accurate "clinical prediction rule" can estimate the pretest probability of renovascular disease (Tables 14.9 and 14.10) based on clinical information gathered at the initial evaluation (56).

The goal of laboratory testing in patients suspected of renovascular hypertension is to demonstrate the presence

Table 14.9 Clinical Information for Estimating the Probability of Renovascular Hypertension

Clinical characteristic	Never smoked	Current or former smoker
Age (years)		
20–29	0	0
30–39	1	4
40–49	2	8
50–59	3	5
60–69	4	5
≥70	5	6
Female gender	2	2
ASCVD[a]	1	1
Hx HTN[b] ≤2 years	1	1
BMI[c] <25 kg/m^2	2	2
Abdominal bruit	3	3
Serum creatinine (mg/dL)		
0.5–0.75	0	0
0.75–1.0	1	1
1.0–1.2	2	2
1.2–1.65	3	3
1.7–2.2	6	6
≥ 2.3	9	9
Hypercholesterolemia (>250 mg/dL or drug-treated)	1	1

[a]ASCVD, signs, symptoms, or clinical evidence of atherosclerotic cardiovascular disease.
[b]Hx HTN, history of hypertension.
[c]BMI, body mass index [weight in kg/(height in cm)^2].
Note: To estimate the prior-probability of renovascular hypertension, compare the sum of the point score from Table 14.9 the points column in Table 14.10.
Source: Adapted from Krijnen P, van Jaarsveld BC, Steyerberg EW et al. A clinical prediction rule for renal artery stenosis. Ann Intern Med 1998; 129:738–740.

Table 14.10 Clinical Prediction Rule for Estimating the Probability of Renovascular Hypertension

Points (from Table 14.9)	Probability of Renovascular Hypertension (95% CI)
≤5	<2 (0–5)
6	3 (1–8)
7	5 (2–10)
8	8 (3–12)
9	11 (5–20)
10	15 (7–28)
11	25 (14–40)
12	37 (18–55)
13	47 (28–65)
14	62 (40–80)
15	72 (46–84)
16	80 (62–86)
17	87 (72–92)
18	89 (78–95)
19	90 (82–97)
20	≥90 (92–100)

Note: CI, confidence interval.

Two newer imaging modalities are of particular importance:

- Ultrasonic visualization of the renal arteries, with interrogation of flow by Doppler measurements, is widely available, but its usefulness varies greatly. When an experienced, dedicated technician examines a properly prepared patient, the sensitivity and specificity of the test are well in excess of 90%, and the cost is reasonable. Unfortunately, in obese patients and those with much intestinal gas, the test is much less useful with the rate of renal artery localization only ~60%. However, some centers still prefer this screening test.
- Magnetic resonance angiography (with gadolinium) may soon become the best choice. It is very accurate with pictures nearly the quality of a standard angiogram, noninvasive, and the patient needs no specific preparation. However, its limited availability and expense currently outweigh these major advantages.

In many centers, the screening test of choice is captopril scintigraphy. Only ACE-inhibitors and ARBs need to be stopped before performing the test, and adverse reactions from the single dose of captopril are rare. Some centers perform a baseline scan without captopril, and then an hour later another with it, which doubles the cost, but it may be more convenient for the patient. A normal captopril scan often precludes the need for further investigation. A "captopril-induced change in the renogram" (especially a change in the distribution of tracer between kidneys)

of renal artery stenosis and also determine whether the lesions are in fact the cause of the patient's hypertension (55). However, before testing, it is useful to discuss with the patient the possible results. Further investigation is probably unwarranted if the patient is unwilling to consider or unsuitable for surgery, which might be required if the renal artery is damaged during angiography. Recent data from the Netherlands and the Mayo Clinic suggest that continued medical therapy (including ACE-inhibitors and ARBs) may be as useful in the long term as revascularization. This suggests that only patients with uncontrolled hypertension need be evaluated. Such individuals with a high (>70%) pretest probability for renovascular hypertension should have an angiogram without a screening test. Screening tests for those at moderate risk should be based on either biochemical or imaging techniques (Table 14.11).

Table 14.11 Screening Tests for Renovascular Hypertension

Type of tests	Sensitivity	Specificity	Invasive?	Availability	Cost[a]
Biochemical tests					
Serum potassium	~70%	~5%	No	Widespread	$20–35
Plasma renin activity (PRA)	~80%	~60%	No	Widespread	$25–155
Captopril challenge test	60–70%	~80%	No	Widespread	$100–300
Renal vein renin activity ratio	~75–90%	~80%	Yes: F[b]; vein	Variable	>$2500
Imaging Tests					
Rapid-sequence intravenous pyelography	74%	80–86%	A[b] or F[b] vein	Widespread	$300
Renal scintigraphy (^{99m}Tc-DTPA)	74%	77%	A[b] vein	Widespread	$350
Renal scintigraphy with captopril (or enalaprilat); ^{99m}Tc-DTPA or MAG-3	85%	90%	A[b] vein	Most major medical centers	$400
Intravenous digital subtraction angiography (DSA)	80%	88%	A[b] vein	Variable	$750
Intra-arterial DSA	95%	99%	F[b]	Limited	$1500
Standard angiography	>99%	>99%	F[b] artery	Widespread	$4000
Duplex ultrasound of renal arteries	Operator-dependent (50–99%)	Operator-dependent (50–99%)	No	Highly variable	$600
MRI	Perhaps ~90%	Perhaps ~90%	No	Limited	$2000

[a]Costs vary over time and from institution to institution. These are approximate and derived from purveyors at RUSH University Medical Center, Chicago, in late 2003.
[b]F, femoral; A, antecubital.

may predict lower blood pressure after revascularization. Most centers use ^{99m}Tc-DTPA, a radioisotope of technicium chelated to diethylenetriaminepenta-acetic acid, but the more expensive MAG-3 is more accurate in detecting bilateral renal artery stenosis. Following femoral artery-approached DSA with angioplasty and stenting successfully opens >95% of stenosed renal arteries, especially those with ostial lesions. Screening high-probability patients with captopril scintigraphy and following with angioplasty and stenting is the most cost-effective approach. One analysis finds that if the pretest probability of renovascular disease is >30%, this approach saves money overall.

2. Pheochromocytoma

Patients with pheochromocytoma are nearly always symptomatic, usually with a cluster of complaints that occur in paroxysms or "spells" (57), the description of which is usually the same in each patient. An attack may be precipitated by eating, pain, postural changes, or urination, and hypertension is often exacerbated during a spell. The most common symptoms include headache, diaphoresis, and palpitations; but others such as anxiety, weakness, and tremulousness are also frequently found. Although most patients do not have a heredo-familial reason for their pheochromocytoma a skin examination and screening for other tumors related to multiple endocrine neoplasia syndromes are recommended.

Diagnostic testing for pheochromocytoma generally involves two steps: demonstrating that excess catecholamines are produced and localizing the tumor (58). Currently, there are multiple possibilities for each step (Table 14.12). Seek biochemical confirmation of an increase in catecholamine production if a pheochromocytoma is suspected. Despite recent enthusiasm for plasma metanephrines in some centers (59), the slightly less sensitive and specific measurement of 24 h urinary excretion of total catecholamines (norepinephrine, epinephrine, and dopamine) or their metabolites (vanillylmandelic acid or metanephrines) costs much less. Whether assaying urine

Table 14.12 Diagnostic Tests for Pheochromocytoma

Biochemical
- Urinary free catecholamines
- Urinary vanillylmandelic acid
- Urinary metanephrines
- Plasma catecholamines (or metanephrines)
- Clonidine suppression test
- Glucagon stimulation test

Imaging Studies
- Computerized axial tomographic (CAT) scan
- Magnetic resonance imaging (especially T_2-weighted images)
- ^{131}I-meta-iodobenzylguanidine
- Abdominal ultrasound
- Adrenal vein or vena caval drainage
- Angiography

or plasma, pay attention to the conditions under which the sample is collected. Measure creatinine in the same urine sample to verify that there was a full 24 h collection. To minimize false-positive results, the patient should be in a nonstressful situation when the sample is obtained.

When urinary values are nondiagnostic, the measurement of plasma catecholamines and/or metanephrines can be very useful (59). If plasma catecholamines (norepinephrine plus epinephrine) levels exceed 2000 pg/mL in the basal state, the presence of a pheochromocytoma is highly likely. If the levels are between 1000 and 2000 pg/mL, a clonidine suppression test is often recommended (57). If plasma catecholamine levels do not suppress after the administration of 0.3 mg of oral clonidine, the patient warrants a more aggressive search for a pheochromocytoma. Individuals with plasma catecholamine levels <1000 pg/mL can undergo glucagon stimulation testing concurrently with α-blockade, which blunts the blood pressure response but not the diagnostic increase in serum norepinephrine.

Choosing which initial imaging procedure to obtain is also controversial. Computed arial tomographic (CAT) scanning is a highly sensitive imaging modality that will locate nearly all pheochromocytomas, especially those in the adrenal gland or in the abdomen. MRI does not require contrast material, which is sometimes necessary with CAT scanning, and is also helpful in localizing nonadrenal or nonabdominal pheochromocytomas. Enhancing MRI T_2-weighted images of pheochromocytomas and adrenal carcinomas helps distinguish adrenal masses that are not biochemically active (incidentalomas) from metabolically active or malignant tumors. Meta-iodobenzylguanidine scanning is particularly helpful when a pheochromocytoma is suspected, but not clearly located with CAT or MRI. This radiopharmaceutical is a guanethidine analog that is concentrated in pheochromocytomas and other neural crest tumors. Total-body scanning helps localize the tumor, if the initial CAT or MRI scans are negative or equivocal. The sensitivity of this test exceeds 90%, but it is not widely available.

3. Mineralocorticoid-Excess States

The symptoms of these forms of secondary hypertension that may help the clinician are related to hypokalemia (60). Usually prominent are muscle weakness, cramps, polyuria, and even nocturia, although many who are just becoming hypokalemic do not have these complaints. Target organ damage is typically less severe and less extensive than often seen with similar levels of blood pressure in primary hypertension. The majority of patients (50–60%) with this syndrome have a benign adrenal adenoma that secretes aldosterone autonomously; some (30–50%) have bilateral (idiopathic) adrenal hyperplasia.

Rarer causes include adrenal carcinomas, glucocorticoid-suppressible hyperaldosteronism, and licorice ingestion. Recent research has shown that both glycyrrhizic acid (the active agent in licorice) and its hydrolyzed product, glycyrrhetinic acid, inhibit peripheral (e.g., intrarenal) 11-β-hydroxysteroid dehydrogenase (the enzyme responsible for inactivation of cortisol to cortisone). This leads to an excessive mineralocorticoid action of cortisol, which has clinical manifestations similar to hyperaldosteronism.

A low serum potassium level discovered as part of the routine evaluation of a hypertensive patient may be the only clue that a mineralocorticoid-excess state is present. Hypokalemia, especially a serum level $\leq$3.2 mEq/L, when not secondary to diuretic therapy suggests that mineralocorticoid-excess hypertension may be present.

There are three major steps in the diagnostic evaluation of primary hyperaldosteronism: demonstrating the autonomous overproduction of mineralocorticoids, distinguishing between the several causes, and monitoring the chosen therapy (61). The best test for identifying patients with normal renal function and primary aldosteronism is the measurement of a 24 h urinary aldosterone excretion during salt loading. After 3 days of salt loading (>200 mEq/day), an excretion rate of >14 mcg of aldosterone within 24 h distinguishes ~93% of patients with primary aldosteronism from those with essential hypertension. Typically, all drugs that interfere with the renin–angiotensin–aldosterone system are discontinued for at least a week before this urine collection. Because ~7–38% of patients with primary aldosteronism do not present with hypokalemia, the plasma aldosterone/renin ratio has been proposed to define the appropriateness of peripheral renin activity (PRA) for the circulating levels of aldosterone. Some authorities recommend this calculation as an initial screening tool, but its specificity as a screening test is low. Direct genetic testing of DNA or a dexamethasone challenge test can diagnose glucocorticoid-suppressible hyperaldosteronism.

Although a number of hormonal tests can distinguish aldosterone-producing adrenal adenomas from bilateral adrenal hyperplasia, a more direct approach is to perform a thin-cut (every 5 mm) adrenal CAT scan. This is simple, noninvasive, and efficient. The success of high resolution CAT scanning for adenomas exceeds 90%, and is close to 100% for those >1.5 cm in diameter, which is slightly better than iodocholesterol scintigraphy. Adrenal venous aldosterone levels are very expensive and risky to obtain by inexperienced hands, and are needed only when the biochemical findings are highly suggestive of an adenoma, but the thin-cut CAT scan is not diagnostic.

Chronic medical therapy is necessary in patients suffering from adrenal hyperplasia, adenoma with high surgical risks, and bilateral adrenal adenomas that may require bilateral adrenalectomy (62). Potassium-sparing diuretics and calcium antagonists are currently the most useful treatments and eplerenone will be very important in the near future. Surgical excision of an aldosterone-producing adenoma usually reverses hypertension and biochemical defects. However, 1 year postoperatively, ~70% of patients are normotensive, and 5 years postoperatively, only 53% remain normotensive. The restoration of normal potassium homeostasis is usually permanent. Patients should receive drug treatment for 8–10 weeks before surgery to decrease blood pressure and correct metabolic abnormalities. Potassium deficiencies must be corrected preoperatively because hypokalemia increases the risk of cardiac dysrhythmias during anesthesia.

4. Other Forms of Secondary Hypertension

Symptoms characteristic of sleep apnea, thyroid disorders, hyperparathyroidism, and Cushing's syndrome should be noted, as these disorders may indicate hypertension that responds to therapy directed at the primary disease.

Physical examination is generally sufficient to exclude acromegaly and coarctation of the aorta, especially if the peripheral pulses are palpated (searching for radio-femoral delay). A thigh blood pressure measurement will exclude this possibility in all newly diagnosed young hypertensive patients. An echocardiogram can identify ~95% of aortic coarctations through the first 8 cm of the descending aorta.

V. FOLLOW-UP

The patient's absolute cardiovascular risk and achievement of blood pressure goals determine the schedule for follow-up visits. The maximum follow-up time for a treated hypertensive should be 6 months, as prescriptions are often not honored >6 months after the date written. Whenever medication is initiated or changed, a return visit in 2–4 weeks is reasonable. Today's long-acting medications take five to seven serum half-lives to achieve a steady state plasma level and probably twice that to attain a stable pharmacodynamic effect. A quicker visit may also send the unwarranted message to the patients that they are at higher risk and that the physician is concerned.

VI. CONCLUSIONS

The diagnosis of hypertension is traditionally based on blood pressure measurements obtained in a physician's office, using a mercury sphygmomanometer. Newer methods are being increasingly used, including home measurements, ambulatory blood pressure monitoring, and alternative devices that do not use liquid mercury. The initial assessment of a hypertensive patient should include a detailed history and physical examination, but a limited number of tests: serum chemistries (including a lipid profile), urinalysis, ECG and hematocrit. Other tests are warranted only when supported by an appropriate clinical suspicion. These measures help limit expensive and possibly dangerous drug therapy to individuals who are most likely to benefit from it.

REFERENCES

1. Chobanian AV, Bakris GL, Black HR, Cushman WC, Green LA, Izzo JL Jr, Jones DW, Materson BJ, Oparil S, Wright JT Jr, Roccella EJ. National Heart, Lung, and Blood Institute; Joint National Committee on Prevention, Detection, Evaluation, and Treatment of High Blood Pressure; National High Blood Pressure Education Program Coordinating Committee; The Seventh Report of the Joint National Committee on Prevention, Detection, Evaluation, and Treatment of High Blood Pressure: The JNC 7 Report. J Am Med Assoc 2003; 9:2560–2572.
2. 2003 European Society of Hypertension—European Cardiology guidelines for the management of arterial hypertension; Guidelines Committee. J Hypertens 2003; 6:1011–1053.
3. Pickering TG, Hall JE, Appel LJ, Falkner BE, Graves J, Hill MN, Jones DW, Kurtz T, Sheps SG, Roccella EJ. Recommendations for blood pressure measurement in humans and experimental animals: Part 1: Blood pressure measurement in humans: a statement for professionals from the Sub-committee of Professional and Public Education of the American Heart Association Council on High Blood Pressure Research. Hypertension 2005; 45:142-161.
4. Yarows SA, Julius S, Pickering TG. Home blood pressure monitoring. Arch Intern Med 2000; 160:1251–1257.
5. White WB, Anwar YA. Evaluation of the overall efficacy of the Omron office digital blood pressure HEM-907 monitor in adults. Blood Press Monit 2001; 6:107–110.
6. Herpin D, Pickering T, Stergiou G, de Leeuw P, Germano G. Consensus conference on self-blood pressure measurement; clinical applications and diagnosis. Blood Press Monit 2000; 5:131–135.
7. Kikuya M, Chonan K, Imai Y, Goto E, Ishii M. Accuracy and reliability of wrist-cuff devices for self-measurement of blood pressure. J Hypertens 2002; 20:629–638.
8. Ohkubo T, Imai Y, Tsuji I, Nagai K, Kato J, Kikuchi N, Nishiyama A, Aihara A, Sekino M, Kikuya M, Ito S, Satoh H, Hisamichi S. Home blood pressure measurement has a stronger predictive power for mortality than does screening blood pressure measurement: A population-based observation in Ohasama, Japan. J Hypertens 1998; 16:971–975.
9. Aylett M, Marples G, Jones K. Home blood pressure monitoring: its effect on the management of hypertension in general practice. Br J Gen Pract 1999; 49:725–728.

10. Broege PA, James GD, Pickering TG. Management of hypertension in the elderly using home blood pressures. Blood Press Monit 2001; 6:139–144.

11. Leeman MJ, Lins RL, Sternon JE, Huberlant BC, Fassotte CE. Effect of antihypertensive treatment on office and self-measured blood pressure: The Autodil study. J Human Hypertens 2000; 14:525–529.

12. Kjeldsen SE, Hedner T, Jamerson K, Julius S, Haley WE, Zabalgoitia M, Butt AR, Rahman SN, Hansson L. Hypertension optimal treatment (HOT) study: Home blood pressure in treated hypertensive subjects. Hypertension 1998; 31:1014–1020.

13. Stergiou GS, Baibas NM, Gantzarou AP, Skeva II, Kalkana CB, Roussias LG, Mountokalakis TD. Reproducibility of home, ambulatory, and clinic blood pressure: implications for design of trials for the assessment of antihypertensive drug efficacy. Am J Hypertens 2002; 15:101–104.

14. O'Brien E, Beevers G, Lip GYH. ABC of hypertension: Blood pressure measurement: part III—automated sphygmomanometry: ambulatory blood pressure measurement. BMJ 2001; 322:1110–1114.

15. Tunis S, Kendall P, Londner M, Whyte J. Medicare Coverage Policy ~ Decisions: Ambulatory Blood Pressure Monitoring (#CAG-00067N): Decision Memorandum. Washington, DC. Health Care Financing Administration, October 17, 2001. Available at: www.hcfa.gov/coverage/8b3-ff2.htm; accessed 01 APR 02 at 18:32 CST.

16. Staessen JA, Thijs L, Fagard R, O'Brien ET, Clement D, de Leeuw PW, Mancia G, Nachev C, Palatini P, Parati G, Tuomilehto J, Webster J. Predicting cardiovascular risk using conventional versus ambulatory blood pressure in older patients with systolic hypertension. J Am Med Assoc 1999; 282:589–596.

17. Verdeccia P. Prognostic value of ambulatory blood pressure. Hypertension 2000; 35:844–851.

18. Kario K, Pickering TG, Matsuo T, Hoshide S, Schwartz JE, Shimada K. Stroke prognosis and abnormal nocturnal blood pressure falls in older hypertensives. Hypertension 2001; 38:852–857.

19. Bur A, Herkner H, Vlcek M, Woisetschläger C, Derhaschnig U, Hirschl MM. Classification of blood pressure levels by ambulatory blood pressure in hypertension. Hypertension 2002; 40:817–822.

20. Kario K, Pickering TG, Umeda Y, Hoshide S, Hoshide Y, Morinari M, Murata M, Kuroda T, Schwartz JE, Shimada K. Morning surge in blood pressure as a predictor of silent and clinical cerebrovascular disease in elderly hypertensives: a prospective study. Circulation 2003; 107:1401–1406.

21. Clement DL, De Buyzere ML, De Bacquer DA, de Leeuw PW, Duprez DA, Fagard RH, Gheeraert PJ, Missault LH, Braun JJ, Six RO, Van Der Niepen P, O'Brien E. Office versus Ambulatory Pressure Study Investigators. Prognostic value of ambulatory blood-pressure recordings in patients with treated hypertension. N Engl J Med 2003; 348:2407–2415.

22. O'Brien E, Coats A, Owens P, Petrie J, Padfield PL, Littler WA, de Swiet M, Mee F. Use and interpretation of ambulatory blood pressure monitoring: Recommendations of the British Hypertension Society. BMJ 2000; 320:1128–1134.

23. Verdecchia P, Schillaci G, Borgioni C, Ciucci A, Telera MP, Pede S, Gattobigio R, Porcellati C. Adverse prognostic value of a blunted circadian rhythm of heart rate in essential hypertension. J Hypertens 1998; 16:1335–1343.

24. Nakano S, Fukuda M, Hotta F, Ito T, Ishii T, Kitazawa M, Nishizawa M, Kigoshi T, Uchida K. Reversed circadian blood pressure rhythm is associated with occurrence of both fatal and nonfatal vascular events in NIDDM subjects. Diabetes 1998; 47:1501–1506.

25. Verdeccia P, Schillaci G, Reboldi G, Franklin SS, Porcellati C. Different prognostic impact of 24 h mean blood pressure and pulse pressure on stroke and coronary artery disease in essential hypertension. Circulation 2001; 103:2579–2584.

26. Verdecchia P, Reboldi G, Porcellati C, Schillaci G, Pede S, Bentivoglio M, Angeli F, Norgiolini S, Ambrosio G. Risk of cardiovascular disease in relation to achieved office and ambulatory blood pressure control in treated hypertensive subjects. J Am Coll Cardiol 2002; 39:878–885.

27. Liu M, Takahashi H, Morita Y, Maruyama S, Mizuno M, Yuzawa Y, Watanabe M, Toriyama T, Kawahara H, Matsuo S. Non-dipping is a potent predictor of cardiovascular mortality and is associated with autonomic dysfunction in haemodialysis patients. Nephrol Dial Transplant 2003; 18:563–569.

28. Lurbe E, Redon J, Kesani A, Pascual JM, Tacons J, Alvarez V, Batlle D. Increase in nocturnal blood pressure and progression to microalbuminuria in type 1 diabetes. N Engl J Med 2002; 347:797–805.

29. Kario K, Eguchi K, Hoshide S, Hoshide Y, Umeda Y, Mitsuhashi T, Shimada K. U-curve relationship between orthostatic blood pressure change and silent cerebrovascular disease in elderly hypertensives: orthostatic hypertension as a new cardiovascular risk factor. J Am Coll Cardiol 2002; 40:133–141.

30. Redon J, Campos C, Narciso ML, Rodicio JL, Pascual JM, Ruilope LM. Prognostic value of ambulatory blood pressure monitoring in refractory hypertension: a prospective study. Hypertension 1998; 31:712–718.

31. Verdeccia P, Staessen JA, White WB, Imai Y, O'Brien ET. Properly defining white coat hypertension. Eur Heart J 2002; 23:106–109.

32. Bellomo G, Narducci PL, Rondoni F, Pastorelli G, Stangoni G, Angeli G, Verdecchia P. Prognostic value of 24 h blood pressure in pregnancy. J Am Med Assoc 1999; 282:1447–1452.

33. Pierdomenico SD, Bucci A, Constantini F, Lapenna D, Cuccurullo F, Mezzetti A. Twenty-four hour autonomic nervous function in sustained and "white coat" hypertension. Am Heart J 2000; 140:672–677.

34. Palatini P, Mormino P, Santonastaso M, Mos L, Dal FM, Zanata G, Pessina AC. For the HARVEST Study Investigators. Target organ damage in stage 1 hypertensive subjects with white coat and sustained hypertension: Results from the HARVEST Study. Hypertension 1998; 31:57–63.

35. Grandi AM, Broggi R, Colombo S, Santillo R, Imperiale D, Bertolini A, Guasti L, Venco A. Left ventricular changes in isolated office hypertension: a blood pressure-matched comparison with normotension and sustained hypertension. Arch Intern Med 2001; 161:2677–2681.

36. Sega R, Trocino G, Lanzarotti A, Carugo S, Cesana G, Schiavina R, Valagussa F, Bombelli M, Giannattasio C, Zanchetti A, Mancia G. Alterations of cardiac structure in patients with isolated office, ambulatory, or home hypertension: Data from the general population (Pressione Arteriose Monitorate E Loro Associazioni [PAMELA] Study). Circulation 2001; 104:1385–1392.

37. Perloff D, Sokolow M, Cowan RM, Juster RP. Prognostic value of ambulatory blood pressure measurements: further analyses. J Hypertens 1989; 7(suppl 3):S3–S10.

38. Verdeccia P, Schillaci G, Borgioni C, Ciucci A, Porcellati C. White-coat hypertension: not guilty when correctly defined. Blood Press Monit 1998; 3:147–152.

39. Moser M. White-coat hypertension—to treat or not to treat: a clinical dilemma [Editorial]. Arch Intern Med 2001; 161:2655–2656.

40. Verdecchia P, Schillaci G, Borgioni C, Ciucci A, Porcellati C. Prognostic significance of the white coat effect. Hypertension 1997; 29:1218–1224.

41. Liu JE, Roman MJ, Pini R, Schwartz JE, Pickering TG, Devereux RB. Cardiac and arterial target organ damage in adults with elevated ambulatory and normal office blood pressure. Ann Intern Med 1999; 131:564–572.

42. Staessen JA, Gasowski J, Wang JG, Thijs L, Den Hond E, Boissel JP, Coope J, Ekbom T, Gueyffier F, Liu L, Kerlikowske K, Pocock S, Fagard RH. Risks of untreated and treated isolated systolic hypertension in the elderly: meta analysis of outcome trials. Lancet 2000; 355:865–872.

43. Prospective Studies Collaborative. Age-specific relevance of usual blood pressure to vascular mortality: a meta-analysis of individual data for one million adults in 61 prospective studies. Lancet 2002; 360:1903–1913.

44. Wallis EJ, Ramsay LE, Ul Haq I, Ghahramani P, Jackson PR, Rowland-Yeo K, Yeo WW. Coronary and cardiovascular risk estimation for primary prevention: Validation of a new Sheffield table in the 1995 Scottish health survey population. Brit Med J 2000; 320:671–676.

45. Wallis EJ, Ramsay LE, Jackson PR. Cardiovascular and coronary risk estimation in hypertension management. Heart 2002; 88:306–312.

46. Verdecchia P, Schillaci G, Borgioni C, Ciucci A, Gattobigio R, Zampi I, Porcellati C. Prognostic significance of serial changes in left ventricular mass in essential hypertension. Circulation 1998; 97:48–54.

47. Redfield MA, Jacobsen SJ, Burnett JC Jr, Mahoney DW, Bailey KR, Rodeheffer RJ. Burden of systolic and diastolic ventricular dysfunction in the community: appreciating the scope of the heart failure epidemic. J Am Med Assoc 2003; 289:194–202.

48. Yusuf S, Pfeffer MA, Swedberg K, Granger CB, Held P, McMurray JJ, Michelson EL, Olofsson B, Ostergren J. CHARM Investigators and Committees. Effects of candesartan in patients with chronic heart failure and preserved left-ventricular ejection fraction: The CHARM-Preserved trial. Lancet 2003; 362:77–781.

49. Dahlof B, Devereux RB, Kjeldsen SE, Julius S, Beevers G, de Faire U, Fyhrquist F, Ibsen H, Kristiansson K, Lederballe-Pedersen O, Lindholm LH, Nieminen MS, Omvik P, Oparil S, Wedel H. LIFE Study Group. Cardiovascular morbidity and mortality in the Losartan Intervention for Endpoint reduction in hypertension study (LIFE): A randomized trial against atenolol. Lancet 2002; 359:995–1003.

50. Gerstein HC, Mann JF, Yi Q, Zinman B, Dinneen SF, Hoogwerf B, Halle JP, Young J, Rashkow A, Joyce C, Nawaz S, Yusuf S. HOPE Study Investigators. Albuminuria and risk of cardiovascular events, death, and heart failure in diabetic and nondiabetic individuals. J Am Med Assoc 2001; 286:421–426.

51. Asmar RG, London GM, O'Rourke ME, Safar ME, for the REASON Project coordinators and investigators. Improvement in blood pressure, arterial stiffness, and wave reflections with a very-low-dose perindopril/indapamide combination in hypertensive patients: a comparison with atenolol. Hypertension 2001; 38:922–926.

52. Blacher J, Asmar R, Djane S, London GM. Aortic pulse wave velocity as a marker of cardiovascular risk in hypertensive patients. Hypertension 1999; 33:1111–1117.

53. Homocysteine Studies Collaboration. Homocyteine and risk of ischemic heart disease and stroke: a meta-analysis. J Am Med Assoc 2002; 288:2015-2022.

54. Ridker PM, Rifai N, Rose L, Buring JE, Cook NR. Comparison of C-reactive protein and low-density lipoprotein cholesterol levels in the prediction of first cardiovascular events. N Engl J Med 2002; 347:1557–1565.

55. Safian RD, Textor SC. Medical progress: renal-artery stenosis. N Engl J Med 2001; 344:431–442.

56. Krijnen P, van Jaarsveld BC, Steyerberg EW, Man in 't Veld AJ, Schalekamp MA, Habbema JD. A clinical prediction rule for renal artery stenosis. Ann Intern Med 1998; 129:738–740.

57. Bravo EL. Pheochromocytoma. Cardiol Rev 2002; 10:44–50.

58. Pacak K, Linehan WM, Eisenhofer G, Walther MM, Goldstein DS. Recent advances in genetics, diagnosis, localization, and treatment of pheochromocytoma. Ann Intern Med 2001; 134:315–329.

59. Lenders JW, Pacak K, Walther MM, Linehan WM, Mannelli M, Friberg P, Keiser HR, Goldstein DS, Eisenhofer G. Biochemical diagnosis of pheochromocytoma: Which test is best? JAMA 2002; 287:1427–1434.

60. Ganguly A. Primary aldosteronism. N Engl J Med 1998; 339:1828–1834.

61. Stewart PM. Mineralocorticoid hypertension. Lancet 1999; 353:1341–1347.

62. Ghose RP, Hall PM, Bravo EL. Medical management of aldosterone-producing adenomas. Ann Intern Med 1999; 131:105–108.

15

The Heart and Investigation of Cardiac Disease in Hypertension

ROBERT J. MACFADYEN

University Department of Medicine and Department of Cardiology, City Hospital, Birmingham, UK

KEYPOINTS

- Exertional pain, breathlessness, palpitations, presyncope or syncope in hypertensive patients are not sensitive markers of concomitant disease but still require further investigation.

- Rest electrocardiography has a poor sensitivity and specificity for cardiac target organ damage in hypertension. Signal-averaged P wave electrocardiography may indicate structural atrial remodeling.

- Voltage left ventricular hypertrophy (LVH) has a separate prognostic impact from echocardiographic LVH.
- Exercise electrocardiography often yields false positive and false negative results. Pharmacological stress echocardiography is more sensitive and specific for identification of coronary disease in hypertensives.
- Symptoms of exercise limitation mandate assessment of ventricular function by echocardiography or radionuclide ventriculography. Echocardiographic back scatter techniques may differentiate hypertensive changes from those seen in obstructive cardiomyopathy.
- Asymptomatic and symptomatic atrial fibrillation is powerfully linked to LVH and poor blood pressure control.
- QT interval dispersion is commonly linked to mortality. However, there is little evidence of a specific linkage of increased QTd to LVH or sudden death in hypertension.

SUMMARY

The investigation of symptoms attributable to heart disease is a critical aspect of hypertension management. The use of various cardiac technologies to define cardiac structure and function and their clinical utility in hypertension is affected by disease specific processes and multiple clinical associations such as ischaemic stroke; coronary artery disease; atrial fibrillation; and diabetes and obesity.

Simple electrocardiography remains a valid technique yet with reduced sensitivity and specificity for the definition of ischemia or past infarction. It retains a role in defining electrocardiographic ventricular hypertrophy. Both signal averaging technology and ambulatory electrocardiography may be under utilised in hypertension. Exercise electrocardiography maintains a basal role, but where available either stress echocardiography or scintigraphy have better utility and are preferred for the definition of myocardial ischemia. Coronary arteriography retains its pivotal role in the definition and management of epicardial coronary disease. Newer MR and PET techniques for ischemia and functional myocardial assessment are still in evolution alongside screening systems such as electron beam calcification. Hypertension specific application of these technologies is limited. Echocardiography maintains its pivotal role in the cardiovascular risk stratification of hypertension. While this remains outside standard assessment of asymptomatic patients it is critical in symptomatic

subjects where imaging must be integrated with quantified functional exercise capacity.

I. INTRODUCTION

The link among the function of the heart, coronary circulation, and hypertension is intimate. The epidemiologist finds many independent statistical associations in population study between the presence of hypertension and cardiac disease. It comes to the individual physician to take these associations and define the presence of cardiac disease in the individual hypertensive patient. It is widely accepted that controlling hypertension can reduce the relative risk of future cardiac events. In particular, the detailed associations between the hypertension and occlusive coronary artery disease have been highlighted ≥ 30 years (1). In this section, we consider the investigation of many of the well-described aspects of cardiac structure and function associated with hypertension, and how these can be best defined in practice. There are several key areas of cardiac function of importance.

A. Coronary Ischemia

The relationship between coronary disease and hypertension is a complex one. Clearly, the sequence of events starts in the pathology of atherosclerosis and vascular degeneration that in the presence of hypertension will generate accelerated symptomatic and asymptomatic coronary artery disease and both fatal and nonfatal coronary events. As coronary disease does not "cause" hypertension, often the onset of symptomatic coronary disease allows the clinical recognition of hypertension at the same time which may have been present in asymptomatic individual patients for many years previously. Thus, the diagnosis or rather recognition of hypertension has a confounding association with the onset of symptomatic coronary artery disease. In a proportion of cases, death from a fatal first coronary occlusion can occur before hypertension is diagnosed or recognized as a primary factor in the development of coronary atherosclerosis in the index case. This is not a new association (2) and the temporal sequence of these critical events has long been a source of concern (3).

B. Valvular Function

There are clear associations of hypertension with degenerative valvular heart disease and, in particular, with left heart valve function and the aortic valve. As with coronary artery atheroma, the coming together of degenerative change in valve structure along with changes in vascular compliance and structure with an increased pressure after load in the arterial system is well accepted as a detrimental phenomenon.

C. Restrictive Myocardial Changes and Ventricular Hypertrophy

Restrictive cardiac filling abnormalities primarily due to myocardial hypertrophy associated with hypertension are a feature which often confused with cardiac muscle disease; the range of hypertrophic cardiomyopathy in particular or clinically with restrictive changes in the pericardium.

D. Ventricular Function Assessment

Systolic contractility of the left ventricle is of great importance and powerfully defines outcome in hypertensive patients. The evolution of hypertensive heart disease from the state of hypertrophic changes with generally preserved systolic contractility is a complex one through to the phase of ventricular dilatation and systolic impairment. Generally, these patients would tend to have unrecognized, untreated or persistently uncontrolled hypertension and individually the progression is not often recognized. The population association of hypertension to systolic ventricular impairment suggests the presence of such a progressive change regardless of intervening coronary occlusion and infarction.

E. Rhythm Assessment

The primary changes in cardiac structure in hypertensive heart disease are associated with changes in cardiac conduction and instability of cardiac rhythm. These can occur with or without the impact of intervening intermittent cardiac ischemia or prior myocardial infarction (MI). Much of the rhythm instability of hypertensive heart disease is asymptomatic until late in the disease where there are major myocardial changes linked to hypertensive left ventricular hypertrophy. Both resting conduction and ambulatory cardiac rhythm need to be considered.

II. SYMPTOMATIC STATE

A. Symptoms in Hypertensive Patients

- Symptoms in hypertension are not sensitive markers of diagnosis or concomitant disease.
- Concomitant symptoms can represent drug adverse events.
- The emergence of typically cardiac symptoms such as exertional pain or breathlessness; palpitation; and presyncope or syncope require a coherent pattern of targeted investigation.

The investigation of the heart in hypertensive patients starts either at the detection of asymptomatic hypertension at chance screening or on the presentation of linked or unlinked cardiac or general symptoms. The presence of symptomatic complaints among patients with hypertension is commonly the subject of population investigation. These do not often indicate a causal link and separating these on the basis of clinical presentation alone can often be problematic. In the interpretation of cardiac symptoms in hypertensive patients', similar problems apply.

A good example is the association between hypertension and headache. Although the association may be more direct in the case of patients with severe uncontrolled or untreated hypertension, most studies have conclusively shown that mild hypertension and headache are not causally associated. However, this is a frequent association by the patient and some clinicians and such a symptom is due to the presence of hypertension. In a large sample of 1763 hypertensive patients, Fuchs et al. (4) used logistic regression models to explore the association between severity of hypertension and pulse pressure with the presence of headache at the point of diagnosis of hypertension while controlling for the potential confounders. Intermittent headache was present in 903 subjects (51.3% of whole sample) and from these 378 of the patients (21.4%) were classified as having moderate to severe hypertension (stage III of the JNC-VI classification system). However, the diagnosis of moderate to severe hypertension was clearly not independently associated with headache [odds ratio (OR) 1.02, 95% confidence intervals (CI) from 0.79 to 1.30] and arterial pulse pressure and headache were inversely associated (OR 0.91, 95% CI from 0.86 to 0.97, for 10 mmHg).

Many studies are directed at the impact of concomitant drug therapy on the symptomatic state of hypertensive patients. In this regard, the quality of life of untreated patients with hypertension is complex and dealt with elsewhere in the book. However, some symptoms due to treatment are of the orthostatic variety (dizziness, postural light-headedness, and presyncope). Syncope is relatively rare but among those with a documented episode of true syncope hypertension is a common co-morbidity representing around the population prevalence of hypertension at ~25% of patients (5). There are simple biological links among syncope, hypertensive vascular disease, and cardiac function. For example, syncope is common among elderly hypertensive patients with pre-existent or coexistent sinus node disease (6) or carotid sinus disease (7). Furthermore, orthostatic symptoms are more common in patients with white coat hypertension yet normal ambulatory blood pressure and receive treatment. In addition, patients with neuro-degenerative diseases affecting the dentate-rubro-spinothalamic pathways that produce a spectrum of disorders from primary autonomic failure through to more mixed effects characterized by supine hypertension and orthostatic hypotension. The individual composition and origin of blood pressure effects in these often elderly patients can, therefore, be complex and require detailed assessment to define autonomic, arterial vasodilator, or cardiogenic (mostly a vagal dromotropic response) elements (8).

The link between chest pain symptoms and hypertension is probably the most important one for the patient and the clinician. There is a worsening outcome for patients with chest pain who have hypertension and a greater prevalence of coronary disease and, underlying myocardial ischemia as a cause of this symptom. There is a clear-cut profile of elevated risk particularly with an acute symptom onset (9). Yet, symptomatic presentation alone is neither sensitive nor specific enough to define the emergence of coronary disease in the hypertensive patient. This is where the investigational aspects of the diagnostic process become essential. The first tool of assessment is the electrocardiograph (ECG/EKG), which can contain many valuable observations but at the same time is inherently a limited test strategy. Although at one point this may have been the start and end of cardiac assessments in "uncomplicated" hypertension (with or without the obligatory yet largely fruitless chest radiograph), this is now rarely the case.

III. INVESTIGATION OF THE HEART IN HYPERTENSIVE PATIENTS

A. Electrocardiography

- Rest electrocardiography has poor sensitivity and specificity for structural or functional change in hypertension.
- Signal averaged P wave electrocardiography may better indicate structural atrial remodelling in HBP.
- QT dispersion does not necessarily improve on the detection of LVH by voltage criteria.
- Voltage LVH has separate prognostic impact from echocardiographic LVH.
- While the prevalence of electrocardiographic LVH varies with ethnicity, the diagnostic sensitivity and specificity is similar.

B. Ischemia Detection in Hypertension

- The sensitivity nor specificity of rest ECG changes in hypertension does not further degrade the utility of exercise electrocardiography.
- False positive and false negative results make alternative diagnostic imaging studies necessary.

- Pharmacological stress echocardiography (by either dobutamine or Dipyridamole) where available is a more sensitive and specific technique for the definition of clinically significant epicardial coronary disease.

The surface electrocardiograph has been a fundamental part of basic cardiac assessment for over a century. Its utility comes from the ease of use and simplicity. Its value is amplified by repeated recordings made in a consistent fashion and particularly where performed during a symptomatic episode either pain or palpitation or breathlessness. In hypertensive patients as in other patient groups, its primary drawback used at rest, continuously or during exercise stress, has been its relatively low sensitivity (failing to identify disease where this is present) and low specificity (suggesting disease when none is present) to define the common cardiac processes. The key aspects in hypertension are to assess reversible ischemia, evolving infarction, or patterns of cardiac hypertrophy. There is no doubt that recent more sensitive and specific tools which are described here have correctly overshadowed its importance. However, increasing this understanding is not a detriment to use this standard test within its limitations and its routine use in the initial assessment of hypertensive patient, whether symptomatic or not, is likely to continue for many decades.

C. Resting Electrocardiogram

The utility of the baseline electrocardiogram (ECG) has been defined in large population surveys. The prevalence of any electrocardiographic abnormality is increased in patients with hypertension compared with normotensive controls. For example, in 1190 hypertensive patients from the WHO Community Control Program for Hypertension in Italy, a standard 12-lead ECG was recorded for all subjects (10). The overall prevalence of any electrocardiographic abnormalities (i.e., all Minnesota codes) was 40.8% with a slightly higher prevalence in males than in females at 42.4% vs. 39.4%. Electrocardiographic left ventricular hypertrophy (discussed succeedingly) was more frequent in males (21.2%) than in females (14.5%) but not for ECG changes indicative of ischemia (4:1–4:3 or 5:1–5:3). The prevalence of ECG abnormalities increased with age with the exception of electrocardiographic criteria suggestive of left ventricular hypertrophy. Predictably younger males in the age class 20–29 years showed these more often 11.1–17.5% (where these findings may represent a false positive finding) of the subjects compared with the frequency in the oldest age group (60–64 years) which were 15.2% and 12.4%, respectively. These are markedly higher than in normotensive well subjects. The prevalence of electrocardiographic abnormalities is in part due to the high rate of nonspecific false positive results for ischemia, infarction, or hypertrophy.

1. P-Wave Changes in Hypertension

P-wave morphology may reflect, in part, atrial dimensions and structure (11), and can therefore readily be seen as a reasonable point of interest on the surface ECG in hypertension, either in sinus rhythm or in the phase, before persistent atrial fibrillation is established in susceptible hypertensive patients. However, studies in hypertension, in general, show a complex link between P-wave morphology on the rest ECG and cardiac structure.

In several surveys of hypertensive patients, the most frequent rest ECG abnormality is an abnormal P-wave (23%). This compares the much lesser prevalence of abnormal repolarization (10%), increased limb lead or chest lead QRS voltage (5.4%), or one or other patterns of abnormal intraventricular conduction (10%) (12). In general, there is no simple correlation between abnormal P-wave and other ECG abnormalities, although patients with an abnormal P-wave are often shown to have higher systolic blood pressure and heart rate. The electrocardiographic findings are, in general, unresponsive to blood pressure treatment although this may simply be due to lack of sensitivity rather than reflecting underlying structural change.

Genovesiebert et al. (13) from Pisa explored the link between abnormal P-waves and structure in 53 untreated hypertensive patients. Although abnormal P-wave conformation was predictably common in their sample, they could not relate simple P-wave morphology (duration and voltage) to left atrial size as measured by echocardiography. However, they did show some relationship between abnormal P-wave morphology and transmitral Doppler indices of left ventricular filling. Thus in patients with hypertension, they suggest that simple P-wave changes indicative of LA abnormality were perhaps more likely to be indicative of increased left atrial work, possibly secondary to an impaired ventricular filling, rather than due to more simple left atrial enlargement.

In order to further address, this lack of sensitivity of the P-wave in hypertension some investigators have turned to the use signal-averaging technology. This is similar in principle to the technology employed for many years in the assessment of ventricular conduction, defining the presence of after potentials on repeatedly averaged and combined high sensitivity ECG recordings, and linking this to susceptibility to ventricular arrhythmia. In this setting, studying a P-wave signal averaged ECG (P-SAelectrocardiogram) has been analyzed in patients with hypertension. In 234 normotensive, 84 white hypertensive and 34 black hypertensive patients undergoing P-SAelectrocardiogram analysis Madu et al. (14) were able to show that mean filtered P-wave duration and total P-wave time–voltage area for normotensives of either ethnic group were similar. However, hypertensive black patients had greater increase in P-wave duration (138 ± 16 vs. 132 ± 12 ms; $P < 0.01$) and total P-wave time–voltage area (922 ± 285 vs. 764 ± 198 µV ms; $P < 0.001$) than white hypertensives. In addition, the P-wave duration and total P-wave voltage integral increased with severity of hypertension.

Thus, the early stages of hypertension are associated with prolonged atrial conduction as defined using a resting P-SAelectrocardiogram and this index may better reflect the electrical remodeling of the atria. The changes seen in black hypertensive patients seem to be greater than those in white patients with hypertension and may link in with the greater cardiac structural changes seen in hypertension in black patients.

The role of the PR interval as an index of autonomic tone reflecting atrial electrical conduction velocity has been confirmed in hypertensive patients (15). However, the role of this in predicting, for example, the degeneration of sinus rhythm to either atrial fibrillation or atrioventricular block has not been tested prospectively.

2. QT Intervals and QT Dispersion

Heart rate-corrected QT interval is another important and well-studied general ECG marker of ventricular repolarization. It is generally susceptible to the prevailing level of autonomic tone in hypertensive patients. Prior to treatment, a prolonged heart rate-corrected QT interval is associated with higher risk of mortality in patients with coronary heart disease and in the general population. Although unaffected by age, there is possibly a confounding effect of female gender (16) on this measure and as with many ECG measures some ethnic variance among patients of African descent (e.g., African-American or Afro-Caribbean) (17). Xiao et al. (18) in a detailed if small cohort of hypertensive patients with pathological ventricular hypertrophy [14/42 due to the effects of hypertension, the remainder due to atrio ventricular defects (AVD) or hypertropic obstructive cardioyopathy (HOCM)] suggested that QRS duration had a bimodal distribution and correlated with measured mass only if the QRS duration was <135 ms.

The association between QRS duration and ventricular mass was lost above that figure and correlated more with the onset of a proximal left bundle branch block and associated uncoordinated left ventricular activation/ contraction. The presence of electrocardiographic intraventricular conduction delay and broad QRS duration is well documented in patients with hypertension. Although these are often automatically associated with the presence of epicardial coronary artery disease and prior infarction, they have a strong association with hypertension in the absence of coronary artery disease (19) and more often with the effect of echocardiographic ventricular hypertrophy on intra ventricular conduction (20). Thus the interpretation of these findings becomes more complex in separating structural change (hypertrophy) from functional changes (ischemia/infarction or intrinsic conduction disease) both of which coexist in the hypertensive population making conclusions from the individual of reduced value in the hypertensive patient.

QT prolongation in the form of an analysis of the spatial dispersion of the QT interval (QT dispersion, corrected QT dispersion, or QT dispersion index) across the heart (most commonly a simple subtraction of maximal and minimal measured QT interval in millisecond across standard chest ECG leads) is a similar marker of adverse risk in hypertension (21,22), heart failure (23), and coronary disease and even in the general population (24,25). The changes in QT dispersion again appear to track with changes in ventricular hypertrophy in hypertension (being elevated in untreated hypertrophy and at least in part reversed by management of ventricular hypertrophy); in the valvular pressure overload of aortic stenosis and in endurance athletes with exercise related ventricular hypertrophy, the latter group being regarded as physiological (26).

However, QT dispersion indices are not better than simple voltage criteria at detecting ventricular hypertrophy (27). The relationship of variability in QT dispersion as with RR interval may be linked to autonomic tone in hypertension and pathological hypertrophic cardiomyopathy (28). A recent small pilot study (29) has suggested that a minor adjustment to record QT interval to peak voltage, rather than the asymptote of the T-wave and the isoelectric line (a strategy previously well analyzed in clinical pharmacology), might improve the ability of QT interval measures to predict left ventricular hypertrophy. This might deserve closer examination in a larger cohort again mostly due to the cost effectiveness and potential for automation and cut-offs afforded by of simple 12-lead ECG analyses. Similarly, the use of time–voltage area measures for the ventricular complex in hypertension particularly that derived from all 12 leads might also afford better sensitivity for the definition of left ventricular hypertrophy from the simple ECG (30).

3. The Definition of Ventricular Hypertrophy Using Electrocardiography in Hypertension

The electrocardiographic definition of ventricular hypertrophy has been well established for many decades and examined closely in population studies because of its ease of use, albeit with varied criteria (31). The patterns seen in hypertensive patients are not easily nor reliably distinguished from patients with coronary artery disease on the basis of the ECG appearance alone. This can be readily appreciated from studies completed in patients who show normal coronary angiographic imaging but marked left ventricular hypertrophy and strain patterns on the rest ECG (32). Notwithstanding this difficulty in interpretation, there is no doubt about the link between electrocardiographic left ventricular hypertrophy and future vascular events in hypertensive patients (33).

Electrocardiographic left ventricular hypertrophy as defined by the most widely used criteria (those of Sokolow Lyon = SV1 + RV5 or RV6 ≥ 35 mm) have been reliably and independently related to untreated clinic blood pressure levels, male gender and Afro-Caribbean racial origin and inversely associated with body mass index (34).

It is accepted that echocardiography and the rest ECG simply give different information with respect to the presence of left ventricular hypertrophy and that their diagnostic reliability (sensitivity and specificity) can be different, whether they are positive or negative. It is clear that ECG defined left ventricular hypertrophy is significantly less sensitive than echocardiographic assessment of left ventricular mass (35) and is also prone to being less specific particularly in younger patients and in nonwhite patients (where false positive results are more common) (36). Just as body fat is associated with high electrical resistance, obesity markedly confounds the accuracy of surface ECG voltage and limits the ability of voltage-based criteria to reliably identify left ventricular hypertrophy (37). A lack of specificity can be particularly problematic where a blood pressure treatment decision is being made on the basis of elevated clinic blood pressure readings and electrocardiographic left ventricular hypertrophy is taken as the sole confirmation of end organ damage.

The prevalence of ECG-left ventricular hypertrophy may be upto six times higher in African-American patients with hypertension than in white patients, depending on the criteria used (given a range of 6–24% in blacks vs. 1–7% in whites). However, this observation is due in part to a lack of specificity as the difference in the prevalence of echocardiographic left ventricular hypertrophy is less striking (26% in blacks and 20% in whites; $P > 0.2$). The sensitivity of the rest ECG is generally low (range, 3–17%) and does not differ significantly between African-Americans and whites for any conventional criteria (Sokolow Lyon; Cornell adjusted score). Specificity is lower in blacks for all criteria (range, 73–94% vs. 95–100% for whites; $P = 0.0001$ to 0.09). The predictive value of an ECG positive for left ventricular hypertrophy is therefore consistently lower in black subjects even outside the USA (38). Black ethnic groups are associated with the strongest independent predictor of decreased ECG specificity in multiple logistic regression analysis considering age, gender, body mass index, left ventricular mass index, and smoking (35).

Recent observations from another UK cohort suggest that the apparent differences in electrocardiographic voltage and the prevalence of left ventricular hypertrophy between ethnic groups may be dependent on the ECG-left ventricular hypertrophy criteria chosen and may simply be secondary to differences in body mass index (39). Unlike Afro-Caribbean patients, South Asians (those of Indian subcontinent origin) do not apparently demonstrate significant differences in ECG voltage compared with Caucasians.

Several attempts have been made to adjust the criteria used to define left ventricular hypertrophy on the basis of rest electrocardiography by modifying the voltage criteria (40) to account for the impact of obesity (41) and/or age (42). In general, these often help improve sensitivity but often leave unacceptably low rates particularly in the elderly and in females. In the CASTEL study of 447 subjects (all of whom shared perfect echocardiography) the sensitivity, specificity, positive and negative predictive value of the most commonly used ECG tests of left ventricular hypertrophy were calculated and compared. All ECG calculations had a very low sensitivity in the elderly (43). Furthermore, except for the Cornell index and the Minnesota code, they were unable to demonstrate the higher prevalence of echocardiographic left ventricular hypertrophy in elderly females in comparison with males. The predictive value of the rest ECG for echo left ventricular hypertrophy appears consistently better in elderly males than females whether negative or positive. Some criteria were more predictive in males, some in females, and in others, equally predictive in both sexes. Overall, these authors felt that the rest ECG, however, a voltage left ventricular hypertrophy calculation is derived is not a reliable method for screening left ventricular hypertrophy in the elderly.

D. Exercise-Based Studies in Hypertensive Patients

Exercise protocols using either step testing, shuttle walking, upright or supine bicycle exercise, or a variety of treadmill-based structures is generally used in many cardiovascular testing protocols. In the hypertensive population, diagnostic exercise stress testing gives information from both the blood pressure and the electrocardiographic aspects of the response to exercise.

The cardiac prognostic significance of exercise blood pressure rise in the hypertensive population has been recognized for some time (44). Blood pressure measurements of course form part of any routine diagnostic exercise testing protocol. Simplified submaximal exercises testing using step tests have been tested in the assessment of hypertensive patients (45). These have the value of added safety where blood pressure overshoot may cause anxiety for patients or technicians supervising tests and appear to have some value showing associations with the presence of endothelial dysfunction (46), predicting levels of ambulatory blood pressure (47), and predicts maximal QT interval dispersion on the rest ECG (discussed earlier) although not left ventricular mass (48). In contrast in a small study of maximal treadmill exercise testing Gottdeiner et al. (49) in Washington in normotensive male subjects suggested that they could demonstrate a correlation between echocardiographic left ventricular mass and a blood pressure over shoot on exercise testing (defined as measured systolic blood pressure >210 mmHg). All these studies suggest a pathological significance to exercise blood pressure loads for the heart in hypertension or pre-hypertensive states and underlines the general utility of exercise-based protocols in the hypertensive population.

However, with respect to the definition of myocardial ischemia in unselected subjects with a blood pressure overshoot during the performance of a maximal exercise perfusion scintigram, Campbell et al. (50) found their subjects with blood pressure over shoot (peak systolic blood pressure ≥ 210 mmHg in men and ≥ 190 mmHg in women) are less likely to have a scintigraphic perfusion defect (transient, fixed, or reversible). Moreover, during 6 years of prospective follow-up, they were able to analyze 283 deaths and in this subset and could find no association between the exercise blood pressure overshoot and any mortality risk. Thus, they felt their larger study suggested that exercise induced blood pressure rises were associated with a lower likelihood of myocardial perfusion abnormalities and thus were not associated with any increased mortality rate.

The limitations of exercise stress electrocardiography for the definition of myocardial ischemia in unselected patients are well recognized and like the rest ECG is summarized by a generally low sensitivity (false negative rates of >30%) and low specificity (false positive rates of >30%) in groups such as the elderly; women and patients with diabetes. An ability to exercise fully is essential although there may be some value in submaximal testing (discussed earlier). Although there is an additional value in other aspects of exercise testing such as the definition of work achieved, heart rate and blood pressure response are the key issues for most subjects, as is the electrocardiographic response, and whether this is indicative of ischemia.

In the hypertensive patient, the presence of electrocardiographic changes at rest (the strain pattern) would be expected to influence the predictive capacity of an exercise test. However, in testing this Marwick et al. (51) recently saw little impact (either positive or negative) on the sensitivity of exercise electrocardiography although specificity was slightly reduced in the presence of ventricular hypertrophy (74% vs. 69%) in a group of 68 hypertensive patients.

Given the frequency of normal epicardial coronary angiographic studies in patients with a positive noninvasive test for ischemia, it is often suggested that hypertension by its association with a poor coronary flow reserve (independent of epicardial coronary artery disease), left ventricular hypertrophy and possibly microvascular disease, would indicate that different diagnostic strategies are required to define tissue ischemia in these patients as compared to epicardial flow limiting stenoses (52). Although stress-induced (physical; mental, or pharmacological) cardiac wall motion abnormalities (e.g., detected at echocardiography) are generally highly specific for angiographic epicardial coronary artery disease, ST segment depression and/or scintigraphic myocardial perfusion abnormalities are often found in the presence of angiographically normal coronary arteries where there is coexistent hypertensive left ventricular hypertrophy or microvascular disease.

The value of exercise stress electrocardiography in hypertensive patients has been portrayed by some as its negative predictive value, which is at least comparable in both normotensive and hypertensive patients. That is where the test is negative for inducible ischemia it reliably defines an absence of epicardial coronary disease. Unfortunately, the overall negative predictive value of exercise electrocardiography in hypertensive patients is poor providing false negative rates in the region of 50% (low sensitivity) even if there is effective blood pressure control (53). Thus, whether exercise-electrocardiography stress test is positive or negative, uninterpretable or ambiguous, generally another imaging stress test is warranted if there is a genuine high level of clinical suspicion of coronary artery disease to reliably identify significant flow limiting epicardial coronary disease and to allow ischemia-guided revascularization.

E.   Continuous Ambulatory Electrocardiogram Studies in the Definition of Ischemia in Hypertension

Despite its general utility in the definition of ambulatory ischemia (54), continuous ST segment monitoring has not been studied greatly in the assessment of patients with hypertension. Pringle et al. (55) have produced the most significant contribution in reporting a detailed assessment of 90 hypertensive patients with left ventricular hypertrophy and abnormal 48 h ambulatory ECG studies suggestive of ischemia. From 68 men and 22 women (mean age 57, range 25–79 years) they completed 48 h ambulatory ST segment monitoring (in all patients), and additional exercise electrocardiography ($n = 79$), stress thallium scintigraphy ($n = 80$), coronary arteriography ($n = 35$) to finalize diagnoses. They found that 48% of their sample (43 patients) had at least one episode of ST segment depression on ambulatory electrocardiographic

monitoring. These were frequent (median number of episodes 16, range 1–84), protracted (median duration of 8.6, range 2–17 min) but in the vast majority asymptomatic. Twenty-six of the patients went on to show positive exercise electrocardiography and 48 patients showed reversible stress thallium perfusion defects despite chest pain having occurred in only five of the patients during exercise. Eighteen of the 35 patients (20%) who progressed to coronary arteriography had clinically significant epicardial coronary artery disease. Of these, seven had given no history of chest pain at any time. Thus, symptomatic and asymptomatic myocardial ischemia were shown to be common in hypertensive patients with left ventricular hypertrophy, even in the absence of epicardial coronary artery disease. These patients could be reliably detected on Holter monitoring and continuous ECG analysis; yet this remains a poorly applied, simple and effective technique in the routine assessment of hypertensive patients.

Similar studies by Asmar et al. (56) in Paris on unselected hypertensive patients looking for ambulatory ischemic change as defined by electrocardiographic criteria (a horizontal or down sloping ST depression (>1 mm and >60 s)) found ST-segment depression together with concomitant blood pressure (blood pressure) and heart rate variations to be common and follow a diurnal variation. In 100 hypertensive patients (male:female ratio $= 1:1$) 23 patients (15 men and 8 women) had 72 episodes of ST depression with two peaks: on awakening and in the late afternoon periods. The mean ambulatory blood pressure load was greater in the patients with ST-segment depression than without for both systolic and diastolic blood pressure (135 ± 14 vs. 129 ± 15 and 84 ± 8 vs. 79 ± 10 mmHg, respectively; $P < 0.01$), plasma glucose (5.83 ± 0.70 vs. 5.46 ± 0.71 mmol/L; $P = 0.04$), and self-rated work-related stress levels (22% vs. 13%; $P = 0.03$) were also higher in patients with ambulatory ST-segment depression regardless of symptoms suggestive of ischemia. There was no difference between the patient groups with or without ambulatory electrocardiographic ischemia on the basis of clinical parameters, left ventricular mass index, and other general cardiovascular risk factors (gender, smoking, lipids, etc.). Thus, this group also found 24 h ambulatory electrocardiographic monitoring to have utility even in unselected hypertensive patients. They suggested that those hypertensive patients showing ambulatory ST depression episodes had a higher ambulatory blood pressure load. Thus, by this technology, electrocardiographic ischemia was common regardless of symptoms or the presence of left ventricular hypertrophy. Finally, Siegel et al. (57) studied the role of diuretic induced potassium depletion in affecting the diagnostic utility of ambulatory ECG studies in 186 male subjects. They treated their patients to ensure repletion of potassium following control of blood pressure using diuretic therapy. Siegel, found a 27% prevalence of silent ambulatory ST segment depression compatible with ischemia. The episodes followed a similar pattern to that seen by both Asmar and Pringle with peaks in the early morning hours between 0000 h (mid-night) and 0600 h (6:00 am).

Thus, ambulatory ECG studies are distinct from rest or exercise studies in the hypertensive population and have a better profile in the assessment of both symptomatic or asymptomatic hypertensive patients regardless of the presence of either electrocardiographic or echocardiographic left ventricular hypertrophy. Why such simple and reliable technology remains poorly applied in the routine assessment of hypertensive patients is unclear, but this may simply relate to the time and effort required to complete such a detailed analysis.

F. Stress Myocardial Perfusion Studies

As stated earlier, a positive exercise electrocardiography test has a low diagnostic specificity in hypertensive patients with or without rest changes and warrants a complementary imaging test to further explore the diagnosis of coronary artery disease. As an initial investigation to supplement symptomatic clinical assessment, nuclear cardiac studies are generally accepted as more sensitive and specific than exercise electrocardiography in the definition of significant epicardial coronary artery disease.

Symptom limited bicycle exercise stress test in conjunction with either 99mTc technetium, sestamibi, or tetrofosmin single photon emission computed tomography (SPECT) imaging provides similar levels of diagnostic accuracy; sensitivity and specificity whether or not the patient is normotensive or hypertensive for the detection of fixed or reversible perfusion defects (58). Abnormal cardiac function in patients with positive exercise electrocardiography and normal coronary angiography is well recognized and hypertension is a common finding (59). However, neither the presence of hypertension *per se* nor hypertensive left ventricular hypertrophy (60) in the absence of coronary disease appears to increase the prevalence of perfusion abnormalities for a given level of cardiovascular risk (61).

Generally, comparative studies in hypertension show that the sensitivity of pharmacological stress perfusion is greater than that achieved by exercise electrocardiography, and result specificity is also improved (62). The features of a false positive test (a perfusion study suggesting ischemia still with a normal coronary angiography) may relate to the presence of small vessel coronary disease visualized as a slow angiographic run off. The optimal agent to provide either flow/vasodilator or rate stress or the best perfusion tracer are not specifically identified for the assessment of hypertensive patients.

G. Stress Echocardiography

In some studies of patients with hypertension, there is evidence to suggest that the incidence of coronary artery disease can be overestimated by both stress electrocardiography and stress perfusion scintigraphy because of false-positive results (symptomatic patients who have test results suggestive of epicardial coronary disease and yet have unequivocally normal coronary angiography). Stress echocardiography has been suggested to be a more sensitive and specific technique than the earlier testing modalities.

This strategy is particularly useful in patients who have limited exercise capacity or in those who cannot (or will not) reach adequate levels of exercise stress to achieve a diagnostic outcome. This technique is clearly more operator dependent than electrocardiography or nuclear scintigraphy and is influenced by the echocardiographic image quality of the patient studied. A similar range of techniques to those used in scintigraphy can be used to place the heart under stress. The key differences are that imaging is generally completed at baseline and immediately after completion of physical exercise and that no graded assessments during exercise are generally possible. The exercise protocols are generally similar to those familiar in exercise electrocardiography. Pharmacological stress commonly using dobutamine (with or without atropine); adenosine; dipyridamole or a range of less commonly used agents has advantages in that patients are not physically moving and graded imaging can be completed during the infusion protocol.

The endpoint of analysis is the detection of stress induced reversible wall motion impairment of contractility. Segmental wall motion analysis allows broad anatomical location of the ischemic response and the definition of these wall motion abnormalities has prognostic significance in terms of subsequent coronary events. Thus, anterior/LAD abnormalities are associated with a significantly increased risk of cardiac death and nonfatal MI. This added prognostic risk of events is independent of the resting left ventricular ejection fraction and the perceived extent of wall motion abnormalities identified during stress echocardiography in hypertension (63).

Echocardiographic imaging is normally acquired by the transthoracic route but can also be completed by the transoesophageal route where either a direct pacing stress or pharmacological stress can be employed with reasonable comparability to pharmacological transthoracic stress echocardiography (64). While pharmacological stress is generally preferred to minimize motion artefact during echocardiography, this is associated with some adverse effects and in early studies safety was an issue particularly for hypertensive patients where an abrupt pressor response is more often seen during pharmacological stress protocols (65,66). As with exercise electrocardiography, there are composite endpoints for the test including symptoms; concomitant electrocardiographic changes and most centrally the definition of reversible regional wall motion abnormalities suggestive of flow limiting myocardial ischemia.

Using an exercise echo technique in hypertensive patients without electrocardiographic left ventricular hypertrophy who had already undergone coronary angiography, Senior et al. (67) from Northwick Park Hospital could show improved sensitivity and specificity even in a relatively small sample of 43 patients of which only 29 had coronary disease. Maltagliati et al. (53) tested the role of exercise echocardiography as an alternative to exercise electrocardiography for coronary artery disease detection in hypertension, before and after adequate blood pressure control. In a parallel group, case–control comparison of 59 hypertensive and normotensive patients undergoing coronary angiography for chest pain, they used upright bicycle exercise ECG and post exercise stress echocardiographic tests in each group. The hypertensive patients had a further test after blood pressure control (in this study using sublingual nifedipine). Coronary artery disease (defined as >1 angiographic lumenal narrowing >50%) was found in 22 hypertensive and 41 normotensive patients. The sensitivity, specificity, and diagnostic accuracy of the two techniques were not statistically different (95%, 94%, and 94%) in hypertensives or (82%, 77%, and 83%) normotensives, but were significantly better than for the exercise ECG test (68%, 70%, and 69%). Blood pressure lowering had little impact on exercise echocardiography slightly decreasing sensitivity (91%), whereas the sensitivity of exercise ECG decreased even more markedly (45%).

In 1164 hypertensive patients, Elhendy et al. (68) from Rotterdam demonstrated the hemodynamic profile, safety, and feasibility of Dobutamine (up to 40 μg/kg per min)-atropine (up to 1 mg) stress echocardiography in patients with "limited exercise capacity" (age, 60 ± 12 years; 761 men). In this large overall study, 446 of the patients were known to have hypertension. Using an 85% of the maximal heart rate cutoff and/or an ischemic end point (new or worsened wall motion abnormalities, ST segment depression, or angina) was achieved. They saw no procedure related MIs or deaths in their sample. Predictably, dobutamine induced a significant increase of heart rate in patients with and without hypertension (59 ± 25 and 63 ± 23 beats per minute, respectively). A hypotensive response (>40 mmHg systolic blood pressure drop) was more frequent in older hypertensive patients with higher baseline blood pressure treated with calcium channel blockers (7% vs. 4%). Protocol related ventricular tachycardia was not infrequent but similar (4.1%) in both normotensive or hypertensive patients and terminated

promptly by intravenous metoprolol administration. This form of testing proved feasible in 91% of patients with and 92% of patients without hypertension. Reasonably, they concluded this technology was safe, effective, and reliable in the assessment of hypertensive patients where evaluation for myocardial ischemia was indicated.

Perfusion imaging has been directly compared with stress echocardiography in other reports. Astarita et al. (69) studies 53 patients with hypertension ($n = 53$), (29 males, aged 58 ± 10 years) and normal left ventricular function with a positive exercise test and further investigated these patients with dipyridamole–atropine stress echocardiography (DASE) and thallium-201 stress/rest myocardial SPECT. All patients had additional coronary angiography. Coronary angiography revealed >50% epicardial coronary artery disease in 23 of the 53 patients (43%). Sensitivity for the detection of coronary artery disease was significantly higher for perfusion scintigraphy compared with echocardiography (DASE = 78% vs. SPECT = 100%, $P < 0.05$) whereas specificity was higher for echo (DASE = 100% vs. SPECT = 47%, $P < 0.00001$). Diagnostic accuracy was also higher for echo (DASE = 91% vs. SPECT = 70%, $P < 0.01$). Thus, this group felt that in the further assessment of hypertensive patients with exercise-induced ST segment depression, as both dipyridamole/atropine stress echo and SPECT perfusion scintigraphy were good diagnostic options, dobutamine–atropine stress echo was characterized by a higher specificity but slightly lower sensitivity than stress perfusion SPECT.

In a later and equally useful comparative study, Elhendy et al. (68) compared their pharmacological stress echocardiography protocol with stress perfusion scintigraphy (by a sestamibi SPECT protocol) in hypertensive patients with or without left ventricular hypertrophy where the presence of coronary stenoses at angiography was defined as more than one >50% lesion. From a total of 88 patients in whom epicardial coronary disease was defined in 66 of these two techniques were largely comparable without statistically significant differences in sensitivity or specificity. Both techniques appeared to lack sensitivity compared with an angiographic standard (63% and 51%, respectively, for echocardiography and scintigraphy). The presence of echocardiographic left ventricular hypertrophy had no impact on either technique.

Dipyridamole echocardiography has similar value in the assessment of hypertensive patients with undiagnosed chest pain symptoms and can give reliable prognostic information. In a relatively small prospective study of 257 hypertensive patients with chest pain (110 men, age 63 ± 9 years), Cortigiani et al. (70) had no major complications with a stepped dipyridamole infusion protocol successfully completed in 98% of symptomatic hypertensive patients. A positive echocardiographic response suggestive of ischemia was found in 72 patients (27 during the low-dose (≤ 0.56 mg/kg) and 45 during the high-dose (> 0.56 mg/kg)) dipyridamole infusion. During follow-up (32 ± 18 months), 27 cardiac events occurred: 3 deaths, 8 infarctions, and 16 cases of unstable angina and 27 patients underwent coronary revascularization. At multivariate analysis, the positive echocardiographic result (OR, 5.5; 95% CI, 1.4–16.6) was the only predictor of cardiac events (death and infarction). A positive stress echocardiographic study (OR, 4.2; 95% CI, 1.8–9.6) and family history of coronary artery disease (OR, 4.2; 95% CI, 1.5–6.9) were both independently associated with prognosis. The 5 year survival rates for the negative and the positive populations were, respectively, 97% and 87% ($P = 0.0019$) for cardiac events. In a more recent study, these same workers assessed the relative value of dipyridamole stress echo or exercise electrocardiography in patients with right bundle branch block and hypertension (35) or normal blood pressure (36). They found less concordance of testing in hypertension (69% cf. 92%) compared with the normotensive patients, although overall sensitivity was similar. The accuracy, positive and negative predictive value was much higher with dipyridamole stress echocardiography (66%, 61%, and 75% for exercise electrocardiography, and 86%, 87%, and 84% for stress echo) (71).

However, this comparability of performance was not found in a further study in 101 patients with hypertension, chest pain, and positive exercise EGG by Fragasso (72) completed in Milan. Using stress/rest SPECT with 99mTc-MIBI, dipyridamole and dobutamine stress echocardiography and coronary angiography in hypertensive patients all of whom had normal global ventricular function (57 had left ventricular hypertrophy). They observed no side-effects during perfusion scintigraphy but dose-limiting side-effects in 5 patients during dipyridamole and 7 patients during dobutamine stress echo. The sensitivity, specificity, accuracy, positive and negative predictive values for angiographic coronary disease were, respectively, 98%, 36%, 71%, 67%, and 94% for perfusion scintigraphy, 61%, 91%, 74%, 90%, and 64% for dipyridamole, and 88%, 80%, 84%, 85%, and 83% for dobutamine stress echocardiography. Thus, dipyridamole performed less well in this series than dobutamine stress applied to symptomatic hypertensive patients.

Marwick et al. (73) have completed and published an important stepwise analytical approach to define the added value of stress echocardiographic assessment from a large study of 2363 hypertensive patients followed up for 10 years. They found that while the majority of their cohort had normal studies (63%), ischemia identified by stress echocardiography independently predicted mortality in those able to complete an treadmill exercise echo protocol (hazard ratio (HR) 2.21; 95% CI, 1.10–4.43,

$P = 0.0001$) as well as those undergoing dobutamine echo (HR, 2.39; 95% CI, 1.53–3.75, $P = 0.0001$). The other major predictors of events were age, the presence of resting left ventricular systolic dysfunction, heart failure symptoms, and the Duke treadmill score. Using a stepwise model to replicate the sequence of clinical evaluation (applied after exercise electrocardiography), stress echocardiography added prognostic power to models based on clinical and stress-testing variables. Thus, they suggested that stress echocardiography (exercise or pharmacological) were an independent predictor of cardiac death in hypertensive patients with known or suspected coronary artery disease incremental to clinical risks and exercise results alone.

If conduction defects are present, these influence interpretation of stress echocardiography, making not quite so straightforward as with stress perfusion scintigraphy. Hypertensive patients with conduction defects undergoing stress echocardiography that do not have studies indicative of ischemia have little excess mortality. However, the combination of RBBB and anterior hemi-block has been associated with adverse outcomes even where the study does not suggest coronary ischemia is present (74). Yuda et al. (75) in a small sample of 161 hypertensive patients stratified on the basis of ventricular geometry have suggested that the accuracy of dobutamine stress echocardiography is reduced in patients with concentric remodeling (61%) compared with hypertensive patients with normal geometry (85%, $P < 0.05$) or concentric hypertrophy (86%, $P < 0.05$). Accuracy with eccentric hypertrophy (64%, $P < 0.05$) was lower than with concentric hypertrophy and similar to that found with concentric remodeling.

Patients with chest pain symptoms and completely normal angiography often remain symptomatic and cause concern. However, Zouridakis et al. (76) in London examined 33 such patients with exertional anginal chest pain, a positive exercise stress ECG, and a completely normal coronary arteriogram. They were often hypertensive (17) and female (14) and relatively young. Conducting ambulatory ECG monitoring, dobutamine stress echocardiography; and thallium-201 SPECT, they found that all patients had normal left ventricular systolic function at rest and none fulfilled echocardiographic criteria for left ventricular hypertrophy. Eight of the normotensive patients and ten of the hypertensive patients had perfusion abnormalities on thallium SPECT ($P = 0.61$). As dobutamine infusion reproduced anginal pain and ST segment changes in some patients, none developed regional wall motion abnormalities indicative of ischemia. They concluded that the high prevalence of scintigraphic perfusion defects in both normotensive and hypertensive groups were in fact false positive results or less likely that dobutamine stress echocardiography is insensitive to ischemia caused by microvascular dysfunction.

H. Coronary Angiography

Coronary angiography is frequently performed in patients with hypertension caused by the presence of equivocal or positive noninvasive testing for myocardial ischemia to define the nature of epicardial coronary flow. It is particularly appropriate in hypertension where the implications of the presence (or indeed absence) of epicardial coronary disease are prognostically important.

Although the appearance at angiography is not equivalent to the absence of subintimal coronary atherosclerosis nor indeed a guarantee of no future coronary disease, there is general agreement that the presence of unequivocally normal coronary arteries is a useful and good prognostic indicator even in the presence of hypertension and/or hypertensive left ventricular hypertrophy (77). Even though the morbidity of patients remains high [many have symptoms of chest pain both typical and atypical of inducible ischemia), mortality (in the absence of a documented MI at any point (78)] is consistently low.

The prognostic significance of nonobstructive coronary disease seen at coronary angiography in hypertensive patients is less easy to predict. In unselected patients with noncritical lesions do have significantly lower (albeit only slightly) 10-year survival rates (85.8%) than those with normal coronary arteries (90.1%). The difference in survival rate in population studies of nonobstructive coronary atheroma detected at angiography is generally attributed to more advanced age, frequent male gender and higher prevalence of cigarette smoking, diabetes mellitus, and most significantly, hypertension. However, the presence of noncritical coronary stenoses is not a statistically significant independent determinant of survival. Long-term survival rates of the patients with one or more critical lesions were equivalent to that of patients with critical stenoses plus one or more noncritical lesions (79).

De Cesare et al. (80) in a relatively small comparative case control study in 320 patients with a positive treadmill exercise test with and 320 without hypertension showed that only in the sixth and seventh decade did the patients with hypertension have a greater prevalence of triple vessel coronary disease (40% and 50% cf. 25% and 31%) than the normotensive comparator group. This appeared unrelated to standard cardiovascular risk factor distribution (age, gender, smoking, lipids, etc.) demographics.

I. Vascular Calcification and Electron Beam Studies in High Blood Pressure

In the last 10 years, the longstanding association of vascular calcification with the process of endo-lumenal stenoses

(81) has been explored using the developing technology of noninvasive electron beam tomography. The measurements have been applied to a variety of sites but the most relevant to the heart of the hypertensive patient is on the assessment of the calcification occurring in association with the coronary circulation (CAC). The improving resolution and data interpretation of this noninvasive technology gives the technique (to some) future potential. It has been suggested to provide independent predictive information on vascular occlusive event rates at least over and above that provided by a traditional demographic cardiovascular risk factor analysis (82).

Although the technique appears to show an independent relationship to the severity of coronary stenosis, there are associations with age, hyperlipidaemia, diabetes, smoking status, and gender. African-American ethnicity and interestingly hypertension do not appear to link coronary disease well with the appearance of coronary calcification using electron beam computed tomography (EBCT) (83). However, in the largest study so far of 30,908 asymptomatic individuals undergoing EBCT, report that for both men and women, all conventional risk factors (including hypertension) were significantly associated with the presence of any detectable CAC and the mean CAC score increased in proportion to the number of coronary artery disease risk factors. In age-adjusted (multivariable) logistic regression analysis, cigarette use, histories of hypercholesterolaemia, diabetes, and hypertension were each significantly associated with mild to extensive CAC scores (≥ 10.0). Thus, they felt that coronary artery calcification scores were associated with presumed higher atherosclerotic plaque burden in both men and women.

In a relatively small early one-to-one case-control study, Megnien et al. (84) did find a relationship of the extent of coronary calcification scoring to the duration of high blood pressure in a sample of 73 male hypertensive patients. However, they found no link with the extent of blood pressure elevation in this cohort. They did show a weak link of CAC scores to age that was demonstrable in other reports at that time in asymptomatic normotensive subjects (81). However, at angiography in subjects with diagnosed coronary artery disease, hypertension is less strongly linked to the extent of coronary calcification or stenosis scoring at angiography, than other conventional atherosclerosis risk factors in some studies (85) and not in others (86).

Turner et al. (87) in Minnesota have recently re-examined the relationship of blood pressure to coronary calcification in a sample of 298 hypertensive patients (male and female) using repeated blood pressure measures in the form of ambulatory blood pressure recordings. In this analysis, they were able to demonstrate a link between ambulatory diastolic blood pressure and CAC scoring. More recently, in a logistic regression analysis of CAC in the presence of hypertensive left ventricular hypertrophy, Altunkan et al. (88) have suggested that body mass index and age were the main independent factors affecting the presence and amount of coronary calcification in patients with left ventricular hypertrophy.

IV. CARDIAC STRUCTURE AND FUNCTION IN HYPERTENSION

A. Assessment of Cardiac Structure and Function in Hypertension

- Systolic ventricular function assessment requires mandatory direct imaging by echocardiography or radionuclide ventriculography in hypertensive patients with symptoms of exercise limitation.
- Echocardiographic abnormalities of diastolic filling in hypertension require careful integration with ventricular composition and structure before concluding symptoms are due to diastolic heart failure.
- Echocardiographic back scatter techniques may differentiate hypertensive changes from those seen in obstructive cardiomyopathy.

Aspects of cardiac structure and function that are most relevant in hypertension are valvular, ventricular, and contractile function.

B. Valvular Associations and Hypertension

There are known associations between cardiac valvular dysfunction and hypertension. Several are confounded by the presence of concomitant disease. For example, secondary valvular dysfunction following ischemia or infarction with or without dilatation of the heart would be a well-accepted but separate pathological process. Left heart valvular function has received the most attention in hypertensive patients.

The coexistence of hypertension and stenosis of the aortic valve is well recognized and a common clinical association in surveys of symptomatic aortic stenosis (32% of symptomatic cases of aortic stenosis in some series (89)). It is readily defined in population surveys of patients who come forward for valve replacement surgery. Recent figures suggesting that hypertension is coexistent in 21% of patients with any grade of aortic stenosis and alternately that aortic stenosis affects 1.1% of hypertensive patients (90). Theoretically, there is a simple hypothesis to link the increased valve shear stress caused by hypertension as a possible mediator or at the very least an accelerating factor in the development of aortic valve stenosis. However, the exact inter-relationship of these two conditions is less clear-cut.

Degenerative aortic valve disease is common in the elderly where hypertension is equally more prevalent. For example, in the 5201 subjects over 65 years enrolled in the Cardiovascular Health Study, echocardiographic aortic valve sclerosis was evident in 26% and aortic valve stenosis in 2% of subjects. In those over 75 years, the prevalence of aortic sclerosis rose to 37% and aortic stenosis rose slightly to 2.6%. On multiple logistic regression analysis, the independent predictors of this change included age (twofold increased risk for each 10 year increase in age), male gender (twofold excess risk), smoking (35% increase in risk), and a history of hypertension (20% increase in risk) (91). However, despite this association, hypertension does not independently influence the natural course of aortic valve disease (92). Although a higher left ventricular outflow tract velocity, common in hypertension (93), is associated with more rapid degeneration in aortic valvular stenosis it is not a statistically independent predictor of progression (94). Studies in patients with the two conditions are not frequent, but recent reports suggest that although there are no significant differences between hypertensive and normotensive aortic stenosis patients with respect to age, gender, symptom class, ventricular function, or remodeling patterns in hypertensive patients, symptoms present with larger aortic valve areas and lower stroke work (89). This may be because of the additional overload due to hypertension.

Data on the spontaneous detection of echocardiographic valvular regurgitation, in general, is not extensive and that with respect to associations with arterial hypertension is scant. However, in the normal population, the presence of regurgitation at the mitral position has been shown to have a weak association with coexistent hypertension in the Framingham longitudinal cardiovascular follow-up project. In 1696 men and 1893 women who had acceptable echocardiographic imaging, a multiple logistic regression analysis defined the association of clinical variables to mitral regurgitation or tricuspid regurgitation (more than or equal to mild severity) and aortic regurgitation (AR) (more than or equal to trace severity). Mitral regurgitation of more than mild severity was seen in 19.0% of men and 19.1% of women, with AR of more than or equal to trace severity in 13.0% of men and 8.5% of women. On statistical testing, the demographic associations with the finding of echocardiographic mitral regurgitation were increased age (OR, 1.3/9.9 years; 95% CI, 1.2–1.5), hypertension (OR, 1.6; 95% CI, 1.2–2.0), and body mass index (OR, 0.8/4.3 kg/m(2); 95% CI, 0.7–0.9). The determinants of AR were only age (OR, 2.3/9.9 years; 95% CI, 2.0–2.7) and male gender (OR, 1.6; 95% CI, 1.2–2.1). In the hypertension genetic epidemiology study (95) conducted in 1496 hypertensive patients free of diabetes, the occurrence of aortic and mitral regurgitation was 246/1496 (16.5%) and 75/1496 (5%), respectively. Thus, this hypertensive patient sample provides an estimate of prevalence of left-sided valvular regurgitation that is not markedly different from the population estimate provided from the Framingham Project. In short, the role of hypertension in the evolution of echocardiographic or symptomatic valvular regurgitation seems to be dependent on factors other than hypertension *per se*.

C. Ventricular Function Assessment

Left ventricular assessment is one of the more crucial aspects of hypertension care both in the definition of hypertrophy and in functional assessment of ventricular contraction and to some extent relaxation.

1. Role of Rest Echocardiography in Routine Management (Asymptomatic)

The most widespread mode of diagnostic assessment for ventricular function is the use of transthoracic echocardiography. The definition of ischemia as a cause of symptoms or in the asymptomatic hypertensive patient can also be addressed at least in part by an echocardiographic technique.

As with chest pain symptoms, there is little evidence to suggest that ventricular function can be adequately addressed by a process of structured symptomatic enquiry whether alone or supplemented by examination; or supplemented by basic tests such as electrocardiography or chest radiography. This is not possible in the assessment of systolic function in normotensive cardiac patients (96) and is, therefore, less likely to be acceptable in hypertension given the more subtle nature of the changes involved in these patients, many of whom do not voice symptoms of any form (97).

The use of a variety of technical assessments in hypertension is the subject of a similar regional and/or national guideline statements. In virtually all of these, echocardiography is not routinely recommended for all hypertensive subjects to stratify cardiovascular risk. However, the application of this technology clearly allows more precise definition of ventricular hypertrophy than would be possible on the basis of examination and routine chest X-ray and electrocardiography.

For example, in 1074 hypertensive patients Cuspidi et al. (98) combined echocardiography with ultrasonographic carotid media thickness assessments and were able to show reclassification of hypertensive patients as defined by population risk scoring alone. The proportion of patients, originally defined as low-risk, decreased to 11.1%, and that of medium risk patients also fell to 35.7%. The largest change was that >50% of the patient sample, previously classified at low risk or medium risk were deemed to be at high risk of subsequent vascular events following the use of these two ultrasonographic technologies to assess left ventricular hypertrophy and IMT. A similar conclusion was reached in a separate study by Schillaci et al. (99) in their in reclassification of 792 untreated adult hypertensive patients with and without echocardiographic data. Again, the main change in classification they saw was that the proportion of low-risk subjects were reclassified as at higher vascular event risk and linked to that were candidates for antihypertensive drug therapy. Thus, echocardiography appears to have a valuable role in the routine and initial assessment of hypertension that has not yet been incorporated into current guidelines statements.

Echocardiographic assessments performed at the diagnostic phase of hypertension assessment may be of value in the classification of a white coat response and in the significance of white coat hypertension by putting blood pressure changes in the context of accurate end organ assessments of the heart.

Furthermore, the spectrum of ventricular change, which can be defined in hypertensive patients, can extend to the period before the appearance of fixed blood pressure elevation. For example, diastolic function appears to become abnormal within a normal blood pressure range in the offspring of hypertensive subjects. Aeschbacher et al. (100) performed serial echocardiographic assessments in normotensive male offspring of hypertensive and normotensive parents. Over a 5 year period, blood pressure had not altered overall, but five offspring of hypertensive parents went on to develop mild sustained hypertension. Although overall left ventricular mass was not different between the two groups at follow-up (92 ± 17 vs. $92 \pm 14 \, g/m^2$) and diastolic assessments had been similar at baseline, at follow-up, mitral E-wave deceleration time and pulmonary vein reverse A-wave duration were both prolonged. These changes were associated with significantly higher transmitral A-wave velocities (54 ± 7 vs. $44 \pm 9 \, cm/s$, hypertensives vs. normotensives, $P < 0.05$), a lower E/A ratio (1.31 ± 0.14 vs. 1.82 ± 0.48, $P < 0.05$), increased systolic-to-diastolic pulmonary vein flow ratio (1.11 ± 0.3 vs. 0.81 ± 0.16, $P < 0.005$), longer myocardial isovolumic relaxation times (157 ± 7 vs. $46 \pm 12 \, ms$, $P < 0.05$) as well as smaller myocardial E-wave velocity (10 ± 1 vs. $13 \pm 2 \, cm/s$, $P < 0.05$) and E/A ratio (1.29 ± 0.25 vs. 1.78 ± 0.43, $P < 0.05$), despite similar left ventricular mass (91 ± 16 vs. $93 \pm 18 \, g/m^2$). Thus, normotensive men with a moderate genetic risk for hypertension, develop echocardiographic alterations of left ventricular diastolic function before any appreciable rise in left ventricular mass.

There is still some debate as to the best means of echocardiographic definition of diastolic relaxation in hypertension. Transmitral Doppler filling indices are commonly abnormal but the independent relationship of these changes to hypertension and/or ventricular remodeling independent of aging is not absolutely clear. It is clear that the aging process and response to hypertension differs depending on gender.

Recent investigations of the utility of ultrasonic tissue backscatter have shown some linkage to structure *in vivo* and suggested that these relate to the abnormal restrictive filling patterns seen in hypertensive heart disease. Maceira et al. (101) defined real-time integrated backscatter analysis in 109 patients with essential hypertension. Backscatter cyclic variation and maximal intensity measured in six regions throughout the left ventricle were compared with transmitral filling patterns and subjects classified as showing normal blood pressure and normal diastolic function (29, group 1), hypertension with normal diastolic function (18, group 2), or hypertension with a delayed relaxation pattern (47, group 3). In addition, they found 11 hypertensive patients with a pseudonormal filling pattern (group 4), and 4 hypertensive patients with a restrictive filling pattern (group 5). The highest cyclic variation was found in group 1 and group 2, the lowest in group 4 and group 5 (5.7 ± 0.2 dB in group 1 and 5.7 ± 0.2 dB in group 2 vs. 2.9 ± 0.3 dB in group 4 and 2.1 ± 0.4 dB in group 5; $P < 0.001$), with intermediate values within group 3 (5.2 ± 0.2 dB). In correlation studies, they found that left ventricular chamber stiffness was inversely related to the cyclic variation of backscatter signals ($P < 0.05$) and directly correlated with mid-wall fractional shortening ($P < 0.02$) in all patients with high blood pressure. These results suggest a link between backscatter indices and diastolic function in hypertensive heart disease. Whether this parameter can be applied in routine assessment of diastolic dysfunction in asymptomatic hypertension has yet to be established; but this seems a very useful approach.

As an alternative, left atrial chamber dimensions or volume estimates can be readily defined by using echocardiography (102). As indicated earlier, electrocardiographic indices of atrial conduction tend to link in best with simple diastolic filling parameters. Thus, atrial echocardiographic assessment might also hold useful indirect indices of diastolic function. Tsang et al. (103) in Minnesota have shown that an echocardiographic atrial volume index has additional value in the retrospective cardiovascular event rate of elderly subjects referred within the Olmstead County survey. In a separate report from 140 subjects showed left atrial volume to correlate closely with age, ventricular dimensions and mass in patients without evidence of atrial arrhythmia or valvular heart disease (104). Left atrial volume appeared to be closely associated with the severity of echocardiographic a range of indices of diastolic dysfunction in these patients.

The white coat effect has little relationship to the structure or function of the left ventricle, (105) although there are changes to transmitral flow reported in some series (106), these are of uncertain clinical significance in the absence of ventricular hypertrophy or changes in systolic function despite signs of vascular dysfunction in these subjects (107).

Studies in normotensive subjects also show small declines in resting left ventricular systolic function and mid-wall contractility with aging. In a cross-sectional study of 272 asymptomatic, adults (25–80-years-old) with untreated hypertension Slotwiner et al. (108) saw no change in endocardial or mid-wall stress-corrected left ventricular fractional shortening. Neither cardiac index nor total peripheral resistance changed with age in either gender as age-related increases in systolic pressure were offset by increased concentric remodeling in the female patients or enhanced systolic contractility in the males. Thus, in mild hypertension, although cardiac index and peripheral resistance change with respect to age alone, there are age-related increases in concentricity of ventricular geometry in women and increased ventricular performance indexes in hypertensive men.

Systolic function in patients with hypertension may also need more detailed assessment in hypertensive patients than in the more straightforward studies designed to define contractility following infarction, to rule out abnormal systolic function as a cause of symptoms in hypertension. Occult ischemia is a common cause of both systolic and diastolic impairment and as a cause of symptoms in the hypertensive population. Long-axis contraction of the left ventricle can be analyzed using a variety of echocardiographic techniques either by using simple M-mode mitral annular movements alone or in conjunction with transmitral color flow studies or by tissue Doppler analyses (109). The more recent application of myocardial tissue Doppler imaging can reveal more subtle long-axis systolic ventricular impairment in patients previously presumed to have diastolic dysfunction (109). By defining the heart in a range of parasternal projections and combining these with studies of annular motion, again from a variety of sites, long-axis function can be quantified. The impact of hypertension is to change long-axis measures of contractility and these appear more sensitive in hypertensive patients than indices based on transmitral filling (110).

The geometric pattern of ventricular remodeling seen in individual patients with hypertension can have an impact on cardiac function by influencing both systolic and diastolic mechanics differently at rest or during exercise. Stroke volume is higher in patients with eccentric hypertrophy (83 mL/beat) and lower in patients with concentric left ventricular hypertrophy (68 mL/beat) compared with matched normotensive adults (73 mL/beat) (111). In keeping with these changes, cardiac output is higher in hypertensive patients with eccentric left ventricular hypertrophy and lower in concentric left ventricular hypertrophy. These changes occur independently of achieved blood pressure. In multivariate analysis, left ventricular mass is predictably independently related to higher systolic pressure, older age, stroke volume, male gender, and body mass index. Stroke volume and cardiac output are lower in patients with low stress-corrected mid-wall shortening (112).

D. Role in Symptomatic Assessment

Although echocardiographic technology is constantly improving, the role of this in routine care has not been frequently addressed in symptomatic hypertensive patients. It is feasible to complete rapid assessment at least of overall systolic function using portable machines. By using a hand-held device and comparing this with a standard fully functional echocardiography platform, Senior et al. (67) found a sensitivity of only 72% and positive and negative predictive values of 73% and 90% in 183 patients reviewed within a community systolic heart failure (SHF) screening project.

The subject of diastolic ventricular impairment in hypertension has been debated for many years. It has been marred by a lack of definitions and importantly a link to demonstrable exercise impairment in patients who voice heart failure symptoms (typically breathlessness on exertion and/or undue fatigue), and who still may have normal systolic (generally short axis echocardiographic) ventricular function. The technical assessment is perhaps the least controversial aspect of this area which is critically important in the assessment of symptoms in hypertensive patients.

There is now general agreement that in the routine assessment of patients with heart failure symptoms of whatever origin that many will have no demonstrable abnormality of systolic function, however, assessed. Some may be accounted for by abnormal long-axis systolic function (discussed earlier) (109), by valvular disease, pulmonary hypertension, intermittent occult arrhythmia by (such as PAF common in conjunction with hypertension), or by parenchymal lung disease. Often diastolic heart failure (DHF) is arrived at by the exclusion of other causes and the presence of indicators of impaired ventricular relaxation in conjunction with symptom. A substantial proportion of these patients are female, many are overweight and specifically there is a clear association with hypertension and echocardiographic left ventricular hypertrophy. In support of this, in the Olmsted County survey those patients ($n = 83$) with a new clinical diagnosis of heart failure and subsequent normal systolic function were generally very elderly (mean age 79 years) female (76%) and had hypertension or coronary disease (85%) (113). Given the age range, it is perhaps not surprising, therefore, that the 3 year mortality rate was high (60%).

However, in this type of report, only half of these patients met broader ESC echocardiographic criteria for an association of the presenting symptoms with a diagnosis of DHF.

Symptomatic heart failure without systolic contractile dysfunction remains an important and for some observers even a dominant form of heart failure presentation particularly in the elderly (114). The knowledge base regarding the epidemiology, pathophysiology, natural history, and therapy of these patients is still limited. There is a complex interaction between a number of age-related changes in the heart and vascular system that predispose to the appearance of the clinical presentation. Some population-based observational studies suggest that >50% of persons over 65 years who have heart failure symptoms will have normal left ventricular systolic function. Of these, roughly half will have no other confounding variables (coronary, valvular, or pulmonary disease) and could meet suggested criteria for isolated DHF. This is substantially more common in older women than men and hypertension with echocardiographic left ventricular hypertrophy are almost invariably present. Although short-term mortality rates are ~50% lower than in SHF in stable patients, in acutely hospitalized or very elderly patients, the mortality rate is similar in both systolic and potential DHF. Furthermore, because of its higher prevalence, the total mortality in the older population attributable to DHF in fact exceeds that of SHF.

Morbidity in DHF is therefore substantial and approaches that of SHF. In the chronic setting, DHF patients can have severe exercise intolerance related to failure of the Frank–Starling mechanism with reduced peak cardiac output, heart rate, and stroke volume and increased left ventricular filling pressure. DHF patients also appear to have increased vascular stiffness, accelerated systolic blood pressure response to exercise, neuroendocrine activation, and reduced quality of life.

It is possible and may be essential to define DHF by showing either impaired weight corrected exercise capacity using expired gas analysis at cardiopulmonary testing (115) or even elevated pulmonary wedge pressures at rest or during exercise in patients with symptomatic patients with echocardiographically normal systolic ventricular function (116).

Stress echocardiographic studies of potential diastolic filling abnormalities in hypertension show that coronary flow reserve (the difference between color tissue Doppler of myocardial segments at baseline and during pharmacological stress), in hypertensive left ventricular hypertrophy is reduced. In one survey of thirty patients free of epicardial coronary disease and after adjusting for the left ventricular mass and body mass transmitral filling indices remained in dependently associated with impaired coronary flow reserve linking the two areas directly (117). This may translate to impaired diastolic filling during subclinical ischemia.

The role of transoesophageal echocardiography (TEE) in the definition of diastolic relaxation is generally complimentary to other techniques. Klein et al. (118) from Cleveland have reported a large sample ($n = 181$) from their practice where TEE was used primarily to assess for potential cause of diastolic dysfunction. A large number in this selected group were found to have unsuspected restrictive cardiomyopathy (71) and a further substantial number (55) were had features consistent with constrictive pericarditis, subsequently confirmed at surgery. Only a minority in this series (32%) had idiopathic diastolic dysfunction and surprisingly only a very small number were found in association with hypertension.

There is no doubt that the technical assessment of diastolic filling has progressed rapidly in recent years since the concept of symptomatic isolated DHF has emerged. The population prevalence of this patient group is under represented by studies in hospital populations, which tend to be dominated by systolic ventricular dysfunction. In community-based surveys, prevalence figures of 15–20% are common in the elderly.

Using only an echocardiographic point of analysis Fischer et al. (119) examining the MONICA cohort in Augsburg used the ESC definitions for DHF which are based on an age dependent impairment of ventricular isovolumic relaxation time (95–105 ms and early and late ventricular filling wave reversal 1–0.5). On this basis, they found a 15.8% prevalence of these characteristics in their patients over 65 years from a sample of 1274 individuals. In this study, these echocardiographic abnormalities were more common in men than women, but they were associated with hypertension; left ventricular hypertrophy, coronary artery disease, high body fat mass/body mass index, and diabetes. Abnormalities of diastolic filling were rare (only 1–4% prevalence) in the absence of these features.

Despite such surveys and prospective follow-up studies, there remains debate as to the validity of diastolic filling abnormalities as the cause of heart failure symptoms in patients with normal ejection fractions, whether hypertensive or normotensive. The optimal means of the contribution of diastolic filling assessment to the definition of these patients does still remain controversial.

As with the assessment of coronary involvement and ischemia invasive measures, calculating the rate of decline in ventricular pressures in early diastole is often regarded as a gold standard by some cardiologists, but in fact one can only reliably evaluate the active process of diastolic relaxation (120). Changes in the more detailed end diastolic pressure volume filling loop is the most detailed physiological measure, but this is generally approximated in clinical practice rather than measured directly.

Estimates of ventricular stiffness can be used as a surrogate for a pressure volume study but this parameter is affected by any condition which will increase in ventricular filling pressure and the assumption that ventricular

hypertrophy is related to changes in passive diastolic filling is not entirely valid. For example, an acute ischemic stress will cause the upward shift in end-diastolic pressure–volume (EDPV) relationships, as will pericardial constriction and abnormal mechanical ventricular interaction. In some surveys of DHF-EDPV curves are normal both at rest and during exercise (121), whereas in others they are abnormal. This divergence of findings has further fuelled questions as to the nature of the abnormality in patients with heart failure symptoms and a preserved ejection fraction (122). The key issue is in the clinical definition of the patients themselves and there is no doubt in almost every published survey in community or hospital clinic setting these patients are predominantly older female hypertensive patients with echocardiographic ventricular hypertrophy (123). The presence of obesity and hypertensive ventricular hypertrophy is common in many surveys. This association alone would seem to draw logic and many clinicians toward a cardiac cause for their symptoms, but it is still unclear if the linkage is indeed causal.

There is no doubt that echocardiographic parameters of diastolic filling and altered wall tension or echo backscatter are different between physiological and pathological hypertrophy and that the latter is what is associated with isolated DHF whereas the former is associated with enhanced physical capacity. In this respect, the eccentric hypertrophic remodeling pattern of hypertensive heart disease should be differentiated from that seen with hypertrophic cardiomyopathy. Although hypertensive eccentric hypertrophy is generally a less severe pattern than concentric remodeling in terms of its prognostic impact (124). Clearly, HOCM has separate prognostic implications and differing molecular mechanisms that are not responsive to measures lowering blood pressure that will predominantly reverse eccentric or concentric hypertensive ventricular remodeling (125). The coexistence of hypertension and HOCM can occur and predictably causes confusion unless based on a molecular analysis. These are generally not available in routine practice.

Recent useful data looking at the value of BNP measurements confirm that this parameter commonly seen as of diagnostic value in the definition of systolic dysfunction is not in itself a good enough marker to allow reliable triage at least of echocardiographic indices of diastolic ventricular function. Mottram et al. (126) in 72 hypertensive patients with heart failure symptoms defined a range of appropriate echocardiographic indices of diastolic filling (including transmitral Doppler; color M-mode flow propagation velocities and pulmonary venous flow and systolic strain rates). They found that, although BNP did relate independently to ventricular and atrial systolic parameters, it was normally only within the high normal range in patients with echocardiographic diastolic dysfunction and therefore has limited positive diagnostic value in patients.

E. Contractile Function and Nonechocardiographic Methods

1. MRI Studies

The role of magnetic resonance and positron emission tomography (PET) studies in the assessment of the hypertensive patient continues to emerge. This powerful technology has been applied to the human heart in hypertensive heart disease and hypertensive ventricular hypertrophy for >10 years. It has paid dividends in a number of areas by linking metabolism to very accurate estimates of structure and function. For example, Akinboboye et al. (127) from Columbia University defined that myocardial oxygen demand in the hypertensive, hypertrophied ventricle is best calculated using 11C-labeled acetate. Using this technique, they found that hypertensive left ventricular hypertrophy was most closely related to the physical wall stress as approximated by the stress mass heart rate product.

The analysis of diastolic function by cardiovascular magnetic resonance can be completed to combine estimates of 3D chamber volume, filling velocity and flow as well as myocardial strain and energy content (128). These technologies can focused on specific regions of the myocardium (e.g., a hypertrophied septum) and provide a real-time analysis of function applicable in clinical practice. Lamb et al. (129) from Leiden, using phosphorus-31 magnetic resonance spectroscopy, were able to readily define impaired left ventricular filling in hypertension by an analysis of wall thinning; peak filling rates with normal systolic contractility. In association with these changes, atropine dobutamine stress levels of myocardial phospocreatinine/ATP ratios were lowered from those values seen in normotensive controls. Although not all studies agree with these observations (130), given the accuracy of the technology and their ability to link energy metabolism with contractile function and much more accurate morphological data than are possible with echocardiography (131) might mean that this is the key area where the origins and significance of diastolic filling abnormalities in hypertension will finally be defined. As echocardiographic measures are strongly correlated to MRI studies in selected echogenic patients, magnetic resonance protocols still allow more accurate planimetry and resultant reduced measurement variance of left ventricular mass estimates by ~40% (21–13%) (132). This reproducibility of assessment on repeated measures is now widely accepted.

PET can similarly map fatty acid oxidation and turnover in the heart accurately. From a group based in St Louis, data has been derived across a range of ventricular remodeling showing that myocardial fatty acid uptake, oxidation, and metabolism can be directly correlated to left ventricular mass in hypertension as well as in other states such as ischemic cardiomyopathy (133).

Equally, coronary blood flow reserve (the maximal rise in coronary blood flow above its resting auto regulated values for a given perfusion pressure) can be accurately measured using N^{13} labeled ammonia in hypertensive patients (134). For example, the impact of blood pressure lowering therapy on the rest or stressed CFR of individual patients can be seen to be improved in response to treatment (135). This type of study is regarded by some as the only truly quantitative noninvasive technique for the definition of coronary flow. These studies do not underestimate flow as occurs with coronary sinus sampling.

2. PET Studies

Gimelli et al. (136) from Pisa used the flexibility of PET studies of [13N]ammonia labeling (both at rest and following dipyridamole flow stress) to study the influence of ventricular hypertrophy on regional perfusion patterns in 50 hypertensive patients. Using this technology, they were able to show that patients with regional defects in perfusion were more likely to have ventricular hypertrophy but that overall myocardial blood flow was not simply related to total ventricular mass estimates. During pharmacological stress hypertensive patients who preserved a homogenous pattern of perfusion showed, however, reduced coronary flow.

In the same way as MRI techniques have differentiated the structure of the septum in HOCM from asymmetrical septal hypertrophy of hypertension, PET studies of glucose uptake show altered metabolism. F^{18} (2), deoxyglucose fractional uptake rations for the septum and posterior left ventricular wall are similar in patients with HOCM or hypertensive heart disease but that the regional uptake is more heterogeneous in HOCM (137).

V. CARDIAC RHYTHM IN HYPERTENSION

A. Cardiac Rhythm Assessment in HBP

- The detection of atrial flutter and atrial fibrillation is critical in hypertension to facilitate appropriate management.
- Symptomatic complaint are not a reliable guide to the presence of significant arrhythmia.
- Asymptomatic and symptomatic atrial fibrillation is powerfully linked to LVH and/or poor blood pressure control.
- While QT interval dispersion is commonly linked to mortality there is little evidence of a specific linkage of increased QTd in hypertension linked to LVH and sudden death in hypertension.

B. Assessment and Relevance of Arrhythmia in Hypertension

The definition of cardiac arrhythmia in asymptomatic and symptomatic patients with hypertension is facilitated by ambulatory recordings either of a continuous nature or intermittent (where patients are symptomatic). This allows a basic link to be made between symptoms (generally of palpitation but more realistically these can be very variably described) and rhythm. The key factor in hypertensive heart disease is an assessment of ventricular structure (generally echocardiographic) allowing both systolic and diastolic contractility; intercurrent valve function and hypertrophy to be established. Although, the presence of baseline conduction abnormalities has been alluded to earlier investigation of these generally relates to the linked processes of defining hypertrophy, ischemia, and valve function described previously. Two major areas require specific mention in the analysis of cardiac rhythm in hypertensive patients, namely, atrial fibrillation and ventricular arrhythmia.

C. Atrial Flutter and Fibrillation

The etiological link between atrial fibrillation, hypertension, and stroke disease is a critical one. Nonrheumatic atrial fibrillation is associated with an approximately five-fold increase in the risk of ischemic stroke and a 5–7% yearly risk that increases with age. In addition, atrial fibrillation is associated with an increased incidence of silent cerebral infarction and increased mortality. Treating hypertensive patients' stroke risk must take into account the definition of atrial fibrillation and to a lesser extent atrial flutter coexistent with hypertension.

Unfortunately, few specific studies of atrial flutter and hypertension and its association to hypertension have been completed. In patients with atrial flutter, there is certainly a lesser prevalence of thromboembolic events, but atrial flutter does not have a benign association with concomitant hypertension. Using multivariate analysis, Seidl et al. (138) (following only 191 patients with atrial flutter) found that the only independent risk factor on multivariate analysis for predicting thromboembolic events was a history of hypertension (OR, 6.5; 95% CI, 1.5–45). Atrial flutter cannot be ignored in the hypertensive patient even if it is asymptomatic.

In population studies, the relative risk ratio for acute atrial fibrillation is strongest at the onset of ischemic heart disease but diminishes in these patients over time. The rate of atrial fibrillation is ~1.42 times increased in hypertensive men compared with normotensive men, and although congestive heart failure, valvular heart disease, and cardiomyopathy are important risk factors for the development of AF, they are relatively uncommon in AF patients (139). Atrial fibrillation and hypertension are prevalent, and frequently coexistent, conditions in the elderly. The incidence of both increases with advancing age and independently they can create significant burden of morbidity and mortality (140). Although the interrelationship of these two conditions has long established (141), the details are not yet well-defined. Hypertension is associated with left ventricular hypertrophy, impaired ventricular filling, left atrial enlargement, and a slowing of atrial conduction velocity. Such simple independent changes in cardiac structure favor the loss of sinus rhythm and the development of atrial fibrillation. They also increase the risk of thromboembolic complications in both states. Left atrial diameter by M-mode echocardiography does not predict stroke in patients with AF (142).

The pathological linkage of atrial fibrillation to hypertension is strong and simple although dependent on a progression of several factors. Multifactorial changes alter left atrial size which in turn alters left atrial conduction and contributes to promoting the onset of paroxysmal atrial fibrillation. This links directly to the presence of increased left ventricular mass in hypertensive atrial fibrillation (143) and as with ventricular arrhythmia is generally unrelated to concomitant epicardial coronary disease (144).

Verdecchia et al. (145) have recently described follow-up in 2482 hypertensive patients all of whom were in sinus rhythm at presentation and excluding subjects with known valvular heart disease, coronary artery disease, ventricular arrhythmia, thyroid, or lung disease. In this large cohort of hypertensive patients, the incidence of a first episode of atrial fibrillation was 0.46 per 100 person-years (61 patients). The affected patients at entry were older (59 vs. 51 years), had higher office and 24 h mean systolic blood pressure (165 and 144 vs. 157 and 137 mmHg, respectively), had a greater left ventricular mass [58 vs. 49 g/height (m) (2.7)], and echocardiographic left atrial diameter (3.89 cm vs. 3.56 cm). In a multivariate logistic regression analysis, only age and left ventricular mass predicted the evolution of a first episode of AF in hypertension. They calculated that for every 1 standard deviation increase in left ventricular mass, the risk of atrial fibrillation was increased 1.20 times (95% CI, 1.07–1.34). Interestingly, atrial fibrillation became chronic in only 33% of the subjects in the study during the follow-up period. Similarly, age, left ventricular mass, and on this occasion left atrial diameter were independent predictors of chronic atrial fibrillation. The ischemic stroke rate was 2.7% and 4.6% per year for paroxysmal and chronic atrial fibrillation, respectively. The interesting aspect of this study was that increased left atrial size predisposed to the degeneration of PAF to chronic or persistent AF. Thus echocardiographic assessment may play a role in this hypertensive patient subgroup.

The general population prevalence of AF in the elderly is associated with clear structural changes in the heart definable at echocardiography. In the Framingham Study, subjects routinely evaluated with M-mode echocardiography ($n = 1924$, age 59–90 years), provided data to analyze the association of echocardiographic features with atrial fibrillation risk after adjustment for age, sex, hypertension, coronary heart disease, congestive heart failure, diabetes, and valvular heart disease (146). Over a mean follow-up of 7.2 years, 154 subjects (8.0%) developed atrial fibrillation. Multivariable stepwise analysis identified left atrial size (HR per 5 mm increment, 1.39; 95% CI, 1.14–1.68), left ventricular fractional shortening (HR per 5% decrement, 1.34; 95% CI, 1.08–1.66), and sum of septal and left ventricular posterior wall thickness (HR per 4 mm increment, 1.28; 95% CI, 1.03–1.60) as independent echocardiographic predictors of atrial fibrillation. The likelihood of atrial fibrillation grew markedly when these changes occurred together giving cumulative 8 year, age-adjusted atrial fibrillation rates were 7.3% and 17.0%, respectively, when one and two or more highest-risk-quartile features were present, compared with 3.7% when none was present. These echocardiographic precursors offer prognostic information beyond that provided by traditional clinical atrial fibrillation risk factors.

Although conventional therapy of AF has focused on interventions to control heart rate and/or rhythm and the prevention of stroke through the use of antithrombotic anticoagulant medications, in patients with hypertension and atrial fibrillation, aggressive management of blood pressure by reversing structural change in the heart, can reduce the likelihood of thromboembolic complications, and retard or prevent the occurrence of atrial fibrillation.

The restoration of sinus rhythm by DC cardioversion is feasible in hypertensive atrial fibrillation but the maintenance of sinus rhythm is lowest in patients with ventricular hypertrophy or concomitant ventricular dysfunction (147). Such former strategies are currently being re-evaluated as the benefits of rhythm control seem limited and the risks may outweigh benefit. Although the management issues will be dealt with elsewhere, the key features for the development of atrial fibrillation are clear. The integrated risk of stroke in the hypertensive patient with atrial fibrillation is such that anticoagulation should be a priority (148).

D. Ventricular Arrhythmia

The presence of significant ventricular arrhythmia in hypertension is well established, as is the increased incidence of sudden death frequently assumed to represent serious ventricular arrhythmia. The key mediators are the involvement of ischemia (silent or symptomatic) prior infarction and left ventricular hypertrophy

(149,150). However, there is often confusion over the sequence of events and the primary mediator in individual hypertensive patients. The link among serious arrhythmia, ventricular hypertrophy, arterial pressure/wall stress, ischemia, and sudden death is clearly complex and interdependent. The co-incident occurrence of silent ischemia and left ventricular hypertrophy is a particularly powerful but independent combination in hypertensive patients for future ventricular arrhythmia (151).

Holter studies of the prevalence of ventricular arrhythmia show simple ectopy to be common (>70%), but this is confounded by age and many other factors leading to little prognostic validity whether applied to uncomplicated or symptomatic patients with hypertension. Complex ventricular arrhythmia is less frequent, again age and pressure dependent, and appears responsive in part to blood pressure control (152). Some studies suggest the frequency of arrhythmia is graded and related to the severity of left ventricular hypertrophy even in the absence of angiographic coronary disease (144). Thus, again the electrocardiographic definition of arrhythmia is perhaps less significant than the definition of ventricular structure, presence of inducible ischemia, and function.

Prospective studies of arrhythmia and sudden death in restricted to hypertensive heart disease are rare. There seems to be little evidence of a link between abnormal QT dispersion in left ventricular hypertrophy and risk of arrhythmia in hypertension (153). This is despite extensive investigations of the utility of QT dispersion over the last 10 years in unselected ischemic cardiomyopathy as a predictor of significant arrhythmia (154). The impact and linkage of QT_c dispersion to ventricular arrhythmia may be stronger in nonischemic dilated cardiomyopathy than in hypertensive left ventricular hypertrophy (155). The lack of association to left ventricular hypertrophy is similar to some studies in hypertension. Saadeh and Vann Jones prospectively found only the left ventricular hypertrophy and documented Holter complex arrhythmia associated with sudden (presumed arrhythmic) death in their cohort of hypertensive patients. Unfortunately, their study was very small with only six sudden deaths from a long-term study of 54 hypertensive patients over nearly 10 years, but it remains a valuable observation.

Thus, a simplistic account of hypertensive left ventricular hypertrophy leading directly to fatal arrhythmia even in patients with documented rhythm abnormalities does not realistically integrate the factors appropriately.

VI. CONCLUSIONS

There is little doubt that patients with hypertension present a challenge to effective diagnostic cardiac evaluation. Hypertention assessment extends beyond the definition of blood pressure alone, particularly in symptomatic patients. In addition, there is some evidence that initial assessment of asymptomatic patients should encompass some routine cardiac assessment beyond simplistic traditions of resting electrocardiography and chest radiology. A variety of factors affect the hypertensive patient population—the impact of aging, obesity, concomitant diabetes and vascular disease, drug therapy, and ethnicity—and complicate cardiac diagnostic evaluation.

Although hypertensive patients are traditionally viewed as asymptomatic, sophisticated investigational assessment using both stress and at-rest studies are required to obtain a true overall cardiac risk assessment. When hypertensive patients start experiencing cardiac symptoms, investigation of the symptoms often is not well served by noninvasive standards of practice. In particular, the definition of symptoms that are a result of impaired diastolic relaxation are focused very clearly in the elderly hypertensive population in the community. The complexity of this patient group may be better analyzed by using the evolving magnetic resonance-based technology than by invasive physiological measurements. However, in the near future in the definition of myocardial ischemia, the confounding impact of hypertension means that noninvasive testing protocols still lag behind a simple approach of progressing rapidly toward invasive angiographic risk stratification, provided that blood pressure control has been achieved and that functional cardiac assessment is not ignored.

REFERENCES

1. Kannel WB. Some lessons in cardiovascular epidemiology from Framingham. Am J Cardiol 1976; 37:269–282.
2. Frank CW, Weinblatt E, Shapiro S, Sager RV. Prognosis of men with coronary heart disease as related to blood pressure. Circulation 1968; 38:432–428.
3. Kuller L. Sudden death in arteriosclerotic heart disease; the case for preventive medicine. Am J Cardiol 1969; 24:617–628.
4. Fuchs FD, Gus M, Moreira LB, Moreira WD, Goncalves SC, Nunes G. Headache is not more frequent among patients with moderate to severe hypertension. J Hum Hypertens 2003; 17:787–790.
5. Sarasin FP, Louis-Simonet M, Carballo D, Slama S, Junod AF, Unger PF. Prevalence of orthostatic hypotension among patients presenting with syncope in the ED. Am J Emerge Med 2002; 20:497–501.
6. O'Mahoney D. Pathophysiology of carotid sinus hypersensitivity in elderly patients. Lancet 1995; 346:950–952.
7. Strasberg B, Sagie A, Erdman S, Kusniec J, Sclarovsky S, Agmon J. Carotid sinus hypersensitivity and the carotis sinus syndrome. Prog Cardiovasc Dis 1989; 31:379–391.
8. Schutzman J, Jaeger F, Maloney J, Fouadtarazi F. Head up tilt and hemodynamic changes during orthostatic hypotension in patients with supine hypertension. J Am Coll Cardiol 1994; 24:454–461.
9. Gazes PC, Mobley EM Jr, Faris HM Jr, Duncan RC, Humphries GB. Preinfarctional (unstable) angina—a prospective study—ten year follow-up. Prognostic significance of electrocardiographic changes. Circulation 1973; 48:331–337.
10. Zamboni S, Ambrosio GB, Stefanini MG, Urbani V, Dissegna L, Mazzucato L, Zahalka T, Dal Palu. Electrocardiographic findings in hypertensive patients of a population sample. Role of sex, age, and antihypertensive treatment. J Clin Hypertens 1987; 3:430–438.
11. Alpert MA, Munuswamy K. Electrocardiographic diagnosis of left atrial enlargement. Arch Intern Med 198; 149:1161–1165.
12. Cristal N, Koren I. Evaluation of the electrocardiogram in hypertensive patients: the LOMIR-MCT-IL study experience. Blood Press Suppl 1994; 1:43–47.
13. Genovesiebert A, Marabotti C, Palombo C, Ghione S. Electrocardiographic signs of atrial overload in hypertensive patients—indexes of abnormality of atrial morphology or function. Am Heart J 1991; 121:1113–1118.
14. Madu EC, Baugh DS, Gbadebo TD, Dhala A, Cardoso S. Phi-Res Multi-Study Group. Effect of ethnicity and hypertension on atrial conduction: evaluation with high-resolution P-wave signal averaging. Clin Cardiol 2001; 24:597–602.
15. Presciuttini B, Duprez D, De Buyzere M, Clement DL. How to study sympatho-vagal balance in arterial hypertension and the effect of antihypertensive drugs? Acta Cardiologica 1998; 53:143–152.
16. Tran H, White CM, Chow MSS, Kluger J. An evaluation of the impact of gender and age on QT dispersion in healthy subjects. Ann Noninv Electrocardiol 2001; 6:129–133.
17. Chapman N, Mayet J, Ozkor M, Foale R, Thom S, Poulter N. Ethnic and gender differences in electrocardiographic QT length and QT dispersion in hypertensive subjects. J Hum Hypertens 2000; 14:403–405.
18. Xiao HB, Brecker SJ, Gibson DG. Relative effects of left ventricular mass and conduction disturbance on activation in patients with pathological left ventricular hypertrophy. Br Heart J 1994; 71:548–553.
19. Rotman M, Triebwasser JH. A clinical and follow-up study of right and left bundle branch block. Circulation 1975; 51:477–484.
20. Sundstrom J, Lind L, Andren B, Lithell H. Left ventricular geometry and function are related to electrocardiographic characteristics and diagnoses. Clin Physiol 1998; 18:463–470.
21. Clarkson PB, Naas AAO, McMahon A, MacLeod C, Struthers AD, MacDonald TMM. QT dispersion in essential hypertension. QJM 1995; 88:327–332.
22. Mayet J, Shahi M, McGrath K, Poulter NR, Sever PS, Foale RA, Thom SAM. Left ventricular hypertrophy and QT dispersion in hypertension. Hypertension 1996; 28:791–796.
23. Barr CS, Naas AAO, Freeman M, Lang CC, Struthers AD. QT dispersion and sudden unexpected death in chronic heart failure. Lancet 1994; 343:327–329.
24. Elming H, Holm E, Jun L, Torp-Pedersen C, Kober L, Kircshoff M, Malik M, Camm J. The prognostic value

of the QT interval and QT interval dispersion in all-cause and cardiac mortality and morbidity in a population of Danish citizens. Eur Heart J 1998; 19:1391–1400.

25. de Bruyne MC, Hoes AW, Kors JA, Hofman A, van Bemmel JH, Grobbee DE. QTc dispersion predicts cardiac mortality in the elderly—The Rotterdam Study. Circulation 1998; 97:467–472.

26. Halle M, Huonker M, Hohnloser SH, Alivertis M, Berg A, Keul J. QT dispersion in exercise-induced myocardial hypertrophy. Am Heart J 1999; 138:309–312.

27. Chapman N, Mayet J, Ozkor M, Lampe FC, Thom SAM, Poulter NR. QT intervals and QT dispersion as measures of left ventricular hypertrophy in an unselected hypertensive population. Am J Hypertens 2001; 14:455–462.

28. Piccirillo G, Germano G, Quaglione R, Nocco M, Lintas F, Lionetti M, Moise A, Ragazzo M, Marigliano V, Cacciafesta M. QT-interval variability and autonomic control in hypertensive subjects with left ventricular hypertrophy. Clin Sci 2002; 102:363–371.

29. Wong KYK, Lim PO, Wong SYS, MacWalter RS, Struthers AD, MacDonald TM. Does a prolonged QT peak identify left ventricular hypertrophy in hypertension? Int J Cardiol 2003; 89:179–186.

30. Okin PM, Roman MJ, Devereux RB, Pickering TG, Borer JS, Kligfield P. Time–voltage QRS area of the 12-lead electrocardiogram—detection of left ventricular hypertrophy. Hypertension 1998; 31:937–942.

31. Kannel WB, Gordon T, Offutt D. Left ventricular hypertrophy by electrocardiogram. Prevalence, incidence, and mortality in the Framingham study. Ann Intern Med 1969; 71:89–105.

32. Huwez FU, Pringle SD, Macfarlane PW. Variable patterns of ST-T abnormalities in patients with left ventricular hypertrophy and normal coronary arteries. Br Heart J 1992; 67:304–307.

33. Verdecchia P, Angeli F, Reboldi G, Carluccio E, Benemio G, Gattobigio R, Borgioni C, Bentivoglio M, Porcellati C, Ambrosio G. Improved cardiovascular risk stratification by a simple electrocardiogram index in hypertension. Am J Hypertens 2003; 16:646–652.

34. Antikainen R, Grodzicki T, Palmer AJ, Beevers DG, Coles EC, Webster J, Bulpitt CJ. The determinants of left ventricular hypertrophy defined by Sokolow Lyon criteria in untreated hypertensive patients. Hypertension 2003; 41:499–504.

35. Devereaux RB, Phillips MC, Casale PN, Eisenberger RR, Kligfeld P. Geometric determinants of electrocardiographic left ventricular hypertrophy. Circulation 1983; 67:907–911.

36. Lee DK, Marantz PR, Devereux RB, Klingfield P, Alderman MH. Left ventricular hypertrophy in black and white hypertensives—standard electrocardiographic criteria overestimate racial differences in prevalence. JAMA 1992; 267:3294–3299.

37. Tochikubo O, Miyajima E, Shigemasa T, Ishii M. Relation between body fat-corrected electrocardiogram voltage and ambulatory blood pressure in patients with essential hypertension. Hypertension 1999; 33:1159–1163.

38. Chapman JN, Mayet J, Chang CL, Foale RA, Thom SAM, Poulter NR. Ethnic differences in the identification of left ventricular hypertrophy in the hypertensive patient. Am J Hypertens 1999; 12:437–442.

39. Spencer C, Beevers DG, Lip GYH. Ethnic differences in left ventricular size and the prevalence of left ventricular hypertrophy among hypertensive patients vary with electrocardiographic criteria. J Hum Hypertens 2004; 18(9):631–636.

40. Okin PM, Roman MJ, Devereux RB, Kligfield P. Electrocardiographic identification of increased left ventricular mass by simple voltage duration products. J Am Coll Cardiol 1995; 25:417–423.

41. Norman JE, Levy D. Adjustment of electrocardiogram left ventricular hypertrophy criteria for body mass index and age improves classification accuracy: the effects of hypertension and obesity. J Electrocardiology 1996; 29:241–247.

42. Okin PM, Roman MJ, Devereux RB, Kligfield P. Electrocardiographic identification of left ventricular hypertrophy: test performance in relation to definition of hypertrophy and presence of obesity. J Am Coll Cardiol 1996; 27:124–131.

43. Casiglia E, Maniati G, Daskalakis C, Colangeli G, Tramontin P, Ginocchio G, Spolaore P. Left-ventricular hypertrophy in the elderly: unreliability of electrocardiogram criteria in 477 subjects aged 65 years or more—The CArdiovascular STudy in the ELderly (CASTEL). Cardiology 1996; 87:429–435.

44. Filipovsky J, Ducimetiere P, Safar ME. Prognostic significance of exercise blood pressure and heart rate in middle aged men. Hypertension 1992; 20:333–339.

45. Jette M, Sidney K, Landry F, Quenneville J. Blood pressure responses to a progressive step test in normotensive males and females. Can J App Physiol 1994; 19:421–431.

46. Lim PO, MacDonald TM. Non-invasive profiling of total peripheral vascular resistance using the Dundee step test. Am J Hypertens 1999; 12:173A.

47. Lim PO, Donnan PT, MacDonald TM. How well do office and exercise blood pressures predict sustained hypertension? A Dundee step test study. J Hum Hypertens 2000; 14:429–433.

48. Lim PO, Rana BS, Struthers AD, MacDonald TM. Exercise blood pressure correlates with the maximum heart rate corrected QT interval in hypertension. J Hum Hypertens 2001; 15:169–172.

49. Gottdiener JS, Brown J, Zoltick J, Fletcher RD. Left ventricular hypertrophy in men with normal blood pressure: relation to exaggerated blood pressure response to exercise. Ann Int Med 1990; 112:161–166.

50. Campbell L, Marwick TH, Pashkow FJ, Snader CE, Lauer MS. Usefulness of an exaggerated systolic blood pressure response to exercise in predicting myocardial perfusion defects in known or suspected coronary artery disease. Am J Cardiol 1999; 84:1304–1310.

51. Marwick TH, Torelli J, Harjai K, Haluska B, Pashkow FJ, Stewart WJ, Thomas JD. Influence of left ventricular hypertrophy on detection of coronary artery disease using exercise echocardiography. J Am Coll Cardiol 1995; 26:1180–1186.

52. Picano E, Palinkas A, Amyot R. Diagnosis of myocardial ischemia in hypertensive patients. J Hypertens 2001; 19:1177–1183.

53. Maltagliati A, Berti M, Muratori M, Tamborini G, Zavalloni D, Berna G, Pepi M. Exercise echocardiography versus exercise electrocardiography in the diagnosis of coronary artery disease in hypertension. Am J Hypertens 2000; 13:796–801.

54. Jespersen CM, Rasmussen V. Detection of myocardial ischemia by transthoracic leads in ambulatory electrocardiographic monitoring. Br Heart J 1992; 68:286–290.

55. Pringle SD, Dunn FG, Tweddel AC, Martin W, MacFarlane PW, McKillop JH, Lorimer AR, Cobbe SM. Symptomatic and silent myocardial ischemia in hypertensive patients with left ventricular hypertrophy. Br Heart J 1992; 67:377–382.

56. Asmar R, Benetos A, Pannier B, Agnes E, Topouchian J, Laloux B, Safar M. Prevalence and circadian variations of ST-segment depression and its concomitant blood pressure changes in asymptomatic systemic hypertension. J Hypertens 2001; 19:1883–1891.

57. Siegel D, Cheitlin MD, Seeley DG, Black DM, Hulley SB. Silent myocardial ischemia in men with systemic hypertension and without clinical evidence of coronary artery disease. Am J Cardiol 1992; 70:86–90.

58. Elhendy A, van Domburg RT, Sozzi FB, Poldermans D, Bax JJ, Roelandt JRTC. Impact of hypertension on the accuracy of exercise stress myocardial perfusion imaging for the diagnosis of coronary artery disease. Heart 2001; 85:655–661.

59. Berger HJ, Sands MJ, Davies RA, Wackers FJT, Alexander J, Lachman AS, Williams BW, Zaret BL. Exercise left ventricular performance in patients with chest pain iscemic appearing exercise electrocardiograms and angiographically normal coronary arteries. Ann Int Med 1981; 94:186–191.

60. Cecil MP, Pilcher MP, Eisner RL, Chu TH, Merlino JD, Patterson RE. Absence of defects in SPECT Th-201 myocardial images in patients with systemic hypertension and left ventricular hypertrophy. Am J Cardiol 1994; 74:43–46.

61. Elhendy A, van Domburg RT, Bax JJ, Ibrahim MM, Roelandt JRTC. Myocardial perfusion abnormalities in treated hypertensive patients without known coronary artery disease. J Hypertens 1999; 17:1601–1606.

62. Schillaci O, Moroni C, Scopinaro F, Tavolaro R, Danieli R, Bossini A, Cassone R, Colella AC. Technetium-99m sestamibi myocardial tomography based on dipyridamole echocardiography testing in hypertensive patients with chest pain. Eur J Nuc Med 1997; 24:774–778.

63. Elhendy A, Mahoney DW, Khandheria BK, Paterick TE, Burger KN, Pellikka PA. Prognostic significance of the location of wall motion abnormalities during exercise echocardiography. J Am Coll Cardiol 2002; 40:1623–1629.

64. Lee CY, Pellikka PA, McCully RB, Mahoney DW, Seward JB. Non-exercise stress transthoracic echocardiography: transoesophageal atrial pacing versus dobutamine stress. J Am Coll Cardiol 1999; 33:506–511.

65. Picano E, Mathias W, Pingitore A, Bigi R, Previtali M. Safety and tolerability of dobutamine atropine stress echocardiography a prospective multi centre study. Lancet 1994; 344:1190–1192.

66. Lee CY, Pellikka PA, Shub C, Sinak LJ, Seward JB. Hypertensive response during dobutamine stress echocardiography. Am J Cardiol 1997; 80:970–976.

67. Senior R, Basu S, Handler C, Raftery EB, Lahiri A. Diagnostic accuracy of dobutamine stress echocardiography for detection of coronary heart disease in hypertensive patients. Eur Heart J 1996; 17: 289–295.

68. Elhendy A, Geleijnse ML, van Domburg RT, Bax JJ, Nierop PR, Beerens SAM, Valkema R, Krenning EP, Ibrahim MM, Roelandt JRTC. Comparison of dobutamine stress echocardiography and technetium-99m sestamibi single-photon emission tomography for the diagnosis of coronary artery disease in hypertensive patients with and without left ventricular hypertrophy. Eur J Nuc Med 1998; 25:69–78.

69. Astarita C, Palinkas A, Nicolai E, Maresca FS, Varga A, Picano E. Dipyridamole-atropine stress echocardiography versus exercise SPECT scintigraphy for detection of coronary artery disease in hypertensives with positive exercise test. J Hypertens 2001; 19:495–502.

70. Cortigiani L, Paolini EA, Nannini E. Dipyridamole stress echocardiography for risk stratification in hypertensive patients with chest pain. Circulation 1998; 98:2855–2859.

71. Cortigiani L, Bigi R, Rigo F, Landi P, Baldini U, Mariani PR, Picano E; On behalf of the EPIC (Echo Persantine International Cooperative) Study Group. Diagnostic value of exercise electrocardiography and dipyridamole stress echocardiography in hypertensive and normotensive chest pain patients with right bundle branch block. J Hypertens 2003; 21:2189–2194.

72. Fragasso G, Lu CZ, Dabrowski P, Pagnotta P, Sheiban I, Chierchia SL. Comparison of stress/rest myocardial perfusion tomography, dipyridamole and dobutamine stress echocardiography for the detection of coronary disease in hypertensive patients with chest pain and positive exercise test. J Am Coll Cardiol 1999; 34:441–447.

73. Marwick TH, Case C, Sawada S, Vasey C, Thomas JD. Prediction of outcomes in hypertensive patients with suspected coronary disease. Hypertension 2002; 39:1113–1118.

74. Cortigiani L, Bigi R, Gigli G, Coletta C, Mariotti E, Dodi C, Astarita C, Picano E. Prognostic implications of intraventricular conduction defects in patients undergoing stress echocardiography for suspected coronary artery disease. Am J Med 2003; 115:12–18.

75. Yuda S, Khoury V, Marwick TH. Influence of wall stress and left ventricular geometry on the accuracy of dobutamine stress echocardiography. J Am Coll Cardiol 2002; 40:1311–1319.

76. Zouridakis EG, Cox ID, Garcia-Moll X, Brown S, Nihoyannopoulos P, Kaski JC. Negative stress echocardiographic responses in normotensive and hypertensive patients with angina pectoris, positive exercise stress testing, and normal coronary arteriograms. Heart 2000; 83:141–146.

77. Bory M, Pierron F, Panagides D, Bonnet JL, Yvorra S, Desfossez L. Coronary artery spasm in patients with

normal or near normal coronary arteries—long-term follow-up of 277 patients. Eur Heart J 1996; 17:1015–1021.

78. Da Costa A, Isaaz K, Faure E, Mourot S, Cerisier A, Lamaud M. Clinical characteristics, aetiological factors and long-term prognosis of myocardial infarction with an absolutely normal coronary angiogram—a 3-year follow-up study of 91 patients. Eur Heart J 2001; 22:1459–1465.

79. Crenshaw JH, Elezeky F, Zwaag RV, Sullivan JM, Ramanathan KB, Mirvis DM. The effect of non-critical coronary artery disease on long term survival. Am J Med Sci 1995; 310:7–13.

80. De Cesare N, Polese A, Cozzi S, Apostolo A, Fabbiocchi F, Loaldi A, Montorsi P, Guazzi MD. Coronary angiographic patterns in hypertensive compared with normotensive patients. Am Heart J 1991; 21:1101–1106.

81. Maher JE, Raz JA, Bielak LF, Sheedy PF, Schwartz RS, Peyser PA. Potential of quantity of coronary artery calcification to identify new risk factors for asymptomatic atherosclerosis Am J Epidemiol 1996; 144:943–953.

82. Shaw LJ, Raggi P, Schisterman E, Berman DS, Callister TQ. Prognostic value of cardiac risk factors and coronary artery calcium screening for all-cause mortality. Radiology 2003; 228:826–833.

83. Khurana C, Rosenbaum CG, Howard BV, Adams-Campbell LL, Detrano RC, Klouj A, Hsia J. Coronary artery calcification in black women and white women. Am Heart J 2003; 145:724–729.

84. Megnien JL, Simon A, Lemariey M, Plainfosse MC, Levenson J. Hypertension promotes coronary calcium deposit in asymptomatic men. Hypertension 1996; 27:949–954.

85. Schmermund A, Baumgart D, Gorge G, Gronemeyer D, Seibel R, Bailey KR, Rumberger JA, Paar D, Erbel R. Measuring the effect of risk factors on coronary atherosclerosis: Coronary calcium score versus angiographic disease severity. J Am Coll Cardiol 1998; 31:1267–1273.

86. Guerci AD, Spadaro LA, Goodman KJ, Lledo-Perez A, Newstein D, Lerner G, Arad Y. Comparison of electron beam computed tomography scanning and conventional risk factor assessment for the prediction of angiographic coronary artery disease. J Am Coll Cardiol 1998; 32:673–679.

87. Turner ST, Bielak LF, Narayana AK, Sheedy PF, Schwartz GL, Peyser PA. Ambulatory blood pressure and coronary artery calcification in middle-aged and younger adults. Am J Hypertens 2002; 15:518–524.

88. Altunkan S, Erdogan N, Altin L, Budoff MJ. Relation of coronary artery calcium to left ventricular mass and geometry in patients with essential hypertension. Blood Press Monitor 2003; 8:9–15.

89. Antonini-Canterin F, Huang GQ, Cervesato E, Faggiano P, Pavan D, Piazza R, Nicolosi GL. Symptomatic aortic stenosis—does systemic hypertension play an additional role? Hypertension 2003; 41:1268–1272.

90. Pate GE. Association between aortic stenosis and hypertension. J Heart Valve Dis 2002; 11:612–614.

91. Stewart BF, Siscovick D, Lind BK, Gardin JM, Gottdiener JS, Smith VE, Kitzman DW, Otto CM. Clinical factors associated with calcific aortic valve disease. J Am Coll Cardiol 1997; 29:630–634.

92. Rosenhek R, Binder T, Porenta G, Lang I, Christ G, Schemper M, Maurer G, Baumgartner H. Predictors of outcome in severe, asymptomatic aortic stenosis. New Eng J Med 2000; 343:611–617.

93. Post WS, Larson MG, Levy D. Hemodynamic predictors of incident hypertension—the Framingham Heart Study. Hypertension 1994; 24:585–590.

94. Palta S, Pai AM, Gill KS, Pai RG. New insights into the progression of aortic stenosis—implications for secondary prevention. Circulation 2000; 101:2497–2502.

95. Palmieri V, Bella JN, Arnett DK, Oberman A, Kitzman DW, Hopkins PN, Rao DC, Roman MJ, Devereux RB. Associations of aortic and mitral regurgitation with body composition and myocardial energy expenditure in adults with hypertension: the Hypertension Genetic Epidemiology Network Study. Am Heart J 2003; 145:1071–1077.

96. Thomas JT, Kelly RF, Thomas SJ, Stamos TD, Albasha K, Parrillo JE, Calvin JE. Utility of history, physical examination, electrocardiogram, and chest radiograph for differentiating normal from decreased systolic function in patients with heart failure. Am J Med 2002; 112:437–445.

97. Lim PO, MacFadyen RJ, Clarkson PBM, MacDonald TM. Impaired exercise tolerance in hypertensive patients. Ann Int Med 1996; 124:41–55.

98. Cuspidi C, Ambrosioni E, Mancia G, Pessina AC, Trimarco B, Zanchetti A. Role of echocardiography and carotid ultrasonography in stratifying risk in patients with essential hypertension: the assessment of prognostic risk observational survey. J Hypertens 2002; 20:1307–1314.

99. Schillaci G, de Simone G, Reboldi G, Porcellati C, Devereux RB, Verdecchia P. Change in cardiovascular risk profile by echocardiography in low- or medium-risk hypertension. J Hypertens 2002; 20:1519–1525.

100. Aeschbacher BC, Hutter D, Fuhrer J, Weidmann P, Delacretaz E, Allemann Y. Diastolic dysfunction precedes myocardial hypertrophy in the development of hypertension. Am J Hypertens 2001; 14:106–113.

101. Maceira AM, Barba J, Beloqui O, Diez J. Ultrasonic backscatter and diastolic function in hypertensive patients. Hypertension 2002; 40:239–243.

102. Clarkson PBM, Wheeldon NM, Lim PO, Pringle SD, MacDonald TM. Left atrial size and function—assessment using echocardiographic automated boundary detection. Br Heart J 1995; 74:664–670.

103. Tsang TS, Barnes ME, Gersh BJ, Takemoto Y, Rosales AG, Bailey KR, Seward JB. Prediction of risk for first age related cardiovascular events in an elderly population: the incremental value of echocardiography. J Am Coll Cardiol 2003; 42:1199–1205.

104. Tsang TS, Barnes ME, Gersh BJ, Bailey KR, Seward JB. Left atrial volume as a morphophysiologic expression of left ventricular diastolic dysfunction and relation to cardiovascular risk burden. Am J Cardiol 2002; 15:1284–1289.

105. Verdecchia P, Schillaci G, Borgioni C, Ciucci A, Zampi I, Gattobigio R, Sacchi N, Porcellati C. White coat

hypertension and white coat effect—similarities and differences. Am J Hypertens 1995; 8:790–798.

106. Soma J, Wideroe TE, Dahl K, Rossvoll O, Skjaerpe T. Left ventricular systolic and diastolic function assessed with two-dimensional and Doppler echocardiography in "white coat" hypertension. J Am Coll Cardiol 1996; 28:190–196.

107. Glen SK, Elliott HL, Curzio JL, Lees KR, Reid JL. White-coat hypertension as a cause of cardiovascular dysfunction. Lancet 1996; 348:654–657.

108. Slotwiner DJ, Devereux RB, Schwartz JE, Pickering TG, de Simone G, Roman MJ. Relation of age to left ventricular function and systemic hemodynamics in uncomplicated mild hypertension. Hypertension 2001; 37:1404–1409.

109. Poulsen SH, Andersen NH, Ivarsen PI, Mogensen CE, Egeblad H. Doppler tissue imaging reveals systolic dysfunction in patients with hypertension and apparent "isolated" diastolic dysfunction. J Am Soc Echocardio 2003; 16:724–731.

110. Pela G, Bruschi G, Cavatorta A, Manca C, Cabassi A, Borghetti A. Doppler tissue echocardiography: myocardial wall motion velocities in essential hypertension. Eur J Echocardiog 2001; 2:108–117.

111. Bella JN, Wachtell K, Palmieri V, Liebson PR, Gerdts E, Ylitalo A, Koren MJ, Pedersen OL, Rokkedal J, Dahlof B, Roman MJ, Devereux RB. Relation of left ventricular geometry and function to systemic hemodynamics in hypertension: the LIFE study. J Hypertens 2001; 19:127–134.

112. Desimone G, Devereux RB, Roman MJ, Ganau A, Saba PS, Alderman MH, Laragh JH. Assessment of left ventricular function by the mid wall fractionbal shortening end systolic stress relation in human hypertension. J Am Coll Cardiol 1994; 23:1444–1451.

113. Chen HH, Lainchbury JG, Senni M, Bailey KR, Redfield MM. Diastolic heart failure in the community: clinical profile, natural history, therapy, and impact of proposed diagnostic criteria. J Cardiac Failure 2002; 8:279–287.

114. Kitzman DW. Diastolic heart failure in the elderly. Heart Fail Rev 2002; 7:17–27.

115. Nodari S, Metra M, Dei Cas L. Beta blocker treatment of patients wit diastolic heart failure and arterial hyper tension: a prospective randomised comparison of the long term effects of atenolol vs. nebivolol. Eur J Heart Failure 2003; 5:621–627.

116. Clarkson PB, Wheeldon NM, MacFadyen RJ, Pringle SD, MacDonald TM. Effcets of brain natriuretic peptide on exercise haemodynamics and neurohormones in isolated diastolic heart failure. Circulation 1996; 93:2037–2042.

117. Galderisi M, Cicala S, Caso P, de Simone L, D'Errico A, Petrocelli A, de Divitiis O. Coronary flow reserve and myocardial diastolic dysfunction in arterial hypertension. Am J Cardiol 2002; 90:860–864.

118. Klein AL, Canale MP, Rajagopalan N, White RD, Murray RD, Wahi S, Arheart KL, Thomas JD. Role of transesophageal echocardiography in assessing diastolic

dysfunction in a large clinical practice: a 9 year experience. Am Heart J 1999; 138:880–889.

119. Fischer M, Baessler A, Hense HW, Hengstenberg C, Muscholl M, Holmer S, Doring A, Broeckel U, Riegger G, Schunkert H. Prevalence of left ventricular diastolic dysfunction in the community. Results from a Doppler echocardiographic based survey of a population sample. Eur Heart J 2003; 24:320–328.

120. Weiss JL, Frederiksen JW, Weisfeldt ML. Hemodynamic determinants of the time course of fall in canine left ventricular pressure. J Clin Invest 1976; 58:751–760.

121. Kawaguchi M, Hay I, Fetics B et al. Combined ventricular and arterial stiffening in patients with heart failure and preserved ejection fraction: implications for systolic and diastolic reserve limitations. Circulation 2003; 107:714–720.

122. Burkhoff D, Maurer MS, Packer M. Heart failure with a normal ejection fraction. Is it really a disorder of diastolic function? Circulation 2003; 107:656–658.

123. Angeja BG, Grossmann W. Evaluation and management of diastolic heart failure. Circulation 2003; 107:659–663.

124. Shimizu M, Ino H, Okeie K, Emoto Y, Yamaguchi M, Yasuda T, Fujino N, Fujii H, Fujita S, Nakajima K, Taki J, Mabuchi H. Cardiac sympathetic activity in the asymmetrically hypertrophied septum in patients with hypertension or hypertrophic cardiomyopathy. Am J Hypertens 1998; 11:1171–1177.

125. Takeda A, Takeda N. Different pathophysiology of cardiac hypertrophy in hypertension and hypertrophic cardiomyopathy. J Mol Cell Cardiol 1997; 29:2161–2165.

126. Mottram PM, Leano R, Marwick TH. Usefullness of B type natriuretic peptide in hypertensive patients with exertional dyspnea and normal left ventricular ejection fraction and correlation with new echocardiographic indices of systolic and diastolic function. Am J Cardiol 2003; 92:1434–1438.

127. Akinboboye OO, Reichek N, Bergmann SR, Chou RL. Correlates of myocardial oxygen demand measured by positron emission tomography in the hypertrophied left ventricle. Am J Hypertens 2003; 16:240–243.

128. Paelinck blood pressure, Lamb HJ, Bax JJ, Van der Wall EE, de Roos A. Assessment of diastolic function by cardiovascular magnetic resonance. Am Heart J 2002; 144:198–205.

129. Lamb HJ, Beyer bacht HP, van der Laarse A, Stoel BC, Doornbos J, van der Wall EE, de Roos A. Diastolic dysfunction in hypertensive heart disease is associated with altered myocardial metabolism. Circulation 1999; 99:2261–2267.

130. Beer M, Seyfarth T, Sandstede J, Landschutz W, Lipke C, Kostler H, von Kienlin M, Harre K, Hahn D, Neubauer S. Absolute concentrations of high-energy phosphate metabolites in normal, hypertrophied, and failing human myocardium measured noninvasively with P-31-SLOOP magnetic resonance spectroscopy. J Am Coll Cardiol 2002; 40:1267–1274.

131. Missouris CG, Forbat SM, Singer DR, Markandu ND, Underwood R, MacGregor GA. Echocardiography

overestimates left ventricular mass: a comparative study with magnetic resonance imaging in patients with hypertension. J Hypertens 1996; 14:1005–1110.

132. Germain P, Roul G, Kastler B, Mossard JM, Bareiss P, Sacrez A. Inter study variuability in left ventricular mass measurement. Comparison between M-Mode echocardiography and MRI. Eur Heart J 1992; 13:1011–1019.

133. De las Fuentes L, Herrero P, Peterson LR, Kelly DP, Gropler RJ, Davila-Roman VG. Myocardial fatty acid metabolism: independent predictor of left ventricular mass in hypertensive heart disease. Hypertension 2002; 15:907–910.

134. Stauer BE, Schjwartzkopff B, Kelm M. Assessing the coronary circulation in hypertension. J Hypertens 1998; 16:1221–1233.

135. Masuda D, Nohara R, Tamaki N et al. Evaluation of coronary flowe reserve by ^{13}N – NH$_3$ positron emission tomography wit dipyridamole in the treatment of hypertension with an ACE inhibitor. Ann Nucl Med 2000; 14:353–360.

136. Gimelli A, Schneider-Eicke J, Neglia D, Sambuceti G, Gioretti A, Bigalli G, Parodi G, Pedrinelli R, Parodi O. Homogeneously reduced versus regionally impaired myocardial blood flow in hypertensive patients: two different patterns of myocardial perfusion associated with degree of hypertrophy. J Am Coll Cardiol 1998; 31:366–373.

137. Shiba N, Kagaya Y, Ishide N, Takeyama D, Yamane Y, Chida M, Otani H, Ido T, Shirato K. Myocardial glucose metabolism is different between hypertrophic cardio-myopathy and hypertensive heart disease associated with asymmetrical septal hypertrophy. Tohoku J Exp Med 1997; 182:125–138.

138. Seidl K, Hauer B, Schwick NG, Zellner D, Zahn R, Senges J. Risk of thromboembolic events in patients with atrial flutter. Am J Cardiol 1998; 82:580–583.

139. Krahn AD, Manfreda J, Tate RB, Mathewson FAL, Cuddy TE. The natural history of atrial fibrillation—incidence, risk factors and prognosis in the Manitoba follow-up study. Am J Med 1995; 98:476–484.

140. Healey JS, Connolly SJ. Atrial fibrillation: hypertension as a causative agent, risk factor for complications, and potential therapeutic target. Am J Cardiol 2003; 22 (suppl 10A):9G–14G.

141. Benjamin EJ, Levy D, Vaziri SM, D'Agostino RB, Belanger AJ, Wolf PA. Independent risk factors for atrial fibrillation in a population based cohort—the Framingham study. J Am Med Assoc 1994; 271:840–844.

142. Ezekowitz M, Laupacis A, Boysen G, Connolly S, Hart R, James K, Kistler P, Koudstaal P, Kronmal R, McBride R, Petersen P, Singer D. Echocardiographic predictors of stroke in patients with atrial fibrillation—a prospective study of 1066 patients from 3 clinical trials. Arch Int Med 1998; 158:1316–1320.

143. Hennersdorf MG, Hafke GJ, Steiner S, Dierkes S, Jansen A, Perings C, Strauer BE. Determinants of paroxysmal atrial fibrillation in patients with arterial hypertension. Zeit Fur Kardiol 2003; 92:370–376.

144. Ghali JK, Kadakia S, Cooper RS, Liao Y. Impact of left ventricular hypertrophy on ventricular arrhythmias in the absence of coronary artery disease. J Am Coll Cardiol 1991; 17:1277–1282.

145. Verdecchia P, Reboldi G, Gattobigio R, Bentivoglio M, Borgioni C, Angeli F, Carluccio E, Sardone MG, Porcellati C. Atrial fibrillation in hypertension—predictors and outcome. Hypertension 2003; 41:218–223.

146. Vaziri SM, Larson MG, Benjamin EJ, Levy D. Echo-cardiographic predictors of non rheumatic atrial fibrillation—the Framingham Heart Study. Circulation 1994; 89:724–730.

147. O'Toole L, Williams A, Shaw TRD, Starkey IR, Northridge DB. Hypertension strongly predicts early relapse after elective cardioversion of atrial fibrillation. J Am Coll Cardiol 1998; 31(suppl):195A–195A.

148. Kerr C, Boone J, Connolly S, Greene M, Klein G, Sheldon R, Talajic M. Follow-up of atrial fibrillation: The initial experience of the Canadian registry of atrial fibrillation. Eur Heart J 1996; 17(suppl C):48–51.

149. McLenachan JM, Henderson E, Morris KI, Dargie HJ. Ventricular arrhythmias in patients with hypertensive left ventricular hypertrophy. New Eng J Med 1987; 317:787–792.

150. Haider AW, Larson MG, Benjamin EJ, Levy D. Increased left ventricular mass and hypertrophy are associated with increased risk for sudden death. J Am Coll Cardiol 1998; 32:1454–1459.

151. Szlachcic J, Tubau JF, O'Kelly B, Ammon S, Daiss K, Massie BM. What is the role of siolent coronary artery disease and left ventricular hypertrophy in the genesis of ventricular arrhythmias in men with essential hypertension? J Am Coll Cardiol 1992; 19:803–808.

152. Schillaci G, Verdecchia P, Borgioni C, Ciucci A, Zampi I, Battistelli M, Gattobigio R, Sacchi N, Porcellati C. Association between persistent pressure overload and ventricular arrhythmias in essential hypertension. Hypertension 1996; 28:284–289.

153. Davey P, Bateman J, Mulligan IP, Forfar JC, Barlow C, Hart G. QT interval dispersion in chronic heart failure and left ventricular hypertrophy—relation to autonomic nervous system and Holter tape abnormalities. Br Heart J 1994; 71:268–273.

154. Glancy JM, Garratt CJ, Woods KL, DeBono DP. QT dispersion and mortality after myocardial infarction. Lancet 1995; 345:945–948.

155. Kluger J, Giedrimiene D, White CM, Verroneau J, Giedrimas E. A comparison of the QT and QTc dispersion among patients with sustained ventricular tachyarrhythmias and different etiologies of heart disease. Ann Noninv Electrocardiol 2001; 6:319–322.

16

The Kidney and Hypertension

MOHAMMED YOUSHAUDDIN, GEORGE L. BAKRIS

Rush University Medical Center, Chicago, Illinois, USA

KEYPOINTS

- Sustained BP $> 140/90$ mmHg over years causes kidney damage.
- Maintenance of BP $< 130/80$ mmHg maximally protects against injuries from high blood pressure or diabetes.
- BP $< 120/80$ mmHg may be needed if proteinuria (≥ 1000 mg/d) is present.
- Kidney disease is an independent risk factor for cardiovascular events and is asymptomatic until $>70\%$ of kidney function is lost. Thus, annual biochemical screening is necessary.

SUMMARY

To optimally protect kidney function in those with hypertension: (a) Achieve goal $<130/80$ mmHg;

<120/80 mmHg if proteinuria (>1000 mg/d) present;
(b) Avoid excessive use of NSAIDs or COX-2 agents;
and (c) Have annual biochemical screening age ≥40 for
kidney function including check for albuminuria.

I. INTRODUCTION

Hypertension affects 50 million individuals in the USA,
and approximately 1 billion worldwide (1). Hypertension
secondary to underlying renal parenchymal disease is by
far the most frequent form of secondary hypertension
and accounts for ~5% of all hypertension (2). There is a
unique and distinctive relationship between the kidney
and blood pressure (BP). On one hand, renal dysfunction
can cause an increase in BP; likewise, high BP can accelerate loss of kidney function. One particularly interesting
observation is that the prevalence of hypertension
increases with decreasing renal function; it is estimated
that 80–90% of patients with end-stage renal disease are
affected with hypertension (3) (Fig. 16.1). Although only
a small proportion of patients with primary hypertension
develop progressive renal insufficiency, the incidence of
renal insufficiency increases progressively with every
10 mmHg increment in systolic pressure (4).

In chronic renal parenchymal disease, hypertension is
often sustained and associated with a greater risk of cardiovascular morbidity and mortality compared with that in
the absence of kidney disease. Hypertension-induced vascular or target organ injury can be prevented or delayed by
reducing systolic arterial pressure in the range
<140 mmHg with a striking benefit observed for those
with any level of proteinuria or macroalbuminuria and
chronic kidney disease, if BP is reduced to levels <130/
80 mmHg. Hypertension in patients with chronic renal
parenchymal disease of either diabetic or nondiabetic
etiology markedly accelerates the loss of renal function,
as well as other processes such as atherosclerosis.

This chapter will cover both the pathogenesis and the
treatment of hypertension in people with kidney disease.
It will discuss how high BP contributes to renal injury as
well as perpetuating injury due to other concomitant diseases such as diabetes.

II. PATHOGENESIS

The mechanisms for BP increase in renoparenchymal
disease are complex and interactive, often comprising of
the following four components.

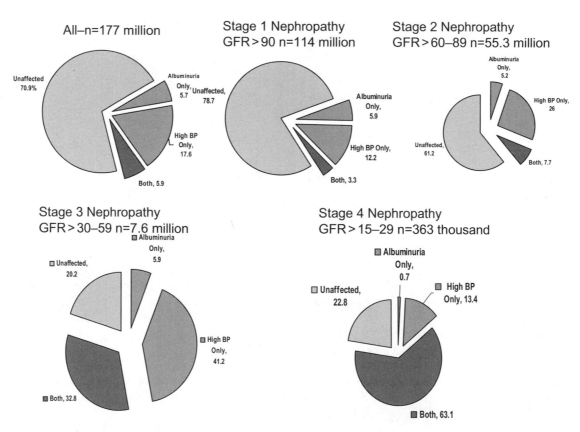

Figure 16.1 Prevalence of albuminuria and high BP in the USA. Data obtained from NHANES III database-numbers represent (%) of
the total group. [Adapted from the KDOQI Blood Pressure Guidelines (63).]

A. Salt Retention

There is a direct correlation between the degree of plasma volume expansion, sodium retention, and the degree of hypertension (5). The progressive loss of functioning nephrons reduces the ability of the diseased kidney to excrete sodium and water. The result is extra cellular fluid (ECF) volume expansion leading to the release of an endogenous ouabain-like hormone (6), which impairs the renal tubular reabsorption of NaCl in an attempt to normalize ECF volume. The inhibition of Na^+/K^+-ATPase in vascular smooth muscle, however, leads to an increase in cytosolic Ca^{2+} with resultant vasoconstriction and an increased sensitivity to circulating vasoactive agents. Hypervolemia occurs in the arterial and venous vascular bed with an increase in the cardiac output and consequent increase in arterial BP.

B. Inappropriate Activity of Sympathetic Nervous System

The sympathetic nervous system is activated in renal failure (7), leading to increased cardiac output, enhanced renal salt retention, an interference of pressure natriuresis, as well as an enhanced systemic and renal vasoconstriction. It has been observed that plasma norepinephrine levels are higher in hypertensive patients with early renal failure compared with normal control subjects or normotensive patients with a similar degree of renal insufficiency (8).

C. Impaired Endothelial Cell-Mediated Vasodilatation

Arterial wall stiffness is increased in chronic renal failure (9). It is hypothesized that, in both essential hypertension and chronic renal failure, there is a defective regulation of systemic and renal vascular tone due to diminished production of an endothelium-relaxing factor (nitric oxide) with an increased production of the endothelium-constricting factor (endothelin) (10–12).

Peripheral resistance can also be increased by reflex vasoconstriction secondary to increased organ flow (13). There is increased vascular responsiveness secondary to thickening of the vascular wall (14) and impairment of the endothelial-vascular smooth muscle paracrine system (10–12). Insulin resistance develops in chronic renal failure, while the higher insulin levels lead to hypertrophy of vascular smooth muscle and renal NaCl retention (15).

D. Abnormal Responses of Renin–Angiotensin–Aldosterone System

Suppression of the renin–angiotensin–aldosterone system (RAAS) in chronic renal failure by ECF volume expansion appears to be impaired (5,16). Thus, plasma renin activity (PRA) levels are inappropriately high for the degree of ECF volume expansion. Furthermore, there is also an increased formation of angiotensin II, which has a strong vasoconstrictive property as well as an increased responsiveness of the vascular smooth muscle to angiotensin II.

III. ROLE OF HYPERTENSION IN PROGRESSION OF RENAL FAILURE

Kidney function declines at different rates depending on the etiology, for example, diabetes mellitus vs. membranous nephropathy vs. IgA nephropathy. Moreover, the timing of achieving BP goal is critically important in the prevention of the catastrophic effect of renal disease progression. Specifically, intervention to a BP goal of <130/80 mmHg during the very early stages of renal dysfunction, that is, glomerular filtration rate (GFR) >85 mL/min, is very likely to stop disease progression, whereas intervention when GFR is <50 mL/min will only slow its progression (Fig. 16.2). Early intervention will impact GFR loss when one looks at the rate of decline in kidney function amongst the various clinical trials (Fig. 16.2). In studies where participants had lost more than half their GFR at the beginning of the study, average rate of loss was in the range of 3–5 mL/min per year, normal being about 1 mL/min per year. In those who had lost ~10–20% at baseline, the average rate of loss was ~1.6–2.5 mL/min per year. Thus, early aggressive BP intervention results in substantial preservation of kidney function.

This concept is exemplified by the results from the Appropriate Blood Pressure Control in Diabetes (ABCD) trial, where the average levels of GFR were >80 mL/min at the start of the trial vs. other diabetes trials where the GFR is generally <50 mL/min at baseline (17). GFR decline was virtually stopped with early BP intervention in the ABCD trial, whereas in other trials of more advanced renal disease GFR, loss occurred at a rate of 2–7 mL/min per year (18). Furthermore, BP levels attained in the ABCD trial averaged <130/80 mmHg. Thus, results of clinical trials among participants with advanced renal disease should not be extrapolated to patients with very early disease, because rates of decline in renal function are not uniformly linear.

An analysis of randomized clinical trials of renal disease progression that included antihypertensive drugs that block the renin angiotensin system, that is, ACE

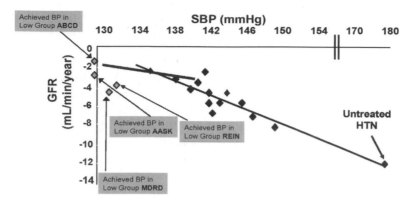

Figure 16.2　Impact of early intervention on decline in kidney function. Four trials were randomized to two levels of BP on kidney outcomes; >a 10 mmHg lower BP slowed progression by 50% between BP 130 and 149 mmHg; and baseline GFR in MDRD, REIN, and AASK (all nondiabetic renal failure studies) was ~45 mL/min whereas in ABCD (diabetic renal disease study) GFR was 84 mL/min. Slowest rate of decline was in group with earliest intervention. (Parving HH et al. Br Med J 1988; 297:1086–1091; Viberti GC et al. JAMA 1994; 271:275–279; Klahr S et al. (MDRD) N Eng J Med 1994; 330:877–884; Lewis EJ et al. N Engl J Med 1993; 329:1456–1462; Hebert L et al. Kidney Int 1994; 46:1688–1693; Lebovitz H et al. Kidney Int 1994; 45:S150–S155; Maschio G et al. (AIPRI) N Engl J Med 1996; 334:939–945; Bakris GL et al. Kidney Int 1996; 50:1641–1650; Bakris GL. Hypertension 1997; 29:744–750; GISEN Group. (REIN) Lancet 1997; 349:1857–1863; Estacio R et al. (ABCD) Diabetes Care 2000; 23(suppl 2):B54–B64; Brenner BM et al. (RENAAL) N Engl J Med 2001; 345:861–869; Lewis EJ et al. (IDNT) N Engl J Med 2001; 345:851–860; Wright JT Jr et al. (AASK) JAMA 2002; 288:2421–2431.)

inhibitors, showed that a rise in serum creatinine limited to 30% given a baseline or initial serum creatinine level of 3 mg/dL (265 mmol/L) and age ≤65 years, within the first 4 months of starting therapy correlated with marked preservation of renal function over a mean follow-up period of ≥3 years (18). In addition, Ramipril Efficacy in Nephropathy (REIN), Angiotensin Converting Enzyme Inhibitor and Progressive Renal Insufficiency (AIPRI), and Modification of Dietary Protein in Renal

Disease (MDRD) trials, as well as other smaller trials, have established the ability of antihypertensive therapy in slowing the progression of renal disease (19–21). These studies and a meta-analysis by Jafar et al. clearly show that level of BP is not only important but also *critical* for patients with proteinuria of >1 g per day, (Fig. 16.3). Thus, attainment of the recommended goal BP < 130/80 mmHg, is critical for the preservation of renal function in such individuals.

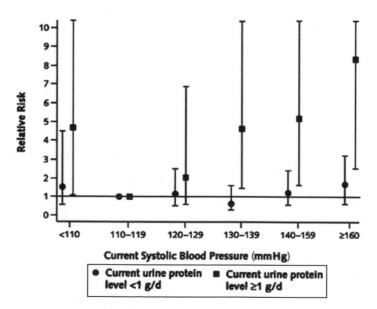

Figure 16.3　Relationship between BP range and relative risk of progression of nondiabetic kidney disease in the context of proteinuria. (From Jafar T et al. Ann Intern Med 2003.)

IV. CAUSES OF RENOPARENCHYMAL HYPERTENSION

A. Primary Renal Disease

Hypertension is much more common and manifests itself earlier in glomerular-vascular disease as compared to tubulointerstitial disease. In one series the frequency of hypertension was 73% for glomerular-vascular disease and 15% for tubulointerstitial disease (22).

1. Glomerulonephritis

The overall incidence of hypertension in primary chronic glomerulonephritis (GN) reported in different series varies from 42% to 62% (23–25). Hypertension is more frequent and severe in patients with sclerotic, proliferative, and extra/endocapillary GN. These patients are more prone to progress to end-stage renal disease in contrast to patients with "minimal change" disease for which hypertension is rare and kidney function is well preserved. In an analysis of 310 cases reported by Danielsen et al. (25), the frequency of hypertension in various types of GN is as shown in Table 16.1.

Renal involvement from multisystemic diseases, for example, scleroderma, systemic lupus, polyarteritis nodosa, hemolytic-uremic syndrome, and atheroembolic renal disease, are classified as secondary glomerulonephritides. The frequency of hypertension in these diseases varies between 10% and 50%.

2. Polycystic Kidney Disease

Hypertension is a common early finding in polycystic kidney disease (PKD), occurring in 50–70% of cases before any significant reduction in GFR or elevation of serum creatinine is seen (26). The changes develop slowly, and they frequently become clinically relevant only in middle age. Hypertension is an important factor in the progression of PKD to end-stage renal disease (27). In advanced stages, the destruction of the renal

Table 16.1 Summary of Glomerular Disease and Frequency of Hypertension

Histological form of glomerulonephritis	Frequency of hypertension (%)
Sclerosing	88
Membranoproliferative	75
Extracapillary	65
Segmental sclerosing	63
Focal proliferative	57
Mesangioproliferative	50
Endocapillary	50

tissue leads to rapid deterioration of renal function, eventually requiring dialysis treatment.

3. Tubulointerstitial Diseases

Hypertension occurs relatively late and sometimes may not appear before end-stage renal disease. In a series of 1921 patients with different nephropathies and hypertension, the incidence of hypertension associated with chronic pyelonephritis was 63% and chronic interstitial nephropathy was 62% (24). Analgesic nephropathy is associated with hypertension in 50% of the cases.

4. Diabetes

Hypertension is common and is closely related to the development of renal disease in patients with diabetes. African-American patients with diabetes have a higher likelihood of developing progressive renal disease than the general population (28). In Type I diabetes, the incidence of hypertension rises from 5% at 10 years to 33% at 20 years, and it is a staggering 70% at 40 years, but hypertension is present in only 2–3% of those without clinically evident renal involvement. Such patients may have underlying essential hypertension. Of the total patients with Type II 30% diabetes have hypertension at the time of diagnosis of diabetes; when nephropathy develops, almost 70% have high BP (29). The relationship between arterial hypertension and diabetic nephropathy in Type II diabetes is not as clear as in Type I diabetes (30). Involvement of the kidney in diabetes is usually asymptomatic.

Patients with diabetes who are at risk of developing nephropathy can be identified by the detection of microalbuminuria (MA). MA is defined as a urinary albumin excretion rate of 30–300 mg per 24 h (or 20–200 μg/mL) on two of three measurements. MA is also a marker of impaired endothelial responsiveness and a predictor of both overall cardiovascular morbidity and risk of kidney disease progression (31–33). BP control using all agents can reduce MA; however, in some studies dihydropyridine calcium antagonists (CA), that is, nifedipine, amlodipine, and others, may not consistently reduce MA (34). MA increases with age and is more common in Type II than in Type I diabetes and is supplanted by macroalbuminuria or proteinuria as nephropathy advances (Fig. 16.1) (35). The prevalence of MA in Type II diabetics is about 20% (range: 12–36%), and is more common ($\sim$30%) in those older than 55 years of age (32,36). The prevalence of MA ranges from 5% to 40% in nondiabetic hypertensives (36) with the degree of MA proportional to the severity of systolic, diastolic, and mean BP elevation as measured by either clinic or 24 h ambulatory BP monitoring (38–40). Circadian abnormalities of BP seen in nondippers, who are known to be at higher risk for cardiovascular events, also have a higher prevalence of MA.

MA is a marker of vascular injury and, quite possibly, inflammation as evidenced by recent findings of a strong correlation between C-reactive protein levels and MA. MA develops secondary to defective podocyte function in the glomerulus coupled with an increased intraglomerular pressure and reflects an enhanced vascular permeability and, hence, altered barrier function of the epithelial/endothelium areas in the kidney (37,73,74). It has been postulated by Remuzzi et al. that MA is pathogenic itself within the kidney and contributes to free radical generation and cytokine production, hence accelerating processes that lead to interstitial fibrosis. Although an attractive hypothesis it remains to be shown in humans. More than 35% of patients with diabetes progress on further to diabetic nephropathy developing macroalbuminuria (>300 mg/day) or proteinuria, a decline in GFR, and an increased arterial pressure. The presence of diabetic nephropathy is associated with increased morbidity and mortality due to both increased cardiovascular events and end-stage renal failure (32). Risk factors for the development of diabetic nephropathy in Type II diabetes include increasing age, long duration of diabetes, poor glycemic control, hypertension, and smoking (35,40).

Those with diabetes and macroalbuminuria are 20 times more likely to die of cardiovascular disease than those without albuminuria. Hence, the treatment should be aimed at both lowering arterial pressure to a stated goal as well as reducing proteinuria by at least 30–50% from baseline (32,41). Patients with diabetes should be started on antihypertensive medications even if the BP is in the high normal range (>135/85 mmHg) because of the heightened cardiovascular and renal risk (1).

Subjects with MA and Type II DM have an annual total mortality and cardiovascular mortality that is about four times higher than those of diabetics without MA (32). In several series, the cardiovascular event and mortality rates in nondiabetic hypertensives with MA was 2–4-fold higher than in those without MA (42,43). MA is also associated with other types of hypertension-related target organ damage (TOD), including left ventricular hypertrophy (LVH). These associations are not as commonly seen in younger individuals, or in those with Stage 1 hypertension, suggesting that the association of MA and LVH may be related to a higher BP load.

B. Unilateral Renal Disease

Hypertension from unilateral renoparenchymal disease is considered to be potentially curable. The most frequent causes of unilateral renal parenchymal disease accompanied by hypertension are for example, reflux nephropathy, hydronephrosis, renal tumors, renal tuberculosis (unilateral), and solitary renal cysts.

C. Evaluation of a Patient with Renal Parenchymal Hypertension

The evaluation of a hypertensive patient with possible renoparenchymal etiology includes a urinalysis, blood urea nitrogen (BUN), serum creatinine, dipstick for proteinuria, spot urine albumin to creatinine ratio reported as milligram of albumin per gram of creatinine (A/C), renal ultrasound, and occasionally renal biopsy.

1. Laboratory Diagnostics

Abnormalities in the urinalysis such as microhematuria, red cell casts in the sediment with concomitant proteinuria, are indicative of GN. Pyuria, bacteuria, and white blood cell casts are seen in pyelonephritis.

Protein excretion >300 mg/day or >200 μg/min represents overt proteinuria (32). The urine dipstick is a relatively insensitive marker for proteinuria, not becoming positive until protein excretion exceeds 300–500 mg/ day. By using a conventional dipstick, which can only detect higher levels of urinary protein (>300 mg/day), the opportunity to characterize a patient's prognosis more precisely, earlier in the disease process, may be missed. Dipsticks that detect MA are now available and fairly inexpensive. It is recommended that all patients with hypertension and "trace" proteinuria by conventional dipstick have a spot urine to quantify urinary protein excretion; this is best assessed by the albumin to creatinine (mg/g) ratio in a spot urine specimen (32). These values have been demonstrated to correlate with 24 h urine collections and are much more practical (44). Routine assessment of MA for diabetic patients is well advised, but in hypertensives without DM, its value is still debatable. In part, this is due to the relatively low prevalence of MA and the uncertainty of the significance of its modification in the nondiabetic population (45).

2. Ultrasonography

Renal ultrasonography is the most important imaging test in cases of suspected renoparenchymal disease. It is useful to compare the renal size, identify cysts, and screen for obstructive uropathy. Small dense "echogenic" kidneys on ultrasound indicate diffuse renoparenchymal disease. In diabetes and amyloidosis, renal size is often increased.

3. Renal Biopsy

Percutaneous renal biopsy should be performed only when the information will contribute to the treatment of the patient (i.e., alter therapy or provide critical prognostic information), for example, when laboratory tests indicate the presence of GN as the cause of hypertension.

V. RENOVASCULAR HYPERTENSION

Renovascular hypertension is the most frequent curable form of hypertension (Table 16.2). Its prevalence is estimated to be between 0.2% and 5% of the entire hypertensive population (2,46). Patients with this form of secondary hypertension often have considerable TOD and are at risk of losing renal function. At least 90% of renovascular hypertension is due to renal artery atherosclerosis, with only 10% being due to fibromuscular dysplasia or unusual causes (47). Atherosclerotic renal artery stenosis is a disease of older individuals and usually involves the ostium, proximal third of main renal artery, and the perirenal aorta (Fig. 16.4). At advanced stages of the disease, segmental and diffuse intrarenal atherosclerosis may be observed, mainly in patients with ischemic nephropathy. Characteristically, these patients develop hypertension after age 50 or have a history of hypertension that had been relatively easy to control and became refractory. Atherosclerotic renal artery stenosis is a progressive disease. A large proportion of these patients are diabetic and frequently have evidence of vascular disease elsewhere (carotids, coronaries, and peripheral circulation, in particular); and the majority are cigarette smokers. Although it is more common in Caucasians, African-Americans also can develop atherosclerotic renovascular hypertension (47). Fibromuscular dysplasia tends to affect young white women in whom BP tends to rise abruptly to Stage 2 during the third decade of life (Fig. 16.5). Abdominal or flank bruits are heard commonly, and renal function is usually normal when the diagnosis is entertained. It frequently involves distal two thirds of the renal artery and its branches, and is characterized by a beaded, aneurysmal appearance on angiogram (47). Clinical hints for renovascular hypertension are summarized in Table 16.3.

A. Pathophysiology of Renovascular Disease

A decrease in renal perfusion pressure activates the renin–angiotensin system, which leads to release of renin and the production of angiotensin II. Angiotensin II elevates the BP by increased aldosterone secretion from adrenal cortex with consequent sodium retention that in turn expands the intravascular volume. Stimulation of sympathetic nervous system, increased intrarenal prostaglandin concentrations, and decreased nitric oxide production are other mechanisms involved in the pathogenesis of renovascular hypertension (48–50).

B. Diagnosis of Renovascular Hypertension

The objective of screening patients suspected of having renovascular hypertension is not only to verify that arterial lesions are present, but also to determine that the lesion discovered is in fact the cause of the patient's hypertension (47). The tests used to confirm the clinical suspicion that a patient has renovascular hypertension are either biochemical or depend on a variety of imaging techniques.

1. Biochemical Test in Renovascular Hypertension

Evidence suggests that increased creatinine or low potassium (indicating hyperreninemia causing hyperaldosteronism)

Table 16.2 Identifiable Secondary Causes of Hypertension and Screening Test Recommended

Diagnosis	Diagnostic test
Chronic kidney disease	Estimated GFR
Coarctation of the aorta	CT Angiography
Cushing's syndrome and other glucocorticoid excess states including chronic steroid therapy	History/dexamethasone suppression test
Drug-induced/related [see Table 17 from ref. (1)]	History; drug screening
Pheochromocytoma	24 h urinary metanephrine and normetanephrine
Primary aldosteronism and other mineralocorticoid excess states	24 h urinary aldosterone level or specific measurements of other mineralocorticoids
Renovascular hypertension[a]	Doppler flow study; MRA
Sleep apnea	Sleep study with O_2 saturation
Thyroid/parathyroid disease	TSH; serum PTH

[a]Most common curable cause of secondary hypertension.
Source: Adapted from JNC 7 (1).

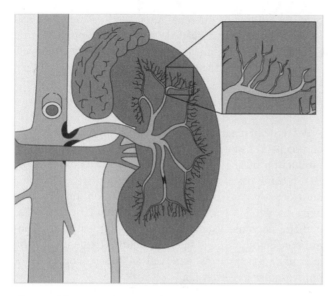

Figure 16.4 Atheromatous lesions of renal artery stenosis. The commonest site effected is at the ostium of the renal artery. [From McLaughlin et al. (70).]

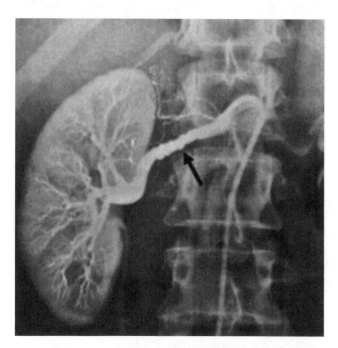

Figure 16.5 Angiogram of renal artery stenosis due to fibromuscular dysplasia of renal artery. Lesions typically affect the main renal artery, are beaded in appearance, and may have multiple stenosis. [From Stimpel M et al. (75).]

Table 16.3 Clinical Features and Pointers to the Diagnosis of Renal Artery Disease

Severe or refractory hypertension
Young hypertensive patients with no family history
   (fibromuscular dysplasia)
Peripheral vascular disease
Deteriorating BP control in compliant, long standing
   hypertensive patients
An acute elevation in serum creatinine after administration of
   ACE inhibitor or angiotensin II receptor blocker
Repeated episodes of flash pulmonary edema
>1.5 cm difference in kidney size on ultrasonography
Secondary hyperaldosteronism (low plasma sodium and
   potassium concentrations)
Systolic–diastolic bruit (not very sensitive)

play no role in case finding for renovascular hypertension because the sensitivity and specificity are too low (51). It is observed that the baseline peripheral PRA is elevated because of the activation of RAS in 50–80% of patients with proven renovascular hypertension. Measurement of the PRA after captopril (captopril test) has a sensitivity of 75% and specificity of 89% although better results have been obtained in some series (52,53), thus not as good as one would want for a diagnostic test. Measuring the concentration and activity of renin simultaneously from each renal vein and computing the renal vein renin ratio was once a very popular approach, but the sensitivity and specificity for detection of renovascular hypertension with this test are both ~75%, unacceptably low for an invasive procedure that requires special expertise and sophisticated measurements. It has been proposed that the accuracy of these measurements can be enhanced by prior administration of an ACE inhibitor, which will increase the renin secretion on the affected side. Renal vein renin ratio may still be useful to help prove that an anatomic lesion is the cause of a patient's hypertension, but should not be used as a screening tool because of relatively high cost and many false negative results (54,55). In short, biochemical screening for renovascular hypertension is not a useful or cost-effective exercise.

2. Imaging for Renovascular Hypertension

Rapid-sequence intravenous pyelography (IVP) was the earliest imaging study used for diagnosing renovascular hypertension. IVP has a sensitivity of 75% and specificity of 86%. Owing to its unreliability in detecting either branch stenosis or bilateral stenosis, together with high dose of dye and radiation exposure, it is not used in the diagnostic approach any longer. Renal duplex ultrasound has the advantage of being noninvasive and widely available. In some laboratories, the sensitivity of this test approaches 90–95% (56,57). However, abdominal gas or fat may make it difficult to visualize the renal arteries, compounded by the fact that this test is very operator-dependent and time-consuming. In many settings, little is gained by using this technique. However, in specialized centers with special expertise and in selected patients, it is a useful test. Gadolinium-enhanced magnetic resonance angiography (MRA) and spiral computed tomography with intravenous contrast (CT angiography) are more expensive approaches for visualization of the renal arteries, becoming more widely available and noninvasive. Both these modalities have sensitivity and specificity of over 90% in detecting stenosis of the main renal arteries but are not as successful at detecting branch lesions (58). Technical improvements are being made to enhance the image quality (59–63). These findings, taken together with the recent 2004 recommendations by the National Kidney Foundation for evaluation of RVH, support the concept that MRA is the diagnostic test of choice to evaluate renal arterial disease (63) (Figs. 16.6 and 16.7). Isotopic renography with labeled diethylenetriamine pentaacetic acid (a measure of glomerular filtration) or MAG-3 (a measure of renal blood flow) with captopril is a minimally invasive test that detects a discrepancy between perfusion and function of the kidneys. The overall sensitivity and specificity are 90% when done carefully, especially in patients whose prior probability of having renovascular hypertension is high (64,65). Only ACE-Is and ARBs need to be discontinued before the test is performed, and adverse reactions from the single dose of captopril are rare. Isotopic renography with captopril also provides functional information. If the time to peak activity is initially normal and becomes abnormal after captopril ("captopril-induced changes"), the likelihood of cure or improvement after revascularization is high.

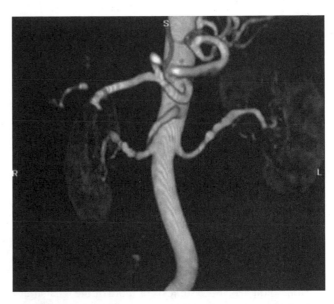

Figure 16.7 Gadolinium-enhanced MR angiogram displays high-resolution illustration of the renal arteries significantly better than duplex ultrasound and captopril nuclear scintigraphy.

Intra-arterial digital subtraction angiography is most frequently performed to define the renal artery anatomy and determine whether an arterial narrowing is present. In addition, the type of lesion (ostial, nonostial, or branch) can be determined. Its disadvantages are the intra-arterial puncture, high cost, and the risk of contrast-induced renal impairment. In many centers, percutaneous renal angioplasty is done at the same time if indicated (Fig. 16.8).

A recent clinical trial and meta-analysis of smaller studies demonstrate little benefit to routine revascularization of renal arteries for treatment of hypertension as compared to medical treatment (66,67). Generally

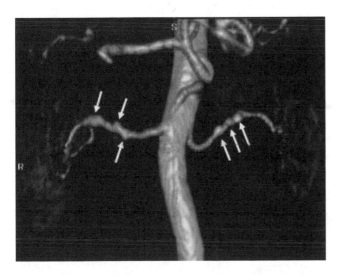

Figure 16.6 Gadolinium-enhanced MR angiogram. Magnified view of the renal arteries shows a "string of beads" appearance (arrows) in the middle-to-distal aspect of both renal arteries characteristic for fibromuscular dysplasia.

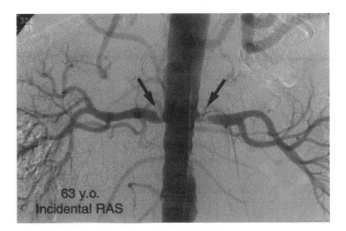

Figure 16.8 Aortogram illustrating relatively high-grade, bilateral atherosclerotic lesions located at the ostia of the renal arteries in a 63-year-old man (76).

Table 16.4   Clues to Viability of the Kidney with Renal Artery
Stenosis

Angiographic evidence of collaterals distal to the occlusion
Kidney size >8.5 cm on US
Biopsy (if available) shows well-preserved glomeruli and
   tubules
Kidney function on isotope renogram
Serum creatinine <4 mg/dL

Source: Adapted from Uzzo RG et al. Transplant Proc 2002;
34(2):723–725.

revascularization is not helpful, unless kidney function is
at risk as evidenced by declining kidney function in spite
of BP control. The criteria for a good outcome in regard
to preservation of renal function are indicated by the
following prognostic factors (Table 16.4).

Note: You need 80% stenosis or more of the renal artery
to affect either function and less clear BP. Stenosis smaller
than this are not associated with declines in kidney function and do NOT merit stenting or angioplasty, in part,
because of the risk of atheroembolic disease.

The presence of anatomic renal artery stenosis does not
mean that the lesion is responsible for the elevation in BP
(functional renal artery stenosis).

When considering whether to proceed with screening
for renovascular disease, the clinician must consider how
the data will be used. At present there is no sufficiently
accurate, noninvasive radiologic or biochemical screening
test that if negative, will completely exclude the presence
of renal artery stenosis (52,68). Thus, clinical index of suspicion and the presence or absence of renal insufficiency
are the primary determinants of the degree and type of
evaluation.

VI.   TREATMENT OF HYPERTENSION IN KIDNEY DISEASE

Management of hypertension in patients with kidney
disease is challenging and should focus not only on lowering BP but also reducing or normalizing MA and/or preventing the development of or a rise in macroalbuminuria
or proteinuria. This generally requires multiple and complementary acting antihypertensive agents to achieve the
recommended BP goal by the JNC 7 guidelines of
<130/80 mmHg. (Figs. 16.9 and 16.10) (1). The most
recent guidelines for management of hypertension in
people with kidney disease are shown in Table 16.5.
These   recommendations   arc   in   concert   with   all

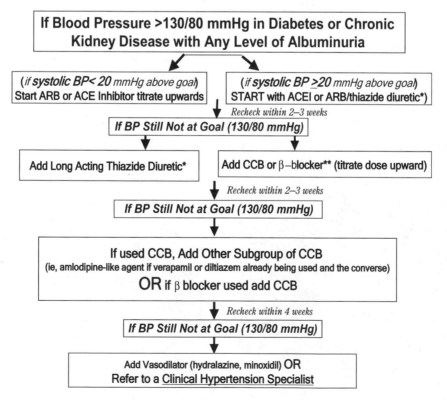

Figure 16.9   Integrated algorithm of American Diabetes Association, 2005; KDOdc-BP guidelines 2004 for treatment of hypertension
in someone with kidney disease or diabetes. *Thiazide diuretic should only be used if eGFR ≥ 50 mL/min otherwise loop diuretic should
be substituted. **The preferred β-blocker is carredilol since it has a neutral metabolic profile compared to other agents in the class.

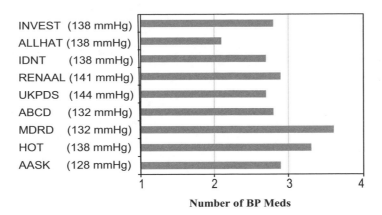

Figure 16.10 Average number of antihypertensive agents needed per patient to achieve target systolic BP goals.

Table 16.5 NKF-K/DOQI Guidelines on Blood Pressure Management and Use of Antihypertensive Agents in Chronic Kidney Disease

Type of kidney disease	Blood pressure target (mmHg)	Recommended agents for CKD, with or without hypertension	Other agents to reduce CVD risk and reach blood pressure target
Diabetic kidney disease	<130/80	ACE Inhibitor or ARB	Diuretics preferred, then BB or CCB
Non-diabetic kidney disease with proteinuria (≥200 mg/g)	<130/80	ACE Inhibitor	Diuretics preferred, then BB or CCB
Non-diabetic kidney disease without proteinuria (<200 mg/g)	<130/80	No preference	Diuretics preferred, then ACE inhibitor, ARB, BB, or CCB
Disease in the kidney transplant	<130/80	No preference	CCB, Diuretic, BB, ACE inhibitor, ARB

international recommendations including the American Diabetes Association, the JNC 7, and the European Guidelines. The goal should be to get to or below 130/80 mmHg to protect against renal and cardiovascular events and reduce organ injury. The data from an analysis of the NHANES III show that only 11% of people being treated for hypertension with diabetic kidney disease achieve the old BP goal of <130/85 mmHg, (69).

A few general rules need to always be considered when treating someone with kidney disease. These include keeping an eye on the BP goal and trying to achieve it; tolerating up to a 30% rise in serum creatinine with ACE inhibitors or ARBs if serum $[K^+]$ is <6 mEq/L and BP is at or close to goal; if diabetes is present, ensure that blood glucose is aggressively controlled with HbA1c <6.5%; all such patients should be on a low dose aspirin 75–150 mg/day along with a statin, if indicated by LDL cholesterol <100 mg/dL. In addition, ARBs or ACE inhibitors should be used as part of the regimen unless prohibited by difficult to manage anemia or potassium in Stage 4 nephropathy, but only after initiation of dialysis. Other blockers of the RAAS as well as beta-blockers and calcium channel antagonists can be used to achieve BP goal.

Lastly, proteinuria or macroalbuminuria should be monitored annually to ensure that reductions are being achieved. One should expect about a 30–35% reduction in proteinuria with an ACE inhibitor or ARB at maximal doses. The addition of an aldosterone receptor antagonist or an ARB to ACE inhibitor or vice versa should provide for another 30–40% reduction in proteinuria independent of further BP reduction (71,72). Use of a dihydropyridine CA is contraindicated in the absence of an ACE inhibitor or ARB in people with advanced disease as it has failed to show a benefit on slowing renal disease progression for those with Stage 3 nephropathy or higher when used in the absence of such agents (63).

This approach taken together with maximizing cardiovascular risk reduction will lead to marked prolongation of kidney function in people with hypertension pharmacology, pitfalls, and dangers.

CONCLUSION

It should be noted that ACE inhibitors and ARBs increase serum potassium in those with renal insufficiency but when used with appropriately dosed diuretics this is minimal. Values of $[K^+]$ upto 5.6 mEq/L should be tolerated. Other concerns include angioedema for this class of agents especially ACE inhibitors, although rare.

REFERENCES

1. Joint National Committee Report on the Diagnosis and the Treatment of Hypertension (JNC-7) Hypertension 2003; 42:1206–1252.

2. Sinclair AM, Isles CG, Brown I, Cameron H, Murray GD, Robertson JW. Secondary hypertension in a BP clinic. Arch Intern Med 1987; 147:1289–1293.

3. Mailloux LU, Haley WE. Hypertension in the ESRD patient: pathophysiology, therapy, outcomes, and future directions. Am J Kidney Dis 1998; 32:705–719.

4. Klag MJ, Whelton PK, Randall BL, Neaton JD, Brancati FL, Ford CE, Shulman NB, Stamler J. BP and end-stage renal disease in men. N Engl J Med 1996; 334:13–18.

5. Beretta-Piccoli C, Weidmann P, De Chatel R, Reubi F. Hypertension associated with early stage kidney disease. Complementary roles of circulating renin, the body sodium/volume state and duration of hypertension. Am J Med 1976; 61:739–746.

6. de Wardener HE, Millett J, Holland S, MacGregor GA, Alaghband-Zadeh J. Ouabainlike Na^+, K^+-ATPase inhibitor in the plasma of normotensive and hypertensive humans and rats. Hypertension 1987; 10:152–156.

7. Converse RL Jr, Jacobsen TN, Toto RD, Jost CM, Cosentino F, Fouad-Tarazi F, Victor RG. Sympathetic overactivity in patients with chronic renal failure. N Engl J Med 1992; 327:1912–1918.

8. Ishii M, Ikeda T, Takagi M, Sugimoto T, Atarashi K, Igari T, Uehara Y, Matsuoka H, Hirata Y, Kimura K, Takeda T, Murao S. Elevated plasma catecholamines in hypertensives with primary glomerular diseases. Hypertension 1983; 5:545–551.

9. Mourad JJ, Girerd X, Boutouyrie P, Laurent S, Safar M, London G. Increased stiffness of radial artery wall material in end-stage renal disease. Hypertension 1997; 30:1425–1430.

10. Aiello S, Remuzzi G, Noris M. Nitric oxide/endothelin balance after nephron reduction. Kidney Int 1998; 53:S63–S67.

11. Kone BC. Nitric oxide in renal health and disease. Am J Kidney Dis 1997; 30:311–333.

12. Remuzzi G, Benigni A. Progression of proteinuric diabetic and nondiabetic renal diseases: A possible role for renal endothelin. Kidney 1997; 51: S66-S68.

13. Ledingham JM, Cohen RD. The role of the heart in the pathogenesis of renal hypertension. Lancet 1993; 2:979–981.

14. Schiffrin EL. Reactivity of small blood vessels in hypertension: relation with structural changes. Hypertension 1992; 19:SII-1–SII-9.

15. Reaven GM. Banting Lecture 1988: Role of insulin resistance in human disease. Diabetes 1988; 37:1595–1607.

16. Davies DL, Beevers DG, Briggs JD, Medina AM, Robertson JI, Schalekamp MA, Brown JJ, Lever AF, Morton JJ, Tree M. Abnormal relation between exchangeable sodium and the renin–angiotensin system in malignant hypertension in hypertension with chronic renal failure. Lancet 1973; 1:683–686.

17. Estacio RO, Gifford N, Jeffers BW, Schrier RW. Effect of BP control on diabetic microvascular complications in patients with hypertension and type 2 diabetes. Diabetes Care 2000; 23:B54-B64.

18. Bakris GL, Weir MR. ACE Inhibitor associated elevations in serum creatinine: is this a cause for concern? Arch Intern Med 2000; 160:685–693.

19. The GISEN group (Gruppo Italiano di Study Epidemiologici in Nefrologia). Randomized placebo controlled trial of effect of Ramipril on decline in glomerular filtration rate and risk of terminal renal failure in proteinuric, nondiabetic nephropathy. Lancet 1997; 349:1857–1863.

20. Maschio G, Alberti D, Janin G, Locatelli F, Mann JF, Motolese M, Ponticelli C, Ritz E, Zucchelli P. Effect of angiotensin converting enzyme inhibitor benazepril on the progression of chronic renal insufficiency. N Engl J Med 1996; 334: 939–945.

21. Peterson JC, Adler S, Burkart JM, Greene T, Hebert LA, Hunsicker LG, King AJ, Klahr S, Massry SG, Seifter JL. BP control, proteinuria and the progression of renal disease. The modification of diet in renal disease study. Ann Intern Med 1995; 123:754–762.

22. Bonomini V, Campieri C, Scolari MP, Vangelista A. Hypertension in acute renal failure. Contrib Nephrol 1987; 54:152–158.

23. Kheder MA, Ben Maiz H, Abderrahim E, el Younsi F, Ben Moussa F, Safar ME, Ben Ayed H. Hypertension in primary chronic glomerulonephritis analysis of 359 cases. Nephron 1993; 63:140–144.

24. Ridao N, Luno J, Garcia de Vinuesa S, Gomez F, Tejedor A, Valderrabano F. Prevalence of hypertension in renal disease. Nephrol Dial Transplant. 2001; 16:70–73.

25. Danielsen H, Kornerup HJ, Olsen S, Posborg V. Arterial hypertension in chronic glomerulonephritis. An analysis of 310 cases. Clin Nephrol 1983; 19:284–287.

26. Bell PE, Hossack KF, Gabow PA, Durr JA, Johnson AM, Schrier RW. Hypertension in autosomal dominant polycystic kidney disease. Kidney Int 1988; 34: 683–690.

27. Gonzalo A, Gallego A, Rivera M, Orte L, Ortuno J. Influence of hypertension on early renal insufficiency in autosomal dominant polycystic kidney disease. Nephron 1996; 72:225–230.

28. Klag MJ, Whelton PK, Randall BL, Neaton JD, Brancati FL, Stamler J. End stage renal disease in African-American and white men. J Am Med Assoc 1997; 227:1293–1298.

29. Mogensen CE. Microalbuminuria, blood pressure and diabetic renal disease: origin and development of ideas. In: Mogensen CE, ed. The Kidney and Hypertension in Diabetes Mellitus. 5th ed. Boston: Kluwer, 2000:655–706.

30. Gall MA, Rossing P, Skott P, Damsbo P, Vaag A, Bech K, Dejgaard A, Lauritzen M, Lauritzen E, Hougaard P. Prevalence of micro- and macroalbuminuria, arterial hypertension, retinopathy and large vessel disease in European type II (NIDDM) diabetic patients. Diabetologia 1991; 34:655–661.

31. Ljungman S, Wikstrand J, Hartford M, Berglund G. Urinary albumin excretion a predictor of risk of cardiovascular disease. Am J Hypertens 1996; 9:770–778.

32. Keane WF, Eknoyan G. Proteinuria, albuminuria, risk, assessment, detection, elimination (PARADE): a position paper of the National Kidney Foundation. Am J Kidney Dis 1999; 33:1004–1010.

33. Bakris GL. Microalbuminuria: prognostic implications. Curr Opin Nephrol Hypertens 1996; 5:219–223.

34. Tarif N, Bakris GL. Preservation of renal function: the spectrum of effects by calcium channel blockers. Nephrol Dial Transplant 1997; 12:2244–2250.

35. Rodby RA. Type II diabetic nephropathy: its clinical course and therapeutic implications. Semin Nephrol 1997; 17:132–147.

36. Dinneen SF, Gerstein HC. The association of microalbuminuria and mortality in non-insulin-dependent diabetes mellitus: a systemic overview of the literature. Arch Intern Med 1997; 157:1413–1418.

37. Pontremoli R, Sofia A, Ravera M, Nicolella C, Viazzi F, Tirotta A, Ruello N, Tomolillo C, Castello C, Grillo G, Sacchi G, Deferrari G. Prevalence and clinical correlates of microalbuminuria in essential hypertension: the MAGIC study. Hypertension 1997; 30:1135–1143.

38. Cirillo M, Senigalliesi L, Laurenzi M, Alfieri R, Stamler J, Stamler R, Panarelli W, De Santo NG. Microalbuminuria in nondiabetic adults: Relation of blood pressure, body mass index, plasma cholesterol levels, and smoking: the Gubbio Population Study. Arch Intern Med 1998; 158:1933–1939.

39. Pedrinelli R, Dell'Omo G, Penno G, Bandinelli S, Bertini A, Di Bello V, Mariani M. Microalbuminuria and pulse pressure in hypertensive and atherosclerotic men. Hypertension. 2000; 35:48–54.

40. Orth SR, Ritz E, Schrier RW. The renal risks of smoking. Kidney Int 1997; 51:1669–1677.

41. Bakris GL, Williams M, Dworkin L, Elliott WJ, Epstein M, Toto R, Tuttle K, Douglas J, Hsueh W, Sowers J. For The National Kidney Foundation Hypertension and Diabetes Executive Committees Working Group. Preserving renal function in adults with hypertension and diabetes: a consensus approach. Am J Kidney Dis 2000; 36:646–661.

42. Gerstein HC, Mann JF, Yi Q, Zinman B, Dinneen SF, Hoogwerf B, Halle JP, Young J, Rashkow A, Joyce C, Nawaz S, Yusuf S; HOPE Study Investigators. Albuminuria and risk of cardiovascular events, death, and heart failure in diabetic and nondiabetic individuals. J Am Med Assoc 2001; 286:421–426.

43. Agewall S, Wikstrand J, Ljungman S, Fagerberg B. Usefulness of microalbuminuria in predicting cardiovascular mortality in treated hypertensive men with and without diabetes mellitus. Am J Cardiol 1997; 80:164–169.

44. Nathan DM, Rosenbaum C, Protasowicki VD. Single-void urine samples can be used to estimate quantitative microalbuminuria. Diabetes Care 1987; 10:414–418.

45. Boulware LE, Jaar BG, Tarver-Carr ME, Brancati FL, Powe NR. Screening for proteinuria in US adults: a cost-effectiveness analysis. J Am Med Assoc 2003; 290:3101–3114.

46. Lewin A, Blaufox MD, Castle H, Entwisle G, Langford H. Apparent prevalence of curable hypertension in the hypertension detection and follow-up program. Arch Intern Med 1985; 145:424–427.

47. Safian RD, Textor SC. Medical progress: renal-artery stenosis. N Engl J Med 2001; 344:431–442.

48. Nakamoto H, Ferrario CM, Fuller SB, Robaczewski DL, Winicov E, Dean RH. Angiotensin-(1–7) and nitric oxide interaction in renovascular hypertension. Hypertension 1995; 25:796–802.

49. An epidemiological approach to describing risk associated with blood pressure levels: final report of the Working Group on Risk and High Blood Pressure. Hypertension 1985; 7:641–651.

50. Miyajima E, Yamada Y, Yoshida Y, Matsukawa T, Shionoiri H, Tochikubo O, Ishii M. Muscle sympathetic nerve activity in renovascular hypertension and primary aldosteronism. Hypertension 1991; 17:1057–1062.

51. Maxwell MH, Bleifer KH, Franklin SS, Varady PD. Cooperative study of renovascular hypertension. Demographic analysis of the study. J Am Med Assoc 1972; 22:1195–1204.

52. Mann SJ, Pickering TG. Detection of renovascular hypertension. State of the art: 1992. Ann Intern Med 1992; 117:845–853.

53. Wilcox CS. Use of angiotensin-converting-enzyme inhibitors for diagnosing renovascular hypertension. Kidney Int 1993; 44:1379–1390.

54. Alcazar JM, Rodicio JL. European Society of Hypertension. How to handle renovascular hypertension. J Hypertens 2001; 19:2109–2111.

55. Roubidoux MA, Dunnick NR, Klotman PE. Renal vein renins: inability to predict response to revascularization in patients with hypertension. Radiology 1991; 178:819–822.

56. Helenon O, Melki P, Correas JM, Boyer JC, Moreau JF. Renovascular disease: Doppler ultrasound. Semin Ultrasound CT MR 1997; 18:136–146.

57. Olin JW, Piedmonte MR, Young JR, DeAnna S, Grubb M, Childs MB. The utility of duplex ultrasound scanning of the renal arteries for diagnosing significant renal artery stenosis. Ann Intern Med 1995; 122:833–838.

58. Vasbinder GB, Nelemans PJ, Kessels AG, Kroon AA, de Leeuw PW, van Engelshoven JM. Diagnostic tests for renal artery stenosis in patients suspected of having renovascular hypertension: a meta-analysis. Ann Intern Med 2001; 135:401–411.

59. Postma CT, Joosten FB, Rosenbusch G, Thien T. Magnetic resonance angiography has a high reliability in the detection of renal artery stenosis. Am J Hypertens 1997; 10:957–963.

60. Rieumont MJ, Kaufman JA, Geller SC, Yucel EK, Cambria RP, Fang LS, Bazari H, Waltman AC. Evaluation of renal artery stenosis with dynamic gadolinium-enhanced MR angiography. AJR Am J Roentgenol 1997; 169:39–44.

61. Olbricht CJ, Paul K, Prokop M, Chavan A, Schaefer-Prokop CM, Jandeleit K, Koch KM, Galanski M. Minimally invasive diagnosis of renal artery stenosis by spiral computed tomography angiography. Kidney Int 1995; 48:1332–1337.

62. Elkohen M, Beregi JP, Deklunder G, Artaud D, Mounier-Vehier C, Carre AG. A prospective study of helical

computed tomography angiography versus angiography for the detection of renal artery stenoses in hypertensive patients. J Hypertens 1996; 14:525–528.

63. Blood Pressure Management Working Group. Blood pressure management in chronic kidney disease (KDOQI) Guidelines. Am J Kidney Dis (Suppl) In Press.

64. van Jaarsveld BC, Krijnen P, Derkx FH, Oei HY, Postma CT, Schalekamp MA. The place of renal scintigraphy in the diagnosis of renal artery stenosis. Fifteen years of clinical experience. Arch Intern Med 1997; 157:1226–1234.

65. Setaro JF, Saddler MC, Chen CC, Hoffer PB, Roer DA, Markowitz DM, Meier GH, Gusberg RJ, Black HR. Simplified captopril renography in diagnosis and treatment of renal artery stenosis. Hypertension 1991; 18:289–298.

66. Chabova V, Schirger A, Stanson AW, McKusick MA, Textor SC. Outcomes of atherosclerotic renal artery stenosis managed without revascularization. Mayo Clin Proc 2000; 75:437–444.

67. van Jaarsveld BC, Krijnen P, Pieterman H, Derkx FH, Deinum J, Postma CT, Dees A, Woittiez AJ, Bartelink AK, Man in 't Veld AJ, Schalekamp MA. The effect of balloon angioplasty on hypertension in atherosclerotic renal-artery stenosis. Dutch Renal Artery Stenosis Intervention Cooperative Study Group. N Engl J Med 2000; 342:1007–1014.

68. Canzanello VJ, Textor SC. Noninvasive diagnosis of renovascular disease. Mayo Clin Proc. 1994; 69:1172–1181.

69. Coresh J, Wei JI, McQuillan G, Brancati FL, Levey AS, Jones C, Klag MJ. Prevalence of high blood pressure and elevated serum creatinine level in the United States: findings from the third National Health and Nutrition Examination Survey (1988–1994). Arch Intern Med 2001; 161:1207–1216.

70. McLaughlin K, Jardine AG, Moss JG. ABC of arterial and venous disease. Renal artery stenosis. Br Med J 2000; 320:1124–1127.

71. Weinberg MS, Kaperonis N, Bakris GL. How high should an ACE inhibitor or angiotensin receptor blocker be dosed in patients with diabetic nephropathy? Curr Hypertens Rep 2003; 5:418–425.

72. Nakao N, Yoshimura A, Morita H, Takada M, Kayano T, Ideura T. Combination treatment of angiotensin-II receptor blocker and angiotensin-converting-enzyme inhibitor in non-diabetic renal disease (COOPERATE): a randomised controlled trial. Lancet 2003; 361:117–124.

73. Pedrinelli R, Bello VD, Catapano G, Talarico L, Materazzi F, Santoro G, Giusti C, Mosca F, Melillo E, Ferrari M. Microalbuminuria is a marker of left ventricular hypertrophy but not hyperinsulinemia in nondiabetic atherosclerotic patients. Arterioscler Thromb 1993; 13:900–906.

74. Erley CM, Risler T. Microalbuminuria in primary hypertension: is it a marker of glomerular damage? Nephrol Dial Transplant 1994; 9:1713–1715.

75. Stimpel M, Groth H, Greminger P, Luscher TF, Vetter H, Vetter W. The spectrum of renovascular hypertension. Cardiology 1985; 72:1–9.

76. Stephen CT. Progressive hypertension in a patient with "incidental" renal artery stenosis. Hypertension 2002; 40:595–600.

17

The Brain and Hypertension

THOMPSON G. ROBINSON

University Hospitals of Leicester NHS Trust, Leicester, UK

KEYPOINTS

- Stroke is the third leading cause of death and a leading cause of disability worldwide.
- Hypertension is the most prevalent modifiable risk factor for both ischemic and hemorrhagic stroke.
- The role of antihypertensive therapy for the primary and secondary prevention of fatal and nonfatal stroke is established.
- Ongoing trials will inform the therapeutic management of acute stroke blood pressure changes.
- Vascular dementia is the second most common cause of dementia worldwide.
- Vascular dementia includes a number of clinical syndromes, including multi-infarct, strategic infarct, white matter, and lacunar disease.
- Midlife hypertension is clearly associated with late-life vascular cognitive impairment and dementia.
- Addressing vascular risk factors, including hypertension, is part of the management of vascular dementia.

SUMMARY

Hypertension is a cause of significant morbidity and mortality as a consequence of its effects on the extracranial and intracranial blood supply. This chapter will focus on two conditions, stroke and dementia, which have important consequences for total and disability-free life expectancy. In particular, the clinical assessment of hypertensive patients with suspected stroke, and dementia will be discussed. Furthermore, the role of antihypertensive therapy in the management of these common conditions will also be considered.

I. INTRODUCTION

Previous chapters have examined the importance of the central nervous system in cardiovascular autonomic control, particularly as it relates to the central control of the afferent and efferent components of the baroreceptor reflex arc and consequent changes in blood pressure level and variability. Despite these changes in systemic blood pressure, the brain has an intrinsic ability to maintain a constant cerebral blood flow over a wide range of perfusion pressures; this is called cerebral autoregulation.

Cerebral autoregulation may occur in the static state, where change in cerebral blood flow follows steady-state alteration in blood pressure, or in the dynamic state, where cerebral blood flow changes in response to an acute (5–10 s) increase or decrease in blood pressure. The changes that hypertension invokes in cerebral blood vessel morphology resulting in altered blood vessel and increased cerebrovascular resistance have also been considered, particularly as they apply to the hypertensive adaptation of the cerebral autoregulatory curve. Nonetheless, in severely hypertensive states above the upper limit of cerebral autoregulation, cerebral blood flow is altered with severe consequences for cerebral function. Hypertensive encephalopathy is the subject of a later chapter.

Hypertension is also important as a risk factor for atherosclerosis. The progression of atherosclerotic plaques in large and medium-sized arteries through a process of necrosis, ulceration, and thrombosis with complete or partial vessel occlusion or distal embolization has also been considered. At the level of smaller arteries, such as the single, deep-perforating end-arteries of the deep cerebral white matter, we have learned that hypertension also produces vessel occlusion by microatheroma and hypertensive lipohyalinosis. Thus, hypertension has important consequences for the brain.

This chapter will focus on the evidence for the role of hypertension, as well as its assessment and management in two common conditions: stroke and vascular dementia.

II. STROKE

The World Health Organization (WHO) defines stroke as the rapid development of clinical signs of focal or global disturbance of cerebral function, with symptoms lasting 24 h or longer or resulting in death from no obvious cause other than a vascular one. It affects nearly 20 million individuals annually worldwide, of whom one-quarter will die, making stroke the third leading cause of death (1). Of the 15 million stroke survivors, one-third will remain disabled and, importantly, more than one in six will suffer recurrent stroke within 5 years.

Hypertension is the most prevalent modifiable risk factor for ischemic and hemorrhagic stroke. This section will focus on its management for both primary and secondary prevention of stroke, as well as in the immediate post-stroke period. However, it is first necessary to discuss the initial clinical assessment of stroke patients.

A. Clinical Assessment

In the clinical assessment of a patient presenting with a suspected stroke or transient ischemic attack, the first priority is to establish whether the symptoms are those of a stroke or whether stroke mimics need to be considered. An accurate clinical history from the patient, caregiver, relative, or witness at the earliest opportunity after symptom onset is vital. Important questions relate to:

Symptom onset: What day and time did the symptoms start? What was the patient doing at the time? Was the onset sudden? Was the neurological deficit maximal at the time of onset or has it progressed or fluctuated?

Symptom location: Which parts of the body were affected?

Symptom nature: What happened—focal or nonfocal? Negative (e.g., loss of power or sensation) or positive (e.g., jerking, hallucinations)?

Symptom association: What else happened—headache, focal or global seizure activity, vomiting, altered conscious level, cardiac symptoms, and so on?

Typically, stroke onset is sudden, although symptoms may or may not worsen gradually or in a stepwise fashion, and focal neurological symptoms result; that is, nonfocal symptoms of faintness, dizziness, confusion, and generalized weakness are unlikely to be caused by a stroke. Although there are many stroke mimics, it is obviously important to exclude conditions that are serious or treatable, for example, hypoglycemia and other metabolic disorders, subdural hemorrhage, benign structural intracranial lesions, infections including encephalitis or abscess, epilepsy, and so on.

The history is supported by a physical examination to define the neurological deficit. A plethora of neurological scales are available. Undoubtedly, the advent of intravenous thrombolysis with rt-PA will result in the increasing use of the National Institutes of Health Stroke Scale, not least because it defines patients unsuitable for thrombolysis but there are also validated teaching packages available for training (2).

There is also merit in using the information gained from the neurological examination to group patients by various constellations of findings into clinical syndromes, such as the total anterior circulation, partial anterior circulation, and lacunar and posterior circulation stroke syndromes of the Oxfordshire Community Stroke Project classification, which correlates well with subsequent neuroradiological findings and guides prognostication (3).

Of course, neuroimaging is the definitive investigation, excluding nonstroke diagnoses and distinguishing an ischemic from hemorrhagic stroke. Although brain computed tomography (CT) is the modality in most widespread use, it is likely to become increasingly displaced by magnetic resonance imaging, with the opportunities that this provides for distinguishing acute and subacute disease and lacunar and white matter disease, as well as for assessing perfusion.

It is important that the medical history, examination, and investigation also focus on defining stroke etiology—at one level, in distinguishing ischemic from hemorrhagic disease, but also another level in establishing large vessel, small vessel, cardioembolic, and other causes of ischemic stroke. This relies on a complete exploration of nonmodifiable (age, gender, genetic) and modifiable (previous stroke or transient ischemic attack, hypertension, dyslipidaemia, cardiac disease including atrial fibrillation, peripheral vascular disease, diabetes, smoking, alcohol, exercise, diet) vascular risk factors on clinical history and examination. It may also indicate the need for more specialist avenues of investigation, such as:

> Hematological (protein C, protein S, antithrombin III, lupus anticoagulant, anticardiolipin antibody).
> Biochemical (homocysteine, drug screen).
> Cardiological (24 h electrocardiography, transthoracic and transoesophageal echocardiography, carotid and transcranial ultrasound).
> Neurological [cerebrospinal fluid (CSF) examination, electroencephalography].

B. Primary Prevention

Confining the discussion to the role of hypertension in stroke, the largest meta-analysis of over 1 million individuals from 61 prospective observational studies has demonstrated a clear relationship between increasing systolic and diastolic blood pressure and stroke mortality (Fig. 17.1). In individuals aged 40–69, each reduction of 20 mmHg systolic blood pressure or 10 mmHg diastolic blood pressure halved the risk of stroke mortality across the blood pressure range 185/115–115/75 mmHg. The risk associated with a 20 mmHg difference in usual systolic blood pressure over the ages of 40–89 was similar worldwide, with age-standardized hazard ratios for stroke mortality of 0.49 (95% confidence level 0.48–0.51) in Europe, 0.50 (0.47–0.53) in the United States or Australia, and 0.42 (0.39–0.46) in Asia. Age-standardized hazard ratios are also similar for hemorrhagic and ischemic stroke (4).

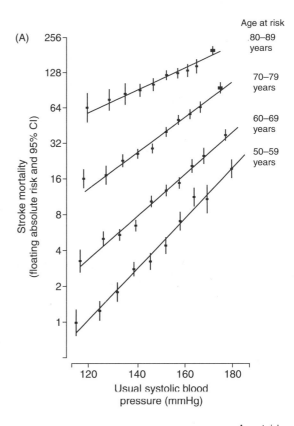

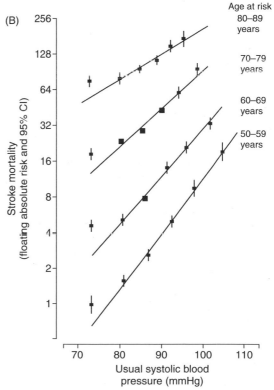

Figure 17.1 Stroke mortality rate in each decade of age vs. usual blood pressure at the start of that decade for: (A) Systolic blood pressure, (B) Diastolic blood pressure. [From Prospective Studies Collaboration (4).]

Isolated systolic hypertension increases in a curvilinear fashion with increasing age. It reflects a rise in systolic blood pressure due to decreased large arterial elasticity, which is not accompanied by a rise in mean arterial pressure or peripheral resistance. Therefore, the best component of blood pressure measurement to predict cardiovascular risk may change across a range of age groups. For example, the Framingham Heart Study found that coronary artery disease risk was best predicted by diastolic blood pressure in individuals younger than 50 and by systolic blood pressure and pulse pressure in individuals over 60, with all three measures being comparable between 50 and 59 years of age (5).

However, there is convincing evidence from many placebo-controlled intervention studies dating back >20 years that pharmacological treatment significantly reduces the risk of fatal and nonfatal stroke in both combined systolic–diastolic and isolated systolic hypertension by 42% (6) and 30% (7), respectively. Furthermore, data from the Systolic Hypertension in the Elderly Program (SHEP) confirms that this benefit is seen in all stroke subtypes, including ischemic, hemorrhagic, and lacunar.

The initiation of pharmacological treatment in hypertensive individuals is based on a combination of blood pressure level and cardiovascular risk. The assessment of blood pressure level is based on a series of readings in an appropriate environment with a validated measurement device over a defined time period. These criteria are clearly laid out in a number of recent guidelines (8,9).

It is noted that consideration may be given to introducing antihypertensive treatment at "normal/prehypertensive" blood pressure levels; for example, systolic levels of 120–139 mmHg and diastolic levels of 80–89 mmHg. This is based on the publication of a number of recent trials highlighting the potential benefits of antihypertensive therapy in normotensive individuals at high cardiovascular risk because of associated stroke [Perindopril pROtection aGainst REcurrent Stroke Study (PROGRESS)], coronary artery disease [Heart Outcomes Prevention Evaluation study (HOPE)], or diabetes (ABCD-Normotensive). Furthermore, the Framingham Heart Study reports that male and female subjects with high normal blood pressure (130–139/85–89 mmHg) have a risk-factor-adjusted hazard ratio for 10 year cardiovascular disease of 1.6 (1.1–2.2) and 2.5 (1.6–4.1), respectively, compared with individuals with optimal blood pressure control (10).

After the exclusion of secondary causes of hypertension, assessing cardiovascular risk depends on the presence of risk factors and the evaluation of target organ damage and associated co-morbid conditions. Cardiovascular disease risk factors include blood pressure level, age, gender, smoking, dyslipidaemia, family history of premature cardiovascular disease, abdominal obesity, and C-reactive protein. Target organ damage is based on the assessment of left ventricular hypertrophy by electrocardiographic voltage criteria or elevated echocardiographic left ventricular mass index, carotid ultrasonographic intima-media thickening or atherosclerotic plaque, elevated serum creatinine, and microalbuminuria. Important co-morbid conditions include diabetes mellitus, cerebrovascular disease, heart disease, renal disease, peripheral vascular disease, and advanced retinopathy.

Depending on the degree of cardiovascular risk determined by the above assessments, a number of treatment strategies are recommended. However, lifestyle measures should be instituted in all patients, including smoking cessation, alcohol moderation (2–4 mmHg), weight reduction (5–20 mmHg/10 kg weight loss), physical exercise (4–9 mmHg), reduced salt intake (2–8 mmHg), and dietary modifications to reduce total and saturated fat and increase fruits and vegetables (8–14 mmHg)— the figures in parentheses relate to approximate systolic blood pressure reduction (9).

Education is also an important component of nonpharmacological management. The Health Survey of England has shown that only 50% of hypertensive patients are aware of their condition, with even poorer uptake of treatment and control (11). Regarding pharmacological treatment, this should be initiated promptly in all high-risk and very high-risk individuals, although a further period of blood pressure observation over at least 3 months is recommended in subjects at moderate or low risk. In those subjects at moderate risk who remain hypertensive (systolic ≥140 mmHg or diastolic ≥90 mmHg), antihypertensive treatment should subsequently be initiated though intervention at other levels may be guided by patient preference and local resource issues.

Of course, the ultimate goal of the therapeutic manipulation of blood pressure is to reduce long-term total cardiovascular morbidity and mortality. Two specific questions arise in relation to stroke prevention:

What is the blood pressure target?
What antihypertensive agents provide the best protection?

1. Blood Pressure Target

There have been only a very few trials that compare intensive vs. less intensive blood-pressure-lowering regimes, and these appear to favor more intensive strategies for blood pressure lowering, particularly in reducing the risk of fatal and nonfatal stroke by 23% (5–37), as well as reducing all major cardiovascular events by 15% (5–24) (12). Assuming the benefits in reduced stroke arise only from the blood pressure level achieved rather than from the antihypertensive agent used, the PROGRESS trial has shown that a blood pressure level of 132/79 mmHg in the active arm compared with 141/83 mmHg in the placebo arm (where 51% of patients received antihypertensive treatment) significantly reduced recurrent stroke rates. In addition, the lower systolic blood pressure achieved in the chlorthalidone-treated subject in the Antihypertensive and Lipid-Lowering Treatment to Prevent Heart Attack Trial (ALLHAT) study compared to either the doxazosin- or lisinopril-treated subjects in this study suggests that levels of 134 mmHg rather than 136 mmHg may be safer in terms of reduced stroke rates.

Overall, more intensive strategies may result in a 23% greater relative reduction in stroke risk, a benefit obtained with relatively moderate additional systolic and diastolic blood pressure reductions of 4/3 mmHg (12). Therefore, current guidelines recommend that blood pressure be lowered to a target of <140/90 mmHg (<130/80 mmHg in diabetics), although they acknowledge that these targets may be difficult to achieve, particularly in the elderly (8,9).

2. Choice of Antihypertensive Agent

More recently, a number of clinical trials have compared different classes of antihypertensive therapy, in particular old (diuretics, β-blockers) vs. new (calcium channel antagonists, angiotensin converting enzyme inhibitors, angiotensin receptor antagonists, α-blockers).

In a recent meta-analysis of nine trials randomizing 67,435 patients, calcium antagonists may provide slightly better protection compared with older drugs, with an odds ratio for fatal and nonfatal stroke of 0.92 (0.84–1.01) (13). In a further analysis of five trials comparing 46,553 patients receiving an angiotensin-converting enzyme (ACE) inhibitor compared to older drugs, slightly less protection was provided by the ACE inhibitor, with an odds ratio of 1.10 (1.01–1.20), although this may have reflected the 40% higher stroke risk in African-American individuals and the lower blood pressure reduction in the lisinopril arm of ALLHAT. However, the Second Australian National Blood Pressure trial found that in Caucasian men on an ACE inhibitor compared to a diuretic-based regime, there were better cardiovascular outcomes, with a hazards ratio of 0.83 (0.71–0.97) (14).

Furthermore, other trials of antihypertensive agents acting on the renin–aldosterone system have published in favor of these agents. The Losartan Intervention for Endpoint (LIFE) reduction in hypertension study reported a significant 25% reduction in fatal and nonfatal stroke in hypertensive patients with left ventricular hypertrophy treated with losartan compared to atenolol over a 4.8 year follow-up period. The Study on Cognition and Prognosis in the Elderly (SCOPE) trial also reported a 28% reduction in nonfatal stroke only in elderly hypertensive patients receiving candesartan compared to a placebo, although 84% of placebo treated patients were receiving antihypertensive therapy (diuretics, β-blockers, or calcium antagonists).

The most recent Blood Pressure Lowering Treatment Trialists' Collaboration of over 162,000 patients has concluded an odds ratio for fatal and nonfatal stroke of 1.09 (1.00–1.18) for ACE inhibitors vs. diuretics or β-blockers, 0.93 (0.86–1.00) for calcium antagonists vs. diuretics/β-blockers, and 1.12 (1.01–1.25) for ACE inhibitors vs. calcium antagonists (12).

In summary, the current guidelines recommend that treatment should be commenced with low-dose monotherapy. Provided the agent is tolerated, it is likely that most patients will require the dose to be increased or alternative therapy added to achieve target blood pressure.

Although specific antihypertensive drug classes may benefit special patient groups—for example, congestive cardiac failure, diabetic and nondiabetic nephropathy, previous cerebrovascular disease—the overriding principle of antihypertensive treatment is that lowering blood pressure *per se* rather than starting with a particular agent is important. In most cases, thiazide-type diuretics should be used in drug treatment for most patients with uncomplicated hypertension, either alone or in combination (8,9).

C. Acute Stroke

Blood pressure changes are a recognized complication of acute stroke, with >50% of patients having hypertensive ($\geq$160 mmHg) levels and ~5% having hypotensive (<120 mmHg) levels (15). In addition, up to 40% of acute stroke patients are already receiving antihypertensive therapy on hospital admission. However, the management of post-stroke blood pressure changes has remained a matter of some debate, and significant differences in clinical practice have been reported, most notably in the continuation of antihypertensive therapy, the initiation of new antihypertensive therapy, and the use of inotropic support.

Nonetheless, post-stroke blood pressure changes may not be benign. The International Stroke Trial Collaborative Group analysed blood pressure data from some 17,398 ischemic stroke patients within 48 h of ictus, and they reported an increased risk of early (2 weeks) death by 17.9% for every 10 mmHg fall in systolic blood pressure <150 mmHg and by 3.8% for every 10 mmHg >150 mmHg.

However, there are theoretical reasons against therapeutic interventions to manipulate blood pressure in the acute stroke period (16). The natural history is for a spontaneous reduction in blood pressure levels over a period of 4–10 days. There are also impairments in dynamic cerebrovascular autoregulation post-stroke, such that cerebral blood flow becomes dependent on systemic blood pressure levels, and any reduction in the latter may have potential adverse consequences for penumbral viability. Finally, there is mounting evidence for impaired autonomic nervous system control of the cardiovascular system following acute stroke, which further adversely affects the physiological responses to systemic blood pressure changes and may again affect penumbral viability. Equally, sustained or therapeutically induced hypertension may also be harmful by increasing cerebral edema and the likelihood of symptomatic hemorrhagic transformation.

Unfortunately, there is currently only limited evidence from controlled clinical trials of blood pressure manipulation in the acute stroke period, and this has been recently reviewed (16–18).

The most extensively examined hypotensive agents are the calcium antagonists, which may have a cerebroprotective effect by limiting post-ischemic intracellular calcium influx, the result of which is increased cerebral blood flow by a preferential vasodilatory action on cerebral blood vessels. Horn et al. identified 47 trials assessing calcium antagonist use in acute ischemic stroke, including 29 trials of 7,665 patients in their systematic review. No effect of calcium antagonists on poor outcome (1.04, 0.98–1.09) or death (1.07, 0.98–1.17) at the end of follow-up was reported (19).

Although β-blockers theoretically may be of benefit by limiting catecholamine-induced cardiac and neurological damage and by reducing the metabolic demands of ischemic brain, in a placebo-controlled trial of 302 patients within 48 h of a stroke, Barer and colleagues reported a nonsignificant increase in mortality and decrease in neurological and functional outcome at 6 months with atenolol and propranolol compared to a placebo.

There is preliminary evidence to support the further assessment of three classes of antihypertensive therapy. Agents acting on the renin–angiotensin system shift the lower limit of cerebrovascular autoregulation and, therefore, can also improve regional cerebral blood flow at low perfusion pressures. The Acute Candesartan Cilexetil Therapy in Stroke Survivors (ACCESS) study evaluated the use of an angiotensin receptor antagonist in hypertensive (>180/105 mmHg) acute ischemic stroke patients, comparing acute (<72 h) vs. delayed (>7 days) intervention. This study reported a significant reduction in 12 month mortality and cardiovascular events in favor of candesartan, odds ratio 0.48 (0.25–0.90) (20). Labetalol, a combined α- and β-adrenergic antagonist, can be administered both intravenously and orally, producing minimal changes in heart rate and cardiac output without rebound hypertension on discontinuation and without producing tachyphylaxis. Preliminary data from the National Institute of Neurological Disorders and Stroke (NINDS) trial reported a significant reduction in the odds ratio of death at 3 months in treated when compared with untreated hypertensive patients ($\geq$185/110 mmHg) in the placebo arm of this intravenous thrombolysis trial (0.1, 0.1–0.7) (21).

Finally, nitrates have many actions that may potentially reverse a number of the detrimental pathophysiological changes associated with acute stroke: cerebral vasodilatation, antiplatelet, antileucocyte, and N-methyl-D-aspartate receptor antagonism. A small study with transdermal nitrate has demonstrated a significant blood pressure reduction when compared with placebo in acute ischemic stroke patients.

These agents are the subjects of ongoing clinical trials (16). The Efficacy of Nitric Oxide in Stroke (ENOS) trial aims to recruit up to 5000 patients within 48 h of ischemic and hemorrhagic stroke. This study will assess the effects of transdermal glyceryl nitrate vs. placebo and the continuation vs. the discontinuation of current antihypertensive therapy during the first week following ictus.

Whether or not current antihypertensive therapy should be continued or stopped, a problem in 40% of acute stroke patients, is also being assessed in the Continue or Stop post-Stroke Antihypertensives Collaborative Study (COSSACS) over a 2 week treatment period. This study aims to recruit 2900 patients within 24 h of the onset of an ischemic or hemorrhagic stroke. The study also will assess the effects of age in two age groups (patients <75 years in age vs. patients >75 years in age).

Finally, the Controlling Hypertension and Hypotension Immediately Post Stroke (CHHIPS) Trail will assess both nondysphagic and dysphagic hypertensive (systolic blood pressure $\geq$160 mmHg) patients recruited within 24 h of ischemic or hemorrhagic stroke onset in a randomized, double-blind, placebo-controlled, step-therapy trial with lisinopril (given orally or sublingually) or labetalol (given orally or intravenously) treatment for a 2 week period. The effects of stroke type, stroke severity, and time to treatment will be assessed.

The CHHIPS trial also will assess the effects of blood pressure elevation on outcome in hypotensive (systolic blood pressure $\leq$140 mmHg) patients recruited within 12 h of nonhemorrhagic stroke and treated with intravenous phenylephrine or placebo for up to 24 h after onset. Although a less common clinical problem, post-stroke hypotension is associated with increased mortality. Induced hypertension is a standard treatment for cerebral ischemia in patients with vasospasm after subarachnoid hemorrhage, and increasing blood pressure levels in stroke patients with low systemic blood pressure could reduce focal cerebral injury by increasing intraluminal hydrostatic pressure, opening collateral channels, and improving perfusion to penumbral ischemic tissue. However, there is limited evidence using hypervolaemia or inotropic therapy with dobutamine, phenylephrine, and noradrenaline in acute stroke patients. In addition, increased odds of combined death and disability have been reported in a placebo-controlled study of 85 patients treated with diaspirin cross-linked hemoglobin to increase blood pressure for 72 h following ischemic stroke (22).

Therefore, current guidelines recommend introducing acute antihypertensive therapy for only a few specific indications following acute stroke (23):

Hypertensive encephalopathy (This condition, whether in the context of acute stroke or not, is a medical emergency. Its management is considered separately in a later chapter).

Cardiac urgencies (e.g., acute myocardial infarction, unstable angina, severe left ventricular failure).

Vascular urgencies (e.g., aortic dissection).

Severe hypertension (>200/120 mmHg) in association with intracerebral hemorrhage.

D. Secondary Prevention

In individuals surviving stroke, the risk of recurrent fatal and nonfatal stroke and other cardiovascular events (cardiovascular death, nonfatal myocardial infarction) is high. In particular, community studies of patients post-stroke have demonstrated that hypertension is associated with an increased risk of stroke recurrence, although other studies have reported either no relationship or a J-shaped relationship. Rodgers et al. (24) reported that each 10 mmHg reduction in systolic blood pressure was associated with a 28% lower risk of stroke in 2435 clinically stable individuals with a history of minor ischemic stroke or transient ischemic attack.

Nonetheless, although the management of acute stroke blood pressure changes remains the subject of ongoing study, the prevention of recurrent stroke by blood pressure reduction has now been clearly established from a number

of trials assessing the relative merits of antihypertensive therapy following stroke (Table 17.1).

Initial studies focused on exclusively hypertensive patients; later studies have included both hypertensive and normotensive stroke survivors. The secondary prevention of recurrent cerebrovascular disease [Fig. 17.2(A)] and other major cardiovascular events [Fig. 17.2(B)] by antihypertensive therapy is increasingly established in both patient groups. The larger, more recent, trials have assessed a number of antihypertensive strategies, including β-blockers alone [the Dutch TIA trial (Dutch TIA), Tenormin after Stroke and TIA study (TEST)], a diuretic alone [Post-Antihypertensive Treatment Study (PATS)], and an ACE inhibitor alone (HOPE, PROGRESS) or an ACE inhibitor with a diuretic (PROGRESS) (16,25).

The PATS study assessed the diuretic indapamide in a placebo-controlled trial of 5665 normotensive and hypertensive Chinese patients >4 weeks after transient ischemic attack (12%), ischemic (71%), or hemorrhagic (16%) stroke onset. Significant reductions were reported: 29% in fatal and nonfatal stroke recurrence and 23% in major cardiovascular events. At this stage, the Individual Data Analysis of Antihypertensive intervention trials (INDANA) Project Collaborators were able to include in their meta-analysis data from stroke and transient ischemic attack patients recruited to a number of hypertension trials, including the European Working Party on High Blood Pressure in the Elderly (EWPHE), Coope & Warrender-1986 (Coope), Hypertension Detection and Follow-up Program (HDFP), Multiple Risk Factor Intervention Trial (MRFIT), SHEP, and Swedish Trial in Old Patients with Hypertension (STOP-Hypertension) trials, as well as the Carter and the Hypertension-Stroke Cooperative Study Group (HSCS) data (26). They concluded that antihypertensive therapy reduced the risk of stroke recurrence

Table 17.1 Placebo-Controlled Trials of Blood Pressure Reduction Following Stroke

Trial	Year	n	Mean entry blood pressure (mmHg)	Time post-stroke (weeks)	Mean blood pressure change (mmHg)	Active treatment	Mean follow-up (years)
Carter	1970	97	>160/110	>2	?	D/MD/GB	4
HSCS	1974	452	167/100	>4	25/12	D/Des	3
Dutch TIA	1993	1473	158/91	>1	8/3	BB	2.6
TEST	1995	720	161/89	>1	4/3	BB	2.3
PATS	1995	5665	154/93	>4	6/3	D	2
HOPE	2000	1013	138/79	>4	3/2	ACE	4.5
PROGRESS	2001	6105	147/86	>4	12/5 (ACE + D) 5/3 (ACEI)	ACE ± D	3.9

Note: TIA, Transient ischemic attack; D, Thiazide diuretic; MD, methyldopa; GB, ganglion blocking agent (debrisoquine, bethanidine); Des, deserpidine; BB, β-blocker; ACE, Angiotensin-converting enzyme inhibitor; Dutch TIA, Dutch transient ishemic attack; HSCS, Hypertension-Stroke Cooperative Study Group; TEST, Tenormin after Stroke and TIA study; PATS, Post-Antihypertensive Treatment Study; HOPE, Heart Outcomes Prevention Evaluation study; PROGRESS, Perindopril pROtection aGainst REcurrent Stroke Study.

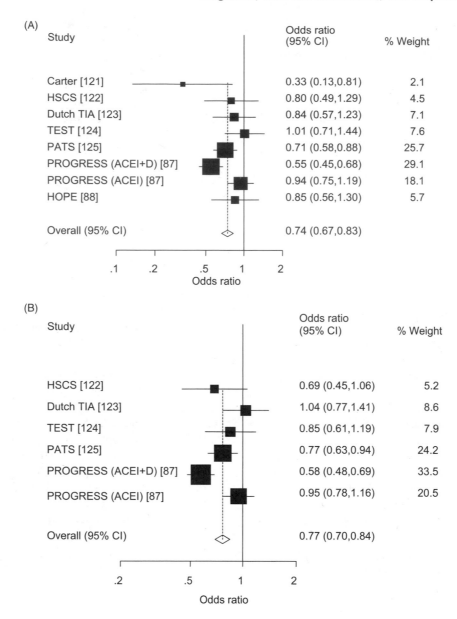

Figure 17.2 Meta-analysis of the effects of antihypertensive therapy following stroke: (A) Fatal and nonfatal stroke recurrence, (B) Major cardiovascular events (nonfatal stroke, nonfatal myocardial infarction, vascular death). [From Robinson and Potter (16) with permission.]

by 28% in stroke survivors, but it was unclear whether such benefit depended on initial blood pressure level.

However, subsequent trials have addressed the issue of managing blood pressure in normotensive stroke survivors, as well as the role of alternative antihypertensive agents. The Dutch TIA trial of 1473 patients who experienced either a transient ischemic attack (32%) or a nondisabling ischemic stroke (68%) assessed the effects of atenolol 50 mg vs. a placebo within 3 months of symptom onset, although only 20% of patients were assigned to active treatment within 1 week of ictus. A nonsignificant 16% reduction was seen in fatal and nonfatal

stroke recurrence, but there was a 4% increase in major cardiovascular events during the mean 2.6 year follow-up period. The TEST study also assessed the effects of 50 mg of atenolol vs. the effect of a placebo on major cardiovascular events and on fatal and nonfatal stroke recurrence in 720 hypertensive (>140/80 mmHg) patients within 3 weeks of ischemic (58%) and hemorrhagic (4%) stroke or transient ischemic attack (19%), reporting a nonsignificant 15% reduction and 1% increase over a mean 2.3 year follow-up period. The PROGRESS trial assessed the ACE inhibitor, perindopril, with or without indapamide compared to placebo in 6105 normotensive and hypertensive patients with ischemic (71%) or hemorrhagic (11%) stroke or transient ischemic attack (22%), although only 25% of patients were recruited within 2 months of the index event. Overall, there was a relative risk reduction of 28% in stroke and 26% in major vascular events during a 4 year period of follow-up. Although these benefits remained significant for important subgroups, including hypertensive vs. nonhypertensive and ischemic vs. hemorrhagic patients, patients who received an ACE inhibitor alone realized only a benefit of a 6% reduction in stroke and a 5% reduction in major cardiovascular events. Similarly, the HOPE study of the ACE inhibitor ramipril demonstrated only a nonsignificant reduction of 15% in fatal and nonfatal stroke recurrence in the subgroup of 1013 patients with a history of stroke >4 weeks previously.

Therefore, a number of trials now point to the singular advantages of agents acting on the renin–angiotensin system in stroke patients. The HOPE study achieved a significant risk reduction in all cardiovascular outcomes in the entire study population, although only modest blood pressure reductions were seen. This observation may be explained by the prevention of angiotensin-II mediated effects on the promotion of atherosclerosis (increased smooth muscle cell lipoxygenase activity, hypertrophy and proliferation, macrophage activation, cytokine production, inflammatory cell adhesion, chemotaxis, fibroblast growth) and thrombosis (increased plasminogen-activator inhibitor type 1 and platelet activation and aggregation), although doubts have been expressed about the timing of blood pressure measurement in relation to treatment within the HOPE study. However, the LIFE and SCOPE studies with the angiotensin receptor antagonists losartan and candesartan, respectively, have similarly reported a 25% all stroke and 28% nonfatal stroke reduction, respectively. PROGRESS, the largest trial that consisted exclusively of stroke patients, clearly indicates the importance of the additional use of a diuretic, with a 6% reduction in total stroke in the group treated with perindopril alone compared with a 45% reduction in the group treated with the perindopril-diuretic combination.

Further trials are ongoing and will provide more evidence regarding specific blood pressure-lowering treatment strategies in stroke patients. The SHARK trial recruited 3883 hemorrhagic and acute-phase stroke patients between 1995 and 1999, although the trial subsequently enrolled only 65 hypertensive patients >1 month after ischemic stroke. Patients received either nilvadipine, cilazapril or no antihypertensive therapy; only four patients had an outcome event by the end of follow-up in 2002. The final data are still unavailable. The ONTARGET™ trial will assess cardiovascular endpoints in 23,400 symptomatic atherothrombotic patients, including stroke patients, randomized to telmisartan (80 mg), ramipril (10 mg), or a combination over a follow-up period of 5.5 years. The sister study of the latter trial, the TRANSCEND™ trial, will examine 6000 patients who are ACE inhibitor-intolerant. The Morbidity and Mortality After Stroke—Eprosartan Compared with Nitrendipine in Secondary Prevention (MOSES) study will assess all cardiovascular outcomes in up to 4000 patients treated with eprosartan or nitrendipine for 2 years and recruited within 24 months of ischemic or hemorrhagic stroke. The PRoFESS® trial started recently; it compares telmisartan to a placebo and aspirin to dipyridamole MR twice daily vs. aspirin and clopidogrel in a randomized, parallel group, double-blind, double-dummy, placebo-controlled study of 15,500 patients recruited within 90 days of ischemic stroke. The primary outcome measure will be the time to first recurrent stroke.

In the light of the results from current trials, it is recommended that patients with a history of stroke or transient ischemic attack should have their blood pressure reduced, provided there is no contraindication to antihypertensive therapy. However, therapy should not be started until at least one week after stroke onset (25). Furthermore, blood pressure reduction should be attempted in both normotensive and hypertensive patients, provided such blood pressure reduction is tolerated by the patient (12). A number of antihypertensive agents have been studied in these clinical trials, but there seems to be particular benefit in the use of a combination of diuretic and ACE inhibitor.

Although it is not the subject of this chapter, it is also important to mention the importance of addressing other risk factors in the secondary prevention of stroke, including lifestyle factors, atrial fibrillation, carotid artery stenosis, dyslipidaemia, and other co-morbidities. In addition, the role of antithrombotic therapy is critically important in the secondary prevention of recurrent stroke in ischemic stroke patients. Readers are referred to the plethora of international and national guidelines on these issues (27).

III. COGNITIVE IMPAIRMENT AND DEMENTIA

The WHO definition of dementia describes "a syndrome due to disease of the brain, usually of a chronic or progressive nature in which there is disturbance of multiple higher cortical function including memory, thinking, orientation, comprehension, calculation, learning capacity, language, and judgment. Consciousness is not clouded. The impairments of cognitive function are commonly accompanied, and occasionally preceded by deterioration in emotional controls, social behavior or motivation." Although this definition has been adapted in various statements and by various associations, it is essential to recognize that dementia has a detrimental influence on activities of daily living, and it is this factor that distinguishes dementia from cognitive impairment *per se*. Furthermore, although there are a number of key elements common to all diagnostic criteria, the importance of some components may differ. For example, disturbances of consciousness may be present in vascular dementia; early cognitive changes may be focal rather than global. Not all cases of dementia progress. However, dementia is one of the leading causes of disability in developed countries, and it is likely to become a significant and increasing burden for health and social service providers with the increasing age of the global population. An estimated 29 million individuals worldwide are affected, with an annual incidence rate of 2.6 million cases (28).

The Framingham Heart Study cohort provided the first clear evidence of a relationship between hypertension and cognition in an aging population. Over a follow-up period of up to 15 years, subjects >75 years of age were more likely to have better cognitive performance if they did not have combined systolic–diastolic hypertension or isolated systolic hypertension (29). These findings have been supported by the 25 year observational Honolulu-Asia Aging Study (HAAS), which confirmed an association between increased midlife systolic blood pressure and late-life cognitive impairment. In a 15 year longitudinal population study of 973 subjects who were 70-year old, Skoog and colleagues (30) were able to comment on the relationship between blood pressure and dementia subtypes. Subjects developing dementia at the ages of 79–85 had higher blood pressure at age 70 than those not developing dementia: 178/101 mmHg vs. 164/92 mmHg, respectively. Furthermore, both subjects developing Alzheimer's disease and vascular dementia exhibited diastolic hypertension compared with those not developing dementia: 101 mmHg at age 70 and 101 mmHg at age 75, respectively. Therefore, longitudinal studies do support an association between mid-life hypertension and late-life cognitive decline.

The role of hypertension as a risk factor for stroke has already been considered; and stroke may be associated with cognitive impairment, dementia, and other psychiatric manifestations (e.g., depression) as a consequence of multiple cortical infarcts, a single "strategic" infarct, or multiple lacunar infarcts. Furthermore, hypertension and, indeed, aging may also produce partial and complete small-vessel occlusion resulting in white matter lesions and lacunar infarcts with associated cognitive impairment and dementia.

In the following sections, we will review the recognized clinical syndromes, in particular the relationship with hypertension, and the clinical assessment of the patient with cognitive impairment. Then we will review the role of antihypertensive therapy in managing cognitive impairment and dementia. Finally, we will briefly consider the role of hypertension and antihypertensive therapy in other dementias, including Alzheimer's disease.

A. Clinical Syndromes

The term vascular cognitive impairment can be used to define cognitive impairment, including vascular dementia, in which vascular pathology either causes or makes a substantial contribution to the cognitive impairment. Vascular dementia is the second most common type of dementia, accounting for some 10–50% of cases depending on geography, patient population, and ascertainment methods. A number of distinct syndromes can then be identified, although the clinical and neuroradiological criteria to distinguish between specific subtypes of vascular cognitive impairment remain the subject of ongoing review and harmonization. However, in all cases, it is important to recognize these syndromes at the earliest possible stage, when modification of risk factors may influence long-term outcome (31).

Multi-infarct dementia reflects the traditional view that stroke-related dementia is a consequence of multiple cortical infarcts [Fig. 17.3(A)]. The typical pattern, originally described by Hachinski et al. (32) is manifested by a sudden onset with a fluctuating course thereafter, with an overall progressive stepwise decline. In particular, there is a history of stroke and vascular risk factors, especially hypertension, with the presence of focal neurological symptoms and signs associated with complaints of nocturnal confusion, depression, and emotional lability, but relative preservation of personality. However, cognitive performance may also be affected following stroke by a single infarct in a brain structure critical for memory, termed a strategic or bottleneck infarct [Fig. 17.3(B)].

More typically, vascular cognitive impairment is related to chronic, diffuse, partial, or occlusive small-vessel disease resulting in predominantly subcortical white matter ischemia [Fig. 17.3(C)], Binswanger type) reflecting areas of focal arteriosclerosis, demyelination, and astrogliosis, which may progress to frank lacunar infarction(s) [Fig. 17.3(D), lacunar state type]. This reflects loss of brain tissue in order of its susceptibility to ischemia: neuron, oligodendrocyte, myelinated axon, astrocyte, and endothelial cell. The clinical onset is frequently insidious, and it is often difficult to define the temporal relationship between symptoms, neuroimaging changes, and stroke. These subcortical changes frequently damage fronto-subcortical circuits, leading to clinical manifestations confined to specific cognitive deficits, such as attention, concentration, and loss of executive function (slowing of motor performance, information processing, decision-making, or self-perception), as well as symptoms and signs of depression, emotional lability,

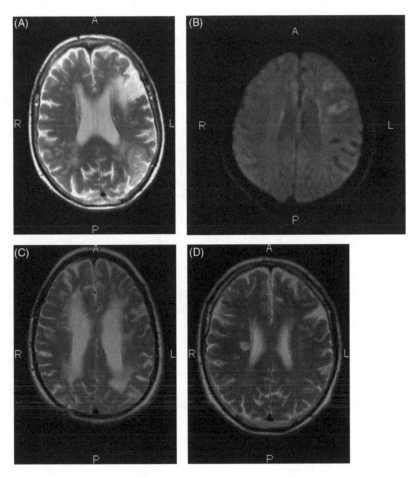

Figure 17.3 Magnetic resonance imaging scans of patients with vascular dementia showing: (Λ) Multiple cortical infarcts (axial T2 sequence), (B) Single "strategic" cortical infarct (axial DWI sequence), (C) Extensive white matter lesions (axial T2 sequence), (D) Lacunar infarction (axial T2 sequence).

and apathy. Episodic memory is often relatively well preserved compared with Alzheimer's disease patients.

It should be noted that white matter lesions are frequently identified on brain magnetic resonance imaging of asymptomatic individuals. The prevalence of such lesions increases dramatically with age, such that they are a common finding in the elderly, where 70% of the population may be affected. Their etiology in this context is unclear, but they often occur in the context of recognized vascular risk factors—for example, hypertension—where they may relate to poorer clinic and 24 h blood pressure control (33) and increase the likelihood of future cognitive impairment (30). They also have important noncognitive consequences, including depression, gait disorder, imbalance, and urinary symptoms.

Hemorrhagic dementias are recognized but uncommon. Hypertensive hemorrhage typically occurs in subcortical regions (basal ganglia, thalamus). The cerebral amyloid angiopathies are characterized by amyloid deposition in the leptomeningeal and cerebral cortical blood vessel wall. Clinical features include recurrent or multiple lobar hemorrhages and cognitive deterioration, with neuroimaging evidence of focal hemorrhagic and ischemic lesions with diffuse white matter changes. Cerebral hypoperfusion, particularly in the context of coronary artery bypass grafting, has also been recognized as a cause of vascular cognitive decline and may affect up to 40% of patients (34). This may be related to reduced cerebral perfusion during cardiac manipulation or to release of microembolic plaque material following aortic unclamping. Finally, mixed dementias, which are characterized by a combination of Alzheimer's disease with stroke often are the rule rather than the exception. These, together with the importance of vascular risk factors in Alzheimer's disease, will be considered later in this chapter.

B. Clinical Assessment

There are two main aspects to the clinical evaluation of patients with vascular cognitive impairment and dementia: the symptomatic diagnosis and the etiological diagnosis. The traditional clinical skills required to undertake a detailed clinical and neurological history and examination are central to evaluating the type and extent of cognitive impairment, the symptomatic diagnosis. These should include an assessment of social functions and personal and domestic activities of daily living, as well as an assessment of psychiatric and behavioral symptoms. In particular, the importance of a history provided by a caregiver or relative cannot be overestimated. However, a more detailed mental state and neuropsychological examination is also clearly indicated. The Folstein Mini-Mental State Examination (MMSE) is commonly used, but it has some limitations because of its emphasis on language and its insensitivity for mild deficits, and it also is influenced by age and education. Other tests commonly recommended are a four- to ten-word memory test with delayed recall, a cube drawing test, a verbal fluency test, and a letter cancellation test. More detailed neuropsychological testing may also be required, which should cover the main cognitive domains of short- and long-term memory, abstract thinking, judgment, aphasia, apraxia, agnosia, orientation, attention, executive functions, and speed of information processing.

Aspects of the clinical history and examination, including neurological and cardiovascular, will also contribute to the evaluation of the vascular cause and related factors, the etiological diagnosis. The calculation of specific scores (e.g., the Hachinski Ischemic Score) has previously been recommended. However, vascular dementia has more causes than a multi-infarct state, and these scores cannot distinguish Alzheimer's disease patients with stroke from vascular dementia; therefore, their utility is increasingly limited. Neuroradiological imaging, preferably with magnetic resonance imaging unless there is a contraindication, is essential as part of the diagnostic work-up. White matter changes include extensive periventricular and deep lesions, typically affecting the genu or anterior limb of the internal capsule, anterior corona radiata, and anterior

centrum semiovale. Lacunar infarcts are typically identified in the caudate nucleus, globus pallidus, thalamus, internal capsule, corona radiata, and frontal white matter. Other routine laboratory tests, including chest radiology and electrocardiography, are important in assessing vascular risk factors, but also to exclude other causes of dementia. Individual cases may require CSF examination, electroencephalography, single photon emission computed tomography, and more detailed cardiac investigation (echocardiography, 24 h electrocardiography, and ultrasound examination of the extra-cranial and intra-cranial arterial circulation).

C. Role of Antihypertensive Therapy in Managing Cognitive Impairment and Dementia

The Framingham Heart Study cohort reported that there was a stronger association between hypertension and cognitive dysfunction in untreated hypertensive subjects than in treated elderly hypertensive subjects after a 20-year follow-up period. The Epidemiology of Vascular Aging (EVA) study observed 1389 patients over a 4-year follow-up period. The study reported that untreated hypertensive subjects were more likely to exhibit cognitive decline, as measured by a greater than four-point deterioration in the MMSE score when, compared with normotensive subjects with a reported relative risk of 4.3 (2.3–8.0). This compared to a relative risk of 1.3 (0.3–3.9) for treated hypertensive subjects compared to normotensive subjects.

Subsequently, a number of placebo-controlled trials have assessed the role of antihypertensive therapy in arresting cognitive decline in hypertensive subjects (Table 17.2). The Systolic Hypertension in Europe (Syst-Eur) trial reported a 50% reduction in dementia cases in the active treatment compared with the placebo group over a 3.9 year follow-up period, quoting a reduction from 7.4 to 3.3/1000 patient-observation years. The Kungsholmen Project also reported a nonsignificant reduction in the

Table 17.2 Placebo-Controlled Trials of the Effects of Blood Pressure Reduction on Cognitive Function

| Study | Year | Number of patients | Entry criteria | | Treatment | Follow-up (years) |
			Age (years)	BP (mmHg)		
SHEP	1994	4736	≥60	≥160/<90	D, BB	5
MRC Older People	1996	2583	≥65	≥160/<115	D, BB	4.5
Kungsholmen Project	1999	1810	≥75	≥160/95	D	3
PROGRESS	2001	6105	No specified criteria		D, ACE	4
Syst-Eur	2002	2418	≥60	≥160/<95	CCB, D, ACE	3.9
SCOPE	2003	4964	≥70	≥160/90	A-II	3.7

Note: MRC Older People, Medical Research Council; SHEP, Systolic Hypertension in the Elderly Program; PROGRESS, Perindopril pROtection aGainst REcurrent Stroke Study; Syst-Eur, Systolic Hypertension in Europe; SCOPE, Study on Cognition and Prognosis in the Elderly; D, Thiazide diuretic; BB, β-blocker; ACE, Angiotensin-converting enzyme inhibitor; CCB, Calcium channel blocker; A-II, Angiotensin receptor antagonist.

relative risk of dementia of 0.6 (0.3–1.2) in active subjects compared to placebo-treated hypertensive patients over a 3 year follow-up period. However, the majority of trials have not demonstrated significant differences in cognitive performance or dementia rates in treated hypertensive subjects compared to placebo controls, although this may reflect the age of subjects who were recruited, the duration of treatment and follow-up, the cognitive tests used, and the blood pressure changes achieved (35).

The effects of diuretic, predominantly thiazide, antihypertensive therapy on cognitive function have been extensively studied in about 8000 patients recruited to 13 trials. However, diuretics were rarely used alone; they were often used in combination with an ACE inhibitor, β-blocker, or calcium antagonist therapy. Although well tolerated, diuretic therapy appeared to have no positive or negative effects on cognitive function and is, therefore, not the antihypertensive drug therapy of choice to prevent cognitive impairment. Similarly, β-blockers have been studied in 13,000 patients in 19 trials without overall significant effect, although some improvement has been noted with selective β-1 therapy and deterioration with propranolol (35). Improvements in MMSE scores were initially reported with angiotensin receptor antagonists in a trial of 69 elderly hypertensive patients comparing losartan with hydrochlorothiazide, although the subsequent assessment of candesartan in the larger placebo-controlled SCOPE trial did not demonstrate the same benefit.

However, the use of other classes of antihypertensive therapy is associated with positive effects on cognitive performance. The calcium antagonists have been assessed in 13 trials of 10,000 patients, and the positive effects of nitrendipine on dementia rates in the Syst-Eur trial have already been discussed. Interestingly, these agents may have positive cognitive effects in nonhypertensive subjects, but the exact mechanisms in both hypertensive patients and nonhypertensive patients require further assessment (36). Finally, the PROGRESS trial has been the largest trial to assess the effects of ACE-inhibitor therapy on cognition in recurrent stroke patients. It reported a 34% reduction in the risk of dementia and a 19% reduction in the risk of severe cognitive decline following recurrent stroke defined by the Diagnostic and Statistical Manual of Mental Disorders (4th Edition) and an MMSE decline by 3 or more points, respectively (37).

At present, it would appear that calcium antagonists and ACE inhibitors are more effective than other antihypertensive agents in their effects on cognitive domains in hypertensive patients, though ongoing trials will provide further insights. In particular, the DEmentia Prevention in HYpertension (DEPHY) trial has been specifically designed to assess the effects of a diuretic vs. a calcium antagonist-based antihypertensive regime in preventing dementia as a primary endpoint in older hypertensive patients (38).

It is also important to briefly consider the role of other treatments. Aspirin has been evaluated in the treatment of vascular dementia. Meyer and colleagues studied 70 multi-infarct dementia patients treated with aspirin 325 mg compared to placebo over a 3-year follow-up period, and found that the aspirin-treated group were more likely to demonstrate improved or stable cognitive function. This may reflect the beneficial effects of aspirin on cerebral perfusion, as trials of other agents (e.g., pentoxyfilline) that improve cerebral perfusion have also reported an improvement in global, intellectual, and cognitive function in vascular dementia patients. However, the most recent Cochrane review suggests that further research is required to investigate the effects of aspirin on cognition, behavior, and quality of life in patients with vascular dementia (39). Finally, cholinergic deficits have been reported in patients with vascular dementia, and there is preliminary evidence of cognitive benefit with the use of cholinesterase inhibitors (31). The use of galantamine, a cholinesterase inhibitor, compared to placebo over a 26 week period was associated with improved cognitive performance, behavioral symptomatology, and activities of daily living in a placebo-controlled trial of probable vascular dementia patients with and without concurrent Alzheimer's disease. Donepezil also improved cognition and global function in a 24 week placebo-controlled trial of patients with possible or probable vascular dementia.

D. Mixed Dementia and Vascular Factors in Alzheimer's Disease

Alzheimer's disease and vascular dementia are the most common causes of dementia, showing similar increases with age; unsurprisingly, there is a considerable overlap between them. There is also evidence of interaction between these two pathologies, not the least of which is that episodes of stroke will precipitate further cognitive decline in known Alzheimer's disease patients and may result in the expression of a dementia syndrome in patients with pre-existing Alzheimer lesions. In addition, up to one-third of vascular dementia patients will have changes consistent with a diagnosis of Alzheimer's disease at post-mortem. Epidemiological studies suggest an association between risk factors linked to stroke in the elderly, increasing the risk of Alzheimer's disease, specifically atherosclerosis (particularly carotid artery plaques), hypertension, smoking, dyslipidaemia, hyperhomocysteinaemia, diabetes, coronary artery disease, and atrial fibrillation (40).

Certainly, genetic factors with vascular effects play an important role in elderly dementia. The APOE ε4 allele is unequivocally linked to nonautosomal dominant forms of Alzheimer's disease, and several-fold increased frequency of this allele has been reported in middle-aged individuals with coronary artery disease and atherosclerosis. ApoE, the product of the APOE gene, has a role in the progression and the regression of atherosclerotic lesions, as well as cholesterol metabolism. Furthermore, APOE $\varepsilon 4$ allele frequency is linked to dementia risk in stroke survivors and to extensive white matter changes on neuroimaging. Interestingly, macro- and microscopic changes consistent with hypertension-related vascular disease have been reported in Alzheimer's disease patients, including large and microcerebral infarcts, periventricular white matter lesions, cerebral amyloid angiopathy, and microvascular degeneration, although it is uncertain whether these changes are incidental or contribute to the pathophysiology of Alzheimer's disease. Further research is needed to assess whether the modification of vascular risk factors will alter the clinical presentation or the progression of Alzheimer's disease directly or only through the prevention of further strokes.

IV. CONCLUSIONS

Hypertension is a cause of significant morbidity and mortality as a consequence of its effects on the extracranial and intracranial blood supply to the brain. This chapter has focused on two conditions, stroke and vascular dementia, which have important consequences for total and disability-free life expectancy. These conditions will remain a significant consumer of health and social services resources, particularly given the increasingly elderly population. However, there is growing evidence for the role of antihypertensive therapy in the primary and secondary prevention of stroke, although questions remain about the management of blood pressure changes common in the acute stroke period. Furthermore, challenges remain to improve the control of hypertension at both an individual and population level. More questions remain in patients with vascular dementia.

The overall control of vascular risk factors superficially appears sensible at a patient level, but significant further research needs to be conducted to better define subtypes of vascular dementia, the role of vascular risk modification on disease progression and regression, the development of disease-modifying therapies, the overlap between Alzheimer's disease and vascular dementia pathologies, and in particular, the benefits of vascular risk modification, including antihypertensive therapy, in preventing the progression to dementia of cognitively impaired patients.

REFERENCES

1. World Health Organisation. The World Health Report 2000. Geneva: World Health Organisation, 2000.

2. The NINDS rt-PA Stroke Study Group. Tissue plasminogen activator for acute ischemic stroke. N Engl J Med 1995; 333:1581–1587.

3. Bamford J, Sandercock P, Dennis M et al. Classification and natural history of clinically identifiable subtypes of cerebral infarction. Lancet 1991; 337:1521–1526.

4. Prospective Studies Collaboration. Age-specific relevance of usual blood pressure to vascular mortality: a meta-analysis of individual data for one million adults in 61 prospective studies. Lancet 2002; 360:1903–1913.

5. Franklin S, Larsen M, Khan S et al. Does the relation of blood pressure to coronary heart disease risk change with aging? The Framingham Heart Study. Circulation 2001; 103:1245–1249.

6. Collins R, Peto R, MacMahon S et al. Blood pressure, stroke and coronary heart disease. Part 2, short-term reductions in blood pressure: overview of randomised drug trials in their epidemiological context. Lancet 1990; 335:827–838.

7. Staessen J, Gasowski J, Wang J et al. Risks of untreated and treated isolated systolic hypertension in the elderly: meta-analysis of outcome trials. Lancet 2000; 355:865–872.

8. Guidelines Committee. 2003 European Society of Hypertension—European Society of Cardiology guidelines for the management of arterial hypertension. J Hypertens 2003; 21:1011–1053.

9. Chobanian A, Bakris G, Black H et al. The Seventh Report of the Joint National Committee on Prevention, Detection, Evaluation, and Treatment of High Blood Pressure: The JNC 7 Report. J Am Med Assoc 2003; 289:2560–2571.

10. Vasan R, Larson M, Leip E et al. Impact of high-normal blood pressure on the risk of cardiovascular disease. N Eng J Med 2001; 345:1291–1297.

11. Primatesta P, Brookes M, Poulter N. Improved hypertension management and control. Results from the Health Survey for England 1998. Hypertension 2001; 38:827–832.

12. Blood Pressure Lowering Treatment Trialists' Collaboration. Effects of different blood-pressure-lowering regimens on major cardiovascular events: results of prospectively-designed overviews of randomised trials. Lancet 2003; 362:1527–1535.

13. Staessen J, Wang J, Thijs L. Cardiovascular prevention and blood pressure reduction: a qualitative overview updated until 1 March 2003. J Hypertens 2003; 21:1055–1076.

14. Wing L, Reid C, Ryan P et al. A comparison of outcomes with angiotensin-converting-enzyme inhibitors and diuretics for hypertension in the elderly. N Engl J Med 2003; 348:583–592.

15. Leonardi-Bee J, Bath P, Phillips S et al. Blood pressure and clinical outcomes in the International Stroke Trial. Stroke 2002; 33:1315–1320.

16. Robinson T, Potter J. Blood pressure in acute stroke. Age and Ageing 2004; 33:6–12.

17. Blood Pressure in Acute Stroke Collaboration. Interventions for deliberately altering blood pressure in acute stroke. The Cochrane Library. Chichester: John Wiley and Sons Ltd, 2003.

18. Blood Pressure in Acute Stroke Collaboration. Vasoactive drugs for acute stroke. The Cochrane Library. Chichester: John Wiley and Sons Ltd, 2003.

19. Horn J, Limburg M. Calcium antagonists for ischemic stroke. A systematic review. Stroke 2001; 32:570–576.

20. Schrader J, Luders S, Kulschewski A et al. The ACCESS Study. Evaluation of acute candesartan cilexetil therapy in stroke survivors. Stroke 2003; 34:1699–1703.

21. Brott T, Lu M, Kothari R et al. Hypertension and its treatment in the NINDS rt-PA stroke trial. Stroke 1998; 29:1504–1509.

22. Saxena R, Wijnhoud A, Man-in-t-Veld A et al. Effect of diaspirin cross-linked haemoglobin on endothelin-1 and blood pressure in acute ischemic stroke in man. J Hypertens 1998; 16:1459–1465.

23. International Society of Hypertension Writing Group. International Society of Hypertension (ISH): Statement on the management of blood pressure in acute stroke. J Hypertens 2003; 21:665–672.

24. Rodgers A, MacMahon S, Gamble G et al. Blood pressure and risk of stroke in patients with cerebrovascular disease. Br Med J 1996; 313:147.

25. Rashid P, Leonardi-Bee J, Bath P. Blood pressure reduction and secondary prevention of stroke and other vascular events. A systematic review. Stroke 2003; 34:2741–2749.

26. The INDANA Project Collaborators. Effect of anti-hypertensive treatment in patients having already suffered from stroke. Gathering the evidence. Stroke 1997; 28:2557–2562.

27. The Intercollegiate Working Party for Stroke. National Clinical Guidelines for Stroke. 2nd ed. London: Royal College of Physicians, 2004.

28. World Health Organisation. The World Health Report, 1998. Geneva: World Health Organisation, 1998.

29. Farmer M, White L, Abbott R et al. Blood pressure and cognitive performance. The Framingham study. Am J Epidemiol 1987; 126:1103–1114.

30. Skoog I, Lernfelt B, Landahl S et al. 15-year longitudinal study of blood pressure and dementia. Lancet 1996; 347:1141–1145.

31. O'Brien J, Erkinjuntti T, Reisberg B et al. Vascular cognitive impairment. Lancet Neurology 2003; 2:89–98.

32. Hachinski V, Lassen N, Marshall J. Multi-infarct dementia: a cause of mental deterioration in the elderly. Lancet 1974; ii:207–210.

33. Sierra C, de la Sierra A, Mercader J et al. Silent cerebral white matter lesions in middle-aged essential hypertensive patients. J Hypertens 2002; 20:519–524.

34. Holdright D. Stroke in the patient with coronary heart disease. Br J Cardiol 2002; 9:163–167.

35. Amenta F, Mignini F, Rabbia F et al. Protective effect of anti-hypertensive treatment on cognitive function in essential hypertension: analysis of published clinical data. J Neurol Sci 2002; 203–204:147–151.

36. Rigaud A, Hanon O, Bouchacourt P et al. Cerebral complications of hypertension in the elderly. Rev Med Int 2000; 22:959–968.

37. Tzourio C, Anderson C, Chapman N et al. Effects of blood pressure lowering with perindopril and indapamide on dementia and cognitive decline in patients with cerebrovascular disease. Arch Intern Med 2003; 163:1069–1075.

38. Birkenhager W, Forette F, Seux M-L et al. Blood pressure, cognitive functions and prevention of dementias in older patients with hypertension. Arch Intern Med 2001; 161:152–156.

39. Williams P, Rands G, Orrel M et al. Aspirin for vascular dementia. The Cochrane Library. Chichester: John Wiley and Sons Ltd, 2003.

40. Kalaria R. The role of cerebral ischaemia in Alzheimer's disease. Neurobiol Aging 2000; 21:321–330.

18

Peripheral Circulation and Hypertension

MARC De BUYZERE, DENIS L. CLEMENT
Ghent University Hospital, Ghent, Belgium

KEYPOINTS

- Evaluation of the peripheral circulation requires simultaneous recordings of blood pressure and flow patterns (e.g., impedance).

- Standardized working definitions to define stiffness indices are mandatory.
- Arterial stiffness indices should be interpreted with caution taking into account actual, local pressure and relevant physiological parameters: aging,

heart rate, stroke volume, body morphology, and reflected waves.

- Arterial stiffness indices do not only reflect intrinsic structural vessel wall characteristics but also changing haemodynamic conditions.
- Cardiovascular interaction (coupling) parameters such as elastance integrate the systemic arterial (peripheral resistance, total compliance) and left ventricle (stroke volume and end-systolic pressure) load.
- A high central pulse pressure and pulse wave velocity seem to have prognostic implications for incident hard cardiovascular endpoints over and above classical risk factors in selected populations of hypertension.
- It is still a matter of debate whether noninvasive estimation of central systolic or pulse pressure starting from peripheral sites requires complex transfer functions.
- Hypertension complicated by peripheral vascular disease implies a worse prognosis vs. uncomplicated hypertension.
- An even borderline reduced ankle to arm systolic blood pressure ratio is associated with a higher incidence of cardiovascular events.

SUMMARY

The peripheral circulation plays a key role in the process of essential hypertension. Blood vessels may be a target organ secondary to longstanding elevated blood pressure, but they also harbor some of the mechanisms causing or accelerating hypertension. In this chapter, we will deal with vessel properties relevant to hypertension. Theoretically, description of the peripheral circulation should imply simultaneously recorded patterns of blood pressure and flow. In part one, we will focus on noninvasive methodologies to define impedance, extending peripheral resistance, and global, regional, and segmental arterial stiffness indices of the peripheral circulation. Potential clinical applications and limitations will be discussed based on a background of technological aspects. For some of the most important stiffness parameters such as pulse pressure, pulse wave velocity, augmentation, the relation with classical risk factors, and relevant physiological parameters such as heart rate, stroke volume, and body morphology will be analysed in more detail. For specific settings of hypertensive populations, evidence that central pulse pressure and pulse wave velocity are prognostic for hard cardiovascular events, even after adjustments for multiple risk factors, will be evaluated. A section will be devoted to the field of cardio-vascular interactions and coupling parameters (e.g., elastance)

integrating systemic *arterial* parameters (resistance and total arterial compliance) and *cardiac* parameters (stroke volume and end-systolic pressure). Additionally, we will address noninvasive estimation of central systolic blood pressure and central pulse pressure starting from peripheral observations.

In part two of this chapter, we will demonstrate that hypertensive patients complicated by atherosclerotic occlusive vascular disease (PVD) are at greater risk and emphasize that arterial stiffness and PVD are by no means equivalent concepts. The bad prognostic implications of an even moderate reduction of the ratio between ankle and brachial systolic blood pressure will be highlighted.

I. INTRODUCTION

Interest in peripheral circulation, particularly palpation of the peripheral arterial pulse, goes back to ancient Chinese medicine and to Galen in the 2nd century A.D. In the 16th and 17th centuries, physicians renewed their interest in palpation of peripheral pulses and it became a core area of medicine. But it was not until the late 19th century that exploration of the peripheral pulses reached the height of its popularity as a result of the development of a device called a sphygmograph. Developed primarily by Marey, Mahomed, Dudgeon, and MacKenzie, this device graphically recorded peripheral pulse data (1). Investigators strove to describe and explain cardiovascular disorders including "hypertension," in terms of "pathologically altered peripheral pulses."

In 1827, William Bright was trying to define "hypertension" in terms of "hardness of the pulse" rather than in terms of the absolute height of blood pressure. The pressure that was needed to extinguish the pulse was a measure of the "hypertension." Between 1872 and 1884, Mahomed was the first to scientifically describe the normal arterial pulse wave at the radial and carotid arteries, and the marked differences existing between them. He associated "hypertension" with morphological changes in the waveforms occurring after the first peak of the curve, but ignoring the information provided by the extremes (top and bottom) of the curve. By the end of the 19th century, insurance companies used the amplitude of this "tidal" wave to identify individuals at high cardiovascular risk.

During the 20th century, it became obvious that Mahomed had been describing the process of "pressure augmentation" and the effect of aging on the morphology of pressure curves.

II. ARTERIAL STIFFNESS

The term *arterial stiffness* is generally used to describe the global buffering properties of the arterial system or regional or local segments of that system. Correct methodologies should contain simultaneous recordings of intraarterial pressure, changes in flow and changes in vessel diameter. The aortic pulse pressure is the simplest indicator of arterial stiffness. Increased aortic pulse pressure together with premature timing of reflected peripheral waves increases the load on the left ventricle and large arteries. This may lead ultimately to ventricular and arterial hypertrophy and fibrosis (5). This abnormal *ventricular–arterial interaction* may help to refine the epidemiological relation between a high brachial artery pulse pressure and cardiovascular morbidity and mortality.

In general, arterial stiffness is considered a dynamic property of peripheral circulation which is determined by the vascular structure (intrinsic vessel wall characteristics) and cardiovascular function (hemodynamic properties, muscle tone, etc.). It is influenced by many physiological conditions such as age, gender, heart rate, blood pressure, and body mass index. In general, high blood pressure is associated with stiffer arteries. Dynamic changes that lead to increased pressure, such as higher ventricular ejection, higher heart rate, greater resistance, and earlier wave reflections, should be taken into account in addition to intrinsic wall properties. Standardized procedures (working definitions) to measure arterial stiffness are imperative. Because arterial stiffness is highly dependent on pressure, the operating pressure should always be clearly defined (4).

All noninvasive methodologies to address stiffness have some significant shortcomings, which makes reliable interpretation difficult. Drawbacks include (a) intrinsic problems with the use of Windkessel (WK) models (see further for global and regional stiffness indices), (b) the incorrect use of brachial rather than local blood pressures, (c) input of not well-validated cardiac output data, (d) no adjustment made for heart rate or contractility parameters, and (e) moreover, there is a nonlinear relationship between vessel diameter and arterial pressure, the influence of smooth muscle tone (autonomic nervous system, endothelium, hormones), the nonhomogeneity of intrinsic arterial properties along the arterial tree (collagen, elastin content), and the spontaneous variability of all physiological parameters (blood pressure, heart rate, vessel diameter); all of them complicating correct interpretation of an arterial stiffness index. Indices of arterial stiffness should be defined under strict working conditions and adjusted for important confounders.

Impedance is defined as the ratio of pressure to flow ($Z = P/Q$, units mmHg s/mL—or in older literature, dyn s/cm^5). When measured at the entrance of the systemic or pulmonary circulation, it is termed *input impedance* (Z_{in}). Under certain conditions, pressure (P) and flow (Q) waves can be decomposed in a Fourier analysis. Z can be considered as consisting of a *steady component*

(mean pressure to mean flow ratio) and a series (Σ) of pulsatile components Z_n (for nth harmonic). Mathematically, P and Q can be represented in their complex "modulus $|Z_n|$ and phase Φ" notation. For a nth harmonic:

$$Z_n = |Z_n|e^{i\Phi_z} \quad \text{with} \quad |Z_n| = \frac{|P_n|}{|Q_n|}$$
$$\text{and} \quad \Phi_z = \Phi_P - \Phi_Q$$

By convention, the steady component (at 0 Hz) is called the *total peripheral resistance* (R, measured in the same units as impedance) and the *fundamental frequency* equals the subject's heart rate. For each measured pressure and flow signal at the entrance of the circulation, a frequency plot of $|Z_{in}|$ and Φ_{Zin} (modulus and phase) can be made. Mostly, for higher harmonics (>3), $|Z_{in}|$ does not vary much and is referred to as the *characteristic impedance* Z_c (sometimes also denoted as Z_o). The physiological meaning of Z_c is the impedance of a heart with a very long, reflection-free aorta of uniform structure. It has been shown by Womersley that under such conditions Z_c is proportional with wave velocity over the aorta and also with blood density, and is inversely proportional with its cross-section. In the laboratory, Z_c is calculated either as the slope of the regression between central (carotid) pressure and aortic flow in early systole or as the average of the moduli of the 4–10th harmonics of input impedance.

Classical biomechanical theories in animal models link abnormal aortic function with accelerated breakdown of elastin, subsequent dilatation of the lumen, and replacement of elastin with the much stiffer collagen. Recently, Mitchell et al. demonstrated that this paradigm should be reconsidered. In systolic hypertension (elevated pulse pressure), they demonstrated that, particularly in women, the elevated pulse pressure was attributable primarily to increased Z_c and a *reduced* effective diameter of the proximal aorta, independent of mean blood pressure (6). Elevation of Z_c was clearly out of proportion to the elevation of pulse wave velocity at comparable mean blood pressures. Their data in systolic hypertension suggested an abnormality in proximal aortic diameter, rather than a difference in the material properties of the aortic wall as an underlying cause of high, central pulse pressure. By using an invasive methodology, Nichols et al. (7) also had previously found increased Z_c in association with hypertension. Moreover, Vasan et al. (8) observed that the aortic root diameter determined through echography was inversely related to systolic blood pressure and brachial pulse pressure in hypertensive subjects from the Framingham Heart Study cohort. The indication is that, particularly in hypertensive women, high pulse pressure is associated with high Z_c and *reduced* effective aorta diameter (rather than aortic root dilatation) despite lower peak flow; thus leading to an abnormal pressure–diameter relationship. Endothelial dysfunction, increased aorta tone, and myocyte hypertrophy, or primary abnormalities of aortic diameters and resting tone may lead to a functional imbalance between aortic flow and diameter. Abnormal large artery function (stiffness) should not always be viewed as an irreversible structural problem because there might also be a reversible hemodynamic aspect of arterial stiffness.

A. Aging Effects on Arterial Stiffness

The complexity and discontinuity of the arterial elastic behavior along the arterial tree may complicate the preceding concepts. The proximal part of the arterial tree (the aorta and major branches) has a relatively low stiffness, particularly at young age. The aorta is composed of vascular smooth muscle cells from the neural crest, which secrete primarily elastin and collagen. The elastin:collagen ratio and its gradient along the aorta are believed by many investigators to determine the proximal aorta elasticity in young subjects. The contractile properties of aorta vascular smooth muscle cells are less important; whereas in the distal parts of the arterial tree, the contractile properties of the vascular smooth muscle cells become very important. These cells are sensitive to many endothelial vasoactive substances.

Although most of the preceding evidence are from animal models, several investigators have extended these relationships to humans. Findings show that in middle-aged controls, the gradient between carotid and radial distensibility is about 25%. As the subjects get older, their central arteries become stiffer, the artery diameters enlarge at the same time pulsatile diameters are reduced, and the extracellular matrix of large arteries increases. Thus for older subjects, both pulse pressure amplification toward the periphery and distensibility gradient between carotid artery and radial artery decrease. On the other hand, central pulse pressure increases as people age. As the aortic diameter becomes greater with age, proximal compliance is less dependent on age than proximal distensibility. From these observations, it seems obvious that age is the most important determinant of arterial stiffness, wave reflection, and pulse pressure in an healthy individual. In the case of hypertension in younger patients, the large arteries also may become stiff because of the high distending blood pressure and the impaired hemodynamics. To allow an inter-subject comparison, the use of *isobaric stiffness indices of central arteries* (or appropriate adjustment for blood pressure) is recommended. Of course, in elderly hypertensive patients, intrinsic vascular wall abnormalities also interfere.

B. Genetic Factors Affecting Arterial Stiffness

Genetic background is becoming a topic of increasing interest with respect to arterial stiffness. Monogenic disorders, such as Marfan disease, are of interest as they allow studying the effects of an isolated gene abnormality. Because age and an elevation in blood pressure are important determinants of arterial stiffness, it is likely that (as for hypertension) the genetic background is polygenic and may involve many genes, polymorphisms, and environmental factors. The interplay among these factors and their effects on blood pressure control mechanisms may be even more important than the classical cardiovascular risk factors.

Durier et al. studied levels of gene expression in aortic specimens in relation to aortic pulse wave velocity in subjects who were undergoing coronary artery bypass grafting (57). The study focused on two groups of transcripts: genes that determine mechanical properties (cytoskeletal–cell membrane–extracellular matrix) and cell signalling genes. They used the Affymetrix GeneChip with U95 Av2 arrays. Thirty-two transcripts in the field of the connection between the cytoskeleton, cell surface, and extracellular matrix were differentially expressed in aortas that were "stiffer." Among them, the integrins α_{2b}, α_6, β_3, and β_5 transcript levels differed, as well as some transcripts of the proteoglycans and related families (decorin, osteomodulin, aggrecan-1, neuroglycan-C, and dermatopontin). Interestingly, osteopontin and vitronectin were not differentially expressed. In addition to the genes that are related to mechanical regulation, a large number of transcripts that are related to signalling/communication or gene expression (PPP1CB, Yotiao, p85-α, synaptojanin, PKCβ_1, and RGS16) were associated with pulse wave velocity. Very importantly, the study also identified many other transcripts of still unknown function that are associated with pulse wave velocity. Thus, we are only at the beginning of an exciting new area and need to conduct further functional genomic studies.

The link between *telomere biology* (mean and individual telomere length and attrition) and biological aging (e.g., vascular aging), as opposed to chronological aging, is becoming a key factor in fundamental research on arterial stiffness. The use of telomere size as a marker of the replicative history of cells has been advocated (58). Telomere length seems to be a molecular record of biological aging. In the study of young twin pairs of the Danish Twin Registry (59), the mean length of the terminal restriction fragments in white blood cells was found to be inversely associated with pulse pressure. The study suggested that both pulse pressure and terminal restriction fragments have a high degree of heritability and individuals with longer telomeres manifest smaller pulse pressures. Benetos et al. (60) studied terminal restriction fragments length in older French subjects, noting age-adjusted longer telomere lengths in women. In both sexes, terminal restriction fragment length decreased with age. In men, age-adjusted shorter telomere length was associated with stiffer arteries (higher pulse pressure and higher pulse wave velocity). Both studies suggest that a subset of the population with shorter telomere length and subsequently stiffer arteries, particularly men with higher pulse pressures, exists with increasing biological age (61).

Important underlying assumptions are that the relationship between telomere length, arterial stiffness, and subsequent higher pulse pressure and pulse wave velocity not only holds true for brachial artery pulse pressure, but also for central pulse pressure, and not only for white blood cell telomeres, but also for all replicating cells. Cell types such as vascular endothelial cells and vascular smooth muscle cells play a pivotal role in blood pressure control and vascular aging. There is also some evidence that the variation in terminal restriction fragment length of subpopulations of somatic cells is smaller than the age-adjusted inter-individual variations. Research is ongoing to authenticate these theories. Accelerated telomere attrition over time is also a point of interest; telomere attrition accelerates in childhood and slows down during adolescence. Whether it increases with vascular aging and arterial stiffness including raised pulse pressure remains to be proven. Attention should further focus on telomere length of individual chromosomes.

In general, large-scale studies using a multivariate setting are needed in healthy subjects, in which genetic, environmental, and cardiovascular risk factors, including aging, are evaluated against hard endpoints (cardiovascular morbidity and mortality). These factors may modulate pulse pressure, arterial stiffness, and wave reflections, or other parameters derived from the complete blood pressure curve.

III. PULSE PRESSURE, WAVE PROPAGATION, AND WAVE REFLECTIONS

In a classic view of physiology, the blood pressure curve is the result of a *steady component* [mean blood pressure (MAP) $\approx$ cardiac output (CO) $\times$ total peripheral resistance (TPR), which remains almost constant over the arterial tree] and a *pulsatile component* (pulse pressure is tracked with ventricular ejections). Pulse pressure is closely related to the cushioning function of large arteries (compliance of primarily aorta and major branches) and to the timing and intensity of reflected waves. Wave reflections are closely related to the (micro)-vascular network which causes peripheral vascular resistance.

Important contributors to the genesis of reflected waves are the geometry and branching (numbers, angles, and diameters) of small muscular arteries and smaller arterioles (resistance vessels), pathological conditions of these vessels comprising hypertrophy, altered matrix composition, remodelling and rarefaction, influences of cations, endothelium-dependent vasodilatation, and vasomotor tone (endothelial and vascular smooth muscle cells). Large arteries do not add significantly to wave reflection unless there are pathological changes such as calcified plaque, tortuosities, or aneurysms. Opinions differ on how far from proximal aorta one or more "functional discrete reflecting site(s)" should be defined, with figures varying from 15 to 75 cm downstream from the heart. Gender differences in wave reflection can be ascribed in part to the length and geometry of the vascular tree and possibly other factors such as hormones (32,33).

Thus, a blood pressure curve can be seen as the sum of forward waves (propagating at a certain pulse wave velocity) and backward (reflected) waves. In young individuals at rest, the reflected wave travels back in the diastolic phase, which leads to a higher peripheral pulse pressure than central pulse pressure. However, as individuals become older and arteries become stiffer, waves travel faster (higher pulse wave velocity) along the arterial tree. The earlier return of reflected waves in older individuals leads to an augmentation of the central (aortic) pressure, which superposes with the forward incident wave during systole, increasing systolic and pulse aortic pressure and somewhat decreasing aortic diastolic pressures. However, ventricular ejection tends to be reduced in the elderly, which leads to some blunting of central PP. In 1980, Murgo defined an "inflection point" on the pulse wave curve (site of interaction between forward and backward waves). Pressure waves could be classified as Murgo type C (young controls) waves with an inflection point after systolic blood pressure and Murgo type A (aged persons) where the inflection points precede systolic blood pressure.

The augmentation index (AIx) is defined as the increment in pressure from the inflection point to the peak pressure of the aortic pressure waveform expressed as a % of the peak pressure. Recently, alternative definitions have been introduced replacing inflection point with the top of the schoulder of the curve. With P_{inf} as the blood pressure at the inflection point (shoulder), AIx is defined as: $AIx = \pm(SBP - P_{inf})/(SBP - DBP)$, where SBP is local systolic blood pressure and DBP is diastolic blood pressure. Conventionally, in a C-type wave, AIx is negative and in an A-type wave, mostly $AIx > 0.12$. Shoulder peak detection is based on zero-crossings of the fourth derivative of the waveforms (first positive-to-negative crossings for A-type waves and second negative-to-positive crossings for C-type waves). Theoretically, true inflection points can be approximated by second derivative cross-overs. In commercial devices, automated detection algorithms for primary and secondary peaks on the curves are based on first- and third-order derivatives.

Following these working definitions, the AIx theoretically should depend on the timing of the reflected wave (most probably related to factors such as gender, height of the individual, amplitude of reflection, and stiffness) and to the shape of the forward wave (which is related to left ventricular outflow and elasticity of the ascending aorta). Factors most likely affecting left ventricular outflow are prolonged ejection, decreased heart rate, reduced contractility, mitral incompetence, and aortic stenosis. Most of these expected determinants of augmentation have been confirmed in observational studies.

Physiological factors that affect augmentation and reflection indices include age, height of the individual, heart rate, and other risk factors.

A. Age

In animal models, aging implies an increase in arterial wall thickness secondary to hyperplasia of the intima and replacement of elastin by collagen in the media. Although, the pathophysiology in humans is less clear, greater augmentation with age has been observed. As people's age and their blood pressure increase, the C-type Murgo wave turns into an A-type Murgo wave—a wave whose inflection point precedes systolic blood pressure. A definition of the AIx is derived from this principle.

Pulse pressure amplification decreases with age as well, and thus elderly people lose the difference between central and peripheral pulse pressure.

B. Height of the Individual

Augmentation and the height of the individual are inversely related. In individuals of shorter stature, the increase of augmentation might be due to the shorter distance from the origin of the waveform to the site of reflections, leading to a quicker return of the reflected wave for a given pulse wave velocity. Thus, height may be in part a surrogate for gender difference in stiffness parameters. Shorter stature is related to other known risks such as decreased forced expiratory volume and peak expiratory flow. Moreover, Elzinga and Westerhof (34) associated reduced length of the arterial tree with faster heart rate, shorter diastolic period, shorter diastolic time constant, and a lower arterial compliance to better match ventricular and arterial loads.

C. Heart Rate

With a faster heart rate, the reflected wave is more likely to arrive in diastole and thus reduce augmentation. In paced heart rates, augmentation decreases by about 4–6% for each 10 beats per min (bpm) increase. This is somewhat counter-intuitive because a reduction in heart rate (e.g., such as the one produced by beta-blocking agents) is expected to be a beneficial matter, but it would in fact be associated with increased augmentation, according to this reasoning. Another statistical observation is that amplification of pulse pressure is less with slower heart rates.

D. Other Risk Factors and Target Organ Damage

Increased augmentation might be expected in populations with prevalent risk factors such as high blood pressure, hypercholesterolemia, and hypertriglyceridemia and in type 2 diabetes mellitus. However, data is scarce and contradictory. For example, no increase in augmentation has been seen in diabetes mellitus type 2 after controlling for confounders. An increase in augmentation not adjusted for heart rate was observed in patients with increased left ventricular mass.

Recently, Nuernberger et al. (35) demonstrated that the AIx derived from carotid applanation tonometry in 216 patients with and without cardiovascular disease was related to age, gender, height of the individual, blood pressure, heart rate, smoking, cholesterol, body mass index, and global risk scores. These include the Framingham Heart Study risk score in subjects without events and SMART (categorical risk), and EPOZ (continuous risk) scores in patients with pre-existing cardiovascular disease (35). Global risk scores (Framingham, SCORE) are a powerful way to target high-risk individuals toward life style changes and drug therapy in primary prevention. Such conditions warrant studies of the role of pulse wave velocity, wave reflection, and augmentation indices in selecting individuals at high risk for cardiovascular disease. Future studies should focus on these parameters as some of them relate to worse outcome in hypertension or in related cardiovascular diseases, beyond the classic risk factors such as systolic and diastolic blood pressure readings.

IV. MEASURES OF ARTERIAL STIFFNESS

The first historical approaches to describe arterial system function used two- or three-element Windkessel (WK) models; these elements included: resistance, capacitance, and impedance. Such models may be realistic in very old and very hypertensive subjects with stiff, inelastic arteries, but in most subjects elastic behavior is distributed along the aorta and all major arteries. Moreover, WK models do not explain wave reflections and frequency-dependence, therefore their value is limited.

More realistic models assume tubes that are more distensible, at the ends of which are resistant elements that create reflected waves. A pressure wave is the resultant of the incident waves from the heart and the reflected waves from the periphery. In very stiff arteries, reflected waves travel faster over the arteries and merge with the systolic instead of the diastolic part of the incident waves, which causes higher blood pressure during systole (*augmentation*) and somewhat lower pressure during diastole (3). Several investigators have tried to derive arterial stiffness parameters from WK models, which will be reviewed later in this chapter.

Another historical evolution came when researchers such as Millar and Drzwiecki developed more accurate and reliable apparatuses than sphygmographs for registering peripheral waves, called *tonometers*, and these are now used in clinical settings. The O'Rourke Group extended peripheral tonometry to "central noninvasive aortic pulse wave analysis." Tonometric signals are recorded at the radial artery and calibrated against brachial artery blood pressure. The resulting radial waveform is then transformed by computer algorithm to a central aortic waveform by using a generalized transfer function (2,3). The algorithm is set to generate calculated values for central pressures, time intervals, and augmentation.

A. Measures of Segmental or Regional Arterial Stiffness

Several noninvasive surrogate parameters of segmental or regional arterial stiffness have been documented and some have been implemented in commercial devices. These parameters are based on three different principles of measurements: methods directly derived from pressure pulse wave morphology, methods based on measurements of pulse transit time, and methods derived from measurements of arterial diameter (changes). In this context, the term compliance (C) is currently used as a surrogate for arterial stiffness, with $C = \Delta V / \Delta P$.

1. Analysis of the Arterial Pressure Pulse

This type of analyses includes stiffness parameters derived from subclavian pulse tracing, proximal and distal compliance from modified WK models, second derivative finger plethysmography, and the AIx.

Subclavian Pulse Tracing

In subclavian pulse tracing (9), compliance is calculated from the pressure, measured with a strain-gauge transducer at the subclavian artery, and from the flow

derived from the aortic annulus diameter and velocity measured by Echo–Doppler.

Proximal and Distal Compliance from a Modified WK Model

Proximal (large artery) and distal (small artery) compliances are calculated from a modified WK model. The input is a radial artery tonometer signal that is calibrated with an oscillometric blood pressure. In older literature, proximal compliance was denoted as "capacitative," and distal compliance denoted as "oscillatory". A recent semi-automated, commercially available device (HDI/PulseWave CR-2000, Research Cardiovascular Profiling System from Hypertension Diagnostics, Inc.) makes use of an algorithm that calculates a large-artery compliance index (C_1) and a small-artery compliance index ($C_2 \ll C_1$). Whether C_1 and C_2 describe clear physiological entities remains a matter of debate. Despite this debate, the CR-2000 has recently been advocated as a screening tool because C_2 might be a marker of functional or structural alterations that occur in early endothelial dysfunction. In this sense, selectively reduced C_2 has been associated with a smoking habit, diabetes mellitus, hypertension, and documented coronary artery disease (10). In addition, C_1 may serve as a marker of vascular aging (11).

Second Derivative Finger Plethysmography

A device from Fukuda Electric Company takes the measure of arterial compliance at the finger. Second derivative finger plethysmography uses the ratio of the second to first inflections of the photoplethysmographic (SDPTG) signal's second derivative (12).

Augmentation Index

An average ascending aorta pressure waveform is mathematically constructed from transformed, tonometer-recorded, peripheral artery waveforms (Millar tonometer), and then a central augmentation index (c-AIx) is calculated (2). The c-AIx is relative to the percentage of the central pulse pressure that can be attributed to the reflected wave and is considered a "global surrogate index of arterial behaviour." It also comprises other factors such as blood pressure, the height of the individual, heart rate, and ventricular arterial coupling. Atcor's Sphygmo-Cor device is commercially available with an in-built generalized transfer function.

2. Calculations from Measurement of the Pulse Transit Time

Calculations from measurement of the pulse transit time rely on the Moens–Korteweg and Bramwell–Hill formulas, which show the relationship between the pulse wave velocity (PWV) and relative changes in volume (ΔV) and pressure (ΔP).

$$[PWV]^2 = \frac{(\Delta PV)}{(\Delta V \rho)}$$

with ρ representing blood density.

Because pulse wave velocity is a velocity, it can be measured as the ratio of a distance (Δx) and a transit time (Δt): $PWV = \Delta x / \Delta t$. The time delay between the feet of the wave front measured at two locations is Δt and the distance measured on the body surface between the two locations is Δx (attention for the true pathway in elderly patients with tortuous arteries!). Another point of care is when the proximal and distal pulse waves are recorded from two different sites where pulse waves propagate in opposite directions. For instance, Δx for carotid-femoral PWV is measured either directly or by subtracting the distance from the carotid location to the sternal notch from the distance between sternal notch to the femoral site or by subtracting it from the total distance. It leads to different reference values! The formula is a rude simplification and supposes among many others assumptions (such as constant velocity and diameters and straight vessels) that the foot of the waveform is not influenced by wave reflections. Wave foot measured by tonometry is seldom influenced by wave reflection because it is made up of components $>10\,Hz$. Lower frequency components ($1-5\,Hz$) are more affected by wave reflection. Theoretically, pulse wave velocity should be minimally affected by changing heart rates. Nevertheless, in a number of studies higher heart rates were associated with higher pulse wave velocities, particularly in males.

With increasing age, the aortic pulse wave velocity increases from about 5 to $12\,m/s$ and the aortic diameter increases by about one-fourth. In general, males have the highest pulse wave velocity, but gender differences are controversial, especially the influence of menopause.

The Δt can be assessed from either recorded arterial pulses or simultaneous recording of Doppler ultrasound patterns. Recorded arterial pulses are taken from dedicated mechanotransducers (for carotid–radial and carotid–femoral sites) or ECG-triggered subtraction of two tonometric signals. The proximal and distal pulses are recorded by means of a high-frequency applanation tonometer, and transit time is related to the R-wave of a stable ECG signal. PWV can be calculated between sites such as the carotid–femoral artery, the subclavian–femoral artery, the subclavian artery–abdominal aorta, the carotid–radial artery, and others. There are several methods that can be used for calculating pulse wave velocity.

The Complior System

Colson has commercialized an automated system which measures pulse wave velocity with dedicated mechanotransducers, called the "Complior System" (13). It selects adequate pressure waves through a built-in quality control system and automatically calculates pulse wave velocity from at least 10 consecutive waveforms. This device is very accurate because it measures beat-to-beat time delay between the two ends of the segment under study. The determination of the waveform foot depends on registration techniques, sampling rate, and so forth, remains a critical step for correct calculation of PWV. Proprietary algorithms in the Complior System therefore try to identify the whole of the rising limb of the pulse wave. In the more recent Complior 2 System, pressure transducers are fixed instead of handheld, which makes the technique even more user-friendly.

The SphygmoCor PWV System

The SphygmoCor PWV System (2) also offers an option to determine transit times. The Millar tonometer records both proximal and distal waveforms, but not simultaneously (which is a disadvantage). The time delay between recorded stable ECG R waves and the proximal (carotid) flow wave feet is subtracted from the time delay between stable ECG R waves and the distal (common femoral) flow wave feet. The apparatus provides us with a choice of four algorithms for a reference point on the curve.

The Doppler Ultrasound Method

In the Doppler ultrasound method (14), the transit time between the root of the left subclavian artery and abdominal aorta bifurcation can be calculated from simultaneous recordings of flow by continuous Doppler probes. Distance is measured from the suprasternal notch to the umbilicus.

The Wall Track System

The Wall Track System (WTS) commercialised by Pie Medical is a high-resolution, echo-tracking device that measures and tracks changes in the internal diameters of superficial arteries at diastole. It also measures intima-media thickness and aortic pulse wave velocity. The vessel wall movement detector system calculates the time delay from the R-top of the ECG to the 10% level of the ascending limb of the distension waveform. The difference between the delay times to the femoral and carotid arteries is used as an estimate of the carotid–femoral transit time (15).

The QKd System

Noninvasive measurement of ambulatory blood pressure by automated inflation of a brachial cuff allows for the calculation of a brachial pulse wave velocity. Transit time is calculated from diastole at the brachial artery and from the onset of ventricular activity (the latter is traced by a cutaneous electrode). Novacor uses this system commercially in their Diasys device.

3. Calculations from Measurements of Changes in Diameter

Various models can be used to calculate related stiffness parameters (beta index, incremental elasticity and other moduli, compliance and distensibility coefficients).

Beta Index Models

The proximal parts of the aorta and large arteries are elastic, and the diameter may change $>10\%$ over one cardiac cycle. There is an "elastic tapering" toward the more distal parts of the artery. Local vasoreactivity is an important confounder in diameter changes during the cycle. The Langewouters et al. (16) studied the mechanical behaviour of aortic segments. The "pressure–area" (A) relation was found to be nonlinear and is described by the arc-tangent model.

$$A(P) = A_m \left[\frac{1}{2} + \frac{1}{\pi} \, \text{tg}^{-1} \left(\frac{P - P_o}{P_1} \right) \right],$$

where A_m, P_o, P_1 parameters are derived from curve-fittings.

An alternative is the "pressure–diameter" (d) relation of Hayashi:

$$P = P_s \, e^{\beta(d_o - d_s)/d_s},$$

with a reference pressure (P_s) and with its associated outer diameter (d_s), and with the outer diameter (d_o) at pressure P, where β is the *beta index*, or stiffness coefficient (17), and for aortas, β may vary between 5 and 20.

When applying beta index models, pressures are obtained from automated brachial oscillometry, and diameters are obtained from ultrasonic, phase-locked, echo-tracking devices at different superficial arteries. The variability of site location for pressure and diameter measurements is a drawback; however, several methodologies have been developed to estimate local pressures. Thoracic aorta stiffness indexes may be defined by using suprasternal echocardiography instead of vascular echography (18).

Echo-tracking Combined with Langewouters' Model

The pressure–diameter relationships between end-diastolic and end-systolic limits can be studied by using high-resolution, ultrasound echo-tracking of the (radial) artery internal diameter and wall thickness, combined with simultaneous finger plethysmography (Finapres). Specific software corrects for time delays between the measurement sites. Compliance and distensibility are calculated according to the Langewouters model. A commercial device was available, the NIUS 2 from Asulab.

Several parameters of intrinsic vascular wall properties can be measured (19,20). The *incremental elasticity modulus* (E_{inc}) is defined from experimental stepwise variation of the pressure and is usually expressed in kilopascal (kPa).

$$E_{inc} \approx 2R_i^2 \frac{(1 - v_p^2)}{(R_o^2 - R_i^2)} \left[\frac{\Delta P}{(\Delta R_o / R_o)} \right],$$

where R_i and R_o represents inner and outer vascular radius and v_p the Poisson ratio of the wall material (≈ 0.5).

As E_{inc} increases with pressure (higher at the periphery than at the aorta), the parameter is usually expressed at a predefined pressure (e.g., 100 mmHg) called the *isobaric E_{inc}*.

The ratio $\Delta P / (\Delta R_o / R_o)$ is termed the *Peterson incremental elasticity modulus*. Such an elasticity modulus is related to the intrinsic mechanical properties of the vascular wall. Historically, the commonly used intrinsic mechanical property parameter has been Young's modulus (E).

$$E = \left(\frac{\Delta P}{\Delta D} \right) D^2 \left[\frac{(1 - v_p^2)}{2h} \right]$$

with diameter changes (ΔD) corresponding to pressure (ΔP) changes and the wall thickness (h).

Echo-Tracking Combined with Local Pulse Pressure Assessment

As mentioned earlier, high-resolution ultrasound echo-tracking of superficial arteries allows the study of pulsatile changes of the internal arterial diameter and intima-media thickness. Local blood pressure can be assessed from either transfer functions or local tonometer signals appropriately calibrated by pressure–time integrals of brachial blood pressures. The WTS delivers diameters (d) and changes in arterial diameter (Δd). Introducing local pulse pressure (ΔP), the following estimates of local arterial stiffness can also be generated: local *arterial compliance coefficient* (CC)

$$CC = \frac{\pi(2d \cdot \Delta d + \Delta d^2)}{4\Delta P},$$

and local *distensibility coefficient* (DC) (15)

$$DC = \frac{(2d \cdot \Delta d + \Delta d^2)}{(\Delta P \cdot d^2)}.$$

CC is the *compliance per unit of length*—the change in cross-sectional area per unit of local pressure. DC is the *relative change* in cross-sectional area per unit of local pressure. Common carotid compliance but not distensibility seems to be gender dependent, with a higher compliance in men. Low compliance in women may lead to lower diastolic pressure.

A modification at the *brachial artery* by using a transmural pressure modulation device and radial artery tonometry has been introduced into the Phase 2 from Biosound Inc. At the digital arteries an index of small artery distensibility has been proposed: time-to-peak divided by total time (PT/TT) on a digital artery pressure curve. It is questionable whether the distensibility of smaller arteries can be adequately measured.

Aortic Stiffness by Transesophageal Echocardiography

Local aortic elastic modulus can be calculated from diameter changes and wall thickness measured by transesophageal echocardiography (21). Subclavian mechanical air transmission against brachial blood pressure calibration is used as "local blood pressure." Measurement of stiffness by cine-magnetic resonance imaging is currently being researched.

Frame Grabber Processing

Off-line measurement on a high-resolution video display of carotid artery diameters and intima-media thickness, combined with local tonometry (22) or even brachial blood pressure (23) has been used to assess stiffness.

B. Measures of Global Arterial Stiffness

Global arterial stiffness (total arterial compliance) can be addressed by different methodologies starting from a simple stroke volume to pulse pressure ratio next to calculations of impedance from lumped parameter WK models or via the pulse pressure method. Other methodologies comprise decay–time curves, and more sophisticated evaluations by input impedance spectra or parameters of cardio-vascular interactions that combine resistance, compliance, and time intervals.

1. Ratio of Stroke Volume to Pulse Pressure

The simplest, although very crude, estimate of total arterial compliance (C_t) is the steady-state ratio of stroke volume (SV) to pulse pressure (PP) ($C_t = SV/PP$) (24). The concept of SV/PP does not take into account the WK principles; it assumes that the complete stroke volume is buffered in the large central elastic arteries and that any flow passes to the peripheral circulation. In fact, the volume increase in the aorta is only a fraction of stroke volume; therefore, SV/PP is an overestimation of true compliance.

2. Lumped Parameter Models

Lumped parameters models can be used to assess arterial compliance. Two- (R, C), three- (R, C, Z_c), and four- (R, C, Z_c, L) element WK models are currently used for the estimation of aortic pressure (P_{est}). R is the total peripheral resistance, C is the total arterial compliance, Z_c is the characteristic impedance, and L is the blood inertia.

Input impedance can be derived from simultaneously measured aortic pressure and flow signals [$Z_{in} = P_{ao}/Q_{ao}$]. C can be estimated by calculating the parameters of a chosen WK model so that modelled and measured Z_{in} matches with each other. Using automated algorithms (e.g., Marquardt–Levenberg), the difference $(P_{est} - P_{ao})^2$ can be minimized by adjusting the parameters of the model to reach an acceptable agreement, resulting in good estimates of total arterial compliance.

3. The Decay–Time Method

In a simplified two-element WK model, the time constant τ of diastolic aortic decay equals RC. Thus, total arterial compliance is approximated as the ratio between time constant and total peripheral resistance ($C = \tau/R$). The parameter τ is mono-exponentially fitted from the last two-thirds of diastolic decay.

This method has been criticized for oversimplification because circulation cannot be viewed as a two-element WK model and pressure decay is not mono-exponential. It shows oscillations at the end.

4. The Area Method

By applying an "area-under-curve" variant of the decay–time method between the dicrotic notch and end diastole on the pressure–time curve (25), C can be calculated as:

$$C = \frac{(\int P dt)}{R(P_{t_1} - P_{t_2})}.$$

R may come from mean flow (cardiac output). The result may vary with the interval ($t_1 - t_2$), and it extends the decay–time method to nonlinear pressure-volume relationships.

5. The Pulse Pressure Method

One of the most useful methodologies is Stergiopulos' pulse pressure method (26); it is an iterative calculation on a two-element (RC) WK model with simultaneously measured instantaneous flow (echo–Doppler) and pulse pressure often measured by appropriately calibrated carotid tonometry (9). R is derived from mean pressure and flow, and C is changed in the RC WK model until measured and predicted pulse pressures satisfactorily agree. Pulse pressure is essentially a low-frequency characteristic of the arterial system and can be reasonably well described by a two-element RC model. Multiple comparisons show that the pulse pressure method generates values of total arterial compliance in agreement with invasive methodologies (27). RC models are relevant to hypertension because both R and C contribute to high arterial load (28).

6. Effective Arterial Elastance

A more precise evaluation of the hydraulic load (left ventricular afterload) requires input impedance spectra or parameters such as the effective arterial elastance (E_a) that incorporates total peripheral resistance, characteristic impedance (Z_c), total lumped arterial compliance, and systolic and diastolic time intervals. The Kass group showed that E_a is impaired in hypertension and can be approximated by the steady-state left ventricular end-systolic pressure/stroke volume ratio or "index of vascular load" (29). E_a tends to lump the steady and pulsatile components of arterial load. Segers et al. (30), using a hydraulic model, observed a mathematical relation between E_a, R, and C by using a four-element WK model with fixed values for inertia (inertance) and characteristic impedance.

$$E_a = 1.023\frac{R}{T} + \frac{0.314}{C} - 0.127,$$

where T is the cardiac cycle length. Recently, Chemla et al. were able to confirm such relationships in both normotensive and hypertensive subjects, and they also found that 0.9 (SAP) was an acceptable estimate of LVESP, leading to a simple estimation of E_a:

$$E_a = 0.9\frac{HR \times SAP}{CI},$$

where HR is the heart rate, SAP represents systolic aortic pressure, and CI represents cardiac index (31).

E_a belongs to the field of *cardiovascular interactions*, the interactions between left ventricle and systemic arterial load. It combines total peripheral resistance and total arterial compliance, and is a ratio of the cardiac parameters end-systolic pressure and stroke volume.

V. RELATIONSHIP OF ARTERIAL STIFFNESS PARAMETERS WITH RISK FACTORS, TARGET–ORGAN DAMAGE, AND HARD ENDPOINTS

Hypertension, particularly in the aged, is associated with higher systolic blood pressure and higher pulse pressure (an elementary marker of stiffer arteries). Several papers also describe stiffer large arteries in hypertensive individuals in general, documented by abnormalities in all of the

earlier-mentioned indices of global, regional, or segmental arterial stiffness. For example, compliance and distensibility at the common carotid artery are reduced and the incremental elasticity modulus higher in hypertensive individuals.

Because high blood pressure is associated with many other generally accepted common risk factors, it is not surprising that significant relationships between stiffness indices and other risk factors have been described as well. A number of these univariate correlations should be viewed with caution. When they are adjusted appropriately for age, height of the individual, heart rate, and other risks or when they are recalculated at isobaric pressure or for comparable wall stress, the differences in large artery stiffness between normotensive and hypertensive patients are minimized or lost.

Thus, when discussing and comparing mechanical properties of large (peripheral) arteries in hypertension along with the intrinsic vascular wall characteristics and hemodynamic properties, such as working pressure and cardiovascular interaction, take into account concomitant risk factors and the nonlinearity of the pressure–volume relations.

Remarkably, in smaller peripheral arteries such as the radial artery, some largely unexplained observations have been made; hypertensive subjects seem to have higher isobaric distensibility and compliance with a lower incremental elasticity modulus (36,37).

A. Pulse Pressure

Increased peripheral pulse pressure has been associated with target-organ damage, particularly with increased intima-media thickness. In the Kuopio study of middle-aged men, the risk factors of age, smoking, higher systolic blood pressure, higher ambulatory pulse pressure, and higher low-density lipoprotein (LDL) cholesterol as well as the presence of diabetes mellitus and a history of ischemic heart disease, were associated with common carotid artery intima-media thickness (38). Until recently, the prognostic value of arterial stiffness for future cardiovascular events was restricted to the pulse pressure recorded at peripheral sites (brachial pulse pressure measured either by casual blood pressure readings or by ambulatory blood pressure readings). In group studies in which blood pressures of subjects were observed over several years, brachial pulse pressure predicted hard endpoints in hypertension (39,40), isolated systolic hypertension (41,42), and in a cohort of French males (43). Only in some of these studies, brachial pulse pressure was a prognostic factor independent of mean blood pressures (40).

As mentioned earlier, brachial pulse pressure may not reflect central (aortic, or its very close surrogate carotid) pulse pressure. A key question is whether central pulse pressure or other noninvasive measures related to stiffness, such as pulse wave velocity, are better indicators of future cardiovascular events than that of peripheral pulse pressure. At this time the answer is uncertain, but some evidence from particular patient settings and selected endpoints has been gathered.

Boutouyrie et al. demonstrated that central pulse pressure (carotid pulse pressure as surrogate marker) was a strong and *independent* determinant of carotid artery enlargement and wall thickening, whereas mean blood pressure and brachial pulse pressure were not. The authors interpreted their data as a contribution of cyclic stretching to pulse–pressure-induced arterial remodeling (44). The Safar group also addressed pathophysiological aspects (45). They found that in end-stage renal disease, the level of carotid pulse pressure (measured by local tonometry without transfer function) and particularly the disappearance of the pulse pressure amplification (the ratio of carotid to brachial pulse pressures) are strong predictors of all-cause mortality, including cardiovascular mortality. After adjusting for age at inclusion, time on dialysis before inclusion and previous cardiovascular events, brachial pulse pressure had no predictive value. However, disappearance of the aortic–brachial pulse pressure amplification was a significant predictor, independent of all standard confounding factors. The authors concluded that the disappearance of pulse pressure amplification is caused principally by an increase in large artery arterial stiffness and wave reflections; thus, by an increased central systolic blood pressure but not by an increase of peripheral systolic blood pressure. As a consequence, the ratio of brachial to carotid pulse pressure will approximately be equal to unity in these patients.

B. Pulse Wave Velocity

The most studied parameter of arterial stiffness after pulse pressure with regard to patient outcomes is pulse wave velocity, which is measured at the aorta or along the aortoiliac pathway. Increased pulse wave velocity is considered a strong indicator of increased pulse pressure. Pulse wave velocity is an independent predictor of future cardiovascular events in end-stage renal disease (46), hypertension (47–49), and in elderly subjects (50).

In a 10-year follow-up of glucose intolerance and type 2 diabetes mellitus, aortic pulse wave velocity was a powerful independent predictor of mortality, displacing systolic blood pressure in Cox Proportional Hazard Models (51). There have been few studies regarding whether treatment (for instance by renin–angiotensin–aldosterone blockers or nitric oxide donors) for reduction of pulse wave velocity influences morbidity and mortality independent of mean blood pressure.

In a study of end-stage renal disease, patients were treated with several drugs including angiotensin-converting enzyme (ACE) inhibitors. Age, left ventricular mass, and pre-existing cardiovascular disease were predictors of mortality independent of blood pressure changes as well as the absence of a decrease in pulse wave velocity in response to a lowering blood pressure. Administration of ACE-inhibitors was positively associated with survival (52).

C. Large-Artery and Small-Artery Compliance Parameters

Cohn et al. has associated selectively reduced C_2 (small artery elasticity index) with smoking, diabetes mellitus, hypertension, and coronary artery disease—conditions all closely related to endothelial dysfunction (53,54). Studies of the prognostic value of C_1 or C_2 are in progress [e.g., Multi-Ethnic Study of Atherosclerosis (MESA)]. Recently, Grey et al. (10) demonstrated that reduced C_2, but not reduced C_1, was a marker of cardiovascular events independent of age in subjects studied at the University of Minnesota; however, this study was not a prospective study.

D. Distensibility Parameters

Significantly reduced large artery *distensibility* (i.e., changes in vessel diameter by pulse pressure normalized for the initial diameter) versus controls has been documented for large and middle-size arteries in hypercholesterolemia, acute smoking, high blood pressure, and in conditions such as type 1 and type 2 diabetes mellitus. In several studies, distensibility was inversely proportional to vessel wall thickness. In congestive heart failure, markedly lower aortic, carotid, and radial distensibility were observed (55). For hypertension, the effect of age is particularly important, even more than the effect of blood pressure. In the Hoorn population of elderly patients, after adjusting for age, gender, and mean blood pressure, type 2 diabetes mellitus was associated with reduced carotid, femoral, and brachial distensibility and reduced compliance coefficients. Impaired glucose metabolism was associated with reduced femoral and brachial distensibility and reduced compliance coefficients (56).

Drug classes such as statins, ACE inhibitors, and angiotensin II receptor antagonists can help reverse distensibility that has been reduced by cardiovascular risk factors (aging, blood pressure, cholesterol, diabetes). In some cases of isolated systolic hypertension, no such reduction is observed.

The whole issue is complicated by repeated observations that smaller artery (such as for the radial artery) distensibility is unchanged or even increased in younger subjects with essential hypertension.

Hypothyroidism is also associated with increased distensibility. In some cases, the vessel may be more distensible even when thickness is increased, particularly when the thickened wall contains mucopolysaccharide material. Physical exercise increases distensibility as well. This is consistent with the visco-elastic behavior of the arterial wall; increased heart rate reduces carotid and radial artery distensibility.

E. Augmentation

Studies on the prognostic value of central augmentation are still lacking, but are planned for future research.

VI. NONINVASIVE ESTIMATION OF CENTRAL AORTIC PRESSURES FROM MEASUREMENTS OF THE PERIPHERAL CIRCULATION

A recent and highly interesting side-effect of the progress made in large artery arterial stiffness is the possibility of noninvasive assessment of central systolic and pulse blood pressure. Under normal conditions and in young individuals, central systolic pressure measured close to the heart (aortic or carotid) is lower than the peripheral pressure at the brachial or radial artery because of the amplification of pulse pressure in peripheral arteries. Still to be determined is whether central and peripheral systolic pressures and pulse pressures are interrelated through simple (approximated by linear or nearly linear algorithms) formulas, or by highly sophisticated complex functions needing phase and amplitude transformations (transfer functions). Several methodologies claim noninvasive estimation of central pressures within acceptable limits.

The Atcor's SphygmoCor tracks tonometer signals on the radial artery, and uses a generalized transfer function to estimate central aortic pressure, but calibrates by brachial artery blood pressure (62). The device shows good inter-observer reproducibility, but it has been recently criticized because of lack of accuracy when compared with catheter-based blood pressure measurements. The apparatus was said to underestimate systolic central blood pressure and to overestimate diastolic central blood pressure vs. invasive measurements. Even noninvasive brachial pressures were closer estimators than the SphymoCor (63). One possible problem might be that pulse pressure amplification from brachial to radial sites is not negligible. Davies et al. (64) evaluated the ability of the transfer function of the SphygmoCor to predict ascending aortic blood pressures. According to these authors, the

transfer function was no better than oscillometric peripheral blood pressure measurements to predict central pressure, and underestimated central systolic and overestimated central diastolic pressures. They question the use of a generalized (or any other) transfer function. Further studies are needed to clarify this.

Chemla et al. (65) demonstrated that using high-fidelity pressure catheters in resting humans, the mean arterial pressure at the aortic root level (MAP$_a$) can be written accurately as:

$$\text{MAP}_a \approx \text{DBP}_a + \frac{\text{PP}_a}{3} + 5\,\text{mmHg},$$

where both DBPa (aortic root diastolic blood pressure) and MAPa are close to peripheral values.

Thus,

$$\frac{\text{PPa}}{3} \approx \text{MAP}_p - \text{DBP}_p - 5\,\text{mmHg}.$$

In peripheral arteries, peripheral mean arterial pressure (MAP$_p$) can be expressed as usual: $\text{MAP}_p \approx \text{DBP}_p + \text{PP}_p/3$, with DBPp denoting peripheral diastolic blood pressure and PP$_p$ denoting pulse pressure.

The Chemla formula agrees with Pauca et al. (66) that radial artery pulse pressure (PP$_p$) is about 15 mmHg higher (pulse pressure amplification) than aortic pulse pressure (PP$_a$). Remarkably, wave reflection parameters (augmentation) and heart rate did not seem to play a major role. One important implication is that because of pressure redundancy, two distinct pressure-powered functions [(systolic blood pressure, diastolic blood pressure) or (pulse pressure, mean arterial pressure)] are enough to characterize the classic four-pressure set. Another implication is that the Chemla formula may be helpful in calibrating carotid artery applanation tonometry. It would offer an easy and elegant way to estimate central aortic pressures.

VII. LOWER LIMB ARTERIAL DISEASE IN HYPERTENSION

Hypertension has been implicated as a risk factor for development of peripheral artery disease. Hypertensive subjects with clinically overt arterial disease of the lower limbs are known to be at considerable risk of future cardiovascular complications. It is generally believed that changes in wave reflection (augmentation) are associated with vascular disease and aging. Vasoactive drugs have little direct effect on large elastic arteries, but they can markedly change wave reflection amplitude and AIx by altering stiffness of the muscular arteries and modifying transmission velocity of the reflected wave from the periphery to the heart (67). The exact role of arterial stiffness in hypertension, which is complicated by lower limb arterial disease, needs further study.

Duprez et al. (68) studied C_1 and C_2 in patients with lower limb arterial disease vs. age and blood pressure matched subjects (elderly with isolated systolic hypertension) without peripheral arterial disease. C_1 and C_2 correlated with peripheral pulse pressure and with the ratio of systolic blood pressure measured respectively at the ankle and at the upper arm (ankle–brachial index discussed subsequently), but did not differ between the groups. In (normotensive) patients with lower limb vascular disease, impaired carotid visco-elastic properties have been described after adjustments for risk factors: lower compliance, and higher Peterson incremental elasticity modulus and beta stiffness index. But at the level of the femoral arteries, no significant differences were observed (69).

Impaired regional (femoral) lower limb stiffness by itself probably is not causing clinical symptoms, unless it is accompanied by a pronounced narrowing of the arterial lumen. Even with significant stenosis or occlusion of the lumen, subjects may remain asymptomatic. If symptoms occur, they are characterized by intermittent claudication (aching pain in the calves or buttocks) while walking, which is relieved when the patients stop walking. At this time, there is no evidence from a controlled trial that hypertensive subjects with impaired lower limb stiffness indices should develop more symptoms of claudication in the future, or be characterized by lower ankle–arm systolic blood pressure index. When treating hypertension that is complicated by lower limb artery disease, the physician should be aware of the importance of local perfusion pressure. In the past, an old controversy regarding the effect of beta-blockers in this type of patient has led physicians to withhold these drugs. Evidence to support this practice is poor. In a recent meta-analysis from the Cochrane group, no definite recommendation with respect to the use or avoidance of drugs could be made for this specific condition.

Ankle–brachial index (ABI), defined as the ratio of noninvasively assessed ankle to brachial (arm) systolic blood pressure, is generally considered a meaningful parameter in the evaluation of peripheral arterial disease (70). When applying the principles of peripheral amplification of systolic and pulse pressure, the ABI ratio should be >1.0 in younger individuals and at least equal unity in elderly subjects. Sensitivity of a resting index of <0.9 approaches 95% in detecting angiogram-confirmed disease. A ratio <0.9 is associated with the presence of ≥50% stenosis in at least one major lower limb vessel. ABI is almost 100% specific in excluding the disease in healthy individuals (71).

In the Cardiovascular Health Study (CHS) Collaborative Research Group that enrolled 5084 elderly (>64-year-old) participants, the modest (asymptomatic) reductions in ABI (0.8–1.0, 16.2% of the group) were associated with increased risk of cardiovascular disease (72). Generally, in subjects initially free of cardiovascular disease, ABI is inversely related to a history of hypertension and to the level of systolic blood pressure, as well as to most other classic cardiovascular risk factors. The association is an inverse dose–response relation for most risk factors. A follow-up of about 6 years showed that an ABI of <0.9 was an independent risk factor (after adjustment for cardiovascular risk factors) for incident cardiovascular mortality. The relative risk was 1.52 (95% CI: 1.05–2.22) for prevalent cardiovascular disease at baseline and even 2.03 (95% CI: 1.22–3.37) with no prevalent cardiovascular disease at baseline (73). In fact, there was a statistically significant decline in survival for each 0.1 reduction in the ABI. Incident clinical (need for hospitalisation) peripheral arterial disease, as expected, is best predicted (even after adjustments for risk factors) by a low ABI (<0.9) at baseline. Relative risk was 6.04 (95% CI: 3.23–11.28) for prevalent cardiovascular disease at baseline and 5.55 (95% CI: 3.08–9.98) with no prevalent cardiovascular disease at baseline. Interestingly, male gender and ABI <0.9, but *not* hypertension, were independent predictors of total and cardiovascular mortality and incident clinical peripheral arterial disease in Cox proportional hazards models, including all relevant risk factors.

In the Systolic Hypertension in the Elderly Program (SHEP) prospective study, an ABI of <0.9 was present in 25.5% of the 1537 subjects and was a major predictor of morbidity and mortality in systolic hypertension. After adjustments for age, gender, classic risk factors, and baseline cardiovascular disease, relative risk for total mortality was 4.1 (95% CI: 2.0–8.3) and 2.4 (95% CI: 1.3–4.4) for all cardiovascular disease (74). In a later ancillary SHEP study of 190 participants at Pittsburgh, the definition of peripheral atherosclerosis was broadened to either low ABI or stenoses at the internal carotid artery by Duplex scanning. Also in the same study, individuals with systolic hypertension and evidence of peripheral atherosclerosis were found to be at high risk for future cardiovascular events (75).

Ankle blood pressure, measured by the Doppler technique, should be interpreted with caution as calcification of the arteries decreases compressibility and thus may lead to overestimation of pressure. This is particularly true in elderly and diabetics with stiff vessels. In addition, one should be aware that changes in ABI often do not reflect the effectiveness of preventive measures or of medical treatment.

These facts indicate that symptomatic and even asymptomatic (characterized by modest decreases in ABI) peripheral vascular disease in combination with hypertension carries important risks for future cardiovascular morbidity and mortality.

VIII. CONCLUSIONS

In this chapter, we first reviewed definitions and technological aspects of some of the most frequently used characteristics of the peripheral circulation: impedance extending peripheral resistance, global, regional and segmental arterial stiffness indices comprising proximal and distal compliance, augmentation indices, pulse wave velocity, distensibility, elasticity moduli, and global compliance derived from mathematical modelling of the arterial circulation. We discussed both limitations inherent to the different technologies and potential clinical applications of the parameters. We tried to interpret stiffness parameters in relation to actual, local blood pressure and physiologically relevant determinants: aging, heart rate, reflected waves and body morphology, and stroke volume. Some of the studied stiffness indices (central pulse pressure, pulse wave velocity) have independent prognostic value for hard cardiovascular endpoints in selected settings of hypertension. The possibility of noninvasive estimation of central systolic or pulse pressure starting from peripheral sites has been explored.

Critical and in-depth analysis of haemodynamics and stiffness indices of the peripheral circulation should encourage investigators to challenge classical pathophysiology of onset of hypertension. Several novel and alternative hypotheses need to be tested, such as the role of a reduced effective aortic diameter in association with increased characteristic impedance in women with essential hypertension. Moreover, there is a strong need of large well-organized community-based studies addressing in a multivariate setting (over and above classical risk indicators) both cross-sectional and longitudinal aspects of well-defined clinically relevant phenotypes integrating cardiac and vascular haemodynamics and stiffness indices characterizing the peripheral circulation and the ventriculo-arterial coupling. The population-based ASKLEPIOS project that has already enrolled more than 2500 subjects in Belgium, is a good example of such a study design. It will help to unravel the complex role of the peripheral circulation in the onset and further evolution of the process of essential hypertension.

REFERENCES

1. O'Rourke M, Pauca A, Jiang X-J. Pulse wave analysis. Br J Clin Pharmacol 2001; 51:507–522.
2. Nichols W, O'Rourke M. Blood Flow in Arteries. 4th ed. London: Arnold, 1998.
3. Karamanuglu M, O'Rourke M, Avolio A et al. An analysis of the relationship between central aortic and peripheral upper limb pressure waves in man. Eur Heart J 1993; 14:160–167.
4. Van Bortel L, Duprez D, Starmans-Kool M et al. Clinical applications of arterial stiffness, Task Force III: recommendations for user procedures. Am J Hypertens 2002; 15:445–452.
5. Saba P, Roman M, Pini R et al. Relation of arterial pressure waveform to left ventricular and carotid anatomy in normotensive subjects. J Am Coll Cardiol 1993; 22:1873–1880.
6. Mitchell G, Lacourcière Y, Ouellet JP et al. Determinants of elevated pulse pressure in middle-aged and older subjects with uncomplicated systolic hypertension. The role of proximal aortic diameter and aortic pressure-flow relationship. Circulation 2003; 108:1592–1598.
7. Nichols W, O'Rourke M, Avolio A et al. Ventricular/vascular interaction in patients with mild systemic hypertension and normal peripheral resistance. Circulation 1986; 74:455–462.
8. Vasan R, Larson M, Levy D. Determinants of the echographic aortic root size: the Framingham Heart Study. Circulation 1995; 91:734–740.
9. Marcus RH, Korcarz C, McCray G et al. Noninvasive method for determination of arterial compliance using Doppler echocardiography and subclavian pulse tracings. Validation and clinical application of a physiological model of the circulation. Circulation 1994; 89:2688–2699.
10. Grey E, Bratelli C, Glasser S et al. Reduced small artery but not large artery elasticity is an independent risk marker for cardiovascular events. Am J Hypertens 2003; 16:265–269.
11. Resnick LM, Militianu D, Cunnings AJ et al. Pulse waveform analysis of arterial compliance: relation to other techniques, age, and metabolic variables. Am J Hypertens 2000; 13:1243–1247.
12. Takazawa K, Tanaka N, Fujita M et al. Assessment of vasoactive agents and vascular aging by the second derivative of photoplethysmogram waveform. Hypertension 1998; 32:365–370.
13. Asmar R, Benetos A, Topouchian J et al. Assessment of arterial distensibility by automatic pulse wave velocity measurement. Validation and clinical application studies. Hypertension 1995; 26:485–490.
14. Lehmann ED, Hopkins KD, Rawesh A et al. Relation between number of cardiovascular risk factors/events and noninvasive Doppler ultrasound assessments of aortic compliance. Hypertension 1998; 32:565–569.
15. van der Heijden-Spek JJ, Staessen JA, Fagard RH et al. Effect of age on brachial artery wall properties differs from the aorta and is gender dependent: a population study. Hypertension 2000; 35:637–642.
16. Langewouters GJ, Wesseling KH, Goedhard WJ. The static elastic properties of 45 human thoracic and 20 abdominal aortas in vitro and the parameters of a new model. J Biomech 1984; 17:425–435.
17. Hayashi K. Experimental approaches on measuring the mechanical properties and constitutive laws of arterial walls. J Biomech Eng 1993; 115:481–488.
18. Dart AM, Lacombe F, Yeoh JK et al. Aortic distensibility in patients with isolated hypercholesterolaemia, coronary artery disease, or cardiac transplant. Lancet 1991; 338:270–273.

19. Bergel H. The properties of blood vessels. In: Fung Y, Perrone N, Anliker M, eds. Biomechanics, Its Foundations and Objectives. New Jersey: Prentice Hall, 1972:105–139.

20. Peterson LH, Jensen RE, Parnell J. Mechanical properties of arteries in vivo. Circ Res 1960; 8:622–639.

21. Lang RM, Cholley BP, Korcarz C et al. Measurement of regional elastic properties of the human aorta. A new application of transesophageal echocardiography with automated border detection and calibrated subclavian pulse tracings. Circulation 1994; 90:1875–1882.

22. Roman MJ, Saba PS, Pini R et al. Parallel cardiac and vascular adaptation in hypertension. Circulation 1992; 86:1909–1918.

23. Liao D, Arnett DK, Tyroler HA et al. Arterial stiffness and the development of hypertension. The ARIC study. Hypertension 1999; 34:201–206.

24. Chemla D, Hebert JL, Coirault C et al. Total arterial compliance estimated by stroke volume-to-aortic pulse pressure ratio in humans. Am J Physiol 1998; 274:H500–H505.

25. Liu Z, Brin KP, Yin FC. Estimation of total arterial compliance: an improved method and evaluation of current methods Am J Physiol 1986; 251:H588–H600.

26. Stergiopulos N, Meister JJ, Westerhof N. Simple and accurate way for estimating total and segmental arterial compliance: the pulse pressure method. Ann Biomed Eng 1994; 22:392–397.

27. Carlier S, Segers P, Pasquet A et al. Non-invasive characterization of total compliance by simultaneous acquisition of pressure and flow: advantages of the pulse pressure method. Comp Cardiol 1998; 25:241–244.

28. Segers P, Stergiopulos N, Westerhof N. Quantification of the contribution of cardiac and arterial remodeling to hypertension. Hypertension 2000; 36:760–765.

29. Kelly RP, Ting CT, Yang TM et al. Effective arterial elastance as index of arterial vascular load in humans. Circulation 1992; 86:513–521.

30. Segers P, Stergiopulos N, Westerhof N. Relation of effective arterial elastance to arterial system properties. Am J Physiol 2002; 282:H1041–H1046.

31. Chemla D, Antony I, Lecarpentier Y et al. Contribution of systemic vascular resistance and total arterial compliance to effective arterial elastance in humans. Am J Physiol 2003; 285:H614–H620.

32. Gatzka CD, Kingwell BA, Cameron JD et al. For the ANBO2 investigators. Australian comparative outcome trial of angiotensin-converting enzyme inhibitor- and diuretic-based treatment of hypertension in the elderly. Gender differences in the timing of arterial wave reflection beyond differences in body height. J Hypertens 2001; 19:2197–2203.

33. O'Rourke MF, Hayward CS. Arterial stiffness, gender and heart rate. J Hypertens 2003; 21:487–490.

34. Elzinga G, Westerhof N. Matching between ventricle and arterial load. An evolutionary process. Circ Res 1991; 68:1495–1500.

35. Nuernberger J, Keflioglu-Scheiber A, Opazo Saez AM et al. Augmentation index is associated with cardiovascular risk. J Hypertens 2002; 20:2407–2414.

36. Laurent S, Hayoz D, Trazzi S et al. Isobaric compliance of the radial artery is increased in patients with essential hypertension. J Hypertens 1993; 11:89–98.

37. Weber R, Stergiopulos N, Brunner HR et al. Contributions of vascular tone and structure to elastic properties of a medium-sized artery. Hypertension 1996; 27:816–822.

38. Salonen R, Salonen JT. Determinants of carotid intima-media thickness: a population-based ultrasonography study in eastern Finnish men. J Intern Med 1991; 22:225–231.

39. Verdecchia P, Schillaci G, Borgioni C et al. Ambulatory pulse pressure: a potent predictor of total cardiovascular risk in hypertension. Hypertension 1998; 32:983–988.

40. Clement DL, De Buyzere ML, De Bacquer DA et al. For the Office versus Ambulatory Pressure Study Investigators. Prognostic value of ambulatory blood-pressure recordings in patients with treated hypertension. N Engl J Med 2003; 348:2407–2415.

41. Domanski MJ, Davis BR, Pfeffer MA et al. Isolated systolic hypertension: prognostic information provided by pulse pressure. Hypertension 1999; 34:375–380.

42. Staessen JA, Thijs L, O'Brien ET et al. For the Syst-Eur Trial Investigators. Ambulatory pulse pressure as predictor of outcome in older patients with systolic hypertension. Am J Hypertens 2002; 15:835–843.

43. Benetos A, Safar M, Rudnichi A et al. Pulse pressure: a predictor of long-term mortality in a French male population. Hypertension 1997; 30:1410–1415.

44. Boutouyrie P, Bussy C, Lacolley P et al. Association between local pulse pressure, mean blood pressure, and large-artery remodeling. Circulation 1999; 100:1387–1393.

45. Safar ME, Blacher J, Pannier B et al. Central pulse pressure and mortality in end-stage renal disease. Hypertension 2002: 39:735–738.

46. Blacher J, Guerin AP, Pannier B et al. Impact of aortic stiffness on survival in end-stage renal disease. Circulation 1999; 99:2434–2439.

47. Laurent S, Boutouyrie P, Asmar R et al. Aortic stiffness is an independent predictor of all-cause and cardiovascular mortality in hypertensive patients. Hypertension 2001; 37:1236–1241.

48. Laurent S, Katsahian S, Fassot C et al. Aortic stiffness is an independent predictor of fatal stroke in essential hypertension. Stroke 2003; 34:1203–1206.

49. Boutouyrie P, Tropeano AI, Asmar R et al. Aortic stiffness is an independent predictor of primary coronary events in hypertensive patients: a longitudinal study. Hypertension 2002; 39:10–15.

50. Meaume S, Benetos A, Henry OF et al. Aortic pulse wave velocity predicts cardiovascular mortality in subjects >70 years of age. Arterioscler Thromb Vasc Biol 2001; 21:2046–2050.

51. Cruickshank K, Riste L, Anderson S, Wright J, Dunn G, Gosling R. Aortic pulse-wave velocity and its relationship to mortality in diabetes and glucose intolerance. An integrated index of vascular function. Circulation 2002; 106:2085–2090.

52. Guerin AP, Blacher J, Pannier B et al. Impact of aortic stiffness attenuation on survival of patients in end-stage renal failure. Circulation 2001; 103:987–992.

53. Cohn JN. Arterial compliance to stratify cardiovascular risk: more precision in therapeutic decision making. Am J Hypertens 2001; 14:258S–263S.

54. McVeigh GE, Bratteli CW, Morgan DJ et al. Age-related abnormalities in arterial compliance identified by pressure pulse contour analysis: aging and arterial compliance. Hypertension 1999; 33:1392–1398.

55. Giannattasio C, Mancia G. Arterial distensibility in humans. Modulating mechanisms, alterations in diseases and effects of treatment (Review). J Hypertens 2002; 20:1889–1899.

56. Henry R, Kostense P, Spijkerman A, Dekker J, Nijpels G, Heine R, Kamp O, Westerhof N, Bouter L, Stehouwer C. Arterial stiffness increases with deteriorating glucose tolerance status. The Hoorn study. Circulation 2003; 107:2089–2095.

57. Durier S, Fassot C, Laurent S et al. Physiological genomics of human arteries: quantitative relationship between gene expression and arterial stiffness. Circulation 2003; 108:1845–1851.

58. Chang E, Harley CB. Telomere length and replicative aging in human vascular tissues. Proc Natl Acad Sci USA 1995; 92:11190–11194.

59. Jeanclos E, Schork NJ, Kyvik KO et al. Telomere length inversely correlates with pulse pressure and is highly familial. Hypertension 2000; 36:195–200.

60. Benetos A, Okuda K, Lajemi M et al. Telomere length as an indicator of biological aging: the gender effect and relation with pulse pressure and pulse wave velocity. Hypertension 2001; 37:381–385.

61. Aviv A. Hypothesis: pulse pressure and human longevity. Hypertension 2001; 37:1060–1066.

62. O'Rourke M. Mechanical principles in arterial disease. Hypertension 1995; 26:2–9.

63. Cloud GC, Rajkumar C, Kooner J et al. Estimation of central aortic pressure by SphygmoCor requires intra-arterial peripheral pressures. Clin Sci (Lond) 2003; 105:219–225.

64. Davies JI, Band MM, Pringle S et al. Peripheral blood pressure measurement is as good as applanation tonometry at predicting ascending aortic blood pressure. J Hypertens 2003; 21:571–576.

65. Chemla D, Hebert JL, Aptecar E et al. Empirical estimates of mean aortic pressure: advantages, drawbacks and implications for pressure redundancy. Clin Sci (Lond) 2002; 103:7–13.

66. Pauca AL, Wallenhaupt SL, Kon ND et al. Does radial artery pressure accurately reflect aortic pressure? Chest 1992; 102:1193–1198.

67. Nichols W, Singh B. Augmentation index as a measure of peripheral vascular disease. Curr Opin Cardiol 2002; 17:543–551.

68. Duprez D, De Buyzere M, De Bruyne L, Clement D, Cohn J. Small and large artery elasticity indices in peripheral arterial occlusive disease (PAOD). Vasc Med 2001; 6:211–214.

69. Cheng K-S, Tiwari A, Baker C, Morris R, Hamilton G, Seifalian A. Impaired carotid and femoral viscoelastic properties and elevated intima-media thickness in peripheral vascular disease. Atherosclerosis 2002; 164:113–120.

70. Clement DL. Diagnostic work-up of patients with intermittent claudication. Acta Cardiol 1979; 34:141–151.

71. Belch JJ, Topol EJ, Agnelli G et al. For the Prevention of Atherothrombotic disease network. Critical issues in peripheral arterial disease detection and management: a call to action. Arch Intern Med 2003; 163:884–892.

72. Newman AB, Siscovick DS, Manolio TA et al. Ankle–arm index as a marker of atherosclerosis in the Cardiovascular Health Study. Cardiovascular Heart Study (CHS) Collaborative Research Group. Circulation 1993; 88:837–845.

73. Newman AB, Shemanski L, Manolio TA et al. Ankle–arm index as a predictor of cardiovascular disease and mortality in the Cardiovascular Health Study. The Cardiovascular Health Study Group. Arterioscler Thromb Vasc Biol 1999; 19:538–545.

74. Newman AB, Sutton-Tyrrell K, Vogt MT et al. Morbidity and mortality in hypertensive adults with a low ankle/arm blood pressure index. J Am Med Assoc 1993; 270:487–489.

75. Sutton-Tyrrell K, Alcorn HG, Herzog H et al. Morbidity, mortality, and antihypertensive treatment effects by extent of atherosclerosis in older adults with isolated systolic hypertension. Stroke 1995; 26:1319–1324.

19

The Eye and Hypertension

PECK-LIN LIP

The Birmingham and Midland Eye Centre and City Hospital, Birmingham, UK

KEYPOINTS

- Hypertensive retinopathy, optic neuropathy, and choroidopathy represent target organ damage in hypertension.
- The recognition of hypertensive retinopathy is important for cardiovascular risk stratification, especially in severe hypertension, hypertensive urgencies/emergencies, and in diabetes.

SUMMARY

Systemic hypertension is a common condition associated with significant morbidity and mortality. Hypertension confers cardiovascular risk by causing target organ damage that includes retinopathy in addition to heart disease, stroke, renal insufficiency, and peripheral vascular disease. The recognition of hypertensive retinopathy is important in cardiovascular risk stratification of hypertensive individuals especially in malignant hypertension.

This chapter re-evaluates the changing perspectives in the pathophysiology, classification, and prognostic significance of the fundal lesions in hypertensives. Other common ocular diseases precipitated by systemic hypertension are also discussed.

I. INTRODUCTION

Hypertension produces cardiovascular risk by causing target-organ damage that includes retinopathy (1). Poorly controlled systemic hypertension causes worsening of microvascular disease of the eye such as diabetic retinopathy (2). In a population of hypertensive patients who had no coexisting systemic vascular disease, the overall incidence of hypertensive retinopathy was ~15%. Specifically, 13% showed arteriolar narrowing, 8% showed retinopathy signs, and 2% showed arterovenous nicking (3).

The prevalence of hypertensive retinopathy is reported to be higher in the women, among Afro-Caribbeans, and in the smoking population (4,5). Recently, there has been speculation that certain specific genotypes are linked with an increased risk of hypertensive retinopathy (6–8). Other hypertension-related complications may also exacerbate retinopathy, such as the presence of microalbuminuria, left ventricular hypertrophy, and renal disease (9–11).

II. PATHOPHYSIOLOGY

Pathologically, the retinal arterioles in hypertensives are narrower, with thickened walls as a result of intimal hyalinization and medial and endothelial hypertrophy. The additional disadvantages are the branching geometry in the retinal vasculature, with reduced circulatory efficiency and microvascular rarefaction (12).

The ocular blood flow is directly related to the perfusion pressure (mean arterial pressure minus intraocular pressure) and inversely related to the resistance to flow (13). Resistance to blood flow depends on the state and caliber of the ocular arteries and is influenced by hypertensive arterial changes and efficiency of the autoregulation of the blood flow (13).

Autoregulation maintains a constant ocular blood flow to tissues during changes in perfusion pressure. Endothelial-derived molecules (i.e., endothelins, thromboxane A2, prostaglandins, and nitric oxide) play a role in autoregulation by modulating vascular tone (14). Breakdown of autoregulation occurs with the rise or fall of perfusion pressure beyond a critical range. In hypertensive individuals, in whom the autoregulation range is set to higher levels, episodic hypotension (spontaneously, as during sleep, or as a result of overtreatment), changes in the tone of the precapillary arterioles (mediated by angiotensin or by antihypertensive drugs), and vascular endothelial changes (leading to reduced nitric oxide synthesis) lead to breakdown of autoregulation (15).

The tight junctions of the retinal endothelium and the retinal pigment epithelium form the inner and outer blood-retinal barriers. Acute hypertension causes disruption of the blood-retinal barriers (13). Unlike the retinal and optic nerve head vascular beds, the choroidal vascular bed has no blood-ocular barrier and, therefore, no autoregulation (13). The retinal vessels are devoid of an autonomic nerve supply, but the choroidal vessels are richly supplied by both sympathetic and parasympathetic nerves. The different anatomical and physiological properties of the retinal, optic nerve head, and choroidal blood vessels, therefore, produce three distinct and unrelated manifestations, that is, retinopathy, optic neuropathy, and choroidopathy.

III. CLASSIFICATIONS OF HYPERTENSIVE RETINOPATHY

The classification of hypertensive retinopathy has proven to be complex because of the interrelationship between hypertensive and arteriosclerotic changes and because of the high variability of clinical findings.

The two most widely accepted classifications are the Keith–Wagener–Barker and Scheie classifications (16,17) (Table 19.1). The Scheie classification defines the hypertensive and arteriosclerotic changes separately. In recent years, attempts had been made to introduce a prognostic-significance classification by using the retinopathy findings for risk stratification and therapeutic decision-making (18). This classification is now commonly adopted in clinical practice and has been simplified to a two-grade classification of retinopathy nonmalignant (nonaccelerated) vs. malignant (accelerated) (the Dodson–Lip classification). This two-grade classification system provides useful correlation between clinical features and prognosis (18,19).

IV. CLINICAL FEATURES

The primary response of the retinal arterioles to systemic hypertension is vasoconstriction. Sustained hypertension leads to disruption of the blood-retinal barrier, increased

Table 19.1 Classifications of Hypertensive Retinopathy

Retinopathy grading		Arteriosclerosis grading	
Grade	Features	Grade	Features
N/A	N/A	0	No changes
I	Mild generalized arteriolar narrowing	1	Barely detectable light reflex changes
II	Definite focal arteriolar narrowing	2	Definite increased light reflex changes
III	Grade II plus retinal hemorrhages, exudates, and cotton–wool spots	3	Grade 2 plus copper wiring of arterioles
IV	Severe grade III and papilloedema	4	Grade 3 plus silver wiring of arterioles

Note: Keith–Wagener–Barker classification (grades I–IV) was based on the level of severity of the retinal findings. Scheie attempted to quantify the changes of both retinopathy (grades I–IV) and arteriolosclerosis (grades 0–4).

vascular permeability, and secondary arteriolosclerosis, which leads to a variety of clinical signs commonly detectable with ophthalmoscopy.

The clinical features of hypertensive retinopathy can be divided into two categories, according to the kinds of changes observed in the eye. Grades I and II hypertensive retinopathy comprise changes in the retinal arterioles. The arterioles show initial generalized narrowing, changing to focal attenuation in more chronic hypertensive damage. Focal arteriolar narrowing is easier to assess clinically than generalized narrowing, but with new computer-assisted quantification, generalized retinal arteriolar narrowing can be ascertained reliably by using standardized photographic grading methods (20).

Grades III and IV hypertensive retinopathy comprise changes that involve the retina, optic disc, and choroids. These include microaneurysms, intraretinal hemorrhages, cotton–wool spots, hard exudates or macular stars [deposition of lipid around the fovea, Fig. 19.1(A)], and papilloedema. Flame-shaped hemorrhage is the hallmark of hypertension [Fig. 19.1(A)], the appearance of which is quite distinct from the dot- and blot-hemorrhages of diabetic retinopathy. In acute hypertension, obstruction of the precapillary arterioles leads to the development of nerve fiber layer infarcts (cotton–wool spots) and papilloedema. Less commonly, macular stars or papilloedema may be the lone presentation (Fig. 19.2) in grade IV hypertensive retinopathy. Complications of severe untreated hypertension include hemorrhagic detachment of the internal limiting membrane of the retina and subhyaloid and vitreous hemorrhages [Fig. 19.1(B)].

Secondary arteriolosclerosis of the common vascular adventitial sheath at the level of the arteriovenous crossing produces compression of the venule. The increased

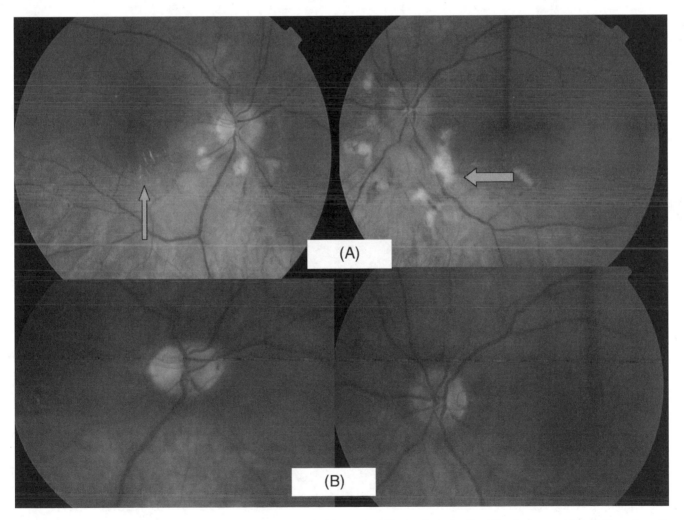

Figure 19.1 (A) A 35-year-old Caucasian woman presented with severe malignant hypertension. Fundoscopy revealed bilateral papilloedema with macular hard exudates (partial macula star, indicated by the thin arrow), cotton–wool spots (indicated by the wide arrows), and flame-shaped retinal hemorrhages. (B) Fundoscopy after 4 months of good blood pressure control, which shows resolution of almost all the retinopathy. Bilateral disc pallor and residual hard exudates remain.

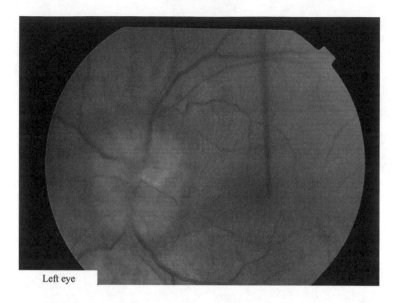

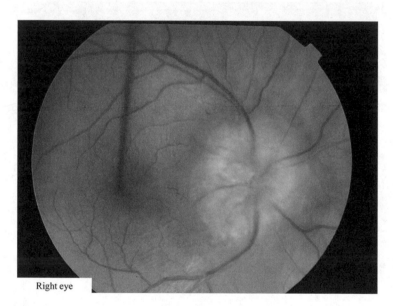

Figure 19.2 Lone papilloedema. A 27-year-old male initially presented with malignant hypertension with gross papilloedema and a blood pressure of 180/130. Following further investigation, he was found to have co-existing benign intracranial hypertension.

arteriolar light reflex correlates with hyalinization of the arteriolar wall. Obscuring of the red blood cell column by the "copper wire" or "silver wire" appearance of the light reflex has classically been described in grade III or grade IV retinopathy, respectively.

V. HYPERTENSIVE OPTIC NEUROPATHY

Papilloedema, or bilateral disc swelling, represents grade IV hypertensive retinopathy. If left untreated, it is considered to be a poor prognostic sign for survival (19).

The pathogenesis of papilloedema secondary to systemic hypertension is controversial. The possible causes include ischemia, raised intracranial pressure, or hypertensive retinopathy or encephalopathy. Experimental studies in animals and clinical studies that used visual evoked potentials and electroretinogram recordings indicated ischemia as the possible underlying mechanism (21).

The World Health Organization (WHO) clinical criterion for malignant hypertension is the presence of severe hypertension in association with bilateral retinal hemorrhages and exudates, with or without papilloedema. Conversely, isolated (lone) papilloedema without retinopathy could represent a variant of malignant hypertension (22). Other differential diagnoses such as neuroretinitis, Leber's stellate maculopathy, papilloedema secondary to increased intracranial pressure, or space-occupying lesions might need to be excluded if there is no resolution of clinical signs following good hypertension control.

Despite the alarming fundal features, patients with malignant hypertension have minimal ocular complaints. Headaches may be the only symptom, and the majority of patients maintain normal visual acuity, with full recovery of color perception and visual field. Most features of acute hypertensive retinopathy regress over 6–12 months with timely antihypertensive therapy. Retinal hemorrhages are likely to resolve first, followed by cotton–wool spots, retinal exudates, and disc swelling. Longstanding chronic hypertension may result in retinal nerve fiber loss and disc pallor. The electroretinogram recordings may remain abnormal for as long as 2–4 years following an acute episode (23).

VI. HYPERTENSIVE CHOROIDOPATHY

Choroidal lesions secondary to elevated blood pressure are less well recognized than retinopathy in the current literature. The underlying mechanism relates to choroidal ischemia and its effects on the retinal pigment epithelium and retina.

The more commonly described features of hypertensive choroidopathy are choroidal vascular sclerosis, Elschnig's spots representing focal areas of degenerative retinal pigment epithelium (Fig. 19.3), and diffuse patchy atrophic retinal pigment epithelial degeneration of chronic hypertension. Siegrist's streaks, linear retinal pigment epithelial changes, are the sequelae of acute hypertensive choroidopathy and generally indicative of a poor prognosis (24).

VII. OCULAR DISEASES SECONDARY TO SYSTEMIC HYPERTENSION

Systemic hypertension is recognized as responsible for a number of ophthalmic complications, potentially leading to blindness. Often, ocular manifestation was

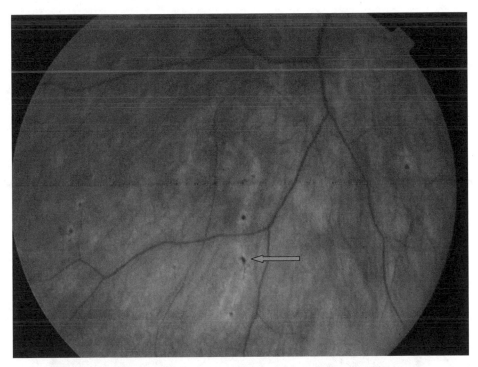

Figure 19.3 Retinal pigment epithelial changes of the peripheral fundus after an episode of malignant hypertension. (Elschnig's spots are indicated by arrow.)

the initial presentation that led to the diagnosis of systemic hypertension. Prompt attention to hypertension control could prevent recurrence or involvement of the other eye.

A.   Retinal Vein Occlusion

Systemic hypertension is associated with an increased risk of developing retinal vein occlusions (57–75%) (24). Other frequent systemic associations are cardiovascular disease and diabetes in the elderly population. In younger patients, the causes for retinal vein occlusions are less clear and require more extensive investigation (25).

The hallmark of an ophthalmoscopy finding of acute retinal vein occlusion is the distribution of superficial flame-shaped hemorrhages along a retinal vascular branch (Fig. 19.4).

The extent and location of involved retina depend on the site of obstruction. The site is almost invariably at an arteriovenous crossing point for branch retinal vein occlusion (involving a quadrant of the retina along a major retinal vascular arcade), at the lamina cribosa for hemispheric vein occlusion (involving the superior or inferior half of the retina), or at the central retinal vein occlusion (involving all four quadrants of retina). Other signs may include engorgement and tortuosity of the obstructive retinal vein, retinal edema, exudation, cotton–wool spots, and disc swelling.

Patients commonly present with sudden painless visual loss of varying degrees depending on the severity of the retinal ischemic changes and the involvement of the foveal region. In the presence of persisting retinal nonperfusion, neovascularization may develop on the disc, the peripheral retina, or the iris. Panretinal scatter photocoagulation is effective therapy in ischemic cases (with established neovascularization) in order to prevent sight-threatening complications such as vitreous hemorrhage and secondary rubeotic glaucoma.

B.   Retinal Arterial Macroaneurysm

Retinal arterial macroaneurysms are acquired focal aneurysmal dilatations of the retinal arterioles, usually occurring in the first three orders of the arteriolar tree (26). They are commonly associated with hypertensive retinopathy, giving rise to star-shaped exudations and are more frequently complicated by retinal, preretinal, or intravitreal hemorrhage. Laser photocoagulation may be applied around a macroaneurysm if spontaneous resolution with thrombosis within the macroaneurysm fails to occur (Fig. 19.5).

C.   Nonarteritic Anterior Ischemic Optic Neuropathy

Nonarteritic anterior ischemic optic neuropathy (AION) is infarction of the optic nerve head. It manifests as a sudden unilateral painless loss of vision. The cause of nonarteritic AION is less clear, but hypertension is associated in ~40%

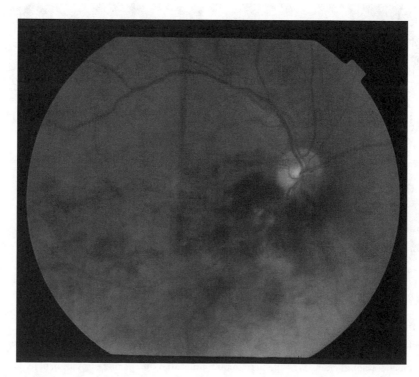

Figure 19.4   Inferior hemispheric retinal vein occlusion with deep, dark retinal hemorrhages (ischemic sign) that involve the inferior half of the fundus.

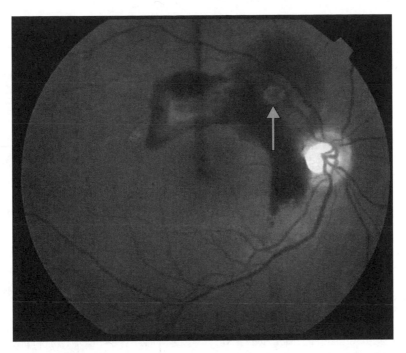

Figure 19.5 Fundoscopy of the right eye showing a macroaneurysm (indicated by arrow) arising from the superotemporal retinal arteriole. The macroaneurysm bled into the surrounding retina.

of all cases (27). The mechanism may be chronic hypoperfusion of the small end-arterial optic nerve head vessels caused by overtreated hypertension or abnormal vascular autoregulation (28).

Vision loss is often partial because only a sector of the optic disc undergoes infarction and edema. Visual field defect is therefore characteristically altitudinal. Spontaneous improvement of vision (partial) may occur in up to 43% of cases, and recurrence is rare. No treatment is proven to be effective (including steroids), but systemic hypertension must be addressed to avoid involvement of the other eye in ~25% of all cases (29).

Patients with nonarteritic AION tend to be younger than patients with giant cell arteritis. The latter may be differentiated from the specific symptoms and signs with abnormal blood tests. In contrast to patients with retinal artery disease (retinal artery occlusion and amaurosis fugax), patients of nonarteritic AION have only a slightly increased incidence of cerebrovascular events, and life expectancy is not significantly shortened (30).

D. Cranial Nerve Palsies

Sudden onset of painless diplopia (pupil-sparing) in middle-aged or elderly patients is almost always secondary to hypertension or diabetes. Often, the patient's medical history suggests microvascular damage as the cause of the pathology. The symptoms may include an isolated palsy or combined palsies and frequently involve the

sixth, third, fourth, and seventh cranial nerves (31). Other ocular examinations, including vision and visual field examinations, are otherwise normal. Neuroimaging may not be indicated in the absence of other neurological signs or pupillary abnormalities. The symptoms usually resolve spontaneously within 3 months.

E. Diabetic Retinopathy

Diabetic retinopathy shows a similar pathological process of microvasculopathy, in which endothelial cell malfunction and impaired regulation of retinal perfusion occur as a result of chronic glucotoxicity. The UKPDS 50 report showed that the incidence of diabetic retinopathy was associated strongly with higher blood pressure (32). Indeed, UKPDS, EUCLID, and other studies have shown retardation in the progression of diabetic retinopathy with improved control of blood pressure. Many studies also have shown that it is both safe and beneficial to further lower blood pressure with ACE inhibitors in patients whose blood pressure is already within the "normal" range but who have known vascular risk factors such as left ventricular dysfunction, hypertension, or diabetic microalbuminuria (33,34).

VIII. CONCLUSIONS

Hypertensive retinopathy, neuropathy, and choroidopathy represent target organ damage in patients with systemic arterial hypertension. Hypertensive retinopathy, in particular, is a recognized cardiovascular risk stratification factor. Prompt recognition and accurate diagnosis of these stages have important implications for both the ocular health and the general health of the individual.

REFERENCES

1. Chobanian A, Bakris G, Black H et al. The seventh report of the Joint National Committee on Prevention, Detection, Evaluation, and Treatment of High Blood Pressure: the JNC 7 Report. J Am Med Assoc 2003; 289:2560–2571.

2. UK Prospective Diabetes Study Group. Tight blood pressure control and risk of macrovascular and microvascular complications in type 2 diabetes: UKPDS 38. Brit Med J 1998; 317:703–713.

3. Klein R, Klein B, Moss S, Wang Q. Hypertension and retinopathy, arteriolar narrowing and arteriovenous nicking in a population. Arch Ophthalmol 1994; 112:92–98.

4. Sharp PS, Chaturvedi N, Wormald R, McKeigue PM, Marmot MG, McHardy S. Young hypertensive retinopathy in Afro-Caribbeans and Europeans: prevalence and risk factor relationships. Hypertension 1995; 25:1322–1325.

5. Bloxham CA, Beevers DG, Walker JM. Malignant hypertension and cigarette smoking. Brit Med J 1979; 1:581–583.

6. Pontremoli R, Sofia A, Tirotta A, Ravera M, Nicolella C, Viazzi F, Bezante GP, Borgia L, Bobola N, Ravazzolo R, Sacchi G, Deferrari G. The deletion polymorphism of the angiotensin I-converting enzyme gene is associated with target organ damage in essential hypertension. J Am Soc Nephrol 1996; 7(12):2550–2558.

7. Yilmaz H, Isbir T, Agachan B, Aydin M. Is epsilon4 allele of apolipoprotein E associated with more severe end-organ damage in essential hypertension? Cell Biochem Funct 2001; 19:191–195.

8. Ravera M, Viazzi F, Berruti V, Leoncini G, Zagami P, Bezante GP, Rosatto N, Ravazzolo R, Pontremoli R, Deferrari G. 5,10-Methylenetetrahydrofolate reductase polymorphism and early organ damage in primary hypertension. Am J Hypertens 2001; 371–376.

9. Biesenbach G, Zazgornik J. High prevalence of hypertensive retinopathy and coronary heart disease in hypertensive patients with persistent microalbuminuria under short intensive antihypertensive therapy. Clin Nephrol 1994; 41:211–218.

10. Pose Reino A, Gonzalez-Juanatey JR, Castroviejo M, Valdes L, Estevez JC, Mendez I, Cabezas-Cerrato J. Relation between left ventricular hypertrophy and retinal vascular changes in mild hypertension. Med Clin (Barc) 1997; 108:281–285.

11. Heidbreder E, Huller U, Schafer B, Heidland A. Severe hypertensive retinopathy. Increased incidence in renoparenchymal hypertension. Am J Nephrol 1987; 7(5):394–400.

12. Stanton AV, Wasan B, Cerutti A, Ford S, Marsh R, Sever PP, Thom SA, Hughes AD. Vascular network changes in the retina with age and hypertension. J Hypertens 1995; 13(12 Pt 2):1724–1728.

13. Hayreh SS. Systemic arterial blood pressure and the eye. Duke–Elder Lecture. Eye 1996; 10:5–28.

14. Haefliger IO, Meyer P, Flammer J, Luescher TF. The vascular endothelium as a regulator of the ocular circulation: new concept in ophthalmology? Surv Ophthalmol 1994; 39:123–132.

15. Luescher TF. The endothelium and cardiovascular disease: a complex relationship. N Engl J Med 1994; 330:1081–1083.

16. Hayreh SS. Classification of hypertensive fundus changes and their order of appearance. Ophthalmologica 1989; 198:247–260.

17. Walsh JB. Hypertensive retinopathy: description, classification and prognosis. Ophthalmology 1982; 8:1127–1131.

18. Hyman BN. The eye as a target organ: an updated classification of hypertensive retinopathy. J Clin Hypertens (Greenich) 2000; 2(3):194–197.

19. Dodson PM, Lip GYH, Eames SM, Gibson JM, Beevers DG. Hypertensive retinopathy: a review of existing classification systems and a suggestion for a simplified grading system. J Hum Hypertens 1996; 10(2):93–98.

20. Couper DJ, Klein R, Hubbard LD, Wong TY, Sorlie PD, Cooper LS, Brothers RJ, Nieto FJ. Reliability of retinal photography in the assessment of retinal microvascular characteristics: the atherosclerosis risk in communities study. Am J Ophthalmol 2002; 133(1):78–88.

21. Kishi S, Tso MOM, Hayreh SS. Fundus lesions in malignant hypertension. II. A pathologic study of experimental hypertensive optic neuropathy. Arch Ophthalmol 1985; 103:1198–1206.

22. Lip GYH, Beevers M, Dodson PM, Beevers DG. Severe hypertension with lone bilateral papilloedema: a variant of malignant hypertension. Blood Press 1995; 4(6):339–342.

23. Talks SJ, Good P, Clough CG, Beevers DG, Dodson PM. The acute and long-term ocular effects of accelerated hypertension: a clinical and electrophysiological study. Eye 1996; 10(Pt 3):321–327.

24. Pohl ML. Siegrist's streaks in hypertensive choroidopathy. J Am Optom Assoc 1988; 59(5):372–376.

25. Central Vein Occlusion Study Group. Natural history and clinical management of central retinal vein occlusion. Arch Ophthalmol 1997; 115:486–491.

26. Panton RW, Goldberg MF, Farber MD. Retinal arterial macroaneurysms: risk factors and natural history. Br J Ophthalmol 1990; 74(10):595–600.

27. Hayreh SS, Joos KM, Podhajsky PA, Long CR. Systemic diseases associated with non-arteritic anterior ischemic optic neuropathy. Am J Ophthalmol 1994; 118:766–780.

28. Hayreh SS, Podhajsky PA, Zimmerman B. Role of nocturnal arterial hypotension in optic nerve head ischemic disorders. Ophthalmologica 1999; 213:76–96.

29. Repka MX, Savino PJ, Schatz NJ et al. Clinical profile and long-term implications of anterior ischemic optic neuropathy. Am J Ophthalmol 1983; 96:478–483.

30. Guyer DR, Miller NR, Auer CL et al. The risk of cerebro-vascular and cardiovascular disease in patients with anterior ischamic optic neuropathy. Arch Ophthalmol 1985; 103:1136–1142.

31. Richards BW, Jones FR Jr, Younge BR. Causes and prognosis in 4,278 cases of paralysis of the oculomotor, trochlear and abducens cranial nerves. Am J Ophthalmol 1992; 113:489–496.

32. Stratton IM, Kohner EM, Aldington SJ, Turner RC, Holman RR, Manley SE, Matthews DR. UKPDS 50: risk factors for incidence and progression of retinopathy in Type II diabetes over 6 years from diagnosis. Diabetologia 2001; 44(2):156–163.

33. Lip GYH, Beevers DG. More evidence on blocking the renin–angiotensin–aldosterone system in cardiovascular disease and the long-term treatment of hypertension: data from recent clinical trials (CHARM, EUROPA, ValHEFT, HOPE-TOO and SYST-EUR2). J Hum Hypertens 2003; 17:747–750

34. Lip GYH, Beevers DG. ACE inhibitors in vascular disease: some PROGRESS, more HOPE. J Hum Hypertens 2001; 15:833–835.

Part D: Management and Treatment in General and in Special Populations

20

Detection, Treatment, and Control of Hypertension in the General Population

PAUL MUNTNER, JIANG HE, PAUL K. WHELTON

Tulane University School of Public Health and Tropical Medicine, New Orleans, Louisiana, USA

KEYPOINTS

- The global burden of hypertension is tremendous.
- Hypertension awareness, treatment, and control in many world regions are low.
- Several domains are in association with higher rates of hypertension awareness, receipt of anti-hypertensive treatment, and blood pressure control.
- Positive trends in hypertension control have been noted in several world regions.
- Implementation of population-based programs aimed at increasing hypertension awareness, treatment, and control may be beneficial.

SUMMARY

Blood pressure control in the context of a patient with hypertension is a function of detection and treatment (pharmacologic and lifestyle modification). While great accomplishments have been made, rates of hypertension control remain low in all world regions. The first step in achieving blood pressure control in the hypertensive patient is disease detection. While rates of hypertension awareness have increased over the past several decades in many countries, awareness remains low. Once hypertension has been detected and the need to initiate treatment has been determined, achieving high rates of treatment is a function of patient monitoring, encouragement, and adherence. Given the success of blood pressure education programs in several countries, similar programs adapted to the need of specific world regions may have a tremendous positive impact in increasing rates of hypertension awareness, treatment and control of hypertension, and reducing the burden of cardiovascular disease.

I. INTRODUCTION

When a patient develops hypertension, controlling it is a function of detection and treatment (pharmacologic and lifestyle modification). Increasing detection and treatment of high blood pressure has been a central focus of blood pressure education programs in the United States for >25 years (1–3). Similar initiatives have been implemented in several countries and have been proposed for enhancing awareness and control of the burden of hypertension in others (4–7). The purpose of this chapter is twofold: first, rates of hypertension awareness, treatment, and control from several national studies are reviewed; second, an overview of factors associated with higher rates of hypertension awareness, treatment, and control is discussed in the context of the hypertensive patient. Although the prevention of hypertension is an essential element in reducing the incidence of cardiovascular disease, increasing the rate of detection, treatment (both pharmacological treatment and lifestyle modification), and control of hypertension is a prerequisite to reduce the burden of cardiovascular disease outcomes that are a result of high blood pressure.

II. DEFINITIONS

The criteria used to define hypertension, and the detection, awareness, and control of hypertension have varied over time and between countries. To provide context for the current chapter and comparability across regions, a common set of definitions were used in collecting and analyzing these data. *Hypertension* was defined as a systolic blood pressure >140 mmHg and/or a diastolic blood pressure >90 mmHg and/or the current use of blood pressure lowering medications. *Hypertension detection* refers to the diagnosis of hypertension by a healthcare provider and *hypertension awareness* refers to the patient's knowledge of this diagnosis. These terms are not synonymous; many patients may have their hypertension detected but remain unaware of this diagnosis. In population-based surveys, limited data are available on the previous detection of hypertension. Therefore, in this chapter, hypertension detection and awareness were used interchangeably and defined as a patients' knowledge (i.e., awareness) of their diagnosis of hypertension. Finally, hypertension control was defined as systolic and diastolic blood pressure <140 mmHg and <90 mmHg, respectively.

III. GLOBAL BURDEN OF HYPERTENSION

Published rates of hypertension prevalence vary widely from 3.4% in rural Indian men and to 72.5% in Polish women (8,9). In most economically developed countries, the prevalence of hypertension is 20–50%. For example, according to data from the United States National Health and Nutrition Examination Survey of 1999–2000, the prevalence of hypertension was 27.1% in men and 30.1% in women in the US general adult population (10). In contrast, the prevalence in the Spanish National Blood Pressure Study was 49.4% in rural and 43.2% in urban residents (11). Although it has been generally thought that the prevalence of hypertension is substantially lower in economically developing regions, recent data show that this is not uniformly true (12,13). Results from the Egyptian National Hypertension Program identified a prevalence of hypertension close to 30% in four of the regions surveyed (13). Data from InterASIA, the most recent national study conducted in China, estimated the prevalence of hypertension among men and women in the age group of 35–74 years to be 28.8% ($N =$ 129,824,000 Chinese persons) among the population aged 35–74 (14). The prevalence of hypertension in South African adults was estimated to be 22.9% in men and 23.4% in women (15). The highest prevalence of hypertension in Sub-Saharan Africa was reported in a study from urban Zimbabwe with rates as high as or higher than those in economically developed countries (15,16).

IV. HYPERTENSION DETECTION (HYPERTENSION AWARENESS)

Hypertension detection, referred to as awareness herein, begins with proper blood pressure measurement. The National High Blood Pressure Education Program of the National Institutes of Health in the United States recommends that blood pressure measurements should be obtained in a standard fashion at each healthcare encounter (3,17). Similar guidelines recommending the measurement of blood pressure at every healthcare encounter have been published by the World Health Organization (6). The goal of this chapter is not to review the recommended techniques for measuring blood pressure as reviews of these methods are provided elsewhere (18). However, a key aspect of the blood pressure measurement is accomplished after the readings have been obtained. Specifically, it is critical for clinicians to communicate the meaning of their patients' blood pressure readings and to advise them of the importance of follow-up visits and future periodic blood pressure readings. The American Heart Association and National Heart, Lung, and Blood Institute of the National Institutes of Health have guidelines for the monitoring of blood pressure in the outpatient setting (1). These guidelines should assist the clinician in detecting, confirming, and monitoring hypertension.

Hypertension detection remains a critical component for reducing the burden of the adverse outcomes of high blood pressure (19). Evidence has overwhelmingly demonstrated that, among patients with hypertension, the incidence of many of these diseases can be lowered through adequate control of blood pressure (20). Only those who are aware of their hypertension are in position to receive treatment and counseling that will enable them to reduce and control their high blood pressure. To raise awareness of the dangers of high blood pressure, programs have been developed in many countries. Although impressive progress has been observed, there is still much room for improvement. For example, although the awareness of hypertension in the USA increased from 51% to 73% between the 12-year interval from NHANES II (1976–1980) and NHANES III (1988–1994), it did not increase any further by NHANES 1999–2000 (10,21). As such, continued and bolstered

efforts are needed to achieve high rates of hypertension awareness.

A. Hypertension Awareness Rates

In previous epidemiological studies and literature reviews, awareness of hypertension has been defined most frequently as a self-report of any prior diagnosis of hypertension by a healthcare professional among the population with hypertension. A recent published review provides the most comprehensive data on the rates of hypertension awareness from world regions (22). The level of hypertension awareness varies considerably between and within world regions (Fig. 20.1) (8–11,13–15,23–37). In economically developed countries, approximately one-half to two-thirds of patients with hypertension are aware of their diagnosis. For example, in the USA in 1999–2000, 68.9% of patients with hypertension, ≥ 18 years, were aware of this diagnosis. In contrast, only 44.5% of patients with hypertension in Spain were aware of their diagnosis of hypertension (10,11). Rates of hypertension awareness were generally, but not always, lower in economically developing countries. In Latin American countries, including the Caribbean, awareness of hypertension was similar to the USA (30). In the other economically developing countries, approximately,

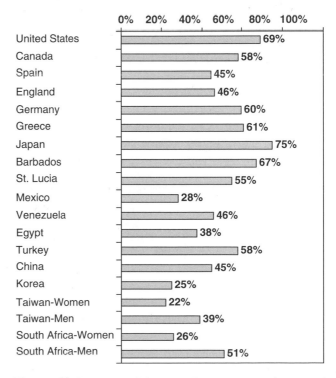

Figure 20.1 Rates of hypertension awareness in several countries.

one-quarter to one-half of patients with hypertension were aware of their diagnosis. For example, data from InterASIA in China indicated a hypertension awareness rate of 44.7% (14).

B. Factors Associated with Higher Hypertension Awareness

Studies from several countries have investigated factors associated with hypertension awareness (11,13,38–40). Although these studies do not uniformly report the same factors to be associated with higher rates of hypertension awareness, common themes have emerged. The following discussion will focus on these common patterns.

1. Geographic Differences

Rates of hypertension awareness not only vary greatly across but also within regions and countries (11,13,37). For example, hypertension awareness has been reported to be higher in urban vs. rural regions of several countries (9,14). Rates of hypertension awareness in urban and rural areas were 46.8% and 39.9%, respectively, in Spain, 52.5% and 44.7%, respectively, in China (11,37). Furthermore, regional variation in rates of awareness is also prominent. Reynolds and colleagues reported higher rates of hypertension awareness in Northern (50.2%) compared with Southern (46.5%) China. In addition, in the Egyptian National Hypertension Project, higher rates of awareness were present in the Coastal Region and Cairo (56.5% and 56.0%, respectively) compared with Northern (20.3%) and Southern (31.8%) Upper Egypt (13).

2. Healthcare

A key factor in the detection of hypertension is access to healthcare. This domain encompasses several facets including health insurance, continuity of care, and frequency of blood pressure measurements. Because each of these characteristics may be more applicable in some countries than others, each component needs to be considered in the context of each independent setting when assessing methods for improving the detection of high blood pressure.

3. Patient Care

Although data from NHANES III indicated that having health insurance and a usual source of healthcare were not associated with higher rates of hypertension awareness, having a physician visit within the previous year was associated with a higher likelihood of being aware of one's hypertension (38,41).

4. Frequency of Blood Pressure Measurement

Several studies have reported higher rates of hypertension awareness among patients with more frequent blood pressure measurements (40,41). Although not directly reported in NHANES III, one can assume the higher rates of hypertension awareness associated with more recent physician visits may be the result of more recent and possibly more frequent blood pressure measurements. More direct data are available from the InterASIA study in China. Specifically, 67.1%, 33.6%, and 6.6% of patients with hypertension who had their blood pressure measured <12 months, 1–5 years, and ≥5 years prior to their study visit, respectively, reported having been previously told of their hypertension diagnosis (40). A strong association was present between a more recent blood pressure measurement and higher hypertension awareness even after adjustment for several potential confounders including age, gender, urban vs. rural, and north vs. south residence. It is worth noting that despite the strong association between more recent blood pressure measurements and a higher likelihood of hypertension awareness, adults in China are substantially less likely to have had their blood pressure measured within the previous year when compared with their counterparts in the USA (Table 20.1) (40).

Among the population age 35–74 years, 32.5% of the Chinese population compared with 3.4% of the US population had not had their blood pressure measured within the past 5 years. To our knowledge, little data from other world regions have been published, and the frequency at which blood pressure measurements are made is not entirely known. In addition, whether the greater frequency of blood pressure measurement explains higher awareness rates has not been directly shown. However, conducting standard blood pressure measurements at every healthcare encounter is a critical component of hypertension detection and may help improve rates of hypertension awareness.

Table 20.1 Patient Awareness and Time Elapsed Since Last Blood Pressure Measurement

Parameters	USA (NHANES)	China (InterASIA)
Subjects aware of their hypertension diagnosis (%)	69.7	43.0
Time elapsed since last blood pressure measurement		
≥5 years	3.4	32.5
1–5 years	16.0	8.0
<12 months	80.6	59.5

Source: From Ref. (40).

5. Cigarette Smoking

Studies from the USA, Europe, and Asia have found cigarette smokers significantly less likely to be aware of their hypertension diagnosis when compared with nonsmokers (11,38,40). For example, data from NHANES III reported that current smokers were 22% less likely to be aware of their hypertension diagnosis when compared with their nonsmoking counterparts ($P = 0.04$). Additionally, data from InterASIA in China showed that after adjustment for age, gender, urban vs. rural, and North vs. South residence, current smokers were 21% less likely to be aware of their diagnosis of hypertension. Whether hypertension detection among smokers is lower than among nonsmokers because of less frequent measurements of blood pressure is not known. In addition, compared with patients who continue to smoke, patients who quit or have never smoked may be more health conscious and visit their physicians more often. In InterASIA, cigarette smokers had less frequent blood pressure measurements. Specifically, current smokers were less likely than never smokers to have had their blood pressure measured in the past 5 years (29% vs. 41%, respectively) and less likely (50% vs. 64%, respectively) to have had their blood pressure measured in the previous 12 months. Unpublished data indicate that the lower rates of hypertension awareness among current smokers are mediated by less frequent blood pressure measurements.

6. Cardiovascular Disease

When individuals with cardiovascular disease are compared with their counterparts who do not have cardiovascular disease, they are substantially more likely to be aware of their hypertension than their counterparts. Studies also have found that people with other major cardiovascular disease risk factors, including obesity, high cholesterol, and diabetes, are more likely to have had their hypertension detected and be aware of this condition. In Spain and China, people who had a body mass index $\geq 30 \, \text{kg/m}^2$ were 1.88 and 2.94 times, respectively, more likely to be aware of their hypertension compared with persons with a body mass index $< 25 \, \text{kg/m}^2$ (each $P < 0.01$). A higher percentage of these patients may be aware of their hypertension because of their more frequent contacts with the healthcare system. Alternatively, physicians may pay more attention to patients with hypertension and other major cardiovascular disease risk factors because these patients are at greater risk for cardiovascular disease. The higher detection of hypertension in overweight or obese patients may represent a "high-risk" approach to the detection of hypertension. Ideally, all patients with hypertension, not just those with other co-existent risk factors, will be aware of their diagnosis of hypertension.

7. Other Factors

Several other factors enable awareness, including having a social support network, a higher education level, and a higher household income. In InterASIA, after adjustment for age, gender, and area of residence, participants who were married were 1.43 times more likely to be aware of their hypertension diagnosis compared with their nonmarried counterparts (40). How being married and having a social support network increases the awareness of hypertension is not entirely known. It has been hypothesized that companionship may increase awareness of health-related issues and attendance at doctor appointments. Household income may increase hypertension awareness through greater access to health care and, in turn, a more recent blood pressure measurement. Finally, InterASIA data show a graded association of higher rates of hypertension awareness at higher education levels. This raises the important question as to whether physicians are communicating the diagnosis of hypertension at a level where patients can understand. Alternative explanations for higher awareness rates among persons with a higher education level include greater access to healthcare and a tendency for patients with a higher education to be more health conscious.

8. Summary

The first step in achieving blood pressure control in the hypertensive patient is disease detection. Even though the rate of hypertension awareness has increased over the past several decades in many countries, awareness remains low (22). Furthermore, rates of hypertension detection are substantially lower in economically developing countries. For example, data from a recent report in China show that hypertension awareness rates in 1999–2000 were similar to those observed in the USA in 1976–1980 (40). In both economically developed and developing countries, a broader population-based approach of identifying all patients with hypertension is needed. Furthermore, methods for physicians to clearly communicate the diagnosis of hypertension to the patient need to be developed and disseminated. Given the high burden of hypertension worldwide, such an approach will provide a mechanism to achieve better care for the large segment of the population that is unaware of their hypertension.

V. TREATMENT FOR HYPERTENSION

Primary prevention of hypertension provides an ideal opportunity to interrupt and prevent the continuing and costly cycle of managing hypertension and its complications (42). However, once present, hypertension needs to be treated with all available means, including lifestyle modification and pharmacological therapy (1). The ultimate goal of any blood pressure lowering treatment is the reduction of cardiovascular and renal disease morbidity and mortality. In clinical trials, pharmacological antihypertensive therapy has been associated with 35–40%, 20–25%, and 50% reductions in stroke, myocardial infarction, and heart failure incidence, respectively (20). In the presence of cardiovascular disease and hypertension, only nine patients need to be treated with antihypertensive therapy to prevent one death (43). The benefits of pharmacologic therapy have been observed in various countries, age, race, gender, and socioeconomic groups and little doubt remains as to the benefit of such treatment.

Although a great emphasis needs to be placed on the primary prevention of hypertension, many of the lifestyle modification approaches recommended for hypertension prevention can and should be applied as first-line and conjunctive treatment of the hypertensive patient. The current discussion will provide an overview of the benefits of several lifestyle modification approaches and pharmacological therapy in treating hypertension, review rates of pharmacological treatment and lifestyle modification usage in the context to the hypertensive patient, and finally discuss factors associated with the receipt of pharmacological treatment of hypertension.

A. Lifestyle Modification

Dozens of clinical trials have documented the blood pressure lowering benefits of lifestyle modification including sodium reduction, weight loss, physical activity, and alcohol reduction. The findings from these trials have been summarized in recent meta-analyses, which provide a means to formally pool and quantify findings from individual trials in a standardized and objective manner (44).

1. Sodium Reduction

Over the past 30 years, more than 80 randomized controlled trials have been conducted to explore the efficacy and effectiveness of reductions in dietary sodium on blood pressure in hypertensive and normotensive patients. The findings from these trials have been summarized in four recent meta-analyses (45–48). When compared with the control groups, the reported mean reduction in blood pressure was −3.9 to −5.9 mmHg for systolic blood pressure and −1.9 to −3.8 mmHg for diastolic blood pressure in hypertensive patients (each $P < 0.05$). Additionally, in the Trial of Nonpharmacologic Interventions in the Elderly, conducted in 875 participants 60–80 years old with well-controlled hypertension, the percentage of persons who were able to discontinue antihypertensive medication and remain drug-free while maintaining their blood pressure <150/90 mmHg and remaining free of a hypertension-related clinical complication was significantly higher among those assigned to a sodium reduction group than in their counterparts who were assigned to the usual care (38% vs. 24%, $P < 0.001$) (49). No safety concerns have been noted with the modest reduction in sodium intake that forms the basis for the national US recommendations and Institute of Medicine's reports (50,51).

2. Weight Loss

A meta-analysis of 25 randomized controlled trials of weight loss and blood pressure that were conducted between 1966 and 2003 was performed to estimate the effect of weight reduction on blood pressure (52). An average net weight reduction of −5.1 kg by means of energy restriction, increased physical activity, or a combined intervention was associated with a significant reduction in systolic blood pressure of −4.44 mmHg (95% CI: −5.93 to −2.95) and a significant reduction in diastolic blood pressure of −3.57 mmHg (95% CI: −4.88 to −2.25). When subgroups were compared on the basis of initial blood pressure level (<140/90 mmHg vs. ≥140/90 mmHg), there was no difference in systolic blood pressure response, but reductions in diastolic blood pressure were approximately twice as great in hypertensive subjects, although this difference was not statistically significant [−4.92 (95% CI: −6.73 to −3.12) vs. −2.35 (95% CI: −4.05 to −0.65)].

3. Physical Activity

Whelton et al. (53) recently published a meta-analysis of 54 trials showing that previously sedentary adults could decrease systolic blood pressure with regular aerobic exercise. Reductions in systolic and diastolic blood pressure associated with regular aerobic exercise were −4.9 (−7.2 to −2.7) mmHg and −3.7 (−5.7 to −1.8) mmHg among patients with hypertension.

4. Alcohol Reduction

Xin et al. (54) conducted a meta-analysis of 15 randomized controlled trials of alcohol reduction conducted between 1984 and 1996. Overall pooled estimates of the effect of alcohol reduction on systolic and diastolic blood pressure were −3.31 (95% CI: −2.52 to −4.10) mmHg and −2.04 (95% CI: −1.49 to −2.58) mmHg, respectively ($P < 0.001$ for both). Reductions in systolic and diastolic blood pressure associated with alcohol reduction were nonsignificantly greater [−3.9 mmHg (95% CI: −5.0 to +0.5) and −2.4 mmHg (−3.3 to −0.4), respectively] among patients with hypertension.

5. Overall Dietary Approach

The Dietary Approaches to Stop Hypertension (DASH) clinical trial randomized 459 adults with systolic blood pressure <160 mmHg and diastolic blood pressure between 80 and 95 mmHg to receive one of three diets: (i) A control diet that was considered to be low in fruits and vegetables with a fat content typical of the American diet; (ii) A diet rich in fruit and vegetables but retaining the same fat intake as the control diet; or (iii) A "combined" diet rich in fruits and vegetables with reduced saturated and total fat (55). Within each of the three study arms, three meals a day, and in-between meal snacks were provided to each study participant (55). Sodium intake and body weight were maintained at constant levels during follow-up. The relative reduction in systolic and diastolic blood pressure was −5.5 (−7.4 to −3.7) and −3.0 (−4.3 to −1.6) mmHg greater for those receiving the "combination" diet when compared with their counterparts receiving the control diet. The effect of these diets was larger in magnitude among persons with hypertension. When compared with hypertensive subjects in the control group, hypertensive subjects who were receiving the fruits and vegetables and "combination" diet had a −7.2 (−11.4 to −3.0) and −11.4 (−15.9 to −6.9) larger reduction in systolic blood pressure and −2.8 (−4.7 to −0.9) and −5.5 (−8.2 to −2.7) larger reductions in diastolic blood pressure (55).

6. Rates of Lifestyle Modification

Despite overwhelming evidence favoring lifestyle modification, only 50.0%, 57.4%, and 43.3% of nonHispanic whites, nonHispanic blacks, and Mexican-Americans, respectively, with hypertension in the USA reported undertaking lifestyle modification as part of their hypertension treatment (41). The most common of these approaches reported was sodium reduction which was undertaken by 43.4%, 53.3%, and 39.9% of nonHispanic whites, nonHispanic blacks, and Mexican-Americans, respectively. In contrast, increased exercise was undertaken by only 10–15% of patients with hypertension. The low rates of lifestyle modification are especially disconcerting given that hypertension control is 6.02 times greater among NHANES III participants who reported undertaking lifestyle modification due to their diagnosis of hypertension (41).

The prevalence of lifestyle modification to lower blood pressure is similar in the USA and China (12). Specifically, in China, 50.2% of InterASIA participants who were aware of their hypertension diagnosis were undertaking lifestyle modification. In China, sodium reduction was the most common lifestyle modification approach to control blood pressure and was undertaken by 33.2% of patients aware of their hypertension diagnosis. Other common lifestyle modifications among patients aware of their hypertension diagnosis reported in InterASIA include weight loss (21.5%), increased exercise (29.2%), and reduced alcohol consumption (32.1%) and other complementary and alternative methods (13.5%) (40).

B. Pharmacological Treatment of Hypertension

Treatment of systolic and diastolic blood pressure to levels <140 mmHg and 90 mmHg, respectively, is associated with a decrease in cardiovascular disease incidence. However, the decision to initiate pharmacologic treatment of hypertension requires consideration of several factors including the degree of blood pressure elevation, the presence of end-organ damage, and the presence of cardiovascular disease risk factors (1). The goal of controlling blood pressure is to reduce cardiovascular disease morbidity and mortality. The JNC7 report from the National Heart Lung and Blood Institute of the USA recommends thiazide-type diuretics be used as initial therapy for most patients with hypertension (56,57). Studies have showed that most patients can achieve adequate blood pressure control (56). However, most patients who are hypertensive will require two or more antihypertensive medications to achieve their blood pressure goals (58). Adoption of a healthy lifestyle by all persons is also critical for the prevention of hypertension-related cardiovascular disease. Combining multiple lifestyle modification approaches and/or lifestyle modification in conjunction with pharmacological blood pressure lowering therapy may increase the likelihood of achieving blood pressure control (49).

1. Rates of Hypertension Treatment

Despite effective therapy, pharmacological therapy for the treatment of hypertension remains under-utilized in essentially all regions of the world (Fig. 20.2) (8–11,13–15,23–37). In economically developed countries, the rates of pharmacological treatment for hypertension ranged from rates of 31.8% of hypertensive patients in UK to 58.4% of those in the USA. The lowest rate of pharmacological treatment of hypertension was observed in Mexico where only 14.6% of women and 6.5% of men (overall rate, 10.7%) with hypertension were receiving pharmacological therapy. On a more positive note, rates of treatment for hypertension have increased in economically developed and developing countries. For example, in the Health Survey for England, the rate of hypertension treatment increased from 31.8% in 1994 to 38.0% in 1998. In China, the rates of hypertension treatment increased from 12.1% in 1991 to 28.2% in 1999–2000.

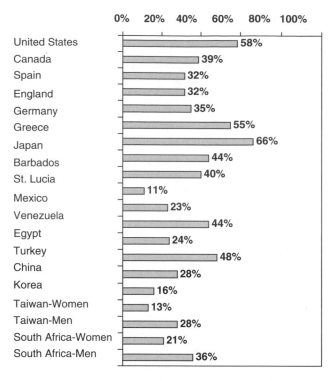

Figure 20.2 Rates of hypertension treatment in several countries.

2. Factors Associated with Treatment

Several studies have investigated factors that increase the likelihood that patients with hypertension will receive blood pressure lowering treatment. In epidemiological studies, several factors have been observed to be associated with a higher likelihood of receiving pharmacological therapy for hypertension.

3. Age

The likelihood of receiving treatment for hypertension is higher at older age. In NHANES III, the mean age of acknowledged and untreated hypertension; acknowledged, treated, and uncontrolled hypertension; and acknowledged, treated, and controlled hypertension was 55.3, 64.9, and 58.6 years of age, respectively. In China, 53%, 64%, and 68% of patients aged <50, 50–64, and ≥65 years, respectively, who aware of their hypertension reported receiving treatment (each $P < 0.001$ comparing older age groups to those 35–49 years of age). Data ascertaining reasons for not treating younger patients with hypertension were not collected in these large national surveys. Given the excess risk of cardiovascular disease risk associated with hypertension, even in these younger age groups, reasons for not treating young- to middle-aged adults need to be investigated.

4. Gender

Data consistently show that men are less likely than women to receive treatment for hypertension. In the USA, only 37–40% of males who acknowledge having hypertension report receiving treatment compared with 54% of women with hypertension report receipt of treatment (10). Similarly, in China, men were 24% less likely than women to receive treatment for their hypertension despite being aware of this condition (12).

5. Access to Healthcare

Not surprisingly, access to healthcare confers a strong advantage for receiving pharmacological treatment for hypertension. However, large cross-sectional studies generally only obtain data about whether the patients have health insurance and about the frequency of physician visits. Although these factors to a certain extent provide an indication of access to healthcare, future studies need to collect data about the ability of patients to talk with their healthcare providers regarding treatment and treatment-related issues. One such tool to collect these data is the GHAA Consumer Satisfaction Survey.

6. Concurrent Risk Factors

Patients with other cardiovascular disease risk factors including diabetes and high cholesterol may be more likely to receive pharmacological therapy for their hypertension diagnosis. In addition, patients with a history of cardiovascular disease are more likely to receive pharmacological therapy for their hypertension.

7. Other Factors

Current smokers have been reported to be less likely and former smokers more likely to receive treatment for hypertension. When compared with patients who continue to smoke, patients who quit smoking may be more health conscious and visit the physician more often after a diagnosis of hypertension. In addition, physicians may pay more attention to patients with hypertension who have taken an active role in their health as indicated by giving up smoking. Chinese adults with hypertension who consume ≥2 alcoholic beverages a day also were 54% less likely to receive treatment for their hypertension.

8. Summary

Treatment of patients with hypertension remains low. Most of the published data on treatment rates of hypertension comes from cross-sectional studies and therefore, whether low treatment rates is a result of never receiving treatment or patient noncompliance, not tolerating treatment, or poor medical follow-up is not known. After hypertension has been detected in a patient and the need to initiate treatment has been determined, achieving high rates of treatment is a function of patient monitoring, encouragement, and adherence. The JNC7 guidelines recommend most patients should be seen within 1–2 months after initiation of therapy to determine the adequacy of hypertension control, the degree of patient adherence, and the presence of adverse effects. Pharmacists also should be encouraged to monitor patients' use of medication.

VI. HYPERTENSION CONTROL

In reporting results, the prevalence of hypertension control is usually presented, separately, for all patients with hypertension and for patients being treated for hypertension. By definition, the rates of hypertension control are higher among patients receiving treatment as this is simply a subgroup of all patients with hypertension. However, even among patients on blood pressure lowering treatment, rates of hypertension control remain low. In this section, we will provide an overview of the rates of hypertension control from different countries and world regions and then discuss factors associated with adequate blood pressure control in the hypertensive patient.

A. Control Among All Hypertensive Patients

Data about the extent of adequate blood pressure control within the population of hypertensive patients are available from several countries. Of patients with hypertension in the USA, 31.0% have achieved adequate blood pressure control (Fig. 20.3) (8–11,13–15,23–37). These reported rates are higher than other countries that comprise the emerging market economies (EME). In other EME countries, rates of controlled hypertension ranged from a low of 5.0% in Spain to a high of 27.0% in Greece (11,26). Large variation in hypertension control rates were observed in Latin American Countries, which included the highest worldwide rates of hypertension control (Barbados, with 38%) and one of the lowest rates (Mexico, with 2.3%) (30,31). In all other world regions (Middle Eastern Crescent, China, Other Asia Islands, and Sub-Saharan Africa), fewer than one in five patients with hypertension achieve adequate blood pressure control (15,34–36).

B. Control Among Hypertensive Patients Treated with Medications

Although hypertension control rates are substantially higher among patients treated for their hypertension,

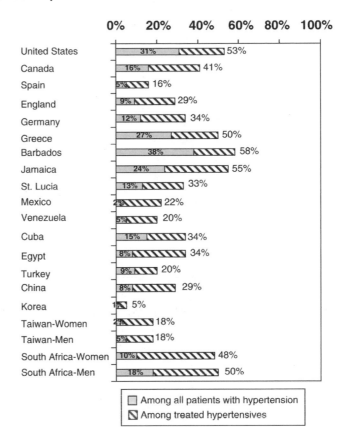

Figure 20.3 Rates of hypertension control in several countries.

compared with all patients with hypertension, only in a few countries did hypertension control rates among this group exceed 50% (Fig. 20.3) (8–11,13–15,23–37). Among the treated population, the highest rates of hypertension control (ranging from 50% to 65%) were reported for the USA, Japan, Barbados, Jamaica, and St. Lucia. In contrast, in several countries hypertension control rates in the treated population was <20%. The lowest rates of hypertension control, among those receiving pharmacological treatment, were reported for Spain, Venezuela, Turkey, Korea, and Taiwan.

C. Trends in Hypertension Control Rates

Although little data are available on the trends in hypertension control, the published literature shows substantial improvements have been made over the past 30 years (Table 20.2). For example, in the USA between NHANES II (1976–1980) and NHANES III (1988–1994), the overall percentage of treated hypertensive patients with controlled blood pressure increased from 32% to 55% (14,21). Improvements in hypertension control have also been reported in economically developing countries. Rates of hypertension control in China

Table 20.2 Trends in the Pharmacological Treatment for Hypertension

Country	Patients receiving pharmacological treatment (%)
USA	
1976–1980 (NHANES II)	31.0
1999–2000 (NHANES 1999–2000)	58.4
UK	
1994 (Health Survey for England)	31.6
1998 (Health Survey for England)	38.0
China	
1991 (Chinese National Hypertension Survey)	8.1
1999–2000 (InterASIA)	28.8

improved significantly between the 1991 Chinese National Hypertension Survey and 1999–2000 InterASIA (14). Specifically, hypertension control among all patients with hypertension increased from 2.8% to 8.1%.

D. Factors Associated with Hypertension Control

Obstacles to the achievement of hypertension control exist and include social and economic factors. Many investigations have studied the association between demographic, socio-economic, clinical, and geographic factors and higher rates of hypertension control. Although the majority of studies have been conducted in economically developed countries, data from economically developing countries are beginning to identify similar themes for the achievement of hypertension control. This section will review the epidemiological evidence regarding factors associated with higher rates of hypertension control.

E. Medication Adherence

Low rates of hypertension control may be a function of poor antihypertensive medication adherence. Approximately, one-half of patients adhere to prescribed medications (59). Although patients on medication with uncontrolled hypertension are often considered to have "refractory hypertension," a significant factor contributing to poor blood pressure control is patient nonadherence to prescribed therapy (60). The asymptomatic and lifelong nature of hypertension are two key factors that undoubtedly contribute to poor patient adherence to drug regimens. Several other modifiable factors impact medication adherence in hypertensive patients: side effects of medication; convenience of drug dosing; cost, number,

and complexity of medications; patients' knowledge, beliefs and attitudes about hypertension and its treatment; patients' involvement with their care; patient demographics; health care system issues (61,62). A recent meta-analysis of six studies and 814 subjects showed that the odds ratio of blood pressure control among patients who adhere to their antihypertensive medication regimens, compared with those who were nonadherent, was 3.44 (95% CI: 1.60 to 7.37) (63).

F. Lifestyle Modification

Studies have found participants aware of their hypertension who undertook lifestyle modification are more likely to have controlled their hypertension to a systolic and diastolic blood pressure <140 mmHg and <90 mmHg, respectively (40,41). The findings of better blood pressure control among persons undertaking lifestyle modification is important but not surprising. As mentioned previously, salt reduction, increased physical activity, potassium supplementation, and moderation in alcohol consumption have been shown to reduce blood pressure in randomized controlled trials. Lifestyle modification is also associated with higher rates of hypertension control in population-based surveys. In InterASIA, the odds ratio of achieving controlled blood pressure was 1.59 for persons undertaking any lifestyle modification and 1.72, 1.64, 1.78, and 1.62 for those attempting to lose weight, reducing their salt intake, exercising, reducing their alcohol consumption, respectively, because of their diagnosis of hypertension (Fig. 20.4) (40). Data from population-based surveys are reassuring because it suggests that these lifestyle modifications are effective in controlling hypertension when applied in settings outside the controlled environment of a randomized trial. Finally, it should be noted that complications from lifestyle modification are minimal and may enfranchise patients to take control of their health (64).

G. Income

In several studies from the USA, socioeconomic status, including higher education and income, have been associated with access to healthcare and hypertension control (65,66). For example, in the Atherosclerosis Risk in Communities Study, lower education and household income were associated with poor blood pressure control (67). In contrast, in the NHANES III, no association was present between education level or higher quartile of income and blood pressure control (41). In China, among all patients with hypertension in InterASIA, higher income was associated with higher rates of hypertension control (40). In contrast, no association was present between higher income and hypertension control when considering

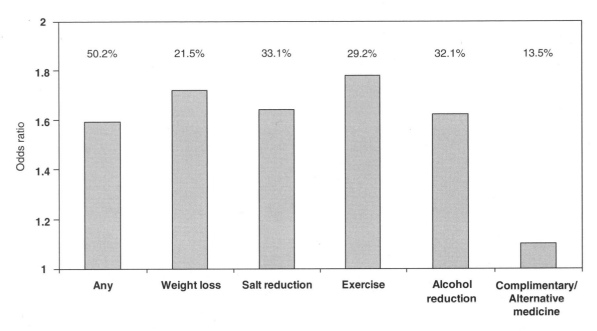

Figure 20.4 Prevalence of lifestyle modification (text in figure) and multivariate adjusted odds ratio of controlled hypertension associated with lifestyle modification from the International Collaborative Study of Cardiovascular Disease in ASIA (InterASIA).

InterASIA participants who were aware of and treated for their diagnosis of hypertension. As such, we can conclude higher income may be a mediator and a marker for greater access to health care and treatment for hypertension.

H. Health Behaviors

Several studies have found that former smokers and light/nondrinkers with hypertension are more likely to have controlled their blood pressure (66,67). Patients who quit smoking may be more health conscious and take a more active in their health when compared with patients who continue to smoke. Additionally, NHANES III and InterASIA patients who were heavy drinkers (three or more drinks in NHANES and two drinks per day in InterASIA) were less likely to have achieved adequate control of their blood pressure (40,41). Although many health behaviors are difficult to change, patients who actively do so may also be more willing to undertake maneuvers that result in blood pressure control (68).

I. Overweight

Among all patients with hypertension, physicians may pay more attention to patients who are overweight or obese because they are at greater risk of cardiovascular disease (69). In a previous report from NHANES III, patients with hypertension who were overweight/obese were more likely to have controlled their hypertension.

Overweight or obese hypertensive patients in InterASIA also were more likely to have achieved adequate hypertension control. In contrast, among InterASIA participants who were aware of their hypertension, rates of hypertension control were lower among patients who were overweight/obese. These results indicate that overweight/obese participants are more likely to achieve hypertension control through higher rates of detection. However, among those aware of their diagnosis the lower rates of hypertension control for overweight/obese patients are consistent with the benefits of weight loss on blood pressure.

J. Healthcare

In the USA, studies report that lack of health insurance is associated with poor hypertension control (41). Specifically, in the NHANES III, persons with private health insurance were 58% more likely to have their hypertension controlled compared with their counterparts with no health insurance. Some researchers have concluded that access to high-quality healthcare may be one of the most important factors for hypertension control in the population.

VII. STRENGTHS AND LIMITATIONS OF THE DATA REPORTED

Most of the population data on awareness, treatment, and control of hypertension have been derived from large cross-sectional surveys. This study design holds strength for understanding the magnitude of the problem of lack of awareness and poor rates of hypertension treatment and control. However, in most cross-sectional studies, blood pressure has been measured during a single visit. According to both World Health Organization and National Institute of Health guidelines, hypertension should be defined on the basis of the average of at least two or more blood pressure readings taken at two or more visits after an initial screening (6,17). Another limitation of data on hypertension awareness, treatment, and control that exists in cross-sectional studies is a lack of longitudinal follow-up. Studies following incident patients would provide more accurate data on rates of hypertension awareness, treatment, and control and a better setting for assessing the mediating factors for increasing rates of hypertension awareness, treatment, and control. Finally, most studies have relied on patient self-reporting in defining the detection of hypertension in large epidemiological studies. Although a chart review of each participant's medical record would provide a more accurate indication of whether hypertension was detected, such methods are time consuming and not feasible in cross-sectional studies that frequently include 10,000–20,000 participants.

On a more positive note, most of the data from cross-sectional studies have been derived from large, representative population-based samples. The studies we have described used sampling techniques that ensure the data collected provided valid estimates for the reference population (usually a country as a whole). Additionally, studies on hypertension awareness, treatment and control are available from several regions of the world. As such, the results are applicable to the general population with hypertension in many world regions. Additional strengths of the data we report here include the use of a standardized protocol with stringent quality control procedures for the measurement of blood pressure in these studies.

VIII. CONCLUSIONS

Acknowledging the global nature of hypertension is required so that healthcare providers routinely screen for and treat elevated blood pressure. The continuing increase in the burden of hypertension in economically developing regions where a majority of the world's population resides is worrisome. Given the success of several population-based programs for raising the awareness, treatment, and control rates of hypertension in economically developed countries, similar programs implemented in world regions currently without such programs may have a tremendous positive impact in reducing the burden of cardiovascular disease.

The public health implications of the low rates of hypertension detection, treatment, and control that currently exist cannot be overstated. Data show that a high-risk strategy for the detection of hypertension is being applied in most countries and world-regions. It appears that the identification of persons with hypertension in many countries is limited to those with additional co-morbid conditions. Furthermore, blood pressure reduction therapies in many countries also are limited to patients with other co-morbid condition, including overweight, high cholesterol levels, and a history of cardiovascular disease. Using this approach (i.e., limiting detection and treatment to those deemed to be at most risk) overlooks the high burden of hypertension and the impact a broad population approach would have in preventing the global burden of cardiovascular disease. Given the success of the National High Blood Pressure Education Program in the USA, similar programs implemented in all world regions may have a tremendous positive impact in increasing rates of hypertension awareness, treatment, and control of hypertension and in reducing the burden of cardiovascular disease.

REFERENCES

1. Chobanian AV, Bakris GL, Black HR, Cushman WC, Green LA, Izzo JL Jr, Jones DW, Materson BJ, Oparil S, Wright JT Jr, Roccella EJ. The Seventh Report of the Joint National Committee on Prevention, Detection, Evaluation, and Treatment of High Blood Pressure: the JNC 7 report. J Am Med Assoc 2003; 289:2560–2572.
2. Roccella EJ, Ward GW. The national high blood pressure education program: a description of its utility as a generic program model. Health Educ Q 1984; 11:225–242.
3. Collaboration in high blood pressure control: among professionals and with the patient. Coordinating Committee of the National High Blood Pressure Education Program. Ann Intern Med 1984; 101:393–395.
4. Campbell NR, Burgess E, Choi BC, Taylor G, Wilson E, Cleroux J, Fodor JG, Leiter LA, Spence D. Lifestyle modifications to prevent and control hypertension. 1. Methods and an overview of the Canadian recommendations. Canadian Hypertension Society, Canadian Coalition for High Blood Pressure Prevention and Control, Laboratory Centre for Disease Control at Health Canada, Heart and Stroke Foundation of Canada. Can Med Assoc J 1999; 160:S1–S6.
5. Ramsay L, Williams B, Johnston G, MacGregor G, Poston L, Potter J, Poulter N, Russell G. Guidelines for management of hypertension: report of the third working party of the British Hypertension Society. J Hum Hypertens 1999; 13:569–592.
6. 2003 World Health Organization (WHO)/International Society of Hypertension (ISH) statement on management of hypertension. J Hypertens 2003; 21:1983–1992.

7. World Hypertension League Statement. Hypertension control in the world: an agenda for the coming decade. Based on the 1995 WHL Ottawa Declaration. J Hum Hyperten 1997; 11:245–247.

8. Rywik SL, Davis CE, Pajak A, Broda G, Folsom AR, Kawalec E, Williams OD. Poland and U.S. collaborative study on cardiovascular epidemiology hypertension in the community: prevalence, awareness, treatment, and control of hypertension in the Pol-MONICA Project and the U.S. Atherosclerosis Risk in Communities Study. Ann Epidemiol 1998; 8:3–13.

9. Singh RB, Sharma JP, Rastogi V, Niaz MA, Singh NK. Prevalence and determinants of hypertension in the Indian social class and heart survey. J Hum Hypertens 1997; 11:51–56.

10. Hajjar IM, Kotchen TA. Trends in prevalence, awareness, treatment, and control of hypertension in the United States, 1988–2000. J Am Med Assoc 2003; 290:199–206.

11. Banegas JR, Rodriguez-Artalejo F, de la Cruz Troca JJ, Guallar-Castillon P, del Rey CJ. Blood pressure in Spain: distribution, awareness, control, and benefits of a reduction in average pressure. Hypertension 1998; 32:998–1002.

12. Gu D, Reynolds K, Wu X, Chen J, Duan X, Muntner P, Huang G, Reynolds RF, Su S, Whelton PK, He J. Prevalence, awareness, treatment, and control of hypertension in china. Hypertension 2002; 40:920–927.

13. Ibrahim MM, Rizk H, Appel LJ, el Aroussy W, Helmy S, Sharaf Y, Ashour Z, Kandil H, Roccella E, Whelton PK. Hypertension prevalence, awareness, treatment, and control in Egypt. Results from the Egyptian National Hypertension Project (NHP). NHP Investigative Team. Hypertension 1995; 26:886–890.

14. Gu D, Reynolds K, Wu X, Chen J, Duan X, Muntner P, Huang G, Reynolds RF, Su S, Whelton PK, He J. Prevalence, awareness, treatment, and control of hypertension in china. Hypertension 2002; 40:920–927.

15. Steyn K, Gaziano TA, Bradshaw D, Laubscher R, Fourie J. Hypertension in South African adults: results from the Demographic and Health Survey, 1998. J Hypertens 2001; 19:1717–1725.

16. Mufunda J, Scott LJ, Chifamba J, Matenga J, Sparks B, Cooper R, Sparks H. Correlates of blood pressure in an urban Zimbabwean population and comparison to other populations of African origin. J Hum Hypertens 2000; 14:65–73.

17. US Department of Health and Human Services. National High Blood Pressure Education Program. 2004. Available at http://www.nhlbi.nih.gov/about/nhbpep/index.htm.

18. Perloff D, Grim CE, Flack JM, Frohlich ED, Hill M, McDonald M, Morgenstern BZ. Human blood pressure determination by sphygmomanometry. Circulation 1993; 88:2460–2470.

19. American Heart Association. Heart and Stroke Statistical Update. Dallas, TX: American Heart Association, 2000.

20. Neal B, MacMahon S, Chapman N. Effects of ACE inhibitors, calcium antagonists, and other blood pressure-lowering drugs: results of prospectively designed overviews of randomised trials. Blood Pressure Lowering Treatment Trialists' Collaboration. Lancet 2000; 356:1955–1964.

21. Burt VL, Cutler JA, Higgins M, Horan MJ, Labarthe D, Whelton P, Brown C, Roccella EJ. Trends in the prevalence, awareness, treatment, and control of hypertension in the adult US population. Data from the health examination surveys, 1960 to 1991. Hypertension 1995; 26:60–69.

22. Kearney PM, Whelton M, Reynolds K, Whelton PK. Worldwide prevalence of hypertension: a systematic review. J Hypertens 2004; 22:11–19.

23. Joffres MR, Ghadirian P, Fodor JG, Petrasovits A, Chockalingam A, Hamet P. Awareness, treatment, and control of hypertension in Canada. Am J Hypertens 1997; 10:1097–1102.

24. Primatesta P, Brookes M, Poulter NR. Improved hypertension management and control: results from the health survey for England 1998. Hypertension 2001; 38:827–832.

25. Thamm M. Blood pressure in Germany—current status and trends. Gesundheitswesen 1999; 61:S90–S93 (in German).

26. Stergiou GS, Thomopoulou GC, Skeva II, Mountokalakis TD. Prevalence, awareness, treatment, and control of hypertension in Greece: the Didima study. Am J Hypertens 1999; 12:959–965.

27. Bennett SA, Magnus P. Trends in cardiovascular risk factors in Australia. Results from the National Heart Foundation's Risk Factor Prevalence Study, 1980–1989. Med J Aust 1994; 161:519–527.

28. Baba S, Pan WH, Ueshima H, Ozawa H, Komachi Y, Stamler R, Ruth K, Stamler J. Blood pressure levels, related factors, and hypertension control status of Japanese and Americans. J Hum Hypertens 1991; 5:317–332.

29. Singh RB, Beegom R, Ghosh S, Niaz MA, Rastogi V, Rastogi SS, Singh NK, Nangia S. Epidemiological study of hypertension and its determinants in an urban population of North India. J Hum Hypertens 1997; 11:679–685.

30. Freeman V, Fraser H, Forrester T, Wilks R, Cruikshank J, Rotimi C, Cooper RA. A comparative study of hypertension prevalence, awareness, treatment and control rates in St. Lucia, Jamaica, and Barbados. J Hypertens 1996; 14:495–501.

31. Arroyo P, Fernandez V, Loria A, Kuri-Morales P, Orozco-Rivadeneyra S, Olaiz G, Tapia-Conyer R. Hypertension in urban Mexico: the 1992–93 national survey of chronic diseases. J Hum Hypertens 1999; 13:671–675.

32. Sulbaran T, Silva E, Calmon G, Vegas A. Epidemiologic aspects of arterial hypertension in Maracaibo, Venezuela. J Hum Hypertens 2000; 14(suppl 1):S6–S9.

33. Ordunez-Garcia PO, Espinosa-Brito AD, Cooper RS, Kaufman JS, Nieto FJ. Hypertension in Cuba: evidence of a narrow black–white difference. J Hum Hypertens 1998; 12:111–116.

34. Sonmez HM, Basak O, Camci C, Baltaci R, Karazeybek HS, Yazgan F, Ertin I, Celik SC. The epidemiology of elevated blood pressure as an estimate for hypertension in Aydin, Turkey. J Hum Hypertens 1999; 13:399–404.

35. Kim JS, Jones DW, Kim SJ, Hong YP. Hypertension in Korea: a national survey. Am J Prev Med 1994; 10:200–204.

36. Pan WH, Chang HY, Yeh WT, Hsiao SY, Hung YT. Prevalence, awareness, treatment and control of hypertension in Taiwan: results of Nutrition and Health Survey in

Taiwan (NAHSIT) 1993–1996. J Hum Hypertens 2001; 15:793–798.

37. Reynolds K, Gu D, Muntner P, Wu X, Chen J, Huang G, Duan X, Whelton PK, He J. Geographic variations in the prevalence, awareness, treatment and control of hypertension in China. J Hypertens 2003; 21:1273–1281.

38. Hyman DJ, Pavlik VN. Characteristics of patients with uncontrolled hypertension in the United States. N Engl J Med 2001; 345:479–486.

39. De Backer G, Myny K, De Henauw S, Doyen Z, Van Oyen H, Tafforeau J, Kornitzer M. Prevalence, awareness, treatment and control of arterial hypertension in an elderly population in Belgium. J Hum Hypertens 1998; 12:701–706.

40. Muntner P, Gu D, Wu X, Duan X, Wenqi G, Whelton PK, He J. Factors associated with hypertension awareness, treatment, and control in a representative sample of the Chinese population. Hypertension 2004; 43:578–585.

41. He J, Muntner P, Chen J, Roccella EJ, Streiffer RH, Whelton PK. Factors associated with hypertension control in the general population of the United States. Arch Intern Med 2002; 162:1051–1058.

42. Krousel-Wood MA, Muntner P, He J, Whelton PK. Primary prevention of essential hypertension. Med Clin North Am 2004; 88:223–238.

43. Ogden LG, He J, Lydick E, Whelton PK. Long-term absolute benefit of lowering blood pressure in hypertensive patients according to the JNC VI risk stratification. Hypertension 2000; 35:539–543.

44. Greenland S. Meta-Analysis. In: Rothman KJ, and Greenland S, eds. Modern Epidemiology, 2nd ed. Philadelphia, PA: Lippincott, Williams & Wilkins, 1998:643–675.

45. He FJ, MacGregor GA. Effect of modest salt reduction on blood pressure: a meta-analysis of randomized trials. Implications for public health. J Hum Hypertens 2002; 16:761–770.

46. Cutler JA, Follmann D, Allender PS. Randomized trials of sodium reduction: an overview. Am J Clin Nutr 1997; 65:643S–651S.

47. Midgley JP, Matthew AG, Greenwood CM, Logan AG. Effect of reduced dietary sodium on blood pressure: a meta-analysis of randomized controlled trials. J Am Med Assoc 1996; 275:1590–1597.

48. Graudal NA, Galloe AM, Garred P. Effects of sodium restriction on blood pressure, renin, aldosterone, catecholamines, cholesterols, and triglyceride: a meta-analysis. J Am Med Assoc 1998; 279:1383–1391.

49. Whelton PK, Appel LJ, Espeland MA, Applegate WB, Ettinger WH Jr, Kostis JB, Kumanyika S, Lacy CR, Johnson KC, Folmar S, Cutler JA. Sodium reduction and weight loss in the treatment of hypertension in older persons: a randomized controlled trial of nonpharmacologic interventions in the elderly (TONE). J Am Med Assoc 1998; 279:839–846.

50. Whelton PK, He J, Appel LJ, Cutler JA, Havas S, Kotchen TA, Roccella EJ, Stout R, Vallbona C, Winston MC, Karimbakas J. Primary prevention of hypertension: clinical and public health advisory from The National High Blood Pressure Education Program. J Am Med Assoc 2002; 288:1882–1888.

51. Appel LJ, Baker DH, Bar-or O, Morris RC Jr, Resnick LM, Sawka MN, Volpe SL, Weinberger MH, Whelton PK. Institute of Medicine Report on Dietary Reference Intakes for Water, Potassium, Sodium, Chloride and Sulfate. In: Rothman KJ and Greenland S. Washington DC: The National Academics Press, 2004:6-1-6.

52. Neter JE, Stam BE, Kok FJ, Grobbee DE, Geleijnse JM. Influence of weight reduction on blood pressure: a meta-analysis of randomized controlled trials. Hypertension 2003; 42:878–884.

53. Whelton SP, Chin A, Xin X, He J. Effect of aerobic exercise on blood pressure: a meta-analysis of randomized, controlled trials. Ann Intern Med 2002; 136:493–503.

54. Xin X, He J, Frontini MG, Ogden LG, Motsamai OI, Whelton PK. Effects of alcohol reduction on blood pressure: a meta-analysis of randomized controlled trials. Hypertension 2001; 38:1112–1117.

55. Appel LJ, Moore TJ, Obarzanek E, Vollmer WM, Svetkey LP, Sacks FM, Bray GA, Vogt TM, Cutler JA, Windhauser MM, Lin PH, Karanja N. A clinical trial of the effects of dietary patterns on blood pressure. DASH Collaborative Research Group. N Engl J Med 1997; 336:1117–1124.

56. Major outcomes in high-risk hypertensive patients randomized to angiotensin-converting enzyme inhibitor or calcium channel blocker vs diuretic: The Antihypertensive and Lipid-Lowering Treatment to Prevent Heart Attack Trial (ALLHAT). J Am Med Assoc 2002; 288:2981–2997.

57. Psaty BM, Lumley T, Furberg CD, Schellenbaum G, Pahor M, Alderman MH, Weiss NS. Health outcomes associated with various antihypertensive therapies used as first-line agents: a network meta-analysis. J Am Med Assoc 2003; 289:2534–2544.

58. Cushman WC, Ford CE, Cutler JA, Margolis KL, Davis BR, Grimm RH, Black HR, Hamilton BP, Holland J, Nwachuku C, Papademetriou V, Probstfield J, Wright JT Jr, Alderman MH, Weiss RJ, Piller L, Bettencourt J, Walsh SM. Success and predictors of blood pressure control in diverse North American settings: the antihypertensive and lipid-lowering treatment to prevent heart attack trial (ALLHAT). J Clin Hypertens (Greenwich) 2002; 4:393–404.

59. Haynes RB, McDonald HP, Garg AX. Helping patients follow prescribed treatment: clinical applications. J Am Med Assoc 2002; 288:2880–2883.

60. Burnier M, Santschi V, Favrat B, Brunner HR. Monitoring compliance in resistant hypertension: an important step in patient management. J Hypertens 2003; 21(suppl 2):S37–S42.

61. Neutel JM, Smith DH. Improving patient compliance: a major goal in the management of hypertension. J Clin Hypertens (Greenwich) 2003; 5:127–132.

62. Marentette MA, Gerth WC, Billings DK, Zarnke KB. Antihypertensive persistence and drug class. Can J Cardiol 2002; 18:649–656.

63. DiMatteo MR, Giordani PJ, Lepper HS, Croghan TW. Patient adherence and medical treatment outcomes: a meta-analysis. Med Care 2002; 40:794–811.

64. Whelton PK, Adams-Campbell LL, Appel LJ. National high blood pressure education program working group

report on primary prevention of hypertension. Arch Intern Med 1993; 153:186–208.

65. Kotchen JM, Shakoor-Abdullah B, Walker WE, Chelius TH, Hoffmann RG, Kotchen TA. Hypertension control and access to medical care in the inner city. Am J Public Health 1998; 88:1696–1699.

66. Lang T. Factors that appear as obstacles to the control of high blood pressure. Ethn Dis 2000; 10:125–130.

67. Nieto FJ, Alonso J, Chambless LE, Zhong M, Ceraso M, Romm FJ, Cooper L, Folsom AR, Szklo M. Population awareness and control of hypertension and hypercholesterolemia. The Atherosclerosis Risk in Communities study. Arch Intern Med 1995; 155:677–684.

68. Egan BM, Lackland DT, Cutler NE. Awareness, knowledge, and attitudes of older Americans about high blood pressure: implications for health care policy, education, and research. Arch Intern Med 2003; 163:681–687.

69. Blackburn H, Grimm R Jr, Luepker RV, Mittelmark M. The primary prevention of high blood pressure: a population approach. Prev Med 1985; 14:466–481.

21

Impact of Treating Blood Pressure

WILLIAM J. ELLIOTT

Rush University Medical Center, Chicago, Illinois, USA

KEYPOINTS

- In meta-analyses, hypertension treatment is associated with significant reductions in cardiovascular mortality (16%), stroke (31%), myocardial infarction (14%), heart failure (46%), major cardiovascular events (22%), and death (10%).
- Several formal cost-effectiveness analyses (which compare costs of treatment with discounted long-term benefits of treatment) in both diabetics and patients with chronic kidney disease have concluded that treating hypertension in these high-risk groups actually saves money overall.

- The cost-effectiveness of treating hypertension could be improved by making sure the initial diagnosis is correct, limiting laboratory testing at diagnosis, choosing inexpensive medications, maximizing adherence to the prescribed drug, and limiting office visits during follow-up.

SUMMARY

In the long-term, treating hypertension reduces major, expensive cardiovascular events; the biggest reductions, from an economic perspective, are for stroke (−31%) and heart failure (−46%). Although hypertension treatment is expensive (about US$88 billion in the USA in 2005), formal cost-effectiveness analyses indicate that for diabetics and people with chronic kidney disease, lowering blood pressure actually saves money overall, because of the eventual reduction in expensive events (including dialysis). The cost-effectiveness of hypertension could be improved by treating only those at high-risk who have truly elevated blood pressures, limiting laboratory expenditures, using only inexpensive drug therapies, ensuring long-term adherence to prescribed drug treatment, and limiting office visits during follow-up.

I. INTRODUCTION

Hypertension (systolic blood pressure ≥ 140 mmHg, diastolic blood pressure ≥ 90 mmHg, or taking drugs to lower blood pressure) is a major reversible risk factor for cardiovascular disease across the world (1,2). According to the World Health Organization (WHO), hypertension is responsible for about two-thirds of strokes and half of the coronary heart disease on earth (3), and its importance in global public health will increase dramatically (3). The human cost of hypertension is therefore great (4), but reliable estimates of the economic costs of hypertension are available only for a few nations. For some developing countries (e.g., Mexico), controlling blood pressure is a challenge because it would require much of the national healthcare budget to be allocated for antihypertensive pills.

II. ECONOMIC IMPACT OF HYPERTENSION AND ITS TREATMENT

Treating hypertension carries a large economic burden worldwide, but the best country-specific data about its costs come from Sweden and United States. In Sweden, nearly all healthcare delivery occurs in a highly organized socialized medical care system, and essentially all costs are borne by the national government. As a result, Swedish public health officials have excellent "real-life" data about the true costs of hypertension. They can estimate (in their population) quite precisely the real costs and the potential benefits of hypertension treatment on the basis of the many randomized clinical trials performed with Swedish research subjects (5).

The United States spends a greater proportion of its gross domestic product on healthcare than any other nation on earth. Much effort is therefore spent to quantify the monies spent for various diagnoses, including hypertension, which (since 1995) is the most common chronic clinical condition for which Americans visit a healthcare provider. In 2005, the United States is expected to spend about US$88 billion on the treatment of hypertension,

~37% of which will be payment for antihypertensive drugs. The diagnosis-specific expenditures for hypertension in the United States derive, in large part, from two voluntary health organizations, which focus on different target organs: the American Heart Association and the US National Kidney Foundation.

A. Costs Associated with Cardiovascular Disease

Each year, the American Heart Association provides an estimate of the expected expenditures for hypertension treatment that is based on an initial study done in 1988 by the Centers for Medicare & Medicaid Services (formerly the Health Care Financing Administration), an agency of the US Department of Health and Human Services. Each year since then, the figures are augmented by the annual inflation rate for each component of medical care. According to this model, in 2005, hypertension costs approximately US$59.7 billion [Fig. 21.1(A)]; the greatest proportion (US$22.3 billion or 37% of the total) was for drug therapy (6).

This sum is of great concern to many, because the rate of increase in expenditures for antihypertensive medications in the United States was about seven times that of inflation from 1997 to 2002 (22% vs. 3%, annualized). In 2005, about US$15.5 billion (26%) was spent on "indirect costs" (disability payments to individuals who survived heart attacks or strokes, social security payments to survivors, and "lost productivity" for individuals who visited physicians' offices for hypertension treatment). About US$10.4 billion (15%) was spent for healthcare provider services and another US$9.9 billion (17%) was paid to hospitals and nursing homes for hypertension-related sequelae. These expenditures pale when compared with expenditures for cardiovascular disease as a whole, which cost about US$393.5 billion in 2005 [Fig. 21.1(B)].

The two largest costs for cardiovascular disease were indirect costs (39%) and hospitals and nursing home care (38%); only 12% went for drug therapy. Because more effective hypertension control has contributed to the recent decrease in cardiovascular deaths, it may be argued that the recent increase in expenditures for antihypertensive drugs has reduced both death and disability from heart disease and stroke (6).

B. Costs Associated with Chronic Kidney Disease

A different accounting system tracks costs related to kidney disease in the United States. By law, the United States Renal Data System (USRDS) reports on annual expenditures for chronic kidney disease (7). The Medicare

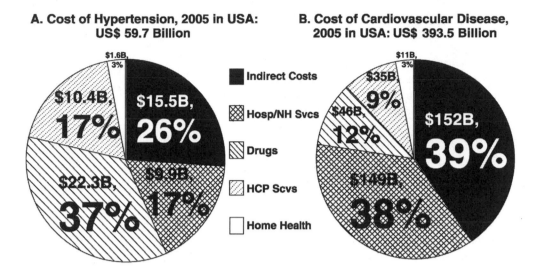

A. Cost of Hypertension, 2005 in USA: US$ 59.7 Billion

$1.6B, 3%
$10.4B, 17%
$15.5B, 26%
$22.3B, 37%
$9.9B, 17%

B. Cost of Cardiovascular Disease, 2005 in USA: US$ 393.5 Billion

$11B, 3%
$35B, 9%
$46B, 12%
$152B, 39%
$149B, 38%

■ Indirect Costs

▨ Hosp/NH Svcs

▧ Drugs

▨ HCP Scvs

□ Home Health

Figure 21.1 Components of the cost of care for hypertension (A) and for cardiovascular disease (B) for the United States in 2005. If these pie charts were drawn to scale, pie chart (A) would be nearly sevenfold smaller in area than that of pie chart (B). These estimates largely exclude the cost of end-stage renal disease because they were compiled by the American Heart Association. [From AHA (6).]

program covers most individuals who begin dialysis or who receive a kidney transplant in the United States; as a result, very precise estimates are available (usually 2–3 years in arrears) for the cost of renal replacement therapy. Unfortunately, even the National Kidney Foundation is unable to provide estimates of the cost of stages 1–4 chronic kidney disease (the stages before dialysis or kidney transplant becomes necessary), so the total amounts are imprecise. Assuming that US$5.0 billion is spent for end-stage renal disease related to hypertension [25.5% of end-stage renal disease was attributed to hypertension in the 2004 USRDS report (7)] and another US$11.6 billion can be attributed to hypertension-related chronic kidney disease that does not yet require renal replacement therapy (7), and the proportion of indirect costs is identical for renal and cardiovascular diseases, the total cost of hypertension-related renal disease in the United States in 2005 would be more than US$28.0 billion. These costs are of great concern to the nation's budget planners, because (since 1991) the number of Americans with end-stage renal disease has increased by 95%, but the expenditures for their care has increased (on a per-patient basis) by 123%. The total cost for hypertension-related cardiovascular and renal disease in 2005 amounted to US$87.7 billion.

C. Costs of Adverse Clinical Events Related to Hypertension

It is useful to consider the estimated costs (in constant 1999 US$) of the most common expensive sequelae of

hypertension. According to the USRDS, hemodialysis costs about US$54,917 per patient per year; kidney transplantation is a little less expensive (US$51,096), but only 5% of end-stage renal disease patients are currently treated with this option (7). According to the American Heart Association (6), a myocardial infarction costs approximately US$10,336 per initial hospitalization, but this is followed by about US$9920 in the first year for direct medical costs (6). The initial hospitalization for stroke is less expensive (US$5692) but has a much higher direct medical cost during the first year (US$28,400), primarily due to the probability of a very expensive rehabilitation or nursing home stay (US$45,000 annually). Heart failure, which costs only US$5456 for the initial hospitalization, adds approximately US$11,210 in direct medical costs for the first year because of increased medication and a high probability of a readmission for heart failure.

D. The Hidden Costs of Hypertension

The estimates reviewed earlier allocate a relatively large percentage of the total expenditures for hypertension to "indirect costs," including the amount of money the patient would have contributed to the economy had it not been necessary to spend time in medical care facilities, at the pharmacy, and for transportation. In addition, several "hidden" costs of hypertension usually are not considered in such analyses. But these hidden costs add to the very high and very real costs of the sequelae of hypertension, apart from the emotional and other human costs. There are five major types of hidden costs of hypertension.

- The cost of healthcare provider visits to evaluate adverse effects of antihypertensive medications, which sometimes transform asymptomatic people into people with "complaints."
- The cost of laboratory studies and tests done to investigate other perceived adverse effects of treatment.
- The administrative costs of healthcare benefit plans (which typically add ~20% to the overall cost in the United States).
- The indirect costs that result from preventable adverse events (including heart attack, stroke, and hospitalization).
- Last, and perhaps specific to the United States, the cost of the tort system used to compensate those who suffer adverse outcomes that can be attributed to a specific source, for example, medication, physician, or hospital.

The population-based (and epidemiologically sound) recommendations of the New Zealand Consensus Committee on the treatment of hypertension work very well in that country, but would likely have major adverse medico-legal consequences in the United States, if it were to be adopted in that country. On the basis of local pharmacoeconomic calculations and other considerations, the New Zealand Expert Panel on Hypertension recommended treatment only if the absolute risk of an adverse event (e.g., stroke, myocardial infarction, and death) exceeded 10% in the next 8 year period (8). All persons with the lower stages of hypertension and insufficient other risk factors have an absolute risk >10% over 8 years were told to adopt lifestyle modifications and not to receive pharmacological therapy. Although this strategy appropriately targets high-risk individuals, there will be about a 1% incidence of cardiovascular events in those from whom drug treatment is withheld. If only 10% of this number were successful in litigation (minimum award of US$3 million per verdict in the United States), it would be far more cost-effective to simply treat all hypertensive patients with medication. The remaining lawsuits could then be defended using this argument: "All that could be done medically was done." In addition to the potential medico-legal costs of denying drug treatment to low-risk patients, the human costs of pain, suffering, and mental and emotional distress to families and patients who suffer cardiovascular events may be even greater. If a monetary value could be assigned to this "utility," one might paraphrase Oscar Wilde, "The only thing worse than the cost of treating hypertension is the cost of not treating hypertension." However, this statement has not been verified by formal cost-effectiveness analyses, which unlike juries, do not affix monetary amounts to human pain and suffering (9).

III. CLINICAL IMPACT OF HYPERTENSION TREATMENT

There is now little doubt that treating hypertension reduces the overall incidence of expensive adverse cardiovascular and renal events (myocardial infarction, stroke, or end-stage renal disease). This has been well substantiated in randomized clinical trials, several observational studies, and even in the vital statistics information of many countries. What is somewhat less clear is the long-term economic value of the clearly beneficial effect of antihypertensive treatment on subclinical endpoints, including left ventricular hypertrophy, doubling of serum creatinine, and proteinuria. Similarly, effective antihypertensive therapy appears to reduce the age-associated increase in blood pressure to some extent, as well as the cost and frequency of visits to healthcare providers, even apart from visits directly related to hypertension (10).

A. Impact on Cardiovascular Disease

Recent overviews have provided useful estimates of the benefits of drug therapy in reducing expensive cardiovascular events in clinical trials (11,12). These trials nearly always underestimate the true benefit of active drug therapy (because some patients decline to take the assigned treatment over the long-term, which reduces the true effectiveness of the active drug, but improves the apparent effectiveness of the placebo). Nonetheless, in a recent meta-analysis, drug therapy was associated with significant reductions in all endpoints (measured as the mean $\pm$ standard deviation) (11): coronary heart disease ($14\% \pm 3\%$), stroke ($31\% \pm 2\%$), heart failure ($46\% \pm 5\%$), major cardiovascular events ($22\% \pm 2\%$), cardiovascular mortality ($16\% \pm 3\%$), and all-cause mortality ($10\% \pm 3\%$).

B. Impact on Chronic Kidney Disease

Unfortunately, there is no corresponding all-inclusive meta-analysis of clinical trials that examines the effect of antihypertensive drugs vs. no treatment on end-stage renal disease. When the results of 11 studies that included 1860 nondiabetic patients with chronic kidney disease randomized to either placebo or angiotensin converting enzyme (ACE)-inhibitor treatment groups were combined, there was a $37\% \pm 8\%$ reduction in end-stage renal disease, but all patients received effective antihypertensive drug therapy in addition to the randomized drug (13). When the results of two recent studies of angiotensin II receptor blockers in type 2 diabetics with chronic kidney disease [Irbesartan Diabetic Nephropathy Trial (IDNT) and Reduction of Endpoints in Non Insulin Dependent Diabetes Mellitus with the Angiotensin II Antagonist Losartan (RENAAL)] are combined in a meta-analysis, the angiotensin receptor blocker was associated with a 27% ± 6% reduction in end-stage renal disease, but again all patients received some blood pressure lowering treatment. For ethical reasons, we do not have data on which to base an estimate of the effectiveness of drugs vs. no treatment to prevent end-stage renal disease. But current estimates indicate that lowering blood pressure to <130/80 mmHg in the "average" American person with stage 2 chronic kidney disease should delay dialysis by ~1.5 years. Given the high annual cost of renal replacement therapy, this is still quite beneficial economically, for the patient, for the health plan, and for the society at large.

IV. COST-EFFECTIVENESS CALCULATIONS IN HYPERTENSION TREATMENT

In simple terms, a cost-effectiveness calculation attempts to determine for a particular treatment the (discounted) cost to save 1 year of life. The cost-effectiveness ratio is the aggregated, discounted cost of treatment, divided by the overall number of years of life saved that are attributed to the treatment strategy. In economics, as in real-life, "discounting" is required because a monetary unit (or a year of life at the current age) is typically "worth" more now (both in purchasing power and in "quality of life" for the individual) than in the future. Cost-effectiveness calculations therefore differ from both "cost-minimization analyses" and "cost-utility analyses." Cost-minimization analysis compares the cost of similar therapies over a defined period of time—for example, the cost of using four initial antihypertensive therapies for a year. Cost-utility analysis is a more complex calculation that attempts to "discount" each year of life gained after a nonfatal adverse event—for example, a year of living after a hemiplegic stroke is valued a good deal less than an identical year without a stroke.

Most cost-effectiveness calculations are performed by using a computerized (or "actuarial") model. In a typical model, a large number of theoretical "patients" are assigned various states of health (e.g., stroke, myocardial infarction, end-stage renal disease, and eventually death); these are based on transition probabilities derived from epidemiological or clinical trial information. The effects of an intervention can be incorporated into the model, and for each time period (usually a year) different numbers of "patients" appear in each health state. Eventually, all "patients" die. Then estimates can be made for the overall number of years of life saved with a given treatment. The cost of treatment also is simultaneously calculated (and discounted for the passage of time). The

uncertainties associated with this type of modeling (variable effectiveness of treatment over time, stability of discount rate, and so on) can be investigated by "sensitivity analyses," in which the "base-case assumptions" are systematically changed and the effects on the cost-effectiveness ratio are examined.

Some cost-effectiveness calculations are solely based on clinical trial information and are somewhat less affected by the discounting process because the time of observation of each patient in a clinical trial is usually short (typical maximum is 5 years). A recent example was the Hypertension Optimal Treatment (HOT) Study, which randomized 18,790 hypertensive patients to one of three diastolic blood pressure targets (14). After 3.8 years of follow-up, those randomized to a diastolic blood pressure target ≤80 mmHg had higher treatment costs (for medications and office visits) by about 3000 Swedish kronor per patient. The overall cost of hospitalizations in this group was also slightly higher (by about 50 Swedish kronor per patient), leading to a negative cost-effectiveness ratio with wide confidence limits. The authors therefore concluded that the extra expense of achieving a diastolic blood pressure of ≤80 mmHg was not economically justified when compared with a target diastolic blood pressure of ≤90 mmHg.

Nearly 30 years ago, Weinstein and Stason published the first of several cost-effectiveness analyses regarding screening and treatment for hypertension. Other investigators have since corroborated their major conclusions by using many different methods. Hypertension treatment has a more attractive cost-effectiveness ratio (i.e., lower cost per year of life saved) for higher risk individuals. This important principle is illustrated in Fig. 21.2, which shows the correlation between absolute risk of stroke and the number of strokes prevented per 1000 patient-years of therapy (a surrogate for cost of treatment). The patients at highest risk for stroke are older [e.g., 76 years, on average in the Swedish Trial in Old Patients with Hypertension (STOP-Hypertension)] or are those with a prior history of a neurological event [Perindopril pROtection aGainst Recurrent Stroke Study (PROGRESS)]. In these high-risk patients, 14 strokes in the STOP-Hypertension and 11 strokes in the PROGRESS were prevented for every 1000 patient-years of therapy. In the younger, low-risk patients of the first Medical Research Council (MRC1) trial, only one stroke was prevented with the same amount of treatment.

A. Cost-Effectiveness Calculations Including All Hypertensive Patients

Because of the high cost of hypertension treatment and the relatively low absolute incidence of expensive major cardiovascular and renal events in the general hypertensive population, the treatment of hypertension costs money

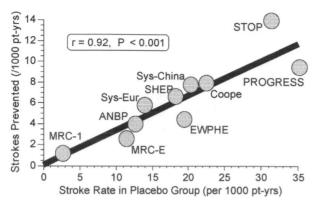

Figure 21.2 Correlation between absolute risk of stroke (stroke rate per 1000 patient-years in the placebo group) and the number of strokes prevented in placebo-controlled trials of antihypertensive drug therapy. pt, Patient; PROGRESS, Perindopril pROtection aGainst REcurrent Stroke Study; STOP, Swedish Trial in Old Patients with Hypertension; Coope, Coope & Warrender; Sys-China, Systolic Hypertension in China; EWPHE, European Working Party on Hypertension in the Elderly; SHEP, Systolic Hypertension in the Elderly Program; Syst-Eur, Systolic Hypertension in Europe; ANBP, Australian National Blood Pressure Trial; MRC-E, Medical Research Council trial in Elderly; MRC-1, Medical Research Council trial of treatment of mild hypertension. The clinical trials included were: Perindopril pROtection aGainst REcurrent Stroke Study (PROGRESS, Lancet 2001; 358:1033–1041); Swedish Trial in Old Patients with Hypertension (STOP, Lancet 1991; 338:1281–1285); Coope & Warrender (Coope, BMJ 1986; 293:1145–1151); Systolic Hypertension in China (Sys-China, J Hypertens 1998; 16:1823–1829); European Working Party on Hypertension in the Elderly (EWPHE, Lancet 1985; 1:1349–1354); Systolic Hypertension in the Elderly Program (SHEP, J Am Med Assoc, 1991; 266:3255–3264); Systolic Hypertension in Europe (Sys-Eur, Lancet 1997; 360:757–764); Australian National Blood Pressure Trial (ANBP, Lancet 1980; 1:1261–1267); Medical Research Council trial in Elderly (MRC-E, BMJ 1992; 304:405–412); Medical Research Council trial of treatment of mild hypertension (MRC-1, BMJ (Clin Res) 1985; 291:97–104).

overall (15). Even nondrug therapies to lower blood pressure seldom result in cost-savings. In several studies, single-patient instruction by nutritionists and exercise physiologists has been more costly than drug treatment. In the recent National Heart, Lung, and Blood Institute PREMIER study, adoption of the Dietary Approaches to Stop Hypertension (DASH) diet for 3 or 6 months did not lower blood pressure significantly better than traditional lifestyle modifications alone (16).

The cost-effectiveness of hypertension treatment in Sweden is the easiest to understand when analyzed by demographic subgroups (Table 21.1). For low-dose diuretics or β-blockers as initial antihypertensive drugs, higher risk individuals (older people with higher diastolic blood pressures) actually have a negative cost-effectiveness ratio, whereas young women with stage 1 hypertension have a very high cost to add a year of life (5).

B.   Cost-Effectiveness Calculations for High-Risk Hypertensive Patients

Many more recent cost-effectiveness analyses have been performed for high-risk patients, who have (by definition) a higher absolute risk for expensive adverse cardiovascular and renal events. In the subset of high-risk individuals (e.g., older people with higher diastolic blood pressures in Table 21.1), overall cost-savings are realized because the cost of antihypertensive drug treatment is outweighed by the reduction in expensive heart attacks, strokes, and end-stage renal disease therapies. In the long run, for both diabetics and people with chronic kidney disease, blood pressure lowering drug therapy prevents more expenditures than it generates.

1.   Diabetes

At least three recent cost-effectiveness analyses of antihypertensive drug therapies for diabetics have reached the

Table 21.1   Cost for Diuretic or β-Blocker Therapy to Add 1 Year of Life

Initial diastolic blood pressure (mmHg)	Cost for men in Sweden (in constant 1992 US$)			Cost for women in Sweden (in constant 1992 US$)		
	Age <45 (years)	Age 45–70 (years)	Age >70 (years)	Age <45 (years)	Age 45–70 (years)	Age >70 (years)
90–94	$118,375	$8500	$3125	$313,250	$26,875	$2625
95–99	$97,500	$4250	$1750	$236,750	$16,625	$875
100–104	$79,500	$8500	$375	$173,500	$7375	—[a]
≥105	$55,000	—[a]	—[a]	$93,250	—[a]	—[a]

[a]Indicates that antihypertensive drug treatment in this group saves money overall.
Source: Johannesson (5).

same conclusion: in general, lowering blood pressure in diabetics saves money overall. The first of these was a cost-effectiveness analysis based on the United Kingdom Prospective Diabetes Study (UKPDS). Despite more use of antihypertensive drugs and more frequent visits for blood pressure monitoring, type 2 diabetics randomized to the lower blood pressure goal (<150/85 mmHg) had 44% fewer strokes, 24% fewer diabetes-related endpoints (including amputations), and 37% fewer microvascular endpoints (including intraocular hemorrhage). The reduction in these expensive clinical endpoints was so great that it more than offset the cost of extra pills and visits to healthcare providers. Even with discounting both costs and benefits, the overall cost-effectiveness ratio was negative (−£720 per year of life gained), meaning that each year of life saved by blood pressure lowering treatment actually saved money overall (17).

A second, independent cost-effectiveness calculation was based on a computerized Markov model that compared blood pressure lowering in diabetics according to the Joint National Committee on the Detection, Evaluation, and Treatment of High Blood Pressure (JNC VI)-recommended target (<130/85 mmHg) and according to the previous and traditional goal keeping the blood pressure at <140/90 mmHg. This analysis used transition probabilities derived from the Framingham Heart Study and clinical trial data and was based on the United States population-based data and costs extant in 1996, with all monetary amounts in stable 1996 US$. The base-case was calculated for a 60-year-old person (the average age of type 2 diabetics in the United States at the time). The lower blood pressure goal (of <130/85 mmHg) was associated with a projected increase in longevity of 0.48 (discounted) years and a cost-savings of −US$3070 per year of life gained (18). When compared with the costs associated with achieving the traditional blood pressure target of <140/90 mmHg, an incremental increase in lifetime expenditures (about US$4000) for more medications plus a 4% increase in the cost of healthcare provider visits for the lower blood pressure goal was outweighed by reduced costs for expensive disease events. The lower blood pressure goal was associated with a 31% projected decrease in stroke costs, a 6% decrease in costs of myocardial infarction, an 18% reduction in the cost of heart failure, and a 15% reduction in the cost of end-stage renal disease. Because economists worry about the critical time-dependence of the amortization of any potential cost-savings, further calculations were done to show that after 6 years of lower blood pressure, the extra cost for pills and office visits to control blood pressure at the lower level were more than offset by the reduced costs for clinical sequelae of hypertension.

The third cost-effectiveness calculation for diabetics was performed by the United States Department of Health and Human Services Centers for Disease Control and Prevention Cost-Effectiveness Group (19). This analysis included a hypothetical population of all United States diabetics >25 years of age and compared treatment of blood pressure, cholesterol, and hyperglycemia. The results were expressed in 1997 US$, and changes in life-expectancy were expressed in quality-adjusted life years, to account for the reduced quality of life associated with survival after cardiovascular events and end-stage renal disease. The authors concluded that intensified blood pressure treatment in diabetics resulted in a prolongation of life of 0.47 (discounted) years (amazingly similar to the previous study!) and a cost-saving of about −US$1959 per quality-adjusted life year gained. In contrast, lipid-lowering and glucose-lowering therapies cost more than US$41,000–52,000 per quality-adjusted year of life gained. These data should reassure those concerned that lowering blood pressure in diabetics to the recently recommended target of <130/80 mmHg is good public policy. It improves the length and quality of life for diabetics and over time decreases total health-care costs.

The UKPDS investigators reached a somewhat different conclusion about the cost-effectiveness of ACE inhibitors in high-risk patients (20). They performed a comparative cost-effectiveness analysis of initial treatment of hypertensive type 2 diabetics with either atenolol or captopril. Overall, there was no significant difference in life expectancy between groups, but the cost of atenolol was much lower than the cost of captopril. In addition, there were significantly fewer and shorter hospital stays in the diabetics randomized to the atenolol treatment group. This economic benefit outweighed the higher cost of more hypoglycemic drugs that were used in the atenolol group, as compared to those used in the captopril group. Overall, the lower initial cost of atenolol led to a significant 14% lower cost of care.

2. Chronic Kidney Disease

Several recent economic analyses of antihypertensive drug therapy in patients with chronic renal impairment also have shown net benefits of different treatment strategies. In general, these calculations compare the costs and benefits of treatment with either an ACE inhibitor or an angiotensin II receptor blocker vs. antihypertensive drug treatment without these drugs.

The first clinical trial that examined the effectiveness of an ACE inhibitor to prevent expensive renal complications was done in type 1 diabetics, comparing captopril with any other antihypertensive drug therapy (excluding an ACE inhibitor; no angiotensin receptor blocker was available at the time). After >3 years of average follow-up, the group receiving captopril had a 50% reduction in death, dialysis, or renal transplantation ($P = 0.006$). On the basis of the results for this clinical trial, the cost-effectiveness ratio for captopril treatment (over 4 years) is −US$30,300 per year of life gained. Approximately US$4850 is saved for each 0.16 years of life saved with captopril because the cost of end-stage renal disease therapy prevented is greater than the cost of captopril and medical care (21). If one calculates the cost per year of life gained off dialysis instead, the cost-effectiveness ratio (for preventing end-stage renal disease, not death) is even better: −US$33,680 per year of life year of dialysis (21). To put it another way, providing captopril to type 1 diabetics with chronic kidney disease reduced the overall cost of care per patient for 4 years by about US$4850 and (with the same treatment) one patient in seven postponed dialysis for a year (21).

A recent cost-effectiveness analysis was based on the Ramipril Efficacy In Nephropathy (REIN) study, in which ramipril was compared with a placebo as initial drug therapy for patients with (mostly) nondiabetic chronic kidney disease (22). The costs and benefits were those extant in Germany in 1999, and the perspective was that of the national health insurance plan. Overall, ramipril therapy for 3 years had a cost-effectiveness ratio of −DM81,900 (about −US$45,000) per patient-year of chronic dialysis that was avoided. Even when extensive sensitivity analyses were performed, varying the baseline conditions over a wide (but reasonable) range, there were major cost-savings with 3 years of ramipril treatment. Because of concerns about large, early costs of extra medication and monitoring visits, the authors calculated the overall cost-effectiveness even at 1 year of treatment; a smaller but still very impressive negative cost-effectiveness ratio was found. The authors concluded that, despite its relatively high cost (compared with other antihypertensive drugs available), ramipril treatment should result in a major cost-savings to the Federal health insurance plan in Germany.

A somewhat similar cost-effectiveness calculation was based on 7 year follow-up in the Angiotensin-Converting Enzyme Inhibition in Progressive Renal Insufficiency (AIPRI) study (23). In the original 3 year clinical trial, only 88 of the 583 European patients reached the primary endpoint (doubling of serum creatinine or end-stage renal disease), but follow-up was continued for a further 3.6 years (on average), resulting in 93 more individuals reaching the primary endpoint. This allowed a more precise, long-term estimate of the absolute benefit of benazepril on delaying the progression of renal disease than had been possible in other studies. The costs, benefits, and utilities related to therapy were based on the United States 1999 estimates from the USRDS. Overall, individuals who received benazepril had a cost-effectiveness ratio of −US$142,000 per quality-adjusted year of life saved, resulting from a lifetime net savings

of US$12,991 per patient and an extension of 0.091 quality-adjusted life years. During the first year of treatment, the costs of drugs and additional office visits outweighed economic benefits, but each year thereafter, the reduction in expensive end-stage renal disease therapy was far greater than the cost of treatment. These conclusions held for many changes to the baseline assumptions about the rates of starting dialysis and other factors that differ between the United States and the Europe.

The importance of the initial lower purchase price of an antihypertensive drug in determining public policy regarding drug choice was probably clearest in the recent Antihypertensive and Lipid-Lowering Treatment to Prevent Heart Attack Trial (ALLHAT). After an average of 4.9 years of follow-up, the group randomized to generically available chlorthalidone had an incident coronary heart disease rate that was not statistically different from the rate for patients randomized to either lisinopril or amlodipine, the most popular ACE inhibitor or calcium antagonist, respectively (24). The ALLHAT investigators therefore concluded that a thiazide-like diuretic should be the preferred first-line choice for hypertension because of its lower cost, although the full cost-effectiveness analysis had not been completed.

However, data from some economic analyses indicate that the cost of the initial drug plays but a small part in the total cost of care. In a now-classic cost-minimization analysis (which compares treatment costs per patient per unit time), there was no significant difference in the total cost of a year's care for hypertension in a large series of patients from Omaha, Nebraska across five initial classes of antihypertensive drugs in 1993 (25). The cheaper initial cost of the generic diuretic was, in this instance, balanced by the greater expenditures for laboratory testing (e.g., serum potassium measurements) and more physician evaluations of perceived adverse effects of the drug. It is unlikely that the comparative cost-effectiveness analysis of the ALLHAT study will include all costs associated with different antihypertensive drug treatments because many of the recommendations for treatment have changed since ALLHAT was designed and that protocol finalized. For example, future drug treatment costs for diabetes that derive from the 41% increased risk of diabetes may or may not be included in the cost-analysis of the chlorthalidone arm. It is unlikely that the analysis will include increased utilization of antihypertensive medications and cholesterol lowering drugs needed to achieve the recommended targets for diabetics (blood pressure <130/80 mmHg and low-density lipoprotein (LDL) cholesterol <100 mg/dL). These lower treatment goals were not in place in 1993–1994, when ALLHAT was designed, and the protocol for cost-effectiveness could not be expected to include them. This difficult issue reinforces previous suggestions that a proper and credible cost-effectiveness analysis must be all-inclusive when determining the overall cost of care.

V. IMPROVING THE COST-EFFECTIVENESS OF HYPERTENSION TREATMENT

Many authors have made different suggestions either for reducing the total cost of care for hypertension or for increasing its effectiveness (26). Some of these recommendations have been incorporated into national or international guidelines. At the local and regional levels, other policies have been implemented primarily by pharmacy benefits managers, who often have the greatest financial stake in reducing prescription drug costs.

A. Ensuring a Correct Diagnosis

Because blood pressure has a large degree of intrinsic variation (Chapter 15), a single blood pressure measurement is usually insufficient for diagnosis and proper assessment of prognosis. The number of low-risk patients needed to be treated for 5 years to prevent one major cardiovascular event is large, meaning that many will take treatment without benefit. One obvious way to make treatment more effective is to be certain that the person committing to therapy really has hypertension and would therefore be more likely to reap the benefits of expensive therapy. Currently, nearly all guidelines recommend multiple blood pressure measurements on different days before instituting long-term drug therapy. Some authors (and some national guidelines) recommend ambulatory blood pressure monitoring as a step in the diagnosis. This procedure typically identifies individuals with white coat hypertension (who appear to be less likely to benefit from long-term drug therapy) and also provides a large number of blood pressure readings throughout the day (thereby minimizing the chance that a diagnosis will be based on one erroneous measurement). More than 10 years ago, several cost-effectiveness analyses of ambulatory blood pressure monitoring in the algorithm for diagnosis of hypertension showed cost-savings overall when ambulatory blood pressure monitoring is used (typically as a last step) in this way. The cost-savings come from the presumption that ~20–25% of individuals with elevated blood pressures in the medical office are really only white coat hypertensives and can avoid treatment if they are properly identified through ambulatory blood pressure monitoring. This was the basis for the decision of the Centers for Medicare & Medicaid Services to approve ambulatory blood pressure monitoring for reimbursement in 2002 (27). It is, however, unlikely that using ambulatory blood pressure monitoring will save money if it is required more than once per year for an individual patient.

Some have advocated a wider role for ambulatory blood pressure monitoring in deciding whether to intensify treatment because office readings are not always representative of everyday levels of blood pressure. One well-done randomized clinical trial compared blood pressure control when treatment decisions were based either on three conventional office blood pressure readings or on a daytime (10 a.m. to 8 p.m.) ambulatory blood pressure monitoring session (28). A physician blinded to the method of blood pressure measurement made decisions about treatment for 419 patients, primarily on the basis of achieving a diastolic blood pressure target of 80–89 mmHg. Over ~6 months of treatment, more patients in the ambulatory blood pressure monitoring group stopped taking drug treatment (26% vs. 7%, $P < 0.001$) and fewer required multiple-drug treatment (27% vs. 43%, $P < 0.001$). At the end of the study, there were no differences in blood pressure (whether measured in the office or by ambulatory blood pressure monitoring), echocardiographically determined left ventricular hypertrophy, or symptom score. Although the cost of treatment was but a secondary endpoint, the cost of ambulatory blood pressure monitoring offset the savings that resulted from fewer physician visits and less intensive drug treatment. This experience suggests that basing treatment decisions solely on ambulatory blood pressure monitoring is too costly and that less expensive methods of routine blood pressure monitoring should be studied.

B. Limiting Testing During the Initial Assessment

Unlike decades ago, when every hypertensive patient had an extensive battery of tests at diagnosis, current guidelines limit initial testing. The JNC7 guidelines suggest that only serum biochemistries (including lipids), a hematocrit, an electrocardiogram, and a urinalysis be included in initial testing. More expensive tests (e.g., echocardiogram) are generally reserved for those rare individuals in whom the results might alter initial therapy. Some groups favor screening all hypertensive patients (particularly diabetics) for microalbuminuria, but this is controversial (29). A recent cost-effectiveness analysis suggested that the most economical approach was simply to treat all diabetics (at diagnosis >50 years of age) with an ACE inhibitor, as long as the annual cost of the drug is lower than US$320 (30). This approach saves the inconvenience and cost of urine collections, costs only US$300 over a lifetime, and results in the greatest gain in quality-adjusted life-years (30).

Screening for secondary hypertension can be recommended when it saves money (typically in younger patients). This requires a sensitive and specific test, a high pre-test probability of the disease, and a high likelihood of saving money after treatment; for example, both adrenalect-omy for primary hyperaldosteronism (31), and captopril renography for screen high-risk individuals for renovascu-lar hypertension (32) can save money in long-term. Additional information about screening tests for diagnosing secondary hypertension is provided in Chapter 14.

C. Choosing the Initial Drug Treatment

Economic considerations are very important in the choice of initial drug therapy because this is a major (and recently increasing) part of the cost of hypertension treatment. When an individual has a "compelling indication" for a specific antihypertensive drug, it makes both clinical and economic sense to use that drug because it is likely to not only lower blood pressure, but also improve prognosis in the second condition. This nearly always costs less than using one drug to lower the blood pressure and a second to treat the second condition.

When there is no compelling indication to use a specific antihypertensive drug, the JNC7 guidelines recommend a thiazide-type diuretic as the drug of first choice "for most people" (1). In ALLHAT, the cheapest drug to pur-chase was chlorthalidone, and outcomes were no worse with this drug than the more expensive alternatives (24). Adopting this recommendation will presumably lower healthcare costs and potentially improve blood pressure control. In the United States Department of Veterans Affairs Medical Centers, healthcare providers were exhorted to adhere to the recommendations of JNC VI, and this resulted in a change in prescribing habits (33). Use of expensive calcium antagonists decreased by 11%; use of inexpensive diuretics increased by 11%; and use of β-blockers increased by 10%. These relatively small changes resulted in an overall US$6 million savings in 1999 and were temporally associated with a major improvement in blood pressure control.

The JNC7 guidelines recommended for the first time that individuals with stage 2 hypertension (blood pressure $\geq 160/100$ mmHg) be treated initially with a two-drug com-bination. This approach should decrease the cost of follow-up visits because two drugs are much more likely than a single drug to control blood pressure. It should also lead to greater use of combination antihypertensive agents, which are generally less expensive to purchase (both for the pharmacy and for the consumer, who pays only a single co-payment) than two separate prescriptions (34).

D. Enhancing Adherence to Medication Regimens

One of the major challenges in the treatment of any chronic condition is that ~50% of people stop taking the recommended therapy after 1 year. Individuals who do not adhere to the prescribed regimen have an infinite cost-benefit ratio—they incur all of the costs of the medi-cation and treatment plan, but enjoy none of the benefits when they stop taking the pills. Approximately 10% of the total cost of care for hypertension in the United States is wasted because of nonadherence to the treatment regimen. According to a recent analysis, the greatest econ-omic benefit in hypertension treatment would derive from improving adherence to the medication regimen rather than stratifying treatment by stage or by routinely using only the least expensive medication (35). The available clinical evidence suggests that current methods of improv-ing adherence to the prescribed medication are inadequate and that new, innovative approaches to assisting patients in taking medication as directed should be developed (36).

E. Choosing a Follow-Up Program

In medicine, as in most businesses, personnel costs typi-cally account for the largest share of expenditures. An appealing target for cost-reduction in hypertension is the outlay for frequent healthcare provider visits for blood pressure monitoring, particularly because other less expensive methods of blood pressure assessment exist. Ambulatory blood pressure monitoring is too expensive to replace routine office blood pressure measurements (28). Home blood pressure monitoring (37), home visits by trained personnel (38), pharmacist visits (39), and other methods (40) have shown promise in some studies and are likely in the near future to play a larger role in determining when medication doses should be titrated.

VI. CONCLUSIONS

Formal cost-effectiveness analyses have shown that, for some groups of high-risk hypertensive patients (especially diabetics and patients with chronic kidney disease), the cost of treating hypertension is less than the cost of pre-vented myocardial infarctions, strokes, heart failure, and end-stage renal disease. Simple methods of improving the cost-effectiveness of hypertension treatment include:

1. Ensuring that the initial diagnosis is correct.
2. Performing limited laboratory studies after diagnosis.
3. Choosing inexpensive medications where possible.
4. Maximizing adherence to the prescribed medi-cation regimen.
5. Limiting the number of office visits during fol-low-up.

REFERENCES

1. Chobanian AV, Bakris GL, Black HR, Cushman WC, Green LA, Izzo JL Jr, Jones DW, Materson BJ, Oparil S, Wright JT Jr, Roccella EJ. National Heart, Lung, and

Blood Institute Joint National Committee on Prevention, Detection, Evaluation, and Treatment of High Blood Pressure. National High Blood Pressure Education Program Coordinating Committee. The seventh report of the Joint National Committee on Prevention, Detection, Evaluation, and Treatment of High Blood Pressure: The JNC 7 report. J Am Med Assoc 2003; 289:2560–2572.

2. 2003 European Society of Hypertension—European Cardiology Society guidelines for the management of arterial hypertension. Guidelines Committee. J Hypertens 2003; 21:1011–1053.

3. Murray CJ, Lauer JA, Hutubessy RC, Niessen L, Tomijima N, Rodgers A, Lawes CM, Evans DB. Effectiveness and costs of intervention to lower systolic blood pressure and cholesterol: A global and regional analysis on reduction of cardiovascular-disease risk. Lancet 2003; 361:717–725.

4. World Hypertension League. Economics of hypertension control. Bull World Health Organ 1995; 73:417–424.

5. Johannesson M. The cost-effectiveness of hypertension treatment in Sweden. Pharmacoeconomics 1995; 7:242–250.

6. American Heart Association. Heart and Stroke Facts: 2005 Statistical Supplement. Dallas, TX, 2004:53.

7. United States Renal Data System. USRDS 2004 Annual Data Report: Atlas of End-Stage Renal Disease in the United States. National Institutes of Health, National Institute of Diabetes and Digestive and Kidney Disease, Bethesda, MD, 2004. Available at: www.usrds.org/adr.htm (accessed 20 Mar 05 at 17:38 CST).

8. Jackson R, Barham P, Bills J, Birch T, McLennan L, MacMahon S, Maling T. Management of raised blood pressure in New Zealand: a discussion document. BMJ 1993; 307:107–110.

9. Swales JD. The costs of not treating hypertension. Blood Press 1999; 8:198–199.

10. Lapuerta P, Simon T, Smitten A, Caro J. CHOICE Study Group. Caring for hypertension on initiation: costs and effectiveness. Assessment of the association between blood pressure control and health care resource use. Clin Ther 2001; 23:1773–1782.

11. Psaty BM, Lumley T, Furberg CD, Schellenbaum G, Pahor M, Alderman MH, Weiss NS. Health outcomes associated with various antihypertensive therapies used as first-line agents: A network meta-analysis. J Am Med Assoc 2003; 289:2534–2544.

12. Turnbull F, Blood Pressure Lowering Treatment Trialists' Collaboration. Effects of different blood-pressure-lowering regimens on major cardiovascular events: Results of prospectively-designed overviews of randomised trials. Lancet 2003; 362:1527–1535.

13. Jafar TH, Schmid CH, Landa M, Giatras I, Toto R, Remuzzi G, Maschio G, Brenner BM, Kamper A, Zucchelli P, Becker G, Himmelmann A, Bannister K, Landais P, Shahinfar S, de Jong PE, de Zeeuw D, Lau J, Levey AS. Angiotensin-converting enzyme inhibitors and progression of nondiabetic renal disease: A meta-analysis of patient-level data. Ann Intern Med 2001; 135:73–87.

14. Jonsson B, Hansson L, Stalhammar NO. Health economics in the Hypertension Optimal Treatment (HOT) study: Costs and cost-effectiveness of intensive blood pressure lowering and low-dose aspirin in patients with hypertension. J Intern Med 2003; 253:453–480.

15. Elliott WJ. The economic impact of hypertension. J Clin Hypertens 2003; 5 (3 suppl 2):3–13.

16. Appel LJ, Champagne CM, Harsha DW, Cooper LS, Obarzanek E, Elmer PJ, Stevens VJ, Vollmer WM, Lin PH, Svetkey LP, Stedman SW, Young DR; Writing Group of the PREMIER Collaborative Research Group. Effects of comprehensive lifestyle modification on blood pressure control: Main results of the PREMIER clinical trial. J Am Med Assoc 2003; 289:2083–2093.

17. Raikou M, Gray A, Briggs A, Stevens R, Cull C, McGuire A, Fenn P, Stratton I, Holman R, Turner R. Cost-effectiveness analysis of improved blood pressure control in hypertensive patients with type 2 diabetes: UKPDS 40. U.K. Prospective Diabetes Study Group. BMJ 1998; 317:720–726.

18. Elliott WJ, Weir DR, Black HR. Cost-effectiveness of the lower treatment goal (of JNC VI) in hypertensive diabetics. Arch Intern Med 2000; 160:1277–1283.

19. CDC Diabetes Cost-effectiveness Group. Cost-effectiveness of intensive glycemic control, intensified hypertension control, and serum cholesterol level reduction for type 2 diabetes. J Am Med Assoc 2002; 287:2542–2551.

20. Gray A, Clarke P, Raikou M, Adler A, Stevens R, Neil A, Cull C, Stratton I, Holman R. An economic evaluation of atenolol vs. captopril in patients with Type 2 diabetes (UKPDS 54). Diabet Med 2001; 18:438–444.

21. Rodby RA, Firth LM, Lewis EJ. For the Collaborative Study Group. An economic analysis of captopril in the treatment of diabetic nephropathy. Diabetes Care 1996; 19:1051–1061.

22. Schadlich PK, Brecht JG, Brunetti M, Pagano E, Rangoonwala B, Huppertz E. Cost-effectiveness of ramipril in patients with non-diabetic nephropathy and hypertension: Economic evaluation of Ramipril Efficacy in Nephropathy (REIN) Study for Germany from the perspective of statutory health insurance. Pharmacoeconomics 2001; 19:497–512.

23. Hogan TJ, Elliott WJ, Seto AH, Bakris GL. Antihypertensive treatment with and without benazepril in patients with chronic renal insufficiency: A US economic evaluation. Pharmacoeconomics 2002; 20:37–47.

24. The ALLHAT Officers and Coordinators for the ALLHAT Collaborative Research Group. The Antihypertensive and Lipid Lowering Treatment to Prevent Heart Attack Trial. Major outcomes in high-risk hypertensive patients randomized to angiotensin-converting enzyme inhibitor or calcium channel blocker vs. diuretic: The Antihypertensive and Lipid Lowering Treatment to Prevent Heart Attack Trial (ALLHAT). J Am Med Assoc 2002; 288:2981–2997.

25. Hilleman DE, Mohiuddin SM, Lucas BD Jr, Stading JA, Stoysich AM, Ryschon K. Cost-minimization analysis of initial antihypertensive therapy in patients with mild-to-moderate essential diastolic hypertension. Clin Ther 1994; 16:88–102.

26. Elliott WJ. Improving the cost-effectiveness of treating hypertension. In: Epstein M, ed. Calcium Antagonists in Clinical Medicine. Chap. 40. 3rd ed. Philadelphia, PA: Hanley & Belfus, Inc., 2002:733–748.

27. Tunis S, Kendall P, Londner M, Whyte J. Medicare Coverage Policy ~ Decisions: Ambulatory Blood Pressure Monitoring (#CAG-00067N): Decision Memorandum. Washington, DC. Health Care Financing Administration, October 17, 2001. Available at: www.hcfa.gov/coverage/8b3-ff2.htm (accessed 01 Apr 02 at 18:32 CST).

28. Staessen JA, Byttebier G, Buntinx F, Celis H, O'Brien ET, Fagard R. Antihypertensive treatment based on conventional or ambulatory blood pressure measurement. A randomized controlled trial. Ambulatory Blood Pressure Monitoring and Treatment of Hypertension Investigators. J Am Med Assoc 1997; 278:1065–1072.

29. Boulware LE, Jaar BG, Tarver-Carr ME, Brancati FL, Powe NR. Screening for proteinuria in US adults: a cost-effectiveness analysis. J Am Med Assoc 2003; 290:3101–3114.

30. Golan L, Birkmeyer JD, Welch HG. The cost-effectiveness of treating all patients with Type 2 diabetes with angiotensin-converting enzyme inhibitors. Ann Intern Med 1999; 131:660–667.

31. Sywak M, Pasieka JL. Long-term follow-up and cost-benefit of adrenalectomy in patients with primary hyperaldosteronism. Br J Surg 2002; 89:1587–1593.

32. Blaufox MD, Middleton ML, Bongiovanni J, Davis BR. Cost efficacy of the diagnosis and therapy of renovascular hypertension. J Nucl Med 1996; 37:171–177.

33. Siegel D, Lopez J, Meier J. Cunningham F. Changes in the pharmacologic treatment of hypertension in the Department of Veterans Affairs 1997–1999: decreased use of calcium antagonists and increased use of β-blockers and thiazide diuretics. Am J Hypertens 2001; 14:957–962.

34. Ambrosioni E. Pharmacoeconomics of hypertension management: the place of combination therapy. Pharmacoeconomics 2001; 19:337–347.

35. Mar J, Rodriguez-Artalejo F. Which is more important for the efficiency of hypertension treatment: hypertension stage, type of drug, or therapeutic compliance? J Hypertens 2001; 19:149–155.

36. Haynes RB, McDonald HP, Garg AX. Helping patients follow prescribed treatment: clinical applications. J Am Med Assoc 2002; 288:2880–2883.

37. Rickerby J. The role of home blood pressure measurement in managing hypertension: an evidence-based review. J Hum Hypertens 2002; 16:469–472.

38. Garcia-Pena C, Thorogood M, Wonderling D, Reyes-Frausto S. Economic analysis of a pragmatic randomised trial of home visits by a nurse to elderly people with hypertension in Mexico. Salud Publica Mexico 2002; 44:14–20.

39. Chabot I, Moisan J, Gregoire JP, Milot A. Pharmacist intervention program for control of hypertension. Ann Pharmacother 2003; 37:1186–1193.

40. Pickering T, Gerin W, Holland JK. Home blood pressure teletransmission for better diagnosis and treatment. Curr Hypertens Rep 1999; 1:489–494.

22

Antihypertensive Treatment Trials: Quality of Life

MARIA I. NUNES, ELLEN R. T. SILVEIRA, CHRISTOPHER J. BULPITT

Imperial College School of Medicine, London, UK

KEYPOINTS

- The choice of drug regimen in mild to moderate hypertension should not affect the patient's well being.
- Overall antihypertensive drugs do not produce any significant improvement in health-related quality of life (HRQoL).
- Angiotensin receptor blockers, ACE inhibitors, newer β-blockers, and low-dose diuretics have few, if any, adverse effects on HRQoL.

SUMMARY

The effectiveness of antihypertensive treatments depends on the need to minimize or avoid symptomatic side effects and to exert positive effects on quality of life (QoL). Since the publication of the pioneering work by Croog et al. (1) on QoL in patients using captopril, propranolol, and methyldopa, many clinical trials have tried to include QoL measures, to examine this domain in greater depth in hypertensive patients. Some of the discrepancies in the effects of antihypertensive agents on QoL in clinical trials may be explained by small numbers of patients, short duration of studies, differences in blood pressure entry criteria, population composition, endpoints chosen, compatibility of QoL measures, and other subjective and objective factors (2). The most recent classes of antihypertensives and some drugs in older classes may have fewer side effects and improve general well-being. This in turn is likely to improve compliance with drug regimens, one of the most decisive factors in evaluations of drug efficacy and QoL. Low-dose diuretics, β-blockers other than propranolol, angiotensin-converting enzyme (ACE) inhibitors, and angiotensin receptor blockers have many trials supporting their short-term benefits in terms of QoL. The same may be true for some calcium channel blockers such as verapamil and amlodipine.

I. INTRODUCTION

Hypertension is a preventable disease, and there is overwhelming evidence from clinical trials which indicates that its treatment is beneficial because it reduces cardiovascular mortality and morbidity at least up to the age of 79 years. A meta-analysis reported a risk reduction of 30% for strokes, 23% for coronary events, and 13% for all-cause mortality (3). Despite this evidence and although awareness about the disease has improved in the last two decades, many people remain untreated in practice and <50% of treated patients are adequately controlled (4).

Many antihypertensive treatments decrease cardiovascular events and mortality to a similar extent. A recent meta-analysis of 15 trials which compares old drugs (diuretics or β-blockers) to new drugs [calcium channel blockers, α-blockers, ACE inhibitors and angiotensin receptor blockers (ARBs)] revealed that both old and new agents offered similar protection against total cardiovascular mortality and nonfatal and fatal myocardial infarction (5). These drugs are safe, well tolerated, and efficacious, which means that outcome indicators of QoL, alongside contra-indications and side effects, should aid and may even determine the choice of medication.

Although 15 years ago little was known about the assessment of QoL, in the past decade not only the interest in QoL has increased sharply, but also it has become a common practice to integrate QoL as part of outcome measures of clinical trials in the drug evaluation process (6,7). According to Sanders et al. (8) reporting on QoL increased during 1980–1997 from 0.63% to 4.2% for trials from all disciplines and from 0.34% to 3.6% for cardiovascular trials.

As hypertension is a chronic disease, which usually requires life-long treatment, the success of treatment will depend on the effects of the drug regimen on the patient's well-being (9). Therefore, the assessment of the therapeutic burden on QoL of hypertensive patients is becoming increasingly more recognized as an important outcome measure in clinical trials (10).

II. ASSESSMENT OF QoL—METHODOLOGICAL CONSIDERATIONS

The concept, QoL, is difficult to define, and also to measure in a scientific way (11). Although no consensus has been achieved regarding an exact definition of QoL, it has been suggested that QoL is the discrepancy between the individual's expectations and the reality (12). It has been argued that it is impossible to provide an exclusive definition of the concept, because QoL as perceived by an individual is not only complex, but also subjective and it is influenced by a multitude of factors (11). Health-related quality of life (HRQoL), a further concept, was created in the 1980s, and this term has been developed to cover certain areas of the concept of QoL; that concerns physical or mental health (13,14). Although no unanimous definition exists for HRQoL, a consensus has been achieved that measures in hypertensive patients should include symptomatic and psychological well-being, activity (work, leisure, sleep, sexual activity, and social participation), cognitive function, and life satisfaction (15).

Within the context of clinical practice, clinicians are usually guided by the findings of clinical trials when choosing medication for the treatment of hypertensive patients. However, it is important when extrapolating data relating to QoL from clinical studies, to bear in mind that the design and duration of the trial, sample size, validity and reliability of the instruments used, and other factors should be considered (16). In terms of ascertainment, measurements of HRQoL should comply with the principles of good design and when comparing differences between treatment groups, a randomized, double-blind trial is to be preferred (17).

To be of value to clinicians, instruments chosen to assess HRQoL should be valid, reliable, and sensitive. There has been a lot of research effort put into developing valid instruments to assess and to quantify the different domains, which comprise the concept of HRQoL. The choice of instruments will depend on the HRQoL dimensions which will be assessed. Other important practical consideration when evaluating HRQoL is how the instrument is going to be administered (17). The instruments developed have been mainly questionnaire-based, either to be self-completed or to be administered by an interviewer. The choice of an instrument and the method to assess HRQoL will depend on different factors such as the cost, the complexity of the study, respondent's burden, among others. It has been argued that self-completion questionnaires are preferable because the input of the person being assessed is mandatory (18); nevertheless, these assessments should be carried out under standard conditions—that is, for hypertensive patients, the questionnaires should be completed in a quiet area at the medical center, before seeing the doctor and having their blood pressure measured. This method would be particularly advantageous to employ in multicenter trials, where it would be costly to train and to organize interviewers. One of the disadvantages of this method is that people who are illiterate are excluded automatically, and some groups of patients, such as the elderly, may not be able to complete self-administered questionnaires because of reduced visual acuity, lack of understanding, or inability to write or draw. Therefore, in these cases interview-administered questionnaires may be preferable (19). However, using an interviewer can introduce bias because it is always possible that the perception of the patient differs from that of the interviewer (16).

Hypertension is a risk factor, rather than a disease *per se* (17), which makes its treatment complex. Clinicians should be aware of the issues discussed earlier, so that they can critically evaluate the findings from clinical studies. The recognition of valid results will aid the choice of treatment for a particular patient.

Many studies have reported on the effects of different antihypertensive treatments on HRQoL, and the results have shown that overall these drugs do not produce any significant improvement in QoL (10). Also, the majority of these studies are characterized by short to moderate duration (12–28 weeks), lack of a placebo group, and a nonrepresentative sample of low-risk hypertensive patients (20). These are some of the limitations and pitfalls of the data available from clinical trials that assess HRQoL; they will be discussed in more detail later in this chapter.

First, we will give an overall view of the evidence accrued from clinical trials of the effects on HRQoL of different antihypertensive drugs. To facilitate this process, the next section has been divided into two subsections: the first describes the findings from long-term clinical trials and the second describes the findings from short-term trials.

III. MONITORING QoL: EVIDENCE FROM CLINICAL TRIALS

A. Long-Term Clinical Trials of Antihypertensive Treatments and the Effects on QoL

There are several long-term trials that have assessed the effects of antihypertensive treatment in reducing cardiovascular morbidity and mortality, but only a few have included the assessment of QoL.

One of the first long-term trials to report on the effects of antihypertensive treatment on QoL was the Systolic Hypertension in the Elderly Program (SHEP). This trial was designed to determine if treatment with a diuretic and a β-blocker-based antihypertensive treatment would satisfactorily control isolated systolic hypertension and, if so, whether it would reduce cardiovascular complications or it would produce new adverse events (21). Of particular concern was the possibility of any antihypertensive medication having a negative impact on cognition or mood in older persons, especially as previous studies, cited by Applegate et al. (22), had shown conflicting findings about the adverse effects of antihypertensive treatment on the QoL and function of older people in comparison to the effects on middle-aged persons.

The trial was a randomized, multicenter, double-blind, placebo-controlled trial of patients 60 years or older with a systolic blood pressure ≥ 160 mmHg/diastolic blood pressure < 90 mmHg. The 4736 participants were randomized to either an actively treatment group or a group given matching placebo and followed up for an average of 5 years in 16 academic clinical trial centers. Active treatment consisted of chlorthalidone (12.5–25 mg), $\pm$ atenolol (25–50 mg), or reserpine (0.05–0.10 mg). The trial was also designed to provide a straightforward look at the effects of a specific drug regimen on measures of cognitive, emotional, and physical function and leisure activities. The behavioral evaluation was administered after randomization and before treatment was started, and cognitive impairment, depression and mood disorders of all participants were assessed twice a year for 20 min, and once a year participants answered questions about their activities of daily living (ADL) and social networks. Additionally, participants in six of the 16 centers ($n = 2034$) received a more detailed assessment of cognitive function every year, which included: psychomotor speed, attention span, visual scanning, mental calculation, expressive language function, verbal memory, and hypothesis testing (21). The questionnaires were administered by behavioral raters, who were centrally trained, and the procedures were standardized.

The findings at baseline showed that there were no differences between active treatment and the placebo groups in cognitive function, depressive symptoms, or mood disorder. Some modest difference was found in the basic and moderate ADLs; more participants in the placebo group had some impairment in these two levels of ADL. However, no differences were noted between the two groups, when all three levels of ADL were taken into account. During the trial there were some small changes in ADL in favor of the treatment group. Also, the changes in cognitive function and depression symptoms, although they were not significant, favored the treatment group (Table 22.1).

In the six centers, where participants did more extensive evaluations, there were no differences in the participant's global assessment of QoL in the two treatment groups. The results also showed a small increase in the active treatment group of some symptoms such as faintness, falls, fatigue, sexual dysfunction, muscle weakness, and trouble with memory (self-reported). The findings from the SHEP trial clearly demonstrated that the chosen drug regimen decreased the incidence of cerebro- and cardiovascular events, without causing deterioration on measures of cognition, emotional state, physical function, or leisure activities (21–22).

The Systolic Hypertension in Europe (Syst-Eur) trial, was a randomized, double-blind, placebo-controlled trial, which also included as a side project the measurement of HRQoL (23). To be included in the trial, patients had to be 60 years and older, with an average sitting systolic blood pressure of 160–219 mmHg, a diastolic blood pressure < 95 mmHg, and a standing systolic pressure of ≥ 140 mmHg. Patients were randomized to either active

Table 22.1   The Systolic Hypertension in the Elderly Program (SHEP)

	Active			Placebo			
	N	Baseline	Last	N	Baseline	Last	Differences
Score							
Cognitive impairment	2317	0.37	0.26	2291	0.37	0.32	+0.05
Depressive symptom	2264	3.13	2.95	2229	3.11	3.09	+0.16
CES-D score	2131	4.13	4.33	2117	4.01	4.59	+0.38
% ≥16	—	4.6	5.5		4.6	6.9	$P = 0.050$ last visit
Activity							
Any basic ADLs	2263/2260	4.5%	18.6%	2205/2200	5.7%	20.1%	+0.20
Any moderate ADLs	2232/2040	11.1%	22.1%	2154/1968	12.4%	23.4%	+0.30
Any advanced ADLs	2260/2203	26.6%	48.6%	2196/2138	27.0%	49.1%	+0.72

Note: Mean cognitive, depressive and center for epidemilogic studies-depression scale (CES-D) scores and activities of daily living (ADL) at baseline and last evaluation by treatment group. ADL: Needs help or unable to do at baseline/any deterioration to last visit. Basic self-care items included: bathing, personal grooming, dressing, eating, ambulation, using the toilet, and transferring from bed to chair. Moderate ADLs included writing/handing small objects, walking up and down the stairs, extending the arms above shoulder level, walking 0.5 mile; whereas advanced ADLs included the ability to perform tasks such as: carrying groceries, moving furniture, lifting and carrying weights (<4.5 kg), pulling or pushing large objects or crouching or kneeling. A positive value indicates that that the result was better in the active treatment group. Although the trend continually favors the active treatment group, the only difference that was statistically significant was in the CES-D score. High scores indicate worse QoL.
Source: Adapted from Appelgate et al. (22).

treatment, which consisted of nitrendipine (10–40 mg daily) plus enalapril (5–20 mg daily) and hydrochlorothiazide (HCTZ) (12.5–25 mg daily) if necessary, or to matching placebos.

A total of 4695 patients were recruited during an 8-year period. The trial was discontinued in February 1997 after the second interim analysis, which showed that the boundary for stroke events was crossed in favor of active treatment (24).

For the QoL side project, 33 centers in 12 countries took part, and a total of 610 patients completed the baseline questionnaire and at least one follow-up assessment. The questionnaire was administered by a trained interviewer under standard conditions, that is, in a quiet area at the medical center before the patient saw the doctor and had his or her blood pressure measured. The questionnaire included cognitive function tests (Reitan Trail Making A and B), the Brief Assessment Index (BAI), which is a measure of depressed mood and four subscales from the Sickness Impact Profile (SIP): ambulation, social interaction, sleep and rest, and housework (25).

For the intention to treat analyses no differences in the SIP and BAI scores were found between the two treatment groups from baseline to the two timepoints: at 6 months and at 2 years (Table 22.2).

Similar results were found for the on randomized treatment analyses. However, when data from all timepoints over the 4 years of follow-up were analyzed, a significant between group difference was found for social interaction where patients in the active treatment group reported problems in this dimension. These may be attributed to the side effects of treatment, such as flushing, edema and headache with nitrendipine, and cough with enalapril. It was reassuring to notice that no adverse effects on measures of depression were found from active treatment (25). In relation to the Reitan Trail Making tests (TMTs), the findings revealed a slower rate of learning for patients in the active treatment group, with the largest difference reported in the first 6 months.

It has been argued that as patients were allocated at random to a drug regimen not to an individual drug, it would be difficult to attribute these negative effects to a particular drug. However, the negative effects reported on Reitan TMTs for the actively treated group may relate to the nitrendipine medication, because 57% of patients were taking this drug alone in the first 6 months.

The findings from the QoL side project of the Syst-Eur trial suggested that when compared with placebo, active treatment had some adverse effect on QoL. However, as pointed out by Fletcher et al. (25), these results have to be considered within the context of the positive benefit from active treatment in reducing stroke by 42% and all cardiovascular endpoints by 31%.

The Treatment of Mild Hypertension Study (TOMHS) was a randomized, double-blind, placebo-controlled clinical trial, which was conducted in four hypertension screening and academic centers in the United States (26). A total of 902 patients, with stage 1 hypertension and without clinical evidence of cardiovascular disease, were followed-up for a minimum of 4 years. Participants between the ages of 45 and 69 years, were randomized to five different antihypertensive drugs: β-blocker (acebutolol), calcium-antagonist (amlodipine maleate), diuretic (chlorthalidone), α-antagonist (doxazosin), and ACE (enalapril) or

Table 22.2 The Systolic Hypertension in Europe (Syst-Eur) Trial

	Differences from baseline at					
	6 months[a]			2 years[a]		
	Placebo (n = 232)	Active treatment (n = 263)	P-Value[b]	Placebo (n = 236)	Active treatment (n = 264)	P-Value
SIP						
Ambulation						
Median	0	0		0	0	0.44
5th−95th PI	−13 to 11	−11 to 13	0.50	−12 to 15	−13 to 15	
Social interaction						
Median	0	0		0	0	0.38
5th−95th PI	−13 to 14	−13 to 7	0.48	−17 to 14	−19 to 9	
Home work						
Median	0	0		0	0	0.46
5th−95th PI	−16 to 11	−13 to 17	0.10	−14 to 16	−13 to 24	
Sleep and rest						
Median	0	0		0	0	0.14
5th−95th PI	−23 to 19	−14 to 14	0.69	−25 to 14	−16 to 14	
BAI						
Median	0	0		0	0	
5th−95th PI	−14 to 10	−14 to 10	0.97	−14 to 14	−19 to 14	0.41

[a]A negative score denotes improvement.
[b]P-Value for difference in medians.
Note: Within-treatment changes in quality of life measures from baseline to 6 months and 2 years (intention-to-treat analysis). SIP, sickness impact profile; BAI, brief assessment index; PI, percentile interval.
Source: Reproduced with permission from Fletcher et al. (25).

placebo. In conjunction with the medication, patients were given lifestyle intervention to reduce weight, dietary sodium intake, and alcohol intake and to increase physical activity.

In order to assess QoL, patients were given a 35-item questionnaire at baseline, at 3 months and thereafter at yearly intervals. The questionnaire comprised seven QoL indexes: general health, energy or fatigue, mental health, general functioning, satisfaction with physical abilities, social functioning, and social contacts

The results showed that at baseline, the mean QoL indexes for the participants were high, which indicated they had good health and functional ability. There were some associations between some of the QoL indexes and gender, sex, age, smoking status, body weight, physical activity, and socioeconomic status. Patients more physically active and less obese had higher QoL. An interesting finding was that older patients (≥55) reported higher QoL for three indexes: energy, mental health, and social functioning than participants <55 years of age.

As a whole, participants reported an improved QoL from baseline, in all randomized groups, including the placebo group, during the 4-year follow-up, except for the general functioning index, which decreased in doxazosin and placebo groups; for social functioning, which decreased on average in the placebo group, and social

contacts which fell in the chlorthalidone group. The results were thought to be directly or indirectly linked to the lifestyle change program and greater improvements were observed for participants with greater weight loss and increase in physical activity. Compared with the placebo group, participants in the actively treated groups reported more favorable changes in most QoL indexes, "with significantly greater relative improvement for mental health, general functioning, and social functioning indexes, and the global statistic" (Table 22.3).

For the general health index, patients in the acebutolol group reported significantly greater QoL than patients on the amlodipine maleate and enalapril maleate (P < 0.01). Similarly, QoL was significantly greater for acebutolol and chlorthalidone groups compared with the enalapril maleate group (P < 0.01) for the mental health index and for the acebutolol group compared with the doxazosin group for the social contacts index. The greater improvement for the active treatment compared with placebo was first observed at 3 months and this was maintained throughout the trial. Also, there was a correlation between the global QoL score and the side effect score, and a lower QoL was associated with more side effects.

The conclusions of the TOMHS trial demonstrated that the treatment of stage I hypertension using one of the five

Table 22.3 The Treatment of Mild Hypertension Study (TOMHS)

QoL index	Acebutolol	Amlodipine maleate	Chlorthalidone	Doxazosin mesylate	Enalapril maleate	Placebo	P-Value[a]
General health	2.17[b]	0.59	1.48	1.19	0.85	0.98	0.02
Energy or fatigue	1.36[b]	0.69	1.45[b]	0.49	0.77	0.67	0.04
Mental health	3.07[b]	1.99	2.72[b]	1.62	1.29	1.43	0.05
General functioning	0.13[b]	0.07	0.14[b]	−0.35	−0.13	−0.32	0.15
Satisfaction with physical abilities	0.40	0.46	0.40	0.26	0.39	0.25	0.30
Social functioning	0.21[b]	0.10	0.17	0.02	0.11	−0.12	0.52
Social contacts	0.10	0.37	−0.21	0.05	0.14	0.15	0.05
Global statistic	479.3[b]	449.8	461.3[b]	422.0	437.9	420.3	0.02
Number of participants	131	126	133	131	132	230	

[a]P-Value comparing 5 drugs.
[b]P < 0.01 for comparing with placebo.
Note: Mean change from baseline in quality of life (QoL) indexes averaged over all follow-up visits by treatment group. The higher the score the better the QoL.
Source: Adapted from Grimm et al. (26).

different antihypertensive drugs used in the trial does not cause deterioration in the QoL indexes assessed. The two drugs that appeared to improve QoL the most were the diuretic and the β-blocker. An important point was that lifestyle changes, especially loss of weight and increase in physical activity were associated with higher QoL scores, and therefore these interventions, not only can assist with blood pressure control, but they have a positive impact on the individual's well-being (26). Unfortunately, this may be due simply to the knowledge that they have lost weight or exercised or lowered their blood pressure, rather than any causative mechanism.

The Medical Research Council Trial in the Elderly was a randomized, placebo-controlled, single-blind trial (27). A total of 4396 patients ranging in age from 65 to 74 years, with a systolic blood pressure between 160 and 209 mmHg and a diastolic blood pressure ≤ 114 mmHg, were randomized to receive a placebo, amiloride hydrochloride with HCTZ, or atenolol. A sub-study was designed to assess cognitive function and 2584 patients were recruited from the 4396, who took part in the main trial. The outcome measures were the rate change in paired associate learning test and the Reitan TMT part A scores. These tests were administered at entry and at 1, 9, 21, and 54 months. The results did not reveal an association between antihypertensive treatment and cognitive outcome over a period of 54 months. No difference was found in the mean learning test coefficients (rate of change of score over time) among the diuretic (-0.31), β-blocker (-0.33), and placebo (-0.30) groups. Similarly, there was no difference in the average Reitan Trail Making coefficients: -2.73, -2.08, -3.01 for diuretic, β-blocker, and placebo, respectively. The conclusion of this sub-study was that the treatment of moderate hypertension in older people does not appear to have an influence, either negative or positive, on cognitive function (27).

Another trial, conducted in Japan, also looked at the effect of antihypertensive treatment on QoL over a 5-year period. However, it did not include a placebo arm; it compared the effects of a calcium antagonist and a diuretic. Patients were recruited from outpatients in 108 medical institutions in Japan. Participants had to be at least 60 years old, with a systolic blood pressure ≥ 160 and < 220 mmHg and a diastolic blood pressure < 115 mmHg. A total of 429 patients were recruited into the trial; 215 were randomized to the nicardipine group and 214 to the trichlormethiazide group (28).

QoL was assessed at baseline and every 6 months for 5 years, and the patients were assessed by an interviewer. The questionnaire included questions on the following domains: physical symptoms, life satisfaction symptoms and well-being, work performance and satisfaction, general symptoms, sleep scale, sexual function, emotional state, cognitive function, and social activity. The results found that the two different antihypertensive drugs had similar effects on the QoL in elderly hypertensive patients, and no deteriorating effect on QoL was observed with either drug. Although there was no significant difference in mean scores in terms of total QoL or in degrees of change between the two groups; a trend to a lower score in three different categories (general symptoms, sleep scale, and sexual function) was observed for the diuretic group. A lower score for cognitive function was observed for the calcium antagonist group (28).

It is important to highlight that apart from the TOMHS trial, all of the other trials mentioned above recruited people who were at least 60 years old, and although there is overwhelming evidence of the benefits of treating hypertension in people aged 60–79 years, the benefit of treating people over the age of 80 years is still not clearly demonstrated. However, clinical trials are being carried out, targeting this age group, including HRQoL measures and should provide a definite answer for or against treatment for the very elderly (29).

B. Short-Term Clinical Trials

In this subsection, common antihypertensive agents including "newer" treatment regimens in trials conducted for a maximum period of 1 year are reviewed to examine the short-term effects of antihypertensive drugs on patients' QoL. Studies on diuretics, β-blockers, calcium channel blockers, ACE inhibitors, and ARBs will be scrutinized for their effects on symptoms, mental health, general functioning, energy and satisfaction with physical abilities, and social contacts.

1. Diuretics

Thiazide diuretics remain one of the most commonly prescribed antihypertensive drugs despite being associated with various biochemical changes (e.g., hypokalaemia, hyperglycaemia, and hyperuricaemia), most of which appear to be dose related (30). Greater sexual dysfunction is a common side effect, in particular in older hypertensive patients taking diuretics compared with placebo (31). Nonetheless, there seems to be general agreement that thiazides do not have marked adverse effects on cognitive function and behavior in hypertensive patients, as shown in studies which have reported no differences in mood, general sense of well-being, social activities, and recreation following diuretic treatment (31,32).

The results of the effects of diuretics on QoL in older hypertensive patients have not been as extensively published as for other types of antihypertensive agents. Thus, conclusions for this age group are not consistent. In some trials, this may in part result from low sensitivity of measures used to tap QoL domains. Trials of multiple

treatment which have compared the effects of different diuretics and diuretics in combination with a β-blocker, ACE inhibitor, or calcium channel blocker have shown identical results in QoL, irrespective of the use of thiazides at various QoL dosages, both lower and higher. A crossover comparison of 6 weeks treatment with HCTZ (25 mg) or clopamide (5 mg) in 17 patients with an average age of 62 years showed similar blood pressure control, plasma biochemical values, and well-being in a comprehensive QoL questionnaire in both treatment groups, despite a significantly expressed preference among patients for clopamide over HCTZ (33). A 1-year maintenance study in patients with mild and moderate hypertension who were receiving placebo or HCTZ (25 mg twice daily or 50 mg once or twice daily), or hydralazine, methyldopa, metoprolol, or reserpine in addition to a diuretic, showed similar improvements on psychometric tests designed to assess cognitive function, motor skills, memory and affect, both in patients whose blood pressure was treated and the placebo–control group (34). The study comprised people over 60 years of age, and the authors concluded that blood pressure reduction *per se* does not seem to affect cognitive and behavioral function in elderly hypertensives, despite the finding of some qualitative differences with respect to side effects between the treatment groups. A further trial that compared HCTZ and doxazosin, an α-1 antagonist, in 107 patients reported no significant differences in overall QoL between treatment groups, despite increased mental health and psychological well-being found in patients taking doxazosin from baseline, and improved energy and decreased fatigue levels in patients on HCTZ (35). However, addition of a diuretic (HCTZ) to three treatment groups (i.e., captopril, methyldopa, and propranolol) was associated with negative effects on various QoL measures in patients from the ages of 21 to 65 years in a 24-week trial. However, these subjects knew that their blood pressure was not well controlled and this may have had an adverse effect on their QoL (1). Given the limitations of short-term clinical trials, data from long-term trials is usually referenced as an indication of a low overall risk of side effects of diuretics and maintenance of QoL in hypertensive patients treated with these drugs.

2. β-Adrenergic Neurone Blockers

Improvements in symptoms, including reduction in anxiety, and other favorable changes in QoL have been reported in patients treated with β-adrenergic blocking drugs. New generation β-blockers show a more consistent enhancement of QoL, including fewer adverse symptoms (15). Propranolol administered to 212 hypertensive male patients with uncomplicated essential hypertension led to a deterioration in general well-being, physical symptoms and sexual dysfunction compared with those 213 receiving an ACE inhibitor over 24 weeks (1). Patients on propranolol showed more favorable changes in work performance than those on methyldopa. However, those on propranolol also had significantly more complaints about shortness of breath and slow heart beat than patients on methyldopa, and complaints of slow heart beat, shortness of breath, and fatigue than patients on captopril. Increased frequency of weak limbs and also headaches and slower walking pace have been reported following propranolol treatment in 47 patients compared with 47 receiving verapamil (36).

Three-hundred and six black patients were randomized to atenolol, captopril, or verapamil over an 8-week treatment period (37). The rate of withdrawal from therapy as a result of adverse effects was low and did not differ by drug treatment or titration level. QoL measures did not differ between the three groups. Vanmolkot et al. (38) did not find any differences in the health index status, total psychiatric morbidity, anxiety, depression, somatic symptoms, and hostility in subjects given bisoprolol (5 mg daily) compared with bendrofluazide (2.5 mg daily) administered to 81 patients for only 8 weeks in a double-blind, two-way crossover trial. The average age of participants was 61 years, with a mean duration of hypertension of 2.9 years. In a larger trial of 24 weeks, significant improvements in tension or anxiety, anger or hostility, vigor and activity, and confusion or bewilderment, as assessed by the Profile of Mood States (39), were found following administration of bisoprolol (5–10 mg) to 368 patients compared with nifedipine retard (40–80 mg) to 379 patients. HCTZ (25 mg) was added in both groups to reach goal pressure (40). There were no significant differences in QoL after 8 weeks of treatment. The SIP and objective tests of cognitive function did not differ statistically between the two groups, and QoL was maintained at a good level in both treatments, with advantages for bisoprolol in certain areas. These included a lower dropout rate and fewer side effects. In their discussion, which included a review of several trials, which had used the same or similar QoL instruments, the authors concluded that bisoprolol had advantages over nifedipine retard in symptomatic and psychological well-being. Some beneficial effects for β-blockers on QoL have also been reported in patients with ischemic heart disease, cardiac arrhythmias, and congestive heart failure (41).

3. Calcium Channel Blockers

High rates of ankle and pedal edema are found in open and double-blind trials following use of calcium channel blockers (42). Some studies show improvements in QoL parameters, and others tend to conclude an absence of adverse effects following reduction in blood pressure with calcium channel blockers (43–45).

In a 4-week clinical trial, 128 patients were randomized to diltiazem (120–360 mg) or metoprolol (50–200 mg as a daily dosage) (46). The authors concluded that diltiazem given as a monotherapy to hypertensive patients did not impair QoL. A study of nifedipine and amlodipine administered to older people during 16 weeks (30–60 and 5–10 mg once daily, respectively) found no significant differences in QoL between these treatments (47). However, nifedipine was associated with more adverse events and a higher discontinuation rate than cilazapril and atenolol in a 6-month, double-blind trial in 540 patients with an average age of 54 years (43). Flushing and edema were the adverse events more often cited as a reason for discontinuation of therapy in the nifedipine group. Coughing was more common with cilazapril, but fatigue was more commonly reported with atenolol (Table 22.4). Serious clinical events were uncommon.

The effects of low-dose, long-acting verapamil on 24 h ambulatory blood pressure and QoL were examined in hypertensive subjects over 60 years of age, in which 28 of whom received 120–240 mg once daily for 8 weeks and 28 received a placebo. As expected, patients treated with verapamil had a significantly lower mean whole-day blood pressure, but no differences were reported in QoL and digit span testing scores (48). Another small study compared verapamil and nifedipine retard in 81 patients with a mean age of 55 years, and it showed a significant increase in flushing and edema and a deterioration in the subjective cognitive score in the nifedipine group (49). A higher HRQoL with verapamil than propranolol treatment also

Table 22.4 The Cilazapril, Atenolol, Nifedipine Trial

Adverse event	Cilazapril ($n = 179$)	Atenolol ($n = 182$)	Nifedipine ($n = 179$)
Cough	11	3	4
Fatigue	7	19	7
Flushing	4	4	30
Headache	10	20	23
Edema	1	5	40
Palpitations—tachycardia	6	1	13
Vertigo	13	14	8
Total events (No)	161	194	242
Total patients with one or more events (No)	93	112	115
Total patients withdrawn due to events (No)	9	15	31

Note: Adverse events spontaneously reported by more than ten patients in any one treatment group.
Source: Adapted from Fletcher et al. (43).

was observed in patients followed up for a longer period (36).

Positive effects for felodipine extended-release (ER) on QoL were found for patients with stage 1 isolated systolic hypertension compared with placebo in a 1-year, double-blind, parallel-group multicenter trial in 171 patients (average age 66 years). Participants on felodipine scored significantly better on anxiety and depression, but not on indices of positive well-being, self-control, health, or total vitality (44). Although the study lacked power to show a significant difference in clinical events between treatments, adverse effects in patients treated with felodipine ER were similar in frequency compared with placebo. However, many authors agree that ankle swelling, headaches, and flushing are frequent side effects of calcium channel blockers. Moreover, compared with other classes of antihypertensive agents, the position of calcium channel blockers with respect to maintenance of QoL in hypertensive patients is uncertain (50–52).

4. ACE Inhibitors

ACE inhibitors are commonly recognized as one of the first-line choices for the treatment of hypertension, despite an increased risk of treatment-associated dry cough and, very rarely, angioedema. One of the earliest randomized double-blind trials on ACE inhibitors in hypertensive males (aged 21–65 years) aimed at determining the comparative effects of captopril, methyldopa, and propranolol on QoL (1) were discussed earlier. The trial showed that patients taking captopril had significantly higher scores on measures of general well-being, fewer adverse effects (i.e., lethargy, dry mouth, dizziness, nausea, and muscle cramps) and better work performance and life satisfaction scores than those on methyldopa. Patients on captopril reported fewer side effects, greater improvement in general well-being, and less sexual dysfunction compared with propranolol after 24 weeks of treatment (Table 22.5). No differences were observed in sleep function, visual memory, and social participation between the groups (1). One crossover trial of captopril and atenolol in 265 patients failed to detect any differences between the groups in QoL measures and concluded that important differences had been excluded (53).

A comparison between captopril and atenolol, propranolol, and enalapril in 360 men with mild to moderate hypertension failed to reveal any differences in QoL in psychometric measures between captopril, atenolol, and enalapril, but did detect a deterioration with propranolol after 4–8 weeks of therapy (54). There were no significant changes in cognitive function. One large trial compared the ACE inhibitor cilazapril with atenolol and nifedipine. The authors concluded that cilazapril and atenolol have equivalent effects on QoL, but nifedipine retard was associated with more symptomatic complaints and a higher discontinuation rate (43).

Reviews on the effects of ACE inhibitors in clinical trials have shown more beneficial or, at least, similar effects on QoL compared with other antihypertensive drugs (15). In particular, ACE inhibitors have been associated with a better QoL than patients receiving methyldopa, propranolol, or nifedipine. These groups do not necessarily represent

Table 22.5 The First Croog et al. Trial

Quality of life measure	Change in patients (%)			P-Value[a]
	Improvement	None	Worsening	
General well-being				
Captopril ($n = 181$)	51.4	17.7	30.9	
Methyldopa ($n = 143$)[b]	39.2	9.8	51.0	<0.01
Propranolol ($n = 161$)[b]	39.1	15.5	45.4	
Physical symptoms				
Captopril ($n = 181$)	29.3	45.3	25.4	
Methyldopa ($n = 142$)[b]	19.7	43.4	36.6	<0.05
Propranolol ($n = 160$)[b]	17.5	45.6	36.9	
Sexual dysfunction				
Captopril ($n = 181$)	18.2	63.0	18.8	
Methyldopa ($n = 141$)[b]	9.2	66.7	24.1	<0.05
Propranolol ($n = 160$)[b]	8.8	65.6	25.6	

[a]P-Value based on chi-square test (3×3) for independence with four degrees of freedom.
[b]Variations in the numbers of subjects in the methyldopa and propranolol treatment groups are due to incomplete responses to the assessment measures.
Note: Changes in quality of life measures in the three treatment groups.
Source: Reproduced with permission from Croog et al. (1). Copyright © 200x (1986) Massachusetts Medical Society.

their pharmacological drug classes. A multicenter, double-blind trial of amlodipine and enalapril in 461 patients, followed up for 52 weeks showed no differences in QoL parameters, tolerability of drugs, and reduction in the risk of coronary heart disease. The major side effects were cough with enalapril and edema with amlodipine, respectively (55). A double-blind, active control randomized trial in 57 Chinese hypertensives (mean age 53 years) showed that the ACE inhibitor captopril (25–50 mg twice daily) and imidapril (5–10 mg daily) given for 12 weeks, induced similarly significant improvements in the mental health component scores in the SF-36 scale from baseline. There were no differences between the two treatments in changes in blood pressure, withdrawal of patients from the study, and frequency of adverse events, despite border-line significance for increased drug-related coughing with captopril (56). However, there is currently no evidence that common side effects of ACE inhibitors (such as cough and sore throat), have a greater impact on QoL than those associated with newer β-blocker agents, namely atenolol (e.g., fatigue, cold fingers) or even calcium channel blockers such as verapamil (e.g., consti-pation). These three groups seemed to be the most effective antihypertensive agents leading to a better QoL and lower rates of discontinuation from therapy as a result of adverse effects in reviews of short-term clinical trials (15).

5. Angiotensin Receptor Blockers

ARBs produce a more complete blockade of the effects of angiotensin II through a combination of ACE-dependent and non-dependent pathways. They lack some of the effects of ACE inhibitors such as inhibition of bradykinin degradation (57). Patients who cannot tolerate ACE inhibi-tors appear to tolerate ARBs relatively well. However, the possibility that use of ARBs may lead to a reduction of morbidity and mortality in patients intolerant to ACE inhibitors is also recently being explored in clinical trials.

Short-term clinical trials have been conducted on the effects of ARBs on QoL. Telmisartan (20–80 mg) was at least as effective as enalapril (5 to 10–20 mg) in lower-ing blood pressure over a 24-h dosing interval, as deter-mined by ambulatory blood pressure monitoring (58) in a 26-week, double-blind, parallel-group trial in 275 patients aged over the age of 65 years who had mild-to-moderate hypertension. Both regimens were well toler-ated, although patients on enalapril had more than double the incidence of drug-related cough. QoL, as assessed by the SF-36, did not change in either group. Breeze et al. (59) included additional QoL measures related to anxiety, self-control, depression, general health, positive well-being, vitality, and incidence of dry persistent cough in hypertensive patients (aged 18 years and over) in a 26-week, double-blind trial following use of eprosar-tan and enalapril for 12 weeks, with the addition of a

thiazide, if needed, for the remaining 14 weeks. The study showed a small improvement in self-control and total psychological well-being scores in enalapril-treated patients, but the use of eprosartan was associated with sig-nificantly less coughing (60). Dahlof et al. (60) random-ized 898 patients to 50–100 mg of losartan, 50 mg of losartan with or without 12.5 mg of HCTZ or 5–10 mg of amlodipine. Dizziness was reported more frequently in patients who were taking the two losartan regimens, and discomfort and swollen ankles in the comparative group of patients taking amlodipine for 12 weeks. The incidence of drug-related adverse events and number of withdrawals from therapy were higher following amlodi-pine than losartan treatment. Similar results on tolerability and adverse reactions were observed in 140 patients, average age 65 years, with diastolic hypertension who were taking losartan with or without added HCTZ or, nifedipine gastro-intestinal therapeutic system during a 12-week, parallel-group trial. The regime with losartan alone or with added HCTZ showed similar efficacy to nife-dipine gastro-intestinal therapeutic system, with greater tol-erability and lesser symptoms of swollen ankles (61). The percentages of patients reaching goal blood pressure (dias-tolic blood pressure <90 mmHg) were comparable in the study, that is, 81% for losartan and 90% for nifedipine.

IV. PITFALLS, DANGERS, AND SIDE EFFECTS

The aim of treating hypertension is to "reduce cardiovas-cular morbidity and mortality by the least intrusive means possible" (62). However, the difficulty in so doing is the fact that for the majority of sufferers the disease has no impact on their HRQoL and all current antihyper-tensive treatments may have a negative impact on patient's HRQoL owing to varying degrees of side effects.

As mentioned earlier, there is a lack of a conceptualiz-ation of HRQoL, which contributes to the inconsistency in selecting the dimensions to be measured. However, this inconsistency may be attributed to the fact that each antihypertensive treatment has different side effects and mechanisms of action, resulting in the need to assess different dimensions and will have an influence on the choice of the instruments to be used. In any case, the choice of dimensions and instruments should happen within a perspective of a HRQL framework (20). It was the need to look at the relationship between the side effects of drug therapy and patient's adherence to treat-ment that generated the interest in the evaluation of HRQoL for patients receiving antihypertensive treatment (63). Patients sometimes discontinue therapy because of a single troublesome side effect such as: edema, cough, constipation, and within this context QoL instruments that can expose the important effects on patient's adherence are particularly relevant (63).

Another important issue that must be highlighted is that assessment of symptoms has been presented as equating to the measurement of HRQoL, and although a symptoms checklist is an important component of the outcome measures of drug intervention, especially considering the side effects of drug therapy, the assessment of HRQoL is much more complex. The choice of instruments also needs careful consideration, and the use of reliable, valid instruments, which evaluate HRQoL domains that are relevant to the patient and to intervention being assessed, is crucial (7). A review of 76 clinical trials looking at the validity, reliability, and QoL domains of instruments used in the evaluation of antihypertensive drug therapy (7) revealed that the information on the psychometric properties of the instruments used was usually inadequate, especially when the instruments used were created specifically for the study. In these cases, only 4% and 13% of the studies offered any information on reliability and validity of the instruments, respectively.

The success in treating hypertension relies on the patient's acceptance of the drug regimen, however, the reality is that although hypertension is a preventable condition and for which treatment is readily available, its management often appears inadequate. Studies in Europe and North America, cited by McInnes (4), have shown that only ~50% of hypertensive patients have their blood pressure controlled. Reasons for this apparent management failure are multifactorial, but nonadherence to treatment, usually caused by deterioration in the patient's QoL as a result of the side effects of the drug regimen, is a major contributor (63). About 50% of the patients who begin treatment for the main antihypertensive drugs, usually drop out of care within 6 months (64). However, as pointed out by McInnes (4), if we look at the evidence from long-term trials, such as the TOMHS, there was a reduction on the incidence of side effects after a 12-month period, so it seems that antihypertensive treatment is not unavoidably related to unfavorable experiences. Also, the findings from the trial revealed that side effects reported by the patients in the treatment group were not more frequent or severe than by those in the placebo group. Similarly, in the Hypertension Optimal Treatment (HOT) study (65), the incidence of side effects was low for the three target groups, also the improvement in well being was better for patients with the lower diastolic blood pressure, which demonstrates that it is possible to achieve blood pressure control without undesirable side effects even if the improvement may have been due to the patient's knowledge of their good pressure control (4).

The assessment of the factors that establish patients' acceptance of treatment is very complex and it has been suggested that the new terminology "concordance"

instead of adherence may better depict what is required for treatment acceptance. In practice, is not easy to assess patient's concordance with treatment and although there are various techniques, none have proven to be accurate (4). In the HOT trial, cited by McInnes (4), a recently developed electronic dispensing method was used to assess the patient's concordance with treatment. The results of a subset analysis showed that concordance was not affected by age or sex, and ~80% of the patients took their medication as prescribed, and no difference was found between groups of patients who reached goal blood pressure and those who did not. This is particularly interesting because it implies that the fact that goal blood pressure is not achieved may not be attributed exclusively to nonconcordance with treatment, but it is more likely due to a reluctance of physicians to increase treatment (4).

Although many clinical trials have investigated the effects of antihypertensive treatment on HRQoL, a recent review (20) of the literature described the process of amalgamating the findings from previous research as challenging, as the results were inconsistent due to the following limitations: a wide variety of instruments used and dimensions studied, small sample sizes, short to moderate duration, and not accounting for missing data. Because of these limitations, short-term trials have relatively low statistical power to test for differences between treatments. Within this context, comparisons are difficult to make for long-term clinical trials because the methods differ in terms of entry criteria, study population, endpoints, and the use of different instruments to assess HRQoL (12).

Another important point is that trials frequently exclude people over 80 years of age and include very few people under 50 years of age, which makes conclusions about the cost/benefit of treatments with antihypertensive agents relevant only to middle-aged and young elderly (2).

From the evidence accrued from clinical long-term trials mentioned earlier, there is no antihypertensive medication that decisively improves QoL, but on the other hand, apart from in the Syst-Eur trial, these medications do not cause any deterioration in QoL. However, in spite of the difficulties in assessing HRQoL, a review by Idler and Beyamini that is cited by Bremner (42) reported that self-rated health in 27 international studies was a strong independent predictor of morbidity and mortality, regardless of the various health status indicators and other covariates that predict mortality.

V. CONCLUSIONS

Mild to moderate hypertension is often asymptomatic and treatment usually is life long, therefore, the choice of drug regimen should not affect patient's well being. Within this context the assessment of HRQoL has become a very important variable in selecting which hypertensive therapy should be used.

A number of long and short-term clinical trials have addressed quality of life issues with different antihypertensives and the results have shown that these drugs are safe, well tolerated and efficacious, but overall they do not produce any significant improvement in HRQoL. In the meantime, ARBs, ACE inhibitors, and newer β-blockers and low-dose diuretics, have few, if any, adverse effects on HRQoL.

REFERENCES

1. Croog SH, Levine S, Testa MA, Brown B, Bulpitt CJ, Jenkins CD, Klerman GL, Williams GH. The effects of antihypertensive therapy on the quality of life. N Engl J Med 1986; 314:1657–1664.
2. Fletcher A, Bulpitt C. Determining the impact of antihypertensive drugs on quality of life. In: Kendall MJ, Kaplan NM, Horton RC, eds. Difficult Hypertension Practical Management and Decision Making. London: Martin Dunitz Publishers, 1995:249–261.
3. Staessen JA, Gasowski J, Wang JG, Thijs L, Den Hond E, Boissel JP, Coope J, Ekbom T, Gueyffier F, Liu L, Kerlikowske K, Pocock S, Fagard RH. Risks of untreated and treated isolated systolic hypertension in the elderly: meta-analysis of outcome trials. Lancet 2000; 355:885–872.
4. McInnes GT. Integrated approaches to management of hypertension: promoting treatment acceptance. Am Heart J 1999; 138:S252–S255.
5. Staessen JA, Wang G, Thijs L. Cardiovascular prevention and blood pressure reduction: a quantitative overview updated until 1 March 2003. J Hypertens 2003; 21:1055–1075.
6. Muldoon MF. What are quality of life measurements measuring? Brit Med J 1998; 316:542–545.
7. Gandhi SK, Kong SX. Quality-of-life measures in the evaluation of antihypertensive drug therapy: reliability, validity and quality-of-life domains. Clin Ther 1996; 18:1276–1295.
8. Sanders C, Egger M, Donavan J, Tallon D, Franked S. Reporting on quality of life in randomised controlled trials: Bibliographic study. Brit Med J 1998; 317:1191–1194.
9. Os I. Quality of life in hypertension. J Hum Hypertens 1994; 8(suppl 1):S27–S30.
10. Nunes MI. The relationship between quality of life and adherence to treatment. Curr Hypertens Rep 2001; 3:462–465.
11. James MA, Potter JF. The effect of antihypertensive treatment on the quality of later years. Drug Therapy 1993; 1:26–39.
12. Calman KC. Quality of life in cancer patients—an hypothesis. J Med Ethics 1984; 10:124–127.
13. McHorney CA. Health status methods assessments for adults: part accomplishments and future challenges. Annu Rev Public Health 1999; 20:309–335.
14. Hennessy CH, Moriarty DG, Zack MM, Scherr PA, Brackbill R. Measuring health-related quality of life for public health surveillance. Public Health Rep 1994; 109:665–672.
15. Bulpitt CJ, Fletcher AE. Quality of life evaluation of antihypertensive drugs. Pharmacoeconomics 1992; 2:95–102.
16. Kittler ME. Elderly hypertensives and quality of life: some methodological considerations. Eur Heart J 1994; 14:113–121.
17. Bulpitt CJ, Fletcher AE. Quality-of-life instruments in hypertension. Parmacoeconomics 1994; 6:523–535.
18. Slevin ML, Plant H, Lynch D, Drinkwater J, Gregory WM. Who should measure quality of life, the doctor or the patient? Br J Cancer 1988; 57:109–112.
19. Bulpitt CJ, Fletcher AE. The measurement of quality of life in hypertensive patients: a practical approach. Br J Clin Pharmacol 1990; 30:353–364.
20. Coyne KS, Davis D, Freech F, Hill MN. Health–related quality of life in patients treated for hypertension: a review of the literature from 1990 to 2000. Clin Ther 2002; 24:142–169.
21. Applegate WB. Quality of life during antihypertensive treatment. Lessons from the Systolic Hypertension in the Elderly Program. Am J Hypertens 1998; 11:57S–61S.
22. Applegate WB, Pressel S, Wittes J, Luhr J, Shekelle RB, Camel GH, Greenlick MR, Hadley E, Moye L, Perry HM Jr. Impact of hypertensive treatment of isolated systolic hypertension on behavioral variables. Results from the Systolic Hypertension in the Elderly Trial. Arch Intern Med 1994; 154:2154–2160.
23. Fletcher AE, Bulpitt CJ, Tuomilehto J, Browne J, Bossini A, Kawecka-Jaszcz K, Kivinen P, O'Brien E, Staessen J, Thijs L, Vanska O, Vanhanen H. Quality of life of elderly patients with isolated systolic hypertension: baseline data from the Syst Eur Trial. J Hypertens 1998; 16:1117–1124.
24. Staessen JA, Fagard R, Thijs L, Celis H, Arabidze GG, Birkenhager WH, Bulpitt CJ, de Leeuw PW, Dollery CT, Fletcher AE, Forette F, Leonetti G, Nachev C, O'Brien ET, Rosenfeld J, Rodicio JL, Tuomilehto J, Zanchetti A. Randomised double-blind comparison of placebo and active treatment for older patients with isolated systolic hypertension. The Systolic Hypertension in Europe (Syst-Eur) Trial Investigators. Lancet 1997; 350:757–764.
25. Fletcher AE, Bulpitt CJ, Thijs L, Tuomilehto J, Antikainen R, Bossini A, Browne J, Duggan J, Kawecka-Jaszcz K, Kivinen P, Sarti C, Terzoli L, Staessen JA; Syst-Eur Trial Investigators. Quality of life on randomised treatment for isolated systolic hypertension: results from the Syst-Eur Trial. J Hypertens 2002; 20:2069–2079.
26. Grimm RH Jr, Grandits GA, Cutler JA, Stewart AL, McDonald RH, Svendsen K, Prineas RJ, Liebson PR. Relationship of quality-of-life measures to long-term lifestyle and drug treatment in the treatment of mild hypertension study. Arch Intern Med 1997; 157:638–648.

27. Prince MJ, Bird AS, Blizard RA, Mann AH. Is the cognitive function of older patients affected by antihypertensive treatment? Results from 54 months of the Medical Research Council's treatment trial of hypertension in older adults. Brit Med J 1996; 312:801–805.

28. Ogihara T, Kuramoto K. Effect of long-term treatment with antihypertensive drugs on quality of life of elderly patients with hypertension: a double-blind comparative study between a calcium antagonist and a diuretic. NICS-EH Study Group. National Intervention Cooperative Study in Elderly Hypertensives. Hypertens Res 2000; 23:33–37.

29. Bulpitt C, Fletcher A, Beckett N, Coope J, Gil-Extremera B, Forette F, Nachev C, Potter J, Sever P, Staessen J, Swift C, Tuomilehto J. Hypertension in the Very Elderly Trial (HYVET): protocol for the Main Trial. Drugs Aging 2001; 18:151–164.

30. Fletcher A, Amery A, Birkenhager W, Bulpitt C, Clement D, de Leeuw P, Deruyterre ML, de Schaepdryver A, Dollery C, Fagard R. Risks and benefits in the trial of the European Working Party on High Blood Pressure in the Elderly. J Hypertens 1991; 9:225–230.

31. Chang SW, Fine R, Siegel D, Chesney M, Black D, Hulley SB. The impact of diuretic therapy on reported sexual function. Arch Intern Med 1991; 151:2402–2408.

32. McCorvey E Jr, Wright JT Jr, Culbert JP, McKenney JM, Proctor JD, Annett MP. Effect of hydrochlorothiazide, enalapril, and propranolol on quality of life and cognitive and motor function in hypertensive patients. Clin Pharm 1993; 12:300–305.

33. Hunter Hypertension Research Group. Well-being and its measurement in hypertension. A randomized, double-blind cross-over comparison of 5 mg clopamide with 25 mg hydrochlorothiazide. Clin Exp Hypertens A 1991; 13:189–195.

34. Goldstein G, Materson BJ, Cushman WC, Reda DJ, Freis ED, Ramirez EA, Talmers FN, White TJ, Nunn S, Chapman RH. Treatment of hypertension in the elderly: II. Cognitive and behavioral function. Results of a Department of Veterans Affairs Cooperative Study. Hypertension 1990; 15:361–369.

35. Grimm RH Jr, Flack JM, Schoenberger JA, Gonzalez NM, Liebson PR. α-blockade and thiazide treatment of hypertension. A double-blind randomized trial comparing doxazosin and hydrochlorothiazide. Am J Hypertens 1996; 9:445–454.

36. Fletcher AE, Chester PC, Hawkins CM, Latham AN, Pike LA, Bulpitt CJ. The effects of verapamil and propranolol on quality of life in hypertension. J Hum Hypertens 1989; 3:125–130.

37. Croog SH, Kong BW, Levine S, Weir MR, Baume RM, Saunders E. Hypertensive black men and women. Quality of life and effects of antihypertensive medications. Black Hypertension Quality of Life Multicenter Trial Group. Arch Intern Med 1990; 150:1733–1741.

38. Vanmolkot FH, de Hoon JN, van de Ven LL, Van Bortel LM. Impact of antihypertensive treatment on quality of life: comparison between bisoprolol and bendrofluazide. J Hum Hypertens 1999; 13:559–563.

39. McNair DM, Lorr M, Doppleman LF. Manual for the profile of mood states. San Diego: San Diego Educational and Industrial Testing Service, 1971.

40. Bulpitt CJ, Connor M, Schulte M, Fletcher AE. Bisoprolol and nifedipine retard in elderly hypertensive patients: effect on quality of life. J Hum Hypertens 2000; 14:205–212.

41. Prisant LM. Fixed low-dose combination in first-line treatment of hypertension. J Hypertens 2002; 20(suppl 1):S11–S19.

42. Bremner AD. Antihypertensive medication and quality of life—silent treatment of a silent killer? Cardiovasc Drugs Ther 2002; 16:353–364

43. Fletcher AE, Bulpitt CJ, Chase DM, Collins WC, Furberg CD, Goggin TK, Hewett AJ, Neiss AM. Quality of life with three antihypertensive treatments. Cilazapril, atenolol, nifedipine. Hypertension 1992; 19:499–507.

44. Black HR, Elliott WJ, Weber MA, Frishman WH, Strom JA, Liebson PR, Hwang CT, Ruff DA, Montoro R, DeQuattro V, Zhang D, Schleman MM, Klibaner MI. One-year study of felodipine or placebo for stage 1 isolated systolic hypertension. Hypertension 2001; 38:1118–1123.

45. Levine JH, Ferdinand KC, Cargo P, Laine H, Lefkowitz M. Additive effects of verapamil and enalapril in the treatment of mild to moderate hypertension. Am J Hypertens 1995; 8:494–499.

46. Dahlof C, Hedner T, Thulin T, Gustafsson S, Olsson SO. Effects of diltiazem and metoprolol on blood pressure, adverse symptoms and general well-being. The Swedish Diltiazem-Metoprolol Multi-Centre Study Group. Eur J Clin Pharmacol 1991; 40:453–460.

47. Pessina AC, Boari L, De Dominicis E, Giusti C, Marchesi M, Marelli G, Mattarei M, Mos L, Novo S, Pirrelli A, Santini M, Santonastaso M, Semeraro S, Uslenghi E, Kilama MO. Efficacy, tolerability and influence on "quality of life" of nifedipine GITS versus amlodipine in elderly patients with mild-moderate hypertension. Blood Press 2001; 10:176–183.

48. Neutel JM, Smith DH, Lefkowitz MP, Cargo P, Alemayehu D, Weber MA. Hypertension in the elderly: 24 h ambulatory blood pressure results from a placebo-controlled trial. J Hum Hypertens 1995; 9:723–727.

49. Palmer A, Fletcher A, Hamilton G, Muriss S, Bulpitt C. A comparison of verapamil and nifedipine on quality of life. Br J Clin Pharmacol 1990; 30:365–370.

50. Fletcher A, Bulpitt C. Quality of life in the treatment of hypertension. The effect of calcium antagonists. Drugs 1992; 44(suppl 1):135–140.

51. Os I, Bratland B, Dahlof B, Gisholt K, Syvertsen JO, Tretli S. Lisinopril and nifedipine in essential hypertension: a Norwegian multicenter study on efficacy, tolerability and quality of life in 828 patients. J Hypertens Suppl 1991; 9:S382–S383.

52. Hollenberg NK, Williams GH, Anderson R, Akhras KS, Bittman RM, Krause SL. Symptoms and the distress they cause: comparison of an aldosterone antagonist and a calcium channel blocking agent in patients with systolic hypertension. Arch Intern Med 2003; 163:1543–1548.

53. Palmer AJ, Fletcher AE, Rudge PJ, Andrews CD, Callaghan TS, Bulpitt CJ. Quality of life in hypertensives treated with atenolol or captopril: a double-blind crossover trial. J Hypertens 1992; 10:1409–1416.

54. Steiner SS, Friedhoff AJ, Wilson BL, Wecker JR, Santo JP. Antihypertensive therapy and quality of life: a comparison of atenolol, captopril, enalapril, and propranolol. J Hum Hypertens 1990; 4:217–225.

55. Omvik P, Thaulow E, Herland OB, Eide I, Midha R, Turner RR. A long-term, double-blind, comparative study on quality of life during treatment with amlodipine or enalapril in mild or moderate hypertensive patients: a multicentre study. Br J Clin Pract Suppl 1994; 73:23–30.

56. Chien KL, Huang PJ, Chen MF, Chiang FT, Lai LP, Lee YT. Assessment of quality of life in a double-blind, randomized clinical trial of imidapril and captopril for hypertensive Chinese in Taiwan. Cardiovasc Drugs Ther 2002; 16:221–226.

57. Unger T. The role of the renin–angiotensin system in the development of cardiovascular disease [Discussion 10A]. Am J Cardiol 2002; 89:3A–9A.

58. Karlberg BE, Lins LE, Hermansson K. Efficacy and safety of telmisartan, a selective AT1 receptor antagonist, compared with enalapril in elderly patients with primary hypertension. TEES Study Group. J Hypertens 1999; 17:293–302.

59. Breeze E, Rake EC, Donoghue MD, Fletcher AE. Comparison of quality of life and cough on eprosartan and enalapril in people with moderate hypertension. J Hum Hypertens 2001; 15:857–862.

60. Dahlof B, Lindholm LH, Carney S, Pentikainen PJ, Ostergren J. Main results of the losartan versus amlodipine (LOA) study on drug tolerability and psychological general well-being. LOA Study Group. J Hypertens 1997; 15:1327–1335.

61. Conlin PR, Elkins M, Liss C, Vrecenak AJ, Barr E, Edelman JM. A study of losartan, alone or with hydrochlorothiazide vs nifedipine GITS in elderly patients with diastolic hypertension. J Hum Hypertens 1998; 12:693–699.

62. The Sixth Report of the Joint National Committee on Prevention, Detection, Evaluation, and Treatment of High Blood Pressure. Arch Intern Med 1997; 314:1657–1664.

63. Testa MA. Methods and applications of quality-of-life measurement during antihypertensive therapy. Curr Hypertens Rep 2000; 2:530–537.

64. Williams GH. Assessing patient wellness: new perspectives on quality of life and compliance. Am J Hypertens 1998; 11:186S–191S.

65. Jones JK, Gorkin L, Lian JF, Staffa JA, Fletcher AP. Discontinuation of and changes in treatment after start of new course of antihypertensive drugs: a study of United Kingdom population. Brit Med J 1995; 311:293–295.

23

Management and Treatment Guidelines

DAVE C. Y. CHUA, GEORGE L. BAKRIS

Rush University Medical Center, Chicago, Illinois, USA

KEYPOINTS

- The blood pressure goal is <140/90 mmHg in all people with hypertension.
- Those with hypertension and either chronic kidney disease and/or diabetes have a blood pressure target of <130/80 mmHg.
- Selection of a blood pressure lowering agent in someone with proteinuria (>300 mg/day) should focus not only on achievement of BP target but also reduction in proteinuria.
- Initial lowering of BP within the first week post stroke needs to be done gingerly and should not be lowered beyond a systolic BP of 160–170 mmHg.
- Initiation of combination antihypertensive therapy should be done in all people who are >20 mmHg, systolic, above the respective goal.

SUMMARY

Use of antihypertensive medications with complementary mechanisms that have proven achievement of BP targets should be preferred initial agents. Physicians should focus on achievement of BP goals by using agents that are least intrusive (very few side effects).

I. INTRODUCTION

Treatment and management guidelines for hypertension have evolved since their inception in the 1970s. The primary purpose of guidelines was to establish a set of general principles that could be applied to the population at large to help reduce cardiovascular morbidity and mortality. However, over the past few decades they have become a sort of "holy grail" for some as the only way to do things. It should be remembered that, in general, the conclusions reached and statements made by such committees are derived from a combination of well designed, published, clinical trials, opinion, derived from experience and knowledge of the specific area and general gestalt. In the end, these ingredients are brought by each of the people on the committee and a consensus is reached and agreed to by all the members. Hence, guidelines are not the stone tablets on Mount Sinai but rather a set of general principles, subject to change over time as more data becomes available.

With that in mind, this chapter reviews the general guidelines in the Western world including those of the Seventh Joint National Committee on Prevention, Detection, Evaluation, and Treatment of High Blood Pressure (JNC-7), the American Diabetes Association, the National Kidney Foundation, the Canadian Guidelines, and the European Hypertension Guidelines. The review focuses on similarities and differences with regard to approach (1–5).

II. COMPARISON OF GUIDELINES FOR MANAGEMENT

In general, all guidelines have a number of principles in common; these are summarized in Table 23.1.

A. Approaches to Treatment

The focus of blood pressure (BP) lowering should be to prevent or reduce the risk of cardiovascular and renal events. To that end, the JNC-7 has tried to alert both patients and physicians to the risks of even small elevations in BP. Individuals with prehypertension defined by a systolic BP of >120 and <140 mmHg should receive lifestyle modifications unless they have diabetes or kidney disease. If either of these conditions is present, treatment with pharmacological agents should be initiated at BP 130/80 mmHg. In all situations, if there is a "compelling indication" for the use of a specific type of antihypertensive drug, it should be utilized, Table 23.2. The reason for a compelling indication is that the drug recommended has been shown in clinical trials to markedly reduce the risk of a specific event(s) in a given disease, such as angiotensin receptor blockers, in diabetic nephropathy (1).

The staging of BP beyond this range remains similar among all guidelines and is divided by 20 mmHg increments in systolic BP and 10 mmHg increments in diastolic BP, as represented by the JNC-7 in Table 23.3. Patients with stage 1 hypertension should receive lifestyle modifications and pharmacologic therapy beginning with a thiazide-type diuretic, if appropriate; unless goal BP is achieved without drugs (1). Patients with confirmed JNC-7, stage 2 hypertension should be strongly considered for initiation with two different antihypertensive medications usually in combination (Tables 23.3 and 23.4).

Table 23.1 Common Principles and Differences Among Various Guidelines

Similarities

  All emphasize achievement of a specific BP goal (<140 mmHg, in the general population and, <130/80 mmHg, if diabetes or chronic kidney disease is present).
  All support use of two or more agents if BP not achieved after reasonable dose adjustment of a single agent.
  All focus on reduction of cardiovascular morbidity and mortality as an endpoint of BP reduction.
  All focus on special populations and specific goals, if any, in those groups.
  All emphasize lifestyle intervention.

Differences

  Definitions of risk for various BP levels differ, especially at the lower end of the scale (pre-hypertension, JNC-7 and other guidelines).
  Approaches to care: although all support use of ACE-Is or angiotensin receptor blockers for those with kidney disease or diabetes and β-blockers for those with CAD, the JNC-7 specifically supports thiazide diuretics as initial agents for achieving goal in most people in the general population, defined as those >55 years of age.

Table 23.2 Clinical Trial and Guideline Basis for Compelling Indications for Individual Drug Classes

Compelling indication[a]	Recommended drugs[b]						Clinical trial basis[c]
	Diuretic	BB	ACE-I	ARB	CCB	Aldo ANT	
Heart failure	•	•	•	•		•	ACC/AHA Heart Failure Guideline, MERIT-HF, COPERNICUS, CIBIS SOLVD, AIRE, TRACE, Val HEFT, RALES, CHARM
Post myocardial infarction		•	•			•	ACC/AHA Post-MI Guideline, BHAT, SAVE, Capricorn, EPHESUS
High coronary disease risk	•	•	•		•		ALLHAT, HOPE, ANBP2, LIFE, CONVINCE, EUROPA, INVEST
Diabetes	•	•	•	•	•		NKF-ADA Guideline, (1) UKPDS, ALLHAT
Chronic kidney disease			•	•			NKF Guideline, Captopril Trial, RENAAL, IDNT, REIN, AASK
Recurrent stroke prevention	•		•				PROGRESS

[a]Compelling indications for antihypertensive drugs are based on benefits from outcome studies or existing clinical guidelines; the compelling indication is managed in parallel with the BP.
[b]Drug abbreviations: BB, β-blocker; ACE-I, angiotensin converting enzyme inhibitor; ARB, angiotensin receptor blocker; CCB, calcium channel blocker; Aldo ANT, aldosterone antagonist.
[c]Conditions for which clinical trials demonstrate benefit of specific classes of antihypertensive drugs used as part of an antihypertensive regimen to achieve BP goal to test outcomes.
Note: A dot in the box means this class of drugs was tested as part of an armamentarium of BP lowering drugs in the given condition. It was shown to reduce either CV events or in the case of kidney disease presence, progression of nephropathy.
Source: Modified from the JNC-7 guidelines (1).

B. Lifestyle Modifications

All guideline statements highlight the need for lifestyle intervention as a primary mode of lowering BP although the adherence and compliance with such measures outside of formal trials has been unsatisfying. This section will briefly highlight the high points of controlled studies on BP of effects of lifestyle modification, which are summarized in Table 23.5.

Most guideline reports recommend weight loss for obese hypertensive patients, modification of dietary sodium intake to ≤ 100 mmol/day (2.4 g sodium or 6.0 g sodium chloride), and modification of alcohol intake to no more than two drinks per day (1,6). In addition, they

Table 23.3 Stages of BP, Risk Stratification, and Treatment Approach

	SBP[a] (mmHg)	DBP[a] (mmHg)	Lifestyle modification	Risk-stratified drug choices	
				No condition specific indication other than hypertension	Other condition specific indications
Normal	<120	OR <80	—		
Prehypertension	120–139	OR 80–89	Yes	No antihypertensive drug indicated	Drug(s) for compelling indications[b]
Hypertension					
Stage 1	140–159	OR 90–99	Yes	To be discussed—three options provided subsequently	Appropriate drug therapy for compelling indication[b] and diuretic
Stage 2	≥160	OR ≥100	Yes	Initiate two drugs for most[c]: diuretic + one of either ACE-I, ARB, BB, or CCB	

[a]Treatment determined by highest BP category.
[b]Compelling indications (Table 23.2).
[c]Consider two drugs or low dose fixed dose therapy (caution in brittle elderly).
Source: Adapted from the JNC-7 (1).

Table 23.4 Fixed-Dose Combination Antihypertensive Drugs

Combination type[a]	Fixed-dose combination[b] (mg)	US trade name
ACE-Is and CCBs	Amlodipine-benazepril hydrochloride (2.5/10, 5/10, 5/20, 10/20)	Lotrel
	Enalapril-felodipine (5/5)	Lexxel
	Trandolapril-verapamil (2/180, 1/240, 2/240, 4/240)	Tarka
ACE-Is and diuretics	Benazepril-hydrochlorothiazide (5/6.25, 10/12.5, 20/12.5, 20/25)	Lotensin HCT
	Captopril-hydrochlorothiazide (25/15, 25/25, 50/15, 50/25)	Capozide
	Enalapril-hydrochlorothiazide (5/12.5, 10/25)	Vaseretic
	Fosinopril-hydrochlorothiazide (10/12.5, 20/12.5)	Monopril/HCT
	Lisinopril-hydrochlorothiazide (10/12.5, 20/12.5, 20/25)	Prinzide, Zestoretic
	Moexipril-hydrochlorothiazide (7.5/12.5, 15/25)	Uniretic
	Quinapril-hydrochlorothiazide (10/12.5, 20/12.5, 20/25)	Accuretic
ARBs and diuretics	Candesartan-hydrochlorothiazide (16/12.5, 32/12.5)	Atacand HCT
	Eprosartan-hydrochlorothiazide (600/12.5, 600/25)	Teveten-HCT
	Irbesartan-hydrochlorothiazide (150/12.5, 300/12.5)	Avalide
	Losartan-hydrochlorothiazide (50/12.5, 100/25)	Hyzaar
	Olmesartan medoxomil-hydrochlorothiazide (20/12.5,40/12.5,40/25)	Benicar HCT
	Telmisartan-hydrochlorothiazide (40/12.5, 80/12.5)	Micardis-HCT
	Valsartan-hydrochlorothiazide (80/12.5, 160/12.5, 160/25)	Diovan-HCT
BBs and diuretics	Atenolol-chlorthalidone (50/25, 100/25)	Tenoretic
	Bisoprolol-hydrochlorothiazide (2.5/6.25, 5/6.25, 10/6.25)	Ziac
	Metoprolol-hydrochlorothiazide (50/25, 100/25)	Lopressor HCT
	Nadolol-bendroflumethiazide (40/5, 80/5)	Corzide
	Propranolol LA-hydrochlorothiazide (40/25, 80/25)	Inderide LA
	Timolol-hydrochlorothiazide (10/25)	Timolide
Centrally acting drug and diuretic	Methyldopa-hydrochlorothiazide (250/15, 250/25, 500/30, 500/50)	Aldoril
	Reserpine-chlothalidone (0.125/25, 0.25/50)	Demi-Regroton, Regroton
	Reserpine-chlorothiazide (0.125/250, 0.25/500)	Diupres
	Reserpine-hydrochlorothiazide (0.125/25, 0.125/50)	Hydropres
Diuretic and diuretic	Amiloride-hydrochlorothiazide (5/50)	Moduretic
	Spironolactone-hydrochlorothiazide (25/25, 50/50)	Aldactazide
	Triamterene-hydrochlorothiazide (37.5/25, 75/50)	Dyazide, Maxzide

[a]Drug abbreviations: BB, β-blocker; ACE-I, angiotensin converting enzyme inhibitor; ARB, angiotensin receptor blocker; CCB, calcium channel blocker.
[b]Some drug combinations are available in multiple fixed doses. Each drug dose is reported in milligrams.
Source: Adapted from the JNC-7 (1).

also recommend an increase in physical activity for all patients with hypertension who have no specific condition that would make such a recommendation not applicable or safe (7). For many patients, however, these suggestions are not feasible or already are being implemented; therefore, drug therapy may be indicated even sooner in these situations.

Three recent studies have combined the two most successful lifestyle modifications (weight loss and Na$^+$ restriction) in prospective, randomized, and well-controlled trials (8–10). The shortest was the PREMIER Clinical Trial that randomized 810 adults with BPs between 120–159 and 80–95 mmHg to one of three intervention groups. After a period of 6 months, those who received a behavioral intervention with exercise, weight loss, and sodium restriction reduced BP by 3.7/1.7 mmHg; $P < 0.001/0.002$, compared with an "advice

only" group. Individuals who received advice about the Dietary Approaches to Stop Hypertension (DASH) diet in addition to their behavioral intervention had an even greater fall in BP (4.3/2.6 mmHg; $P < 0.001/0.001$) (9).

In an earlier, but longer term trial, the Trials of Hypertension Prevention-2 (TOHP-2) studied the value of weight loss and Na$^+$ restriction in a 2×2 factorial design against usual care (10). At 6 months, the group assigned to both Na$^+$ reduction and weight loss did the best (BP fell 4.0/2.8 mmHg, with usual care subtracted), whereas those receiving a single modality did not experience as much of a BP reduction (3.7/2.7 mmHg for the weight loss only group, 2.9/1.6 mmHg for the Na$^+$ reduction only group, also usual care subtracted). During the 3 year follow-up, however, BP reductions were greatly attenuated; the combined treatment had a BP reduction of only 1.1/0.6 mmHg. This finding highlights

Table 23.5 Summary of Lifestyle Modifications to Prevent and Manage Hypertension[a]

Modification	Recommendation	Approximate SBP reduction (range)[b]
Weight reduction	Maintain normal body weight (body mass index 18.5–24.9 kg/m^2)	5–20 mmHg/10 kg
Adopt DASH eating plan	Consume a diet rich in fruits, vegetables, and low-fat dairy products with a reduced content of saturated and total fat	8–14 mmHg (74)
Dietary sodium reduction	Reduce dietary sodium intake to no >100 mmol/day (2.4 g sodium or 6 g sodium chloride)	2–8 mmHg (74)
Physical activity	Engage in regular aerobic physical activity such as brisk walking (at least 30 min/day, most days of the week)	4–9 mmHg
Moderation of alcohol consumption	Limit consumption to no more than two drinks; (e.g., 24 oz beer, 10 oz wine, or 3 oz 80-proof whiskey) per day in most men and to no more than one drink per day in women and lighter weight persons	2–4 mmHg

[a]For overall cardiovascular risk reduction, stop smoking.
[b]The effects of implementing these modifications are dose and time dependent and could be greater for some individuals.
Note: DASH, Dietary approaches to stop hypertension.
Source: Adapted from JNC-7 (1).

another difficulty with lifestyle modifications; the high recidivism rate seen in virtually all long-term studies.

A second long-term, randomized, and well-controlled study directly assessing the value of lifestyle modifications was the Trial of Nonpharmacologic Interventions in the Elderly (TONE) (8). This study also evaluated the efficacy of weight loss and Na$^+$ reduction, but in a different population and with a somewhat different objective. Only hypertensive patients 60–80 years of age were enrolled, and all were already taking single-drug pharmacologic treatment. The objective of TONE was to see whether the imposition of a formal lifestyle approach, again taught by highly trained professionals, would allow hypertensives to stay healthy and go off their medications. The results were equally disappointing. After 30 months when the study ended, 44% of the actively treated subjects were able to stay well without antihypertensive drugs when compared with 38% of those not receiving active lifestyle modifications. Although this was statistically significant ($P < 0.001$), it means that 56% of successfully treated hypertensives needed to resume drug therapy, even when given the best possible lifestyle regimen available administered by experts.

The value of alcohol reduction and consumption on BP has been addressed in a number of studies (11,12). A reduction in alcohol intake to two drinks per day, from five to six drinks, markedly reduces the BP (1). A recent meta-analysis of trials of alcohol reduction on BP concluded that the effect size is smaller than weight reduction, dietary sodium restriction, and physical activity, but is statistically significant ~2.5–4.0/0.9–1.2 mmHg (13).

Appel et al. (14) showed in the DASH trial that a diet rich in fruit and vegetables lowered BP by 2.8/1.1 mmHg more

than did the control diet. The fruit and vegetable diet was designed to contain K$^+$ and Mg^{2+} at the 75th percentile of the usual American diet, whereas the control diet was at the 25th percentile. The "combination" diet also contained foods rich in Ca^{2+} and was lower in total and saturated fat content, lowering BP by 5.5/3.0 mmHg more than did the control diet. In hypertensive subjects in DASH ($n = 133$ of 459), the BP reduction was impressive (11.4/5.5 mmHg). Although this study was only 8 weeks short and may not be generalizable to the population as it was carried out in four centers with special expertise, this approach offers great promise for using nutritional management to prevent hypertension in individuals with high-normal BP. The DASH diet provides high amounts of K$^+$, Mg^{2+}, and Ca^{2+} in the food eaten, not as supplements, and also limits the dietary fat and saturated fat intake. Even more impressive results were obtained in the DASH-Sodium Study (15). Those who received the low-salt control diet also had a very significant 6.7/2.5 mmHg lower BP than those randomized to the high-salt control diet; for the DASH diet, the difference was smaller, 3.0/1.6 mmHg. Further studies done over longer periods in a less highly selected cohort will be needed to verify these results and determine whether the DASH and/or DASH-sodium diets will be valuable therapeutic tools for the general population.

All recommendations for lifestyle modifications include smoking cessation and tobacco avoidance (1,16). The reason for inclusion of this recommendation was improvement of CV health, rather than proven direct relationship between smoking and hypertension. No direct relationship between smoking and BP has been demonstrated in epidemiologic studies; of note, BP is lower in smokers than in nonsmokers (17). It is now clear, however, that cigarette smoking increases BP and HR transiently (~15 min) and this effect is gone by 30 min. This mediated via an increase in catecholamine secretion induced by smoking. As the authors recommend that office readings be taken no sooner than 30 min after smoking or caffeine ingestion (another substance that transiently raises BP), one may very well miss the elevation of BP caused by smoking if it is measured when the patient has not smoked. Indeed, ABPM studies have shown that smokers have significantly higher BP on days when they smoke compared with days when they do not (18).

Perhaps, the most important long-term clinical trial that included lifestyle modifications as a randomized choice was the Treatment of Mild Hypertension Study (TOMHS) (19). This study compared five classes of antihypertensive agents (diuretics, CAs, ACE-inhibitors (Is), α-blockers, and β-blockers) to placebo in middle-aged subjects with only minimal elevations of BP (average BP of 140/91 mmHg when the study started) and superimposed these pharmacologic treatments on a comprehensive lifestyle regimen that included weight loss, Na^+ restriction, alcohol reduction, and exercise. One arm of the study received lifestyle modifications and a placebo (i.e., no drug therapy). In TOMHS, the nutritional advice and the exercise program were monitored by certified nutritionists and trained exercise physiologists. Subjects were seen frequently in both group and individual sessions. The placebo group reduced BP from 140/91 to 132/82 mmHg (a reduction of 9.1/8.6 mmHg) and sustained that level for the 4.4 years of study follow-up, even though the reduction in Na^+ intake, amount of weight loss, and increase in exercise diminished over time. Perhaps, the most important finding in TOMHS was the statistically significantly fewer number of CV events ($P < 0.03$), in the group given pharmacologic treatment plus lifestyle modifications, compared with those who received no active drug. Those who received drug therapy, in aggregate, achieved an average BP of 125/79 mmHg, a reduction of 16/12 mmHg. Even though the lifestyle modifications were successful in reducing BP, the group given drugs had significantly fewer CV events, probably because their BP was lower. The inevitable conclusion from this trial is that even successful lifestyle modifications that bring BP to goal do not reduce morbidity and probably mortality as well as the combination of drugs and therapeutic lifestyle changes that lower BP even further.

The lack of proof for lifestyle modifications to reduce CV events does not mean that physicians should abandon nondrug treatments. The suggested lifestyle changes may well prevent or delay the virtually inevitable rise in BP that occurs especially in those over age 40 who are prehypertensive (systolic BP > 120 < 139 mmHg).

These recommendations also apply to many hypertensives who will be able potentially to reduce BP further than might be achieved with drugs alone.

C. Therapeutic Approaches

The ultimate goal of hypertension treatment is to reduce cardiovascular and renal morbidity and mortality; the short-term goal is to achieve the recommended goal BP by using the least intrusive means possible. Intrusive has several interpretations: economic, office visits, adverse effects, and convenience. The choice of the drug with which to begin therapy is probably the most important decision, the clinician must make when treating hypertensive patients. Approximately, one-third of patients will respond to the first choice and can tolerate most rational options. The remainder, however, will need additional or different treatment. The "preferred" first-line antihypertensive drug class for most patients has now been defined by data from clinical trials (1).

D. Classification of Antihypertensive Agents

Antihypertensive agents are classified by pharmacologic class and their defined primary mechanism of action, Table 23.6. There are more than 100 effective antihypertensive drugs and 50 fixed-dose combinations from which to choose, Table 23.4 (1).

1. Surrogate vs. Clinical Endpoints

Physicians should no longer be willing to simply look at the degree of BP reduction when making the choice about antihypertensive therapy. Clinical endpoints are the events that physicians are ultimately trying to prevent in treating hypertension. The so-called surrogate (or intermediate) endpoints are factors that may contribute to clinical endpoints and can be affected either favorably or unfavorably by treatment. Some surrogate endpoints do not correlate well with mortality/morbidity endpoints, such as changes in serum lipid values or glucose or cholesterol changes (20). BP reduction is a surrogate or intermediate endpoint, because the primary purpose for treating hypertension is to reduce the morbidity and mortality associated with elevated BP and not simply to lower BP. Data from large, prospective clinical trials designed to evaluate the ability of a drug to reduce hypertension-related CV events as well as or better than an otherwise reasonably alternative drug are the most reliable means to use in choosing from among the, otherwise, bewildering number of options.

Table 23.6 Oral Antihypertensive Drugs[a]

Class	Drug (Trade name)	Usual dose range in mg/day	Usual daily frequency[a]
Thiazide diuretics	Chlorothiazide (Diuril)	125–500	1–2
	Chlorthalidone (generic)	12.5–25	1
	Hydrochlorothiazide (Microzide, HydroDIURIL[b])	12.5–50	1
	Polythiazide (Renese)	2–4	1
	Indapamide (Lozol[b])	1.25–2.5	1
	Metolazone (Mykrox)	0.5–1.0	1
	Metolazone (Zaroxolyn)	2.5–5	1
Loop diuretics	Bumetanide (Bumex[b])	0.5–2	2
	Furosemide (Lasix[b])	20–80	2
	Torsemide (Demadex[b])	2.5–10	1
Potassium-sparing diuretics	Amiloride (Midamor[b])	5–10	1–2
	Triamterene (Dyrenium)	50–100	1–2
Aldosterone receptor blockers	Eplerenone (Inspra)	50–100	1
	Spironolactone (Aldactone[b])	25–50	1
BBs	Atenolol (Tenormin[b])	25–100	1
	Betaxolol (Kerlone[b])	5–20	1
	Bisoprolol (Zebeta[b])	2.5–10	1
	Metoprolol (Lopressor[b])	50–100	1–2
	Metoprolol extended release (Toprol XL)	50–100	1
	Nadolol (Corgard[b])	40–120	1
	Propranolol (Inderal[b])	40–160	2
	Propranolol long-acting (Inderal LA[b])	60–180	1
	Timolol (Blocadren[b])	20–40	2
BBs with intrinsic sympathomimetic activity	Acebutolol (Sectral[b])	200–800	2
	Penbutolol (Levatol)	10–40	1
	Pindolol (generic)	10–40	2
Combined α- and β-blockers	Carvedilol (Coreg)	12.5–50	2
	Labetalol (Normodyne, Trandate[b])	200–800	2
ACE-Is	Benazepril (Lotensin[b])	10–40	1
	Captopril (Capoten[b])	25–100	2
	Enalapril (Vasotec[b])	5–40	1–2
	Fosinopril (Monopril)	10–40	1
	Lisinopril (Prinivil, Zestril[b])	10–40	1
	Moexipril (Univasc)	7.5–30	1
	Perindopril (Aceon)	4–8	1
	Quinapril (Accupril)	10–80	1
	Ramipril (Altace)	2.5–20	1–2
	Trandolapril (Mavik)	1–4	1
Angiotensin II antagonists	Candesartan (Atacand)	8–32	1
	Eprosartan (Teveten)	400–800	1–2
	Irbesartan (Avapro)	150–300	1
	Losartan (Cozaar)	25–100	1–2
	Olmesartan (Benicar)	20–40	1
	Telmisartan (Micardis)	20–80	1
	Valsartan (Diovan)	80–320	1–2
CCBs-non-DHPs	Diltiazem extended release (Cardizem CD, Dilacor XR, Tiazac[b])	180–420	1
	Diltiazem extended release (Cardizem LA)	120–540	1
	Verapamil immediate release (Calan, Isoptin[b])	80–320	2

(*continued*)

Table 23.6 *Continued*

Class	Drug (Trade name)	Usual dose range in mg/day	Usual daily frequency[a]
	Verapamil long acting (Calan SR, Isoptin SR[b])	120–480	1–2
	Verapamil—Coer, Covera HS, Verelan PM	120–360	1
CCBs-DHPs	Amlodipine (Norvasc)	2.5–10	1
	Felodipine (Plendil)	2.5–20	1
	Isradipine (Dynacirc CR)	2.5–10	2
	Nicardipine sustained release (Cardene SR)	60–120	2
	Nifedipine long-acting (Adalat CC, Procardia XL)	30–60	1
	Nisoldipine (Sular)	10–40	1
α-1 blockers	Doxazosin (Cardura)	1–16	1
	Prazosin (Minipress[b])	2–20	2–3
	Terazosin (Hytrin)	1–20	1–2
Central α-2 agonists and	Clonidine (Catapres[b])	0.1–0.8	2
other centrally acting drugs	Clonidine patch (Catapres-TTS)	0.1–0.3	1 weekly
	Methyldopa (Aldomet[b])	250–1000	2
	Reserpine (generic)	0.1–0.25	1
	Guanfacine (Tenex[b])	0.5–2	1
Direct vasodilators	Hydralazine (Apresoline[b])	25–100	2
	Minoxidil (Loniten[b])	2.5–80	1–2

[a]In some patients treated once daily, the antihypertensive effect may diminish toward the end of the dosing interval (trough effect). BP should be measured just prior to dosing to determine if satisfactory BP control is obtained. Accordingly, an increase in dosage or frequency may need to be considered. These dosages may vary from those listed in the "Physicians' Desk Reference, 57th ed."
[b]Available now or soon to become available in generic preparations.
Source: Physicians' Desk Reference. Medical Economics. 57th ed. New Jersey: Oradell, 2003.

E. An Approach to Treatment

A general approach to achieve BP goals has been put forth by all guideline committees. A summary paradigm for those with kidney disease or diabetes is shown in Fig. 23.1. Otherwise, a paradigm put forth by the JNC-7 is certainly appropriate for people age 50 or older, Table 23.3. In younger populations, a recent meta-analysis clearly demonstrates that use of any antihypertensive drug class lowers cardiovascular risk as long as it achieves BP goals (21).

III. SPECIFIC INDICATIONS FOR PHARMACOLOGICAL AGENTS: COMPELLING INDICATIONS

All guidelines recognize that hypertensive patients often present with concomitant illnesses or conditions that benefit from therapy with specific antihypertensive drugs. Agents used to lower BP with such conditions have been derived from clinical trials and are shown in Table 23.2.

A. Efficacy vs. Placebo in Preventing Events

Prior to 1997, only initial diuretics and β-blockers have been shown to reduce morbidity and mortality in clinical

trials against placebo in hypertension. Dihydropyridine calcium antagonists (DHPCA) were later added to this list after the Syst-EUR trial was completed (22). This trial used the DHPCA, nitrendipine, followed by enalapril (or captopril), and then hydrochlorothiazide (if needed) to get BP to goal. An initial ACE-I ($\pm$ diuretic) was more effective than an initial placebo (or two) for reducing CV events in the perindopril pROtection aGainst REcurrent Stroke Study (PROGRESS) (23). An initial ARB was more effective in preventing a composite renal endpoint than an initial placebo in both the Irbesartan Diabetic Nephropathy Trial (IDNT) and the Reduction of Endpoints in Noninsulin Dependent Diabetes Mellitus with the Angiotensin II Antagonist Losartan (RENAAL) studies (24,25). For stroke risk reduction, initial treatment with a β-blocker was significantly more effective than placebo/no treatment in preventing only stroke; a similar conclusion was reached in an earlier and smaller meta-analysis of trials involving only older patients (21).

B. Efficacy of Different Classes of Initial Drugs in Preventing Events

Only a very important few of the recent clinical trials about different initial antihypertensive treatments involving

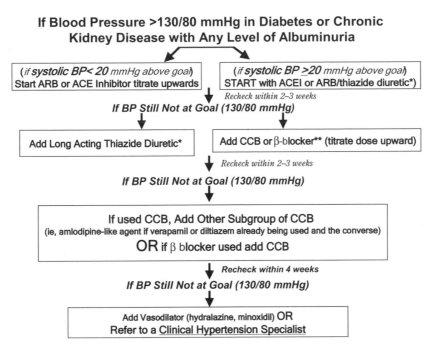

If Blood Pressure >130/80 mmHg in Diabetes or Chronic Kidney Disease with Any Level of Albuminuria

(*if systolic BP< 20* mmHg above goal)
Start ARB or ACE Inhibitor titrate upwards

(*if systolic BP ≥20* mmHg above goal)
START with ACEI or ARB/thiazide diuretic*)

Recheck within 2–3 weeks

If BP Still Not at Goal (130/80 mmHg)

Add Long Acting Thiazide Diuretic*

Add CCB or β-blocker** (titrate dose upward)

Recheck within 2–3 weeks

If BP Still Not at Goal (130/80 mmHg)

If used CCB, Add Other Subgroup of CCB
(ie, amlodipine-like agent if verapamil or diltiazem already being used and the converse)
OR if β blocker used add CCB

Recheck within 4 weeks

If BP Still Not at Goal (130/80 mmHg)

Add Vasodilator (hydralazine, minoxidil) **OR**
Refer to a <u>Clinical Hypertension Specialist</u>

Figure 23.1 Algorithm for treating patients with diabetes or kidney disease to goal BP of <130/80 mmHg. This figure represents an integration of the National Kidney Foundation-BP, JNC-7 and American Diabetes Association guidelines. *Refers to thiazide-type diuretics, specifically chlorthalidone as this is the agent used in the majority of outcome trials showing benefit of diuretics. Note use of two different subclasses of CAs well documented to have additive/synergistic effects on BP lowering (55,79).

ACE-Is or CAs showed significant differences between initial drug strategies in preventing major adverse CV events. To summarize these data, many meta-analyses have been published (21). A recent paper suggested a slight benefit with CAs on stroke, but an increased risk for MI and HF (22). Perhaps most importantly, this paper also contains the results of a meta-regression analysis across 27 trials involving 136,124 patients, suggesting that the differences among the drug classes could be easily explained by achieved differences in systolic BP.

The major problem with the interpretation of large clinical trials involving comparisons across drug classes involves the attribution of the observed difference(s) in endpoints. When there are differences in achieved BPs across randomized groups, most authors attribute this to an inferiority of the drug, rather than its BP-lowering ability, as the "cause" of the poor results. Fairer and easier comparisons result when the BP-lowering effect is equivalent across randomized treatments. When a particular strategy starting with a specific drug is found to be inferior (in either BP-lowering efficacy or CV endpoints) to another, we can more easily adopt the strategy with better results. Five clinical trials are of special interest because of their size and importance of findings. In the Second Australian National Blood Pressure Trial, an initial ACE-I was not significantly better in preventing the first cardiovascular event or death when compared with an initial diuretic (26). An initial ARB (±diuretic) was superior to an initial β-blocker (±diuretic) in patients

with left venticular hypertrophy (LVH) for reducing major cardiovascular events in the Losartan Intervention For Endpoint reduction (LIFE) trial, although the group given losartan had both lower systolic BP and a major reduction in stroke, but not in CHD events or death (27). Two separate trials with a combined participant cohort of over 38,000 dealt with the issue of noninferiority in CV outcomes between a β-blocker and a non-DHPCA, verapamil. The Controlled ONset Verapamil INvestigation of Cardiovascular Endpoints (CONVINCE) trial was stopped prematurely, and failed to demonstrate "equivalence" for a regimen beginning with a novel formulation of verapamil to a traditional regimen beginning with the physician's choice of either a diuretic or a β-blocker (28). The International verapamil/trandolapril Study (INVEST) looked at over 22,000 participants with hypertension and documented coronary artery disease (CAD) and found after a mean follow-up of 2.7 years that no difference in CV outcomes existed between initial therapy with verapamil vs. atenolol (29). Moreover, the incidence of new-onset diabetes was significantly lower in the verapamil group.

Perhaps most importantly, the recent ALLHAT study directly compared the thiazide-like diuretic, chlorthalidone, with three newer antihypertensive drugs: amlodipine (a CA), doxazosin (an α-blocker), and lisinopril (an ACE-I). The doxazosin arm was stopped early, as it showed a significant increase (compared with the diuretic) in CVD, an endpoint that included CHD, heart failure, and peripheral arterial disease (30). Although there were no significant differences between the diuretic and either of the two remaining newer drugs in the primary endpoint (CHD death or nonfatal MI), chlorthalidone was significantly better at preventing heart failure than the other two drugs, and also better in reducing BP, stroke, and CV events than lisinopril (20). Because of its superiority in preventing one or more CV complication of hypertension in people over the age of 55 years and its lower cost, a thiazide-type diuretic was recommended as initial antihypertensive drug therapy by JNC-7 for most people with stage 1 hypertension and without compelling indications for other agents.

Although there are many possible confounders and interpretations of the ALLHAT data, it is difficult to overlook the many strengths of this large, randomized, double-blind and well-done study. It is likely that, for individuals without any specific medical reason to use another antihypertensive agent, a thiazide-type diuretic should be the first choice for patients over 55 years of age. Whether the benefits of the diuretic used in ALLHAT (chlorthalidone) are applicable to others in the class, such as hydrochlorothiazide, cannot be answered definitively, but is likely to be true. However, it clears that they have different pharmacodynamic and kinetic properties that distinguish chlorthalidone from other thiazide diuretics (31). Thus, "hydrochlorothiazide is not your mothers" chlorthalidone.

It should be noted that in the recent World Health Organization/International Society of Hypertension's Blood Pressure Lowering Treatment Trialists' Collaboration meta-analysis of all clinical CV outcome trials, including the ALLHAT, demonstrate that the diuretic, ACE-I, ARB, and CA classes of antihypertensive agents all reduce CV events and one class is not superior to the others—it is the level of BP reduction achieved that influences outcome (21), Fig. 23.2.

C. Sequence of Additional Drugs in "Antihypertensive Cocktail"

For those older individuals started on a diuretic, most people would consider an ACE-I, ARB, β-blocker, or CA to be a reasonable second choice. β-blockers have been the conventional second-line treatment in many previous clinical trials that used a diuretic as the initial treatment. An ARB (candesartan) was more effective than placebo and/or other treatments (not including an ACE-I) following the initial diuretic in the recently completed Study on COgnition and Prognosis in the Elderly (SCOPE) trial, which showed significant stroke reduction (SCOPE) (32). The most successful trial of ACE-I therapy in CV event protection was the Heart Outcomes Prevention Evaluation (HOPE), for which ramipril or placebo was given in addition to other required antihypertensive therapy (i.e., as "add-on" treatment) (33). Although the overall BP reduction with ramipril was said to be only 3/2 mmHg when compared with placebo, some patients were not hypertensive at enrollment, and this (as well as

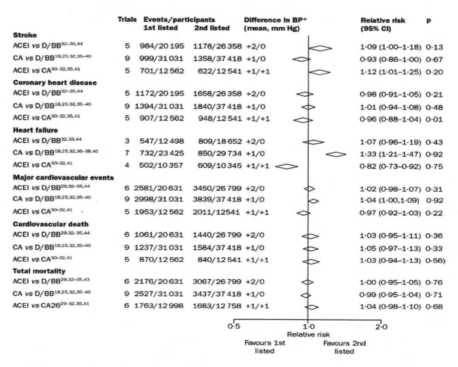

Figure 23.2 Meta-analysis comparing various drug regimens on a variety of cardiovascular outcomes. [From Turnbull et al. (21).]

the possible addition of other antihypertensive drugs to the placebo arm) may have diluted the BP changes. A recent report on the major BP differences across randomized groups in a small subset of patients who underwent ambulatory BP monitoring suggests a much larger BP difference between the groups, especially at night (34). Nonetheless, this trial showed significant reductions in the composite CV endpoint (stroke, MI, or CV death), as well as in each its individual components, in both diabetics and nondiabetics.

A number of fixed-dose combinations with diuretics exist including those with β-blockers, ACE-Is, and ARBs such combinations, either the individual agents or in fixed-dose are suggested as second-line therapy by all major guideline groups (1,3). Moreover, although there are no outcome trials with such combinations, as yet, the JNC-7 and guidelines by the American Diabetes Association and National Kidney Foundation recommends their use for those who are >20/10 mmHg above the BP goal. The first data from a CV outcome trial to compare two different fixed dose combinations will be completed in 2008, the ACCOMPLISH trial.

D. BP Goal

In a majority of hypertensive patients, the goal should be a SBP <140 mmHg and a DBP <90 mmHg. The primary clinical trial evidence for the recommendation for 140/90 mmHg comes from the Hypertension Optimal Treatment (HOT) Study, which randomized 18,790 hypertensives to three different diastolic BP targets; the optimal achieved BP to reduce major CV events was 138.5/82.6 mmHg. No significant CV benefit was obtained with further BP reduction, whereas the number and cost of extra pills were greater (35).

For patients with diabetes, the recommended goal is lower (SBP <130 mmHg and DBP <80 mmHg) (1,36). This is based on results of multiple studies including the United Kingdom Prospective Diabetes Study (UKPDS), which randomized 1148 Type-2 diabetics to a BP of either <180/105 or <150/85 mmHg. After an average follow-up of 8.4 years, those treated to the lower BP goal had an average BP that was 10/5 mmHg lower than subjects randomized to the higher goal, with a significant 24% reduction in diabetes-related endpoints, as well as other major CV benefits (37). In addition, many retrospective analyses demonstrate a marked reduction in risk of CV events and kidney disease progression in those with diabetes when a lower BP, that is, <130 mmHg, systolic is achieved, Fig. 23.3 (38).

This lower level of BP can lead to major cost savings as noted in a cost-effectiveness analysis of American epidemiological and clinical trial data concluded that, for

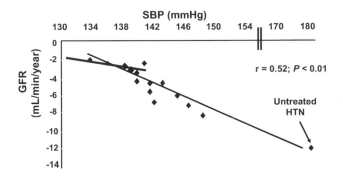

Figure 23.3 Association between level of systolic BP achieved in clinical outcome trials with renal endpoints and rate of kidney function loss. Note ideal achieved range between 130 and 139 mmHg.

diabetics over age 60, achieving a BP goal of <130/85 mmHg saved money overall, as long as the annual cost to lower BP from 140/90 mmHg was less than $414. Again this was due to a reduction in high-cost complications of hypertension, including MI, stroke, ESRD, and HF (39). The recommendation to achieve a diastolic BP <80 mmHg in diabetics is supported by the HOT study, in which the best reductions in major CV events was seen in those patients randomized to the diastolic BP target of ≤80 mmHg.

For patients with kidney disease, JNC-7 also recommends the BP target of <130/80 mmHg. Data from meta-analyses of people with nondiabetic kidney disease, especially those with albuminuria >300 mg/day demonstrate that achieving a systolic BP of <130 mmHg is associated with optimal preservation of kidney function, Fig. 23.4. This relationship is not as strong for people with stage 1 or 2 kidney disease and microalbuminuria,

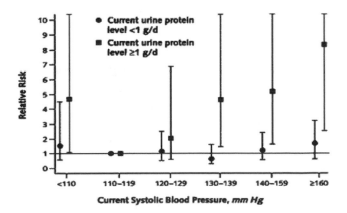

Figure 23.4 Relative risk for progression of nondiabetic kidney disease progression based on current levels of systolic BP and urine protein excretion. [From Jafar et al. (43).] Note that the current recommended BP level of <130 mmHg is very much supported for those with >1 g of proteinuria.

in which case a BP level between 130 and 139 mmHg is quiet reasonable based on data from the African-American Study of Kidney Disease (AASK) and Appropriate Blood pressure Control in Diabetes (ABCD) Study (40,41).

One of the perceived limitations to achieving these lower levels of BP was the fear that lowering BP too far might be harmful, the concept of the "J" curve. Several investigators had pointed out that subjects treated to diastolic BP level <85 mmHg had higher rates of MI than those whose on-treatment diastolic BP was between 85 and 90 mmHg. An increased risk with low diastolic BP is also evident in populations and in the placebo groups of several trials. Furthermore, the Systolic Hypertension in the Elderly Program (SHEP) treated individuals to an average diastolic BP of 67 mmHg and prevented MIs compared with those treated to an average of 71 mmHg. Similarly, analysis of SHEP provided no evidence for an increase in the risk of stroke with decreasing levels of on-treatment systolic BPs (42). Moreover, both HOT and UKPDS 38 studies provided proof that intensive BP lowering was not harmful.

This "J curve" effect is also present for kidney disease especially for those with markedly increased levels of proteinuria. A systolic BP of >110 mmHg, but <130 mmHg should be maintained in such individuals or the benefits of lower BP are diminished (43), Fig. 23.4.

IV. FACTORS TO CONSIDER WHEN CONSTRUCTING AN ANTIHYPERTENSIVE DRUG REGIMEN

The following factors should always be considered when antihypertensive drug therapy is chosen: efficacy, comorbidities, safety, patient demographics, special situations (e.g., pregnancy), dosing schedule, drug interactions, adherence, mechanism(s) of action, and cost. These considerations are important not only in choice of initial therapy, but also for subsequent antihypertensive agents. In recent clinical trials, most patients required a minimum of two and in many cases three drugs to achieve goal BP; a recent meta-regression analysis suggested that there is only a 2.5% chance of achieving target BP with monotherapy when the initial DBP is >10 mmHg higher than goal.

A. Efficacy

Five classes of medications (thiazide diuretics, β-blockers, long-acting CAs, ACE-Is, and ARBs) have been shown to reduce CV or renal endpoints when used as initial therapy as part of a group of medications to lower BP in appropriately designed and implemented clinical trials. Other drugs, such as peripheral sympatholytics (reserpine

and guanethidine), centrally acting α-agonists (α-methyldopa), and vasodilators (hydralazine), have also been used in clinical trials as the second, third, or even fourth agent added to achieve BP control. None of these medications is an option for initial therapy because they are relatively poorly tolerated or need to be taken together with other drugs to lower BP effectively in the long term. α-blockers are valuable adjunctive therapy, but not as initial therapy, based on the findings of ALLHAT (30). α/β-blockers are well tolerated and effective as monotherapy, but have yet to be shown to reduce clinical endpoints in hypertensive patients without heart failure.

B. Comorbidities and Other Risk Factors

The results of event trials conducted in subjects with hypertension and other medical conditions led to the genesis of compelling indications in the JNC-7, Table 23.2. The JNC Committee recognized that individual patients may have certain comorbid conditions for which a specific agent may be appropriate, even though no clinical trial data exist to prove it. These "specific" indications try to codify clinical judgment, which any reasonable clinician would use to care for all the health needs of his or her patients. For the most part, these recommendations do not add classes of drugs to the list of those that are already favored because of a reduction in clinical endpoints, but instead alter the choice of which class should be selected for initial therapy. Thus, other risk factors and active clinical problems can sometimes influence the choice of specific therapy for individual patients. This approach, differently stated, was also adopted by the British Hypertension Society in their guidelines (44).

1. Dyslipidemia

Hypertensive patients with lipid abnormalities (which may represent as many as 50% of treated hypertensives) may also wish to avoid drugs that worsen their particular dyslipidemia. Although it has not been proven that changes in serum lipids caused by certain classes of antihypertensive agents are harmful, it is certainly reasonable to choose a drug that, all things being equal, is lipid-neutral or may improve the lipid profile. In large doses (>25 mg/day), thiazide diuretics and related compounds, such as chlorthalidone, raise total cholesterol (TC) and LDL-C 5–10% and may increase serum triglycerides 15–30%, whereas lowering HDL-C 2–4%. With currently recommended doses (up to 25 mg of chlorthalidone or equivalent), the long-term changes are less troublesome (20). β-blockers that do not have intrinsic sympathomimetic activity lower HDL-C even more (10%) and also raise triglycerides ($\sim$20%) without affecting TC or LDL. β-Blockers that have intrinsic sympathomimetic activity and α-/β-blockers are lipid-neutral. α-blockers reduce TC and LDL cholesterol ~8–10%, triglycerides 15%, and HDL-C 10–15%. Other sympatholytics do not affect the lipid profile, whereas direct vasodilators (e.g., hydralazine) raise HDL-C and lower triglycerides and TG, even when combined with thiazide diuretics. ACE-Is generally do not affect serum lipids. ARBs and CAs are also lipid-neutral (45).

Glucose, Insulin, and New-Onset Diabetes Mellitus

Some antihypertensive drugs, namely, diuretics and β-blockers, affect glucose handling and can either worsen or improve insulin sensitivity (30,46,47). The magnitude and direction of the drug-induced changes seen in glucose and insulin are very similar to what occurs with lipids. Peripheral α-blockers and some ACE-Is (captopril, enalapril, trandolapril, and perindopril) improve insulin sensitivity (48,49). Every ACE-I and ARB so far studied reduces urinary protein excretion, which may potentially contribute to the renal benefit seen in diabetic patients treated with these drugs. In HOPE, the Captopril Primary Prevention Project (CAPPP), LIFE and ALLHAT, incident diabetes was less common when an ACE-I or ARB was the randomized choice (20,27,50). Patients at high risk of developing diabetes, that is, those who are obese with glucose intolerance or other components of the metabolic syndrome, may reduce their risk of new-onset diabetes using ACE-I or ARB treatment.

Hypertensives with Diabetes Mellitus

As discussed earlier, the combination of hypertension and DM confers a much greater risk for CV events and renal failure than either one alone. According to all guideline statements, Type-1 diabetics with renal impairment and proteinuria should receive a blocker of the renin–angiotensin system, which reduces ESRD by 50%. Little other information is available about optimal treatment of hypertension in Type-1 diabetes (1,3,36).

All recently published guidelines for treatment of hypertension in Type-2 diabetics, which include a lower-than-usual goal for BP during treatment (<130/ 80 mmHg, as discussed earlier), and a recommendation for a blocker of the renin–angiotensin system to be a component of the antihypertensive drug regimen (i.e., initial drug therapy) (1,3,36). An ARB has been beneficial in two studies with renal endpoints (IDNT, RENAAL) and for CV event prevention in the diabetic subset of LIFE (24,25,27). An ACE-I provided impressive CV event reduction in micro-HOPE, although the number of subjects reaching ESRD was only 18, and the data from outcome studies in people with established nephropathy is restricted to surrogate markers (51,52). In UKPDS 38,

there was no significant difference between captopril and atenolol as initial therapy, whereas the group achieving the lower BP did much better. These results must also be viewed in the context of achievement of BP goal. Some argue that BP control, rather than how it is accomplished, is the key factor in reducing CV and renal events in patients with Type-2 diabetes.

The role of CAs in treatment of hypertension in diabetic patients has been controversial although some clear information is now available. The following statements about CA use in diabetes are defensible. First, differences in outcome exist between the two subclasses of CAs. Use of DHPCAs in the absence of ACE-Is or ARBs to reduce CV risk in people with normal kidney function in those diabetes is warranted as evidenced by data from ALLHAT and in the subgroup of those with diabetes and stage 2 nephropathy, that is, GFR 60–89 mL/min, in Syst-Eur (53). However, in those with advance nephropathy, that is, stage 3 and beyond, GFR <60 mL/min, DHPCAs were significantly less effective in reducing renal events (but not CV events) when compared with an ARB in IDNT. This has also been observed in *post hoc* analyses of other clinical trials (54). Use of DHPCAs, however, if used with an ACE-I or ARB does not distract from the benefit of the renin–angiotensin system blocking agents and further lowers BP with resultant benefit of stroke reduction. Both the National Kidney Foundation and the American Diabetes Association recommend that DHPCA be used as third-line therapy after a diuretic and either an ACE-I or an ARB (36,38), favoring non-DHPCAs over DHPCAs, because they reduce proteinuria and slow the progression of diabetic nephropathy (54).

In those with diabetes, reducing BP to goal may be a more important factor in reducing mortality and preserving renal function than the initial drug chosen to do so, as it usually takes several drugs to achieve the target BP <130/80 mmHg.

Left Ventricular Hypertrophy

LVH results from chronic elevations in arterial pressure that cause cardiac myocyte hypertrophy and remodeling of the coronary resistance vessels. This leads to perivascular fibrosis of the intramyocardial arteries and arterioles. Over time, these changes in the myocardium contribute to the development of ventricular wall stiffness and diastolic dysfunction. LVH is a robust independent risk factor for CV and premature mortality, probably because it reflects the degree of BP control over the long-term. It is especially common in the elderly, particularly in elderly women, and is often associated with diastolic dysfunction. All antihypertensive agents except direct vasodilators reduce LV mass. In meta-analyses, agents that block the renin–angiotensin–aldosterone system reduce LV mass better or quicker than other antihypertensive agents. However, both the TOMHS and the Veterans Administration (VA) study of monotherapy found no differences among antihypertensive agents in their ability to regress LVH. Moreover, in TOMHS, nutritional hygienic measures, such as weight loss, reduced Na^+ and alcohol intake, and exercise, were effective by themselves in regressing LV mass. Perhaps, the most important factor responsible for regression of LVH is the prolonged reduction of systolic BP.

So far, the only completed clinical trial to enroll only patients with LVH was the LIFE study. The group randomized to losartan ($\pm$ diuretic) had a significant reduction in LVH and composite CV events (mostly due to stroke) when compared with the group receiving atenolol ($\pm$ diuretic), despite a BP difference between groups of only 1.3/0.4 mmHg. Significant differences in cardiac events among randomized groups were seen best in diabetics. These are the first randomized, prospective data to suggest that reducing LVH prevents CV events.

Heart Failure

Hypertension is also a major risk factor for the subsequent development of HF, typically many years later (55). For many under- or untreated hypertensives, LVH is an important intermediate step, resulting in "hypertensive heart disease" with impaired LV filling and increased ventricular stiffness. This type of HF (commonly seen in up to 40% of hospitalized patients with an antecedent history of hypertension) is now called HF with preserved systolic function (56). The more common type of "systolic dysfunction" associated with a reduced LV ejection fraction is often due to previous MI (for which hypertension is also an important risk factor). In a meta-analysis of placebo-controlled clinical trials in hypertension, there was a 42% reduction in HF incidence among hypertensives randomized to either a low-dose diuretic or a β-blocker (57).

Distinguishing between the two subtypes of HF is most easily done by estimation of the LV ejection fraction with the results dictating therapy (58). Patients with low ejection fractions (systolic HF) improve both their BP and long-term prognosis with ACE-Is and diuretics, to which can be added β-blockers, spironolactone, and/or other drugs, as needed (59,60). Two trials directly comparing an ARB with an ACE-I showed significant differences mainly in better tolerability of the ARB. In the valsartan in heart failure (Val-HeFT) trial, an ARB or placebo was given to HF patients taking "conventional therapy" (which included an ACE-I in 93%, but a β-blocker in only 13%). Although there were no differences between the randomized groups in terms of mortality, the group receiving valsartan had a significant 13% reduction in

HF-related morbidity or mortality, mostly due to a 27% reduction in HF hospitalization (61). Valsartan received FDA approval for HF because of the very significant reduction in morbidity and mortality in the 366 patients who did not take an ACE-I in Val-HeFT. However, for patients who took a β-blocker in addition to the ACE-I, valsartan had a significantly higher morbidity or mortality rate. This limits the enthusiasm for valsartan as a third-line HF drug. The recently completed Candesartan in Heart failure Assessment of Reduction in Mortality and morbidity (CHARM), candesartan demonstrated a hazard ratio of 0.77 for CV death and CHF hospitalization when compared with placebo for patients with symptomatic chronic heart failure and intolerance of ACE-I (62). Effects of candesartan in patients with chronic heart failure and reduced left-ventricular systolic function intolerant to ACE-Is: the CHARM-Alternative trial. Similarly in the Valsartan in acute myocardial infarction trial (VALIANT), valsartan was as effective as captopril or their combination in myocardial infarction complicated by heart failure, left ventricular dysfunction, or both (63). The utilization of DHPCAs in the absence of ACE-Is or ARBs while appropriate remains controversial as no study has shown a benefit in heart failure or kidney disease progression outcomes with DHPCAs in the absence of an ACE-I or ARB (64). Moreover, the DHPCAs are associated with the highest incidence of new HF in hypertension trials (19). Hydralazine is used in conjunction with nitrates for the treatment of CHF due to systolic dysfunction in patients who cannot tolerate ACE-Is or ARB. It confers a favorable effect on LV function and mortality. Authorities recommend these drugs as adjunctive therapy (after diuretics, maximum doses of ACE-Is and/or ARBs, a β-blocker, and sometimes spironolactone), if BP continues to be elevated.

The treatment of hypertension in patients with HF and preserved systolic function has not been as well studied, and with the exception of the CHARM trial, which trended but failed to show a benefit of the ARB, no specific therapy is recommended. Most authorities recommend using drugs that reduce HR, increase diastolic filling time, and allow the heart muscle to relax more fully: β-blockers or non-DHP-CAs. In the third arm of the CHARM trial (CHARM-Preserved) evaluating CHF patients with EF >40%, data suggested that candesartan can prevent CHF hospitalizations and the development of diabetes mellitus with a hazard ratio of 0.89 (62).

2. Microalbuminuria and Proteinuria

MA is an independent predictor of CV risk in patients with diabetes, Table 23.7. Achievement of BP goal with all commonly prescribed first-line drugs tends to reduce MA; however, ACE-Is and ARBs have the most data

Table 23.7 Cardiovascular Risk Factors

Major risk factors
Hypertension*
Age (older than 55 for men, 65 for women)[‡]
Diabetes mellitus*
Elevated LDL (or total) cholesterol or low HDL cholesterol*
Estimated GFR <60 mL/min
Family history of premature cardiovascular disease (men < age 55 or women < age 65)
Microalbuminuria
Obesity* (body mass index ≥ 30 kg/m^2)
Physical inactivity
Tobacco usage, particularly cigarettes

*Components of the metabolic syndrome.
Source: Adapted from JNC-7 (1).

showing reductions in MA and delaying its progression to proteinuria (1,52). Both ACE-Is and non-DHPCAs reduce albuminuria and together have additive anti-albuminuric effects (65,66). The effects of different classes of antihypertensive agents on proteinuria in the context on kidney disease progression are summarized in Table 23.8.

The ACE-Is and ARBs are the antihypertensive agents that most consistently reduce proteinuria. A high Na$^+$ intake blunts the antiproteinuric and antihypertensive effects of ACE-Is and diltiazem, so restricting dietary Na$^+$ is recommended for patients with MA or proteinuria (67).

Kidney Dysfunction

Lowering BP will slow the progression of nephropathy, but the recommended target BP is controversial. The recent African-American Study of Kidney disease and hypertension showed no additional benefit to lowering systolic BP to <130 mmHg for nondiabetic renal disease, when compared with <140 mmHg, but many of these people had MA not proteinuria. On the basis of current guidelines, the greater the level of proteinuria, the more important it is to achieve the currently recommended BP goal. ARBs and ACE-Is will slow the progression of diabetic and nondiabetic nephropathy, assuming they are

Table 23.8 Relationship Between Changes in Proteinuria and Kidney Disease Progression with BP Treatment

Increased time to dialysis (30–35% proteinuria reduction)	No change in time to dialysis (no proteinuria reduction)
Captopril trial	DHPCCB arm-IDNT
AASK trial	DHPCCB arm-AASK
RENAAL	
IDNT	
COOPERATE trial	

given with sufficient other drugs to reduce BP <140/90 mmHg as has been in shown in the RENAAL trial (64).

In spite of the preponderance of evidence from many long-term clinical trials, there is a general hesitancy among some clinicians to prescribe ACE-Is (or ARBs) for patients with serum creatinine >1.4 mg/dL, because it often rises after the drug is given. Analysis of long-term clinical trials has confirmed that this reduction in renal function plateaus within a month (68). If the serum creatinine increases by >30% or continues to rise after 3 months of therapy, volume depletion, unsuspected LV dysfunction, or bilateral renal artery stenosis should be considered. There are also concerns about hyperkalemia associated with an ACE-I or ARB; this should be worrisome only if the serum K$^+$ rises ≥ 0.5 mEq/L and the baseline level is already >5 mEq/L.

Thus, although any class of antihypertensive agent may be used to achieve this new recommended lower level of BP to preserve renal function, certain principles should be kept in mind.

- BP will seldom, if ever, be controlled adequately in patients with significant renal impairment (serum creatinine >1.8 mg/dL) without the use of a loop diuretic.
- A long-acting loop diuretic (such as torsemide) is preferred; furosemide or bumetanide should given twice daily.
- Combinations of antihypertensive medications will be needed to achieve goal BP. One of these drugs should be an ACE-I or ARB. Some authors recommend both an ACE-I and an ARB simultaneously, but this has been shown to consistently further lower proteinuria not further lower BP if maximal doses of both are used.

Coronary Artery Disease

As hypertension is a major risk factor for CAD, it is not surprising that a large number of patients have both conditions. It is unlikely on ethical grounds that a placebo-controlled trial will be done with any single antihypertensive drug in such patients. The presence of CAD in a patient with hypertension is likely to influence both the choice of drugs used to treat the patient and the BP goal to be achieved. Because both β-blockers and CAs are effective antihypertensive agents with major anti-anginal efficacy, they are often the preferred agents for initial treatment, especially in the common setting of unstable angina pectoris (69). A recent meta-analysis suggested that the former are more effective, although the latter are more commonly used (70). The recent HOPE trial showed a large survival benefit for high-risk hypertensives (most of whom had known CAD) treated with ramipril. None of the participants in HOPE had known HF at enrollment, for which this degree of benefit would have been expected. Likewise in the EURopean trial On reduction of cardiac endpoints with Perindopril in stable CAD (EUROPA), the perindopril group had a relative risk reduction of 20% in the primary endpoint of composite CV death, nonfatal MI, and cardiac arrest with successful resuscitation (71). These findings have been interpreted by some as evidence in favor for this class of medications in the management of all hypertensive patients with CAD.

The issue of how low to reduce BP in the setting of CAD has been controversial until the results of the INVEST. In this trial, a strategy of a non-DHP-CA, verapamil was compared to a β-blocker, atenolol, for CV events and death. Both received ACE-Is, although the verapamil group received significantly greater percentage of trandolapril. The results demonstrated no difference in outcome with lower morbidity and less new-onset diabetes in the verapamil group. As coronary artery filling occurs during diastole, reducing perfusion pressure at this time might increase coronary ischemia, thus agents such as verapamil or β-blocker in concert with an ACE-I should be included in the antihypertensive regimen of such patients. Lastly, sildenafil citrate (Viagra) appears to have no major interactions with any antihypertensive drugs, but all nitrate-containing preparations are contraindicated.

3. Post Stroke

Although hypertension is the risk factor for stroke with the highest population-attributable risk, and "clinically evident cerebrovascular disease is an indication for antihypertensive treatment," optimal BP management depends on the nature, cause, and chronology of the neurologic symptoms. In the immediate setting of acute stroke, most neurologists avoid antihypertensive drugs unless is very high (e.g., BP > 185/110 mmHg). If treatment is necessary, a short-acting intravenously administered drug is preferred because it can be discontinued quickly if a patient's neurologic condition deteriorates acutely.

The PROGRESS proved that lowering BP in people who had suffered a prior stroke or TIA was beneficial not only in preventing recurrent stroke but also in reducing CV events (23). Although a significant benefit was seen only in the group receiving both the ACE-I, perindopril, and the diuretic, indapamide (and not in those whose physicians chose to give them only perindopril), there was benefit in everyone, regardless of baseline BP. There should no longer be fear in lowering BP in patients who survive a stroke or TIA, once the acute phase has passed.

C. Safety (Adverse Reactions and Side Effects)

The two primary types of adverse reactions and side effects that occur with antihypertensive therapy are clinical and biochemical. Clinical side effects are directly evident to the patient and are perceived by the patient or the clinician to be related to the drug. The appearance of adverse reactions requires that the drug be stopped, the dose be reduced, or the patient must be willing to remain on therapy until they become able to tolerate the side effect or until the side effect disappears. Generally, ARBs, ACE-Is, and CAs are better tolerated than other classes with ARBs having a side effect profile similar to placebo.

Biochemical side effects may lead to clinically evident adverse reactions (e.g., hypokalemia from thiazide diuretics causing muscle weakness, palpitations, nocturia, or polyuria); but these are usually are more troublesome to the clinician than they are to the patient. The importance of biochemical side effects is usually not that they result in clinically evident problems, but the danger that these drug-related changes in lipids, glucose, or insulin may aggravate other risk factors and accelerate the clinical impact of dyslipidemias, glucose intolerance, or insulin resistance. It is unlikely that the relatively minor changes in glucose, triglycerides, HDL-C, or TG that result from therapy with thiazides or β-blockers are responsible for an increase in ischemic heart disease; the exact opposite has been seen in secondary MI prevention studies with several β-blockers. In ALLHAT, the biochemical profile of the group receiving the α-blocker seemed more favorable (lower cholesterol, TG, and glucose and higher K^+) compared with the group on chlorthalidone, yet the diuretic prevented CV events more successfully. Similarly, chlorthalidone prevented at least one or more serious forms of CVD when compared with either amlodipine or lisinopril, despite a significantly lower serum potassium, and higher glucose and cholesterol at 4 years.

At the doses that are now recommended, these changes and the electrolyte disturbances noted with thiazide diuretics are quite modest, although it is still possible that at high doses, thiazides could reduce serum K^+ sufficiently to cause sudden cardiac death. Whether the increases in insulin resistance seen with thiazide diuretics and β-blockers and the hypokalemia associated with thiazides would have precipitated DM sooner in patients who would not otherwise have become diabetic is uncertain. It may be more prudent to select another option for treatment in patients with DM or dyslipidemia, so long as BP is reduced to goal. Certain types of dual therapy also may ameliorate biochemical adverse reactions. Thiazides and either ACE-Is or ARBs, when given together, produce few, if any, of the metabolic abnormalities associated with thiazides alone. Several fixed-dose combinations of these classes of drugs are available and may be appropriate as initial therapy (7) (Table 23.4).

The incidence of clinical side effects tends to rise with increasing doses with all classes of drugs, with the exception of ACE-Is and ARBs. Patients who develop an adverse reaction on a high dose of a drug or on a dose that they previously tolerated do not necessarily need to have the drug discontinued. Instead, the dose can be lowered and another antihypertensive agent can be added. The primary problems with ACE-Is are cough and angioedema, both of which tend to be idiosyncratic and occur with all representatives from that class of agents. Reducing the dose or changing to a different ACE-I is rarely helpful. ACE-Is should be increased to the maximum recommended dose before therapy is abandoned or another agent is added unless a low-dose combination is felt to be more appropriate. ARBs are the best tolerated of all currently available antihypertensive medications, and patients persist in taking them at higher rates than other drugs.

D. Demographic Considerations

1. Blacks and Other Ethnic Minorities

Some classes of antihypertensive agents reduce BP more or less effectively in certain ethnic groups. Thiazide diuretics, for example, are more effective in blacks than in whites; in whites, ACE-Is, ARBs, and β-blockers are more effective at lower doses. Peripheral α-blockers, α-/β-blockers, and CAs are equally effective across all ethnic groups. In general, the response rates to antihypertensive agents in Hispanics are intermediate to that seen in whites and blacks, whereas east Asians, but not necessarily south Asians (patients from the Indian subcontinent), often need lower doses than do whites.

African-Americans bear a larger population burden of hypertension with a higher risk for hypertensive complications than whites. Because data on the benefits of treatment were limited, a larger sample than was present in the US population was recruited for ALLHAT. The significantly poorer stroke, HF, and combined CVD rates in blacks treated with lisinopril (compared with chlorthalidone) may be due to the relative ineffectiveness of the ACE-I in reducing BP, when a diuretic cannot be added to the regimen. However, the importance of ACE-I therapy in blacks was shown in AASK when diuretics were used in nearly all patients. In AASK, patients randomized to ramipril did much better both in loss of GFR and in clinical events than those on either amlodipine or metoprolol (41). Despite the slightly higher risk of angioedema and cough, there is no reason to avoid ACE-I in black hypertensive patients, but perhaps more reason to consider concomitant therapy with a diuretic.

2. The Elderly

All classes of antihypertensive agents lower BP effectively in older persons, although the doses needed to reach goal are often lower than necessary for young- and middle-aged hypertensive patients. However, certain drugs and certain classes of drugs should be used with caution in older hypertensives. These include agents, such as peripheral α-blockers, which can exacerbate the postural fall in BP seen more frequently in older individuals with baroreceptor dysfunction; non-DHPCAs and β-blockers that may aggravate subtle or subclinical conduction defects or precipitate systolic dysfunction and HF, and verapamil, which may not be well tolerated in some older persons already bothered by constipation. Cough from an ACE-I is more common in older women. When compared with placebo, both diuretics and DHPCAs reduce morbidity and mortality in older persons with stage 2 isolated systolic hypertension (72) incidentally, chlorthalidone was more effective than amlodipine in preventing HF in ALLHAT and is much less expensive. The benefits of effective treatment are more evident in older hypertensives as they have a higher absolute risk of CV events than younger counterparts. Even hypertensive patients >80 years of age garner significant benefit from treatment, especially in stroke prevention. Therapy should not be withheld from the elderly for fear of toxicity or lack of efficacy.

V. SPECIAL SITUATIONS

A. Pregnancy

Hypertension is found in ∼10% of pregnancies and is the major cause of perinatal morbidity and mortality in most developed countries. Because of the unique patient population, hypertension in pregnancy has a special definition, four specific types, and a treatment algorithm that recognizes the need to assess outcomes for both mother and baby. Although most pregnancies are primarily managed by obstetricians, the majority of authoritative pronouncements about this condition have been advanced by expert panels drawn from that discipline (73). In the USA, hypertension in pregnancy is defined as either BP >140/90 mmHg on two measurements at least 4 h apart or diastolic BP >110 mmHg at any time during pregnancy or up to 6 weeks postpartum.

The classification of hypertension in pregnancy typically requires some knowledge of BP status before conception. If there was preexisting hypertension, the patient is said to have "chronic hypertension," which can be diagnosed before 20 weeks gestation and persists at least 42 days postpartum. Preeclampsia is hypertension appearing after 20 weeks gestation, with associated proteinuria (at least 300 mg per 24 h collection or 1+ on a random dipstick without urinary tract infection), which typically resolves within 42 days after delivery. Other criteria help to make the diagnosis more likely. Preeclampsia with superimposed chronic hypertension is a combination of the two. Gestational hypertension is diagnosed when and if the BP returns to normal within 42 days after delivery.

A large number of demographic, genetic, laboratory parameters, and other factors have been associated with a higher risk of preeclampsia, but none has been accepted as the "underlying cause." Despite many smaller studies that low-dose aspirin or Ca^{2+} supplementation prevented preeclampsia in high-risk women, large NIH-sponsored mega trials have been unsuccessful in showing benefit from these inexpensive preventive measures. Although aspirin tends to delay parturition and increase the likelihood of bleeding, few obstetricians routinely recommend it. Treatment of elevated BP during pregnancy traditionally begins with bed rest, followed by methyldopa as the primary drug, based on its long history of efficacy and lack of adverse effects on babies. However, DHPCAs and if edema is severe diuretics have been suggested for use. For severe hypertension (BP >160/109 mmHg) in outpatients that are not controlled with these measures or a diastolic BP between 90 and 100 mmHg, hydralazine is used as a first-line agent with doses recommended at 5–10 mg IV every 20–30 min. Labetalol and nifedipine are routinely added for additional BP control in succession.

ACE-Is and ARBs are contraindicated because of renal abnormalities in the fetus. It is important to achieve good BP control at the onset of symptoms as poor maternal outcomes are related to complications, such as cerebral hemorrhage and seizures, if eclampsia develops. For intrapartum management, until delivery can be achieved intravenous magnesium sulfate has been a mainstay for the progression of preecalmpsia to seizures and other more serious complications.

Hypertension during pregnancy also carries prognostic significance for future health problems as the woman ages. Sixty percent of women with early-onset preeclampsia have abnormalities on renal biopsy and a higher risk of persistent hypertension after delivery. Women who develop hypertension during pregnancy are not only at higher risk for hypertension later in life, but also have a roughly twofold increase in the risk of death from CAD.

B. Hypertensive Emergencies and Urgencies

Although rare, hypertensive crises are still seen in physicians' offices and emergency rooms. Fortunately, there are now excellent medications available for both acute, in-hospital treatment, and outpatient management; these improvements have led to a decrease in the 1 year mortality rate after a hypertensive emergency from 80% (1928) to 50% (1955) to <10%, Table 23.9.

The primary pathophysiologic abnormality in patients who experience hypertensive crises is via an alteration of the autoregulation in certain vascular beds (especially cerebral and renal), which often is followed by frank arteritis and ischemia of vital organs (74). Autoregulation is the ability of blood vessels to dilate or constrict in order to maintain normal organ perfusion. Normal arteries from normotensive individuals can maintain flow over a wide range of mean arterial pressures, usually 60–150 mmHg. Chronic elevations of BP cause compensatory functional and structural changes in the arterial circulation and shift the autoregulatory curve to the right; this allows hypertensive patients to maintain normal perfusion and avoid excessive blood flow at higher BP levels. When BP increases above the autoregulatory range, tissue damage occurs. An understanding of autoregulation is also important for therapy, as the sudden lowering of BP to a range that would otherwise be considered normal may reduce BP below the autoregulatory capacity of the hypertensive circulation and can thereby lead to inadequate tissue perfusion. In the later stages of a hypertensive crisis, pathologists have demonstrated cerebral edema in both acute and chronic inflammations of the medium- and small-arteries and arterioles, with associated necrosis.

Hypertensive crises occur in a variety of clinical settings (74). The most common is a chronic and often untreated patient with stage 3 essential hypertension (i.e., usual BP ≥180/110 mmHg) whose BP rises above the autoregulatory range, triggering the pathophysiologic sequence outlined earlier. However, identical crises can occur any time there is an acute or rapid rise in BP in a normotensive or minimally hypertensive individual, such as a child or a woman during pregnancy. Hypertensive crises are most easily recognized by the association of an extremely elevated BP with physical examination or laboratory findings that indicate acute tissue organ damage (TOD), although the actual levels of BP are of little import.

The initial evaluation of a severely hypertensive patient includes a thorough inspection of the optic fundi (looking for acute hemorrhages, exudates, or papilledema); a mental status assessment; careful cardiac, pulmonary, and neurologic examination; a quick search for clues that might indicate secondary hypertension (e.g., abdominal bruit, striae, radial–femoral delay); and laboratory studies to assess renal function (dipstick and microscopic urinalysis, serum creatinine).

There are several different types of common clinical presentations of hypertensive emergencies; the neurologic crises are the most difficult to distinguish from one another. Hypertensive encephalopathy is typically a diagnosis of exclusion; hemorrhagic and thrombotic strokes are usually diagnosed after focal neurologic deficits that are corroborated by CT. Subarachnoid hemorrhage is diagnosed by the typical findings on lumbar puncture. The management of each of these conditions is somewhat different in that nimodipine may be the drug of choice

Table 23.9 Drugs Used for Hypertensive Emergencies[a]

Drug	Dose[b]	Onset of action	Duration of action	Adverse effects[c]	Special indications
Vasodilators					
Sodium nitroprusside	0.25–10 μg/kg per min IV infusion[d]	Immediate	1–2 min	Nausea, vomiting, muscle twitching, sweating, thiocynate, and cyanide intoxication	Most hypertensive emergencies; caution with high intracranial pressure or azotemia
Nicardipine hydrochloride	5–15 mg/h IV	5–10 min	15–30 min, may exceed 4 h	Tachycardia, headache, flushing, local phlebitis	Most hypertensive emergencies except acute heart failure; caution with coronary ischemia
Fenoldopam mesylate	0.1–0.3 μg/kg per min IV infusion	<5 min	30 min	Tachycardia, headache, nausea, flushing	Most hypertensive emergencies; caution with glaucoma
Nitroglycerin	5–100 μg/min as IV infusion[d]	2–5 min	5–10 min	Headache, vomiting, methemoglobinemia, tolerance with prolonged use	Coronary ischemia
Enalaprilat	1.25–5 mg every 6 h IV	15–30 min	6–12 h	Precipitous fall in pressure in high-renin states; variable response	Acute left ventricular failure; avoid in acute myocardial infarction
Hydralazine hydrochloride	10–20 mg IV 10–40 mg IM	10–20 min IV 20–30 min IM	1–4 h IV 4–6 h IM	Tachycardia, flushing, headache, vomiting, aggravation of angina	Eclampsia
Adrenergic inhibitors					
Labetalol hydrochloride	20–80 mg IV bolus every 10 min 0.5–2.0 mg/min IV infusion	5–10 min	3–6 h	Vomiting, scalp tingling, bronchoconstriction, dizziness, nausea, heart block, orthostatic hypotension	Most hypertensive emergencies except acute heart failure
Esmolol hydrochloride	250–500 μg/kg per min IV bolus, then 50–100 μg/kg per min by infusion; may repeat bolus after 5 min or increase infusion to 300 μg/min	1–2 min	10–30 min	Hypotension, nausea, asthma, first degree heart block, HF	Aortic dissection, perioperative
Phentolamine	5–15 mg IV bolus	1–2 min	10–30 min	Tachycardia, flushing, headache	Catecholamine excess

[a]These doses may vary from those in the Physicians' Desk Reference, 51st ed.
[b]IV indicates intravenous; IM, intramuscular.
[c]Hypotension may occur with all agents.
[d]Require special delivery system.

for most neurologic crises, because of its antihypertensive and anti-ischemic effects. Many physicians still prefer nitroprusside or another intravenous vasodilator, such as hydralazine, because it can be discontinued rapidly if BP goes very low. Hydralazine causes a preferential decrease in the vascular resistance in the coronary, cerebral, and renal vascular beds when compared with skin and muscular beds. Because of preferential dilatation of arterioles over veins, postural hypotension is not a common problem. Goal BP also depends on the presenting diagnosis and is usually lower for encephalopathy than it is for acute stroke in evolution, Table 23.10. For hemorrhagic stroke and subarachnoid hemorrhage, BP lowering is usually not recommended unless the BP is "very high" (>180/105 mmHg).

Patients who present with hypertensive crises involving cardiac ischemia/infarction or pulmonary edema can be managed with either nitroglycerin or nitroprusside, although typically a combination of drugs (including an ACE-I when there is HF) is used in these settings. Efforts to preserve myocardium and open the obstructed coronary artery (by thrombolysis, angioplasty, or surgery) are also indicated.

Patients with aortic dissection are managed in a somewhat different fashion (75). A β-blocker is added to the intravenous vasodilator, and the goal BP is much lower: typically 120 mmHg systolic is recommended, but 100 mmHg systolic may be even better. Pharmacologic therapy is only a temporary adjunct to definitive surgical therapy, which should be planned with dispatch, although long-term medical therapy may be more appropriate in some patients.

Hypertensive crises, involving the kidney, are commonly followed by a further deterioration in renal function even when BP is lowered properly. Some physicians prefer fenoldopam to nicardipine or nitroprusside in this setting, because of its lack of toxic metabolites and specific renal vasodilating effects (76). BP should be reduced ~10% during the first hour and a further 10–15% during the next 1–3 h. The necessity for acute dialysis often is precipitated by BP reduction, but many patients are able to avoid dialysis in the long term if BP is carefully and well controlled during follow-up.

Hypertensive crises resulting from catecholamine excess states (pheochromocytoma, monoamine oxidase inhibitor crisis, cocaine intoxication, etc.) are best managed with an intravenous α-blocker (phentolamine), with a β-blocker added later, if needed. Many patients with severe hypertension caused by the sudden withdrawal of antihypertensive agents (e.g., clonidine) can be easily managed by reinstituting the previous therapy.

Table 23.10   Types of Hypertensive Crises with Suggested Drug Therapy and BP Targets

Types of crises	Drug of choice	BP target
Neurological		
Hypertensive encephalopathy	Nitroprusside[a]	25% reduction in mean arterial pressure >2–3 h
Intracranial hemorrhage or Acute stroke in evolution	Nitroprusside[a] (controversial)	0–25% reduction in mean arterial pressure >6–12 h (controversial)
Acute head injury/trauma	Nitroprusside[a]	0–25% reduction in mean arterial pressure >2–3 h (controversial)
Subarachnoid hemorrhage	Nimodipine	Up to 25% reduction in mean arterial pressure in previously hypertensive patients, 130–160 mmHg systolic in normotensive patients
Cardiac		
Ischemial/infaction	Nitroglycerin or nicardipine	Reduction in ischemia
Heart failure	Nitroprusside[a] or nitroglycerin	Improvement in failure (typically 10–15% decrease in BP)
Aortic dissection	β-blocker + nitroprusside[a]	120 mmHg systolic in 30 min (if possible)
Renal		
Hematuria or acute renal impairment	Fenoldopam	0–25% reduction in mean arterial pressure >1–12 h
Catecholamine excess states		
Pheochromocytoma	Phentolamine	To control paroxysms
Drug withdrawal	Drug withdrawn	Typically only one dose necessary
Pregnancy-related		
Eclampsia	MgSO$_4$, methyldopa, hydralazine	Typically <90 mmHg diastolic, but often lower

[a]Some physicians prefer an intravenous infusion of either fenoldopam or nicardipine, neither of which has potentially toxic metabolites, over nitroprusside. Recent studies have also shown improvements in renal function during therapy with the former when compared with nitroprusside.
Source: Adapted from Elliott (74).

Hypertensive crises during pregnancy must be managed in a more careful and conservative manner because of the presence of the fetus. Magnesium sulfate, methyldopa, and hydralazine are the drugs of choice, with oral labetalol and nifedipine being drugs of second choice in the United States. Delivery of the infant often assists in the management of hypertension in pregnancy and often is hastened by the obstetrician under these conditions.

Hypertensive urgencies are situations in which acute TOD is not present; they require somewhat less aggressive management and can nearly always be treated with oral antihypertensive agents without hospital admission. Nifedipine, clonidine, captopril, labetalol, and several other short-acting antihypertensive drugs have been used for this problem. Nifedipine has been reported to cause precipitous hypotension, stroke, MI, and death, according to the US Food and Drug Administration, and "should be used with great caution, if at all." None of these drugs seems to have a major advantage over all the others, and all are effective in most patients (77). The most important aspect of managing a hypertensive urgency is to assure adherence to antihypertensive therapy during long-term follow-up.

Patients presenting with a hypertensive emergency should be diagnosed quickly and started promptly on effective parenteral therapy (often nitroprusside 0.5 μg or μg/kg per min) in an intensive care unit. BP should be reduced ~25% gradually >2–3 h. Oral antihypertensive therapy should be instituted after 6–12 h of parenteral therapy; evaluation for secondary causes of hypertension may be considered after transfer from the intensive care unit. Because of advances in antihypertensive therapy and management, "malignant hypertension" should be malignant no longer. For refractory hypertension, both hydralazine and minoxidil have been used for treatment in conjunction with a β-blocker and a diuretic.

VI. DRUGS INTERACTIONS

The selection of the initial agent to treat hypertension must be done with the understanding that many hypertensive patients may not reach goal BP on that agent alone and will very likely need additional antihypertensive therapy. Furthermore, many hypertensive patients need to take chronic medications for other conditions and so drug–drug interactions are of concern.

Certain combinations of antihypertensive agents are particularly effective, such as thiazide diuretics with β-blockers, ACE-Is, or ARBs. Combinations of ACE-Is with CAs (both DHP and non-DHP) are also effective. Moreover, combinations of the two subtypes of CAs are synergistic with regard to BP reduction. DHPCAs and β-blockers are also very effective combinations. Most importantly, non-DHPCAs and β-blockers should not be used together because of the risk of excessive bradycardia and conduction defects. Thiazide diuretics are effective with all other antihypertensive drugs, including CAs, and always should be included in a triple-drug regimen. Little is known about the efficacy of combining α-blockers with central and peripheral sympatholytics or with ACE-Is or ARBs.

Over the past decade, a series of low-dose combinations have been introduced that have fewer clinical side-effects than when the components are used as monotherapy, Table 23.4. The best example is the combination of a DHPCA with an ACE-I. These fixed-dose combinations have a significantly lower incidence of edema than that seen when a DHPCA is given alone. However, the incidence of cough is not lessened when these drugs are combined. The appeal of a low-dose fixed-dose combination is that BP can be reduced more quickly and effectively, with fewer adverse reactions using two drugs at lower doses than might occur when one or the other component is pushed to the maximum dose. The added advantage is that the patient needs to take fewer pills to get BP to goal and so adherence to the regimen tends to improve (discussed subsequently).

The most commonly used antihypertensives do not have any serious drug–drug interactions with anticoagulants, platelet inhibitors, or antibiotics. Non-DHPCAs, β-blockers, and telmisartan (an ARB) must be used with care in patients who are taking digoxin. Nonsteroidal anti-inflammatory agents may raise BP and can interfere with the activity of all antihypertensive agents; it is still controversial whether the specific inhibitors of cyclooxygenase-2 interfere as much or as widely as the older cyclooxygenase-1 inhibitors.

A. Medication Adherence

Overall, fewer than 50% of patients continue taking the initially prescribed antihypertensive drug therapy for 4 years (78). The proportion who properly adhere to therapy improves only modestly when the drugs and medical care are provided free of charge (20). About 10% of the overall expenditures on hypertension in the United States are wasted because of nonadherence to medical advice and antihypertensive drug therapy. Patients who do not follow the advice of their physicians and do not take their medications correctly have an infinite cost/benefit ratio because they incur all the cost associated with the therapy, but derive none of the benefits of treatment.

Some medications induce physical signs that are absent in those who have not recently taken them, for example, bradycardia with β-blockers; orthostatic BP change with α-blockers; and an increase in serum urate with diuretics. A telephone call to the patients pharmacy generally will reveal how many times the prescribed medications have been refilled during the last year. Several interventions have been advocated to improve adherence with medications, Table 23.9.

VII. CONCLUSIONS

Drug therapy is indicated in all hypertensive patients, if goal BP is not reached with lifestyle modifications alone. The following steps are recommended for choosing a regimen and then altering it until the goal is reached: (a) deal with the cost first. If the patient is unable to afford any but the least expensive drugs or cannot pay for the one that is selected, price becomes the primary issue; (b) ascertain whether other risk factors or comorbidity is present. Avoid drugs that may worsen these factors or conditions and choose the ones that may improve them; (c) find out what clinical adverse reactions the patient would or did find most troublesome and avoid agents that are likely to cause or exacerbate these problems. Some patients are not concerned by certain side effects that are very troublesome to others; (d) consider demographic issues and select the drug class with a higher probability of success if options are available; (e) start with the lowest effective dose and plan to see the patient within 4 weeks unless the severity of the patient's hypertension or another problem warrants an earlier visit. Carry out appropriate biochemical monitoring when necessary. Start with a fixed-dose combination when appropriate (e.g., stage 2 hypertension); (f) increase the dose if goal BP has not been reached or if there has been only a sub-optimal response. Do not increase the first dose or any dose prematurely. Give each dose adequate time to be fully effective. If intolerable side effects occur and are drug-related or if no BP lowering response to the medication has occurred, only then switch to another appropriate agent as monotherapy; (g) continue the process of dose titration and monitoring until the maximum recommended dose has been reached. Stopping before the full dose has been reached leads to a situation in which the patient is treated with multiple agents at sub-therapeutic doses when only one or two drugs may be necessary; (h) if the maximum-tolerated dose of the first drug fails to reduce BP to goal, add a second agent that has a different mechanism of action and is known to have additive antihypertensive effects to the first-choice agent. A fixed-dose combination that combines two drugs in the desired doses also could be used at this time; (i) titrate the second drug to the full dose, as was done for the first drug, and continue appropriate monitoring. If the two-drug combination fails, consider a specific cause for the patient's refractory hypertension, and if none is evident, add a third drug, being sure that a diuretic is part of the regimen. Consider a referral to a hypertension specialist; (j) plan to see a patient who is at goal at least once every 3 months to be sure that BP control is sustained; and (k) reinforce the need for adherence to the regimen (including lifestyle modifications) and inquire about adverse reactions. Although some patients will not reach goal with this approach even with the many available treatment options, most will come under control or close to it. Patients who do this can anticipate substantial long-term benefit with an extended life expectancy and a markedly reduced risk of stroke, ischemic heart disease, HF, and probably renal failure and quite possibly, dementia.

REFERENCES

1. Chobanian AV, Bakris GL, Black HR, Cushman WC, Green LA, Izzo JL Jr, Jones DW, Materson BJ, Oparil S, Wright JT Jr, Roccella EJ. Joint National Committee on Prevention, Detection, Evaluation, and Treatment of High Blood Pressure. National Heart, Lung, and Blood Institute; National High Blood Pressure Education Program Coordinating Committee. Seventh report of the Joint National Committee on Prevention, Detection, Evaluation, and Treatment of High Blood Pressure. Hypertension 2003; 42:1206–1252.
2. American Diabetes Association: clinical practice recommendations 2002. Diabetes Care 2002; 25:S1–S147.
3. 2003 European Society of Hypertension-European Society of Cardiology guidelines for the management of arterial hypertension. J Hypertens 2003; 21:1011–1053.
4. Campbell NR. The 2001 Canadian Hypertension Recommendations—What is new and what is old but still important. Can J Cardiol 2002; 18:591–603.
5. K/DOQI clinical practice guidelines for chronic kidney disease: evaluation, classification, and stratification. Kidney disease outcome quality initiative. Am J Kidney Dis 2002; 39:S1–S246.
6. He J, Whelton PK, Appel LJ, Charleston J, Klag MJ. Long-term effects of weight loss and dietary sodium reduction on incidence of hypertension. Hypertension 2000; 35:544–549.
7. Whelton SP, Chin A, Xin X, He J. Effect of aerobic exercise on blood pressure: a meta-analysis of randomized, controlled trials. Ann Intern Med 2002; 136:493–503.
8. Whelton PK, Appel LJ, Espeland MA, Applegate WB, Ettinger WH Jr, Kostis JB, Kumanyika S, Lacy CR, Johnson KC, Folmar S, Cutler JA. Sodium reduction and weight loss in the treatment of hypertension in older persons: a randomized controlled trial of nonpharmacologic interventions in the elderly (TONE). TONE Collaborative Research Group. J Am Med Assoc 1998; 279:839–846.
9. Appel LJ, Champagne CM, Harsha DW, Cooper LS, Obarzanek E, Elmer PJ, Stevens VJ, Vollmer WM, Lin PH, Svetkey LP, Stedman SW, Young DR. Writing Group of the PREMIER Collaborative Research Group. Effects of comprehensive lifestyle modification on blood pressure

control: main results of the PREMIER clinical trial. J Am Med Assoc 2003; 289:2083–2093.

10. Effects of weight loss and sodium reduction intervention on blood pressure and hypertension incidence in overweight people with high-normal blood pressure. The Trials of Hypertension Prevention, phase II. The Trials of Hypertension Prevention Collaborative Research Group. Arch Intern Med 1997; 157:657–667.

11. Kawano Y, Pontes CS, Abe H, Takishita S, Omae T. Effects of alcohol consumption and restriction on home blood pressure in hypertensive patients: serial changes in the morning and evening records. Clin Exp Hypertens 2002; 24:33–39.

12. Saito K, Yokoyama T, Yoshiike N, Date C, Yamamoto A, Muramatsu M, Tanaka H. Do the ethanol metabolizing enzymes modify the relationship between alcohol consumption and blood pressure? J Hypertens 2003; 21:1097–1105.

13. Xin X, He J, Frontini MG, Ogden LG, Motsamai OI, Whelton PK. Effects of alcohol reduction on blood pressure: a meta-analysis of randomized controlled trials. Hypertension 2001; 38:1112–1117.

14. Appel LJ, Moore TJ, Obarzanek E, Vollmer WM, Svetkey LP, Sacks FM, Bray GA, Vogt TM, Cutler JA, Windhauser MM, Lin PH, Karanja N. A clinical trial of the effects of dietary patterns on blood pressure. DASH Collaborative Research Group. N Engl J Med 1997; 336:1117–1124.

15. Sacks FM, Svetkey LP, Vollmer WM, Appel LJ, Bray GA, Harsha D, Obarzanek E, Conlin PR, Miller ER III, Simons-Morton DG, Karanja N, Lin PH, DASH-Sodium Collaborative Research Group. Effects on blood pressure of reduced dietary sodium and the Dietary Approaches to Stop Hypertension (DASH) diet. N Engl J Med 2001; 344:3–10.

16. 2003 European Society of Hypertension-European Society of Cardiology guidelines for the management of arterial hypertension. J Hypertens 2003; 21:1011–1053.

17. Minami J, Ishimitsu T, Matsuoka H. Effects of smoking cessation on blood pressure and heart rate variability in habitual smokers. Hypertension 1999; 33:586–590.

18. Bolinder G, de Faire U. Ambulatory 24 h blood pressure monitoring in healthy, middle-aged smokeless tobacco users, smokers, and nontobacco users. Am J Hypertens 1998; 11:1153–1163.

19. Elmer PJ, Grimm R Jr, Laing B, Grandits G, Svendsen K, Van Heel N, Betz E, Raines J, Link M, Stamler J. Lifestyle intervention: results of the Treatment of Mild Hypertension Study (TOMHS). Prev Med 1995; 24:378–388.

20. Major outcomes in high-risk hypertensive patients randomized to angiotensin-converting enzyme inhibitor or calcium channel blocker vs diuretic: The Antihypertensive and Lipid-Lowering Treatment to Prevent Heart Attack Trial (ALLHAT). J Am Med Assoc 2002; 288:2981–2997.

21. Turnbull F. Effects of different blood-pressure-lowering regimens on major cardiovascular events: results of prospectively-designed overviews of randomised trials. Lancet 2003; 362:1527–1535.

22. Staessen JA, Wang JG, Thijs L. Cardiovascular protection and blood pressure reduction: a meta-analysis. Lancet 2001; 358:1305–1315.

23. Randomised trial of a perindopril-based blood-pressure-lowering regimen among 6,105 individuals with previous stroke or transient ischaemic attack. Lancet 2001; 358:1033–1041.

24. Brenner BM, Cooper ME, de Zeeuw D, Keane WF, Mitch WE, Parving HH, Remuzzi G, Snapinn SM, Zhang Z, Shahinfar S, RENAAL Study Investigators. Effects of losartan on renal and cardiovascular outcomes in patients with type 2 diabetes and nephropathy. N Engl J Med 2001; 345:861–869.

25. Lewis EJ, Hunsicker LG, Clarke WR, Berl T, Pohl MA, Lewis JB, Ritz E, Atkins RC, Rohde R, Raz I, Collaborative Study Group. Renoprotective effect of the angiotensin-receptor antagonist irbesartan in patients with nephropathy due to type 2 diabetes. N Engl J Med 2001; 345:851–860.

26. Wing LM, Reid CM, Ryan P, Beilin LJ, Brown MA, Jennings GL, Johnston CI, McNeil JJ, Macdonald GJ, Marley JE, Morgan TO, West MJ, Second Australian National Blood Pressure Study Group. A comparison of outcomes with angiotensin-converting—enzyme inhibitors and diuretics for hypertension in the elderly. N Engl J Med 2003; 348:583–592.

27. Dahlof B, Devereux RB, Kjeldsen SE, Julius S, Beevers G, de Faire U, Fyhrquist F, Ibsen H, Kristiansson K, Lederballe-Pedersen O, Lindholm LH, Nieminen MS, Omvik P, Oparil S, Wedel H, LIFE Study Group. Cardiovascular morbidity and mortality in the Losartan Intervention For Endpoint reduction in hypertension study (LIFE): a randomised trial against atenolol. Lancet 2002; 359:995–1003.

28. Black HR, Elliott WJ, Grandits G, Grambsch P, Lucente T, White WB, Neaton JD, Grimm RH Jr, Hansson L, Lacourciere Y, Muller J, Sleight P, Weber MA, Williams G, Wittes J, Zanchetti A, Anders RJ, CONVINCE Research Group. Principal results of the Controlled Onset Verapamil Investigation of Cardiovascular End Points (CONVINCE) trial. J Am Med Assoc 2003; 289:2073–2082.

29. Pepine CJ, Handberg EM, Cooper-DeHoff RM, Marks RG, Kowey P, Messerli FH, Mancia G, Cangiano JL, Garcia-Barreto D, Keltai M, Erdine S, Bristol HA, Kolb HR, Bakris GL, Cohen JD, Parmley WW, INVEST Investigators. A Calcium Antagonist vs a Noncalcium Antagonist Hypertension Treatment Strategy for Patients With Coronary Artery Disease. The International Verapamil-Trandolapril Study (INVEST): a Randomized Controlled Trial. J Am Med Assoc 2003; 290:2805–2816.

30. Major cardiovascular events in hypertensive patients randomized to doxazosin vs chlorthalidone: the antihypertensive and lipid-lowering treatment to prevent heart attack trial (ALLHAT). ALLHAT Collaborative Research Group. J Am Med Assoc 2000; 283:1967–1975.

31. Carter BL, Ernst ME, Cohen JD. Hydrochlorothiazide versus chlorthalidone: evidence supporting their interchangeability. Hypertension 2004; 43:4–9.

32. Lithell H, Hansson L, Skoog I, Elmfeldt D, Hofman A, Olofsson B, Trenkwalder P, Zanchetti A. SCOPE Study Group. The Study on Cognition and Prognosis in the Elderly (SCOPE): principal results of a randomized

double-blind intervention trial. J Hypertens 2003; 21:875–886.

33. Heart Outcomes Prevention Evaluation Study Investigators. Effects of ramipril on cardiovascular and microvascular outcomes in people with diabetes mellitus: results of the HOPE study and MICRO-HOPE substudy. Lancet 2000; 355:253–259.

34. Svensson P, de Faire U, Sleight P, Yusuf S, Ostergren J. Comparative effects of ramipril on ambulatory and office blood pressures: a HOPE Substudy. Hypertension 2001; 38:E28–E32.

35. Hansson L, Zanchetti A, Carruthers SG, Dahlof B, Elmfeldt D, Julius S, Menard J, Rahn KH, Wedel H, Westerling S. Effects of intensive blood-pressure lowering and low-dose aspirin in patients with hypertension: principal results of the Hypertension Optimal Treatment (HOT) randomised trial. HOT Study Group. Lancet 1998; 351:1755–1762.

36. Summary of Revisions for the 2004. Clinical Practice Recommendations. Diabetes Care 2004; 27:S1–S146.

37. UK Prospective Diabetes Study Group. Tight blood pressure control and risk of macrovascular and microvascular complications in type 2 diabetes: UKPDS 38. Brit Med J 1998; 317:703–713.

38. Bakris GL, Williams M, Dworkin L, Elliott WJ, Epstein M, Toto R, Tuttle K, Douglas J, Hsueh W, Sowers J. Preserving renal function in adults with hypertension and diabetes: a consensus approach. National Kidney Foundation Hypertension and Diabetes Executive Committees Working Group. Am J Kidney Dis 2000; 36:646–661.

39. Elliott WJ, Weir DR, Black HR. Cost-effectiveness of the lower treatment goal (of JNC VI) for diabetic hypertensive patients. Joint National Committee on Prevention, Detection, Evaluation, and Treatment of High Blood Pressure. Arch Intern Med 2000; 160:1277–1283.

40. Schrier RW, Estacio RO, Esler A, Mehler P. Effects of aggressive blood pressure control in normotensive type 2 diabetic patients on albuminuria, retinopathy and strokes. Kidney Int 2002; 61:1086–1097.

41. Wright JT Jr, Bakris G, Greene T, Agodoa LY, Appel LJ, Charleston J, Cheek D, Douglas-Baltimore JG, Gassman J, Glassock R, Hebert L, Jamerson K, Lewis J, Phillips RA, Toto RD, Middleton JP, Rostand SG, African American Study of Kidney Disease and Hypertension Study Group. Effect of blood pressure lowering and antihypertensive drug class on progression of hypertensive kidney disease: results from the AASK trial. J Am Med Assoc 2002; 288:2421–2431.

42. Perry HM Jr, Davis BR, Price TR, Applegate WB, Fields WS, Guralnik JM, Kuller L, Pressel S, Stamler J, Probstfield JL. Effect of treating isolated systolic hypertension on the risk of developing various types and subtypes of stroke: the Systolic Hypertension in the Elderly Program (SHEP). J Am Med Assoc 2000; 284:465–471.

43. Jafar TH, Stark PC, Schmid CH, Landa M, Maschio G, de Jong PE, de Zeeuw D, Shahinfar S, Toto R, Levey AS, AIPRD Study Group. Progression of chronic kidney disease: the role of blood pressure control, proteinuria, and angiotensin-converting enzyme inhibition: a patient-level meta-analysis. Ann Intern Med 2003; 139:244–252.

44. Ramsay LE, Williams B, Johnston GD, MacGregor GA, Poston L, Potter JF, Poulter NR, Russell G. British Hypertension Society guidelines for hypertension management 1999: summary. Brit Med J 1999; 319:630–635.

45. Major outcomes in moderately hypercholesterolemic, hypertensive patients randomized to pravastatin vs usual care: The Antihypertensive and Lipid-Lowering Treatment to Prevent Heart Attack Trial (ALLHAT-LLT). J Am Med Assoc 2002; 288:2998–3007.

46. Gress TW, Nieto FJ, Shahar E, Wofford MR, Brancati FL. Hypertension and antihypertensive therapy as risk factors for type 2 diabetes mellitus. Atherosclerosis Risk in Communities Study. N Engl J Med 2000; 342:905–912.

47. Sowers JR, Bakris GL. Antihypertensive therapy and the risk of type 2 diabetes mellitus. N Engl J Med 2000; 342:969–970.

48. Elisaf MS, Theodorou J, Pappas H, Papagalanis N, Katopodis K, Kalaitzidis R, Siamopoulos KC. Effectiveness and metabolic effects of perindopril and diuretics combination in primary hypertension. J Hum Hypertens 1999; 13:787–791.

49. Grimm RH Jr, Flack JM, Grandits GA, Elmer PJ, Neaton JD, Cutler JA, Lewis C, McDonald R, Schoenberger J, Stamler J. Long-term effects on plasma lipids of diet and drugs to treat hypertension. Treatment of Mild Hypertension Study (TOMHS) Research Group. J Am Med Assoc 1996; 275:1549–1556.

50. Hansson L, Lindholm LH, Niskanen L, Lanke J, Hedner T, Niklason A, Luomanmaki K, Dahlof B, de Faire U, Morlin C, Karlberg BE, Wester PO, Bjorck JE. Effect of angiotensin-converting-enzyme inhibition compared with conventional therapy on cardiovascular morbidity and mortality in hypertension: the Captopril Prevention Project (CAPPP) randomised trial. Lancet 1999; 353:611–616.

51. Gerstein HC. Reduction of cardiovascular events and microvascular complications in diabetes with ACE inhibitor treatment: HOPE and MICRO-HOPE. Diabetes Metab Res Rev 2002; 18:S82–S85.

52. Bakris GL, Weir M. ACE inhibitors and protection against kidney disease progression in patients with type 2 diabetes: what's the evidence. J Clin Hypertens (Greenwich) 2002; 4:420–423.

53. Voyaki SM, Staessen JA, Thijs L, Wang JG, Efstratopoulos AD, Birkenhager WH et al. Follow-up of renal function in treated and untreated older patients with isolated systolic hypertension. Systolic Hypertension in Europe (Syst-Eur) Trial Investigators. J Hypertens 2001; 19:511–519.

54. Koshy S, Bakris GL. Therapeutic approaches to achieve desired blood pressure goals: focus on calcium channel blockers. Cardiovasc Drugs Ther 2000; 14:295–301.

55. Levy D, Larson MG, Vasan RS, Kannel WB, Ho KK. The progression from hypertension to congestive heart failure. J Am Med Assoc 1996; 275:1557–1562.

56. Kitzman DW, Little WC, Brubaker PH, Anderson RT, Hundley WG, Marburger CT, Brosnihan B, Morgan TM, Stewart KP. Pathophysiological characterization of isolated

diastolic heart failure in comparison to systolic heart failure. J Am Med Assoc 2002; 288:2144–2150.

57. Psaty BM, Smith NL, Siscovick DS, Koepsell TD, Weiss NS, Heckbert SR, Lemaitre RN, Wagner EH, Furberg CD. Health outcomes associated with antihypertensive therapies used as first-line agents. A systematic review and meta-analysis. J Am Med Assoc 1997; 277:739–745.

58. Gomberg-Maitland M, Baran DA, Fuster V. Treatment of congestive heart failure: guidelines for the primary care physician and the heart failure specialist. Arch Intern Med 2001; 161:342–352.

59. Pitt B, Zannad F, Remme WJ, Cody R, Castaigne A, Perez A, Palensky J, Wittes J. The effect of spironolactone on morbidity and mortality in patients with severe heart failure. Randomized Aldactone Evaluation Study Investigators. N Engl J Med 1999; 341:709–717.

60. Pitt B, Williams G, Remme W, Martinez F, Lopez-Sendon J, Zannad F, Neaton J, Roniker B, Hurley S, Burns D, Bittman R, Kleiman J. The EPHESUS trial: eplerenone in patients with heart failure due to systolic dysfunction complicating acute myocardial infarction. Eplerenone Post-AMI Heart Failure Efficacy and Survival Study. Cardiovasc Drugs Ther 2001; 15:79–87.

61. Cohn JN, Tognoni G. A randomized trial of the angiotensin-receptor blocker valsartan in chronic heart failure. N Engl J Med 2001; 345:1667–1675.

62. Pfeffer MA, Swedberg K, Granger CB, Held P, McMurray JJ, Michelson EL, Olofsson B, Ostergren J, Yusuf S, Pocock S, CHARM Investigators and Committees. Effects of candesartan on mortality and morbidity in patients with chronic heart failure: the CHARM-Overall programme. Lancet 2003; 362:759–766.

63. Pfeffer MA, McMurray JJ, Velazquez EJ, Rouleau JL, Kober L, Maggioni AP, Solomon SD, Swedberg K, Van de Werf F, White H, Leimberger JD, Henis M, Edwards S, Zelenkofske S, Sellers MA, Califf RM, Valsartan in Acute Myocardial Infarction Trial Investigators. Valsartan, captopril, or both in myocardial infarction complicated by heart failure, left ventricular dysfunction, or both. N Engl J Med 2003; 349:1893–1906.

64. Bakris GL, Weir MR, Shanifar S, Zhang Z, Douglas J, van Dijk DJ, Brenner BM, RENAAL Study Group. Effects of blood pressure level on progression of diabetic nephropathy: results from the RENAAL study. Arch Intern Med 2003; 163:1555–1565.

65. Bakris GL, Weir MR, DeQuattro V, McMahon FG. Effects of an ACE inhibitor/calcium antagonist combination on proteinuria in diabetic nephropathy. Kidney Int 1998; 54:1283–1289.

66. Boero R, Rollino C, Massara C, Berto IM, Perosa P, Vagelli G, Lanfranco G, Quarello F. The verapamil versus amlodipine in nondiabetic nephropathies treated with trandolapril (VVANNTT) study. Am J Kidney Dis 2003; 42:67–75.

67. Bakris GL, Weir MR. Salt intake and reductions in arterial pressure and proteinuria. Is there a direct link? Am J Hypertens 1996; 9:200S–206S.

68. Bakris GL, Weir MR. Angiotensin-converting enzyme inhibitor-associated elevations in serum creatinine: is this a cause for concern? Arch Intern Med 2000; 160:685–693.

69. Yeghiazarians Y, Braunstein JB, Askari A, Stone PH. Unstable angina pectoris. N Engl J Med 2000; 342:101–114.

70. Heidenreich PA, McDonald KM, Hastie T, Fadel B, Hagan V, Lee BK, Hlatky MA. Meta-analysis of trials comparing β-blockers, calcium antagonists, and nitrates for stable angina. J Am Med Assoc 1999; 281:1927–1936.

71. Fox KM. Efficacy of perindopril in reduction of cardiovascular events among patients with stable coronary artery disease: randomised, double-blind, placebo-controlled, multicentre trial (the EUROPA study). Lancet 2003; 362:782–788.

72. Staessen JA, Gasowski J, Wang JG, Thijs L, Den Hond E, Boissel JP, Coope J, Ekbom T, Gueyffier F, Liu L, Kerlikowske K, Pocock S, Fagard RH. Risks of untreated and treated isolated systolic hypertension in the elderly: meta-analysis of outcome trials. Lancet 2000; 355:865–872.

73. Guidelines, Hypertension in Pregnancy. http://www.nhlbi. nih.gov/health/prof/heart/hbp/hbp_preg.htm accessed on 3/30/05, 2004.

74. Elliott WJ. Hypertensive emergencies. Crit Care Clin 2001; 17:435–451.

75. Dmowski AT, Carcy MJ. Aortic dissection. Am J Emerg Med 1999; 17:372–375.

76. Murphy MB, Murray C, Shorten GD. Fenoldopam: a selective peripheral dopamine-receptor agonist for the treatment of severe hypertension. N Engl J Med 2001; 345:1548–1557.

77. Grossman E, Ironi AN, Messerli FH. Comparative tolerability profile of hypertensive crisis treatments. Drug Saf 1998; 19:99–122.

78. Conlin PR, Gerth WC, Fox J, Roehm JB, Boccuzzi SJ. Four-Year persistence patterns among patients initiating therapy with the angiotensin II receptor antagonist losartan versus other artihypertensive drug classes. Clin Ther 2001; 23:1999–2010.

79. Saseen JJ, Carter BL, Brown TE, Elliott WJ, Black HR. Comparison of nifedipine alone and with diltiazem or verapamil in hypertension. Hypertension 1996; 28:109–114.

24

Lifestyle Modifications and Value of Nondrug Therapy

FRANCESCO P. CAPPUCCIO, GABRIELA B. GOMEZ
St. George's Hospital Medical School, London, UK

KEYPOINTS

- Lifestyle modifications are helpful measures in the management and treatment of hypertension.
- Not all lifestyle modifications that may be recommended have equally valuable evidence base.
- The principal lifestyle modifications that should be recommended are:
  o Dietary salt reduction.
  o Increase of dietary potassium.
  o Weight loss if overweight.
  o Smoking cessation, moderate alcohol drinking and regular physical exercise.

SUMMARY

Lifestyles modifications and non-drug therapies are a vast group of measures essential to the prevention and management of hypertension. International experts unanimously recommend some of them. However, not all measures are equally valuable or have the same evidence base. The first step in the management of patients of any age who have hypertension should be a reduction in salt intake (from 9 to 6 g/day), either alone or in combination with drug therapy, to which is often additive. A high potassium diet achieved with an increase in the consumption of fruit, vegetables and pulses is also recommended. Weight reduction, regular dynamic exercise and reduction of alcohol consumption should be included in management plans for the prevention and non-pharmacological treatment of hypertension. Limited evidence supports the role of calcium and magnesium, or stress management for the prevention and management of hypertension.

I. INTRODUCTION

It is widely accepted that changes in diet and lifestyle do lower blood pressure and reduce cardiovascular risk. They represent valuable tools for the prevention and

Table 24.1 Summary of Lifestyle Changes to Improve the Control of Hypertension

Lose weight if overweight
Reduce your sodium intake: not more than 5 g of salt per day
Follow a diet with a high consumption of fruit, vegetables, and
　pulses
Moderate alcohol consumption: not more than 2 or 3 units
　per day
Regular and dynamic exercise
Stop smoking

management of hypertension. Although these lifestyle measures are remarkably useful because of their low cost, their effectiveness is related to the patient's ability and motivation to change and to maintain this change.

International experts recommend a series of nonpharmacological measures on the basis of the evidence currently available (Table 24.1). They consistently insist on the importance of weight reduction, if overweight, restriction of dietary salt intake, limitation of alcohol consumption, and regular and dynamic exercise. A diet that increases vegetables, fruit and low-fat or fat-free dairy product consumption (therefore, rich in fiber, potassium, calcium, and magnesium) is also part of the unanimously accepted recommendations. In this chapter, we will review the evidence available supporting these measures and other behavioral measures, such as smoking cessation and relaxation, which may have an impact on blood pressure control.

II. WEIGHT REDUCTION

The burden of obesity in societies is increasing. The prevalence of obesity in the United States, defined as body mass index (BMI) $\geq 30 \text{ kg/m}^2$, by the year 2000 was $\sim 20\%$ of the adult population and overweight or obese (BMI $\geq 25 \text{ kg/m}^2$) was over 60% (1). In the United Kingdom, the progression of obesity has followed the same direction. In 1980, 8% of women and 6% of men were obese, whereas currently half of women and two-thirds of men are overweight or obese (BMI $\geq 25 \text{ kg/m}^2$) (2). Following this tendency, the risk of co-morbidity increases proportionally to the increase in body weight and so do the cardiovascular risk factors such as dyslipidemia, diabetes mellitus, and hypertension. Moreover, obesity is also an independent risk factor for coronary heart disease and total cardiovascular morbidity and mortality.

Over the past decades, many studies have investigated the relationship between blood pressure and obesity. An early review published by MacMahon et al. shows a linear, positive, and independent relation between BMI

or body weight and systolic and diastolic blood pressure (3). Obesity may account for one-third of the prevalence of hypertension. Although, this association is present in all subgroups by age, sex, or ethnic group, the results suggested it to be stronger in whites than in people of black African origin and to diminish with age.

In overweight subjects, the distribution of body fat seems to affect the risk of cardiovascular disease and hypertension. The prospective study of "men born in 1913" showed a significant association between waist-to-hip circumference ratio and stroke, ischemic heart disease, and death from all causes (4). Furthermore, the influence of central adiposity on hypertension has been suggested in different studies in men, women, whites, and people of black African origin (5–9). However, as the methods used to measure waist-to-hip ratio have lacked standardization and suffer from large observer bias, the National Institutes of Health Clinical Guidelines on the Identification, Evaluation, and Treatment of Overweight and Obesity in Adults proposed the waist circumference as a reference measure of central adiposity (10). The results from the Olivetti Heart Study show that, in middle aged men, waist circumference is a strong predictor of high blood pressure independently of BMI and insulin resistance (6).

Considering the relationship between weight and blood pressure, weight reduction has been proposed as a measure to reduce blood pressure in overweight subjects. The results of the Trials of Hypertension Prevention (TOHP), Phase I and II, multicenter, randomized clinical interventions, indicate that both short and long-term weight loss interventions are successful in reducing blood pressure (11,12). In TOHP I, an 18-month intervention was significantly associated with 77% reduction in the incidence of hypertension after a 7-year follow-up. In TOHP II, a longer-term intervention of 36 months resulted, equally, in significant reductions in systolic and diastolic blood pressures and in a lower incidence of hypertension.

The latest published meta-analysis of 25 randomized controlled trials between 1978 and 2002—including only weight reduction by means of energy restriction, increased physical activity, or both—showed a blood pressure reduction of 4.4/3.6 mmHg for a 5 kg weight loss (13). [Fig. 24.1(A) and (B)]. A dose-response was observed, that is, the greater the weight loss, the greater the blood pressure reduction. Furthermore, the beneficial effect of weight reduction on blood pressure was independent of age, gender, and initial BMI, although the effect appeared greater in patients on antihypertensive therapy. This meta-analysis also highlights the problem of lack of compliance during long-term interventions because the maximal effect was reached before the end of the trials. A previous Cochrane review also associated a modest weight loss to a modest blood pressure reduction and finally recommended a weight loss program as part of a nondrug

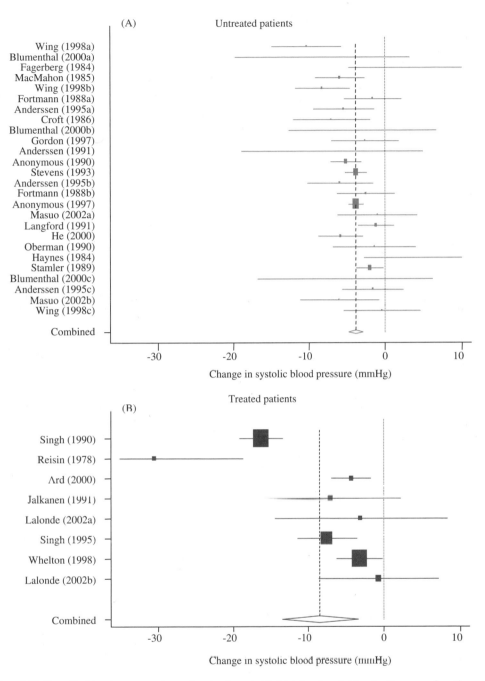

Figure 24.1 (A and B) Systolic blood pressure in randomized controlled trials of weight reduction as a function of whether patients follow antihypertensive treatment.

intervention or as adjunctive to drug therapy, as it decreases the dosage of antihypertensive therapy needed to reach blood pressure control (14).

Moreover, the Trial of Nonpharmacologic Interventions in Elderly (TONE) showed that a combined intervention reducing average body weight by ~3.5 kg and sodium intake by ~40 mmol/day in elderly patients (60–80 years) was associated with a 30% reduction in blood pressure (equivalent to that achieved with antihypertensive

medication) (15). Likewise, the Diet, Exercise, and Weight Loss Intervention Trial (DEW-IT), a recent controlled trial, has confirmed that weight loss and changes in lifestyle do lower blood pressure in obese participants taking a stable dose of a single antihypertensive drug. The participants were randomized into two groups: a control group and a lifestyle group that was fed a hypocaloric and low-salt version of the Dietary Approaches to Stop Hypertension (DASH) diet and followed a fitness program. The mean weight loss in the lifestyle group was 4.9 kg and the blood pressure reduction observed during this trial was similar to that achieved with pharmacotherapy: $-12/-6$ mmHg (16).

An exploratory prospective analysis of the cohort of middle aged men in the Chicago Western Electric study, a long-term prospective study, confirms a positive relationship between weight gain and average annual change in blood pressure (17).

The biological mechanisms involved in the effect of weight reduction on blood pressure are not fully understood, but at least three different pathways must be considered: first, an effect mediated through inhibition of an overactive renin–angiotensin–aldosterone system in obese subjects; secondly, a stimulation of the natriuretic peptides system with vasodilatation and natriuresis; and thirdly, a reduction in insulin resistance and hyperinsulinemia (13–18).

In conclusion, weight loss is a widely accepted recommendation for overweight or obese patients (19,20). The complete available evidence shows the significant benefits related to this lifestyle modification and its importance when managing and preventing hypertension. Therefore, physicians and health professionals should constantly insist on the importance of weight loss, underlining the related health benefits of this measure alone and as part of a combination therapy, including salt reduction, moderation in alcohol consumption, and increased physical activity, for additive blood pressure reductions.

III. DIETARY SODIUM REDUCTION

There is a large body of evidence supporting the view that high salt intake contributes to elevated blood pressure. Indeed, the reduction of dietary sodium intake is one of the most important and effective lifestyle modifications to reduce blood pressure and to control hypertension. Although the nonvascular health effects of a reduction of salt intake in the long term are less clear, the value of the public health recommendations in the management and prevention of hypertension and other cardiovascular diseases is beyond doubt.

The direct relationship between blood pressure and dietary salt intake has been shown consistently in the past decades. The INTERSALT study, an epidemiological, standardized international study included 10,079 men and women, aged 20–59 years old in 52 centers from 32 different countries (21). The analyses were performed at two levels. First, the intra-center results showed a significant, positive, independent, and linear association between the two principal outcomes of this trial: 24 h urinary sodium excretion reflecting the amount of sodium intake and systolic blood pressure. A 100 mmol/day higher sodium

intake would predict a 3–6 mmHg higher systolic and up to 3 mmHg higher diastolic blood pressure. These results were valid in the different subgroups analyzed: men, women, young, elderly, and for 8344 participants with normal blood pressure.

The cross-population analysis, including 52 centers, also showed a significant, independent relationship between 24 h urinary sodium excretion and median systolic and diastolic blood pressure. Furthermore, there was an association between systolic and diastolic blood pressure and the prevalence of hypertension, and an increase with age of systolic and diastolic blood pressure also was observed.

These results are corroborated by the Multiple Risk Factor Intervention Trial (MRFIT). In this cohort of more than 11,000 participants and a follow-up of 6 years, sodium intake (assessed by dietary records) was significantly, directly, and independently related to systolic and diastolic blood pressure in both those receiving and not receiving antihypertensive medication (22). This relationship was detected even though the authors may have underestimated the effect of dietary sodium by calculating sodium intake only from reported foods consumed and not taking into account any discretionary salt added in the kitchen or at the table. Although the literature shows that most of the salt consumed in western societies comes from processed food, a correction for systematic bias was introduced in the analysis to reduce this error (23).

A moderate reduction in salt intake reduces blood pressure. Different meta-analyses show a significant blood pressure reduction in response to a reduction in sodium intake in hypertensive patients. In the latest published meta-analysis of 40 trials, an average reduction in urinary sodium excretion of 77 mmol/24 h is associated with a reduction in blood pressure of 2.54/1.96 mmHg (24). Previous meta-analyses published concordant results. When analyzing data in normotensive patients, some reported significant reductions in blood pressure following a reduction in sodium intake and others argued for a nonsignificant effect in this population (25). The controversy has, in part, been encouraged by sections of the food industry (and particularly by their public relation companies protecting the interests of salt manufacturers) to avoid a population-wide reduction in salt intake with devastating effects on their profits (26).

A moderate reduction in sodium intake lowers blood pressure and is beneficial in preventing hypertension. In the Trial of Hypertension Prevention Phase II, a sodium reduction of 100 mmol/day (equivalent to 6 g of salt/day) alone or combined with weight loss prevents hypertension by 20%. The TONE trial reported a 30% decrease in the need for antihypertensive medication by reducing the average sodium intake by ∼40 mmol/day (15).

Finally, in the DASH study, the authors argued that even lower sodium intakes should be recommended (27). Although blood pressure could be lowered by reducing sodium intake from 140 to 100 mmol/day (the 6 g salt threshold recommended by international guidelines), a further reduction of sodium intake from 100 to 65 mmol/day (to ~3 g of salt) caused a further decrease in blood pressure. The effect of salt reduction is, therefore, dose-dependent. It lasts as long as the reduction is sustained with no evidence of an adaptation effect, from periods of several weeks to a few years (28). Two recent meta-analyses (29,30) and studies in the UK (31) and in the US (32,33) support the role of a moderate reduction in sodium intake to lower blood pressure.

The effect of salt reduction on blood pressure in children and adolescents has also been studied. In a double-blind, randomized controlled trial conducted in 1980 among 476 newborn infants, Hofman et al. (34) showed that infants fed with a diet lower in salt had lower blood pressure in the first 6 months of life. Furthermore, a follow-up of this cohort 15 years later showed that the two groups had significantly different blood pressures. The children who were assigned to the lower salt intake during the intervention had lower systolic blood pressure (35). A recent review of a limited number of observational and interventional studies suggested an association between blood pressure and salt consumption in children and adolescents (36).

Long-term effects or health benefits remain to be studied. Graudal et al. (37) claimed possible hormonal and metabolic hazards of reducing the consumption of sodium to very low levels. The levels of renin and aldosterone were increased by 3.6-fold and 3.2-fold, respectively. They argued that a reduced sodium intake should be used as a supplementary treatment in hypertensives only. However, in another study, Meade et al. (38) concluded that plasma renin was not associated with cardiovascular disease.

The size of the reduction in blood pressure related to a reduction in sodium intake varies according to age, level of the initial blood pressure, and sharpness of the response of the renin angiotensin system. Irrespective of the initial blood pressure, a modest reduction in salt intake in people over the age of 60 induces a significant reduction in blood pressure, without untoward effect (39). These findings are supported by several trials showing larger reductions in blood pressure in response to sodium restriction in older patients (25,40). The TONE trial included 975 men and women aged 60–80 years with a blood pressure <145/85 mmHg while receiving treatment with a single antihypertensive medication (15). This study in an elderly population concluded that in hypertensives, it is feasible to achieve and maintain moderate decreases in sodium intake and body weight. These changes result in important reductions in blood pressure and a reduction

in the need for antihypertensive drugs. People of black African origin are another group that shows greater effect in blood pressure when dietary salt is reduced (27,41). The renin–angiotensin system is the metabolic response to a reduction in salt intake. The more efficient this compensatory response is, the smaller the blood pressure reduction following a decrease in sodium intake (42). This phenomenon explains why, for instance, the effect is larger in hypertensives and amongst the elderly. These groups have weaker responses of the renin–angiotensin system to a change in the amount of sodium ingested, showing a greater blood pressure fall. Similarly, "low-renin" black populations respond more than white populations to the same degree of salt restriction (43).

Considering these mechanisms, some additive effects of salt restriction and drugs blocking the renin–angiotensin system would be predicted. Indeed, angiotensin-converting enzyme inhibitors, β-blockers, and angiotensin II receptor antagonists have an additive effect on blood pressure in those already on a reduced sodium intake (44). Furthermore, the reduction in sodium intake associated with any of the above classes of drugs is as effective as adding a low-dose thiazide diuretic.

There is a great interest in the genetic determinants of the blood pressure sensitivity to salt and its ethnic variations (45). Genes involved in the regulation of the renin–angiotensin pathway, in transmembrane ion exchange, and in the modulation of sympathetic activity have been a focus of intense research. The Olivetti Heart Study involving a large population sample of middle aged men showed an association between the Gly40Ser mutation of the glucagon receptor gene and an increased sodium reabsorption at the proximal tubule (46). The study indicates a possible genetic contributor to the blood pressure sensitivity to salt. However, this genetic variant is almost absent in other ethnic groups, particularly in those of black African origin who are known to be most salt sensitive (47). In contrast, the C(-344)T polymorphic variant of the aldosterone synthase gene (CYP11B2) modulates the relationship of blood pressure and plasma aldosterone levels with age (48). The associations between functional mutations associated with altered renal sodium handling and changes in sodium intake have not been clearly explained yet. A reasonable hypothesis seems to be that each functional mutation has an influence in the individual response of blood pressure to sodium intake.

Reduced salt intake has other benefits as well as blood pressure reduction, for instance, it is recommended in conditions of sodium and fluid retention. It is associated with a reduction of urinary calcium excretion and risk of kidney stones, reduction in bone mineral loss with age, and osteoporosis (49–51). It seems to protect against stomach cancer, stroke, and asthma attacks (52).

Table 24.2 How to Reduce Salt Intake: A Practical Advice

Target daily salt intake should not exceed 5 g/day

1. Never add salt to a meal

You should not

   Use rock salt or sea salt. They are the same as table salt!

   Add sauces, most of them contain salt (i.e., tomato ketchup, soy sauce, HP sauce)

Instead

Use pepper, garlic, lemon, and herbs

2. Do not add salt to the cooking

You should not

   Use stock cubes, gravy browning, soy sauce, or salted dry fish

   Use curry powders and prepared mustards, some of them are high in salt

Instead

Try other flavorings!

   Any fresh, frozen, or dried herbs

   All spices

   Lemon or lime. Vinegar

   Wine, beer, or cider

   Onions, garlic, shallots, ginger, and chillies

3. Avoid manufactured or processed foods with added salt

Food labeling

   Salt is sodium chloride. At the moment, most food labels only report sodium as grams per 100 g of food. To convert to salt multiply by 2.5 (1 g of sodium per 100 g of food is the equivalent to the saltiness of seawater!)

Beware

   Most breads are high in salt

   Many cereals contain too much salt

   All ready soups, all processed meats, take-away pizzas, Chinese take-away, and some ready-made foods are often very high in salt

   Some mineral waters also are high in salt

Ideally

Only chose food items with no more than 0.3 g of sodium per 100 g of food (equivalent to ~0.75 g of salt per 100 g of food)

Reduction of dietary salt intake is one of the most important nonpharmacological lifestyle modifications recommended by international organizations (19,20) (Table 24.2). This reduction will be only effective in western societies if negotiations with the food industry start and manufacturers decrease the amount of salt added to processed food. In these societies, a large proportion of sodium intake (~77%) comes from processed food and bread (21). On the contrary, in developing countries where the prevalence of hypertension continues to increase, more traditional health promotion strategies would be applicable and nutritional education might have an important effect in these societies (53,54).

Another approach to lower salt intake is the use of salt substitutes. The American Heart Association recommends the use of nonchloride salts of sodium because they do not increase blood pressure (55). In a double-blind, randomized placebo-controlled trial that includes 100 men and women 55–75 years old with untreated mild-to-moderate hypertension, Geleijnse et al. (56) showed a significant decrease in blood pressure of 7.6/3.3 mmHg when using a mineral salt substitute (sodium:potassium:magnesium, 8:6:1). The effect was sustained as long as the patients used the salt subtitute.

In conclusion, there is enough evidence to recommend a decrease of dietary salt intake (from 9 to 6 g/day) as an effective measure to lower blood pressure in hypertensive patients. At a population level, the issue is more complex. The expected benefits of a modest reduction in blood pressure across the whole population would be significant, especially on stroke, coronary heart disease, and all other cardiovascular conditions for which high blood pressure is a causative risk factor. The benefits would be greater in the elderly. They have a much higher stroke incidence (greater absolute risk), and the majority of strokes occur at levels of blood pressure not always requiring drug therapy (more stroke events attributable to the effect of blood pressure).

IV. INFLUENCE OF OTHER MICRONUTRIENTS ON BLOOD PRESSURE

A. Potassium

Several factors seem to be involved in the regulation of blood pressure and nutritional factors are the most important environmental elements influencing it. In particular, the association between potassium intake and blood pressure had raised substantial interest.

Two large prospective studies have shown an inverse association between dietary potassium intake and prevalence of hypertension. Ascherio et al. (57) analyzed a cohort of 30,681 United States male professionals, 40–75 years old, without diagnosed hypertension for a follow-up period of 4 years. A significant inverse association was found between potassium intake and risk of hypertension after adjustment for energy intake, age, relative weight, and alcohol consumption. When adjusted additionally for dietary fiber and magnesium intake, the association was no longer significant. The same result was observed before in a large cohort of women, the Nurses' Health Study cohort (58). Although there is a significant association between potassium and hypertension, there is also an important correlation between potassium, calcium, and magnesium intake as they are present simultaneously in foods such as fruits, nuts, vegetables, cereals, and dairy products—hence the difficulty to differentiate the importance of the potassium effect when adjusted to the other micronutrients in these prospective studies (59).

The INTERSALT co-operative study also estimated the effect of potassium in blood pressure. A reduction in systolic and diastolic blood pressure of 3.36/1.87 mmHg was related to a higher potassium intake of 50 mmol/day (60). Other cross-sectional studies also have shown this inverse relationship between potassium intake and blood pressure. Accordingly, a recent meta-analysis by Geleijnse et al. (24) including 27 potassium trials showed a similar association between the increase of potassium intake (median: 44 mmol/24 h) and a decrease in systolic and diastolic blood pressure of 2.42 mmHg (95% CI, 1.08–3.75) and 1.57 mmHg (0.50–2.65) respectively.

Furthermore, in the TOHP phase I trial, a double-blind, randomized controlled trial, Whelton et al. (61) showed that there was a significant, independent, dose-response relationship between the variations of both 24 h urinary potassium excretion and urinary sodium potassium ratio and the corresponding change in diastolic blood pressure.

The relation between high potassium intake and lower blood pressure has been widely shown and it appears to be the same in women and men. However, Grim et al. (62) presented results showing a difference between African-Americans and whites in their response to changes in potassium intake. At similar levels of sodium intake and with low potassium intake, the prevalence of hypertension was higher in African-Americans. Two different intervention trials in participants from this ethnic group published a substantial reduction in blood pressure after potassium supplementation (63,64).

Two major meta-analyses that included randomized controlled trials, where the effect of potassium supplementation on blood pressure was tested, showed similar results. In an early meta-analysis, the review of 19 clinical trials (586 patients including 412 hypertensive patients) showed an overall effect of potassium supplementation of −5.9 mmHg (95% CI, −6.6 to −5.2) and −3.4 mmHg (95% CI, −4.0 to −2.8) for systolic and diastolic blood pressure, respectively. The lowering effect of potassium supplementation was greater in hypertensives, and the longer the duration of the supplementation, more pronounced the effect observed (65). In a more recent meta-analysis including 2609 participants in 33 randomized controlled trials, Whelton et al. (66) published similar effects of potassium supplementation (Fig. 24.2). Furthermore, they concluded that the effect of potassium supplementation on blood pressure appeared to be enhanced in studies including patients with a high sodium intake.

In a "potassium-deprivation" intervention trial by Krishna et al. (67), 10 healthy normotensive and hypertensive patients were randomized to an isocaloric diet consisting of an equal sodium intake and either low (10 mmol/day) or normal potassium (90 mmol/day) intake. Both mean arterial blood pressure and diastolic blood pressure were significantly higher in the low potassium diet. They argued in a latter publication that potassium depletion in humans is accompanied by sodium retention and calcium depletion and also by an altered response to vasoactive hormones. These metabolic effects together with the direct vasoconstrictive effects of hypokalemia might be the cause of the augmentation in blood pressure during a decrease of potassium intake (68).

Nevertheless, the mechanisms responsible for the hypotensive effect of increased potassium intake have not been

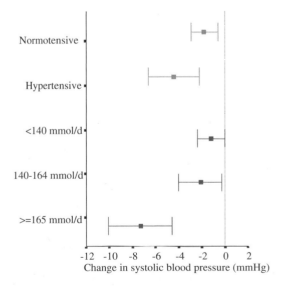

Figure 24.2 Difference in systolic blood pressure after potassium supplementation as a function of the hypertension status and urinary sodium (marker of salt intake).

fully understood. Several hypotheses have been put forward. High potassium intake might reduce the development of atherosclerosis, therefore, having a vascular protective effect. It may also reduce arteriolar thickening in the kidney. Moreover, potassium infusion increases acetylcholine-induced vasodilatation, and this effect is inhibited by the consequent infusion of the nitric oxide synthase inhibitor L-NMMA (l-nitromonomethylarginine). This suggests that through a nitric oxide-dependent vasodilatation, potassium could lower blood pressure.

The main sources of dietary potassium in the form of inorganic or organic salts are fruits, vegetables, pulses, and nuts. The results of a recent randomized controlled trial conducted in 59 volunteers suggested that mean arterial blood pressure was reduced by an average of 7.01 mmHg as a result of a low-dose potassium supplementation (24 mmol of slow-release potassium chloride per day) equivalent to the content of 5 portions of fresh fruits and vegetables (69).

Not only does the increase in dietary potassium help to reduce blood pressure, but also, it is a feasible and effective measure to reduce antihypertensive drug treatment. In 1991, Siani et al. (70) showed that after dietary advice, the intervention group increased their potassium intake compared with the control group. Consequently, blood pressure could be controlled using <50% of the initial therapy in 81% of the patients in this group compared with 29% of the patients in the control group. For instance, high potassium intake in patients with diuretic-induced hypokalemia improves blood pressure control (71).

Currently, the existing evidence supports the notion that a diet which provides a sufficient amount of potassium (as much as five portions of fresh fruits and vegetables a day) is an effective nonpharmacological measure to improve blood pressure control in hypertensives and to reduce the risk of hypertension in the general population (Table 24.3). Although potassium supplementation cannot be considered as a fully nonpharmacological intervention, it should be included as part of the recommendations for treatment and prevention of hypertension because of its significant benefits in this group.

B. Calcium

The potential effect of dietary calcium on blood pressure has been the focus of a considerable amount of research because calcium intake can be increased by simple dietary measures at low cost.

Several observational studies investigating the association between calcium intake and blood pressure have been published. However, they show inconsistent results. Potential explanations of this inconsistency are the differences in the design of the studies, the methods used to assess calcium intake, and the sample characteristics and

Table 24.3   Foods Rich in Potassium Classified by Descending Content

Fresh fruits	Pulses (legumes)	Vegetables
Foods with 5 mmol or more of elemental potassium per 100 g		
Banana	Bean (dry)	Mushroom
Apricot	Broad bean (dry)	Potatoes
Plum	Chickpeas (dry)	Spinach
Cherries	Lentils (dry)	Artichoke
Grapefruit	Broad bean (fresh)	Broccoli
Grapes		Cauliflower
Oranges		Chicory
Peaches		Asparagus
		Cabbage
		Fennel
		Lettuce
		Prickly lettuce
		String beans
		Raw tomatoes
		Turnip
Other foods: 2–5 mmol of elemental potassium per 100 g		
Orange juice	Canned beans	Carrots
Pear	Canned lentils	Green tomatoes
Apple	Peas (fresh)	Aubergine
	Peas (frozen)	Radicchio
		Green peppers
		Peppers

sizes. Altogether, these studies indicate that for 1 g higher calcium intake there would be a reduction in systolic blood pressure from −0.34 to −0.01 mmHg in men, from −0.16 to −0.15 mmHg in women, and from −0.39 to −0.06 mmHg in both groups combined. The corresponding reduction in diastolic blood pressure would be from −0.22 to −0.01 in men, from −0.06 to −0.05 in women, and from −0.35 to −0.06 in the groups combined (72,73). In conclusion, there may be a significant inverse association between calcium and blood pressure. However, the size of these estimates and the lack of causality do not justify an increase in calcium intake above the Recommended Dietary Allowance at population level for the prevention and treatment of high blood pressure.

Intervention trials are more likely to prove a causal relationship. Two large meta-analyses of randomized controlled trials have been published analyzing the blood pressure lowering effect of calcium supplementation (Fig. 24.3).

In 1996, Allender et al. (74) pooled 22 trials including a total of 1231 participants. They estimated a reduction of −0.89 and −0.18 mmHg of, respectively, systolic and diastolic blood pressure in the overall sample. An analysis of two subgroups of trials, carried out in hypertensive patients and normotensive patients, respectively, showed a higher reduction of −1.68 mmHg in systolic blood

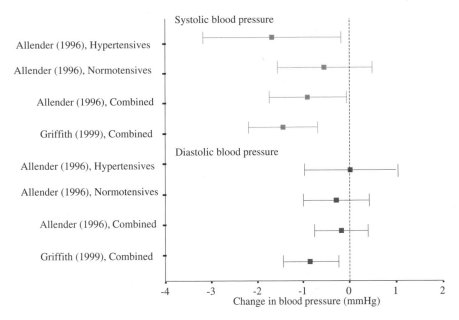

Figure 24.3 Change in blood pressure after an average calcium supplementation of 1 g/day.

pressure for trials of hypertensive than that for normotensive persons (-0.53 mmHg). However, the diastolic blood pressure was not significantly affected by the supplementation in either of the subgroups. In 1999, Griffith et al. (75) updated the 1996 meta-analysis by adding 10 studies to the 32 original trials. They confirmed the previous results by showing a small significant reduction of systolic blood pressure of -1.44 mmHg and diastolic blood pressure of -0.84 mmHg.

Although these two meta-analysis consistently concluded that a small reduction in blood pressure was achieved following the interventions, the evidence is insufficient to support the use of calcium supplementation for the prevention and treatment of hypertension. However, calcium deficiency should be avoided. Hamet et al. (76) argued that calcium may have an influence on the effect of sodium intake on blood pressure by showing that higher blood pressure was associated with high sodium intake among people at low calcium intake. The so-called "Calcium Antihypertension Theory" was put forward just to divert the attention from the evidence that a reduced salt intake has a beneficial effect on health (77).

An inverse relationship has been described in early observational studies between calcium intake and gestational hypertension and preeclampsia (78). Calcium supplementation may be beneficial only for women at high risk of gestational hypertension and with low dietary calcium intake. However, these benefits were only found in small trials (79).

The Trial of Calcium for Preeclampsia Prevention (CPEP) included 4589 healthy, nulliparous women and randomly assigned them to either 2 g of elemental calcium or to a placebo during their pregnancies (80). The results showed neither a significant reduction in the incidence or severity of preeclampsia nor a delay in its onset. Furthermore, there was no difference between the prevalence of gestational hypertension or adverse perinatal outcomes observed in the intervention group compared to the placebo group. Calcium supplementation may only be beneficial in women at high risk of hypertension during pregnancy and low calcium intake. However, the optimum dosage requires further investigation (81).

In conclusion, there is insufficient evidence to recommend high intake of calcium or use of calcium supplementation for the prevention or treatment of hypertension. Calcium deficiency should be avoided, especially during pregnancy. Calcium supplementation during pregnancy does not prevent preeclampsia or gestational hypertension in healthy nulliparous women whose calcium intake is not low (82).

C. Magnesium

The possible association between dietary intake of magnesium and blood pressure has also been the focus of interest (78). A qualitative review of 29 observational studies on the association between magnesium and blood pressure included the majority of cross-sectional studies (83). However, the studies employed a large number of tools to assess dietary intake of magnesium, which makes the interpretation of the results difficult. Nevertheless, it was suggested, that a 100 mg increase in magnesium could be associated with a 0.81 mmHg (95% CI 0.72–0.91) lower systolic and a 0.60 mmHg (95% CI 0.53–0.67) lower diastolic blood pressure.

The overall antihypertensive response to magnesium supplementation among hypertensive individuals is small, and several trials have failed to show a significant effect of magnesium supplementation on blood pressure (84). For example, in a small crossover trial, Cappuccio et al. (85) showed no change in blood pressure after 4 weeks of treatment with magnesium aspartate (15 mmol magnesium per day). Also, in the larger Trial of Hypertension Prevention (TOHP), 227 patients were randomized to receive either 15 mmol of magnesium per day or placebo for 6 months (86). No blood pressure lowering effect due to the magnesium supplementation was detected. Moreover, Sacks et al. (87) recruited 300 normotensive women in the Nurses' Health Study II, whose intake of potassium, magnesium, and calcium was low. They were randomized into different treatment groups, one of which included a supplement of 14 mmol of magnesium per day for 16 weeks. The results did not show any effect on blood pressure.

Nevertheless, Witteman et al. (88) in a double-blind randomized controlled trial of 91 untreated middle-aged and elderly women with mild-to-moderate hypertension found that magnesium supplementation (20 mmol/day) for 6 months significantly lowered diastolic (−3.4 mmHg) but not systolic blood pressure.

In conclusion, there is no consistent evidence to support magnesium supplementation for the prevention and treatment of hypertension.

D. Vitamins

There has been interest in the possible role of vitamins in blood pressure regulation. For instance, the possible negative regulation of the renin–angiotensin system by 1.25 (OH) vitamin D has been described (89). Antioxidant vitamins have been of particular interest. In a randomized, double-blind, cross-over controlled trial including 38 treated hypertensive patients, Galley et al. (90) reported a significant reduction in systolic blood pressure following a short-term oral high-dose combination antioxidant therapy (200 mg of zinc sulphate, 500 mg of ascorbic acid, 600 mg of α-tocopherol, and 30 mg of β-carotene daily).

The Third National Health and Nutrition Examination Survey ($n = 15,317$ men and women aged over 20 years old) indicated in multivariate adjusted models a positive and significant association between vitamins A and E and both systolic and diastolic blood pressure (91). However, a significant inverse association of α-carotene and β-carotene with blood pressure was only identified

with systolic blood pressure. In addition, vitamin C was only associated with diastolic pressure.

In a systematic review, Ness et al. (92) found a consistent association between higher vitamin C intake and lower blood pressure. However, there was no real control for confounding factors in the majority of the studies included in this review. Since then, several intervention trials have reported an inverse association between vitamin C and blood pressure. However, these studies are small and it is not clear whether the effect is sustainable in the long term (93–97).

V. IMPORTANCE OF DIETARY PATTERNS

A. Vegetarian Diet

In randomized controlled trials, a lower blood pressure has been observed in people on vegetarian diets, independently of body weight, sodium, or potassium intake (98). The main characteristics of a vegetarian diet include a higher intake of fiber, calcium, magnesium, polyunsaturated, and monounsaturated fatty acids and lower intake of animal protein and saturated fats. A high intake of fiber has recently been shown to account for a moderate but significant reduction in blood pressure (99–101). These are changes that are consistent with the international recommendations to increase fruit and vegetables intake and to reduce intake of saturated fats.

B. Dietary Approach to Stop Hypertension Diet

Lifestyle changes and nonpharmacological approaches to prevent and treat hypertension are now part of national and international guidelines. The current evidence shows a wide range of dietary factors that influence blood pressure. However, the effect of a single nutrient on blood pressure may be difficult to detect in trials, whereas the cumulative effect of several nutrients consumed together as part of a diet should be different and more detectable. Following this hypothesis, the dietary approach to stop hypertension (DASH) diet tested the effects on blood pressure of a change in dietary patterns.

The DASH diet trial was an 11-week feeding program including 459 adults with untreated mild hypertension (102). For 3 weeks, participants followed a control diet that was low in fruit, vegetable, and dairy products. The fat content was representative of the average consumption in the United States. Then, for the next 8 weeks, the participants were separated randomly in three groups and each group was fed three different diets. One group was fed the same control diet, the second a diet richer in fruit and vegetables but similar to the control diet for other nutrients, and the third group was fed the DASH diet. The DASH

Table 24.4 The DASH Diet: Eating Plan for 2000 Calories Per Day

Food group	Daily servings	Serving sizes	Significance to the DASH diet
Grains and grain products	7–8	1 slice bread 1 oz dry cereal 1/2 cup cooked rice, pasta, or cereal	Major sources of energy and fiber
Vegetables	4–5	1 cup raw leafy vegetable 1/2 cup cooked vegetable 6 oz vegetable juice	Rich sources of potassium, magnesium, and fiber
Fruits	4–5	6 oz fruit juice 1 medium fruit 1/4 cup dried fruit 1/2 cup fresh, frozen, or canned fruit	Important sources of potassium, magnesium, and fiber
Low fat or fat free dairy	2–3	8 oz milk 1 cup yoghurt 1/2 oz cheese	Major sources of calcium and protein
Meats, poultry, or fish	2 or less	3 oz cooked meats, poultry, or fish	Rich sources of protein and magnesium
Nuts, seeds, and dry beans	4–5 per week	1/3 cup or 11/2 oz nuts 2 tbsp or 1/2 oz seeds 1/2 cup cooked dry beans	Rich sources of energy, magnesium, potassium, protein, and fibre
Fats and oils	2–3	1 tsp vegetable oil 2 tbsp light salad dressing 1 tsp soft margarine 1 tbsp low fat mayonnaise	DASH has 27% of calories as fat, including fat in or added to foods
Sweets	5 per week	1 tbsp sugar 1 tbsp jelly or jam 1/2 oz jelly beans	Sweets should be low in fat

Note: After "Facts about the DASH Eating Plan" fact sheet. US Department of Health and Human Services. National Institutes of Health, National Heart, Lung, and Blood Institute. NIH publication no. 03-4082. 24 pages (available online at http://www.nhlbi.nih.gov/health/public/heart/hbp/dash).

diet was a diet rich in fruit and vegetables, low-fat or fat-free dairy products, and reduced saturated and total fat content, in other words, a high potassium, magnesium, calcium, fiber, and protein diet (Table 24.4). The sodium intake was kept constant in the three groups. Alcohol intake and weight did not change during the trial or between the groups.

There was a gradient in the reduction in blood pressure between the diets. The DASH diet reduced blood pressure on average by 5.5/3.0 mmHg compared with the control diet, whereas the "fruit and vegetables" diet reduced it by 2.8/1.1 mmHg. Among subjects with hypertension, the blood pressure reductions in the DASH group were more pronounced, on average 11.4/5.5 mmHg.

In 2001, a second trial involving the DASH diet was published, extending the evidence to the additional importance of salt intake (27). In this second trial, 412 participants were randomly allocated to two dietary groups, one following a control diet representative of the average diet in the United States and the other following the DASH diet. Within these groups, participants were randomly assigned to three groups with increasing amounts of salt consumption (~3, 6, and 10 g of salt per

day) (Fig. 24.4). The difference of systolic blood pressure between the DASH-low sodium group and the control-high sodium group was an impressive reduction of 7.1 mmHg in participants without hypertension and 11.5 mmHg in participants with hypertension.

The public health implications of these findings are important considering that these results represent an alternative to drug therapy for those patients with mild hypertension and willing to comply with these dietary changes.

VI. ALCOHOL REDUCTION

Cross-sectional and prospective studies have consistently reported a significant and direct association between blood pressure and alcohol intake independent of age, gender, ethnic group, smoking status, and other potential cofounders (57), which indicates that high alcohol consumption is one of the most important modifiable risk factors for hypertension (22,103–106).

The strength of the association depends on both the quantity and the pattern of alcohol consumption. For

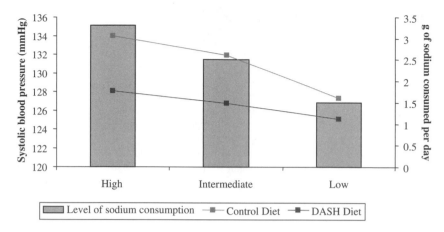

Figure 24.4 Systolic blood pressure reduction after following the DASH diet and a reduction of salt intake.

example, a consumption of three or more drinks per day is related to higher systolic and diastolic blood pressure and also to higher prevalence of hypertension, which shows that alcohol consumption is a strong predictor of the development of hypertension in men (57,105) and women (105,107). The INTERSALT study, an international multicenter study that includes 50 centers world-wide and 4844 men and 4837 women 20–59 years old, presented an average increase in systolic and diastolic blood pressure in men and women as a function of their alcohol intake. For men who drank 300–499 mL alcohol per week, a difference of 2.7/1.6 mmHg was observed compared with nondrinkers. Men who drank >500 mL alcohol per week showed a greater difference of 4.6/3.0 mmHg. In women, the difference in blood pressure between nondrinkers and women who drank >300 mL alcohol per week was 3.9/3.1 mmHg (106). In the Framingham cohort of 5203 white men and women with no hypertension and a follow-up of 20 years, blood pressure was higher in nondrinkers than among light drinkers but among drinkers blood pressure was higher at higher consumption levels (104). Furthermore, in another cohort study with a 6 years follow-up and 8334 participants, middle aged (45–64 years old) subjects and no hypertension at baseline, higher levels of alcohol consumption were associated with a higher risk of hypertension (103). These results were consistent throughout all ethnic groups studied (black ethnic minority and whites), men or women.

The relationship between alcohol consumption and blood pressure is similar for all types of alcoholic beverages (wine, beer, or spirits) in both women (107) and men (108).

The nature of this association is less understood. There is no agreement on whether it is linear, J, or U shape. Klatsky et al. (105) studied the blood pressure in relation to known drinking habits in over 80,000 men and women. They found a threshold at three or more drinks per day. In particular, men consuming alcohol up to that

level had similar blood pressures compared to nondrinkers, whereas women consuming up to two drinks per day had slightly lower blood pressures than those of nondrinkers. Similar results in women were published by Witteman et al. (107). Equally, in the Framingham Heart Study, there was a threshold showing that in men and women blood pressure was higher in nondrinkers than in light drinkers (95). Contrasting results have also been published. The INTERSALT study, for instance, suggested a continuous relationship between alcohol consumption and blood pressure in men and, if anything, a weaker relation at levels <300 mL/week (106).

Altogether, moderate drinking is associated with a reduced risk whereas heavy drinking is definitely associated with an increased risk. The threshold effect could be placed at two or three units per day in both men and women in all ethnic groups (one unit is equal to half a pint of beer, one glass of wine, or one measure of spirits).

Although the effect of alcohol on blood pressure is related to the amount consumed, it is not the only factor involved. The pattern of consumption may play a role as well. A study investigating the consequences of binge drinking in 1154 men and women 18–54 years old showed that consumption of eight or more drinks at one sitting presented a significant risk for coronary heart disease and hypertension compared with usual drinking (109). However, no effect on the risk of other cardiovascular disease was observed. Episodic drinking produces greater differences in blood pressure compared with regular drinking. This result is corroborated by the conclusions of the INTERSALT study (106). Additionally, the effects of daily heavy drinking on blood pressure are more prominent than those of week-end heavy drinking (110).

Potters and Beevers (111) first showed the direct response of blood pressure to variations of alcohol intake. They showed that in a group of patients, the withdrawal of alcohol consumption was accompanied with a reduction in blood pressure and the following reintroduction of alcohol was accompanied by an increase in blood pressure. Inversely, in another group, the continuation of alcohol consumption sustained the rise in blood pressure. The following withdrawal led to a decrease in blood pressure. Since then, prospective observational studies have indicated a reduction in blood pressure following a reduction in alcohol intake compatible with that observed in intervention trials.

A recent meta-analysis by Xin et al. (112) estimated a reduction in systolic and diastolic blood pressure of 3.31/2.04 mmHg, respectively, for an average 76% reduction in alcohol consumption from a baseline of three to six drinks per day (Fig. 24.5). The findings also suggested that the reduction in blood pressure following a reduction in alcohol intake could be sustained over time. This reinforces recommendations for moderation of alcohol consumption to prevent and treat hypertension. However, in 1998, the Prevention and Treatment of Hypertension Study (PATHS) randomized controlled trial showed a lack of significant effect on blood pressure after alcohol reduction (113). These results suggested that although moderation in alcohol intake as part of a multifactorial intervention should be recommended, it is not suitable as a sole approach to the prevention and management of hypertension.

In conclusion, moderation in alcohol intake to a threshold of two drinks per day as recommended by the British Hypertension Society and the Joint National Committee (JNC) on the detection, evaluation, and treatment of high blood pressure is an accurate and beneficial position (19,20). Extended recommendations under this threshold remain a subject of debate, as the balance between risk and benefit of further reducing alcohol consumption is not well understood.

VII. REGULAR AND DYNAMIC EXERCISE

Increasing the level of physical activity is one of the most widely accepted lifestyle measures to reduce cardiovascular risk and blood pressure (19,20). It includes mainly the "dynamic" or "aerobic" exercise that consists of activities like walking, running, cycling, or swimming. In contrast, isometric exercise (e.g., weight training or body building) is not recommended, because it is associated with higher blood pressure levels.

In a recent meta-analysis of 54 randomized controlled trials including 2419 participants, aerobic exercise was associated with a reduction in blood pressure of 3.84/2.58 mmHg (114). The association between exercise and blood pressure was independent from weight change. Although all forms

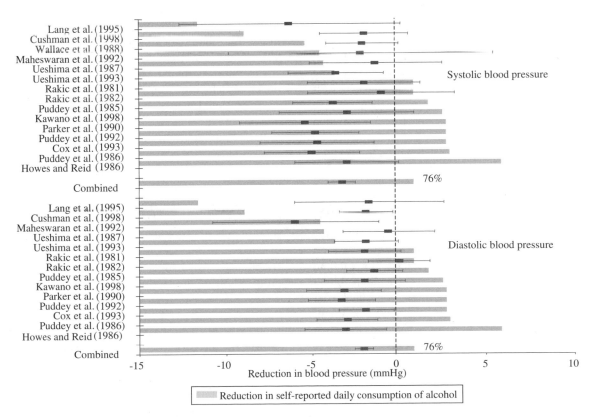

Figure 24.5 Effect of alcohol reduction on systolic and diastolic blood pressure.

of dynamic exercise seem to be effective in reducing blood pressure, adherence to the intervention program is essential to be successful in achieving and maintaining the benefit. Such a moderate reduction in blood pressure constitutes a valuable strategy for the prevention and management of hypertension. A modest reduction in the population's blood pressure would translate into a significant decrease in the incidence of cardiovascular disease.

The changes in blood pressure associated with exercise could be due to different mechanisms. First, a hemodynamic mechanism would involve the reduction of both resting cardiac output and peripheral vascular resistance. Secondly, a humoral mechanism includes the reduction of the activity of the renin–angiotensin–aldosterone system and of the sympathetic nervous system activity and an increase in prostaglandins with vasodilator effect.

Particular attention should be paid to people at high cardiovascular risk and to persons aged 40 years or older and with sedentary lifestyles who want to start exercise programs. The relatively frequent cases of sudden death during exercise are more likely due to a predisposition of this group and an undetected left ventricular hypertrophy related to hypertension. Therefore, an exercise ECG testing is recommended for these patients before starting any exercise program.

There is no optimal recommendation for the intensity or frequency of a "regular" dynamic exercise. However, at least 30 min of exercise at 40–60% maximum working capacity three to four times per week seems a reasonable suggestion.

Additionally, a recent randomized controlled trial assessed the efficacy of simultaneously implementing exercise recommendations as part of a comprehensive lifestyle modification program (16). Forty-four hypertensive overweight adults on mono-therapy for hypertension were randomly allocated to either a control group or an intervention group. The latter was fed with a low-sodium and hypocaloric version of the DASH diet and they participated in a supervised exercise program three times per week. The control group received no intervention. The average total weight loss was 4.9 kg and the difference in daytime blood pressure was 12.1/6.6 mmHg. This trial showed that a comprehensive lifestyle modification improves hypertension control in patients, proving an invaluable tool to prevent and manage high blood pressure. Finally, a recent randomised controlled trial suggests that moderate intensity resistance training might not be contraindicated in hypertensive patients (115).

VIII. SMOKING CESSATION

Smoking is a risk factor for cardiovascular diseases including atherosclerosis, coronary heart disease, acute myocardial infarction, as well as sudden death (116). In a prospective study of 22,444 middle aged men with 17 years follow-up, the association between systolic blood pressure and risk of cardiovascular events was modulated by smoking (117). The risk of coronary heart disease in hypertensives was increased two to three-fold by smoking, even though coronary heart disease is already the commonest cause of death in hypertensives (118).

Furthermore, the impact of smoking on cardiovascular health is the same in old men with a follow-up of 20 years, which showed that smoking had more impact than high blood pressure on coronary heart disease, cardiovascular, and all-cause mortality, given a low cholesterol level (119). In addition, the combination of high blood pressure and smoking was associated with higher risk of coronary heart disease, cardiovascular, and all-cause of mortality among people with low or high cholesterol levels.

Thus, smoking cessation is a recommended lifestyle modification for a more comprehensive nonpharmacological approach to the overall reduction of cardiovascular risk.

Although the effects of nicotine on hemostasis, arterial stiffness, vessel wall damage, and dyslipidemia, may contribute to an overall increased cardiovascular risk in smokers, the mechanisms involved in the observed acute effects of smoking (tachycardia, pressor, and vasoconstrictive response) is not completely understood (120). The association between salivary cotinine and blood pressure suggests that a long-term nicotine exposure might be related to an increase in blood pressure in smokers (121). Moreover, the stimulation of the sympathetic nervous system by nicotine or other smoking products has already been observed. This acute effect of smoking could partly be due to an alteration in the nervous regulation of blood pressure, which with time will promote the development of arterial hypertension (122).

Smokers tend to be undertreated and they have a higher daytime blood pressure than nonsmokers do. This difference is not detected by office blood pressure (123). Data from the Health Survey for England 1994 showed that smokers are, indeed, less likely to be aware of their high blood pressure or to be treated (124). Additionally, when treated, smokers do not receive full protection from the antihypertensive treatment compared with nonsmokers. An early analysis of five hypertension intervention trials (HDFP, MRFIT, Australian National Blood Pressure Trial (ANBP), IPPPSH, MRC) uniformly showed that the protective effect of treatment in hypertensives was diminished by smoking. The HDFP smokers had twice the mortality rates compared with nonsmokers, regardless of the treatment group to which they were randomized. The placebo nonsmokers group in the Australian Study had a lower incidence of events than

Table 24.5 Recommendations for Physicians on Smoking Cessation

1. Ask and record patient's smoking status
2. Advice smokers to quit
3. Assess their motivation to do so

If motivated to quit	If not motivated to quit
Offer behavioural support (i.e., leaflets)	Pros and cons of smoking and smoking cessation
Offer pharmacotherapy	Discuss risks of smoking and passive smoking
Referrals to cessation resources	Identify barriers for quitting
Arrange a follow-up visit	Offer help to stop smoking
	Follow-up during next visit

Note: After West et al. Smoking cessation guidelines for health professionals: an update. Thorax 2000; 55:987–999.

in smokers under active therapy. The results of the MRFIT showed that the coronary death rates were up to ten times higher in smoking hypertensives with high cholesterol than in nonsmokers with lower cholesterol levels. The beneficial effect of β-blockers was absent in smokers in both the MRC and the IPPPSH (125). These findings were corroborated by two other studies, where the efficacy of β-blockers in the treatment of mild hypertension was significantly decreased in smokers (120,126).

Smoking cessation is, therefore, a very effective lifestyle modification that hypertensive patients should implement to reduce their cardiovascular risk and to improve their blood pressure control through antihypertensive drugs. Physicians should counsel their patients about smoking cessation and information should be available about smoking cessation programs and aids (18,19). (Table 24.5). The small amounts of nicotine in smoking cessation aids usually will not raise blood pressure and may be used with appropriate counseling (Table 24.6). Moreover, the cardiovascular benefits of smoking cessation can be seen within a year in all age groups (19).

Attention should be paid to the tendency to weight gain when trying to stop smoking as smoking cessation leads almost invariably to it (116). Counseling and measures to prevent weight gain are often needed.

IX. RELAXATION

A popular perception in western societies is that stress and psychosocial factors play an important role in the development and course of hypertension. Hence, the focus of the debate and study in the past decades is on relaxation, behavioral, and cognitive interventions to control blood pressure.

In a recent systematic review published by the Expert Working Group of the National Heart Foundation of Australia, different psychosocial factors were included in the definition of stress and their influence to coronary heart disease and blood pressure analyzed separately. They concluded that there is evidence to support the hypothesis of an independent causal association between depression, social isolation, lack of quality social support, causes and prognosis of coronary heart disease, and hypertension (127). Although there is growing support to the

Table 24.6 Pharmacotherapy Available for Smoking Cessation Treatment

Drug	Duration of treatment	Dose
First line		
NRT[a] patches	8 weeks	Starting dose 21 mg/day, unless weight <45.5 kg or <10 cigarettes/day then 14 mg/day. During 4 weeks then reduce until stopped
NRT[a] gum	8–12 weeks	1 piece/h
NRT[a] inhaler	3–6 months	6–16 cartridges/day
NRT[a] spray	3–6 months	1–2 doses/h
Bupropion	7–12 weeks (up to 6 months to maintain abstinence)	150 mg/day for 3 days then 150 mg twice a day Should start 1 week before quitting date
Second line		
Nortriptyline	12 weeks	75–100 mg/day. Should be started 10–28 days before quitting date at a dose of 25 mg/day
Clonidine	3–10 weeks	0.1–0.3 mg twice a day

[a]Nicotine Replacement Therapy.
Note: After West et al. Smoking cessation guidelines for health professionals: an update. Thorax 2000; 55:987–999.

idea that stress causes high blood pressure, the results of intervention studies on stress management are inconsistent.

An early meta-analysis explored the efficacy of cognitive behavioral techniques (biofeedback as a self-motivated control of blood pressure) when treating hypertension (128). Although the authors searched all the studies published between 1970 and 1991 involving cognitive behavioral techniques in the treatment of adult patients with mild-to-moderate hypertension, only 26 trials met the entry criteria and several methodological issues were identified during the qualitative analysis. During the meta-analysis, 16 studies were included with patients ($n = 368$) assigned to either a cognitive therapy or a placebo intervention (sham biofeedback, "pseudo-meditation"). Blood pressure decreased by 2.8 (95% CI, -0.8 to 6.4)/1.3 mmHg (95% CI, -1.3 to 3.8) with intervention. These changes were neither statistically nor clinically significant. They demonstrated that cognitive interventions were more effective than no therapy at all but the effect is not significant when compared with a control group. Furthermore, no single cognitive behavioral technique appears to be more effective than any other.

A randomized controlled trial involving 35 subjects aged 20–60 years treated for hypertension, tested an intervention on the basis of relaxation techniques lasting 1 h/week for 8 weeks, then once a month over a 1-year follow-up (129). The control group used nonspecific counseling. The effects on blood pressure of one year's daily muscle relaxation and yoga exercises were identical with those observed in a control group that did not take exercise.

Conversely, Paran et al. (130) included 20 mild hypertensive patients into the study and subjected them to a mental arithmetic stress test before and 6 months after completing biofeedback-assisted relaxation therapy including ten sessions of biofeedback-assisted relaxation instruction and continuous home practice. They showed an attenuation of blood pressure responses to stress in the intervention group compared with the control group. More recently, Henderson et al. (131) randomly allocated 30 mild untreated hypertensives to active treatment ($n = 16$) or placebo ($n = 14$). In the laboratory, they found no difference between the responses of those with active therapy and placebo in agreement with the results of the earlier meta-analysis. However, they found a significant biofeedback lowering activity after 4 weeks of home training compared with the placebo group.

Two recent meta-analyses suggested that biofeedback was more effective in reducing blood pressure in patients with essential hypertension than those with no intervention. However, the treatment was only found to be superior to other behavioral interventions when combined with other relaxation techniques (132,133).

The available evidence to support stress management techniques or cognitive interventions is inconsistent.

Consequently, various international groups are cautious in recommending approaches in this area for the prevention and treatment of hypertension (19,20).

REFERENCES

1. Mokdad AH, Bowman BA, Ford ES, Vinicor F, Marks JS, Koplan JP. The continuing epidemics of obesity and diabetes in the United States. JAMA 2001; 286:1195–1200.
2. Campbell I. The obesity epidemic: can we turn the tide? Heart 2003; 89:ii22–ii24.
3. MacMahon S, Cutler J, Brittain E, Higgins M. Obesity and hypertension: epidemiological and clinical issues. Eur Heart J 1987; 8:57–70.
4. Larsson B, Svardsudd K, Welin L, Wilhelmsen L, Bjorntorp P, Tibblin G. Abdominal adipose tissue distribution, obesity, and risk of cardiovascular disease and death: 13 year follow-up of participants in the study of men born in 1913. Br Med J (Clin Res Ed) 1984; 288:1401–1404.
5. Welborn TA, Dhaliwal SS, Bennett SA. Waist-hip ratio is the dominant risk factor predicting cardiovascular death in Australia. Med J Aust 2003; 179:580–585.
6. Siani A, Cappuccio FP, Barba G, Trevisan M, Farinaro E, Lacone R, Russo O, Russo P, Mancini M, Strazzullo P. The relationship of waist circumference to blood pressure: the Olivetti heart study. Am J Hypertens 2002; 15:780–786.
7. Croft JB, Strogatz DS, Keenan NL, James SA, Malarcher AM, Garrett JM. The independent effects of obesity and body fat distribution on blood pressure in black adults: the Pitt County study. Int J Obes Relat Metab Disord 1993; 17:391–397.
8. Cassano PA, Segal MR, Vokonas PS, Weiss ST. Body fat distribution, blood pressure, and hypertension. A prospective cohort study of men in the normative aging study. Ann Epidemiol 1990; 1:33–48.
9. Folsom AR, Prineas RJ, Kaye SA, Munger RG. Incidence of hypertension and stroke in relation to body fat distribution and other risk factors in older women. Stroke 1990; 21:701–706.
10. National Institutes of Health. Clinical guidelines on the identification, evaluation, and treatment of overweight and obesity in adults—the evidence report. Obes Res 1998; 6:51S–209S.
11. He J, Whelton PK, Appel LJ, Charleston J, Klag MJ. Long-term effects of weight loss and dietary sodium reduction on incidence of hypertension. Hypertension 2000; 35:544–549.
12. Stevens VJ, Obarzanek E, Cook NR, Lee IM, Appel LJ, Smith West D, Milas NC, Mattfeldt-Beman M, Belden L, Bragg C, Millstone M, Raczynski J, Brewer A, Singh B, Cohen J, Trials for the Hypertension Prevention Research Group. Long-term weight loss and changes in blood pressure: results of the trials of hypertension prevention, phase II. Ann Intern Med 2001; 134:1–11.

13. Neter JE, Stam BE, Kok FJ, Grobbee DE, Geleijnse JM. Influence of weight reduction on blood pressure: a meta-analysis of randomized controlled trials. Hypertension 2003; 42:878–884.

14. Mulrow CD, Chiquette E, Angel L, Cornell J, Summerbell C, Anagnostelis B, Grimm R Jr, Brand MB. Dieting to reduce body weight for controlling hypertension in adults. Cochrane Database Syst Rev 2000; CD000484.

15. Whelton PK, Appel LJ, Espeland MA, Applegate WB, Ettinger WH Jr, Kostis JB, Kumanyika S, Lacy CR, Johnson KC, Folmar S, Cutler JA. Sodium reduction and weight loss in the treatment of hypertension in older persons: a randomized controlled trial of nonpharmacologic interventions in the elderly (TONE). TONE Collaborative Research Group. JAMA 1998; 279:839–846.

16. Miller ER III, Erlinger TP, Young DR, Jehn M, Charleston J, Rhodes D, Wasan SK, Appel LJ. Results of the Diet, Exercise, and Weight Loss Intervention Trial (DEW-IT). Hypertension 2002; 40:612–618.

17. Stamler J, Liu K, Ruth KJ, Pryer J, Greenland P. Eight-year blood pressure change in middle-aged men: relationship to multiple nutrients. Hypertension 2002; 39:1000–1006.

18. Engeli S, Bohnke J, Gorzelniak K, Janke J, Sching P, Bader M, Luft FC, Sharma AM. Weight loss and the renin-angiotensin-aldosterone system. Hypertension 2005; 45:356–362.

19. Joint National Committee. The sixth report of the Joint National Committee on prevention, detection, evaluation, and treatment of high blood pressure. Arch Intern Med 1997; 157:2413–2446.

20. Ramsay L, Williams B, Johnston G, MacGregor G, Poston L, Potter J, Poulter N, Russell G. Guidelines for management of hypertension: report of the third working party of the British hypertension society. J Hum Hypertens 1999; 13:569–592.

21. Stamler J. The INTERSALT study: background, methods, findings, and implications. Am J Clin Nutr 1997; 65:626S–642S.

22. Stamler J, Caggiula AW, Grandits GA. Relation of body mass and alcohol, nutrient, fiber, and caffeine intakes to blood pressure in the special intervention and usual care groups in the multiple risk factor intervention trial. Am J Clin Nutr 1997; 65:338S–365S.

23. Mattes RD, Donnelly D. Relative contributions of dietary sodium sources. J Am Coll Nutr 1991; 10:383–393.

24. Geleijnse JM, Kok FJ, Grobbee DE. Blood pressure response to changes in sodium and potassium intake: a metaregression analysis of randomised trials. J Hum Hypertens 2003; 17:471–480.

25. Midgley JP, Matthew AG, Greenwood CM, Logan AG. Effect of reduced dietary sodium on blood pressure: a meta-analysis of randomized controlled trials. JAMA 1996; 275:1590–1597.

26. MacGregor GA, de Wardener HE. Salt, diet, and health. Cambridge University Press, 1998; 1–233.

27. Sacks FM, Svetkey LP, Vollmer WM, Appel LJ, Bray GA, Harsha D, Obarzanek E, Conlin PR, Miller ER III, Simons-Morton DG, Karanja N, Lin PH; DASH-Sodium Collaborative Research Group. Effects on blood pressure of reduced dietary sodium and the Dietary Approaches to Stop Hypertension (DASH) diet. DASH-Sodium Collaborative Research Group. N Engl J Med 2001; 344:3–10.

28. Cutler JA, Follmann D, Allender PS. Randomized trials of sodium reduction: an overview. Am J Clin Nutr 1997; 65:643S–651S.

29. Hooper L, Bartlett C, Davey Smith G, Ebrahim S. Systematic review of long term effects of advice to reduce dietary salt in adults. Br Med J 2002; 325:628–632.

30. He FJ, MacGregor GA. How far should salt intake be reduced? Hypertension 2003; 42:1093–1099.

31. Khaw KT, Bingham S, Welch A, Luben R, O'Brien E, Wareham N, Day N. Blood pressure and urinary sodium in men and women: the Norfolk Cohort of the European Prospective Investigation into Cancer (EPIC-Norfolk). Am J Clin Nutr 2004; 80:1397–1403.

32. Kumanyika SK, Cook NR, Cutler JA, Belden L, Brewer A, Cohen JD, Hebert PR, Lasser VI, Raines J, Raczynski J, Shepek L, Diller L, Whelton PK, Yamamoto M. Sodium reduction for hypertension prevention in overweight adults: further results from the Trials of Hypertension Prevention Phase II. J Hum Hypertens 2005; 19:33–45.

33. Cook NR, Kumanyika SK, Cutler JA, Whelton PK. Dose-response of sodium excretion and blood pressure change among overweight nonhypertensive adults in a 3-year dietary intervention study. J Hum Hypertens 2005; 19:47–54.

34. Hofman A, Hazebroek A, Valkenburg HA. A randomized trial of sodium intake and blood pressure in newborn infants. JAMA 1983; 250:370–373.

35. Geleijnse JM, Hofman A, Witteman JC, Hazebroek AA, Valkenburg HA, Grobbee DE. Long-term effects of neonatal sodium restriction on blood pressure. Hypertension 1997; 29:913–917.

36. Simons-Morton DG, Obarzanek E. Diet and blood pressure in children and adolescents. Pediatr Nephrol 1997; 11:244–249.

37. Graudal NA, Galloe AM, Garred P. Effects of sodium restriction on blood pressure, renin, aldosterone, catecholamines, cholesterols, and triglyceride: a meta-analysis. JAMA 1998; 279:1383–1391.

38. Meade TW, Cooper JA, Peart WS. Plasma renin activity and ischemic heart disease. N Engl J Med 1993; 329:616–619.

39. Cappuccio FP, Markandu ND, Carney C, Sagnella GA, MacGregor GA. Double-blind randomised trial of modest salt restriction in older people. Lancet 1997; 350:850–854.

40. McCarron DA. The dietary guideline for sodium: should we shake it up? Yes! Am J Clin Nutr 2000; 71:1013–1019.

41. Vollmer WM, Sacks FM, Ard J, Appel LJ, Bray GA, Simons-Morton DG, Conlin PR, Svetkey LP, Erlinger TP, Moore TJ, Karanja N, DASH-Sodium Trial Collaborative Research Group. Effects of diet and sodium intake on blood pressure: subgroup analysis of the DASH-sodium trial. Ann Intern Med 2001; 135:1019–1028.

42. Cappuccio FP, Markandu ND, Sagnella GA, MacGregor GA. Sodium restriction lowers high blood pressure through a decreased response of the renin system—direct evidence using saralasin. J Hypertens 1985; 3:243–247.

43. He FJ, Markandu ND, Sagnella GA, MacGregor GA. Importance of the renin system in determining blood pressure fall with salt restriction in black and white hypertensives. Hypertension 1998; 32:820–824.

44. Cappuccio FP, MacGregor GA. Combination therapy in hypertension. In: Laragh JH, Brenner BH, eds. Hypertension. Pathophysiology, Diagnosis, and Management. New York: Raven Press Publishers, 1995:2969–2983.

45. Grim CE, Luft FC, Weinberger MH, Miller JZ, Rose RJ, Christian JC. Genetic, familial and racial influences on blood pressure control systems in man. Aust NZ J Med 1984; 14:453–457.

46. Strazzullo P, Iacone R, Siani A, Barba G, Russo O, Russo P, Barbato A, D'Elia L, Farinaro E, Cappuccio FP. Altered renal sodium handling and hypertension in men carrying the glucagon receptor gene (Gly40Ser) variant. J Mol Med 2001; 79:574–580.

47. Barbato A, Russo P, Venezia A, Strazzullo V, Siani A, Cappuccio FP. Analysis of Gly40Ser polymorphism of the glucagon receptor (GCGR) gene in different ethnic groups. J Hum Hypertens 2004; 17:577–579.

48. Russo P, Siani A, Venezia A, Iacone R, Russo O, Barba G, D'Elia L, Cappuccio FP, Strazzullo P. Interaction between the C(-344)T polymorphism of CYP11B2 and age in the regulation of blood pressure and plasma aldosterone levels: cross-sectional and longitudinal findings of the Olivetti prospective heart study. J Hypertens 2002; 20:1785–1792.

49. Strazzullo P, Cappuccio FP. Hypertension and kidney stones: hypotheses and implications. Semin Nephrol 1995; 15:519–525.

50. Cappuccio FP, Siani A, Barba G, Mellone MC, Russo L, Farinaro E, Trevisan M, Mancini M, Strazzullo P. A prospective study of hypertension and the incidence of kidney stones in men. J Hypertens 1999; 17:1017–1022.

51. Cappuccio FP, Kalaitzidis R, Duneclift S, Eastwood JB. Unravelling the links between calcium excretion, salt intake, hypertension, kidney stones, and bone metabolism. J Nephrol 2000; 13:169–177.

52. Cappuccio FP, MacGregor GA. Dietary salt restriction: benefits for cardiovascular disease and beyond. Curr Opin Nephrol Hypertens 1997; 6:477–482.

53. Cappuccio FP, Plange-Rhule J, Eastwood JB. Prevention of hypertension and stroke in Africa. Lancet 2000; 356:677–678.

54. Cappuccio FP, Micah FB, Emmett L, Kerry SM, Antwi S, Martin-Peprah R, Phillips RO, Plange-Rhule J, Eastwood JB. Prevalence, detection, management, and control of hypertension in Ashanti, West Africa. Hypertension 2004; 43:1017–1022.

55. Kotchen TA, McCarron DA. Dietary electrolytes and blood pressure: a statement for healthcare professionals from the American Heart Association Nutrition Committee. Circulation 1998; 98:613–617.

56. Geleijnse JM, Witteman JC, Bak AA, den Breeijen JH, Grobbee DE. Reduction in blood pressure with a low sodium, high potassium, high magnesium salt in older subjects with mild to moderate hypertension. BMJ 1994; 309:436–440.

57. Ascherio A, Rimm EB, Giovannucci EL, Colditz GA, Rosner B, Willett WC, Sacks F, Stampfer MJ. A prospective study of nutritional factors and hypertension among US men. Circulation 1992; 86:1475–1484.

58. Witteman JC, Willett WC, Stampfer MJ, Colditz GA, Sacks FM, Speizer FE, Rosner B, Hennekens CH. A prospective study of nutritional factors and hypertension among US women. Circulation 1989; 80:1320–1327.

59. Cappuccio FP. The epidemiology of diet and blood pressure. Circulation 1992; 86:1651–1653.

60. Elliott P, Dyer A, Stamler R. The INTERSALT study: results for 24 h sodium and potassium, by age and sex. INTERSALT co-operative research group. J Hum Hypertens 1989; 3:323–330.

61. Whelton PK, Buring J, Borhani NO, Cohen JD, Cook N, Cutler JA, Kiley JE, Kuller LH, Satterfield S, Sacks FM et al. The effect of potassium supplementation in persons with a high-normal blood pressure. Results from phase I of the Trials of Hypertension Prevention (TOHP). Trials of Hypertension Prevention (TOHP) Collaborative Research Group. Ann Epidemiol 1995; 5:85–95.

62. Grim CE, Luft FC, Miller JZ, Meneely GR, Battarbee HD, Hames CG, Dahl LK. Racial differences in blood pressure in Evans County, Georgia: relationship to sodium and potassium intake and plasma renin activity. J Chronic Dis 1980; 33:87–94.

63. Brancati FL, Appel LJ, Seidler AJ, Whelton PK. Effect of potassium supplementation on blood pressure in African Americans on a low-potassium diet. A randomized, double-blind, placebo-controlled trial. Arch Intern Med 1996; 156:61–67.

64. Matlou SM, Isles CG, Higgs A, Milne FJ, Murray GD, Schultz E, Starke IF. Potassium supplementation in blacks with mild to moderate essential hypertension. J Hypertens 1986; 4:61–64.

65. Cappuccio FP, MacGregor GA. Does potassium supplementation lower blood pressure? A meta-analysis of published trials. J Hypertens 1991; 9:465–473.

66. Whelton PK, He J, Cutler JA, Brancati FL, Appel LJ, Follmann D, Klag MJ. Effects of oral potassium on blood pressure. Meta-analysis of randomized controlled clinical trials. JAMA 1997; 277:1624–1632.

67. Krishna GG, Miller E, Kapoor S. Increased blood pressure during potassium depletion in normotensive men. N Engl J Med 1989; 320:1177–1182.

68. Krishna GG. Role of potassium in the pathogenesis of hypertension. Am J Med Sci 1994; 307:S21–S25.

69. Naismith DJ, Braschi A. The effect of low-dose potassium supplementation on blood pressure in apparently healthy volunteers. Br J Nutr 2003; 90:53–60.

70. Siani A, Strazzullo P, Giacco A, Pacioni D, Celentano E, Mancini M. Increasing the dietary potassium intake reduces the need for antihypertensive medication. Ann Intern Med 1991; 115:753–759.

71. Barri YM, Wingo CS. The effects of potassium depletion and supplementation on blood pressure: a clinical review. Am J Med Sci 1997; 314:37–40.

72. Birkett NJ. Comments on a meta-analysis of the relation between dietary calcium intake and blood pressure. Am J Epidemiol 1998; 148:223–228.

73. Cappuccio FP, Elliott P, Allender PS, Pryer J, Follman DA, Cutler JA. Epidemiologic association between dietary calcium intake and blood pressure: a meta-analysis of published data. Am J Epidemiol 1995; 142:935–945.

74. Allender PS, Cutler JA, Follmann D, Cappuccio FP, Pryer J, Elliott P. Dietary calcium and blood pressure: a meta-analysis of randomized clinical trials. Ann Intern Med 1996; 124:825–831.

75. Griffith LE, Guyatt GH, Cook RJ, Bucher HC, Cook DJ. The influence of dietary and nondietary calcium supplementation on blood pressure: an updated meta-analysis of randomized controlled trials. Am J Hypertens 1999; 12:84–92.

76. Hamet P, Mongeau E, Lambert J, Bellavance F, Daignault-Gelinas M, Ledoux M, Whissell-Cambiotti L. Interactions among calcium, sodium, and alcohol intake as determinants of blood pressure. Hypertension 1991; 17:I150–I154.

77. Cappuccio FP. The "calcium antihypertension theory." Am J Hypertens 1999; 12:93–95.

78. Cappuccio FP. Calcium and magnesium supplementation. In: Whelton PK, He J, Louis GT, eds. Lifestyle Modification for the Prevention and Treatment of Hypertension. New York: Marcel Dekker Inc., 2003:227–242.

79. Hofmeyr GJ, Roodt A, Atallah AN, Duley L. Calcium supplementation to prevent pre-eclampsia—a systematic review. S Afr Med J 2003; 93:224–228.

80. Levine RJ, Hauth JC, Curet LB, Sibai BM, Catalano PM, Morris CD, DerSimonian R, Esterlitz JR, Raymond EG, Bild DE, Clemens JD, Cutler JA. Trial of calcium to prevent preeclampsia. N Engl J Med 1997; 337:69–76.

81. Atallah AN, Hofmeyr GJ, Duley L. Calcium supplementation during pregnancy for preventing hypertensive disorders and related problems. Cochrane Database Syst Rev 2002; CD001059.

82. Krauss RM, Eckel RH, Howard B, Appel LJ, Daniels SR, Deckelbaum RJ, Erdman JW Jr, Kris-Etherton P, Goldberg IJ, Kotchen TA, Lichtenstein AH, Mitch WE, Mullis R, Robinson K, Wylie-Rosett J, St Jeor S, Suttie J, Tribble DL, Bazzarre TL. Revision 2000: a statement for healthcare professionals from the Nutrition Committee of the American Heart Association. J Nutr 2001; 131:132–146.

83. Mizushima S, Cappuccio FP, Nichols R, Elliott P. Dietary magnesium intake and blood pressure: a qualitative overview of the observational studies. J Hum Hypertens 1998; 12:447–453.

84. Harlan WR, Harlan LC. Blood pressure and calcium and magnesium intake. In: Laragh JH, Brenner BH, eds. Hypertension: Pathophysiology, Diagnosis, and Management. New York: Raven Press Publishers, 1995:1143–1154.

85. Cappuccio FP, Markandu ND, Beynon GW, Shore AC, Sampson B, MacGregor GA. Lack of effect of oral magnesium on high blood pressure: a double blind study. Br Med J (Clin Res Ed) 1985; 291:235–238.

86. Yamamoto ME, Applegate WB, Klag MJ, Borhani NO, Cohen JD, Kirchner KA, Lakatos E, Sacks FM, Taylor JO, Hennekens CH. Lack of blood pressure effect with calcium and magnesium supplementation in adults with high-normal blood pressure. Results from phase I of the Trials of Hypertension Prevention (TOHP). Trials of Hypertension Prevention (TOHP) Collaborative Research Group. Ann Epidemiol 1995; 5:96–107.

87. Sacks FM, Willett WC, Smith A, Brown LE, Rosner B, Moore TJ. Effect on blood pressure of potassium, calcium, and magnesium in women with low habitual intake. Hypertension 1998; 31:131–138.

88. Witteman JC, Grobbee DE, Derkx FH, Bouillon R, de Bruijn AM, Hofman A. Reduction of blood pressure with oral magnesium supplementation in women with mild to moderate hypertension. Am J Clin Nutr 1994; 60:129–135.

89. Li YC. Vitamin D regulation of the renin–angiotensin system. J Cell Biochem 2003; 88:327–331.

90. Galley HF, Thornton J, Howdle PD, Walker BE, Webster NR. Combination oral antioxidant supplementation reduces blood pressure. Clin Sci (Lond) 1997; 92:361–365.

91. Chen J, He J, Hamm L, Batuman V, Whelton PK. Serum antioxidant vitamins and blood pressure in the United States population. Hypertension 2002; 40:810–816.

92. Ness AR, Chee D, Elliott P. Vitamin C and blood pressure—an overview. J Hum Hypertens 1997; 11:343–350.

93. Bates CJ, Walmsley CM, Prentice A, Finch S. Does vitamin C reduce blood pressure? Results of a large study of people aged 65 or older. J Hypertens 1998; 16:925–932.

94. Block G, Mangels AR, Norkus EP, Patterson BH, Levander OA, Taylor PR. Ascorbic acid status and subsequent diastolic and systolic blood pressure. Hypertension 2001; 37:261–267.

95. Duffy SJ, Gokce N, Holbrook M et al. Treatment of hypertension with ascorbic acid. Lancet 1999; 354:2048–2049.

96. Fotherby MD, Williams JC, Forster LA, Craner P, Ferns GA. Effect of vitamin C on ambulatory blood pressure and plasma lipids in older persons. J Hypertens 2000; 18:411–415.

97. Hajjar IM, George V, Sasse EA, Kochar MS. A randomized, double-blind, controlled trial of vitamin C in the management of hypertension and lipids. Am J Ther 2002; 9:289–293.

98. Margetts BM, Beilin LJ, Vandongen R, Armstrong BK. Vegetarian diet in mild hypertension: a randomised controlled trial. Br Med J (Clin Res Ed) 1986; 293:1468–1471.

99. He J, Streiffer RH, Munter P, Krousel-Wood MA, Whelton PK. Effect of dietary fiber intake on blood pressure: a randomized, double-blind, placebo-controlled trial. J Hypertens 2004; 22:73–80.

100. Streppel MT, Arends LR, van't Veer P, Grobbee DE, Geleijnse JM. Dietary fiber and blood pressure: a meta-analysis of randomized placebo-controlled trials. Arch Intern Med 2005; 165:150–156.

101. Whelton SP, Hyre AD, Pedersen B, Yi Y, Whelton PK, He J. Effect of dietary fiber intake on blood pressure: a meta-analysis of randomized, controlled clinical trials. J Hypertens 2005; 23:475–481.

102. Appel LJ, Moore TJ, Obarzanek E, Vollmer WM, Svetkey LP, Sacks FM, Bray GA, Vogt TM, Cutler JA, Windhauser MM, Lin PH, Karanja N. A clinical trial of the effects of dietary patterns on blood pressure. DASH Collaborative Research Group. N Engl J Med 1997; 336:1117–1124.

103. Fuchs FD, Chambless LE, Whelton PK, Nieto FJ, Heiss G. Alcohol consumption and the incidence of hypertension: The Atherosclerosis Risk in Communities Study. Hypertension 2001; 37:1242–1250.

104. Gordon T, Kannel WB. Drinking and its relation to smoking, BP, blood lipids, and uric acid. The Framingham study. Arch Intern Med 1983; 143:1366–1374.

105. Klatsky AL, Friedman GD, Siegelaub AB, Gerard MJ. Alcohol consumption and blood pressure Kaiser-Permanente Multiphasic Health Examination data. N Engl J Med 1977; 296:1194–1200.

106. Marmot MG, Elliott P, Shipley MJ, Dyer AR, Ueshima H, Beevers DG, Stamler R, Kesteloot H, Rose G, Stamler J. Alcohol and blood pressure: the INTERSALT study. BMJ 1994; 308:1263–1267.

107. Witteman JC, Willett WC, Stampfer MJ, Colditz GA, Kok FJ, Sacks FM, Speizer FE, Rosner B, Hennekens CH. Relation of moderate alcohol consumption and risk of systemic hypertension in women. Am J Cardiol 1990; 65:633–637.

108. Arkwright PD, Beilin LJ, Rouse I, Armstrong BK, Vandongen R. Effects of alcohol use and other aspects of lifestyle on blood pressure levels and prevalence of hypertension in a working population. Circulation 1982; 66:60–66.

109. Murray RP, Connett JE, Tyas SL, Bond R, Ekuma O, Silversides CK, Barnes GE. Alcohol volume, drinking pattern, and cardiovascular disease morbidity and mortality: is there a U-shaped function? Am J Epidemiol 2002; 155:242–248.

110. Seppa K, Laippala P, Sillanaukee P. Drinking pattern and blood pressure. Am J Hypertens 1994; 7:249–254.

111. Potter JF, Beevers DG. Pressor effect of alcohol in hypertension. Lancet 1984; 1:119–122.

112. Xin X, He J, Frontini MG, Ogden LG, Motsamai OI, Whelton PK. Effects of alcohol reduction on blood pressure: a meta-analysis of randomized controlled trials. Hypertension 2001; 38:1112–1117.

113. Cushman WC, Cutler JA, Hanna E, Bingham SF, Follmann D, Harford T, Dubbert P, Allender PS, Dufour M, Collins JF, Walsh SM, Kirk GF, Burg M, Felicetta JV, Hamilton BP, Katz LA, Perry HM Jr, Willenbring ML, Lakshman R, Hamburger RJ. Prevention and Treatment of Hypertension Study (PATHS): effects of an alcohol treatment program on blood pressure. Arch Intern Med 1998; 158:1197–1207.

114. Whelton SP, Chin A, Xin X, He J. Effect of aerobic exercise on blood pressure: a meta-analysis of randomized, controlled trials. Ann Intern Med 2002; 136:493–503.

115. Cornelissen VA, Fagard RH. Effect of resistance training on resting blood pressure: a meta-analysis of randomised controlled trials. J Hypertens 2005; 23:251–259.

116. Halimi JM, Giraudeau B, Vol S, Caces E, Nivet H, Tichet J. The risk of hypertension in men: direct and indirect effects of chronic smoking. J Hypertens 2002; 20:187–193.

117. Khalili P, Nilsson PM, Nilsson JA, Berglund G. Smoking as a modifier of the systolic blood pressure-induced risk of cardiovascular events and mortality: a population-based prospective study of middle-aged men. J Hypertens 2002; 20:1759–1764.

118. Sleight P. Smoking and hypertension. Clin Exp Hypertens 1993; 15:1181–1192.

119. Houterman S, Verschuren WM, Kromhout D. Smoking, blood pressure, and serum cholesterol-effects on 20-year mortality. Epidemiology 2003; 14:24–29.

120. Kochar MS, Bindra RS. The additive effects of smoking and hypertension. More reasons to help your patients kick the habit. Postgrad Med 1996; 100:147–159.

121. Istvan JA, Lee WW, Buist AS, Connett JE. Relation of salivary cotinine to blood pressure in middle-aged cigarette smokers. Am Heart J 1999; 137:928–931.

122. Gerhardt U, Hans U, Hohage H. Influence of smoking on baroreceptor function: 24 h measurements. J Hypertens 1999; 17:941–946.

123. Bang LE, Buttenschon L, Kristensen KS, Svendsen TL. Do we undertreat hypertensive smokers? A comparison between smoking and non-smoking hypertensives. Blood Press Monit 2000; 5:271–274.

124. Gulliford MC. Low rates of detection and treatment of hypertension among current cigarette smokers. J Hum Hypertens 2001; 15:771–773.

125. Heyden S, Schneider KA, Fodor JG. Smoking habits and antihypertensive treatment. Nephron 1987; 1:99–103.

126. Greenberg G, Thompson SG, Brennan PJ. The relationship between smoking and the response to antihypertensive treatment in mild hypertensives in the Medical Research Council's trial of treatment. Int J Epidemiol 1987; 16:25–30.

127. Bunker SJ, Colquhoun DM, Esler MD, Hickie IB, Hunt D, Jelinek VM, Oldenburg BF, Peach HG, Ruth D, Tennant CC, Tonkin AM. "Stress" and coronary heart disease: psychosocial risk factors. Med J Aust 2003; 178:272–276.

128. Eisenberg DM, Delbanco TL, Berkey CS, Kaptchuk TJ, Kupelnick B, Kuhl J, Chalmers TC. Cognitive behavioral techniques for hypertension: are they effective? Ann Intern Med 1993; 118:964–972.

129. van Montfrans GA, Karemaker JM, Wieling W, Dunning AJ. Relaxation therapy and continuous ambulatory blood pressure in mild hypertension: a controlled study. BMJ 1990; 300:1368–1372.

130. Paran E, Amir M, Yaniv N. Evaluating the response of mild hypertensives to biofeedback-assisted relaxation using a mental stress test. J Behav Ther Exp Psychiatry 1996; 27:157–167.

131. Henderson RJ, Hart MG, Lal SK, Hunyor SN. The effect of home training with direct blood pressure biofeedback of hypertensives: a placebo-controlled study. J Hypertens 1998; 16:771–778.

132. Nakao M, Yano E, Nomura S, Kuboki T. Blood pressure-lowering effects of biofeedback treatment in hypertension: a meta-analysis of randomized controlled trials. Hypertens Res 2003; 26:37–46.

133. Yucha CB, Clark L, Smith M, Uris P, LaFleur B, Duval S. The effect of biofeedback in hypertension. Appl Nurs Res 2001; 14:29–35.

25

Principles of Individualized Hypertension Management

TREFOR MORGAN

University of Melbourne, Melbourne and Hypertension Clinic, Austin Health, Heidelberg, Australia

KEYPOINTS

- It is important to determine that a person has hypertension before they must embark on a lifetime of therapy.
- Control of blood pressure should be maintained consistently over 24 h. Particular attention needs to be paid to night time and awakening blood pressure.
- Drugs can be titrated at 2-week or 4-week intervals. When it appears that control of blood pressure has been achieved, it is important to ensure that this control is maintained >24 h.

- The patient must be educated with respect to the disease and to the other factors that increase risk. The whole person must be treated, not just the blood pressure.
- Lowering of blood pressure with any antihypertensive drug improves morbidity and mortality rates, but the extent of the improvement depends on the severity of the initial disease.
- Therapies that are based on diuretics, β-blockers, angiotensin-converting enzyme (ACE) inhibitors, angiotensin receptor blockers (ARBs), and calcium blockers improve the outcome in mild hypertension.

SUMMARY

Large clinical trials provide the guidelines on which therapy for hypertension should be based. There are usually no definitive trials that address how individual patients should be treated. The disease status and end organ damage of patients varies markedly and affects the choice of therapy. The key to success is reduction of blood pressure with any drug or combination of drugs. The effectiveness of blood pressure reduction is much greater than potential adverse or beneficial effects of specific agents. The response in blood pressure reduction and morbidity and mortality is affected by age, gender, race, environment, and damage to organs caused by hypertension or other diseases. Blood pressure, systolic and diastolic, needs to be controlled using any of the major drug classes. However usually more than one drug will be required. Combinations should be chosen that have additive blood pressure lowering and reduction of adverse events.

I. INTRODUCTION

Males and females respond similarly to most drugs that are used in the treatment of hypertension, although women appear to experience more side effects. The choice of drugs to use for premenopausal women is influenced by the drug's potential effect on the fetus if a woman becomes pregnant.

The response to drugs in older and younger patients differs. Older patients respond better to calcium blockers and diuretics; younger patients respond better to angiotensin-converting enzyme (ACE) inhibitors and β-blockers. The control rate achieved with monotherapy is <30%, so two or more drugs are usually required to achieve control.

African-Americans appear to respond better to calcium blockers and diuretics than to the other drug classes, but including ACE inhibitors in the therapy improves the outcome.

If there is associated cardiovascular disease, the drugs that are chosen to treat hypertension must take into account their specific effects on type of cardiovascular disease. Blood pressure control is essential, but the choice of treatment might be β-blockers in the case of angina, ACE inhibitors in the case of cardiac hypertrophy, and diuretics and ACE inhibitors in the case of cardiac failure.

In diabetic patients and patients with the metabolic syndrome, it appears preferable to use ACE inhibitors or angiotensin receptor blockers (ARBs) because of the adverse effects of thiazide diuretics and β-blockers on glucose metabolism and lipid profile. Many of these patients require more than one drug, and an ACE inhibitor or ARB should be included.

Most patients with renal disease and hypertension also require two or more drugs to achieve adequate blood pressure control. The rate of progression is slowed best by a therapy regimen that includes an ACE inhibitor or ARB. In these patients, excellent control is necessary.

Patients with a degree of sodium retention and a subsequent low renin level—which includes patients with renal disease, the elderly with systolic hypertension, African-American, and patients on nonsteroidal anti-inflammatory drugs (NSAIDs)—respond better to calcium channel blockers and diuretics. However, for many of these patients, the outcome is better if the patient is on drugs that block the renin angiotensin system (RAS), emphasizing the need for combination therapy.

II. DIAGNOSING HYPERTENSION CORRECTLY

The most important aspect of patient management is to ensure that the person actually has a blood pressure level that requires treatment. Blood pressure that is measured at the initial clinic visit is usually higher than it is on subsequent visits; it may take up to seven visits before the basal level is obtained (1). If treatment is based on clinic measurements, it is suggested that initially nonpharmacological (lifestyle and diet) therapy be introduced, that appropriate tests be performed when indicated by concomitant conditions or patient medical history, and that the patient be seen on three or four occasions (with blood pressure being measured three times at each visit) before drug therapy is started. This assumes that the blood pressure is not excessively high and that there is little or no end organ damage. The level of blood pressure can be assessed more rapidly initially by monitoring it over a 24 h period, which on its first application provides a reading only 1–2 mmHg higher than on subsequent measurements (2,3), or by performing home blood pressure recording over 1 to 2 weeks. It is important to determine whether treatment is essential because if hypertension is diagnosed, a lifetime of therapy will probably be necessary.

III. BLOOD PRESSURE VARIATION

Blood pressure follows a circadian pattern with a sleep trough, a peak upon awakening in the morning, and a drop during the day, with a second peak in the afternoon and then a gradual decline to the sleep trough (4). The variation between the morning peak and the usual daytime level is usually ∼7 mmHg systolic in normotensive people and may be much higher in hypertensive people. Thus, the time of day at which blood pressure is taken may influence who should be treated. If the patient is seen at different times of the day, spurious effects of treatment may be observed. The patient should be seen at a similar time on each visit. The level of clinic blood pressure at which treatment is indicated is 140/90 mmHg (5), although in certain groups (e.g., people with diabetes or renal disease), treatment is indicated at lower levels. The goal of therapy for patients with no other medical complications is a systolic blood pressure <140 mmHg and diastolic blood pressure <90 mmHg. However, for patients with complications, the goal is <130/80 mmHg. If ambulatory blood pressure monitoring (ABPM) is used, a daytime value of >135/85 mmHg and a sleep value >120/75 mmHg probably indicates that treatment is needed. ABPM values measured during the process of diagnosis correlate better with subsequent outcome than do clinic values, and there is evidence both experimentally (6) and clinically (7,8) that sleep blood pressure has the greatest prognostic importance.

IV. TREATMENT

After the decision is made to begin drug treatment, it is important to evaluate the patient's response to therapy. It is also important to determine whether blood pressure is controlled consistently over 24 h. There is some merit to see the patient in the early morning, between 8 and 10 a.m. This is a time of higher blood pressure, and because patients usually take their medication in the morning, they can be asked not to take their medication on the day of the clinic visit. If a patient is seen later in the day, the person usually would have taken the blood pressure medication in the morning and thus is seen at the time of peak response. In this case, the blood pressure may appear to be controlled, but the control may not extend over 24 h, particularly through the sleep period and the awakening hours (morning surge), when mortality from cardiovascular events is highest. This under-titration is common with a number of ACE inhibitors which control blood pressure for 3–8 h after a dose but do not extend for 24 h (Table 25.1) (9,10). When a patient is seen in the

afternoon, it may not be feasible to exclude the morning dose of the drug because the next dose would then be taken 32–36 h after the previous dose.

To complicate the issue, some classes of drugs appear to act more effectively at different times of the day. Thus, β-blockers administered in the morning may lower blood pressure during the day but have little effect when the patient is asleep (11). Conversely, ACE inhibitors and ARBs have a greater effect during sleep than during waking periods, even when given in the morning, which means that the blood pressure level was less during the sleep period (11,12). Diuretics and calcium blockers appear to work evenly over a 24 h period. Thus, to determine whether blood pressure is truly controlled throughout the day, ABPM may be critical. This variation in responsiveness over a 24 h period is another reason why combination therapy may be useful.

A. Titration of Drugs

Hypertension therapy should be started with a low dose of the drug of choice. However, with ACE inhibitors, the starting dose of many of the drugs will not give 24 h control (9,10). Therefore, a low dose should be administered on the first or second occasion but it should be increased to effective levels for 24 h control prior to the next visit (Table 25.1). The incidence of dose-related side effects for ACE inhibitors and ARBs is small, and the evidence is that higher doses may have effects in addition to lowering blood pressure (13–15). The majority of drugs exert most of their effect within 2 weeks, and therapy can be titrated at 2–4 week intervals depending on the severity of the hypertension.

When the patient is seen after taking medication, a careful assessment needs to be made not only of the blood pressure response but also of any side effects. If there has been some response to a drug, but the response is not adequate, a greater effect is usually achieved by adding a second drug rather than by doubling the dose of the initial drug (16,17). However, this may not apply if the patient is taking a drug dosage that does not have 24 h duration in most people (e.g., enalapril, 5 or 10 mg; ramipril, 1.25 or 2.5 mg; lisinopril, 10 mg; felodipine, 2.5 mg). The rationale for adding an appropriate second drug is that this provides a greater blood pressure reduction and reduces side effects when compared with doubling the dose of the first drug (16,17).

B. Control Over a 24 h Period

As mentioned earlier, 24 h blood pressure control is important to achieve the best outcome. This can be determined by choosing a drug in a dose known to work for 24 h after it is administered; by stopping the medication on the

Table 25.1 Different Duration of Blood Pressure Response (10)

| Drug | Dose (mg) | Systolic and diastolic blood pressure (mmHg) | |
		3 h postdose	24 h postdose
Enalapril	5	157/92	171/102
	10	156/90	167/101
	20	158/92	164/98
	40	154/89	161/95
Perindopril	2	155/94	163/100
	4	151/87	168/92
	8	148/86	158/90

day of the clinic visit; or by ABPM (18,19). When control appears to be achieved in the clinic, it is worthwhile to repeat the ABPM. This is the only way to detect whether a patient has an elevated sleep blood pressure that may require modifying the therapy. If control of blood pressure is not achieved in the clinic, a 24 h monitor is also a valuable asset. This is particularly important when patients develop symptoms suggestive of hypotension on different drug therapies, even though the clinic blood pressure is high. Twenty-four hour monitoring may indeed indicate that the patient develops hypotension after drug administration but has white coat hypertension.

C. Other Treatment Measures

During this initial management period, it is important to educate patients about their disease so that they realize the importance of controlling blood pressure as well as controlling other risk factors. If this is done, compliance with the medication protocol is likely to improve. For some patients, particularly for those with white coat hypertension, home blood-pressure monitoring may be essential. In addition, other risk factors should be addressed. The importance of lifestyle modification and diet must be emphasized and encouraged at each visit (see Chapter 25). The treatment must include not only control of the blood pressure, but also well being of the entire patient.

From the treatment guidelines, we know who to treat and what drugs can be used, but our aim is to find the best drug to use for each patient.

V. MORBIDITY AND MORTALITY

Antihypertensive drugs of all classes probably improve the morbidity and mortality rates associated with hypertension, although the benefits of some of the older classes of drugs may be clearly evident only in severe hypertension and not necessarily evident in milder forms of the disease (20–24). Lowering of blood pressure is the first criterion on which to base the use of an antihypertensive agent. Without a reduction in blood pressure, it is unlikely that the full benefit of any drug can be gained. However, other effects, either beneficial or adverse, are associated with drug use, and this translates into effects on morbidity and mortality rates that are of extreme importance. Outcome trials are not necessarily a predictor of the outcome in individual care because the drug usually is continued even when there is no reduction in blood pressure. Conversely, in clinical care the drug is stopped and replaced by another drug when no reduction in blood pressure is evident. The third criterion on which the choice of therapy is based is the side-effect profile in the group of patients, particularly for an individual.

The following sections will discuss the choice of a drug for use in different groups of patients, but it should be emphasized that the data on which these choices are based is incomplete and is frequently derived from data in studies that were designed for other purposes.

A. Population Choice of Drugs

Most drugs probably lower blood pressure to a similar extent in the overall hypertensive population, although different subgroups may respond differently. Diuretics (21,22), calcium channel blockers (25), ACE inhibitors (26), and angiotensin I (AT_1) receptor blockers (27) have all been shown to improve the prognosis even in mild hypertension. The evidence for β-blockers (22,28) is less clear; in the two large Medical Research Council (MRC) trials in which diuretics, β-blockers, and a placebo were compared, β-blockers did not improve the outcome compared with the placebo. Used in combination with diuretics, there was an improved outcome (23,29). However, in a number of these studies, particularly in studies of the elderly, most of the blood pressure-lowering effect and possibly the improvement in morbidity and mortality rates was due to the diuretic (29). There is no conclusive evidence that therapy based on one drug is better than therapy based on another, although the Second Australian National Blood Pressure Study (ANBP2) study (26) and the Losartan Intervention for Endpoint (LIFE) reduction in hypertension study (27) suggest that ACE inhibitor-based therapy is better than diuretic-based therapy (26), and that AT_1 receptor blocker therapy is better than β-blocker therapy (27). The Antihypertensive and Lipid-Lowering Treatment to Prevent Heart Attack Trial (ALLHAT) provided a large amount of data (30). However there were no differences in the primary end point among the drugs and, thus, on primary endpoint data, the drugs should be considered equal. Most people in that study and other studies stopped their previous therapy when they entered the study. This would lead to selection bias because in the ALLHAT study diuretics were probably the most frequently discontinued drug. Specific evidence is not available, and this could have led to results that were correct in the study but are not applicable to patients with previously untreated hypertension.

In the ALLHAT study, cardiac failure was more frequent in patients who received a vasodilator (doxazosin), a calcium channel blocker (amlodipine), or an ACE inhibitor (lisinopril) than in those who received chlorthalidone. This difference in reported heart failure did not translate into a difference in mortality rate. Most people required more than one drug to control blood pressure, and diuretics were a drug class that could not be added to the other groups of drugs in the study. Therefore, the study outcome may be due principally to the trial design. The general conclusion is probably that drugs from diuretic, ACE inhibitor, ARB, and calcium blocker classes all can be used to initiate therapy, with the expectation that most people will require additional agents to fully control blood pressure.

B. Choice of Drugs Based on Gender

Few studies have been designed to determine whether there is a difference in response between males and females, although most evaluation trials provide a gender breakdown, in which the comment usually is that there was no difference in response. Some trials have failed to show significant improvement in prognosis in females but have shown a significant improvement in males. This may be due to the lower frequencies of adverse outcomes in women (particularly young women), and, thus, the trials did not have sufficient power to show an effect greater than that of placebo. A meta analysis of trials indicates that there is little difference in the relative benefits of antihypertensive therapy in men and women (31). In the recent ANBP2 study (26), ACE inhibitor-based therapy improved the trial outcome measure compared with diuretic-based therapy (0.89; $P = 0.05$). However, when men and women were compared, all of the improvement took place in men (0.83; $P = 0.02$); there was no difference in the women. This study included only older patients and may not necessarily apply to younger patients.

There is little evidence for basing the choice of drug class for treatment on response rate and on mortality and morbidity rates. However, there is evidence for basing the choice on differences in side-effect profiles. In the Treatment of Mild Hypertension Study (TOMHS) study (32), women had more adverse effects than men had and were more likely to develop hypokalaemia while on a diuretic. Women also developed more coughing on ACE inhibitors and complained more often of swollen ankles when on a calcium channel blocker. Men were more likely to develop gout (32) and impotence when on a diuretic (22), although these effects may be less common with the lower doses that are now used.

In premenopausal women, there is a particular problem (Table 25.2). Few of the more modern class of drugs have

Table 25.2 Choice of Antihypertensive Medication in Women

Life stage of the woman	Recommended drug
Postmenopause	Any drug
Premenopause, adequate contraception	Any drug
Premenopause, pregnancy risk	α methyl dopa
	Labelatol
	? Diuretics
Early pregnancy	α methyl dopa

been used by patients during pregnancy. If a woman has had children, does not plan to become pregnant and have a child and is taking appropriate contraceptive measures, any drug class can be used. However, if she plans to become pregnant, drugs should not be used that may have teratogenic effects on the fetus (calcium channel blockers), that may affect fetal growth (ACE inhibitors, AT_1 receptor blockers, and β-blockers), or that cause problems such as oligohydramnios (ACE inhibitors and AT_1 receptor blockers) (33). Thus, for women who want to become pregnant or who are in the early stages of pregnancy, there are relatively few drugs from which to choose. After 12 weeks of pregnancy, when the teratogenic risk is reduced, there is a wider choice. In a young woman who is not planning to become pregnant at the time treatment is required, adequate contraceptive measures should be employed and blood pressure controlled as well as possible with drugs from any of the drug classes. When the patient wants to become pregnant, drugs with possible adverse outcomes on the fetus should be discontinued and blood pressure control maintained with a limited range of drugs and lifestyle measures.

The drugs that are recommended to control blood pressure either before a patient becomes pregnant or during the early stages of pregnancy are α methyl dopa or labetalol (34). Diuretics are frequently said to be contraindicated, but a broad analysis has shown no adverse fetal outcome when the mother is taking diuretics (35). However, of particular concern is evidence that there is a linear relationship between a reduction in blood pressure that is induced by treatment of mild forms of hypertension and the proportion of babies born small to these mothers. Thus, in cases of mild hypertension it may be preferable to discontinue medication and simply observe the mother closely. However, if the mother's blood pressure increases significantly, it must be reduced to improve fetal survival. Later in pregnancy, the choice of drugs is wider, although ACE inhibitors and ARBs still should be avoided because they interfere with fetal development. Although there are problems with the choice of drugs for premenopausal women, elevated blood pressure does need to be reduced both before and during pregnancy.

C. Choice of Drugs Related to Aging

Choosing the appropriate drugs for older people is complex. Older people have a mixture of isolated systolic hypertension and combined systolic and diastolic hypertension, although in the latter group, the pulse pressure is usually large, which indicates vascular stiffness. In younger people, isolated systolic hypertension is relatively uncommon; we generally see combined systolic and diastolic hypertension. Thus, the problem of choosing an appropriate

Table 25.3 Response to the Different Antihypertensive Drugs

	Young (37) S–DBP	Old (36) SBP
β-blockers	↑↑↑	↑
ACE inhibitors	↑↑↑	↑
Vasodilators	↑↑↑	not tested
Diuretics	↑↑	↑↑↑
Calcium blockers	↑	↑↑↑

Note: S–DBP, systolic and diastolic blood pressure; SBP, systolic blood pressure.

drug may not necessarily be one based only on the age of the patient, but on the nature of the hypertension.

Two studies have investigated the response to monotherapy in previously untreated hypertensive patients (Table 25.3). The first study, by Morgan et al. (36), used a double-blind crossover design to compare two doses of the four major groups of antihypertensive drugs with a placebo in people >65 years old. The reduction in blood pressure and control achieved were greatest with dihydropyridine calcium blockers and diuretics, which were approximately equal, followed by ACE inhibitors and β-blockers, which were approximately equal, followed by the placebo. The placebo and β-blockers had more side effects than the other treatments, and more people in those groups did not proceed to the higher dose of the drug. The second study, by Deary et al. (37), covered previously untreated younger people who had diastolic hypertension. The order of responsiveness in this study was almost the reverse of the previously mentioned studies, with β-blockers and ACE inhibitors causing the greater reduction in blood pressure. Thus, the age of the person or, possibly more correctly, the nature of the hypertensive process determines the responsiveness. However, this is not consistently true for every patient. Some older people may respond to β-blockers and ACE inhibitors, and some younger people may respond to diuretics and calcium channel blockers.

A study by Materson et al. (38) in the United States also looked at the response rate to the various drugs. The results are slightly different than those discussed previously, but the study was performed in previously treated subjects whose medication was discontinued, and this could have led to bias in the results. Overall, the response rate was greater for calcium blockers, atenolol, clonidine, hydrochlorothiazide, captopril, and prazosin than for placebo, but the response in African-American and Caucasian males differed. The Caucasian subjects responded better to atenolol and captopril than did the African-American subjects, and the younger Caucasian subjects responded better to captopril than did the older ones.

Geriatricians are reluctant to use diuretics or β-blockers to treat hypertension in the elderly. It is thought that diuretics make people more prone to postural hypotension with associated falls and that this is more common with systolic hypertension. Another concern is that β-blockers also appear to reduce the ability of elderly people to cope physically and reduce their mobility.

An argument can be made for the use of thiazide diuretics in elderly women with osteoporosis because these drugs reduce calcium excretion by the kidney and increase bone density, which may be associated with a reduction in fractures of the neck of the femur (39). Although there are related contraindications against the use of diuretics and β-blockers in elderly hypertensive patients, these drugs clearly need to be used when indicated. Thus, people with associated angina should receive β-blockers and people with cardiac failure frequently need a diuretic.

A number of studies have examined the drugs with which patients were still being treated successfully after 1 year. The study by Bloom (40) compared the different drug classes. Drugs were discontinued if there were side effects or the response rate was poor. The patients in this study were observed over a 12-month period. During this period, there was a progressive decline in taking all medications, but the largest decline was in taking diuretics, whose use fell to 38%. AT_1 receptor blockers were continued longer than the other drugs tested (Table 25.4).

A discussion of monotherapy is too simplistic. In the studies previously mentioned, the response rate or control rate when corrected for the placebo was <30% (36–38). Thus, most patients will need two or more drugs. The decision that is required is what combinations of drugs lower blood pressure most effectively and reduce morbidity and mortality rates in different age groups. Unfortunately, no data on this is available.

D. Ethnicity

Different racial groups respond differently to the various drug classes. What is not certain is whether this difference is related to differences in genetic makeup or to different environmental conditions. The reality is probably a combination of these two factors. The differences in response usually have not been studied formally, but there is a large amount of data available from many outcome

Table 25.4 Patients Taking the Same Drug after 1 Year (40)

Drug used	%
AT_1 blockers	64
ACE inhibitors	58
Calcium blockers	50
β-Blockers	43
Diuretics	48

studies. In particular, the ALLHAT study compared the effect of different drugs on morbidity and mortality rates and included a large number of African-Americans (30). The Perindopril Protection Against Recurrent Stroke Study (PROGRESS) included a large number of Asians (Chinese and Japanese) who can be compared with the Caucasians in the study (41).

The generally accepted view is that African-Americans are relatively resistant to β-blockers and ACE inhibitors and respond better to diuretics and calcium channel blockers. This is thought to be due to a relatively sodium-overloaded state and low renin levels. A study reported by Materson et al. (38) (Table 25.5) showed that younger African-Americans responded better to captopril and atenolol than did older African-Americans, and that older African-Americans responded better to diuretics than did younger African-Americans. This is similar to the response seen in the studies by Morgan et al. (36) and Deary et al. (37). However, the placebo-corrected response rates for all drugs except diltiazem were <40%, and most were <30%.

The ALLHAT study allowed a comparison between African-Americans and Caucasians (30). In African-American patients, the reduction in systolic blood pressure was greater with diuretic-based therapy than with ACE inhibitor-based therapy by 4 mmHg. This appeared to translate into a reduction in the incident rate of strokes. This improvement in the stroke rate comparing lisinopril with chlorthalidone was seen only in the African-American population and not in the other populations included in the study. Amlodipine and chlorthalidone showed similar effectiveness in the African-American group, and there was no difference in outcome between African-Americans and the other populations. Most patients needed multiple therapies, and, thus, this study suggests that diuretics (or calcium blockers, or both) are an essential component in the treatment of African-American patients to prevent strokes.

A second large study in African-Americans was in patients with hypertension and renal disease who received

Table 25.5 Response Rate in African-American Patients

| Drug | % Response | |
	<60 years	>60 years
Captopril	14	4
Atenolol	29	14
Clonidine	27	25
Hydrochlorthiazide	22	38
Prazosin	19	18
Diltiazem	46	44

Note: The values are corrected for the response in the placebo group (38).

an ACE inhibitor, a β-blocker, or a dihydropyridine as basic therapy, with other drugs, including frusemide, to achieve blood pressure control (42). The group treated with the ACE inhibitor had a marked reduction in the number of cardiac events compared with those on amlodipine or metoprolol. Thus, despite using a drug which by itself is less effective at reducing blood pressure, there was a marked improvement in outcome. This is probably due to the concomitant use of a diuretic.

Thus, in African-Americans, diuretics and calcium blockers produce the better reduction in blood pressure. However, to prevent complications, an ACE inhibitor is more effective than amlodipine when the ACE inhibitor is used in association with a diuretic.

In the PROGRESS study (41), although the majority of the patients were Caucasian, a significant number of patients were from China and Japan. The mortality profile of patients in China and Japan differed from the Caucasians. There was a less frequent use of diuretics in Japan, but the response pattern to the different drugs in the different populations has not yet been analysed.

VI. CARDIAC DISEASE

Cardiac disease is a common sequelae of hypertension, and normalization of blood pressure would probably prevent its development. The primary problems are cardiac hypertrophy and atherosclerosis of the coronary arteries. Both of these, if untreated, will lead to cardiac failure—in the first situation, principally diastolic failure; in the second situation, systolic dysfunction due to loss of muscle cells and impaired contractility. Another important factor is the stiffness of blood vessels that occurs with age, which is accelerated by hypertension (43). The stiffness of the larger blood vessels alters the time at which reflected waves return from the periphery, causing increased central aortic augmentation of systolic blood pressure. This causes increased cardiac work and may be important in cardiac hypertrophy (44). Reducing the patient's blood pressure is the most important goal, but different drug classes used for treating hypertension also have beneficial effects on other specific problems (Table 25.6).

A. Angina

For a person with angina, the first goal is to decrease blood pressure. This reduces cardiac work and by itself causes resolution of the angina. In addition, β-blockers reduce catecholamine effects on the heart, which leads to more efficient oxygen use and, thus, to a reduction in angina in addition to the blood pressure-lowering effect (45). Calcium blockers cause dilatation of the coronary arteries

Table 25.6 Drug Choice when Hypertension is Associated with Cardiovascular Disease

Associated cardiovascular condition	Preferred drug choices
Angina	β-Blocker; calcium blocker
Cardiac hypertrophy	Angiotensin-converting enzyme I; angiotensin receptor blocker; diuretic
Vascular stiffness	Angiotensin-converting enzyme; calcium blocker; angiotensin receptor blocker
Cardiac failure	Diuretic; angiotensin-converting enzyme I; angiotensin receptor blocker; β-blocker
Atherosclerosis	Angiotensin-converting enzyme I; angiotensin receptor blocker; calcium blocker

Note: For all conditions, it is important to achieve blood pressure control. Any of the drug classes may be used. Combination therapy is often required.

in addition to lowering blood pressure and are indicated in particular where there is a vasospastic element associated with the angina. More fundamentally, ACE inhibitors, ARBs, and calcium blockers—at least experimentally (46)—can all reduce atherosclerosis or prevent its progression and can restore endothelial function toward normal. Thus, all of the major groups of drugs have specific attributes to offer in people with coronary artery disease and angina.

B. Hypertrophy

For people with cardiac hypertrophy, the focus has been on drugs that prevent angiotensin II activity. ACE inhibitors and ARBs reduce cardiac hypertrophy more than the other drug groups and improve the prognosis (47–49). A lesser effect on cardiac hypertrophy is observed with β-blockers, despite similar blood pressure control (27). This may be due to a failure to cause reduction of the stiffness of the blood vessel, and, thus, central aortic systolic blood pressure stays high (50). In addition, β-blockers do not adequately reduce sleep blood pressure (10), which experimentally and clinically has a strong association with left ventricular hypertrophy and morbidity (6, 8,51–53). The reduction in left ventricular hypertrophy is important because it reduces cardiovascular risk (54). The question is not simply the blockade of the RAS, because diuretic-based therapy does reduce left ventricular hypertropy (49,55,56), and therapy based on a low dose of an ACE inhibitor and a diuretic is very effective (57). A high sodium chloride intake can prevent the effect of complete blocking of the RAS; thus, there is an important

interaction between sodium intake, angiotensin II levels, blood pressure, and cardiac hypertrophy (58,59). It is suggested that the most effective therapy is an ARB or an ACE inhibitor coupled with sodium restriction or a low-dose diuretic. This is very effective at lowering blood pressure, and in addition, appears to have an additional effect on left ventricular hypertrophy.

C. Stiff Blood Vessels

Stiff blood vessels cause an increased pulse pressure and an increase in central aortic systolic blood pressure augmentation (43). ACE inhibitors, dihydropyridine calcium channel blockers, and diuretics all cause an acute reduction in central aortic systolic blood pressure, the reduction with β-blockers is much less (50). Chronic treatment with ACE inhibitors also allows structural improvement in the small blood vessel structure (60). Thus, in a person with a large pulse pressure, ACE inhibitors have a theoretical advantage. However, in many people with predominantly systolic hypertension, ACE inhibitors are less effective at reducing branchial artery blood pressure compared with calcium channel blockers (36). Thus, therapy that is based on a diuretic or on a calcium channel-blocker is most effective at lowering brachial artery systolic blood pressure, but an ACE inhibitor appears to have an additional effect in unloading the heart. For the same level of brachial artery blood pressure control, β-blockers do not reduce the central aortic augmentation index (50) and do not improve the function of small arteries (60). Thus, therapy should probably be based on a diuretic or on a dihydropyridine calcium channel blockers with an ACE inhibitor (probably an AT_1 receptor blocker) added to maximize the benefit.

D. Cardiac Failure

The key to treating cardiac failure is prevention, which involves early and complete management of the patient to prevent left ventricular hypertropy and atherosclerosis. If cardiac failure is present, there are three aspects of the condition that determine its management and the outcome:

* Significant fluid retention. If there is significant fluid retention that is causing symptoms, treatment with sodium restriction or diuretic, or both, and probably with a potassium sparing diuretic added is preferable (61).
* Reduction in cardiac output and tissue perfusion. Excessive diuretic therapy may reduce cardiac output and tissue perfusion. Thus, unloading the heart through vasodilator therapy will improve the performance of a person and increase perfusion of the tissues. Therapy based on either an ACE

inhibitor or an ARB, or both, is usually preferred because this type of therapy blocks the humoral component of vasoconstriction and is associated with less sodium retention than standard vasodilatation therapy. It also improves the prognosis (62,63).

- Excessive neurohumoral activation. Patients with cardiac failure also die suddenly, possibly because of excessive neurohumoral activation. Therapy with a β-blocker drug with (64) or without (65) vasodilatory activity improves the outcome.

Therefore, in hypertension with cardiac failure, it is important to use a diuretic to relieve symptoms, an ACE inhibitor or an ARB to improve cardiac performance, and a β-blocker to prevent sudden death. If the use of an ACE inhibitor or an ARB or a β-blocker is contraindicated, then a calcium channel blocker may be essential.

VII. METABOLIC SYNDROME

Hypertension is often associated with obesity, abnormal lipids, hyperuricemia, and diabetes—that is, the metabolic syndrome. Both men (66) and women (67) with the full metabolic syndrome or various components have a marked increase in risk. The key to management is to alter the diet and lifestyle; if the change in diet and lifestyle is unsuccessful, drug therapy to treat hypertension and other components is essential (Table 25.7).

Diuretics elevate uric acid. Diuretics and β-blockers also have adverse effects on the lipid profile. And possibly more important, the incidence of new diabetics in a hypertensive patient population may be influenced by the choice of drugs to treat the hypertension. In the Heart Outcomes and Evaluation (HOPE) study (68), fewer new diabetics were seen in the nondiabetic group treated with an ACE inhibitor. In both the ALLHAT (30) and the ANBP2 (26) studies, more new diabetics were detected in the diuretic-treated subjects than in the subjects who were treated with an ACE inhibitor. The outcome of cardiovascular events was improved by diuretics, but the effect on

Table 25.7 Effects of Different Drugs on Metabolic Syndrome Components

Drug class	Effect
Diuretics	Increase in uric acid
	Adverse lipid effects
	Abnormal glucose values
	Increase in diabetic rate
β-Blockers	Adverse lipid effects
ACE inhibitors and ARBs	Decrease in diabetic rate
	Decrease in uric acid

glucose metabolism leading to more cases of diabetes implies that ACE inhibitor-based therapy is preferable to diuretic-based therapy.

VIII. DIABETIC PATIENTS

If high blood pressure is present in a diabetic patient, the important issue is to reduce blood pressure to <130/ 80 mmHg. It has been demonstrated that a reduction in blood pressure with most, if not all, agents slows the rate of progression of renal disease (69,70). There is evidence that ACE inhibitors and AT_1 receptor blockers may have additional benefits over and above the blood pressure-lowering effect, improving the outcome (68,71). Thus, in the treatment of elevated blood pressure that is associated with diabetes, either an ACE inhibitor or an AT_1 receptor blocker should be the first drug used. If there is no response or inadequate response to this treatment, it is essential to control blood pressure with a drug from any of the other drug classes.

Diuretics in the older high-dose regimes were relatively contraindicated in diabetic patients because the high doses could cause loss of diabetic control. In general, diuretics would not be used as first-line therapy, but they can be added in low doses to ACE inhibitors or to AT_1 receptor blockers, with little effect on diabetic control. ACE inhibitors and AT_1 receptor blockers reduce the rate of progression of renal disease and also reduce proteinuria. This effect is seen even in the absence of hypertension and without a major reduction in blood pressure, which has led to the belief that this effect is due specifically to blocking of the RAS (68,69,71). However, in the United Kingdom Prospective Diabetes Study (UKPDS), captopril and atenolol had a similar effect (70). Also, in a recent study, a small dose of a diuretic in conjunction with a small dose of an ACE inhibitor reduced proteinuria more than a high dose of an ACE inhibitor (72).

There is a specific problem with dihydropyridine calcium channel blocker therapy. This therapy may be necessary to control blood pressure, either alone or in combination with other drugs, and is often effective. However, if proteinuria is present, despite good reduction in blood pressure proteinuria may not be reduced and actually may increase (73). In such circumstances, it may be useful to add an ACE inhibitor or an AT_1 receptor blocker for the additional benefit this may have on proteinuria, possibly independent of blood pressure reduction.

In patients with marked proteinuria, there is some evidence that AT_1 receptor blockers in doses higher than those used for blood pressure control may reduce proteinuria. There is also some evidence that in these circumstances, the combination of an ACE inhibitor and an AT_1 receptor blocker may have incremental effects on the proteinuria, although there is only a small additional effect on blood pressure control (74,75).

IX. RENAL DISEASE

In people with renal disease, the essential step is to normalize the blood pressure. This is rarely achieved with one drug, three or four drugs frequently are required (69,76). The hypertension that is associated with renal disease is due largely to the retention of sodium chloride in the body, and the first line of management should be a reduction in sodium chloride intake. This may reduce blood pressure sufficiently, but even if it does not, reducing sodium chloride intake makes patients more sensitive to most antihypertensive agents.

When antihypertensive agents are given to patients with impaired renal function, the effects on renal function, acutely and chronically, may differ. For example, administration of a dihydropyridine calcium blocker not only reduces blood pressure but also frequently causes a small increase in glomerular filtration rate, which may stay above baseline for up to 6 months (77). Subsequently, renal function deteriorates. In contrast, when an ACE inhibitor (and probably an AT_1 receptor blocker) is given, renal function may deteriorate acutely and serum creatinine rise frequently giving cause for alarm. However, persistence with the drug and long-term management lead to a reduction in the rate of renal function deterioration and have long-term benefits that help prevent renal failure (69,76–78).

From the clinical trials, ACE inhibitors and AT_1 receptor blockers appear consistently to improve morbidity and mortality rates compared with other agents and, thus, should be the first drugs chosen. However, if blood pressure is not reduced to $>130/80$ mmHg or even lower, other drugs should be added as required to achieve this goal. Diuretics are a sensible second drug to add to the ACE inhibitor or AT_1 receptor blocker. In most hypertensive patients, the diuretic that is used is usually a thiazide or thiazide-like diuretic administered in relatively small doses. These small doses of a thiazide have relatively little effect in patients with impaired renal function (e.g., creatinine >0.15 mol/L), and even higher doses are relatively ineffective. Therefore, if a diuretic is used, a loop diuretic usually is required. The effectiveness of the diuretic in reducing blood pressure is improved if sodium chloride intake and thus the load of sodium to be excreted by the kidney is reduced.

Renal failure may also affect the required dose of the drug used to treat hypertension because many of the agents are excreted in the urine. This is not a major problem given that the response and safety range of many of the drugs are wide and that the dose of the drug will be titrated according to the blood pressure response. However, it needs to be recognized because occasionally it can lead to problems. Among the ACE inhibitors, fosinopril has a potential advantage because it combines renal excretion and liver metabolism and because its blood concentration for a given dose stays relatively consistent despite renal failure (79).

X. RENOVASCULAR HYPERTENSION

It is often stated that ACE inhibitors and AT_1 receptor blockers are contraindicated in renal artery stenosis, causing hypertension because of the risk of necrosis of the stenosed kidney. This is particularly true if there is a bilateral stenosis or stenosis in a solitary kidney. In these circumstances, and for most people with functional renal artery stenosis, the preferred treatment is to restore circulation either by dilatation and a stent or surgery (80). If surgery is contraindicated, then in a person with two kidneys, one of which is stenosed, the preferred treatment is a drug that blocks the RAS. These are the groups of drugs that will provide the best blood pressure control, and by treating blood pressure, they may prevent progression of the disease in the nonstenosed kidney adequately.

XI. ARTHRITIS

Most antihypertensive drugs are effective in arthritic patients, but the use of NSAIDs may cause a loss of blood pressure control in some patients. This is probably because of an effect on prostaglandins that alters sodium excretion and leads to sodium retention (81). The effect of most antihypertensive drugs, except for that of calcium antagonists (82), is blunted by sodium retention and, thus, blood pressure control is lost. This is particularly relevant for ACE inhibitors. In a study (83) that compared the effect of indomethacin given to people whose blood pressure was controlled on enalapril or amlodipine, there was an increase of 12 mmHg/5 mmHg in patients on enalapril and an increase of 1 mmHg/0 mmHg in patients on amlodipine. All antihypertensive drugs can be used in arthritic patients, but if NSAID use is intermittent, it appears to be preferable to base therapy on a calcium channel blocker.

XII. SCIENTIFIC BASIS FOR DIFFERENT RESPONSES TO DRUGS

A simple test to determine the most appropriate drug for a patient would simplify management. It has been claimed (84) that renin profiling allows a rational choice of therapy. The hypothesis is that in people with a relatively high renin, blocking of the RAS by ACE inhibitors or AT_1 receptor blockers or by prevention of renin secretion by β-blockers provides a good response. Conversely, patients with a relatively low renin have a good response to diuretics and calcium channel blockers. There is evidence to suggest that when this hypothesis is applied to groups, there is merit in this proposal. African-American patients, elderly patients, and patients with renal disease have sodium retention and relatively low renin, so these groups respond better to calcium channel blockers and diuretics than to β-blockers and blocking of the RAS. However, although the group data support this hypothesis, when the hypothesis is applied to an individual, the predictive value is much weaker. Some elderly people with a low renin have an excellent response to an ACE inhibitor or a β-blocker, so the classification is only a guide to initial selection.

XIII. ACHIEVEMENT OF THE BLOOD PRESSURE GOAL

In recent years, the goal has been to reduce blood pressure to an ideal level of <130 mmHg systolic and <80 mmHg diastolic. In most people who have a systolic blood pressure >160 mmHg, this goal will not be achieved with monotherapy. This raises the questions of how many drugs need to be prescribed to achieve this goal and how high the dosages should be. The Hypertension Optimal Treatment study (85) showed that aggressive therapy did improve the outcome in some subgroups, but there is no data available to indicate how much of the improvement is related to the first drug, the second drug, the third drug, and so on. In particular, if blood pressure was not controlled, was there a negative effect of the additional drugs as assessed by such factors as morbidity, mortality, financial cost, and lifestyle. Although it is preferable to reach the stated ideal goals for blood pressure levels, treatment regimens must be tempered by common sense, and the goal for individual patients may be relaxed as more drugs are used. In the elderly, it is particularly difficult to reach systolic blood pressure goals (Table 25.8). In many cases this will require a multiple drug regimen.

Suggested indicators for choosing a particular regimen are shown in Table 25.9.

All drugs do have side effects, some of which are related to the mechanism of action. For a number of drug classes (diuretics, β-blockers, calcium blockers, vasodilators), side effects increase as drug doses increase. However, the side-effect profiles of most ACE inhibitors and AT_1 receptor blockers in doses that are effective for 24 h are relatively dose independent. Another important factor is that a much greater response usually is obtained by adding a second drug than by doubling the dose of

Table 25.8 Recommendations for Treating Systolic Hypertension in the Elderly

Number of drugs used at one time	Systolic blood pressure (mmHg)	Recommendation
One	<130	Great success; continue
	<135	Accept
	≥135	Add a second drug
Two	<135	Continue
	<140	Accept
	≥140	Add a third drug
Three	<140	Continue
	<150	Accept
	≥150	Add a fourth drug
Four	<160	Accept
	≥160	What to do? unknown

Note: This is assuming an initial systolic blood pressure of ≥150 mmHg. If the reduction in blood pressure is <10 mmHg after initial therapy, try a different drug class.

the first drug (86). Thus, the guiding principle for what follows is that appropriate second drug should be added rather than titrating to the maximum doses of the initial drugs, and in the case of ACE inhibitors and AT_1 receptor blockers, start with a moderately high dose. Some of the more useful combinations are as follows:

- ACE inhibitors and diuretics;
- β-blockers and diuretics;
- AT1 receptor blockers and diuretics;
- vasodilators and diuretics;
- ACE inhibitors and dihydropyridines;
- AT1 receptor blockers and dihydropyridines;
- dihydropyridines and β-blockers.

These combinations are useful and, in most cases, are additive in their effects or in reducing the side-effect profile, or both. In many of the above combinations, a diuretic is the second drug used, and this diuretic usually can be in a dose range where the dose of the diuretic, by itself, is relatively ineffective but in combination with another class of drug has a positive additive effect.

Combinations that are less than additive in their effects include the following:

- ACE inhibitors and β-blockers;
- ACE inhibitors and AT_1 receptor blockers;
- dihydropyridines and diuretics.

However, in certain circumstances there may be a specific indication for their use.

Although statements can be made about the effectiveness of different drug treatment combinations, there is little conclusive data regarding whether some combinations are better than others at improving the outcome.

Table 25.9 Choice of Drug for Specific Situations

Specific patient characteristic or disease condition	Recommended drug classes for the situation	Contraindicated drugs for the situation
Young patient	ACE inhibitor; β-blocker	
Older patient	Calcium blocker; diuretic	
Diastolic hypertension	ACE inhibitor; β-blocker	
Systolic hypertension	Calcium blocker; diuretic	
African-American	Calcium blocker; diuretic	
Diabetic	ACE inhibitor; angiotensin receptor blocker	
Metabolic syndrome	ACE inhibitor; angiotensin receptor blocker	Diuretic; β-blocker
Renal disease	ACE; ARB	
Obstructive airway disease		β-Blocker
High salt intake	Calcium blocker; diuretic	
NSAID use	Calcium blocker	Angiotensin-converting enzyme inhibitor; angiotensin receptor blocker
High pulse rate	β-Blocker	
Cardiovascular disease		
Angina	β-Blocker; calcium blocker	
Cardiac failure	Diuretic; ACE inhibitor; ARB; β-blocker	
Stiff blood vessels	ACE inhibitor; calcium blocker	
Cardiac hypertrophy	ACE inhibitor; ARB; diuretic	

Note: This refers to drugs used as monotherapy. Frequently, a diuretic needs to be added to allow full expression of the effect of another drug.

XIV. CONCLUSION

Large clinical trials provide objective information about the effect of drugs on morbidity and mortality rates, and they provide general guidelines that are related to overall outcome. However, such studies are inflexible, and patients continue on their assigned drugs even if they have no effect on blood pressure levels. In addition, patients with complications were excluded in many of the earlier studies, although this is less frequently the case in more recent studies.

By tailoring the therapy to the patient (Table 25.9), it should be possible to obtain better results in individual patients than those indicated in the clinical trials. Drugs can be used to which the patient responds; and drugs can be discontinued if there is no response or the response is inadequate. Other disorders that affect the morbidity and mortality rates can be treated at the same time hypertension is being treated. Better treatment compliance can be obtained through individual management and encouragement. Only if all risk factors associated with an adverse outcome are managed will success be possible in reducing morbidity and mortality rates back to the rates for people who do not have hypertension.

REFERENCES

1. Chalmers J, Morgan TO, Doyle AE, Dickson B, Hopper J, Matthews J, Matthews G, Moulds R, Myers J, Nowson C et al. Australian National Health and Medical Research Council dietary salt study in mild hypertension. J Hypertens 1986; 4(suppl 6):S629–S637.

2. Mancia G, Omboni S, Parati G, Ravogli A, Villani A, Zanchetti A. Lack of placebo effect on ambulatory BP. Am J Hypertens 1995; 8:311–315.

3. Staessen JA, Thijs L, Bieniaszewski L, O'Brien ET, Palatini P, Davidson C, Dobovisek J, Jaaskivi M, Laks T, Lehtonen A, Vanhanen H, Webster J, Fagard R. Ambulatory monitoring uncorrected for placebo overestimates long-term antihypertensive action. Hypertension 1996; 27:414–420.

4. Kario K, Pickering TG, Umeda Y, Hoshide S, Hoshide Y, Morinari M, Murata M, Kuroda T, Schwartz JE, Shimada K. Morning surge in blood pressure as a predictor of silent and clinical cerebrovascular disease in elderly hypertensives: a prospective study. Circulation 2003; 107:1401–1406.

5. Chobanian AV, Bakris GL, Black HR, Cushman WC, Green LA, Izzo JL Jr, Jones DW, Materson BJ, Oparil S, Wright JT Jr, Roccella EJ and the National High Blood Pressure. Education Program Coordinating Committee. Seventh report of the Joint National Committee on prevention, detection, evaluation and treatment of high blood pressure. Hypertension 2003; 42:1206–1252.

6. Morgan TO, Brunner HR, Aubert J-F, Wang Q, Griffiths C, Delbridge L. Cardiac hypertrophy depends upon sleep blood pressure: a study in rats. J Hypertens 2000; 18:445–451.

7. Clement DL, De Buyzere ML, De Bacquer DA, de Leeuw PW, Duprez DA, Fagard RH, Gheeraert PJ, Missault LH, Braun JJ, Six RO, Van Der Niepen P, O'Brien E. Prognostic

value of ambulatory blood-pressure recordings in patients with treated hypertension. N Engl J Med 2003; 348:2407–2415.

8. Wing LMH, Reid CM, Ryan P, Beilin LJ, Brown MA for Management Committee, High Blood Pressure Research Council of Australia. Night ambulatory blood pressure predicts outcome in the Second Australian National Blood Pressure Study (ANBP2). (Abstract) J Hypertens 2004; 22(suppl 2):S12.

9. Anderson A, Morgan O, Morgan TO. Effectiveness of blood pressure control with once daily administration of enalapril and perindopril. Am J Hypertens 1994; 7:371–373.

10. Morgan TO, Morgan O, Anderson A. Effect of dose on trough peak ratio of antihypertensive drugs in elderly hypertensive males. CEPP 1995; 2:778–780.

11. Morgan TO, Anderson A. Different drug classes have variable effects on blood pressure depending on the time of day. Am J Hypertens 2003; 16:46–50.

12. Morgan T, Anderson A, Jones E. The effect on 24 h blood pressure control of an angiotensin converting enzyme inhibitor (perindopril) administered in the morning or at night. J Hypertens 1997; 15:205–211.

13. Mancia G, Seravalle G, Grassi G. Tolerability and treatment compliance with angiotensin II receptor antagonists. Am J Hypertens 2003; 16:1066–1073.

14. Mazzolai L, Burnier M. Comparative safety and tolerability of angiotensin II receptor antagonists. Drug Saf 1999; 21:23–33.

15. Gregoire JP, Moisan J, Guibert R, Ciampi A, Milot A, Cote I, Gaudet M. Tolerability of antihypertensive drugs in a community-based setting. Clin Ther 2001; 23:715–726.

16. Morgan TO, Anderson A, Jones E. Comparison and interaction of low dose felodipine (ER) and enalapril in the treatment of essential hypertension in elderly patients. Am J Hypertens 1992; 5:238–243.

17. Sica DA. Rationale for fixed-dose combinations in the treatment of hypertension: the cycle repeats. Drugs 2002; 62:443–462.

18. Morgan T, Ménard J, Brunner H. Twenty-four hour blood pressure control and trough to peak ratio: who, when, how and why? J Hum Hypertens 1998; 12:45–48.

19. Morgan T, Ménard J, Brunner H. Trough to peak ratio as a guide to BP control: measurement and calculation. J Hum Hypertens 1998; 12:49–53.

20. VA Cooperative Study Group. Effects of treatment on morbidity in hypertension. Results in patients with diastolic blood pressures averaging 115 through 129 mmHg. J Am Med Assoc 1967; 202:1028–1034.

21. Management Committee. The Australian therapeutic trial in mild hypertension. Lancet 1980; 1:1261–1267.

22. Medical Research Council Working Party. MRC trial of treatment of mild hypertension: principal results. Br Med J (Clin Res Ed) 1985; 291:97–104.

23. SHEP Cooperative Research Group. Prevention of stroke by antihypertensive drug treatment in older persons with isolated systolic hypertension. Final results of the Systolic Hypertension in the Elderly Program (SHEP). J Am Med Assoc 1991; 265:3255–3264.

24. Neal B, MacMahon S, Chapman N. Effects of ACE inhibitors, calcium antagonists, and other blood-pressure-lowering drugs: results of prospectively designed overviews of randomised trials. Blood pressure Lowering Treatment Trialists' Collaboration. Lancet 2000; 356:1955–1964.

25. Staessen JA, Fagard R, Thijs L, Celis H, Arabidze GG, Birkenhager WH, Bulpitt CJ, de Leeuw PW, Dollery CT, Fletcher AE, Forette F, Leonetti G, Nachev C, O'Brien ET, Rosenfeld J, Rodicio JL, Tuomilehto J, Zanchetti A. Randomised double-blind comparison of placebo and active treatment for older patients with isolated systolic hypertension. The Systolic Hypertension in Europe (Syst-Eur) Trial Investigators. Lancet 1997; 350:757–764.

26. Wing LM, Reid CM, Ryan P, Beilin LJ, Brown MA, Jennings GL, Johnston CI, McNeil JJ, Macdonald GJ, Marley JE, Morgan TO, West MJ. A comparison of outcomes with angiotensin-converting-enzyme inhibitors and diuretics for hypertension in the elderly. N Engl J Med 2003; 348:583–592.

27. Dahlöf B, Devereux RB, Kjeldsen SE, Julius S, Beevers G, Faire U, Fyhrquist F, Ibsen H, Kristiansson K, Lederballe-Pedersen O, Lindholm LH, Nieminen MS, Omvik P, Oparil S, Wedel H. Cardiovascular morbidity and mortality in the Losartan Intervention For Endpoint reduction in hypertension study (LIFE): a randomised trial against atenolol. Lancet 2002; 359:995–1003.

28. Medical Research Council Working Party. Medical Research Council trial of treatment of hypertension in older adults: principal results. Brit Med J 1992; 304:405–412.

29. Dahlöf B, Lindholm LH, Hansson L, Scherstén B, Ekbom T, Wester P-O. Morbidity and mortality in the Swedish Trial in Old Patients with Hypertension (STOP-Hypertension). Lancet 1991; 338:1281–1285.

30. The ALLHAT Officers and Coordinators for the ALLHAT Collaborative Research Group. Major outcomes in high-risk hypertensive patients randomized to angiotensin-converting enzyme inhibitor or calcium channel blocker vs diuretic: the Antihypertensive and Lipid-Lowering Treatment to Prevent Heart Attack Trial (ALLHAT). J Am Med Assoc 2002; 288:2981–2997.

31. Gueyffier F, Boutitie F, Boissel JP, Pocock S, Coope J, Cutler J, kbom T, Fagard R, Friedman L, Perry M, Prineas R, Schron E. Effect of antihypertensive drug treatment on cardiovascular outcomes in women and men : a meta-analysis of individual patient data from randomized, controlled trials. The INDANA Investigators. Ann Intern Med 1997; 126:761–767.

32. Lewis CE, Grandits A, Flack J, McDonald R, Elmer PH. Efficacy and tolerance of antihypertensive treatment in men and women with stage 1 diastolic hypertension: results of the Treatment of Mild Hypertension Study. Arch Intern Med 1996; 156:377–385.

33. Brown MA, Whitworth JA. Pregnancy. In: Bennett WM, McCarron DA, eds. Contemporary Issues in Nephrology: Pharmacology and Management of Hypertension. Vol. 28. New York: Churchill Livingstone, 1994:89–116.

34. Sibai BM. Treatment of hypertension in pregnant women. N Engl J Med 1996; 335:257–265.

35. Collins R, Yusuf S, Peto R. Overview of randomised trials of diuretics in pregnancy. Brit Med J Clin Res Ed 1985; 290:17–23.

36. Morgan TO, Anderson AIE, MacInnis RJ. ACE inhibitors, β blocking drugs, calcium channel blocking drugs and diuretics for the control of elevated systolic blood pressure in the elderly. Am J Hypertens 2001; 14(3):241–247.

37. Deary AJ, Schumann AL, Murfet H, Haydock SF, Foo RS-Y, Brown MH. Double blind, placebo-controlled crossover comparison of five classes of antihypertensive drugs. J Hypertens 2002; 20:771–777.

38. Materson BJ, Reda DJ, Cushman WC, Massie BM, Freis ED, Kochar MS, Hamburger RJ, Fye C, Lakshman R, Gottdiener J et al. Single-drug therapy for hypertension in men: a comparison of six antihypertensive agents with placebo. The Department of Veterans Affairs Cooperative Study Group on Antihypertensive Agents. N Engl J Med 1993; 328:914–921.

39. Feskanich D, Willett WC, Stampfer MJ, Colditz GA. A prospective study of thiazide use and fractures in women. Osteoporos Int 1997; 7:79–84.

40. Bloom BS. Continuation of initial antihypertensive medication after 1 year of therapy. Clin Ther 1998; 20:671–681.

41. PROGRESS Collaborative Group. Randomised trial of a perindopril-based blood-pressure-lowering regimen among 6,105 individuals with previous stroke or transient ischaemic attack. Lancet 2001; 358:1033–1041.

42. Wright JT Jr, Bakris G, Greene T, Agodoa LY, Appel LJ, Charleston J, Cheek D, Douglas-Baltimore JG, Gassman J, Glassock R, Hebert L, Jamerson K, Lewis J, Phillips RA, Toto RD, Middleton JP, Rostand SG. Effect of blood pressure lowering and antihypertensive drug class on progression of hypertensive kidney disease: results from the AASK trial. J Am Med Assoc 2002; 288:2421–2431.

43. O'Rourke MF. From theory into practice: arterial haemodynamics in clinical hypertension. J Hypertens 2002; 20:1901–1915.

44. Gatzka CD, Cameron JD, Kingwell BA, Dart AM. Relation between coronary artery disease, aortic stiffness and left ventricular structure in a population sample. Hypertension 1998; 32:575–578.

45. Gibbons RJ, Abrams J, Chatterjee K, Daley J, Deedwania PC, Douglas JS, Ferguson TB Jr, Fihn SD, Fraker TD Jr, Gardin JM, O'Rourke RA, Pasternak RC, Williams SV. ACC/AHA 2002 guideline update for the management of patients with chronic stable angina—summary article: a report of the American College of Cardiology/American Heart Association Task Force on practice guidelines (Committee on the Management of Patients with Chronic Stable Angina). J Am Coll Cardiol 2003; 41:159–168.

46. Matsumoto K, Morishita R, Moriguchi A, Tomita N, Aoki M, Sakonjo H, Matsumoto K, Nakamura T, Higaki J, Ogihara T. Inhibition of neointima by angiotensin-converting enzyme inhibitor in porcine coronary artery balloon-injury model. Hypertension 2001; 37:270–274.

47. Dahlöf B, Pennert K, Hansson L. Reversal of left ventricular hypertrophy in hypertensive patients. A metaanalysis of 109 treatment studies. Am J Hypertens 1992; 5:95–110.

48. Schmieder RE, Schlaich MP, Klingbeil AU, Martus P. Update on reversal of left ventricular hypertrophy in essential hypertension (a meta-analysis of all randomized double-blind studies until December 1996). Nephrol Dial Transplant 1998; 13:564–569.

49. Gottdiener JS, Reda DJ, Massie BM, Materson BJ, Williams DW, Anderson RJ. Effect of single-drug therapy on reduction of left ventricular mass in mild to moderate hypertension: comparison of six antihypertensive agents. The Department of Veterans Affairs Cooperative Study Group on Antihypertensive Agents. Circulation 1997; 95:2007–2014.

50. Morgan T, Lauri J, Bertram D, Anderson A. Effect of different antihypertensive drug classes on central aortic pressure. Am J Hypertens 2004; 17:118–123.

51. Verdecchia P. Prognostic value of ambulatory blood pressure: current evidence and clinical implications. Hypertension 2000; 35:844–851.

52. Wing LMH, Reid CM, Beilin LJ, Brown MA for ANBP2 Management Committee. Outcome related to clinic and ambulatory blood pressure in the Second Australian National Blood Pressure Study (ANBP2). (Abstract) International Society of Hypertension meeting, Feb 2004.

53. Cicconetti P, Morelli S, Ottaviani L, Chiarotti F, De Serra C, De Marzio P, Costarella M, Sgreccia A, Ciotti V, Marigliano V. Blunted nocturnal fall in blood pressure and left ventricular mass in elderly individuals with recently diagnosed isolated systolic hypertension. Am J Hypertens 2003; 16:900–905.

54. Verdecchia P, Angeli F, Borgioni C, Gattobogio R, de Simone G, Devereux RB, Porcellati C. Changes in cardiovascular risk by reduction of left ventricular mass in hypertension: a meta-analysis. Am J Hypertens 2003; 16:895–899.

55. Gosse P, Sheridan DJ, Zannad F, Dubourg O, Gueret P, Karpov Y, de Leeuw PW, Palma-Gamiz JL, Pessina A, Motz W, Degaute JP, Chastang C. Regression of left ventricular hypertrophy in hypertensive patients treated with indapamide SR 1.5 mg versus enalapril 20 mg: the LIVE study. J Hypertens 2000; 18:1465–1475.

56. Liebson PR, Grandits GA, Dianzumba S, Prineas RJ, Grimm RJ Jr, Neaton JD, Stamler J. Comparison of five antihypertensive monotherapies and placebo for change in left ventricular mass in patients receiving nutritional-hygienic therapy in the Treatment of Mild Hypertension Study (TOMHS). Circulation 1995; 91:698–706.

57. Asmar RG, London GM, O'Rourke MF, Mallion JM, Romero R, Rahn KH, Trimarco B, Fitzgerald D, Hedner T, Duprez D, De Leeuw PW, Sever P, Battegay E, Hitzenberger G, de Luca N, Polonia P, Benetos A, Chastang C, Ollivier JP, Safar ME, on behalf of the REASON Project investigators. Amelioration of arterial properties with a perindopril–indapamide very-low-dose combination. J Hypertens 2001; 19(suppl 4):S15–S20.

58. Abro E, Griffiths CD, Morgan TO, Delbridge LMD. Regression of cardiac hypertrophy in the SHR by combined renin–angiotensin system blockade and dietary sodium restriction. JRAAS 2001; 2(suppl 1):S148–S153.

59. Griffiths CD, Morgan TO, Delbridge LMD. Effects of combined administration of ACE inhibitor and angiotensin II receptor antagonist are prevented by a high NaCl intake. J Hypertens 2001; 19(11):2087–2095.

60. Schiffrin EL, Deng LY, Larochelle P. Progressive improvement in the structure of resistance arteries of hypertensive patients after 2 years of treatment with an angiotensin I-converting enzyme inhibitor: comparison with effects of a β-blocker. Am J Hypertens 1995; 8:229–236.

61. Pitt B, Zannad F, Remme WJ, Cody R, Castaigne A, Perez A, Palensky J, Wittes J. The effect of spironolactone on morbidity and mortality in patients with severe heart failure. Randomized Aldactone Evaluation Study Investigators. N Engl J Med 1999; 341:709–717.

62. Pfeffer MA, Braunwald E, Moye LA, Basta L, Brown EJ Jr, Cuddy TE, Davis BR, Geltman EM, Goldman S, Flaker GC et al., for the SAVE Investigators. Effect of captopril on mortality and morbidity in patients with left ventricular dysfunction and myocardial infarction: results of the Survival and Ventricular Enlargement Trial. N Engl J Med 1992; 337:669–677.

63. The European Trial on Reducation of Cardiac Events with Perindopril in Stable Coronary Artery Disease investigators. Efficacy of perindopril in reduction of cardiovascular events among patients with stable coronary artery disease: randomised, double-blind, placebo-controlled, multi-centre trial (the EUROPA study). Lancet 2003; 362:782–788.

64. Poole-Wilson PA, Swedberg K, Cleland JGF, Di Lenarda A, Hanrath P, Komajda M, Lubsen J, Lutiger B, Metra M, Remme WJ, Torp-Pedersen C, Scherhag A, Skene A; for the COMET Investigators. Comparison of carvedilol and metoprolol on clinical outcomes in patients with chronic heart failure in the Carvedilol Or Metoprolol European Trial (COMET): randomised controlled trial. Lancet 2003; 362:7–13.

65. Hjalmarson A, Goldstein S, Fagerberg B, Wedel H, Waagstein F, Kjekshus J, Wikstrand J, El Allaf D, Vitovec J, Aldershvile J, Halinen M, Dietz R, Neuhaus KL, Janosi A, Thorgeirsson G, Dunselman PH, Gullestad L, Kuch J, Herlitz J, Rickenbacher P, Ball S, Gottlieb S, Deedwania P. Effects of controlled-release metoprolol on total mortality, hospitalizations, and well-being in patients with heart failure: the Metoprolol CR/XL Randomized Intervention Trial in congestive heart failure (MERIT-HF). MERIT-HF Study Group. J Am Med Assoc 2000; 283:1295–1302.

66. Lakka HM, Laaksonen DE, Lakka TA, Niskanen LK, Kumpusalo E, Tuomilehto J, Salonen JT. The metabolic syndrome and total and cardiovascular disease mortality in middle-aged men. J Am Med Assoc 2002; 288:2709–2716.

67. Hsia J, Bittner V, Tripputi M, Howard BV. Metabolic syndrome and coronary angiographic disease progression: the Women's Angiographic Vitamin & Estrogen trial. Am Heart J 2003; 146:439–445.

68. Heart Outcomes Prevention Evaluation Study Investigators. Effects of an angiotensin-converting-enzyme inhibitor, ramipril, on cardiovascular events in high risk patients. N Engl J Med 2000; 342:145–153.

69. Jafar TH, Stark PC, Schmid CH, Landa M, Maschio G, de Jong PE, de Zeeuw D, Shahinfar S, Toto R, Levey AS. Progression of chronic kidney disease: the role of blood pressure control, proteinuria, and angiotensin-converting enzyme inhibition: a patient-level meta-analysis. Ann Intern Med 2003; 139:244–252.

70. UKPDS 38. Tight blood pressure control and risk of macrovascular and microvascular complications in type 2 diabetes UKPDS 38. UK Prospective Diabetes Study Group. Brit Med J 1998; 317:703–713.

71. Heart Outcomes Prevention Evaluation Study Investigators. Effects of ramipril on cardiovascular and microvascular outcomes in people with diabetes mellitus: results of the HOPE study and MICRO-HOPE substudy. Lancet 2000; 355:253–259.

72. Mogensen CE, Viberti G, Halimi S, Ritz E, Riulope L, Jermendy G, Widimsky J, Sareli P, Taton J, Rull J, Erdogan G, De Leeuw PW, Ribeiro A, Sanchez R, Mechmeche R, Nolan J, Sirotiakova J, Hamani A, Scheen A, Hess B, Luger A, Thomas SM. Effect of low-dose perindopril/indapamide on albuminuria in diabetes. Preterax in albuminuria regression: PREMIER. Hypertension 2003; 41:1063–1071.

73. Morgan T, Anderson A. A comparison of candesartan, felodipine and their combination in the treatment of elderly patients with systolic hypertension. Am J Hypertens 2002; 15(6):544–549.

74. Mogensen CE, Neldam S, Tikkanen I, Oren S, Viskoper R, Watts RW, Cooper ME. Randomised controlled trial of dual blockade of renin–angiotensin system in patients with hypertension, microalbuminuria, and non-insulin dependent diabetes: the candesartan and lisinopril microalbuminuria (CALM) study. Brit Med J 2000; 321:1440–1444.

75. Morgan T, Anderson A, Bertram D, MacInnis R. Effect of candesartan and lisinopril alone and in combination on blood pressure and microalbuminuria. Submitted to JRAAS.

76. Jafar TH, Schmid CH, Landa M, Giatras I, Toto R, Remuzzi G, Maschio G, Brenner BM, Kamper A, Zucchelli P, Becker G, Himmelmann A, Bannister K, Landais P, Shahinfar S, de Jong PE, de Zeeuw D, Lau J, Levey AS. Angiotensin-converting enzyme inhibitors and progression of nondiabetic renal disease: a meta-analysis of patient-level data. Ann Intern Med 2001; 135:73–87.

77. Agodoa LY, Appel L, Bakris GL, Beck G, Bourgoignie J, Briggs JP, Charleston J, Cheek D, Cleveland W, Douglas JG, Douglas M, Dowie D, Faulkner M, Gabriel A, Gassman J, Greene T, Hall Y, Hebert L, Hiremath L, Jamerson K, Johnson CJ, Kopple J, Kusek J, Lash J, Lea J, Lewis JB, Lipkowitz M, Massry S, Middleton J, Miller ER III, Norris K, O'Connor D, Ojo A, Phillips RA, Pogue V, Rahman M, Randall OS, Rostand S, Schulman G, Smith W, Thornley-Brown D, Tisher CC, Toto RD, Wright JT Jr, Xu S. Effect of ramipril vs amlodipine on renal outcomes in hypertensive nephrosclerosis: a randomized controlled trial. J Am Med Assoc 2001; 285:2719–2728.

78. Peterson JC, Adler S, Bukart JM, Greene T, Hebert LA, Hunsicker LG, King AJ, Klahr S, Massry SG, Seifter JL, for the Modification of Diet in Renal Disease (MDRD) Study Group. Blood pressure control, proteinuria and the progression of renal disease. Ann Intern Med 1995; 123:754–762.

79. Mancia G, Giannattasio C, Grassi G. Treatment of heart failure with fosinopril: an angiotensin converting enzyme inhibitor with a dual and compensatory route of excretion. Am J Hypertens 1997; 10:236S–241S.

80. Textor SC. Revascularization in atherosclerotic renal artery disease. Kidney Int 1998; 53:799–811.

81. Whelton A. Nephrotoxicity of nonsteroidal anti-inflammatory drugs: physiologic foundations and clinical implications. Am J Med 1999; 106:13S–24S.

82. Morgan TO, Anderson A, Wilson D, Myers J, Murphy J, Nowson C. Paradoxical effect of sodium restriction on blood pressure in people on slow channel calcium blocking drugs. Lancet 1986; 1:793.

83. Morgan TO, Anderson A, Bertram D. Effect of indomethacin on blood pressure in elderly people with essential hypertension well controlled on amlodipine or enalapril. Am J Hypertens 2000; 13:1161–1167.

84. Laragh J. Laragh's lessons in pathophysiology and clinical pearls for treating hypertension. AJH 2001; 14:837–854.

85. Hansson L, Zanchetti A, Carruthers SG, Dahlöf B, Elmfeldt D, Menard J, Rahn KH, Wedel H, Westerling S, for the HOT Study Group. Effects of intensive blood pressure lowering and low-dose aspirin in patients with hypertension: principal results of the Hypertension Optimal Treatment (HOT) randomised trial. Lancet 1998; 351:1755–1762.

86. Law MR, Wald NJ, Morris JK, Jordan RE. Value of low dose combination treatment with blood pressure lowering drugs: analysis of 354 randomized trials. Brit Med J 2003; 326:1427–1434.

26

Diuretic Therapy in Cardiovascular Disease

DOMENIC A. SICA

Virginia Commonwealth University, Richmond, Virginia, USA

KEYPOINTS

- There exist multiple diuretic classes, each with distinctive pharmacodynamic features.
- Diuretics are used for control of volume in sodium-retaining states as well as to reduce blood pressure. Blood pressure reduction with diuretic therapy is the result of both volume removal and a direct vasodilator effect with these compounds. Thiazide-type diuretics reduce blood pressure more effectively than do loop diuretics unless the loop diuretic is being used for volume removal.

- Diuretics compare favorably with most medication classes in establishing blood pressure control in mild-to-moderate forms of hypertension. Diuretics are also useful adjunctive therapy for most antihypertensive medication classes.
- Outcomes data are positive with thiazide-type diuretics particularly as relates to the incidence rate of stroke.
- The most prominent diuretic related side-effects are electrolyte in nature. Thiazide and loop diuretics will increase urinary losses of potassium and magnesium; conversely, potassium-sparing diuretics

reduce urinary losses of both potassium and magnesium. New-onset diabetes and sexual dysfunction are side-effects also seen with thiazide-type diuretics.

SUMMARY

Diuretics have been available for more than a half-century and have become mainstays of therapy for edematous states and/or hypertension. Considerable pharmacologic heterogeneity is present amongst the members of the various classes of diuretics. Diuretics have an important role in the management of hypertension either as monotherapy or as adjuncts to other antihypertensive medication classes. Thiazide-type diuretics can be distinguished from loop diuretics in that they are more efficient in reducing blood pressure but less effective as pure diuretic agents. Diuretic-related side-effects are typically electrolyte in nature and are linked in their severity with the duration and site of action of respective diuretics.

I. INTRODUCTION

Modern diuretic therapy grew out of two apparently unrelated events in the 1930s: the development of sulfanilamide, which was the first effective antibacterial drug, and the characterization of the enzyme carbonic anhydrase. Clinical experience with sulfanilamide showed that this drug increased urine flow as well as sodium and potassium excretion. The recognition that sulfanilamide inhibited carbonic anhydrase catalyzed attempts to synthesize compounds that might more specifically inhibit carbonic anhydrase. The compound acetazolamide was discovered in the process. The diuretic effect of acetazolamide proved to be short-lived, which led to a search for more potent diuretic compounds with greater long-term effectiveness. The first of this more potent kind of diuretics was chlorothiazide, and its advent in 1958 ushered in the modern era of diuretic therapy (1).

Diuretics are important therapeutic tools because they effectively reduce blood pressure and at the same time decrease the morbidity and mortality that result from hypertension. Diuretics are currently recommended by the Joint National Committee on Detection, Evaluation, and Treatment of Hypertension in its seventh report (JNC7) as first-line therapy for the treatment of hypertension (2). In addition, diuretics remain an important aspect of congestive heart failure treatment because they improve the congestive symptomatology that typifies the more advanced stages of congestive heart failure. This chapter reviews the mechanism of action of the various diuretic classes and the physiologic adaptations that accompany

the use of these drugs, establishes the basis for their use in the treatment of hypertension and congestive heart failure, and reviews commonly encountered side effects.

II. CLASSES OF DIURETICS

The predominant nephron action site(s) of various diuretic classes are represented in Fig. 26.1. All available diuretic classes have distinctive pharmacokinetics and, in many instances, differing pharmacodynamic responses that depends on both the nature and stage of the underlying disease being treated (Table 26.1) (3).

A. Carbonic Anhydrase Inhibitors

The administration of a carbonic anhydrase inhibitor ordinarily produces a brisk alkaline diuresis. Although carbonic anhydrase inhibitors work at the proximal tubule level, where the bulk of sodium reabsorption occurs, their final diuretic effect is typically rather modest, being blunted by reabsorption in more distal nephron segments (4). Acetazolamide is the only carbonic anhydrase inhibitor with relevant diuretic effects. Acetazolamide is readily absorbed and is eliminated by tubular secretion. Its use is limited because of its transient action and because prolonged administration leads to metabolic acidosis. But in contrast, acetazolamide (250–500 mg daily) also can correct the metabolic alkalosis that occasionally occurs with thiazide or loop diuretic therapy.

B. Loop Diuretics

Loop diuretics act predominately at the apical membrane in the thick ascending limb of the loop of Henle, where they compete with chloride for binding to the sodium/potassium/chloride co-transporter, thereby inhibiting sodium and chloride reabsorption (5). Loop diuretics also have a mixture of effects on sodium and chloride reabsorption within other nephron segments, but these appear to be quantitatively minor compared with their effects on the thick ascending limb. Other clinically important effects of loop diuretics include a block of both free water excretion during water loading and free water absorption during dehydration (6), a 30% increase in fractional calcium excretion (7), a substantial increase in magnesium excretion (8), and a transient increase followed by an ultimate decrease in uric acid excretion (9). Loop diuretics are also capable of increasing renal prostaglandin synthesis, particularly that of the vasodilatory prostaglandin E_2 (10). Angiotensin II, generated following the administration of intravenous loop diuretics, coupled with an increased synthesis of prostaglandin E_2 is the likely reason that loop diuretics shift renal blood flow from the inner to the outer

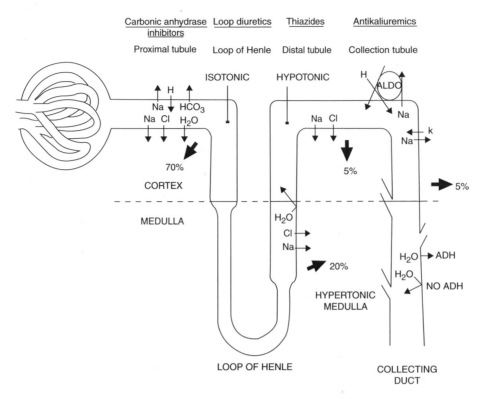

Figure 26.1 Schematic of the nephron illustrating the handling of water and electrolytes by the different segments and the major nephron sites of diuretic action. (Heavy arrows represent the approximate percentage of sodium that is reabsorbed by the various nephron segments.)

Table 26.1 Pharmacokinetics of Diuretics

		Half-life of drug (h)		
Diuretic	Bioavailability (%)	Normal subjects	Subjects with renal failure	Subjects with congestive heart failure
Loop				
Furosemide	10–100	1.5–2	2.8	2.7
Bumetanide	80–100	1	1.6	1.3
Torsemide	80–100	3–4	4–5	6
Thiazide				
Bendroflumethazide	ND	2–5	ND	ND
Chlorthalidone	64	24–55	ND	ND
Chlorothiazide	30–50	1.5	ND	ND
Hydrochlorothiazide	65–75	2.5	Increased	ND
Indapamide	93	15–25	ND	ND
Polythiazide	ND	26	ND	ND
Trichlormethiazide	ND	1–4	5–10	ND
Distal or collecting duct				
Amiloride	?	17–26	100	ND
Triamterene	>80	2–5	Prolonged	ND
Spironolactone	?	1.5	No change	ND
Eplerenone				

Note: ND, not determined.

cortex of the kidney (10). Despite this redeployment of renal blood flow, both total renal blood flow and glomerular filtration rate are maintained after loop diuretic administration to normal subjects (11).

The available loop diuretics include bumetanide, ethacrynic acid, furosemide, and torsemide. These compounds are heavily protein bound and, therefore, must gain access to the tubular lumen (site of action) by tubular secretion. Tubular secretion of these compounds occurs by way of organic anion transporters that are contained within the proximal tubule. Thiazide-type diuretics also access the tubular compartment this way before they are conveyed to their site of action in the course of urine flowing more distally (12). Urinary diuretic concentrations are a useful indicator of the rate of drug delivery to the medullary thick ascending limb in that they correlate with the diuretic-related natriuretic response (3,12).

Furosemide is the most widely used diuretic in this class (13). It is unpredictably absorbed with a bioavailability of $49 \pm 17\%$ (range of 12–112%) (14). The coefficients of absorption variation for different furosemide products vary from 25% to 43%; thus, switching between furosemide formulations will not standardize patient absorption and thus response to oral furosemide (14). Bumetanide and (to an even greater degree) torsemide are both more predictably absorbed than is furosemide. The predictability of torsemide absorption is a consideration when loop diuretic therapy is called for in a patient with heart failure (15,16). Compared with patients treated with furosemide, patients treated with torsemide are typically less fatigued and less apt to be readmitted for congestive heart failure or for any cardiovascular–renal causes (16).

All loop diuretics circulate as organic anions, highly bound to albumin, that access the tubular lumen through a probenecid-sensitive proximal tubular secretory mechanism. Loop diuretic protein binding may be decreased by uremic toxins or fatty acids, although the basis for altered drug effect has been inadequately explored (17). Secretion of furosemide and other loop diuretics may be slowed in the presence of elevated levels of endogenous organic acids, such as in the case of chronic kidney disease, and may be slowed by drugs that share the same transporter, such as salicylates and nonsteroidal anti-inflammatory drugs (NSAIDs).

The three loop diuretics most commonly used—furosemide, bumetanide, and torsemide—exhibit decreased renal clearance in the chronic kidney disease patient. This change evolves parallel with the degree of change in renal function. In general, furosemide pharmacokinetics are more significantly changed than other loop diuretics used in treating chronic kidney disease because both the renal clearance and the metabolism of this compound are altered (18). Bumetanide and torsemide undergo

significant hepatic metabolism, hence there is predictably less change in their pharmacokinetic profile in chronic kidney disease (Table 26.1) (19,20).

The relationship between urinary furosemide excretion (and also excretion of other loop diuretics) and the natriuretic effect takes the form of a sigmoidal shaped dose–response curve (Fig. 26.2) (3,12,21). A normal dose–response relationship (typically seen in the untreated hypertensive patient) can be distorted downward and rightward by a number of clinical conditions, ranging from volume depletion (braking phenomenon) to heart failure or nephrotic syndrome (disease-state alterations), to various drug therapies (22,23). The NSAID indomethacin reworks the dose–response relationship through its inhibition of prostaglandin synthesis (24), which, in turn, modifies renal blood flow and tubular sodium handling. Although the normality of this relationship can falter in the setting of nephrotic-range proteinuria, it is not because of urinary protein binding of loop diuretics (25).

C. Thiazide Diuretics

The major action site of thiazide diuretics is the early distal convoluted tubule where the coupled reabsorption of sodium and chloride is inhibited (Fig. 26.1) (26). In addition to effects on sodium excretion, thiazide diuretics also impair urinary diluting capacity while preserving urinary concentrating mechanisms (27), reduce calcium and uric acid excretion (28,29), and increase magnesium excretion (30). The latter is particularly prominent in treatment with long-acting thiazide-type diuretics such as chlorthalidone (30).

Hydrochlorothiazide is the most widely utilized drug in this diuretic class. It is well absorbed, with a bioavailability of ~70%. The onset of diuresis with

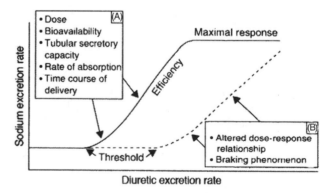

Figure 26.2 Pharmacokinetic (A) and pharmacodynamic (B) determinants of loop diuretic response. (The broken line represents an altered dose–response relationship, as observed in a typical diuretic-resistant state.) The diuretic delivery necessary to achieve a threshold response can vary substantially in the presence of diuretic resistance.

hydrochlorothiazide is rapid (within 2 h), peaking at 3–6 h, and continuing for as long as 12 h. However, of the total natriuretic response following a single dose, only a small fraction is gained >6 h of dosing. The diuretic effect of hydrochlorothiazide can be extended by administering higher doses (50–200 mg) than the doses conventionally used. Alternatively, if a more prolonged natriuresis is desired, a longer-acting thiazide-type diuretic, such as chlorthalidone or metolazone, can be considered (31,32).

The half-life of hydrochlorothiazide (and other thiazide diuretics) is prolonged in patients with decompensated congestive heart failure or renal insufficiency (32). Large doses of thiazide-type compounds (100–200 mg/day) can be diuretic in patients with chronic kidney disease despite the often-cited belief that these drugs are ineffective in advanced-stage chronic kidney disease (33). However, the magnitude of the diuretic response is controlled by two factors: the reduced glomerular filtration rate, which means that the filtered load is low, and the nephron site at which a thiazide diuretic is active, which is a site where only a modest diuretic response should be expected when sodium reabsorption is blocked (33,34).

Metolazone is a quinazoline diuretic with a major site of action in the distal tubule and a minor inhibitory effect on proximal sodium reabsorption through a carbonic anhydrase-independent mechanism (35,36). Metolazone is fairly lipid soluble, with a wide volume of distribution (V_D) and a prolonged duration of action. These properties facilitate its tubular delivery in the setting of renal insufficiency and support its effectiveness in diuretic-resistant situations when combined with a loop diuretic (37,38). Metolazone absorption is slow and erratic, which presents an interpretive problem in a "diuretic-resistant" patient. That is, the failure to respond to a metolazone-based regimen is usually taken to signify a worsening of the primary volume-retaining state, but the failure to respond to the drug may simply be the offshoot of poor drug absorption (12,38).

D. Distal Potassium-Sparing Diuretics

There are two classes of potassium-sparing diuretics: competitive antagonists of aldosterone, such as spironolactone, and compounds that do not interact with aldosterone receptors, such as amiloride and triamterene. These agents inhibit active sodium absorption in the late distal tubule and the collecting duct. In the process, basolateral sodium-potassium-ATPase activity falls, and intracellular potassium concentration is reduced. The resulting fall in the electrochemical gradient for both potassium and hydrogen cations reduces their secretion (39,40). Because these drugs are capable of only a modest

natriuresis, their usefulness resides more in their ability to reduce the excretion of potassium and hydrogen cations, especially in states of hyperaldosteronism or when more proximally acting diuretics increase distal delivery (41). Potassium-sparing diuretics also reduce calcium and magnesium excretion (8).

Spironolactone is a lipid-soluble potassium-sparing diuretic that is well absorbed and highly protein bound. It has a 20 h half-life and can take 24–48 h to reach maximal effectiveness. (42,43) Spironolactone undergoes extensive metabolism. 7-α-thiomethylspirolactone and canrenone are two important metabolites of spironolactone that are responsible for much of its anti-mineralocorticoid activity (44). Spironolactone can be particularly useful in states of reduced renal function because it can gain access to its site of action independent of filtration; however, its propensity to cause hyperkalemia limits its use in chronic kidney disease patients (45).

Eplerenone is an aldosterone receptor antagonist whose molecular structure affords selectivity for the aldosterone receptor. Accordingly, its lesser affinity for androgen and progesterone receptors results in its causing gynecomastia less frequently than is the case for spironolactone (46). Under most circumstances, eplerenone is a very mild diuretic; thus, its antihypertensive effects derive from the nondiuretic aspects of its actions. These actions result in a level of blood pressure reduction that compares favorably to the reduction seen with other drug classes such as angiotensin-converting enzyme (ACE) inhibitors and calcium channel blockers (47,48). Eplerenone also effectively regresses left ventricular hypertrophy, either by itself or when combined with an ACE inhibitor (49), and the drug has a prominent anti-proteinuric effect (48). It is worth noting that eplerenone in combination with optimal medical therapy reduces morbidity and mortality among patients with acute myocardial infarction complicated by left ventricular dysfunction and heart failure (46).

Amiloride is a potassium-sparing diuretic, which is actively secreted by proximal tubular cationic transporters (50). Amiloride blocks epithelial sodium channels in the luminal membrane of the collecting duct, so that a modest natriuretic response can be anticipated with its use. Amiloride undergoes extensive renal clearance and will accumulate (with repetitive dosing) in the cases of chronic kidney disease or senescence-related reduction in renal function (51). It is advisable to either reduce the dose of amiloride or decrease its frequency of dosing in chronic kidney disease (glomerular filtration rate <50 cc/min) to minimize the risk of hyperkalemia.

Triamterene is another potassium-sparing diuretic, which does not act by the way of aldosterone antagonism. Triamterene is metabolized to an active phase-II sulfate conjugated metabolite. Both triamterene and its sulfated metabolite gain access to their intraluminal site of action by proximal tubular secretion. Triamterene and its metabolite will accumulate upon repetitive dosing in cases of chronic kidney disease, with an inherent tendency to cause hyperkalemia. Therefore, in those rare circumstances where its use is contemplated in cases of chronic kidney disease empiric dosage adjustment is advisable (52). Because of its weak blood-pressure-lowering properties, triamterene is seldom used as monotherapy for hypertension. Instead, it is used in combination with thiazide-type diuretics in a variety of strengths for each component. The premise behind such a combination of two diuretics is for triamterene as a potassium-sparing diuretic to reduce the potassium and magnesium losses that might accompany thiazide therapy (53). Triamterene given together with NSAIDs has been reported to cause acute renal failure, occasionally lasting several days (54). The mechanism behind this acute renal failure is unclear, but it may relate to two factors: first, there is as much as a 30% fall in renal blood flow observed with triamterene and second, this compound increases urinary excretion of the vasodilator prostaglandins E_2 and $F_{2\alpha}$ (53,55).

III. RESPONSES TO DIURETICS

In addition to responses to specific diuretics, two general types of responses may be encountered during treatment with diuretics.

A. Adaptation to Diuretic Therapy

Diuretic-induced inhibition of sodium reabsorption in one nephron segment elicits important adaptations in other nephron segments, which not only limits their antihypertensive and fluid-depleting actions but also contributes to treatment side effects. Although a portion of this diuretic resistance is a normal consequence of diuretic use, profound diuretic resistance from such adaptations can be encountered in patients who have other clinical disorders such as congestive heart failure, cirrhosis, or renal insufficiency. An understanding of the mechanisms comprising adaptation to diuretic therapy is necessary to minimize this process and limit side effects.

The initial dose of a diuretic ordinarily manufactures a brisk diuresis, which in most cases ends with a net negative sodium balance. The new equilibrium state established is one where body weight stabilizes at a reduced value because adaptive processes intervene and preclude an unremitting volume loss. In nonedematous patients who are given either a thiazide or a loop diuretic, this adaptation, or *braking phenomenon*, occurs within a matter of days and limits weight loss to 1–2 kg (22). This braking phenomenon has been convincingly demonstrated in normal subjects administered the loop diuretics furosemide

or bumetanide (56–58). Furosemide administered to subjects who ingest a high-salt diet (270 mmol/24 h) produced a brisk natriuresis, which resulted in a negative sodium balance for the first 6 h. This was followed by an 18 h period when sodium excretion was reduced to amounts considerably below the level of intake. This post-diuresis sodium retention corrected for initial sodium losses, with the result that at the end of the day, a neutral sodium balance state existed, with no net weight loss. In fact, this same pattern of sodium loss and compensatory retention persists even after a month of furosemide administration (11). Sodium intake, prior to and after diuretic dosing, will adjust the outcome through the braking phenomenon. If sodium intake is kept low, sodium balance will remain negative in the hours after the initial natriuresis and permit a net reduction in body weight.

The pathophysiology of the braking phenomenon is complex. In part, the relationship between natriuresis and the rate of loop diuretic excretion depends on the level of sodium intake. In subjects who are receiving a low-sodium diet, the response curve for a diuretic is typically shifted rightward, which is indicative of a blunting of the tubular responsiveness to the diuretic (Fig. 26.2) (56–58). Extracellular fluid volume depletion is an important factor in the genesis of post-diuretic sodium retention. Using lithium clearance methodology (as a marker of proximal sodium handling) in the post-diuretic period, overall sodium retention has been ascribed to both an increase in proximal and distal sodium absorption. It has been suggested that this heightened sodium reabsorption may be being prompted by α-stimulation or renin–angiotensin–aldosterone system activation; however, the administration of α-adrenergic antagonists and blockers of the renin–angiotensin–aldosterone system do not seem to modify the braking phenomenon in a meaningful manner (11,56,57). Moreover, a volume-independent component to the process has been suggested, which may be structural (11,59–61). Structural hypertrophy in the distal nephron has been demonstrated in rats receiving prolonged infusions of loop diuretics (60,61). These structural changes are associated with enhanced rates of distal nephron sodium and chloride absorption and increased secretion of potassium, a sequence that is independent of aldosterone (62). These nephron adaptations may contribute to post-diuretic sodium retention and to diuretic tolerance in humans and are one possible explanation for the sodium retention that can persist for up to 2 weeks after diuretic therapy is discontinued (11,63).

B. Neurohumoral Response to Diuretics

Neurohumoral activation by diuretics remains an important consideration in the overall effectiveness of diuretics in hypertension and congestive heart failure. The neurohumoral response to diuretics depends on both the route of administration as well as the extent of drug exposure. Intravenous loop diuretics have an immediate (within minutes) stimulatory effect on the renin–angiotensin–aldosterone system arising at the macula densa that is independent of volume depletion or sympathetic nervous system activation (64). This first wave of neurohumoral effects with an intravenous loop diuretic is short-lived, but it can be of sufficient magnitude to increase afterload (in a dose-dependent manner) and for a short time may diminish the effectiveness of a diuretic (65). This sequence of events may provide an explanation for the restoration of a diuretic response in a diuretic-resistant patient (one who has not responded to bolus loop diuretic therapy) when loop diuretics are administered in an infusion (66). A second response of increased renal prostaglandin production is triggered within 5–15 min of intravenous loop diuretic administration (64). This secondary response offers a likely explanation for the reduction in preload and ventricular filling pressures that takes place shortly after intravenous loop diuretic administration (67).

Both intravenous and oral diuretics can be involved with the next stage of neurohumoral activation, which occurs with excess volume removal. Volume removal can chronically activate the renin–angiotensin–aldosterone system and in so doing increase concentrations of both angiotensin II and aldosterone, each of which independently can stimulate sodium absorption in proximal and distal tubular locations, respectively. The role of aldosterone excess in electrolyte depletion or persistent hypertension in a patient being treated with diuretics is underappreciated. Low-dose spironolactone provides significant additive blood pressure reduction in diuretic-treated patients with resistant hypertension (68).

IV. DIURETICS IN TREATMENT OF HYPERTENSION

In nondiabetic patients, hypertension is defined as a systolic and diastolic blood pressure of ≥ 140 and ≥ 90 mmHg, respectively (2). Hypertension and the newly defined pre-hypertension state are widely prevalent in the USA, with over 100 million people affected with one or the other of these disorders (69). Worldwide prevalence estimates for hypertension may be as much as 1 billion individuals, with $\sim$7.1 million deaths per year possibly attributable to it (70). Cardiovascular (CVR) and cerebrovascular events, renal failure progression, and all-cause mortality each increase in a continuous fashion with increasing diastolic or systolic blood pressure or both. The beneficial effects of blood-pressure-lowering treatment on the risks of major cardiovascular and renal events are not disputed. What has been questioned is the comparative effects of

regimens that are based on different drug classes or regimens that target different blood pressure goals. To answer this question, a recent analysis was conducted by the Blood Pressure Lowering Treatment Trialists' Collaboration; the results showed no significant differences in total major CVR events between regimens that are based on ACE inhibitors, calcium channel blockers, diuretics, or β-blockers (71).

Analyses such as this tend to shift the argument from what should be the preferred first drug in the treatment of hypertension to what compound or combination of drugs is the most cost-effective treatment. In this regard, diuretic therapy as first-step treatment or as a component of multi-drug therapy has an established and widely accepted position. All of the prior Joint National Committee on the Detection, Evaluation, and Treatment of High Blood Pressure (JNC) documents (dating to 1977) and the most recent guidelines, the seventh report (JNC7), favor the early use of diuretic therapy in the management of hypertension, often in a "stepped-care" approach to hypertension management (2).

A. Mechanism of Action

Thiazide-type diuretics have been used in the treatment of hypertension for almost 50 years. But despite the enormous treatment experience with these compounds, a number of uncertainties remain concerning their use. Of the unanswered questions concerning thiazide-type diuretics, three are particularly relevant: first, to what degree is a persistent reduction in extracellular fluid volume a prerequisite for continuing blood pressure reduction with these compounds? Secondly, do thiazide-type diuretics provide better blood pressure reduction than loop diuretics? Thirdly, are all thiazide-type diuretics the same in their blood-pressure-reducing effect (have a "class effect")?

The exact means by which thiazide-type diuretics lower blood pressure is unclear. Their effect on blood pressure may be divided into three sequential phases: *acute*, *subacute*, and *chronic*, corresponding to periods of up to 2 weeks, several weeks, and several months, respectively (Fig. 26.3) (72). In the acute response phase, the blood-pressure-lowering effect of a diuretic is coupled to a reduction in extracellular fluid volume and a corresponding drop in cardiac output. The early response (the first 2–4 days of treatment) to a thiazide-type diuretic, in the setting of a "no salt added" diet (100–150 mmol/day), results in a net sodium loss of 100–300 mmol, which translates into a 1–2 L decrease in extracellular fluid volume. Plasma sodium concentrations are unchanged in the process.

Direct measurements of extracellular fluid volume in thiazide diuretic-treated hypertensive patients in the acute response phase show a 12% decrease (73). There

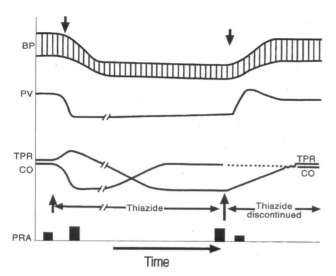

Figure 26.3 Effects of thiazide administration in an "idealized" patient. (BP, blood pressure; PRA, plasma renin activity; TPR, total peripheral resistance; CO, cardiac output; PV, plasma volume.)

is a similar reduction in plasma volume, which suggests that this acute volume loss arises proportionally from both the plasma and the interstitial compartments (74). This decrease in plasma volume reduces venous return and diminishes cardiac output, providing the basis for the initial drop in blood pressure with a thiazide diuretic (75). This change in plasma volume can stimulate both the sympathetic nervous and renin–angiotensin–aldosterone systems, with the degree to which these systems activate governing the magnitude of the acute blood pressure decrease observed with diuretics (72,73).

In due course, thiazide diuretic effects on volume and cardiac output lessen in importance, although blood pressure remains lowered. During the subacute phase of a treatment response (the first few weeks), plasma volume returns to slightly less than pretreatment levels, despite the continued administration of a diuretic (74). The subacute response phase with thiazide-type diuretics is a transitional period, during which both volume and resistance factors contribute to the blood pressure reduction (75,76).

B. Blood Pressure Reduction

In the chronic response phase of therapy, the vasodepressor influence of a diuretic develops into a process mechanistically driven by a reduction in total peripheral resistance. There is no simple explanation for the drop in total peripheral resistance that accompanies long-term diuretic use. This decrease has been attributed to several factors, including changes in the ionic content of vascular smooth-muscle cells, altered ion gradients across smooth-muscle cells, or potassium-channel activation, and changes in membrane-bound ATPase activity. The ability of thiazide-type diuretics to reduce blood pressure seems to be critically linked to the presence of functioning renal tissue; thus, these drugs will not reduce blood pressure in patients undergoing maintenance hemodialysis (77).

A mechanistic understanding of both diuretic action and countervailing forces triggered by diuresis provide for a well-reasoned approach to the treatment of hypertension. The early action of diuretics to reduce extracellular fluid volume is optimized if dietary sodium is restricted at the beginning of therapy. This limits the repercussions of the braking phenomenon, which is an inevitable occurrence with continuous diuretic use (12). Some limitation in dietary sodium intake also may be relevant to how diuretics chronically reduce total peripheral resistance. It is thought that adjustments in sodium–calcium balance in vascular smooth muscle cells come about with the acute volume contraction observed during the first several days of thiazide diuretic therapy. How this phenomenon of volume contraction translates specifically into a reduction in total peripheral resistance remains unclear (72,73). Whatever the mechanism, it can be quite long-lived because a residual blood pressure reduction can be seen several weeks after the withdrawal of thiazide diuretics (even without interposing nonpharmacologic treatments for maintenance of blood pressure control) (78,79). However, this residual blood pressure-reducing effect of thiazide-type diuretics has not been compared carefully to that observed with other antihypertensive medication drug classes (79).

Another consideration in the chronic blood pressure reduction with a diuretic relates to the duration of a natriuretic response. For example, when long-term responses to hydrochlorothiazide and furosemide are compared in hypertensive patients, diastolic blood pressure and even more so systolic blood pressure are more consistently reduced with hydrochlorothiazide (80,81). This difference has been attributed to the more gradual and prolonged diuresis with a thiazide diuretic (with a less profound braking phenomenon) compared to the brisk and early diuretic response with a loop diuretic (more significant braking phenomenon). During the acute phase of response, a thiazide diuretic may be able to maintain a mild state of volume contraction more effectively than a loop diuretic (12). It is thought that this pattern of volume removal with a thiazide-type diuretic lends itself to a greater downward shift in total peripheral resistance. A direct vasodilator effect of hydrochlorothiazide has been postulated but in reality is quite small, only occurring at high local concentrations when experimentally infused into the human forearm (82).

C. Diuretic Class Effect

The concept of "class effect" has been applied to both loop diuretics and thiazide-type diuretics with respect to the management of hypertension. In this regard, the loop diuretic effect on blood pressure is a function of at least two processes: the manner in which volume removal is effected with these compounds and their capacity to independently decrease total peripheral resistance. It has been observed that small doses of the long-acting loop diuretic torsemide may cause significant blood pressure reduction in patients with essential hypertension. This process, which is not demonstrable with subdiuretic doses of furosemide, seems to be independent of the observed degree of diuresis (83). Notably, furosemide does not directly dilate human forearm arterial vessels even at supratherapeutic concentrations (84); however, given in bioequivalent doses, furosemide is equally as effective in reducing 24 h ambulatory blood pressure as torsemide in patients with stage 1–3 chronic kidney disease (85). Until comparison studies among loop diuretics are conducted in diverse populations, it is premature to presume that compounds are distinguishable (independent of volume removal) in their blood-pressure-reducing ability.

The idea of a class effect for thiazide-type diuretics is one promulgated by many, but one that has only minimal experimental support (2). Much of the recent debate has centered on the similarities (or lack thereof) between chlorthalidone and hydrochlorothiazide (86). The concept of class effect with thiazide-type diuretics needs to be considered in two ways: first, with respect to a drop in blood pressure, and secondly, with respect to event-rate reduction. These two compounds are fundamentally different diuretics; chlorthalidone has a considerably longer duration of diuretic action than hydrochlorothiazide. This does not necessarily mean that chlorthalidone is a better antihypertensive compound, although it is likely that the longer duration of diuretic action with chlorthalidone makes it a milligram-to-milligram stronger antihypertensive compound than hydrochlorothiazide. The exact dose equivalence between the two compounds is a matter of some debate and one that will not be easily resolved. Chlorthalidone has had a more consistent pattern of favorable outcomes than hydrochlorothiazide (86–89). However, although it is tempting to assume that chlorthalidone is a better outcome drug, it cannot be verified until this has been prospectively studied.

D. Diuretics in Clinical Trials

By the mid-1990s, evidence of the effects of blood-pressure-lowering regimens that are based primarily on diuretics and β-blockers was available from a series of randomized controlled clinical trials that involved >47,000 hypertensive patients (90–94). Systematic overviews and meta-analyses of these trials showed that within just a few years of beginning therapy, reductions in blood pressure of 10–12 mmHg systolic and 5–6 mmHg diastolic provided relative risk reductions for stroke and coronary heart disease of 38% and 16%, respectively (90–94). These effects were similar in major subgroups of patients and seemed to be largely independent of differences in disease event rates among study patients. The few studies that directly compared diuretics and β-blockers detected no obvious differences in the risk of either stroke or coronary artery disease; however, differences between these two therapies may be more likely to be detected in specific patient groups. For example, in an overview of treatment outcomes in elderly patients it has been shown that first-line diuretic therapy was superior to β-blockade in preventing cerebrovascular events, fatal stroke, coronary heart disease, CVR mortality, and all-cause mortality. In contrast, β-blocker therapy reduced only the odds for cerebrovascular events and was ineffective in preventing coronary heart disease, cardiovascular mortality, and all-cause mortality (95).

In 1995, a number of studies of blood-pressure-lowering drugs were known to be planned or were ongoing with completion anticipated in the near future. Most of these trials had been designed to detect large differences in relative risk and had insufficient power to detect small to moderate differences between the regimens being studied. To maximize the information acquired by these and future trials, a collaborative program of prospectively designed overviews was developed. The first of these overviews became available in the year 2000 (96).

The overview of trials in hypertensive patients that compared ACE inhibitor-based regimens with diuretic-based or β-blocker-based regimens does not show that the endpoint benefits of ACE inhibitors are any different than those provided by diuretics or β-blockers (Fig. 26.4) (96). The overview of trials comparing calcium channel blockers therapy with diuretic-based or β-blocker-based regimens provides some evidence of difference in the effects of the two regimens on cause-specific outcomes, with the risk for stroke being significantly less with calcium channel blockers than with diuretics (Fig. 26.5) (96). There was no evidence of differences between the treatment effects of calcium channel blocker regimens on the basis of whether dihydropyridine or nondihydropyridine calcium channel blockers were compared to diuretic/β-blocker regimens (97–99).

The most recent trial of note that provides information on the issue of diuretic therapy and outcomes is the Antihypertensive and Lipid-Lowering Treatment to Prevent Heart Attack Trial (ALLHAT) (89). A total of 33,357 participants aged 55 years or older (35% African-Americans)

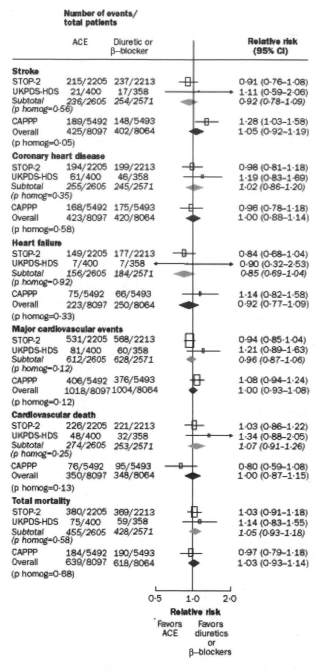

Figure 26.4 Comparisons of ACE-inhibitor-based therapy with diuretic-based or β-blocker-based therapy. (ACE, angiotensin-converting enzyme inhibitor; p HOMOG, *P* value from χ^2 test for homogeneity; CI, confidence level; STOP-2, Second Swedish Trial in Old Patients with Hypertension; UKPDS, United Kingdom Prospective Diabetes Study; HDS, Hypertension in Diabetes Study; CAPPP, Captopril Prevention Project.)

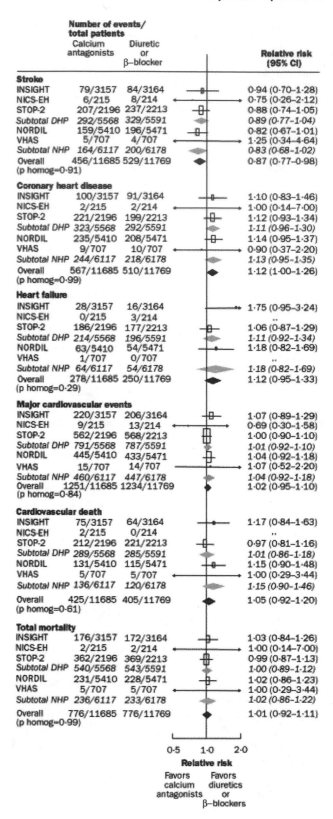

Figure 26.5 Comparisons of calcium-antagonist-based therapy with diuretic-based or β-blocker-based therapy. (DHP, Dihydropyridine; NHP, Nondihydropyridine; p HOMOG, *P* value from χ^2 test for homogeneity.)

with hypertension and at least one other coronary heart disease risk factor were enrolled in ALLHAT. ALLHAT originally set out to study ACE inhibition (lisinopril), calcium channel blocker therapy (amlodipine), and peripheral α-antagonism (doxazosin) compared to therapy with the diuretic chlorthalidone with regard to differences in a composite primary outcome of fatal coronary heart disease or nonfatal myocardial infarction. Although the primary outcome in ALLHAT was comparable for both the chlorthalidone and the doxazosin treatment groups, the doxazosin treatment was terminated early because of an increased risk of stroke and combined cardiovascular disease (of which heart failure was a component) when compared with chlorthalidone (100).

In ALLHAT, no significant difference was observed between chlorthalidone and either amlodipine or lisinopril in the primary outcome; however, the secondary outcome findings showed a smaller reduction in total major CVR events, stroke, and heart failure with lisinopril than with chlorthalidone (89). This difference in event rates was largely attributable to worse outcomes in the African-American cohort in ALLHAT and may have related to the smaller blood pressure reduction with the ACE-inhibitor-based regimen in that subgroup. This difference in blood pressure control among primary drug classes was not unexpected, given the stated purpose and design of the study, and it limits the ability to generalize the positive findings with diuretics in ALLHAT.

E. Responsive Patient Populations

When used alone in the nonedematous patient, thiazide diuretics are as effective as most other antihypertensive drug classes, an observation which is independent of body mass index (101,102). Although it is erroneous to make universal recommendations about antihypertensive care on the basis of race, age, or gender, this still happens rather routinely. That being said, African-American, elderly, and female hypertensive patients typically respond better to diuretics than do non-African-American or younger patients, who are more likely to be salt-sensitive (101,103,104). The same can be said for other salt-sensitive forms of hypertension, such as the form that is characteristic of the hypertensive diabetic. However, the basis for the majority of the interindividual variability in response to a thiazide diuretic continues to go unexplained despite the earlier cited patient characteristics (African-American ethnicity and female gender) offering some measure of predictability of response by category (104).

1. Elderly Populations

A number of studies that used diuretic-based regimens have been conducted specifically in the elderly hypertensive population (>60 years in age): the Systolic Hypertension in Elderly Program (SHEP) (105), the Swedish Trial in Old Patients with Hypertension (STOP-Hypertension) (106), the Medical Research Council trial in the treatment

of older adults (MRC2) (107), the European Working Party on High Blood Pressure in the Elderly (EWPHE), (108) and the Coope and Warrender randomized trial of treatment of hypertension in elderly patients in primary care (103). Significant reductions in stroke, similar to those observed in younger patients, and greater benefits in terms of protection from myocardial infarction and congestive heart failure were demonstrated in these older patients (109). Each of these trials found significant reductions in cardiovascular and cerebrovascular morbidity and mortality associated with diuretic or β-blocker therapy.

As an example of these trials, we will highlight the SHEP trial—a double-blind, placebo-controlled trial that consisted of 4736 men and women with isolated systolic hypertension who were older than 60 years of age (105,112). Patients were randomized to receive a low-dose of the diuretic chlorthalidone (12.5–25.0 mg/day) as initial therapy; a β-blocker (atenolol 25–50 mg/day) or reserpine (0.05–0.10 mg/day) was then added as needed to reach the goal blood pressure—a systolic blood pressure <160 mmHg or at least a 20 mmHg decrease in systolic blood pressure.

At the end of the 5 year follow-up period, 46% of the subjects had adequate blood pressure control using only a low dose of chlorthalidone, and blood pressure was equally well-controlled irrespective of the serum creatinine (range 35–212 mmo/L) (Fig. 26.6) (105,112).

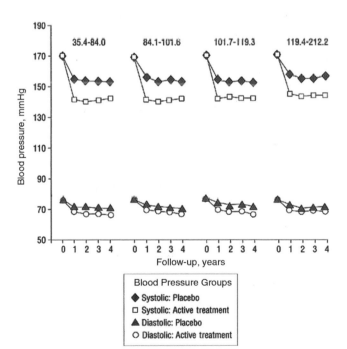

Figure 26.6 Variations of mean systolic and diastolic blood pressures during follow-up according to treatment and baseline serum creatinine levels in the SHEP. (The graph has been truncated >4 years.)

Another 23% of patients were controlled with the addition of a β-blocker. Outcomes included both a statistically significant 36% reduction in fatal and nonfatal strokes and nonstatistically significant reductions in myocardial infarction of 27% and overall mortality of 13%. However, these positive outcome benefits were negated when hypokalemia (serum potassium <3.5 mmol/L) occurred in these chlorthalidone-treated patients (113).

In addition, four clinical trials, with a total of almost 35,000 patients, have compared diuretics with β-blockers: the International Prospective Primary Prevention Study in Hypertension (IPPPSH) (110), Heart Attack Primary Prevention in Hypertension (HAPPHY) trial (111), Medical Research Council trials one and two (MRC and MRC2) (107). In these comparative trials, β-blocker therapy was comparable to diuretic therapy with regard to the incidence of stroke, although this observation has been disputed (109). Findings were mixed with regard to myocardial infarction, with two studies favoring either diuretics or β-blockers over the other, although differences between these classes were quite small.

Overall, the results of these trials clearly establish the benefit of low-dose diuretics or β-blockers, or both together, for the treatment of isolated systolic hypertension in the elderly. They have been the basis for current treatment recommendations advocating diuretic therapy in uncomplicated forms of hypertension, strengthened by the ALLHAT findings (89,100).

2. Black Populations

In black patients, hypertension is more prevalent at a younger age, is usually more severe, and is associated with a greater incidence of cardiac, central nervous system, and renal complications that occur in white patients (114). Although the pathogenesis of hypertension has not been clearly defined, the majority of blacks fall into the low-renin category. This low-renin status cannot be explained by volume expansion alone because no consistent relationship between these two factors has been detected in this population (115). In addition, the INTERSALT study, a multi-center, cross-sectional study that evaluated the relationship between electrolytes and blood pressure, was unable to correlate excessive salt intake with the development of hypertension in blacks (116). Although this issue is not yet fully resolved, there appears to be an important emerging role for potassium intake in the blood pressure patterns expressed in normotensive and hypertensive blacks (117,118).

Nonetheless, black patients respond very well to diuretic therapy, with 40–67% of young and 58–80% of elderly blacks responding to diuretic monotherapy (119–121). However, the absolute blood pressure reduction (−12/ 8 mmHg) in black patients, although more predictable

than in cases where other drug classes are administered as monotherapy (such as ACE inhibitors, β-blockers, or angiotensin receptor blockers), is often insufficient to bring blood pressure to the goal level (22). Consequently, diuretics often need to be administered together with other antihypertensive drug classes in blacks if the goal blood pressure is to be reached. This practice of administering multiple antihypertensive drugs (including a diuretic) to blacks can be undertaken with the diuretic as the beginning therapy or with the diuretic therapy added on to other drug classes, such as ACE inhibitors or β-blockers (123).

Diuretic therapy has been associated with reductions in morbidity and mortality in blacks. (89,124,125) Black patients made up approximately half of the study participants in the Veterans Administration Cooperative study and the Hypertension Detection and Follow-up Program (HDFP), both of which were diuretic-based studies (124,125). In the Veterans Administration study, hydrochlorothiazide treatment compared to a placebo was associated with a reduction in morbid events from 26% to 10% in black patients (124). In the HDFP study, there was an 18.5% reduction in mortality for black men and a 27.8% reduction in mortality for black women (125). In ALLHAT, diuretic therapy reduced the primary outcome of fatal coronary heart disease and nonfatal myocardial infarction comparably to lisinopril and amlodipine (89). However, the ability of diuretics to delay or prevent renal dysfunction in hypertensive blacks was put into question by the Multiple Risk Factor Intervention Trial (MRFIT), which did not show a benefit in this regard (126). More recently in ALLHAT, diuretic therapy did not seem to adversely impact renal function (development of end-stage renal disease) within the limits of its determination in this trial (89). It has been speculated that diuretic therapy might negatively influence renal function if the renin–angiotensin–aldosterone system becomes overly activated; however, because an ACE inhibitor or an angiotensin receptor blocker is generally co-administered with a diuretic in most chronic kidney disease patients, this is less of an issue.

F. Regression of Left Ventricular Hypertrophy with Diuretic Therapy

Left ventricular mass has been recognized as a powerful independent risk factor for CVR morbidity (127). Antihypertensive therapy, with the exception of direct vasodilators, is effective in regressing left ventricular hypertrophy (128). In 1991, Moser and Setaro (129) compiled an overview of all studies that evaluated left ventricular hypertrophy regression in diuretic-treated hypertensive patients; this overview supports the effectiveness of diuretics in regressing left ventricular mass. Several meta-analyses have also been undertaken specifically to examine left ventricular hypertrophy regression with different classes of antihypertensive agents (128,130,131). Using echocardiography, Dahlof et al. (130) analyzed 109 studies comprising 2357 patients and found diuretics to be associated with an 11.3% reduction in left ventricular mass; however, this finding was in large measure the result of a reduction in left ventricular volume. Alternatively, the reduction of left ventricular mass associated with ACE inhibitor therapy was 15%, β-blocker 8%, and calcium channel blocker treatment 8.5%, with structural changes largely reflected by a decrease in posterior and intraventricular septal thickness. In another meta-analysis (comprising 39 qualifying trials) of ACE inhibitors, calcium channel blockers, β-blockers, and diuretics, it was observed that both the decrease in left ventricular mass index and wall thickness were correlated with the treatment-induced decline in blood pressure, and, in particular, the fall in systolic blood pressure. Reductions in left ventricular mass of 13%, 9%, 6%, and 7% occurred with ACE inhibitors, calcium channel blockers, β-blockers, and diuretics, respectively (131). Accordingly, diuretics are not remarkably dissimilar to most other drug classes in their ability to regress left ventricular mass (128,130,131).

G. Future of Diuretics in Hypertension Treatment

Diuretics are likely to find their major future use as "priming" agents. Their primary mode of sensitization derives from volume depletion-related neurohumoral or sympathetic nervous system activation. In this regard, even subtle degrees of volume contraction (or renin–angiotensin–aldosterone system activation), as produced by low-dose thiazide-type diuretic therapy, establishes a basis for an enhanced effect of coadministered antihypertensive compounds (123). This additive effect has revived interest in the use of low-dose diuretic fixed-combination antihypertensive therapy in the primary management of essential hypertension (123). The idea of using two drugs at low doses for blood pressure control is not recent. It has, however, gathered new support because it is increasingly evident that most patients who receive such treatment achieve their target blood pressure with a minimum of side effects (132,133).

The dose–response relationship for the antihypertensive effect of diuretics has been more completely characterized over the past 20 years. In the process, many of the negative effects earlier attributed to diuretics have been shown to be less so than was first thought. In the early days of diuretic use, doses were unnecessarily high with dosing driven by the belief that "if a little is good, more is better." Over time, it was recognized that the blood pressure response to the dose for a thiazide-type diuretic (such as hydrochlorothiazide) was relatively flat

above a daily dose of 25 mg and that much of the negative metabolic experience with diuretics occurred at only very high doses (100–200 mg/day) (123,134). At lower doses (12.5–25.0 mg of hydrochlorothiazide), the metabolic mischief became less of a concern, with the possible exception of patients with new-onset diabetes (134). Recent observations suggest that new-onset diabetes that results from diuretic therapy carries the same negative CVR risk, which exists for the diabetic population in general (135).

Although positive outcome data for diuretic therapy exists, the exact positioning of diuretic therapy in treatment algorithms is still actively argued. Treatment guidelines such as JNC7 offer perspective (2) with the choice of the term "thiazide-type diuretics for most" to describe treatment recommendations for stage 1 hypertension. This prudently infers that thiazide-type diuretics are not the only available choice for intial treatment of all stage 1 hypertensive patients, leaving the choice of an initial agent discretionary. In stage 2 hypertension and for individuals with compelling indications for specific therapies, diuretics should be used with some regularity but more in a supporting role to improve the effectiveness of the nondiuretic antihypertensive therapies.

V. ADVERSE EFFECTS OF DIURETICS

A. Hyponatremia

Hyponatremia can prove to be a serious complication of diuretic therapy (136,137), with thiazide diuretics more likely to cause hyponatremia than loop diuretics. Loop diuretics inhibit sodium transport in the renal medulla and preclude the generation of a maximal osmotic gradient, thus impairing the ability of the kidney to concentrate urine. Thiazide-type diuretics increase sodium excretion and preclude maximal urine dilution while preserving the kidney's innate capacity to concentrate urine. When diuretic-related hyponatremia occurs, it is typically in elderly females and usually happens shortly after therapy begins (within the first 2 weeks) (138). Multiple factors contribute to the predisposition of elderly females to diuretic-related hyponatremia, including an exaggerated natriuretic response to a thiazide diuretic, a diminished capacity to excrete free water, and a low solute intake (Fig. 26.7).

Mild asymptomatic diuretic-related hyponatremia (typically a plasma sodium level of 125–135 mmol/L) can be treated in a number of ways, sometimes in combination, including restricting free water intake, restoring potassium losses, withholding diuretics, or converting to loop diuretic therapy (139,140). Severe, symptomatic hyponatremia (generally below a concentration of 125 mmol/L), complicated by seizures or other active

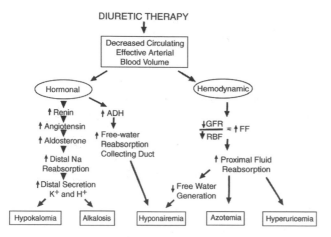

Figure 26.7 Adaptive changes to conserve salt and water in states of extracellular volume depletion that result in diuretic-related side effects.

neurologic sequelae, represents a true medical emergency. A drop in serum sodium to this degree calls for intensive therapy; however, symptomatic hyponatremia should not be corrected too rapidly because an osmotic demyelinating syndrome can occur under these circumstances. The risks of ongoing hyponatremia must be weighed against the risks of too rapid a correction; current recommendations are that plasma sodium should be corrected by no more than 0.5 mmol/h in the first 24 h of treatment (141,142). Initial treatment efforts should be halted once a mildly hyponatremic serum sodium range has been reached (~125–130 mmol/L). The acuity (≤48 h) of the hyponatremia also influences the rate at which hyponatremia should be corrected. Several aspects of hyponatremia therapy are still controversial.

B. Hypokalemia and Hyperkalemia

A serum potassium value of <3.5 mmol/L, which is the most common criterion for a diagnosis of hypokalemia, is a common finding in patients treated with loop or thiazide diuretics (143). During the first several days of thiazide diuretic therapy, plasma potassium levels decrease by an average of 0.6 mmol/L (in a dose-dependent manner) in subjects who are not taking potassium supplements, compared with a 0.3 mmol/L drop in plasma potassium in subjects who are being treated with furosemide (143). However, it is unusual for serum potassium values to settle <3.0 mmol/L in diuretic-treated outpatients, unless the patients have a high dietary sodium intake or are being treated with a long-acting diuretic (as is the case with chlorthalidone). Mechanisms that contribute to the onset of hypokalemia during diuretic use include increased flow-dependent distal nephron potassium secretion (more commonly observed with a high sodium

intake), a fall in distal tubule luminal chloride concentration, metabolic alkalosis, and secondary hyperaldosteronism (Fig. 26.7) (144,145).

The cardiac implications of diuretic-induced hypokalemia remain controversial. It would seem logical to infer that arrhythmia-related event rates are connected to the degree of hypokalemia, but it is not a clear relationship (at least in an outpatient setting). This connection is confused by several factors, including the inconstant relationship between serum potassium concentrations and total body potassium deficits during diuretic therapy. This theme is confused by several factors including: the inconstant relationship between serum K^+ concentrations and total body K^+ deficits in the face of diuretic therapy; the fact that in most clinical trials evaluating arrhythmia risk (and/or sudden cardiac death) serum K^+ values have not been measured frequently enough or under sufficiently standardized conditions to allow for anything more than an educated guess as to the "average" K^+ value at the time of an event; that the range of serum K^+ values most commonly associated with increased ventricular ectopy is very small—typically between 3.0–3.5-mmol/ L and finally the issue of whether hypokalemia produced by transcellular shifts of K^+ carries the same risk as a reduced serum K^+ on the basis of body losses.

Even mild degrees of diuretic-induced hypokalemia can be associated with ventricular ectopy (146,147). For example, the MRFIT trial found a significant inverse relationship between the concentration of serum potassium and the frequency of premature ventricular contractions (147). However, this relationship has not been detected in all studies, possibly because of the short duration of many of these trials (148,149). For example, in the MRC study, 287 of 324 patients with mild hypertension underwent ambulatory electrocardiogram (ECG) monitoring. In the short term (8 weeks), there was not an increased frequency of premature ventricular contractions. However, after 24 months, a significant difference (correlated with serum potassium concentrations) emerged in the premature ventricular contraction rate (20% in patients treated with a diuretic vs. 9% in patients treated with a placebo) (149).

The hazards central to diuretic-related hypokalemia are most apparent in patients with left ventricular hypertrophy, congestive heart failure, or myocardial ischemia, particularly when they become acutely ill and require hospitalization (150–153). As mentioned previously, outpatient forms of diuretic-related hypokalemia are seldom severe enough to require urgent attention. However, even these mildly lowered serum potassium values create a basis for more significant degrees of hypokalemia when transcellular shifts of potassium are interposed (e.g., during stressful circumstances, which are marked by high endogenous epinephrine levels) (154). This is one of the major at-risk scenarios of diuretic-related hypokalemia.

Despite a sometimes tedious level of concern with diuretic therapy about CVR risk as opposed to its benefits (in part because of its associated electrolyte abnormalities), several clinical trials, including SHEP, STOP-Hypertension, and MRC, have shown that low-dose diuretic therapy reduces CVR event rates by 20–25% (105,106,108). Perhaps the use of lower doses of thiazides or the combination of thiazides with a potassium-sparing diuretic explains these favorable results when compared with results of earlier trials, such as MRFIT, in which higher doses of diuretics were used and premature ventricular contractions were more frequent. However, in the SHEP trial, patients with hypokalemia (serum potassium <3.5 mmol/L) did not experience the treatment benefit recognized in similarly-treated normokalemic patients (113).

Two additional treatment issues exist for diuretic-related hypokalemia: the hemodynamic benefit of normalizing serum potassium, and the consequences of different doses, combinations of diuretics or potassium-sparing diuretics, or both, on sudden cardiac death (155–157). In the case of normalizing serum potassium, potassium supplementation (average increase in serum potassium of 0.56 mmol/L) in hypokalemic (serum potassium values <3.5 mmol/L) diuretic-treated patients has been associated with a 5.5 mmHg average drop in mean arterial pressure (155). In the case of effects of dose levels or combinations of doses on sudden cardiac death, the risk of sudden cardiac death among patients receiving combined thiazide and potassium-sparing diuretic therapy has been shown to be lower than the risk found in patients treated with thiazides alone; the odds ratios for a cardiovascular death event increase significantly when hydrochlorothiazide doses are in 25–100 mg/day range. Adding potassium supplements to thiazide therapy had little effect on the risk of sudden cardiac death (Fig. 26.8).

Distal potassium-sparing diuretics (such as triamterene and amiloride) and aldosterone-receptor antagonists (such as spironolactone and eplerenone) can cause significant degrees of hyperkalemia. Hyperkalemia is usually encountered in patients with an existing reduction in their glomerular filtration rate (especially the elderly or in patients given potassium chloride supplements or salt substitutes), in patients being treated with an ACE inhibitor or angiotensin receptor blocker, or both, or with a NSAID, or in patients in other situations that predispose them to hyperkalemia, such as metabolic acidosis, hyporeninemic hypoaldosteronism, or heparin therapy (including subcutaneous heparin regimens) (158).

C. Acid–Base Changes

Mild metabolic alkalosis is a somewhat common feature of thiazide-type diuretic therapy. Severe metabolic alkalosis is much less frequent, occurring more so in association

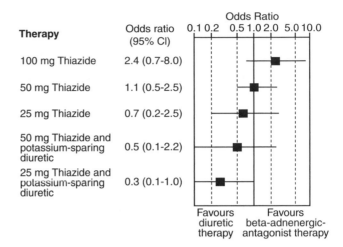

Figure 26.8 Risk of primary cardiac arrest that is associated with thiazide therapy, with and without potassium-sparing diuretic therapy, compared to β-adrenergic-antagonist therapy among patients treated with a single antihypertensive drug. Odds ratios are adjusted for age, gender, pretreatment systolic blood pressure and heart rate, duration of hypertension, current smoking habits, and concurrent diabetes mellitus. (CI, Confidence interval.)

with the use of a loop diuretic. The generation of a metabolic alkalosis with diuretic therapy is primarily due to contraction of the extracellular fluid space caused by urinary losses of a relatively bicarbonate-free fluid (159). Diuretic-induced metabolic alkalosis is best managed by the administration of potassium chloride or sodium chloride, or both, although sodium chloride administration may be problematic in patients for whom volume expansion is already an issue (such as those with congestive heart failure). In such cases, a potassium-sparing diuretic or a carbonic anhydrase inhibitor, such as acetazolamide, may be considered. Metabolic alkalosis also impairs the natriuretic response to loop diuretics and may contribute to diuretic resistance in the congestive heart failure patient (160). All potassium-sparing diuretics can cause hyperkalemic metabolic acidosis, which in elderly patients or those with renal impairment or congestive heart failure can reach a life-threatening level (161).

D. Hypomagnesemia

Both thiazide and loop diuretics increase urine magnesium excretion. Potassium-sparing diuretics, including spironolactone, diminish the magnesuria that accompanies the use of a thiazide or loop diuretic (7,8).

Prolonged therapy with thiazide and loop diuretics reduces plasma magnesium concentration an average of 5–10%, although patients can develop more severe hypomagnesemia (162). Cellular magnesium depletion occurs in up to 50% of patients during thiazide therapy and can exist despite normal serum magnesium concentrations. Hypomagnesemia occurs more frequently in the elderly and in patients who are receiving prolonged, high-dose diuretic therapy (such as heart failure patients) (163). Hypomagnesemia often coexists with hyponatremia and hypokalemia, with one study finding 41% of patients with hypokalemia to also have low serum magnesium concentrations (164). Concurrent electrolyte disorders such as these (including refractory hypocalcemia) cannot be fully reversed until the underlying magnesium deficit is corrected (165).

The measurement of serum magnesium concentration continues to be the routine test for detection of hypomagnesemia (166,167). However, the presence of hypomagnesemia can be suspected from characteristic ECG and neurologic or neuromuscular findings. When the patient is monitored with ECG, hypomagnesemia can present as prolongation of the Q–T and P–R intervals, widening of the QRS complex, ST segment depression, and low T waves, as well as supraventricular and ventricular tachyarrhythmias (168). The neurological changes with hypomagnesemia are nonspecific and confined to mental changes or neuromuscular irritability. Tetany, one of the most striking and better known manifestations of magnesium deficiency, is only rarely found; instead, less specific signs such as tremor, muscle twitching, peculiar movements, focal seizures, generalized convulsions, delirium, or coma are more common (169).

Although it is helpful to know when the serum magnesium level is low, which is typically indicative of low intracellular stores, normal serum magnesium values can still be observed in the face of a significant body deficiency of magnesium; thus, serum magnesium determinations are an unreliable measure of total body magnesium balance (170). Intracellular magnesium measurements, as well as other technologies, are available to assess magnesium balance, but they remain clinically impractical. A more practical measure of magnesium balance is the "magnesium loading test," which is at the same time both therapeutic and diagnostic. This test consists of the parenteral administration of magnesium sulfate and an assessment of urinary magnesium retention over a specific time interval. This can be accomplished on an outpatient basis in as short a time interval as 1 h. Individuals with a normal magnesium balance eliminate at least 75% of an administered magnesium load in this interval (171).

Several theoretical reasons exist for treating diuretic-related hypomagnesemia, beyond simple empirical correction to normalize a laboratory value. These include improvement in blood pressure control, a positive effect on deterring development of arrhythmias, and resolution of co-existing electrolyte or neuromuscular symptoms. Although there appears to be little additional reduction in blood pressure when magnesium deficiency is corrected, there is evidence of some measure of blood pressure reduction when magnesium supplementation occurs in a nondeficient state. The available studies on this issue are sufficiently indeterminate to preclude a specific recommendation for magnesium supplementation as a mode of therapy for hypertension.

Identifying magnesium deficiency is recommended in all patients in whom hypomagnesemia is suspected, but particularly in patients with ischemic heart disease or known cardiac arrhythmias. In mild deficiency states, magnesium balance often can be reestablished by limiting diuretic and sodium intake and allowing the magnesium content in a normal diet to correct the deficit. Parenteral magnesium administration, however, is the most effective way to correct a hypomagnesemic state and should be the route used when replacement is an emergency situation. Total body deficits of magnesium in the depleted patient are typically on the order of 1–2 mEq/kg per body weight. One commonly employed empirical regimen administers 2 g of magnesium sulfate (16.3 mEq) intravenously over 30 min, followed by a constant infusion providing 32–64 mEq/day until the deficit is presumed corrected.

A variety of oral magnesium salts are available for clinical use. Magnesium oxide is commonly used, but this salt is poorly soluble and acts as a cathartic, thereby decreasing absorption. Magnesium gluconate is the preferred salt form for oral therapy because it is very soluble and causes minimal diarrhea. Magnesium carbonate is poorly soluble and does not appear to be as effective in reversing hypomagnesemia as the gluconate salt. Oral magnesium is not recommended for therapy during acute situations because the high doses that would be necessary almost always cause significant diarrhea. The intramuscular route for magnesium administration is a useful but a painful means of delivery and should be avoided as long as intravenous access is available (166).

E. Hyperuricemia

Thiazide diuretic therapy increases serum urate concentrations by as much as 35%, an effect that is related to decreased renal clearance of urate and is most prominent in those with the highest pretherapy urate clearance values (172). Decreased urate clearance may be related to increased reabsorption secondary to diuretic-related extracellular fluid volume depletion or to competition for tubular secretion. This is because both thiazide diuretics and urate undergo tubular secretion by the same organic anion transporter pathway (29,173). Diuretic-related hyperuricemia is dose-dependent and does not typically precipitate a gout attack unless the patient has an underlying tendency to gout or the serum urate concentrations exceed 12 mg/dL (173). In the MRC trial, patients who were receiving thiazide diuretics had significantly more withdrawals from treatment because of gout than did placebo-treated patients (4.4 vs. 0.1/1000 patient-years) (108).

If a gouty attack occurs in a diuretic-treated patient, the diuretic in question should be discontinued. If this is not feasible, then the lowest effective dose should be given with careful attention to avoidance of excessive volume contraction. An alternative in the patient with gout who requires diuretic therapy is that of the xanthine oxidase inhibitor allopurinol. However, allopurinol should be used cautiously (dose adjusted according to renal function level) in patients receiving a thiazide-type diuretic because the incidence of allopurinol hypersensitivity reactions increases with this combination (174). Moreover, allopurinol should not be started routinely for diuretic-related asymptomatic hyperuricemia, as is often done (175).

F. Metabolic Abnormalities

Two types of metabolic abnormalities can result from diuretic therapy: hyperglycemia or hyperlipidemia.

1. Hyperglycemia

Prolonged thiazide diuretic therapy impairs glucose tolerance and may occasionally precipitate diabetes mellitus (89,135,176–178). Short-term metabolic studies, epidemiological studies, and a variety of clinical trials suggest a causal link between the use of thiazide diuretics and subsequent development of type 2 diabetes. However, it should be noted that many of these studies involved small numbers of patients, relatively limited follow-up periods, varying definitions of "new-onset diabetes," inadequate comparison groups, selection criteria that limit the ability to generalize the findings, and study designs that precluded interclass comparisons among antihypertensive drug classes (179).

Hyperglycemia and carbohydrate intolerance have been linked to diuretic-induced hypokalemia, which inhibits insulin secretion by β cells. However, diuretic-induced changes in glucose metabolism are not conclusively related to altered potassium homeostasis, and impaired glucose tolerance occurs even when thiazide-type diuretics in relatively low doses are combined with potassium-sparing agents. The glucose intolerance seen with diuretic therapy can be compounded by increases in sympathetic nervous system activity, which also decreases peripheral glucose utilization. Diuretic-associated glucose intolerance appears to be dose-related, less common with loop diuretics and not present with spironolactone, and reversible upon withdrawal of the agent. Although the data on reversibility in hydrochlorothiazide-treated patients is inconsistent (177), a review of this issue found that in several studies glucose homeostasis was variably

affected by low-dose hydrochlorothiazide (12.5–50 mg/day) (180).

Recently, a large prospective cohort study (12,550 nondiabetic adults 45–64 years old) concluded, after appropriate adjustment for confounders, that hypertensive patients taking thiazide diuretics were not at greater risk for subsequent diabetes development than patients who were not receiving antihypertensive therapy. However, the diuretic doses were not reported in this cohort study. Because of the perceived variability of the effect on glucose tolerance, blood glucose should be monitored during thiazide therapy, particularly in patients with either existing diabetes or the metabolic syndrome (181). This is particularly necessary because the CVR risk with new-onset diuretic-related diabetes appears similar to that observed in patients with existing diabetes (135).

2. Hyperlipidemia

Short-term thiazide diuretic therapy can cause a dose-dependent elevation in serum total cholesterol levels, a modest increase in low-density lipoprotein (LDL) cholesterol levels, raised triglyceride levels, but little change in high-density lipoprotein (HDL) cholesterol (182–185). The lipid effects have been reported to be more apparent in black persons, males, and diabetic patients (185). All diuretics, including loop diuretics, cause these lipid changes, with the possible exception of indapamide (184). The mechanisms behind diuretic-induced dyslipidemia remain unclear, but they have been related to worsened insulin sensitivity and to reflex activation of the renin–angiotensin–aldosterone system and sympathetic nervous system in tandem with volume contraction. Supporting this latter relationship is the fact that low doses of diuretics do not tend to cause lipid alterations; in contrast, higher doses are more likely to be associated with reflex sympathetic activation. However, long-term clinical trials have reported unchanged cholesterol levels after 1 year of diuretic therapy (183,184). Moreover, data from the HDFP study indicate that hypertensive subjects with baseline cholesterol values of >250 mg/dL who are treated with diuretics, experience a decline in cholesterol levels from the second to the fifth years of diuretic treatment (125).

G. Impotence

Adverse effects of thiazide and thiazide-like diuretics on male sexual function, including decreased libido, erectile dysfunction, and ejaculation difficulties, have been reported in several studies with an incidence that varies from 3% to 32% (176,186,187). In the MRC trial, in which 15,000 hypertensive subjects received either a placebo, thiazide (bendrofluazide), or a β-blocker (propranolol) for 5 years, impotence was 22-fold higher with thiazide over a placebo and four-fold higher with a β-blocker over a placebo (176). In this trial, impotence was the most frequent reason for withdrawal from antihypertensive therapy. Another smaller trial in patients receiving a thiazide that was reported by Chang et al. (188) confirmed a higher frequency of decreased libido, of difficulty in gaining and sustaining an erection, and of difficulty in ejaculating (188). Multivariate analysis suggested that the findings were not mediated by low serum potassium levels or by the drop in blood pressure.

In the study by Wassertheil-Smoller et al., problems with sexual interest, erection, and orgasm were greater among men receiving chlorthalidone than among those given placebo or atenolol (189). Interestingly, in this trial weight loss ameliorated the problem of chlorthalidone-induced sexual dysfunction (187). Combined use of a diuretic and other antihypertensive agents has been reported to be associated with a higher incidence of sexual dysfunction symptoms than with the use of a diuretic agent alone. The mechanism by which thiazides affect erectile function or libido is unclear, but it has been suggested that these drugs wield a direct effect on vascular smooth muscle cells or decrease the response to catecholamines, or both. However, patients with diuretic-related impotence can respond favorably to sildenafil without any associated additional drop in blood pressure (190).

Impotence and decreased libido are the more frequent sexual side effects of spironolactone (186). Gynecomastia, another fairly frequent complication of spironolactone therapy, may be associated with mastodynia and is typically bilateral. The sexual side effects of spironolactone have been attributed to endocrine dysfunction/spironolactone is structurally similar to sex hormones and inhibits the binding of dihydrotestosterone to androgen receptors, thus producing an increased clearance of testosterone (191). Eplerenone is another aldosterone receptor antagonist that is more selective and does not have the sexual side effects of spironolactone (192).

H. Drug Allergy

Photosensitivity dermatitis occurs rarely during thiazide or furosemide therapy (193). Hydrochlorothiazide causes photosensitivity more often than do the other thiazides (194). Diuretics may occasionally cause a more serious generalized dermatitis and, at times, even a necrotizing vasculitis. Cross-sensitivity with sulfonamide drugs may occur with all diuretics, with the exception of ethacrynic acid. Severe necrotizing pancreatitis is an additional serious, life-threatening complication of thiazide therapy (195). Acute allergic interstitial nephritis with fever, rash, and eosinophilia, although an uncommon complication of diuretics, is a condition that may result in permanent renal failure if the drug exposure is prolonged (196).

It may develop abruptly or some months after therapy is begun with a thiazide diuretic or, less commonly, with furosemide (197). Ethacrynic acid is chemically dissimilar from the other loop diuretics and can be safely substituted in diuretic-treated patients who experience a number of these allergic complications.

I. Carcinogenesis

Twelve clinical studies, three cohort studies (1,226,229 patients with 802 cases of renal cell carcinoma), and nine case-controlled studies (4185 cases of renal cell carcinoma and 6010 controls) have evaluated the association between the use of diuretics and renal cell carcinoma. In all case-controlled studies, the odds were greater for patients being treated with diuretics to develop renal cell carcinoma with an average odds ratio of 1:55. The risk of renal cell carcinoma appeared to be related to the duration of the diuretic treatment in several studies, although the average daily dose of the diuretic seemed to carry less risk for the development of renal cell carcinoma. Unlike the association between diuretics and renal cell carcinoma, no association has been found between diuretic therapy and breast cancer. The issue of renal cell carcinoma occurring with diuretic therapy at the current time remains one that is incompletely resolved (198–200).

J. Adverse Drug Interactions

Loop diuretics can potentiate aminoglycoside nephrotoxicity (201). By causing hypokalemia, diuretics increase the risk of digitalis toxicity (202). Plasma lithium concentrations can increase with thiazide therapy with significant volume contraction due to the associated increase in lithium absorption (203). However, some diuretics, such as chlorothiazide or furosemide, with significant carbonic anhydrase inhibitory effects, can increase lithium clearance, leading to a drop in blood levels (204,205). Whole-blood lithium should be closely monitored in patients administered lithium in conjunction with diuretics. NSAIDs can both antagonize the effects of diuretics and predispose diuretic-treated patients to a form of functional renal insufficiency. The combination of indomethacin and triamterene may be particularly dangerous because it can precipitate acute renal failure (206).

VI. CONCLUSIONS

Diuretics remain an important component of any management plan for hypertension. Of the several diuretics that exist, the thiazide-type diuretic is the one most commonly used in the treatment of hypertension. The safe and effective use of diuretics in the treatment of hypertension and edema requires a thorough understanding of their pharmacokinetics and pharmacodynamics. With such an understanding in hand, these compounds can be used deftly enough to effect significant blood pressure reduction with a minimum of side effects.

REFERENCES

1. Dustan H, Roccella EJ, Garrison H. Controlling hypertension. A research success story. Arch Intern Med 1996; 156:1926–1935.
2. Chobanian AV, Bakris GL, Black HR, Cushman WC, Green LA, Izzo JL Jr, Jones DW, Materson BJ, Oparil S, Wright JT Jr, Roccella EJ, Joint National Committee on Prevention, Detection, Evaluation, and Treatment of High blood pressure. National Heart, Lung, and Blood Institute; National High blood pressure Education Program Coordinating Committee. Seventh Report of the Joint National Committee on Prevention, Detection, Evaluation, and Treatment of High blood pressure. Hypertension 2003; 42:1206–1252.
3. Brater DC. Diuretic therapy. N Engl J Med 1998; 339:387–395.
4. Eveloff J, Warnock DG. Renal carbonic anhydrase. In: Dirks JH, Sutton RA, eds. Diuretics: Physiology, Pharmacology and Clinical Use. Philadelphia: WB Saunders, 1986:49–65.
5. O'Grady SM, Palfrey HC, Field M. Characteristics and function of $Na^+/K^+/2Cl^-$ cotransport in epithelial tissues. Am J Physiol 1987; 252:C177–C192.
6. Earley LE, Friedler RM. Renal tubular effects of ethacrynic acid. J Clin Invest 1964; 43:1495–1506.
7. White MG, van Gelder J, Eastes G. The effect of loop diuretics on the excretion of Na^+, Ca^{2+}, Mg^{2+}, and Cl^-. J Clin Pharmacol 1981; 21:610–614.
8. Ryan MP, Devane J, Ryan MG, Counihan TB. Effects of diuretics on the renal handling of magnesium. Drugs 1984; 28:167–181.
9. Steele TH, Oppenheimer S. Factors affecting urate excretion following diuretic administration in man. Am J Med 1969; 47:564–574.
10. Gerber JG. Role of prostaglandins in the hemodynamic and tubular effects of furosemide. Fed Proc 1983; 42:1707–1710.
11. Loon NR, Wilcox CS, Unwin RJ. Mechanism of impaired natriuretic response to furosemide during prolonged therapy. Kidney Int 1989; 36:682–689.
12. Sica DA, Gehr TWB. Diuretic combinations in refractory edema states: pharmacokinetic–pharmacodynamic relationships. Clin Pharmacokinet 1996; 30:229–249.
13. Benet LZ. Pharmacokinetics/pharmacodynamics of furosemide in man: a review. J Pharmacokinet Biopharm 1979; 7:1–27.
14. Murray MD, Haag KM, Black PK, Hall SD, Brater DC. Variable furosemide absorption and poor predictability of response in elderly patients. Pharmacotherapy 1997; 17:98–106.
15. Vargo DL, Kramer WG, Black PK, Smith WB, Serpas T, Brater DC. Bioavailability, pharmacokinetics, and pharmacodynamics of torsemide and furosemide in patients with congestive heart failure. Clin Pharmacol Ther 1995; 57:601–609.
16. Murray MD, Deer MM, Ferguson JA, Dexter PR, Bennett SJ, Perkins SM, Smith FE, Lane KA, Adams LD, Tierney WM, Brater DC. Open-label randomized trial of torsemide compared with furosemide therapy for patients with heart failure. Am J Med 2001; 111:513–520.
17. Chennavasin P, Seiwell R, Brater DC, Liang WM. Pharmacodynamic analysis of the furosemide-probenecid interaction in man. Kidney Int 1979; 16:187–195.
18. Voelker JR, Cartwright-Brown D, Anderson S, Leinfelder J, Sica DA, Kokko JP, Brater DC. Comparison of furosemide to bumetanide in chronic renal insufficiency. Kidney Int 1987; 32:572–578.
19. Rudy DW, Gehr TW, Matzke GR, Kramer WG, Sica DA, Brater DC. The pharmacodynamics of intravenous and oral torsemide in patients with chronic renal insufficiency. Clin Pharmacol Ther 1994; 56:39–47.
20. Rose JH, O'Malley K, Pruitt AW. Depression of renal clearance of furosemide in man by azotemia. Clin Pharmacol Ther 1976; 21:141–146.
21. Takamura N, Maruyama T, Otagiri M. Effects of uremic toxins and fatty acids on serum protein binding of furosemide: possible mechanism of the binding defect in uremia. Clin Chem 1997; 43:2274–2280.
22. Wilcox CS, Mitch WE, Kelly RA, Skorecki K, Meyer TW, Friedman PA, Souney PF. Response of the kidney to furosemide. I. Effects of salt intake and renal compensation. J Lab Clin Med 1983; 102:450–458.
23. Brater DC, Day B, Burdette A, Anderson S. Bumetanide and furosemide in heart failure. Kidney Int 1984; 26:183–189.
24. Chennavasin P, Seiwell R, Brater DC. Pharmacokinetic-dynamic analysis of the indomethacin-furosemide interaction in man. J Pharmacol Exp Ther 1980; 215:77–81.
25. Agarwal R, Gorski JC, Sundblad K, Brater DC. Urinary protein binding does not affect response to furosemide in patients with nephrotic syndrome. J Am Soc Nephrol 2000; 11:1100–1105.
26. Ellison DH, Velazquez H, Wright FS. Thiazide-sensitive sodium chloride cotransport in early distal tubule. Am J Physiol 1987; 253:F546–F554.
27. Seldin DW, Eknoyan G, Suki WN, Rector FC Jr. Localization of diuretic action from the pattern of water and electrolyte excretion. Ann N Y Acad Sci 1966; 139:328–343.
28. Giles TD, Sander GE, Roffidal LE, Quiroz AC, Mazzu AL. Comparative effects of nitrendipine and hydrochlorothiazide on calciotropic hormones and bone density in hypertensive patients. Am J Hypertens 1992; 5:875–879.
29. Weinman EJ, Eknoyan G, Suki WN. The influence of the extracellular fluid volume on the tubular reabsorption of uric acid. J Clin Invest 1975; 55:283–291.
30. Leary WP, Reyes AJ. Diuretic-induced magnesium losses. Drugs 1984; 28:182–187.
31. Welling PG. Pharmacokinetics of the thiazide diuretics. Biopharm Drug Dispos 1986; 7:501–535.

32. Beermann B, Groschinsky-Grind M. Clinical pharmacokinetics of diuretics. Clin Pharmacokinet 1980; 5:221–245.

33. Knauf H, Mutschler E. Diuretic effectiveness of hydrochlorothiazide and furosemide alone and in combination in chronic renal failure. J Cardiovasc Pharmacol 1995; 26:394–400.

34. Sica DA, Gehr TWB. Diuretic use in stage 5 chronic kidney disease (chronic kidney disease) and end-stage renal disease. Curr Opin Nephrol Hypertens 2003; 12:483–490.

35. Stern A. Metolazone, a diuretic agent. Am Heart J 1976; 91:262–263.

36. Suki WN, Dawoud F, Eknoyan G et al. Effects of metolazone on renal function in normal man. J Pharmacol Exp Ther 1972; 180:6–12.

37. Craswell PW, Ezzat E, Kopstein J, Varghese Z, Moorhead JF. Use of metolazone, a new diuretic, in patients with renal disease. Nephron 1974; 12:63–73.

38. Sica DA. Pharmacotherapy in congestive heart failure: metolazone and its role in edema management. Cong Heart Fail 2003; 9:100–105.

39. Wingo CS. Cortical collecting tubule potassium secretion: effect of amiloride, ouabain, and luminal sodium concentration. Kidney Int 1985; 27:886–891.

40. Wingo CS. Potassium secretion by the cortical collecting tubule: effect of Cl gradients and ouabain. Am J Physiol 1989; 256:F306–F313.

41. Netzer T, Knauf H, Mutschler E. Modulation of electrolyte excretion by potassium retaining diuretics. Eur Heart J 1992; 13:G22–G27.

42. McInnes GT. Relative potency of amiloride and spironolactone in healthy man. Clin Pharmacol Ther 1982; 31:472–477.

43. Rahn KH. Clinical pharmacology of diuretics. Clin Exp Hypertens 1983; 5:157–166.

44. Gardiner P, Schrode K, Quinlan D, Martin BK, Boreham DR, Rogers MS, Stubbs K, Smith M, Karim A. Spironolactone metabolism: steady-state serum levels of the sulfur-containing metabolites. J Clin Pharmacol 1989; 29:342–347.

45. McLaughlin N, Gehr TWB, Sica DA. Aldosterone receptor antagonism in end-stage renal disease. Current Hypertension Reports 2004; 6:327–330.

46. Pitt B, Remme W, Zannad F, Neaton J, Martinez F, Roniker B, Bittman R, Hurley S, Kleiman J, Gatlin M, Eplerenone Post-Acute Myocardial Infarction Heart Failure Efficacy and Survival Study Investigators. Eplerenone, a selective aldosterone blocker, in patients with left ventricular dysfunction after myocardial infarction. N Engl J Med 2003; 348:1309–1321.

47. Williams GH, Burgess E, Kolloch RE, Ruilope LM, Niegowska J, Kipnes MS, Roniker B, Patrick JL, Krause SL. Efficacy of eplerenone versus enalapril as monotherapy in systemic hypertension. Am J Cardiol 2004; 93:990–996.

48. White WB, Duprez D, St Hillaire R, Krause S, Roniker B, Kuse-Hamilton J, Weber MA. Effects of the selective aldosterone blocker eplerenone versus the calcium antagonist amlodipine in systolic hypertension. Hypertension 2003; 41:1021–1026.

49. Pitt B, Reichek N, Willenbrock R, Zannad F, Phillips RA, Roniker B, Kleiman J, Krause S, Burns D, Williams GH. Effects of eplerenone, enalapril, and eplerenone/enalapril in patients with essential hypertension and left ventricular hypertrophy: the 4E-left ventricular hypertrophy study. Circulation 2003; 108:1831–1838.

50. Somogyi AA, Hovens CM, Muirhead MR, Bochner F. Renal tubular secretion of amiloride and its inhibition by cimetidine in humans and in an animal model. Drug Metab Dispos 1989; 17:190–196.

51. Somogyi A, Hewson D, Muirhead M, Bochner F. Amiloride disposition in geriatric patients: importance of renal function. Br J Clin Pharmacol 1990; 29:1–8.

52. Knauf H, Mohrke W, Mutschler E. Delayed elimination of triamterene and its active metabolite in chronic renal failure. Eur J Clin Pharmacol 1983; 24:453–456.

53. Sica DA, Gehr TW. Triamterene and the kidney. Nephron 1989; 51:454–461.

54. Favre L, Glasson P, Vallotton MB. Reversible acute renal failure from combined triamterene and indomethacin: a study in healthy subjects. Ann Intern Med 1982; 96:317–320.

55. Favre L, Glasson P, Riondel A, Vallotton MB. Interaction of diuretics and non-steroidal anti-inflammatory drugs in man. Clin Sci (Lond) 1983; 64:407–415.

56. Kelly RA, Wilcox CS, Mitch WE, Meyer TW, Souney PF, Rayment CM, Friedman PA, Swartz SL. Response of the kidney to furosemide. II. Effect of captopril on sodium balance. Kidney Int 1983; 24:233–239.

57. Wilcox CS, Guzman NJ, Mitch WE, Kelly RA, Maroni BJ, Souney PF, Rayment CM, Braun L, Colucci R, Loon NR. Na+ and blood pressure homeostasis in man during furosemide: Effects of prazosin and captopril. Kidney Int 1987; 31:135–141.

58. Wilcox CS, Loon NR, Ameer B, Limacher MC. Renal and hemodynamic responses to bumetanide in hypertension: effects of nitrendipine. Kidney Int 1989; 36:719–725.

59. Almeshari K, Ahlstrom NG, Capraro FE, Wilcox CS. A volume-independent component to post-diuretic sodium retention in man. J Am Soc Nephrol 1993; 3:1878–1883.

60. Ellison DH, Velazquez H, Wright FS. Adaptation of the distal convoluted tubule of the rat. Structural and functional effects of dietary salt intake and chronic diuretic infusion. J Clin Invest 1989; 83:113–126.

61. Kim J, Welch WJ, Cannon JK, Tisher CC, Madsen KM. Immunocytochemical response of type A and type B intercalated cells to increased sodium chloride delivery. Am J Physiol 1992; 262:F288–F302.

62. Stanton BA, Kaissling B. Adaptation of distal tubule and collecting duct to increase Na$^+$ delivery. II. Na$^+$ and K$^+$ transport. Am J Physiol 1988; 255:F1269–F1275.

63. Idiopathic edema: Role of diuretic abuse. Kidney Int 1981; 19:881–891.

64. Wilson TW, Loadholt CB, Privitera PJ, Halushka PV. Furosemide increases urine 6-keto-prostaglandin F1α.

Relation to natriuresis, vasodilation, and renin release. Hypertension 1982; 4:634–641.

65. Kraus PA, Lipman J, Becker PJ. Acute preload effects of furosemide. Chest 1990; 98:124–128.

66. Pivac N, Rumboldt Z, Sardelic S, Bagatin J, Polic S, Ljutic D, Naranca M, Capkun V. Diuretic effects of furosemide infusion versus bolus injection in congestive heart failure. Int J Clin Pharmacol Res 1998; 18:121–128.

67. Dikshit K, Vyden JK, Forrester JS, Chatterjee K, Prakash R, Swan HJ. Renal and extrarenal hemodynamic effects of furosemide in congestive heart failure after acute myocardial infarction. N Engl J Med 1973; 288:1087–1090.

68. Nishizaka MK, Zaman MA, Calhoun DA. Efficacy of low-dose spironolactone in subjects with resistant hypertension. Am J Hypertens 2003; 16:925–930.

69. Hajjar I, Kotchen TA. Trends in prevalence, awareness, treatment, and control of hypertension in the United States, 1988–2000. J Am Med Assoc 2003; 290:199–206.

70. World Health Report 2002: Reducing risks, promoting healthy life. Geneva, Switzerland: World Health Organization, 2002. http://www.who.int/whr/2002.

71. Turnbull F. Blood Pressure Lowering Treatment Trialists' Collaboration. Effects of different blood-pressure-lowering regimens on major cardiovascular events: results of prospectively-designed overviews of randomised trials. Lancet 2003; 362:1527–1535.

72. Roos JC, Boer P, Koomans HA, Geyskes GG, Dorhout Mees EJ. Haemodynamic and hormonal changes during acute and chronic diuretic treatment in essential hypertension. Eur J Clin Pharmacol 1981; 19:107–112.

73. Van Brummelen P, Man in't Veld AJ, Schalekamp MA. Hemodynamic changes during long-term thiazide treatment of essential hypertension in responders and non-responders. Clin Pharmacol Ther 1980; 27:328.

74. Tarazi RC, Dustan HP, Frohlich ED. Long-term thiazide therapy in essential hypertension. Circulation 1970; 41:709–717.

75. Conway J, Lauwers P. Hemodynamic and hypotensive effects of long-term therapy with chlorothiazide. Circulation 1960; 21:21–27.

76. Shah S, Khatri I, Freis ED. Mechanism of antihypertensive effect of thiazide diuretics. Am Heart J 1978; 95:611–618.

77. Bennett WM, McDonald WJ, Kuehnel E, Hartnett MN, Porter GA. Do diuretics have antihypertensive properties independent of natriuresis? Clin Pharmacol Ther 1977; 22:499–504.

78. Nelson MR, Reid CM, Krum H, Ryan P, Wing LM, McNeil JJ. Management Committee, Second Australian National Blood Pressure Study. Short-term predictors of maintenance of normotension after withdrawal of antihypertensive drugs in the second Australian National blood pressure Study (ANBP2). Am J Hypertens 2003; 16:39–45.

79. Levinson PD, Khatri IM, Freis ED. Persistence of normal blood pressure after withdrawal of drug treatment in mild hypertension. Arch Intern Med 1982; 142:2265–2268.

80. Holland OB, Gomez-Sanchez CE, Kuhnert LV, Poindexter C, Pak CY. Antihypertensive comparison of furosemide with hydrochlorothiazide for black patients. Arch Intern Med 1979; 139:1015–1021.

81. Araoye MA, Chang MY, Khatri IM, Freis ED. Furosemide compared with hydrochlorothiazide. Long-term treatment of hypertension. J Am Med Assoc 1978; 240:1863–1866.

82. Pickkers P, Hughes AD, Russel FG, Thien T, Smits P. Thiazide-induced vasodilation in humans is mediated by potassium channel activation. Hypertension 1998; 32:1071–1076.

83. Dunn CJ, Fitton A, Brogden RN. Torasemide. An update of its pharmacological properties and therapeutic efficacy. Drugs 1995; 49:121–142.

84. Pickkers P, Dormans TP, Russel FG, Hughes AD, Thien T, Schaper N, Smits P. Direct vascular effects of furosemide in humans. Circulation 1997; 96:1847–1852.

85. Vasavada N, Saha C, Agarwal R. A double-blind randomized crossover trial of two loop diuretics in chronic kidney disease. Kidney Int 2003; 64:632–640.

86. Carter BL, Ernst ME, Cohen JD. Hydrochlorothiazide versus chlorthalidone: evidence supporting their interchangeability. Hypertension 2004; 43:4–9.

87. Mortality after 10 1/2 years for hypertensive participants in the Multiple Risk Factor Intervention Trial. Circulation 1990; 82:1616–1628.

88. Prevention of stroke by antihypertensive drug treatment in older persons with isolated systolic hypertension: final results of the Systolic Hypertension in the Elderly Program (SHEP). SHEP Cooperative Research Group. J Am Med Assoc 1991; 265:3255–3264.

89. Major outcomes in high-risk hypertensive patients randomized to angiotensin-converting enzyme inhibitor or calcium channel blocker vs diuretic: the Antihypertensive and Lipid-Lowering Treatment to Prevent Heart Attack Trial (ALLHAT). J Am Med Assoc 2002; 288:2981–2997.

90. Collins R, Peto R, MacMahon S, Hebert P, Fiebach NH, Eberlein KA, Godwin J, Qizilbash N, Taylor JO, Hennekens CH. Blood pressure, stroke, and coronary heart disease. Part 2: Short-term reductions in blood pressure: Overview of randomised drug trials in their epidemiological context. Lancet 1990; 335:827–838.

91. Collins R, MacMahon S. Blood pressure, antihypertensive drug treatment and the risks of stroke and of coronary heart disease. Br Med Bull 1994; 50:272.

92. Gueyffier F, Boutitie F, Boissel JP, Pocock S, Coope J, Cutler J, Ekbom T, Fagard R, Friedman L, Perry M, Prineas R, Schron E. Effect of antihypertensive drug treatment on cardiovascular outcomes in women and men: a meta-analysis of individual patient data from randomised controlled trials. Ann Intern Med 1997; 126:761–767.

93. Psaty BM, Smith NL, Siscovick DS, Koepsell TD, Weiss NS, Heckbert SR, Lemaitre RN, Wagner EH, Furberg CD. Health outcomes associated with antihypertensive therapies used as first-line agents: a systematic review and meta-analysis. J Am Med Assoc 1997; 277:739–745.

94. Wright JM, Lee CH, Chambers GK. Systematic review of antihypertensive therapies: Does the evidence assist in choosing a first-line drug? CMAJ 1999; 161:25–32.

95. Messerli FH, Gorssman E, Goldbourt U. Are β blockers efficacious as first-line therapy for hypertension in the elderly? A systematic review. J Am Med Assoc 1998; 279:1903–1907.

96. Blood Pressure Lowering Treatment Trialists Collaboration. Effects of ACE inhibitors, calcium antagonists, and other blood-pressure-lowering drugs: results of prospectively designed overviews of randomised trials. Lancet 2000; 355:1955–1964.

97. Hansson L, Lindholm LH, Ekbom T, Dahlof B, Lanke J, Schersten B, Wester PO, Hedner T, de Faire U. Randomised trial of old and new antihypertensive drugs in elderly patients: Cardiovascular mortality and morbidity the Swedish Trial in Old Patients with Hypertension-2 study. Lancet 1999; 354:1751–1756.

98. Brown MJ, Palmer CR, Castaigne A, de Leeuw PW, Mancia G, Rosenthal T, Ruilope LM. Morbidity and mortality in patients randomised to double-blind treatment with a long-acting calcium-channel blocker or diuretic in the International Nifedipine GITS study: Intervention as a Goal in Hypertension Treatment (INSIGHT). Lancet 2000; 356:366–372.

99. Hansson L, Hedner T, Lund-Johansen P, Kjeldsen SE, Lindholm LH, Syvertsen JO, Lanke J, de Faire U, Dahlof B, Karlberg BE. Randomised trial of effects of calcium antagonists compared with diuretics and β-blockers on cardiovascular morbidity and mortality in hypertension: The Nordic Diltiazem (NORDIL) study. Lancet 2000; 356:359–365.

100. Antihypertensive and Lipid-Lowering Treatment to Prevent Heart Attack Trial Collaborative Research Group. Diuretic versus α-blocker as first-step antihypertensive therapy: final results from the Antihypertensive and Lipid-Lowering Treatment to Prevent Heart Attack Trial (ALLHAT). Hypertension 2003; 42:239–246.

101. Materson BJ, Reda DJ, Cushman WC, Massie BM, Freis ED, Kochar MS, Hamburger RJ, Fye C, Lakshman R, Gottdiener J, et al. Single-drug therapy for hypertension in men. A comparison of six antihypertensive agents with placebo. N Engl J Med 1993; 328:914–921.

102. Materson BJ, Williams DW, Reda DJ, Cushman WC, Veterans Affairs Cooperative Study Group on Antihypertensive Agents. Response to six classes of antihypertensive medications by body mass index in a randomized controlled trial. J Clin Hypertens (Greenwich) 2003; 5:197–201.

103. Coope J, Warrender TS. Randomized trial of treatment of hypertension in elderly patients in primary care. Br Med J 1986; 293:1145–1151.

104. Chapman AB, Schwartz GL, Boerwinkle E, Turner ST. Predictors of antihypertensive response to a standard dose of hydrochlorothiazide for essential hypertension. Kidney Int 2002; 61:1047–1055.

105. SHEP Cooperative Research Group. Prevention of stroke by antihypertensive drug treatment in older patients with isolated systolic hypertension. Final results of the Systolic Hypertension in the Elderly Program (SHEP). J Am Med Assoc 1991; 265:3255–3264.

106. Dahlof B, Lindholm LH, Hansson L, Schersten B, Ekbom T, Wester PO. Morbidity and mortality in the Swedish Trial in Old Patients with Hypertension (STOP-Hypertension). Lancet 1991; 338:1281–1285.

107. Amery A, Birkenhager W, Brixko P, Bulpitt C, Clement D, Deruyttere M, De Schaepdryver A, Dollery C, Fagard R, Forette F. Mortality and morbidity results from the European Working Party on High blood pressure in the Elderly Trial. Lancet 1985; 1:1349–1354.

108. MRC Working Party. Medical Research Council trial of treatment of hypertension in older adults: principal results. Brit Med J 1992; 304:405–412.

109. Messerli F, Grossman E, Lever AF. Do thiazide diuretics confer protection against stroke? Arch Int Med 2003; 163:2557–2560.

110. The IPPPSH Collaborative Group. Cardiovascular risk and risk factors in a randomised trial of treatment based on the β blocker oxprenolol: The International Prospective Primary Prevention Study in Hypertension (IPPPSH). J Hypertens 1985; 3:379–392.

111. Wilhelmsen L, Berglund G, Elmfeldt D, Fitzsimons T, Holzgreve H, Hosie J, Hornkvist PE, Pennert K, Tuomilehto J, Wedel H. β-blockers versus diuretics in hypertensive men: Main results from the HAPPHY trial. J Hypertens 1987; 5:561–572.

112. Pahor M, Shorr RI, Somes GW, Cushman WC, Ferrucci L, Bailey JE, Elam JT, Applegate WB. Diuretic-based treatment and cardiovascular events in patients with mild renal dysfunction enrolled in the Systolic Hypertension in the Elderly Program. Arch Intern Med 1998; 158:1340–1345.

113. Franse LV, Pahor M, Di Bari M, Somes GW, Cushman WC, Applegate WB. Hypokalemia associated with diuretic use and cardiovascular events in the Systolic Hypertension in the Elderly Program. Hypertension 2000; 35:1025–1030.

114. Douglas JG, Bakris GL, Epstein M, Ferdinand KC, Ferrario C, Flack JM, Jamerson KA, Jones WE, Haywood J, Maxey R, Ofili EO, Saunders E, Schiffrin EL, Sica DA, Sowers JR, Vidt DG, Hypertension in African Americans Working Group of the International Society on Hypertension in Blacks. Management of high blood pressure in African Americans: consensus statement of the Hypertension in African Americans Working Group of the International Society on Hypertension in Blacks. Arch Intern Med 2003; 163:525–541.

115. Chrysant SG, Danisa K, Kem DC, Dillard BL, Smith WJ, Frohlich ED. Racial differences in pressure, volume and renin interrelationships in essential hypertension. Hypertension 1979; 1:136–141.

116. INTERSALT Cooperative Research Group. INTERSALT: An international study of electrolyte excretion and blood pressure. Results of 24 h urinary sodium and potassium excretion. Brit Med J 1988; 297:319–328.

117. Wilson DK, Sica DA, Miller SB. Effects of potassium on blood pressure in salt sensitive and salt-resistant black adolescents. Hypertension 1999; 34:181–186.

118. Whelton PK, He J, Cutler JA, Brancati FL, Appel LJ, Follmann D, Klag MJ. Effects of oral potassium on

blood pressure. Meta-analysis of randomized controlled clinical trials. J Am Med Assoc 1997; 277:1624–1632.

119. Freis ED. Age and antihypertensive medication (hydrochlorothiazide, bendroflumethiazide, nadolol and captopril). Am J Cardiol 1988; 61:117–121.

120. Veterans Administration Cooperative Study Group on Antihypertensive Drugs. Comparison of propranolol and hydrochlorothiazide for the initial treatment of hypertension. I. Results of short term titration with emphasis on racial differences in response. J Am Med Assoc 1982; 248:1996–2003.

121. Moser M, Lunn J. Responses to captopril and hydrochlorothiazide in black patients with hypertension. Clin Pharmacol Ther 1982; 32:307–312.

122. Sareli P, Radevski IV, Valtchanova ZP, Libhaber E, Candy GP, Den Hond E, Libhaber C, Skudicky D, Wang JG, Staessen JA. Efficacy of different drug classes used to initiate antihypertensive treatment in black subjects: results of a randomized trial in Johannesburg, South Africa. Arch Intern Med 2001; 161:965–971.

123. Sica DA. Rationale for fixed-dose combinations in the treatment of hypertension: the cycle repeats. Drugs 2002; 62:443–462.

124. Veterans Administration Cooperative Study Group on Antihypertensive Agents. Effects of treatment on morbidity in hypertension. II. Results in patients with diastolic blood pressure averaging 90 through 114 mm Hg. J Am Med Assoc 1970; 213:1143–1152.

125. Hypertension Detection and Follow Up Program Cooperation Group. Five-year findings of the Hypertension Detection and follow up program. I. Reduction in mortality of patients with high blood pressure, including mild hypertension. J Am Med Assoc 1979; 242:2562–2571.

126. Walker WG, Neaton JD, Cutler JA, Neuwirth R, Cohen JD. Renal function change in hypertensive members of the Multiple Risk Factor Intervention Trial: racial and treatment effects. J Am Med Assoc 1992; 268:3085–3091.

127. Levy D, Garrison RJ, Savage DD, Kannel WB, Castelli WP. Prognostic implications of echocardiographically determined left ventricular mass in the Framingham Heart Study. N Engl J Med 1990; 322:1561–1566.

128. Klingbeil AU, Schneider M, Martus P, Messerli FH, Schmieder RE. A meta-analysis of the effects of treatment on left ventricular mass in essential hypertension. Am J Med 2003; 115:41–46.

129. Moser M, Setaro JF. Antihypertensive drug therapy and regression of left ventricular hypertrophy: a review with a focus on diuretics. Eur Heart J 1991; 12:1034–1039.

130. Dahlof B, Pennert K, Hansson L. Reversal of left ventricular hypertrophy in hypertensive patients. A meta-analysis of 109 treatment studies. Am J Hypertens 1992; 5:95–110.

131. Schmieder RE, Martus P, Klingbeil A. Reversal of left ventricular hypertrophy in essential hypertension. J Am Med Assoc 1996; 275:1507–1513.

132. Hansson L, Zanchetti A, Carruthers SG, Dahlof B, Elmfeldt D, Julius S, Menard J, Rahn KH, Wedel H, Westerling S. Effect of intensive blood-pressure lowering and low-dose aspirin in patients with hypertension: principal results of the Hypertension Optimal Treatment (HOT) randomised trial. Lancet 1998; 351:1755–1762.

133. Frishman WH, Bryzinski BS, Coulson LR, DeQuattro VL, Vlachakis ND, Mroczek WJ, Dukart G, Goldberg JD, Alemayehu D, Koury K. A multifactorial trial design to assess combination therapy in hypertension: treatment with bisoprolol and hydrochlorothiazide. Arch Intern Med 1994; 154:1461–1468.

134. Moser M. Why are physicians not prescribing diuretics more frequently in the management of hypertension? J Am Med Assoc 1998; 270:1813–1816.

135. Verdecchia P, Reboldi G, Angeli F, Borgioni C, Gattobigio R, Filippucci L, Norgiolini S, Bracco C, Porcellati C. Adverse prognostic significance of new diabetes in treated hypertensive subjects. Hypertension 2004; 43:963–969.

136. Ayus JC. Diuretic-induced hyponatremia. Arch Intern Med 1986; 146:1295–1296.

137. Chow KM, Szeto CC, Wong TY, Leung CB, Li PK. Risk factors for thiazide-induced hyponatraemia. QJM 2003; 96:911–917.

138. Ashraf N, Locksley R, Arieff AI. Thiazide-induced hyponatremia associated with death or neurologic damage in outpatients. Am J Mcd 1981; 70:1163–1168.

139. Szatalowicz VL, Miller PD, Lacher JW, Gordon JA, Schrier RW. Comparative effect of diuretics on renal water excretion in hyponatraemic oedematous disorders. Clin Sci (Lond) 1982; 62:235–238.

140. Sonnenblick M, Friedlander Y, Rosin AJ. Diuretic-induced severe hyponatremia. Review and analysis of 129 reported patients. Chest 1993; 103:601–606.

141. Gross P, Reimann D, Neidel J, Doke C, Prospert F, Decaux G, Verbalis J, Schrier RW. The initial treatment of severe hyponatremia. Kidney Int Suppl 1998; 64:S6–S11.

142. Decaux G, Soupart A. Treatment of symptomatic hyponatremia. Am J Med Sci 2004; 326:25–30.

143. Morgan DB, Davidson C. Hypokalemia and diuretics: an analysis of publications. Br Med J 1980; 280:905–908.

144. Khuri RN, Strieder WN, Giebisch G. Effects of flow rate and potassium intake on distal tubular potassium transfer. Am J Physiol 1975; 228:1249–1261.

145. Velazquez H, Wright FS. Control by drugs of renal potassium handling. Ann Rev Pharmacol Toxicol 1986; 26:293–309.

146. Holland OB, Nixon JV, Kuhnert L. Diuretic-induced ventricular ectopic activity. Am J Med 1981; 70:762–768.

147. MacMahon S, Collins G, Rautaharju P, Cutler J, Neaton J, Prineas R, Crow R, Stamler J. Electrocardiographic left ventricular hypertrophy and effects of antihypertensive drug therapy in hypertensive patients in the Multiple Risk Factor Intervention Trial. Am J Cardiol 1989; 63:202–210.

148. Madias J, Madias N, Gavras H. Nonarrhythmogenicity of diuretic-induced hypokalemia: Its evidence in patients with uncomplicated essential hypertension. Arch Intern Med 1984; 144:2171–2176.

149. Medical Research Council, Working Party on Mild to Moderate Hypertension. Ventricular extrasystole during thiazide treatment: substudy of MRC Mild Hypertension Trial. Br Med J 1983; 287:1249–1253.

150. Kafka H, Langevin L, Armstrong P. Serum magnesium and potassium in acute myocardial infarction: influences on ventricular arrhythmia. Arch Intern Med 1987; 147:465–469.

151. Packer M. Potential role of potassium as a determinant of morbidity and mortality in patients with systemic hypertension and congestive heart failure. Am J Cardiol 1990; 65:45E–51E.

152. Dargie HJ, Cleland JG, Leckie BJ, Inglis CG, East BW, Ford I. Relation of arrhythmias and electrolyte abnormalities to survival in patients with severe chronic heart failure. Circulation 1987; 75:IV98–IV107.

153. Macdonald JE, Struthers AD. What is the optimal serum potassium level in cardiovascular patients? J Am Coll Cardiol 2004; 43:155–161.

154. Sica DA, Struthers AD, Cushman WC, Wood M, Banas JS Jr, Epstein M. Importance of potassium in cardiovascular disease. J Clin Hypertens 2002; 4:198–206.

155. Kaplan NM, Carnegie A, Raskin P, Heller JA, Simmons M. Potassium supplementation in hypertensive patients with diuretic-induced hypokalemia. N Engl J Med 1985; 312:746–749.

156. Siscovick DS, Raghunathan TE, Psaty BM, Koepsell TD, Wicklund KG, Lin X, Cobb L, Rautaharju PM, Copass MK, Wagner EH. Diuretic therapy and the risk of primary cardiac arrest. N Engl J Med 1994; 330:1852–1857.

157. Cooper HA, Dries DL, Davis CE, Shen YL, Domanski MJ. Diuretics and risk of arrhythmic death in patients with left ventricular dysfunction. Circulation 1999; 100:1311–1315.

158. Sica DA, Gehr TWB, Yancy C. Hyperkalemia, congestive heart failure, and aldosterone receptor antagonism. Congest Heart Fail 2003; 9:224–229.

159. Cannon PJ, Heinemann HO, Albert MS, Laragh JH, Winters RW. "Contraction" alkalosis after diuresis of edematous patients with ethacrynic acid. Ann Intern Med 1965; 62:979–990.

160. Loon NR, Wilcox CS, Nelson R, Mounts M. Metabolic alkalosis impairs the response to bumetanide. Kidney Int 1988; 33:200A.

161. O'Connell JE, Colledge NR. Type IV renal tubular acidosis and spironolactone therapy in the elderly. Postgrad Med J 1993; 69:887–889.

162. Kroenke K, Wood DR, Hanley JF. The value of serum magnesium determination in hypertensive patients receiving diuretics. Arch Intern Med 1987; 147:1553–1556.

163. Petri M, Cumber P, Grimes L, Treby D, Bryant R, Rawlins D, Ising H. The metabolic effects of thiazide therapy in the elderly: a population study. Age Aging 1986; 15:151–155.

164. Whang R, Oei TO, Aikawa JK, Watanabe A, Vannatta J, Fryer A, Markanich M. Predictors of clinical hypomagnesemia, hypokalemia, hypophosphatemia, hyponatremia, and hypocalcemia. Arch Intern Med 1984; 144:1794–1796.

165. Dyckner T, Wester PO. Effects of magnesium infusions in diuretic induced hyponatraemia. Lancet 1981; 1:585–586.

166. Sica DA, Frishman WH, Cavusoglu E. Magnesium, potassium, and calcium as potential cardiovascular disease therapies. In: Frishman W, Sonnenblick E, Sica DA, eds. Cardiovascular Pharmacotherapeutics. New York: McGraw-Hill, 2003:177–190.

167. Saris NE, Mervaala E, Karppanen H, Khawaja JA, Lewenstam A. Magnesium. An update on physiological, clinical, and analytical aspects. Clin Chim Acta 2000; 294:1–26.

168. Chen WC, Fu XX, Pan ZJ, Qian SZ. ECG changes in early stage of magnesium deficiency. Am Heart J 1982; 104:1115–1116.

169. Kingston ME, Al'Siba'i MB, Skooge WC. Clinical manifestations of hypomagnesemia. Crit Care Med 1986; 14:950–954.

170. Reinhart RA. Magnesium metabolism: a review with special reference to the relationship between intracellular content and serum levels. Arch Int Med 1988; 148:2415–2420.

171. Rob PM, Dick K, Bley N, Seyfert T, Brinckmann C, Hollriegel V, Friedrich HJ, Dibbelt L, Seelig MS. Can one really measure magnesium deficiency using the short-term magnesium loading test? J Intern Med 1999; 246:373–378.

172. Ljunghall S, Backman U, Danielson BG, Fellstrom B, Johansson G, Odlind B, Wikstrom B. Effects of bendroflumethiazide on urate metabolism during treatment of patients with renal stones. J Urol 1982; 127:1207–1210.

173. Sica DA, Schoolwerth A. Renal handing of organic anions and cations and renal excretion of uric acid. In: Brenner B, Rector F, eds. The Kidney. 7th ed. Philadelphia, PA: WB Saunders, 2004:637–662.

174. Young JL Jr, Boswell RB, Nies AS. Severe allopurinol hypersensitivity. Association with thiazides and prior renal compromise. Arch Intern Med 1974; 134:553–558.

175. Gurwitz JH, Kalish SC, Bohn RL, Glynn RJ, Monane M, Mogun H, Avorn J. Thiazide diuretics and the initiation of anti-gout therapy. J Clin Epidemiol 1997; 50:953–959.

176. Adverse reactions to bendrofluazide and propranolol for the treatment of mild hypertension. Report of Medical Research Council Working Party on Mild to Moderate Hypertension. Lancet 1981; 2:539–543.

177. Furman BL. Impairment of glucose intolerance produced by diuretics and other drugs. Pharmacol Ther 1981; 12:613–649.

178. Dornhorst A, Powell SH, Pensky J. Aggravation by propranolol of hyperglycaemic effect of hydrochlorothiazide in type II diabetics without alteration of insulin secretion. Lancet 1985; 1:123–126.

179. Sowers JR, Bakris GL. Antihypertensive therapy and the risk of type 2 diabetes mellitus. N Engl J Med 2000; 342:969–970.

180. Ramsay LE, Yeo WW, Jackson PR. Influence of diuretics calcium antagonists and α-blockers on insulin sensitivity and glucose tolerance in hypertensive patients. J Cardiovasc Pharmacol 1992; 20:S49–S53.

181. Gress TW, Nieto FJ, Shahar E, Wofford MR, Brancati FL. Hypertension and antihypertensive therapy as risk factors for type 2 diabetes mellitus. N Engl J Med 2000; 342:905–912.

182. Ruppert M, Overlack A, Kolloch R, Kraft K, Gobel B, Stumpe KO. Neurohormonal and metabolic effects of severe and moderate salt restriction in non-obese normotensive adults. J Hypertens 1993; 11:743–749.

183. Mantel-Teeuwisse AK, Kloosterman JM, Maitland-van der Zee AH, Klungel OH, Porsius AJ, de Boer A. Drug-Induced lipid changes: a review of the unintended effects of some commonly used drugs on serum lipid levels. Drug Saf 2001; 24:443–456.

184. Lakshman MR, Reda DJ, Materson BJ, Cushman WC, Freis ED. Diuretics and β blockers do not have adverse effects at 1 year on plasma lipid and lipoprotein profiles in men with hypertension. Arch Intern Med 1999; 159:551–558.

185. Kasiske BL, Ma JZ, Kalil RS, Louis TA. Effects of antihypertensive therapy on serum lipids. Ann Intern Med 1995; 122:133–141.

186. Bansal S. Sexual dysfunction in hypertensive men. A critical review of the literature. Hypertension 1998; 12:1–10.

187. Grimm RH Jr, Grandits GA, Prineas RJ, McDonald RH, Lewis CE, Flack JM, Yunis C, Svendsen K, Liebson PR, Elmer PJ. Long-term effects on sexual function of five antihypertensive Drugs and Nutritional Hygienic Treatment in hypertensive Men and Women. Treatment of Mild Hypertension Study (TOMHS). Hypertension 1997; 29:8–14.

188. Chang SW, Fine R, Siegel D, Chesney M, Black D, Hulley SB. The impact of diuretic therapy on reported sexual function. Arch Intern Med 1991; 151:2402–2408.

189. Wassertheil-Smoller S, Blaufox MD, Oberman A, Davis BR, Swencionis C, Knerr MO, Hawkins CM, Langford HG. Effect of antihypertensives on sexual function and quality of life: the TAIM study. Arch Intern Med 1991; 114:613–620.

190. Kloner RA, Brown M, Prisant LM, Collins M. Effect of sildenafil in patients with erectile dysfunction taking antihypertensive therapy. Sildenafil Study Group. Am J Hypertens 2001; 14:70–73.

191. Spironolactone and endocrine dysfunction. Ann Intern Med 1976; 85:630–636.

192. Williams GH, Burgess E, Kolloch RE, Ruilope LM, Niegowska J, Kipnes MS, Roniker B, Patrick JL, Krause SL. Efficacy of eplerenone versus enalapril as monotherapy in systemic hypertension. Am J Cardiol 2004; 93:990–996.

193. Addo HA, Ferguson J, Frain Bell. Thiazide-induced photosensitivity: a study of 33 subjects. Br J Dermatol 1987; 116:749–760.

194. Diffey BL, Langtry J. Phototoxic potential of thiazide diuretics in normal subjects. Arch Dermatol 1989; 125:1355–1358.

195. Frommer JP, Wesson DE, Eknoyan G. Side effects and complications of diuretic therapy. In: Eknoyan G, Martinez-Maldonado M, eds. The Physiological Basis of Diuretic Therapy in Clinical Medicine. Orlando, FL: Grune & Stratton, 1986:293–309.

196. Schwarz A, Krause PH, Kunzendorf U, Keller F, Distler A. The outcome of acute interstitial nephritis: Risk factors for the transition from acute to chronic interstitial nephritis. Clin Nephrol 2000; 54:179–190.

197. Magil AB, Ballon HS, Cameron EC, Rae A. Acute interstitial nephritis associated with thiazide diuretics. Clinical and pathologic observations in three cases. Am J Med 1980; 69:939–943.

198. Grossman E, Messerli FH, Goldbourt U. Does diuretic therapy increase the risk of renal cell carcinoma? Am J Cardiol 1999; 83:1090–1093.

199. Tenenbaum A, Grossman E, Fisman EZ, Adler Y, Boyko V, Jonas M, Behar S, Motro M, Reicher-Reiss H. Long-term diuretic therapy in patients with coronary disease: increased colon cancer-related mortality over a 5-year follow up. J Hum Hypertens 2001; 15:373–379.

200. Grossman E, Messerli FH, Goldbourt U. Carcinogenicity of cardiovascular drugs. Curr Hypertens 1999; Rep 1:212–218.

201. Lawson DH, Macadam RF, Singh MH, Gavras H, Hartz S, Turnbull D, Linton AL. Effect of furosemide on antibiotic-induced renal damage in rats. J Infect Dis 1972; 126:593–600.

202. Shapiro S, Slone D, Lewis GP, Jick H. The epidemiology of digoxin toxicity. A study in three Boston hospitals. J Chronic Dis 1969; 22:361–371.

203. Petersen V, Hvidt S, Thomsen K, Schou M. Effect of prolonged thiazide treatment on renal lithium clearance. Br Med J 1974; 3:143–145.

204. Boer WH, Loomans HA, Dorhout Mees EJ. Effects of thiazides with and without carbonic-anhydrase inhibiting activity on free water and lithium clearance. In: Puschett J, Greenberg A, eds. Diuretics III: Chemistry, Pharmacology, and Clinical Applications. New York: Elsevier Science Publishing, 1990:31–33.

205. Shirley DG, Walter SJ, Sampson B. A micropuncture study of renal lithium reabsorption: effects of amiloride and furosemide. Am J Physiol 1992; 263:F1128–1133.

206. Favre L, Glasson P, Vallotton MB. Reversible acute renal failure from combined triamterene and indomethacin: a study in healthy subjects. Ann Intern Med 1982; 96:317–320.

27

β-Adrenergic Receptor Blockers in Hypertension

NIALL S. COLWELL, MICHAEL B. MURPHY
University College Cork, Cork, Ireland

KEYPOINTS

- β-blockers have an extensive and largely affirmative track record in the management of hypertension.
- Trial evidence and meta-analyses show that β-blockers are on average, as effective as other classes of antihypertensives at lowering blood pressure.
- β-blockers are potent cardiovascular preventative agents, which are under-utilized, perhaps because of undue focus on surrogate, rather than clinical cardiovascular end-points in trials (19).
- Newer third generation β-blockers may have a lower side effect profile conferring improved compliance. These, together with adjuvant actions, for example, anti-proliferative effects, NO release, and so on, may confer additional benefits, though further clinical evidence in hypertension is awaited.

SUMMARY

Beta-adrenergic receptor antagonists (β-blockers) have a long and distinguished history, in the effective management of hypertension. The JNC VI and VII guidelines cite diuretics and β-blockers as first choice agents in the initial therapy of hypertension. European guidelines allow for more latitude in allowing the selection of the agent appropriate to the clinical setting.

Nonselective β-blocker may be associated with more side effects than newer antihypertensive therapies (e.g., ARBs), but the advent of more cardioselective β-blockers with ancilliary properties and lower side effect profiles have redressed this imbalance to a considerable extent. Although they are effective antihypertensives, their indication for use is enhanced by the presence of other conditions requiring β-blocker therapy in addition to hypertension. These indications include postmyocardial infarction, systolic and diastolic heart failure, hypertrophic cardiomyopathy, arrhythmias, palpitations, tremor, migraine, diabetes, perioperatively, noncritical peripheral vascular disease, and in those at high cardiovascular risk including diabetics.

Meta-analyses have shown no substantive difference between the various classes of cardiovascular drugs commonly used in hypertension at reducing cardiovascular end-points. Future meta-analyses addressing the blood pressure independent effects of antihypertensive drug classes are awaited with interest.

The ability to administer β-blockers either orally or intravenously, to have ultra-short to long-acting agents, and β-adrenergic antagonists with a range of ancillary properties, broadens the armamentarium of the clinician. In clinical trials and other studies, β-blockers have been used as initial therapy or as add-on treatment to effectively lower blood pressure and have been shown to significantly reduce cardiovascular events. When β-blockers have been compared with other agents in meta-analyses they have shown equal antihypertensive efficacy. In the case of the MRC trials however, diuretics were superior to β-blockade, and in hypertensive patients with ECG evidence of left ventricular hypertrophy, losartan was superior to atenolol. Therefore, β-blockers may not always be regarded as first-line treatment of hypertension when compared with diuretics or losartan in these clinical settings. Nevertheless, trials of β-blockers in hypertension included both young and older patients, men and women, and in aggregate with diuretics showed a 38% reduction in fatal/nonfatal strokes, whereas studies that used β-blocker based treatment reduced stroke 29%.

The majority of patients with hypertension will require more than one drug treatment to achieve blood pressure goals (57), especially in patients with diabetes and renal disease. β-blockers can be used with all other classes of antihypertensives, especially diuretics and dihydropyridine calcium channel blockers. Concerns about metabolic surrogate end-points and the higher side effect profile of nonselective β-blockers compared with newer antihypertensives have led some to question their leading role in

hypertension management. But the advent of newer more cardioselective agents with a lower overall side effect profile has largely redressed this imbalance. β-blockers remain an important, inexpensive, and effective therapeutic class in the physician's armamentarium in controlling hypertension.

I. INTRODUCTION

Hypertension is a leading risk factor for cardiovascular diseases, which cause $\sim$40% of deaths annually in the developed world. Approximately 1 billion people are considered to have hypertension worldwide. Blood pressure reduction significantly lowers cardiovascular events, but despite this only 34% of subjects with hypertension are adequately controlled in the United States and figures from other countries are no better.

Consequently, the use of combination therapy in the majority of patients with hypertension is required to achieve satisfactory blood pressure reductions. In six large randomized controlled trials of antihypertensive therapy, between 2.5 and 4 drugs were needed per patient to control hypertension.

Compelling indications for the use of β-blockade according to JNC VII guidelines include patients who are post-MI, or in heart failure, those with diabetes mellitus, and those at otherwise high cardiovascular risk (1).

β-Receptor antagonists have a long and distinguished history in the treatment of hypertension (2). Many reviews are written on the subject (3,4), and the primary focus of this chapter is to give an overview of the current role of β-blockers in the management of hypertension.

A. What are β-Blockers?

β-Blockers are reversible inhibitors of β-adrenergic receptors, and so block the effects of cathecolamines (e.g., adrenaline and noradrenaline) and pharmacologic agents (isoprenaline) by inhibiting their binding to the receptor.

II. HISTORY

Cathecolamines are neurohormonal agonists that transmit their signals to cells by reversibly binding to cell-surface β-adrenergic receptors. A seminal breakthrough in our understanding of the adrenergic nervous system was work performed by Ahlquist (5) in 1948 in which he demonstrated the existence of two forms of cathecolamine receptor termed alpha (α) and beta (β). These receptors mediated the effects of cathecolamines by transducing a signal into the cell. In his work, Ahlquist noted that the order of potency of cathecolamines in eliciting smooth muscle *contraction* was noradrenaline > adrenaline > isoprenaline and he termed these effects "alpha." Whereas smooth muscle *relaxation*, cardiac chronotropy and inotropy were elicited by a cathecolamine order of potency of isoprenaline > adrenaline > noradrenaline. These effects were ascribed to a different set of receptors termed "beta." Thus, he postulated the existence of two types of adrenergic receptors based on the patterns of cathecolamine agonist specificity. An important criterion of a specific receptor-mediated event is the selectivity of blockade by an antagonist. This led to the discovery of dichloroisoproterenol (a partial agonist) and later to the first therapeutic *β*-blocker propranolol by Black in 1962. *β*-Receptors were further classified as *β*1 or *β*2; the former predominate in the heart, whereas the latter in bronchi and blood vessels. The discovery of propranalol opened the vista of *β*-blockers in therapeutic medicine. The search by pharmaceutical companies for cardioselective (*β*1 > *β*2) blockade followed, and numerous agents came on to the market with varying properties. They were originally used to treat angina and tachyarrhythmias. Later their effect on the treatment of hypertension was elucidated.

A. Mode of Action

β-Blockers are reversible antagonists of 7-transmembrane *β*-receptors, and prevent binding of their physiologic agonists noradrenaline and adrenaline. On binding their physiologic ligand, *β*-receptors undergo a conformational change and activate G-proteins. Upstream negative regulators of *β*-receptors include the *β*-Arrestins and G-protein-coupled receptor kinase, whereas the downstream effector is Gs, which stimulates adenyl cyclase. This enzyme converts ATP into cAMP, a pivotal second messenger involved in the activation of protein kinases. Thence *β*-adrenergic receptors are members of the G-protein-coupled receptor super-family, linked to kinases (6). G-protein-coupled receptor kinase functions to uncouple the *β*-adrenergic receptor and thus deactivate this signaling cascade (7). In models of hypertension, there are alterations in *β*-receptor density and responsiveness. *β*-Adrenoreceptors have been cloned (8) and knockout mice have been constructed. Mice deficient in *β*-adrenoreceptors are predisposed to obesity.

β-Adrenoreceptor blocking drugs are characterized by their binding affinity to *β*-adrenergic receptors. Blockade prevents these receptors from binding their endogenous ligands (adrenaline and noradrenaline) at drug concentrations that generally do not cause substantive side effects. In doing so, *β*-blockers avert the desensitization and down-regulation of *β*$_1$-receptors in conditions such as heart failure. They block renin release, which contributes to their antihypertensive effect.

In general, *β*-blockers have a relatively flat dose-response curve, such that the response to twice daily low-dose propranolol and atenolol is approaching the antihypertensive effect of higher doses of the same medicines (9). At usually prescribed doses, the antihypertensive effects of *β*-blockers are similar, but the effect is additive to that of low-dose diuretics. Thence the combination of low-dose bisoprolol and hydrochlorthiazide is an effective antihypertensive with minimal adverse metabolic effects associated with higher doses of either agent alone (10).

The half-life of many *β*-blockers is such that they may not provide 24 h blood pressure coverage. This may lead to the unopposed surge of blood pressure on awakening, a time when acute cardiovascular events are more prevalent. Metoprolol and acebutolol blunted this rise in blood pressure, whereas atenolol and pindolol did not (11).

Although the molecular mechanism of *β*-blocker action is substantially understood, the means by which blood pressure reduction is achieved is more complex. Factors involved in lowering blood pressure include a reduction in heart rate (negative chronotropy) and stroke volume (negative inotropy). This leads to a fall in cardiac output by ~15–20% (except with pindolol due to high ISA), which combined with decreased renin release, central sympathetic output, presynaptic blockade, and altered peripheral vascular resistance may lower blood pressure further.

The effect of the oral agents is not immediate, due in part to counter-regulatory mechanisms and alteration in peripheral vascular resistance. Moreover, nonvasodilating *β*-blockers initially raise peripheral vascular resistance, which changes over time, so that chronically peripheral vascular resistance may be reduced. Cathecolamine levels in the setting of *β*-blockade are increased because of reduced drug clearance and baroreflex-mediated sympathetic activation.

The effects of *β*-blockade include reduction in exercise and anxiety-related tachycardia, with a reduction in tremor due to anxiety, hypoglycemia, and thyrotoxicosis. Conversely, because of the blockade of *β*$_2$-receptors *β*-blockers generally and non-selective agents in particular may have ancillary or unwanted effects. These include bronchoconstriction and exacerbation of asthma, hypoglycemia due to reduced gluconeogenesis, vivid dreams, and hallucinosis. Another potential drawback of *β*-blockade in middle age (45–64 years) is the potential to increase the risk of developing diabetes, an increase of 28%, when compared with ACE inhibitors, low-dose thiazides, and calcium channel blockers (12).

However, not all *β*-blockers are the same in their effect on disease states. For example, carvedilol was superior to metoprolol in the COMET heart failure study (13) and metoprolol was superior to atenolol in preventing sudden cardiac death (14).

B. β-Blocker Classification

Classification may be according to relative β-receptor selectivity, solubility, antagonist action, duration of action, and the presence of adjunctive actions (15).

β-Blockers can be *selective* or *nonselective* depending on their relative selectivity for β_1 as opposed to β_2 receptors. Currently nebivolol has the highest β_1 selectivity, whereas propranolol is the prototype agent for non-selective β-blockers. β_2-receptors occur in the peripheral circulation, the bronchi, and the pancreas. As no cardio-selective β-blocker is absolutely specific for β_1-receptors, the potential for β_2-receptor binding and side effects are present, especially at higher doses. This can lead to bronchospasm through β_2-receptor blockade in bronchi, vasoconstriction from β_2 blockade in peripheral vessels, which can exacerbate peripheral vascular disease, especially given the drop in cardiac output and reduction in limb blood flow mediated by β_1-receptor blockade. Moreover, β-blockers by masking the symptoms of hypoglycemia can exacerbate the effect of insulin and oral hypoglycemic agents in this regard, and slow the recovery from hypoglcaemic episodes. These adverse effects are more likely with nonselective than selective agents.

β-blockers may also be classified based on physico-chemical properties as *hydrophilic* (atenolol and nadolol) or *lipophilic* (metoprolol and propranolol). Hydrophilic agents undergo less first-pass metabolism and therefore have more predictable steady-state levels than lipophilic counterparts. Hydrophilic agents avoid substantial first-pass metabolism and therefore have longer durations of action, and are less likely to cross the blood–brain barrier and cause CNS side effects. They are principally renally excreted and therefore, may require dose adjust-ment in patients with renal insufficiency. Lipophilic agents, such as metoprolol, propranolol, and labetalol undergo hepatic metabolism as compared to hydrophilic agents, atenolol, sotalol, and nadolol. Intermediate between these extremes is bisoprolol and celiprolol.

They may also be classified as pure antagonists or partial agonist with intrinsic sympathomimetic activity (ISA). Agents which are pure antagonists include meto-prolol, whereas agents with ISA include acebutalol and especially pindolol. There is little clinical end-point data to suggest that these agents confer a benefit over complete antagonists. They have a niche use in patients who may develop profound bradycardia or bronchospasm, because in the resting state they act as agonists, whereas when the sympathetic activity is high they act as antagonists. They may also be preferable in patients with peripheral vascular disease, diabetes, and dyslipidaemia.

Classification may be in terms of the duration of action of the β-blocker: ultra-short acting (Esmolol, $t_{1/2} = 9$ min), short-acting (metoprolol $t_{1/2} = 4$ h), intermediate (atenolol = 6–8 h), and long-acting agents [Acebutolol (diacetolol) = 12 h].

Adjunctive actions include alpha receptor antagonism (labetalol and carvedilol), nitric oxide release (nebivolol), vasodilator actions, antioxidant properties (carvedilol) and interaction with other targets such as the potassium channel antagonist activity of the (+) enantiomer of sotalol. Membrane stabilization effects of β-blockers tend to occur only at supra-therapeutic doses and are there-fore only of relevance in overdose situations.

C. β-Blockers have Additional Indications for Use Other Than Hypertension

It seems reasonable that where an ancillary condition exists which is amenable to treatment with β-blockade, in a patient who also has hypertension there should be heightened con-sideration for use of a β-blocker. A list of these indications is shown in Table 27.1. Some are approved indications, whereas other are unapproved (∗). Such is the importance of β-blockers as cardiovascular agents in the treatment of hypertension that they are included as "essential medicines" on the WHO Model list of drugs. β-Blockers are particularly useful in patients who have hypertension and are at high cardiovascular risk, such as those who are postmyocardial infarction, in congestive cardiac failure, with diabetes, and stable peripheral vascular disease.

D. Combined α and β-Receptor Blockers and Third Generation β-Blockers

These include labetalol, carvedilol, celiprolol, and nebivo-lol. Labetalol is lipohilic, rapidly absorbed, and is ∼33% bioavailable. Bioavailability increases with age. Carvedilol is rapidly absorbed and ∼25% bioavailable. Both are non-selective β-blockers which are given twice a day. Labetalol also blocks α-receptors but at a potency of 1:4 that of β-receptors, and carvedilol has a lesser α-receptor potency.

Labetalol is useful in treating malignant hypertension as it can be given intravenously for a rapid onset of action. It can also be used in treating hypertension in preg-nancy where first-line agents α-methyldopa and calcium channel blockers, such as nifedipine, are ineffective or not tolerated. It can be used orally to treat all grades of hypertension, for the treatment of angina with hyperten-sion, and for management of phaeochromocytoma or for a hypotensive effect during anesthesia.

Carvedilol has been shown to be superior to equivalent dose metoprolol in treating heart failure, and so has a niche use in hypertensives with congestive failure (13). It blocks β_1, β_2, and $\alpha 1$ receptors and has antioxidant and anti-atherosclerotic actions.

Nebivolol has a vasodilating effect in part attributable to NO release. It has a lesser bradyarrhythmic effect than pure β_1 receptor antagonists, such as atenolol, and

Table 27.1 Indications for *β*-Blocker Use

Cardiovascular

Hypertension: For most patients with hypertension use of a *β*-blocker for treatment is reasonable (16). Caution is needed, however, in patients who are suspected of having a phaeochromocytoma, in whom unopposed *α*-receptor stimulation in the presence of *β*-blockade could result in a hypertensive crisis.

Angina: *β*-Blockade is a mainstay symptomatic therapy for stable angina pectoris.

β-Blockade reduces re-infarction and ischemia and improves survival.

Acute coronary syndromes: Oral or intravenous *β*-blockade can be used in hospitalized acutely ill patients, that can then be up-titrated to maintain the resting heart rate between 50–60, provided there are no contraindications.

Myocardial infarction treatment and prophylaxis: Intravenous *β*-blockade has been shown to be effective in the setting of acute MI, whereas cardioselective lipophilic agents without ISA, such as metoprolol, are preferred for secondary prevention.

Treatment of tachyarrhythmias (Sinus Tachycardia, Supraventricular tachycardia, atrial flutter, atrial fibrillation and ventricular tachycardia): Rate control of atrial fibrillation as an approach to therapy in patients over 65 has been shown to be equivalent in outcome to an approach based on rhythm control.

Congestive heart failure (low-dose and titrate upward) Where formerly *β*-blockade was contraindicated in heart failure, now it is a standard treatment when carefully instituted. In studies with bisoprolol, extended-release metoprolol and carvedilol, *β*-blockade was shown to reduce all-cause mortality (34–35%); all-cause hospitalizations (18–20%), and sudden cardiac death (41–44%) in patients with heart failure (17). In the elderly with heart failure, nebivolol reduced mortality and morbidity (hospitalization) 14%.

Hypertrophic cardiomyopathy (with and without outflow obstruction): *β*-Blockers improve symptoms and exercise tolerance in hypertrophic cardiomyopathy, both with and without obstruction. Their main indication is for those with symptoms or with outflow gradients during exertion (18,19).

Diastolic dysfunction*

Prevention of sudden cardiac death: But is inferior to implantable cardioverter defibrillator.

Hypertensive crisis. Intravenous Labetalol is particularly suited for this purpose.

Hypotension induction* Labetalol has been used for this and intravenous esmolol in cases of aortic aneurysm prerupture.

Miscellaneous (19): Mitral valve prolapse, myocardial bridging, Long QT (20) syndrome, cathecolaminergic polymorphic ventricular tachycardia, in patients with a pacemaker or an implantable defibrillator.

Endocrine

Diabetes: Patients benefit from *β*-blockade if tolerated (21). Thyrotoxicosis: treats tachycardia and sympathetic symptoms, and a non-selective agent is preferable.

Phaeochromocytoma in addition to an *α*-blocker—to avoid unopposed *β*-receptor stimulation and hypertensive crisis.

CNS

Tremor*

Migraine: In the prophylaxis against migraine.

Anxiety: *β*-Blockers can be used to treat general anxiety disorder as a second-line therapeutic approach. They are useful in suppressing somatic symptoms especially tachycardia (22).

GI

Esohageal varices, prevention of bleeding (23).

Portal hypertension*

Ethanol withdrawal*

Ophthalmology

Glaucoma; used in treating open-angle glaucoma. There can be an additive effect of orally prescribed *β*-blockers to those prescribed topically for this purpose.

Surgery

Perioperatively in patients at high cardiovascular risk (24), and those suffering from burns (25).

Nephrology

Scleroderma renal crisis* and diabetic renal disease (26).

*Unapproved use of *β*-blockade.

therefore is less likely to induce heart block. Additionally, it has a mild pressor effect on standing when tested in patients >60 years after 5 min supine and 1 min standing. This could have an advantage in older patients who are more predisposed to orthosatic hypotension (26). Nebivolol is effective in treating heart failure in the elderly (27).

Celiprolol is a long-acting cardioselective *β*-blocker with vasodilator actions. It has β_2-receptor agonist activity and may act through nitric oxide release. Like other agents mentioned it has anti-inflammatoy effects and lacks the peripheral vasocontrictor effects of pure β_1-receptor antagonists (28). Certain foods and medication can affect its plasma concentration (29–31).

Other *β*-blockers with ancilliary actions include sotalol, which has type III antiarrhythmic activity and bucindolol, which has vasodilator actions and mild ISA activity.

Bucindolol unlike other β-blockers did not reduce mortality in heart failure (32) but reduced nonfatal myocardial infarction (33).

III. CHOOSING AND USING A β-BLOCKER

There are over a hundred manufactured β-blockers, over thirty of which are marketed world-wide (15). In general, a hydrophilic cardioselective β-blocker with intrinsic sympathomimetic activity is least likely to cause side effects. However, in high-risk patients or in those with known coronary heart disease the lipophilic cardioselective non-ISA agents confer the best protection, for example, metoprolol.

Co-morbid conditions influence the choice of β-blocker in hypertensive patients. β-blockers have a lesser degree of effectiveness in African-Americans, but the suggestion of decreased effectiveness in the elderly appears incorrect. The dose of β-blocker should be halved in the elderly. The elderly or those with minor conducting system abnormalities may be cautiously tried on low-dose β-blockade, and agents with a lesser bradycardic effect are preferred.

The clinical setting dictates the choice of β-blocker. In hospital, where a patient's condition may fluctuate, use of a shorter acting β-blocker such as metoprolol 25 mg three times daily is reasonable, as one may require to adjust therapy abruptly. In the outpatient setting, a longer acting agent or an extended release form of a short-acting variety is preferred (e.g., bisoprolol or metoprolol XL). Lipophilic agents are used in renal failure, whereas hydrophilic β-blockers are used in hepatic insufficiency.

If the blood pressure is elevated $>20/10$, combination therapy is indicated, and β-blockers can be usefully combined with a thiazide diuretic or a dihydropyridine calcium channel blocker. Supplying these combinations in a single pill is now feasible and likely improves compliance. For hypertensive emergencies, intravenous labetalol is effective and may be switched to oral therapy later.

It is usual to start with a low-dose of a β-blocker and titrate the dose upward, as this may achieve the desired effect and minimize adverse reactions. The choice of β-blocker is influenced by additional indications in addition to hypertension. For example, a patient with hypertension who is also prone to tachyarrythmias may derive benefit from sotalol. A β-blocker should be withdrawn gradually to avoid rebound hypertension, and caution must be exercised when used in conjunction with other bradyarrhythmic medications.

IV. SIDE EFFECTS

Side effects may be dose related or dose independent. The principal side effects, which often pertain to the cardio-respiratory system are listed in Table 27.2. Patients with chronic obstructive airways disease are not entirely excluded from therapy with β-blockade (34). Abrupt withdrawal of β-blockade should be avoided because of the risk of rebound hypertension, and precipitation of angina, myocardial infarction, or stroke.

Major side effects include, decrease in heart rate, AV nodal conduction and contractility can lead to severe bradycardia, sinus arrest, heart failure and advanced/complete heart block and in overdose asystole. Deaths have been reported in overdose (2).

In a setting where conduction abnormalities may arise, use of an agent with ISA activity or a third generation highly selective β-blocker, such a nebivolol, may lessen the likelihood of such events.

Central effects include insomnia, depression, nightmares, hallucinations, impotence, and fatigue, although

Table 27.2 β-Blocker Side Effects

System	Side effect
Cardiac	AV and SA block, angina, cardiac arrest, orthostatic hypotension, peripheral vasoconstriction, peripheral edema, exacerbate or precipitate heart failure. Relatively contraindicated in Wolff–Parkinson White and Bradycardia–Tachycardia syndromes
Dermatological	Alopecia, exfoliative dermatitis, pruritis
GI	Diarrhea, Dyspepsia, Abnormal LFTs, Jaundice, Hepatic necrosis, nausea, and vomiting
Respiratory	Dyspnoea, bronchospasm—avoid in asthma
CNS	Depression, dizziness, hallucinations, headache, nightmares, insomnia, parasthesiae
Rheumatological	Arthralgia, myalgia
Constitutional	Fatigue, diaphoresis, asthenia,
Ophthalmic	Xerosis, ocular irritation, lacrimation
Genitourinary	Impotence, decreased libido, priapism, ejaculatory dysfunction
Metabolic	Hyperglycemia, hypoglycemia
Hematologic	Agranulocytosis
Immunologic	Anaphylaxis: exacerbation of

the latter may be due to a reduction in cardiac output. In general, lipophilic *β*-blockers are more prone to central effects than hydrophilic agents.

Bronchoconstriction, due to *β*₂ receptor blockade, so that in general, these agents are contraindicated in patients with asthma. This is especially so for nonselective agents, although recent evidence suggests that the more cardioselective agents, for example, bisoprolol and nebivolol; may be used with caution in patients with mild reactive airways disease.

Nonselective agents may exacerbate symptoms in patients with peripheral vascular disease and Raynauds phenomenon. This is likely however, only in advanced disease and like patients with diabetes, patients with milder forms of peripheral vascular disease benefit from *β*-blockade. Patients should not be deprived of these agents unless there is a clear clinical indication to avoid them, such as critical limb ischemia.

Nonselective agents may mask the sympathetically mediated symptoms of hypoglycemia in diabetes mellitus and delay the recovery of blood sugar levels. This may result in hypoglycemic coma.

β-Blockers generally can exacerbate the hyperlipidaemic state. Nonselective agents raise triglycerides and lower HDL-cholesterol values.

β-Blockers with ISA tend to cause lesser or no effect, whereas Celiprolol may raise HDL-cholesterol.

A. Medical Conditions

Systemic side effects can influence CNS, peripheral circulation, lung, hepatic, and renal function. *β*-blockers can reduce sexual function and exercise capacity, alter mental state, skin, connective tissue, and electrolyte levels. Toxicity can result from overdose, abrupt cessation and drug–drug interaction, or allergy. *β*-Blocker withdrawal can exacerbate allergy to another agent.

B. Phaeochromocytoma

Caution is advised as there may be unopposed *α*-adrenergic stimulation and hypertensive crisis. Raynaud's phenomenon may be exacerbated especially by nonselective *β*-blockers. Prinzmetal angina may be worsened by *β*-blockers due to unopposed *α*-adrenergic stimulation. Rapid withdrawal of a *β*-blocker can result in rebound hypertension, angina, stroke, and myocardial infarction. If patients need to discontinue *β*-blockers, they should do so by weaning the therapy gradually over 7–10 days.

C. Pregnancy and Lactation

There have been few placebo-controlled trials with *β*-blockers in the treatment of hypertension in pregnancy.

The safety of *β*-blockers in pregnancy is questioned especially when given before 24 weeks gestation, as they are associated with intrauterine growth retardation (35). They are not associated with teratogenic effects. *β*-Blockade may be continued during delivery and cardioselective *β*-blockers without an effect on uterine contraction are preferred. Labetalol is of similar efficacy and maternal side effect profile to methyldopa. It is used as second-line oral therapy for hypertension in pregnancy and in hypertensive crises. Atenolol and metoprolol achieve higher levels in breast milk than labetalol and propranolol (36).

D. Overdose

Overdose has resulted in fatalities but usually responds to *β*-agonist therapy. Heart block, bradycardia, profound hypotension, seizures, and coma can occur.

Of historical interest is that practolol predisposed to cataracts and xamoterol, which was used in heart failure treatment, increased mortality when compared with controls, probably because of its high intrinsic sympathomimmetic activity. Therefore, one should use agents with intrinsic sympathomimmetic activity in patients with known coronary disease with caution. Moreover, unlike bisoprolol, metoprolol, and carvedilol, bucindolol failed to reduce cardiovascular end-points in heart failure underscoring the principle that not all *β*-blockers are of equal benefit.

Overall tolerability of *β*-blocker is reasonable, but up to 16% of patients in a recent study reported symptoms with *β*-blockers, half of which were avoidable or ameliorable (37). Erectile dysfunction after *β*-blockade may not be as common as previously suggested. Recently it was found that erectile dysfunction is related to knowledge of side effects and is reversed by placebo (38).

V. DRUG–DRUG INTERACTIONS (39)

Aluminum and bile acid sequestrants can reduce *β*-blocker absorption. *β*-Blocker metabolism may be altered by certain drugs. Cimetidine decreases first-pass metabolism of propranolol and may increase plasma concentrations fourfold.

Other drugs influencing propranolol metabolism includes flecainide, propafenone (increases metoprolol levels twofold), quinidine, and tricyclic antidepressants, fluoxetine, paroxetine, and fluvoxamine. Conversely drugs concentrations may be altered by *β*-blockers; these drugs include antiarrhythmics (flecanide, lignocaine, and dihydropyridine calcium channel blockers (nifedipine and nisoldipine).

Special caution is advised against the use of *β*-blockers with nondihydropyridine calcium channel blockers, such as verapamil and diltiazem, because of the risk of complete heart block, especially in patients with conduction abnormalities, left ventricular dysfunction, and the elderly.

Hypoglycemic agents: Nonselective agents are more prone to cause a fall in blood glucose than selective β-blockers. β-blockers can mask the symptoms of hypoglycemia and delay the recovery from it.

General anesthetic agents: Some agents can have an additive negative inotropic effect in combination with β-blockade (e.g., cyclopropane, diethyl ether, and methoxyflurane) and anesthetists need to take this into account at induction.

Favorable interactions include the combination of a β-blocker with a low-dose thiazide diuretic or a dihydropyridine calcium channel blocker in treating hypertension.

VI. TRIAL EVIDENCE FOR β-BLOCKER USE IN HYPERTENSION

There are few large placebo-controlled β-blocker end-point trials in hypertension. Trials can be separated into primary and secondary prevention. A trial list is shown in Tables 27.3 and 27.4, with the penultimate four being meta-analyses and the final reference is a consensus document on β-blockade (Table 27.3).

A. Primary Prevention Trials: UKPDS, ANBP, MRC, HAPPHY, and IPPPSH

In general, β-blockers have a negative profile of surrogate end-points as they can increase glucose levels, insulin resistance, triglycerides, and body weight and decrease HDL and are often regarded as relatively contraindicated in diabetes mellitus (Table 27.2). However, this approach is largely debunked by the results of the UKPDS study of atenolol and captopril in control of hypertension in type II diabetes mellitus (19). In this 9 year primary prevention study of 1148 subjects with type II diabetes and hypertension, tight blood pressure control was favored over less tight control for any of the clinical end-points. But in the tight control group, the event rate for clinical end-points tended to be less in the atenolol compared with the

Table 27.3 Large End-Point Trials and Meta-analyses Involving β-Blockers in Hypertension, and a Recent Consensus Statement

AASK	African American Study of Kidney Disease and Hypertension 2002
ANBPS	Australian National Blood Pressure Study 1980–1984
ARIC	Atherosclerosis Risk In Communities 2000
ASCOT	Anglo-Scandanavian Cardiac Outcomes Trial 2003
BHAT	Beta Blocker Heart Attack Trial 1984
CAPPP	CAPTOPRIL PREVENTION PROJECT 1999
CONVINCE	Controlled Onset Verapamil Investigation of Cardiovascular Trial Endpoints Trial 2003
Coope and Warrender	Treatment of hypertension in elderly in primary care 1986
ELSA	European Lacidipine Study of Atherosclerosis 2000
HAPPHY	Heart Attack Primary Prevention in Hypertensives Trial 1987
HDS	Hypertension in Diabetes Study 1993
IPPPSH	International Prospective Primary Prevention Study in Hypertension 1985
INVEST	International Verapamil–Trandolopril Study 2003
LIFE	Losartan Intervention For Endpoint reduction in hypertension study 2002; LIFE Diabetic 2002; LIFE LVH 2002.
Metoprolol Atherosclerosis in Hypertensive Study	1988
MRC	MRC Trial of Treatment in Mild Hypertension 1985
MRC-O	MRC Trial of Treatment of Hypertension in older adults 1992
NORDIL	Nordic Diltiazem Study 2000
SAFE	Safety After Fifty Evaluation 1992
SHEP	Systolic hypertension in the elderly program 1991
STOP-HTN	Swedish Trial in Old Patients with Hypertension 1991
STOP-2	Swedish Trial in Old Patients with Hypertension 2 1998
TOMHS	Treatment of Mild Hypertension Study 1993
UKPDS	UK Prospective Diabetes Study Group 1998
BPLTTC1[a]	Blood Pressure Lowering Treatment Trialists' Collaboration 1 2000
BPLTTC2[a]	Blood Pressure Lowering Treatment Trialists' Collaboration 2 2003
Gueyffier[a]	1997
Psaty BM[a]	2003
ESC	ESC Expert Consensus Document on β-adrenergic Receptor Blockade 2004

[a]Meta-analyses.

Table 27.4 β-Blocker Trials in Hypertension

Trial	n, age, sex, BP	Trial design, Rx	End-point	Time (years)	Result	%RRR
ANBP	n = 3931 30–69 years M&F DBP >95 DBP <110 SBP <200	Randomized, prospective, SB, placebo-controlled, mild hypertension. CTZ 500 mg–1 g, pindolol propranolol, other	Fatal CVD or other nonfatal CVA, TIA MI, Angina CCF, AAARF, Eye	3	All + fatal TEP reduced	~30%
MRC	n = 17,354 35–64 years M&F DBP 90–109	Randomized Prospective, SB, placebo-controlled, bendrofluazide propranolol other (methldopa, guanethidine)	Stroke, Coronary All CVD	5	All CVD events decreased decrease in stroke in men and women on diuretic, not β-blocker	~40% stroke in both sexes
HAPPHY	n = 6569 40–64 years M DBP > 100	Comparison trial, not randomized atenolol or metoprolol vs. benrofluazide or hydrochlorthiazide Add hydralazine Spironolactone	Death MI Stroke	5	No difference CHD mortality or event rates	NS
IPPSH	n = 6357 M&F DBP 100–125	Double-blind randomized, prospective trial Oxprenolol vs. non-β-blocker therapy	MI, SCD. CVA. Effectiveness	4	No difference in outcome	NS
MAPHY	n = 3234 40–64 years M DBP > 100	Age stratified, randomized, open label, controlled primary prevention study metoprolol vs. diuretic	Death, sudden cardiac death, combined coronary events, stroke	5	Mortality lower for metoprolol than thiazide due to reduced risk of SCD	22% 1st coronary event; 35% SCD; 20% total mortality
STOP-HTN trial	n = 1627 70–84 years M&F SBP >180 DBP >90:or DBP >105	Atenolol HCTZ metoprolol pindolol	Stroke MI CV death	4	Reduced primary end-point CVA Total mortality	38% RR primary end-points
SHEP trial	n = 4736 Age >60 M&F SBP 160–219 DBP <90	Placebo-controlled diuretic, add atenolol, (reserpine)	Fatal, nonfatal stroke. Many secondary outcomes	>5	Reduced Stroke MI LVF CVD	36% for stroke; 27% overall CHD
MRC older	n = 4396 65–74 years M&F SBP 160–219 DBP <115	Randomized, prospective,SB, placebo-controlled amiloride/ HCTZ Atenolol +/−nifedipine	Death Stroke Coronary event	5.8	Benefits greater ++ with diuretic than β-blocker	Stroke 25% and all CV events 17%

(continued)

Table 27.4 *Continued*

Trial	n, age, sex, BP	Trial design, Rx	End-point	Time (years)	Result	%RRR
TOMHS	n = 902 Age 45–69 M&F DBP 90–99	Prospective, block randomization placebo-controlled, acebutolol (n = 132), chlorthalidone Doxazosin Amlodipine enalopril	Death from CHD; CVD; and all-causes. 11 Nonfatal end-points	4–5.5	All rx lowered BP No difference between rx	31% in combined events relative to placebo
VA Mono-Therapy	n = 1292 >21 years M DBP 95–109	Atenolol 25–100 Clonidine Captopril Diltiazem-SR Prazosin HCTZ	BP control Age race Obesity LVH regression Systolic function LA size Lipids Heart rate	4	Authors concluded HCTZ or atenolol is reasonable first choice agent to treat Hypertension	Less reduction in LVH with atenolol than HCTZ. Both at low doses had a side effect rate less than placebo
HOT	n = 18,790 50–80 years M&F DBP >100 <115	Felodipine +/− β-blocker ACE inhibitor +/− HCTZ Aim DBP <90; <85; <80 +/− low-dose ASA	Major CVD Events related to DBP	3.8	Maximum risk reduction achieved at DBP <85 ASA reduced risk of MI and MCE	15% major CVD by ASA. In all groups except females; 36% MI; 51% DM for DBP <80
BHAT	n = 3837 30–69 years M&F 40.8% HTN	Randomized prospective placebo-controlled trial of Propranolol Post-MI Secondary prevention	Total mortality, CHD mortality SCD Nonfatal MI + CHD death	3	Significant lowered total mortality and fatal event + nonfatal MI	Total mortality (26%) and CV. Events. In both HTN (31%) non-HTN (15%) groups
STOP HTN-2	n = 6614 70–84 years M&F DBP >104 SBP >179	Prospective intervention PROBE trial. Atenolol metoprolol CR pindolol Amiloride, CTZ vs. CCB or ACE inhibitor	Fatal CVD, fatal+ nonfatal CVD, DM, A. Fib, CHF	5	No difference in fatal events	No difference in total or CVD morbidity
LIFE	n = 9193 55–80 M&F BP: 160–200/95–115	Double-blind, randomized parallel group trial of losartan vs. atenolol. In patients who have ECG with LVH	CV death Nonfatal MI Nonfatal CVA	>4	Despite similar lowering BP Losartan reduced CVD events more than atenolol	25% reduction in stroke and 11% CVD for losartan. Reduction in new onset DM, and side effects

Note: M, male; F, female; TEP, trial end-points; SB, single-blind; CVD, cardiovascular disease; *n*, number; DBP, diastolic blood pressure; SBP, systolic blood pressure; CTZ, chlorthiazide; HCTZ, hydrochlorthiazide; CVA, cerebrovascular accident; TIA, transient ischaemic attack; MI, myocardial infarction; CCF, congestive cardiac failure; AAA, abdominal aortic aneurysm; RF, renal failure; SCD, sudden cardiac death; RRR, relative risk reduction; DM, diabetes mellitus; ASA, aspirin.

captopril group. Thus, it seems that the focus on surrogate end-points can be misleading and the clinical benefits of atenolol may be attributable to the antiarhythmic, antiatherosclerotic effects, and the inhibition of renin release by *β*-blockers. Additionally, a highly cardioselective *β*-blocker has a better effect on nocturnal dipping of blood pressure than less selective agents, which could add to their benefit (40).

Nonselective agents can block both β_1 and peripheral β_2 receptors in insulin dependent patients and cause a paradoxical increase in blood pressure due to unopposed alpha stimulation. Therefore in IDDM, highly β_1 selective agents are preferable to nonselective *β*-blockers.

A potential difficulty in current studies on hypertension is that they are of ethical necessity designed with a comparison therapeutic arm, but lack a placebo control group. Any difference between treatment arms may then suggest that one treatment is superior to another. But to obtain identical blood pressure reductions, which are accurately measured, throughout the 24 h period on each treatment is difficult. Differences may therefore be explained at least in part by small differences in blood pressure alone. The lack of a placebo arm can raise doubts as to the efficacy of *β*-blockers generally in hypertension, as there are few large prospective randomized end-point placebo-controlled studies of *β*-blockers in hypertension. Instead they were used in combination with other medications, especially thiazides. In the Australian National Blood Pressure Study (ANBP), chlorthiazide, pindolol, and propranolol (methyldopa, clonidine, and hydrallazine) were used (41). In this trial, a significant reduction in total trial end-points (stroke, MI, and other cardiovascular events) and fatal trial end-points was noted. A significant reduction in trial end-points was noted for men (67 events on treatment vs. 91; $P < 0.05$), women (24 on treatment vs. 36; $P < 0.044$), and for persons >50 years (69 vs. 96; $P < 0.025$).

The Medical Research Council trial showed a highly significant proportionate benefit in stroke reduction (42), but because a priori risk was low in the population, the absolute benefit was also low (NNT 850 to prevent one stroke). Although thiazide therapy faired better in reducing event rates than propranolol, the blood pressure lowering with the diuretic was superior to that of propranolol. Therefore, at least part of the explanation for the difference could be due to the effect of the drug on blood pressure. Interestingly, propranolol reduced stroke in nonsmokers but not in smokers; therefore, the reduced effect of propranolol may be due to its diminished effectiveness in smokers and/or to an interaction effect between propranolol and smoking. Smoking by increasing cathecolamines may increase blood pressure by unopposed *α*-adrenergic stimulation. A similar finding to this occurred in the IPPPSH trial but not in HAPPHY study, and may be due to *post hoc* subgroup analysis.

In the Heart Attack Primary Prevention in Hypertensives (HAPPHY) trial (43), the aim was to establish whether *β*-blockers were superior to thiazide diuretics in preventing nonfatal MI, mortality from CHD and total mortality in men at high risk of developing CHD. The result for the *β*-blocker (metoprolol and atenolol) was similar to the thiazide arm; an effect seen with oxprenolol in the International Primary Prevention Study in Hypertension (44).

Nevertheless, treatment arms in trials have yielded differences in outcome, which cannot readily be explained by differences in blood pressure. In the ALLHAT study (45), the doxazosin arm was withdrawn early because of an increased cardiovascular event rate when compared with an ACE inhibitor, diuretic, and calcium channel blocker. Germane to *β*-blockers, the LIFE study (46) showed that losartan for similar blood pressure lowering had a lower CV event rate when compared with atenolol in patients with ECG evidence for LVH. Substantial cerebrovascular benefit was obtained in patients across the spectrum of cardiovascular risk (47). Therefore, in patients with ECG evidence for LVH, it is reasonable to choose losartan in preference to atenolol.

In the Metoprolol Atherosclerosis in Hypertensives (MAPHY) primary prevention study (14), a significant effect was noted for treatment of men whose diastolic blood pressure was >100 mmHg with metoprolol compared to atenolol in prevention of sudden cardiac death. Additionally, as compared to atenolol in the MRC and HAPPHY studies (48), the metoprolol group had a significantly lower total or coronary mortality, and first coronary event rate than the thiazide-treated group.

In treatment of mild hypertension (TOMHS) (49), acebutolol 400 mg od/bd was well tolerated >4–5.5 years, but did not lower blood pressure in blacks as well as nonblacks. Nevertheless, treatment of blood pressure in this trial was effective at significantly lowering total cardiovascular events compared to placebo ($P < 0.031$).

In the AASK trial (50), ACE inhibition was found to be superior to metoprolol in slowing glomerular filtration rate decline in this African-American group, the authors suggest that *β*-blockers may be better than amlodipine in this regard, especially for those with minimal renal dysfunction ($P = 0.003$).

B. Secondary Prevention *β*-Blocker Trials or Those Including Patients with a Prior History of a Cardiovascular Event: STOP-Hypertension, SHEP, BHAT, ACTION

The STOP-Hypertension trial was a primary/secondary prevention trial in elderly men and women who had systo-diastolic hypertension (51). Treatment was either diuretic or *β*-blocker (metoprolol, atenolol, and pindolol) with addition of the other agents as needed. The active treatment groups had a significant reduction in primary end-point (stroke, MI, or other cardiovascular death), fatal and nonfatal stroke, and death compared with placebo. Similarly, the SHEP study, in which atenolol was added as a second-line agent to chlorthalidone in persons >60 years with systolic hypertension, showed a significant reduction in fatal and nonfatal strokes compared with placebo (52). In the MRC trial in older adults, amiloride/hydrochlorthiazide was compared with atenolol and each group with their placebo arm (53). Nifedipine was added if needed. The systolic blood pressure reduction was virtually identical for the diuretic and β-blocker, but the diastolic was reduced more in the diuretic arm. There was a significant increase in side effects compared with control (results per thousand patient years: dyspnoea (22.9 vs. 1.1), Raynaud's phenomenon (11.3 vs. 1.1), lethargy (19.1 vs. 2.0), headache (7.2 vs. 1.1), and dizziness (10.6 vs. 1.2) in the β-blocker. Side effects and withdrawal rate were greater for atenolol than the diuretic group. The benefits were also greater in the diuretic group for stroke, coronary event reduction, and decreasing all cardiovascular events.

In beta-blocker Heart Attack trial (BHAT), 40.8% of patients had a history of hypertension, 29.4% of participants had treated hypertension, and 11.4% untreated (54). In this prospective trial of men and women, postmyocardial infarction, all-cause mortality (AR reduction 1.2%; $P < 0.004$), cardiovascular (ARR 1.1%; $P < 0.009$) and atherosclerotic death (ARR 0.006; $P < 0.006$), and sudden death (ARR 0.6; $P < 0.04$) were significantly reduced by propranolol therapy compared with placebo. Additionally, coronary incidence was decreased (ARR 1.4; $P < 0.004$). Thus, there is a more potent reduction in cardiovascular events in this secondary prevention trial by β-blockade when compared with primary prevention studies. The benefit of β-blockers reducing cardiovascular events depends considerably on the a priori risk of the population studied. The cumulative mortality of hypertensives postmyocardial infarction treated with propranolol was significantly less than placebo but equivalent to the nonhypertensive placebo group and higher than the nonhypertensive treatment group. Therefore, the deleterious effect of hypertension was ameliorated by those taking propranolol. In the Action trial, 80% of subjects who were enrolled with stable angina pectoris were on β-blockade. Addition of nifedipine to hypertensives reduced combined cardiovascular end-points 13%, stroke or transient ischaemic attack 30%, coronary angiography 16%, new overt heart failure by 38%, and debilitating stroke 33%. This underscores the effectiveness of combination treatment in lowering cardiovascular events in hypertensives (55), and indeed in preserving cognitive function (56).

C. Literature Reviews and Meta-Analyses

The most recent Blood Pressure Lowering Treatment Trialists' Collaboration study found no substantive difference between trials of β-blockade and other agents (ACE inhibitors, diuretics, or calcium channel blockers) in cardiovascular outcomes, even when β-blockers were compared alone or in combination with diuretic treatment (57). This mirrors the earlier review where again no substantive difference was found between traditional (β-blocker or diuretic therapy) and newer agents (ACE inhibitors and calcium channel blockers), although newer agents were superior to placebo (58).

These studies reinforce previous meta-analyses (59,60) as to the utility of β-blockers in treating hypertension. However, Calcium channel blockers are superior to β-blockers and other antihypertensive classes as initial therapy in black adults (61).

VII. STRENGTHS AND WEAKNESSES OF β-BLOCKADE

Many trials have focused on testing the superiority of one drug over another agent from a different class. This is germane only to a proportion of patients with hypertension, a majority needing at least two or more agents to control their blood pressure. The relative safety and efficacy of β-blockers in treating hypertension, coupled with the additive effect when combined with other agents, such as diuretics and dihydropyridine calcium channel blockers, make them a reasonable choice for the treatment of hypertension in most instances. When most of the benefits of hypertensive therapy are derived from the degree of blood pressure reduction achieved, the cost effectiveness of these agents also makes them attractive. Once blood pressure control is achieved, the addition of aspirin confers extra benefit (62). The many potential side effects of these agents have led some to question their usefulness (63), but the advent of newer more cardioselective agents has gone some way toward addressing these concerns (64). Nebivolol, for example, has a side effect profile equivalent to angiotensin II receptor antagonists and placebo. The concern over side effects is obvious, given that up to 9% of patients attending an ambulatory care setting were documented as having β-blocker related side effects (37). The authors correctly cautioned that without a control group the side effects may be an over-estimate. Only 2% of patients were withdrawn from the HAPPHY study due to side effects of β-blockade which supports this notion.

Certainly β-blockers are of additional benefit in patients postmyocardial infarction, in congestive heart failure or LV dysfunction, and in diabetes mellitus patients who are at high cardiovascular risk (1). The JNC VII guidelines indicate use of diuretics as the initial drug of choice in the treatment of hypertension, differs somewhat from the European guidelines, which allow the clinician to choose the initial form of therapy (65). Recent results from the Blood Pressure Lowering Treatment Trialists' Collaboration which compared the effect of different treatment regimens on cardiovascular events rates, found no convincing evidence that newer agents (ACE inhibitors, angiotensin II receptor antagonists, or calcium channel blockers) were superior to conventional treatments with either diuretic or *β*-blocker. In this regard, there was no heterogeneity for any outcome when the results of *β*-blocker alone was compared with those of diuretic alone or those of *β*-blocker or diuretic combined.

Drug regimens may differ in their effect on patient subgroups, such as those with diabetic nephopathy, left ventricular hypertrophy, renal failure, or the subsequent occurrence of new onset diabetes. These are currently under review (57), but form a minority of patients compared to the many who have undiagnosed or under-treated hypertension. Therefore *β*-blockers, along with diuretics, calcium channel blockers, ACE inhibitors, and angiotensin II receptor blockers, are reasonable choices in the management of hypertension. The newer cardioselective agents are less likely to cause unwanted side effects, which should help improve compliance with therapy.

VIII. CONCLUSIONS

β-Blockers have a long and distinguished history in the effective management of hypertension. Their use is enhanced by the presence of any of the additional indications for their administration, for example, postmyocardial infarction, congestive heart failure, and so on.

Concern about side effects have often limited their use in patients at high risk, for example, in hypertensive patients with diabetes. However, the advent of newer more cardioselective *β*-blockers or agents with ancillary actions have resulted in a substantive drop in adverse effects, and improved outcomes.

Recent trial data of the superiority of Losartan over Atenolol at reducing cardiovascular events in a patient subset with ECG evidence of left ventricular hypertrophy, should not detract from meta- analyses showing that no single drug class is superior to another in the management of hypertension. These meta-analyses indicate that blood pressure reduction *per se* is the most important element in managing hypertension (66).

A substantial proportion of patients with hypertension require more than one medication (67). *β*-Blockers can readily be combined with nondihydropyridine calcium channel blockers, diuretics, and *α*-blockers, and with

ACE inhibitors or angiotensin receptor blockers, despite reduced efficiency with the latter.

Novel actions of third generation *β*-blockers including *α*-blockade (Carvedilol and Labetolol), nitric oxide release (Nebivolol), antiproliferative, and antioxidant effects, may further elaborate upon the clinical usefulness of these antihypertensives, through blood pressure independent effects. Future trials and meta-analyses assessing the blood pressure independent effects of antihypertensives are awaited with interest (68).

REFERENCES

1. Chobanian AV, Bakris GL, Black HR, Cushman WC, Green LA, Izzo JL Jr, Jones DW, Materson BJ, Oparil S, Wright JT Jr, Roccella EJ; National Heart, Lung, and Blood Institute Joint National Committee on Prevention, Detection, Evaluation, and Treatment of High Blood Pressure; National High Blood Pressure Education Program Coordinating Committee. The Seventh Report of the Joint National Committee on Prevention, Detection, Evaluation, and Treatment of High Blood Pressure: the JNC 7 report. JAMA 2003; 289:2560–2572.
2. Frishman WH. Clinical Pharmacology of the b-Adrenoreceptor Blocking Drugs. Vol. 1. Norwalk, CT: Appleton-Century-Crofts, 1984:501.
3. Moser M, Setaro J. Continued importance of diuretics and beta-adrenergic blockers in the management of hypertension. Med Clin North Am 2004; 88:167–187.
4. Prichard BC, Cruickshank JM. Beta blockade in hypertension. In: Mancia GC, Julius S, Saruta, T, Weber M, Ferrari A, Wilkinson I, eds. Manual of Hypertension. Vol. 1. Edinburgh: Churchill Livingstone, 2002:317–337.
5. Ahlquist R. A study of the adrenotropic receptors. Am J Physiol 1948; 155:586–600.
6. Xiang Y, Kobilka BK. Myocyte adrenoceptor signaling pathways. Science 2003; 300:1530–1532.
7. Hata JA, Koch WJ. Phosphorylation of G protein-coupled receptors: GPCR kinases in heart disease. Mol Interv 2003; 3:264–272.
8. Frielle T, Collins S, Daniel KW, Caron MG, Lefkowitz RJ, Kobilka BK. Cloning of the cDNA for the human beta 1-adrenergic receptor. Proc Natl Acad Sci USA 1987; 84:7920–7924.
9. Kaplan N. Treatment of hypertension: drug therapy. In: Kaplan N, ed. Clinical Hypertension. Vol. 1. Baltimore: Williams and Wilkins, 1998:205–214.
10. Frishman WH, Bryzinski BS, Coulson LR, DeQuattro VL, Vlachakis ND, Mroczek WJ, Dukart G, Goldberg JD, Alemayehu D, Koury K. A multifactorial trial design to assess combination therapy in hypertension. Treatment with bisoprolol and hydrochlorothiazide. Arch Intern Med 1994; 154:1461–1468.
11. Raftery EB, Carrageta MO. Hypertension and *β*-blockers. Are they all the same? Int J Cardiol 1985; 7:337–346.
12. Gress TW, Nieto FJ, Shahar E, Wofford MR, Brancati FL. Hypertension and antihypertensive therapy as risk

factors for type 2 diabetes mellitus. Atherosclerosis Risk in Communities Study. N Engl J Med 2000; 342:905–912.

13. Poole-Wilson PA, Swedberg K, Cleland JG, Di Lenarda A, Hanrath P, Komajda M, Lubsen J, Lutiger B, Metra M, Remme WJ, Torp-Pedersen C, Scherhag A, Skene A; Carvedilol Or Metoprolol European Trial Investigators. Comparison of carvedilol and metoprolol on clinical outcomes in patients with chronic heart failure in the Carvedilol Or Metoprolol European Trial (COMET): randomised controlled trial. Lancet 2003; 362:7–13.

14. Wikstrand J, Warnold I, Olsson G, Tuomilehto J, Elmfeldt D, Berglund G. Primary prevention with metoprolol in patients with hypertension. Mortality results from the MAPHY study. JAMA 1988; 259:1976–1982.

15. Frishman WH. Alpha- and beta-adrenergic blocking drugs. In: Frishman WH, Sonnenblick EH, Sica D, eds. Cardiovascular Pharmacotherapeutics. Vol. 1. New York: McGraw-Hill, 2003:67–97.

16. Wikstrand J. Primary prevention with beta-blockade in patients with hypertension: review of results and clinical implications. J Cardiovasc Pharmacol 1990; 16(suppl 5): S64–S75.

17. Di Lenarda A, Sabbadini G, Sinagra G. Do pharmacological differences among beta-blockers affect their clinical efficacy in heart failure? Cardiovasc Drugs Ther 2004; 18:91–93.

18. Maron BJ, McKenna WJ, Danielson GK et al. American College of Cardiology/European Society of Cardiology Clinical Expert Consensus Document on Hypertrophic Cardiomyopathy. A report of the American College of Cardiology Foundation Task Force on Clinical Expert Consensus Documents and the European Society of Cardiology Committee for Practice Guidelines. Eur Heart J 2003; 24:1965–1991.

19. Lopez-Sendon J, Swedberg K, McMurray J, Tamargo J, Maggioni AP, Dargie H, Tendera M, Waagstein F, Kjekshus J, Lechat P, Torp-Pedersen C; Task Force On β-Blockers of the European Society of Cardiology. Expert consensus document on beta-adrenergic receptor blockers. Eur Heart J 2004; 25:1341–1362.

20. Tight blood pressure control and risk of macrovascular and microvascular complications in type 2 diabetes: UKPDS 38. UK Prospective Diabetes Study Group. BMJ 1998; 317:703–713.

21. Taylor D, Paton C. The Maudsley 2003 Prescribing Guidelines. In: Taylor D, Kerwin R, eds. Vol. 1. London: Martin Dunitz, 2003:160.

22. Merkel C, Marin R, Angeli P, Zanella P, Felder M, Bernardinello E, Cavallarin G, Bolognesi M, Donada C, Bellini B, Torboli P, Gatta A; Gruppo Triveneto per l'Ipertensione Portale. A placebo-controlled clinical trial of nadolol in the prophylaxis of growth of small esophageal varices in cirrhosis. Gastroenterology 2004; 127:476–484.

23. Fleisher LA, Eagle KA. Clinical practice. Lowering cardiac risk in noncardiac surgery. N Engl J Med 2001; 345:1677–1682.

24. Abramowicz M. Prevention and treatment of heat injury. Med Lett Drugs Ther 2003; 45:58–60.

25. Bakris GL. Role for beta-blockers in the management of diabetic kidney disease. Am J Hypertens 2003; 16:7S–12S.

26. Cleophas TJ, Grabowsky I, Niemeyer MG, Makel WM, van der Wall EE. Paradoxical pressor effects of beta-blockers in standing elderly patients with mild hypertension: a beneficial side effect. Circulation 2002; 105:1669–1671.

27. Flather MD, Shibata MC, Coats AJ et al. Randomized trial to determine the effect of nebivolol on mortality and cardiovascular hospital admission in elderly patients with heart failure (SENIORS). Eur Heart J 2005; 26:215–225.

28. Heusser K, Schobel HP, Adamidis A, Fischer T, Frank H. Cardiovascular effects of beta-blockers with and without intrinsic sympathomimetic activity. A comparison between celiprolol and metoprolol. Kidney Blood Press Res 2002; 25:34–41.

29. Lilja JJ, Backman JT, Laitila J, Luurila H, Neuvonen PJ. Itraconazole increases but grapefruit juice greatly decreases plasma concentrations of celiprolol. Clin Pharmacol Ther 2003; 73:192–198.

30. Lilja JJ, Juntti-Patinen L, Neuvonen PJ. Orange juice substantially reduces the bioavailability of the β-adrenergic-blocking agent celiprolol. Clin Pharmacol Ther 2004; 75:184–190.

31. Lilja JJ, Niemi M, Neuvonen PJ. Rifampicin reduces plasma concentrations of celiprolol. Eur J Clin Pharmacol 2004; 59:819–824.

32. Eichhorn EJ, Domanski MJ, Krause-Steinrauf H, Bristow MR. A trial of the beta-blocker bucindolol in patients with advanced chronic heart failure. N Engl J Med 2001; 344:1659–1667.

33. O'Connor CM, Gottlieb S, Bourque JM et al. Impact of nonfatal myocardial infarction on outcomes in patients with advanced heart failure and the effect of bucindolol therapy. Am J Cardiol 2005; 95:558–564.

34. Salpeter SR, Ormiston TM, Salpeter EE. Cardioselective beta-blockers in patients with reactive airway disease: a meta-analysis. Ann Intern Med 2002; 137:715–725.

35. August P, Lindheimer MD. Chronic hypertension and pregnancy. In: Lindheimer MD, Roberts JM, Cunningham FG, eds. Chesley's Hypertensive Disorders in Pregnancy. Stamford, CT: Appleton and Lange, 1999:625–628.

36. Beardmore KS, Morris JM, Gallery ED. Excretion of antihypertensive medication into human breast milk: a systematic review. Hypertens Pregnancy 2002; 21:85–95.

37. Gandhi TK, Weingart SN, Borus J, Seger AC, Peterson J, Burdick E, Seger DL, Shu K, Federico F, Leape LL, Bates DW. Adverse drug events in ambulatory care. N Engl J Med 2003; 348:1556–1564.

38. Silvestri A, Galetta P, Cerquetani E, Marazzi G, Patrizi R, Fini M, Rosano GM. Report of erectile dysfunction after therapy with beta-blockers is related to patient knowledge of side effects and is reversed by placebo. Eur Heart J 2003; 24:1928–1932.

39. Auer J. Cardiovascular drugs. In: Mozayani A, Raymon L, eds. Handbook of Drug Interactions. Vol. 1. Totowa, NJ: Humana Press, 2004:233–238.

40. Neutel JM, Smith DH, Ram CV et al. Application of ambulatory blood pressure monitoring in differentiating

between antihypertensive agents. Am J Med 1993; 94:181–187.

41. Reader R, Bauer GE, Doyle AE, Edmondson KW, Hunyor S, Hurley TH, Korner PI, Leighton PW, Lovell RRH, McCall MG, McPhie JM, Rand MJ, Whyte HM. The Australian Therapeutic Trial in Mild Hypertension. Lancet 1980; I:1261–1267.

42. Medical Research Council Working Party. MRC trial of treatment of mild hypertension: principal results. Br Med J (Clin Res Ed) 1985; 291:97–104.

43. Wilhelmsen L, Berglund G, Elmfeldt D, Fitzsimons T, Holzgreve H, Hosie J, Hornkvist PE, Pennert K, Tuomilehto J, Wedel H. Beta-blockers versus diuretics in hypertensive men: main results from the HAPPHY trial. J Hypertens 1987; 5:561–572.

44. The IPPPSH Collaborative Group. The international prospective primary prevention study in hypertension (IPPPSH): objectives and methods. Eur J Clin Pharmacol 1984; 27:379–391.

45. ALLHAT Collaborative Research Group. Major cardiovascular events in hypertensive patients randomized to doxazosin vs chlorthalidone: the antihypertensive and lipid-lowering treatment to prevent heart attack trial (ALLHAT). JAMA 2000; 283:1967–1975.

46. Dahlof B, Devereux RB, Kjeldsen SE, Julius S, Beevers G, de Faire U, Fyhrquist F, Ibsen H, Kristiansson K, Lederballe-Pedersen O, Lindholm LH, Nieminen MS, Omvik P, Oparil S, Wedel H; LIFE Study Group. Cardiovascular morbidity and mortality in the Losartan Intervention For Endpoint reduction in hypertension study (LIFE): a randomised trial against atenolol. Lancet 2002; 359:995–1003.

47. Kizer JR, Dahlof B, Kjeldsen SE et al. Stroke reduction in hypertensive adults with cardiac hypertrophy randomized to losartan versus atenolol: the Losartan Intervention for Endpoint reduction in hypertension study. Hypertension 2005; 45:46–52.

48. Berglund G. Beta-blockers and diuretics. The HAPPHY and MAPHY studies. Clin Exp Hypertens A 1989; 11:1137–1148.

49. Neaton JD, Grimm RH Jr, Prineas RJ, Stamler J, Grandits GA, Elmer PJ, Cutler JA, Flack JM, Schoenberger JA, McDonald R. Treatment of Mild Hypertension Study. Final results. Treatment of Mild Hypertension Study Research Group. JAMA 1993; 270:713–724.

50. Wright JT Jr, Bakris G, Greene T, Agodoa LY, Appel LJ, Charleston J, Cheek D, Douglas-Baltimore JG, Gassman J, Glassock R, Hebert L, Jamerson K, Lewis J, Phillips RA, Toto RD, Middleton JP, Rostand SG; African American Study of Kidney Disease and Hypertension Study Group. Effect of blood pressure lowering and antihypertensive drug class on progression of hypertensive kidney disease: results from the AASK trial. JAMA 2002; 288:2421–2431.

51. Dahlof B, Lindholm LH, Hansson L, Schersten B, Ekbom T, Wester PO. Morbidity and mortality in the Swedish Trial in Old Patients with Hypertension (STOP-Hypertension). Lancet 1991; 338:1281–1285.

52. SHEP Cooperative Research Group. Prevention of stroke by antihypertensive drug treatment in older persons with isolated systolic hypertension. Final results of the Systolic Hypertension in the Elderly Program (SHEP). JAMA 1991; 265:3255–3564.

53. MRC Working Party. Medical Research Council trial of treatment of hypertension in older adults: principal results. BMJ 1992; 304:405–412.

54. Byington RP. Beta-blocker heart attack trial: design, methods, and baseline results. Beta-blocker heart attack trial research group. Control Clin Trials 1984; 5:382–437.

55. Lubsen J, Wagener G, Kirwan BA, Brouwer S, Poole-Wilson PA. Effect of long-acting nifedipine on mortality and cardiovascular morbidity in patients with symptomatic stable angina and hypertension: the ACTION trial. J Hypertens 2005; 23:641–648.

56. Papademetriou V. Hypertension and cognitive function. Blood pressure regulation and cognitive function: a review of the literature. Geriatrics 2005; 60:20–22, 24.

57. Turnbull F. Effects of different blood-pressure-lowering regimens on major cardiovascular events: results of prospectively-designed overviews of randomised trials. Lancet 2003; 362:1527–1535.

58. Neal B, MacMahon S, Chapman N. Effects of ACE inhibitors, calcium antagonists, and other blood-pressure-lowering drugs: results of prospectively designed overviews of randomised trials. Blood Pressure Lowering Treatment Trialists' Collaboration. Lancet 2000; 356:1955–1964.

59. Gueyffier F, Boutitie F, Boissel JP, Pocock S, Coope J, Cutler J, Ekbom T, Fagard R, Friedman L, Perry M, Prineas R, Schron E. Effect of antihypertensive drug treatment on cardiovascular outcomes in women and men. A meta-analysis of individual patient data from randomized, controlled trials. The INDANA Investigators. Ann Intern Med 1997; 126:761–767.

60. Psaty BM, Smith NL, Siscovick DS, Koepsell TD, Weiss NS, Heckbert SR, Lemaitre RN, Wagner EH, Furberg CD. Health outcomes associated with antihypertensive therapies used as first-line agents. A systematic review and meta-analysis. JAMA 1997; 277:739–745.

61. Brewster L, Kleijnen J, Montfrans G. Effect of antihypertensive drugs on mortality, morbidity and blood pressure in blacks. Cochrane Database Syst Rev 2005:CD005183.

62. Hansson L, Zanchetti A, Carruthers SG, Dahlof B, Elmfeldt D, Julius S, Menard J, Rahn KH, Wedel H, Westerling S. Effects of intensive blood-pressure lowering and low-dose aspirin in patients with hypertension: principal results of the Hypertension Optimal Treatment (HOT) randomised trial. HOT Study Group. Lancet 1998; 351:1755–1762.

63. Messerli FH, Beevers DG, Franklin SS, Pickering TG. *β*-Blockers in hypertension-the emperor has no clothes: an open letter to present and prospective drafters of new guidelines for the treatment of hypertension. Am J Hypertens 2003; 16:870–873.

64. Messerli FH, Grossman E. β-Blockers in hypertension: is carvedilol different? Am J Cardiol 2004; 93:7B–12B.

65. Zanchetti A, Cifkova R, Fagard R, Kjeldsen S, Mancia G, Poulter N, Rahn KH, Rodicio JL, Ruilope LM, Staessen J, van Zwieten P, Waeber B, Williams B. European Society of Hypertension–European Society of Cardiology guidelines for the management of arterial hypertension. J Hypertens 2003; 21:1011–1053.

66. Puddey IB. Large multicentre hypertension trials. Curr Opin Nephrol Hypertens 2000; 9:285–292.

67. Basile JN. Optimizing antihypertensive treatment in clinical practice. Am J Hypertens 2003; 16:13S–17S.

68. Bakris GL, Bell DS, Fonseca V et al. The rationale and design of the Glycemic Effects in Diabetes Mellitus Carvedilol-Metoprolol Comparison in Hypertensives (GEMINI) trial. J Diabetes Complications 2005; 19:74–79.

28

α_1-Receptor Inhibitory Drugs in the Treatment of Hypertension

BRIAN N. C. PRICHARD
University College London, London, UK

PIETER A. VAN ZWIETEN
Universiteit van Amsterdam, Amsterdam, The Netherlands

KEYPOINTS

- α_1-Inhibitory drugs reduce blood pressure by reducing vasoconstrictor tone.
- Dosage must not be excessive to prevent reflex adjustments for example, to erect posture.
- Care is needed to avoid a first dose effect, particularly when added on to pre-existing treatment.
- Increments should be small to increase patient tolerance.
- Other than excessive falls of blood pressures, particularly postural, side effect profile is favourable,

insulin sensitivity is increased and effect on lipid profile is favourable.
- They reduce benign prostatic hypertrophy and drugs more specific for prostatic alpha receptors have been developed.

SUMMARY

The final common pathway for the sympathetic control of blood vessels is the α_1 adrenoceptor. The hormones adrenaline and noradrenaline exert their vasoconstrictor activity at this site. The α_1 receptor is crucial in the reflex control of blood pressure. Most notably, increased α_1-mediated vasoconstriction is essential in the cardio-vascular responses to the erect positive. Competitive inhibitors of the α receptor, such as prazosin, trimazosin, and doxazosin, must be given in amounts that allow some overcoming of the α blockade in the erect posture so that an excessive drop in blood pressure, postural hypo-tension, does not occur from the effect of gravity. A noncompetitive inhibitor, such as phenoxybenzamine, is therefore not suitable for the treatment of hypertension, with the exception of pheochromocytoma.

The first-dose phenomenon was a problem with the early use of prazosin. It is advisable with all α_1-blocking drugs to start with a small dose because initially as with an α_1-blocker, the cardiovascular system is sensitive to the increased vascular capacity from the inhibition of vaso-constrictor tone that later declines. This is probably due to a later modest increase in vascular volume, although evidence is not strong. The first-dose phenomena is more likely if the patient is already taking an antihypertensive drug such as a diuretic or a β-blocker. As with all antihy-pertensive drugs, it is best to keep subsequent increments small unless urgency dictated by the height of the blood pressure level indicates otherwise.

Not withstanding some evidence of a favorable effect on surrogate endpoints, such as a modest improvement in lipid profile and an improvement in insulin sensitivity, major outcome studies have been disappointing. In the ALLHAT study, doxazosin was associated with an increase in stroke and heart failure compared with treat-ment with a diuretic, although the former situation may be a function of a 2.3 mmHg lower systolic blood pressure with chlorthalidone and the latter situation at least partly a result of discontinuing a diuretic prior to admission to the study, which possibly unmasks latent heart failure. The recent guidelines of the European Society of Hypertension–European Society of Cardiology advise

that α_1-blockers no longer be regarded as first-line agents, although they are valuable in combination with other drugs. Multiple drugs are now being used in most patients for adequate control of blood pressure.

I. INTRODUCTION

The α adrenoceptor mediates neuronal vasoconstriction and is crucial to the control of blood pressure. Drugs that inhibit the innervation of the α adrenoceptor at various sites—on the central sympathetic control centers, sympath-etic ganglia, adrenergic nerve endings, and the α receptor itself—have been important since effective antihyperten-sive drugs were discovered.

II. α RECEPTORS

The α adrenoceptors have been divided into α_1 receptors and α_2 receptors and then further subdivided by cloning experiments and according to their responses to various agonists and antagonists (1) (Table 28.1). Adrenaline or noradrenaline, "the first messenger," interacts with the adrenergic receptor of the target cell. The stimulation of the α_1 receptor involves coupling to the Gq_{11} protein, which stimulates phospholipase C and leads to intracellu-lar calcium release. The α_2 receptors are coupled predomi-nantly to inhibitory the GTP-binding protein to inhibit adenylyl cyclase and, thus, inhibit the opening of voltage-gated calcium channels (1).

Phenylephrine is selective, methoxamine is the most selective stimulant for the α_1 receptor, and clonidine is an example of a drug that exerts its therapeutic effect by central α_2-receptor stimulation, although it also has α_1 properties. Azepexole (B-HT 933) is a selective α_2 agonist (2). Adrenaline and noradrenaline stimulate both receptor subtypes. Prazosin, doxazosin, and trimazosin are competitive antagonists at the α_1 receptors; yohimbine,

Table 28.1 α Adrenoceptors

Type of receptor block	Type of effect	Stimulation	Blockade
α_1	Postjunctional Vascular smooth muscle	Noradrenaline Adrenaline Phenylephrine Methoxamine Clonidine (secondary)	Prazosin Doxazosin Trimazosin Phentolamine
α_2	Prejunctional Postjunctional e.g., saphenous vein	Noradrenaline Adrenaline Clonidine (primary) Oxymetazoline Azepexole	Yohimbine Rauwolscine Idazoxan Phentolamine

Note: α_1 receptor subdivisions: α_{1A} (previously α_{1C}), α_{1B}, α_{1D} (previously $\alpha_{1a/d}$); α_2 receptor subdivisions: $\alpha_{2A/D}$, α_{2B}, α_{2C}.

rauwolscine, and the more selective idazoxan inhibit α_2 receptors, whereas phentolamine inhibits both α_1 receptors and α_2 receptors.

Postsynaptically the α_1 receptors predominate in most vascular smooth muscle, but α_2 receptors are also important. There is considerable species variation; in the human forearm, both α_1 receptors and α_2 receptors are present. Vascular smooth muscle has postsynaptic α_1 receptors that are involved in the mediation of the nerve impulse and, therefore, mediate vasoconstrictor control of blood vessels in both arteries and veins. The α_2 receptors are extrasynaptic; both subtypes of α receptors mediate contraction in response to hormonal stimulation. Presynaptic α_2 receptors are also present; these inhibit neuronal release of noradrenaline and, thus, are a negative feedback mechanism. The α_1 receptors in vascular smooth muscle appear to be found in the adventitial layer, whereas the α_2 receptors are found closer to the interior, where they respond to circulatory catecholamines (3,4).

In the central nervous system, α_2 receptors are the predominant α receptor subtype, although α_1 receptors have been demonstrated by receptor binding techniques and are involved in baroreceptor reflex function. Stimulation of central α_2 receptors is important in the antihypertensive effect of methyldopa and clonidine. The more recently described imidazoline I_1-receptors are also important in the antihypertensive effect of clonidine, and more so with agents that bind selectively for the imidazoline I_1-receptor compared to their α_2-receptor binding such as moxonidine and rilmenidine (5).

III. CONTROL OF BLOOD PRESSURE

Blood pressure control in both normotensive and hypertensive subjects is complex. Although the autonomic nervous system plays a major part in the moment-to-moment regulation of blood pressure, hormonal and renal factors are important in the long-term regulation of blood pressure. As Guyton has stressed, the volume adjustment by the kidney would readily compensate for the pressor effect from sympathetic vasoconstriction (6). There are, however, many ways in which the nervous system can influence renal function (7).

The sympathetic neurones that supply the heart and blood vessels originate in the vasomotor center, which is located in the lateral part of the reticular formation and the bulbar zone of the brain stem. Axons from the neurones of the vasomotor center form the bulbospinal tract that descends in the interomedial lateral columns to the preganglionic cells that are situated in the arteriolateral columns. The control of vasomotor tone is achieved by the balance of stimulation and inhibition, which modulates the number of impulses traveling by the final common pathway, the

preganglionic neurone. This neurone synapses in paravertebral ganglia (sympathetic ganglia), which liberate acetylcholine, to activate the postganglionic neurone. Vasoconstriction of resistance vessels and veins results from the stimulation of these nerves. Neuronal vasodilation is largely achieved by fewer vasoconstrictor impulses (8). Unlike the importance of sympathetic tone in blood vessels, at rest the parasympathetic tone of the heart is dominant. However even at rest in the supine position, however, sympathetic tone in the heart, if not dominant, is also significant. The dose-dependent reduction in resting supine heart rate that results from the administration of a β-adrenoreceptor-blocking drug illustrates this point.

The peripheral α_1 receptors that mediate sympathetic tone and reflexes are crucial to blood pressure control. Any drug that inhibits the innervation of the α receptor, regardless of the site of action, can be expected to produce a greater effect when physiological conditions require increased α-mediated sympathetic activity to maintain blood pressure. There is the potential for a drop in blood pressure when a person stands up because of the effect of gravity on the system. Venous return is reduced, despite some compensatory venoconstriction, by ~20% even under normal circumstances, that is, without any α_1 receptor inhibition. Thus, cardiac output decreases. Exercise, a very warm environment, and digestion all are physiological events that lead to local vasodilation, which then requires venoconstriction elsewhere to maintain systemic blood pressure. Likewise, a reduced blood volume means that vasoconstriction is required to maintain systemic blood pressure. The α-mediated tone needs to be reduced at low rates of sympathetic stimulation (e.g., resting in a supine position) in order to lower the blood pressure. It is important, however, that high rates of sympathetic activity should not be inhibited excessively so that the higher rates of sympathetic nerve traffic from cardiovascular stress (e.g., exercise in an upright position in a very warm environment or after eating in the early hours of the morning—the "dinner dance syndrome") can result in adequate vasoconstriction to maintain an adequate blood pressure for cerebral perfusion. Adequate inhibition of the α_1 receptor at a low rate of sympathetic nerve activity, without excessive inhibition at high rates of sympathetic nerve activity, can be achieved with appropriate adjustment of dosage by a drug that competitively inhibits the α_1 receptor such as prazosin, terazosin, doxazosin, or urapidil. High rates of sympathetic nerve activity will partly reverse the α_1 block to minimize any excessive drop in blood pressure. However, the effect of a noncompetitive α-receptor inhibitor in essential hypertension, as seen with phenoxybenzamine, is totally postural, no effect being observed on supine position blood pressure. It is, therefore, not a useful general antihypertensive agent. Although a postural drop in blood pressure with an α_1 receptor blocker is not often a clinical problem, a tendency for a lower pressure when standing than when supine is often seen in patients who are being treated with α_1-blocking drugs. Symptoms of postural hypotension, such as dizziness, may necessitate discontinuing treatment with prazosin (9), terazosin (10), doxazosin (11), and indoramin (12) and possibly to a lesser extent also with urapidil (13).

IV. α-ADRENERGIC BLOCKING DRUGS

Drugs that inhibit the α-adrenergic receptors can be divided into several types (14) (Table 28.2). Phenoyxbenzamine is a nonselective drug that blocks both α_1 and α_2 receptors. Its action is noncompetitive, and thus increased sympathetic impulses observed in the erect posture do not reverse the blockade; at tolerated doses, there is no useful effect on supine position blood pressure. Phenoyxbenzamine is only used in pheochromocytoma. Phentolamine is also nonselective; it has a very short action and, in addition, has a direct vasodilator effect and also sympathetic and parasympathetic actions.

Nonselective α blockade means that presynaptic α_2 receptors, which reduce the release of noradrenaline, are inhibited because the negative feedback mechanism is blocked. There is, therefore, an increase in noradrenaline release, which attenuates the desired α_1 blockade and

Table 28.2   Types of α-Adrenergic-Blocking Drugs

Nonselective $\alpha_1 + \alpha_2$ blockade
   Phenoxybenzamine
   Phentolamine
Selective α_1 blocking drugs
   Prazosin
   Terazosin
   Doxazosin
   Urapidil
   Indoramin
Selective α_{1a} blocking drugs
   Tamulosin
Selective α_2-blocking drugs
   Yohimbine
Combined α-blockers and β-blockers
   Labetalol
   Carvedilol
Drugs with α-blocking properties unrelated to clinical use
   Amiodarone
   Bromocriptine
   Chlorpromazine
   Haloperidol
   Ketanserine
   Quinidine

Source: Frishman and Kotob (14).

also leads to increased β-mediated stimulation, that is, tachycardia and increased renin release. Some acute studies with α_1-blocking drugs, however, also have shown an increase in heart rate because vagal withdrawal in response to a drop in blood pressure is not reduced (9–11,15,16).

The selective α_1-blockers, quinazoline derivatives such as prazosin (9,15), doxazosin (11,16), and terazosin (10), represent the α-blockers that are most widely used in hypertension treatment. Indoramin, in addition to its α_1-blocking activity, results in a relatively high incidence of sedation and dry mouth (12); urapidil stimulates central $5HT_{1A}$ receptors, reducing sympathetic nerve activity that therefore supplements its peripheral α_1-receptor action in lowering blood pressure (13). Their pharmacokinetic properties are summarized in Table 28.3.

Tamsulosin is a specific α_{1A}-receptor-blocking drug and is, therefore, of special value in treating benign prostate hyperplasia (17). Yohimbine is a specific α_2-blocking drug; labetalol and carvedilol are both α-blocking and β-blocking agents. Finally, there are several drugs which, although they possess α-blocking activity, this does not contribute to their clinical use, for example, chlorpromazine, imipramine, haloperidol, and bromocriptine (14).

V.   HYPERTENSION AND α-MEDIATED VASOCONSTRICTION

Genetic and environmental influences are responsible for the development of essential hypertension. There is evidence of the central role of the sympathetic nervous system. This involves both influence on vascular α receptors and influence on the release and action of insulin. Patients with early hypertension have a hyperdynamic circulation with an increase in noradrenaline levels. There is an increase in sympathetic nerve activity as evidenced by increased nerve impulses measured in the peroneal nerve. There may be an initial increase in venous return from increased vascular tone, and thus cardiac output is increased. Over a number of years there is a gradual transformation in these patients to established hypertension with increased peripheral resistance and a normal cardiac output, as has been shown in repeated studies in a group of patients over 20 years (18).

The inhibition of α receptor innervation and the consequent reduction of peripheral resistance represent the action of a group of drugs that reverse the most prominent hemodynamic change of hypertension. The vascular tone of both arteries and veins is inhibited. The arteriolar dilation tends to increase cardiac output, whereas venous dilation results in venous pooling and a reduction in venous return, this being an effect that reduces cardiac

Table 28.3 Pharmacokinetic Properties of α-Blockers

Drug [source of data]	Bioavailability (%)	Effect of food on response	T_{max} (h)	Plasma protein binding (%)	Volume of distribution (L/kg)	Metabolism	$T_{1/2}$ (h)
Prazosin [Stanaszek et al. 1983 (9)]	[a]55–82 (E: 48)	No effect	1–3	92	0.6 (E: 0.9)	6 and 7 dealkylation 10% unchanged	2.55–2.9 (E: 3.23)
Doxazosin [Fulton et al. (16)]	62–69	Delays T_{max} 1 h C_{max} not affected	1.7–3.6	98–99	0.97–1.69	O-demethylation hydroxylation 5% unchanged	16–22
Terazosin [Titmarsh and Monk (10)]	90	No significant effect	1–2	90–94	0.25–0.98	O-demethylation hydroxylation 2–8% unchanged	10–18
Indoramin [Holmes and Sorkin (12)]	31	Delays T_{max} 0.4 h	1–2	86	2.4	Conjugation hydroxylation 5% unchanged	2.6–4.6 (E: 14.7)
Urapidil [Dooley and Goa (13)]	72	May delay T_{max} Increase C_{max}	0.5–6	75–80	0.6–0.8	O-demethylation hydroxylation Uracil-N-demethylation	2.0–4.8

E elderly >65 years;
[a]First-pass metabolism.

output. The net effect of α blockade is that cardiac output is usually unchanged (19).

VI. EXERCISE

Perhaps due to the absence or relative absence of increased tachycardia, presumably the result of there being no presynaptic α_2 blockade and also the reduction in after load from α_1 blockade, prazosin has been shown to reduce myocardial oxygen consumption on exercise with no alteration in exercising heart rate. The exercise performance of hypertensive joggers was not reduced by α_1 blockade with prazosin. At lower levels of exercise, diastolic pressure was reduced, whereas the response of systolic blood pressure was not altered in contrast with atenolol, which also reduces exercise performance (20).

VII. FIRST-DOSE PHENOMENON

Drugs such as the α_1 receptor-blocking drugs that act by interfering with vasoconstrictor tone have the possibility that even with competitive agents there is sufficient α_1 blockade to inhibit reflex responses to such a degree that there is an excessive drop in blood pressure. This is seen with first-dose phenomenon, that is, an excessive drop in blood pressure with the initial dose of the drug, in which the circulation is especially sensitive to α_1 blockade, and excessive drops in blood pressure may occur, particularly upon standing up from a supine or seated position, with doses that are easily tolerated with chronic administration because there is subsequently some shift of fluid into the intravascular compartment. A significant first-dose phenomenon can be avoided by initially giving a very small dose of an α_1-blocking drug. This is particularly important if the α-blocker has been added to other antihypertensive drugs that also are being prescribed, which will usually be the case (4).

VIII. RENAL AND OTHER EFFECTS

Clinically apparent fluid retention rarely occurs with prazosin. Renal vascular resistance is reduced to balance the drop in blood pressure from prazosin so that renal blood flow and glomerular filtration rate are maintained. Similar findings have been reported with the use of urapidil. An increase in blood volume and extracellular volume and a reduction in blood viscosity have been reported with prazosin. Some investigators have observed an increase in body weight that has been associated with a smaller drop in blood pressure with prazosin (21), although others have not found this effect.

Some investigations of acute conditions with α_1 treatment show an increase in renin and noradrenaline, which is in contrast with the absence of these effects with prolonged administration. Plasma noradrenaline has been reported to be elevated with urapidil, but larger doses appear to reduce catecholamine excretion (4).

IX. LEFT VENTRICULAR HYPERTROPHY

An important consequence of hypertension is the development of left ventricular hypertrophy. The development of left ventricular hypertrophy is associated with a worsened prognosis. The evidence that α_1-blocking drugs reduce left ventricular hypertrophy is less convincing than that for the other major classes of antihypertensive drugs currently in use. In one meta-analysis, an average of 15.6 months administration of α_1-blocking drugs were reported to reduce left ventricular mass by 10.6%, similar to results for other antihypertensive drugs. However, the confidence limits (-2.2 to 23.4, the minus sign indicates an increase) crossed zero (22). This was very possibly due to the fact that there were fewer studies that included α_1-blocking drugs. However, in the Veterans Administration Study, prazosin showed no reduction at all on left ventricular mass in patients with the highest tertile of baseline left ventricular mass, in contrast to the significant reduction in mass reported for patients treated with hydrochlorothiazide, captopril, or atenolol (23).

X. CLINICAL USE OF α_1 INHIBITORS IN TREATING HYPERTENSION

α_1-Blocking drugs are no longer regarded as first-choice agents (24), even though monotherapy with α_1-inhibiting drugs suggests that in about one-half of patients with mild hypertension, blood pressure can be controlled by using these agents. Prazosin was the original drug of this group to be used for treating mild hypertension. But it has to be used with multiple daily dosing (9,15) unless a delayed-release preparation is used. Subsequently, α_1 receptor-blocking drugs were introduced that had a longer half-life (Table 28.3) and were thus suitable for once-a-day dosing. Doxazosin (11,16) is the most evaluated example with a half-life 16–22 h; terazosin has a half-life of ~12 h, which also is suitable for once-daily dosing (10). Indoramin, however, has a shorter half-life (5 h) and must be taken two to three times a day, and it is associated with a high incidence of sedation (12). Urapidil also has a half-life that is too short (under 5 h) for once-daily administration (13).

XI. COMPARATIVE STUDIES

There do not appear to be any important differences between the various α_1-blocking drugs in the control of hypertension, provided that dosage is sufficiently frequent with the shorter acting drugs.

In the 4 year Treatment of Mild Hypertension Study (TOMHS), the control of blood pressure with doxazosin was compared with control achieved by a drug from each of the other major drug classes (Fig. 28.1). Rather more patients in the doxazosin, (21.5%) enalapril (20.2%), and chlorthalidone (17.9%) groups required additional drugs to achieve a diastolic blood pressure of <95 mmHg than patients in the acebutolol (11.4%) or amlodipine (11.4%) groups. The dosages for chlorthalidone were up to 30 mg, the dosages for acebutolol were up to 800 mg, and the dosages for amlodipine were up to 10 mg. However, the maximum doses of doxazosin (4 mg) and enalapril (10 mg) used were substantially less than the maximum doses that can be administered (25).

Materson et al. (26,27) reported a large monotherapy comparison in 1292 men. This was a double-blind, randomized parallel group study, with 178–188 patients in each drug group. Blood pressure control was defined as 90 mmHg sitting diastolic in the dose titration period and ≤95 mmHg at 1 year follow-up. This control was achieved in 54% of the patients with prazosin (4–20 mg) given twice a day, 50% of the patients with captopril, 55% of the patients with hydrochlorothiazide, 60% of the patients with atenolol, and 72% of the patients with diltiazem (27). Control with prazosin was better in older patients (≥60 years) than in patients <60 years of age on prazosin, both in whites (69% vs. 55%) and in blacks (49% vs. 42%).

The Antihypertensive and Lipid-Lowering Treatment to Prevent Heart Attack Trial (ALLHAT) was a large outcome study that compared chlorthalidone, doxazosin, amlodipine, and lisinopril. The doxazosin segment of the study was terminated prematurely because its use was associated with increased cardiovascular endpoints (28,29). Doxazosin (2–8 mg, $n = 9067$) was compared with chlorthalidone (12.5–25 mg, $n = 15,268$) for an average of 3.3 years. If blood pressure remained at $\geq140/90$ mmHg, other drugs, most often atenolol, could be added. In those patients who were followed for 4 years, 35% of the chlorthalidone group and 37% of the doxazosin group had dual medication. A diuretic was used in 23% of the doxazosin group; an α-blocker was used in 4% of the chlorthalidone group. Three or more drugs were used in 19% of the chlorthalidone-treated patients and in 27% of the doxazosin-treated patients. After 2 years treatment, average blood pressures were 136/78 mmHg with the chlorthalidone-based regimen and 138/78 mmHg with the doxazosin-based regimen.

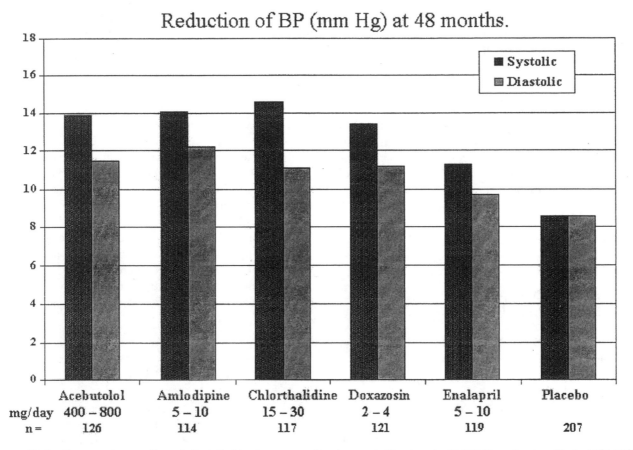

Figure 28.1   Decrease in systolic and diastolic blood pressure after 4 years in Treatment of Mild Hypertension Study (TOMHS). [After Neaton et al. (25).]

Throughout the study, systolic blood pressures averaged 2.3 mmHg less in patients on chlorthalidone compared with doxazosin, which would account for at least part of the less favorable outcome with doxazosin. There was no difference in the primary outcome of fatal or nonfatal myocardial infarction, or all-cause mortality. There was a 19% excess stroke incidence with doxazosin ($P = 0.001$) and a highly significant increase (25%) in combined cardiovascular disease ($P < 0.001$), which included coronary heart disease death, nonfatal myocardial infarction, and fatal and nonfatal stroke, angina, coronary vascularization operation, heart failure, and peripheral vascular disease. There was an increase of 66% in fatal or hospitalized heart failure in the doxazosin group, which, therefore, makes it a major contribution to the excess combined cardiovascular disease. The excess on doxazosin in combined cardiovascular disease was found regardless of age (both under 65 years and 65 and older), or race, or the presence or absence of diabetes, although blacks showed a 28% excess in combined cardiovascular disease compared with whites 16% (29).

It should be pointed out that ∼90% of the patients in the ALLHAT study were previously on antihypertensive treatment, so that the high incidence of heart failure on doxazosin might be at least partly due to diuretic withdrawal unmasking occult heart failure rather than to any effect of doxazosin (30). In support of this view, the rates of heart failure on doxazosin and chlorthalidone diverge very early and thereafter are parallel (31).

Because of the results of the ALLHAT study, α-blockers are no longer recommended as initial monotherapy for the management of hypertension (24). Although determining an appropriate monotherapy is regarded as less important now because combining drugs so often is required to satisfactorily control blood pressure, an exception to combining drugs might be controlling blood pressure in patients with mild hypertension and co-existing prostatic hyperplasia.

XII. COMBINATION OF α_1-BLOCKERS WITH OTHER ANTIHYPERTENSIVES

Although α_1-blockers are no longer regarded as first-choice antihypertensive agents in uncomplicated hypertension, they have a useful place in combination with other antihypertensive drugs in cases of more resistant hypertension (32). Brown et al. (33), in their discussion of combination therapy, suggested α_1-receptor-blocking drugs as a fourth-step option for resistant–hypertension control. One interesting study demonstrated that the use of amlodipine (5 or 10 mg daily) in combination with doxazosin (2–4 mg daily) resulted in a drop in blood pressure ($-20/13$ mmHg) that was significantly greater than the sum of the individual drops in blood pressure with amlodipine ($-10/4$ mmHg) or doxazosin ($-2/2$ mmHg) (34). Another investigation found that lower doses of doxazosin (1–4 mg) combined with the selective β-blocker betaxolol achieved better blood pressure control than monotherapy with the angiotensin-converting enzyme (ACE) inhibitor quinapril or with hydrochlorthiazide (35).

XIII. EFFECT OF α_1-BLOCKERS IN ELDERLY PATIENTS

Doxazosin controls blood pressure in patients >65 years old; in one study, it reduced average levels by 23/15 mmHg compared with 21/14 mmHg in younger patients. Dizziness was more frequent (10.9% vs. 5.1%) in the elderly, possibly due to the overall increase in frequency of this complaint, in general, in older patients rather than it being a side effect of doxozosin (36). The Veterans Administration Study with prazosin also showed a trend for blood pressure in older patients (≥ 60 years) to be better controlled with α_1-blockers (27).

XIV. EFFECT OF α_1-BLOCKERS ON LIPID PROFILE AND INSULIN RESISTANCE

The α_1 antagonists are unique among the classes of antihypertensive drugs because they have a moderate but favorable effect on lipid profile and other risk factors (37). They modestly reduce both total and low-density lipoprotein (LDL) cholesterol and also result in a modest increase in high-density lipoprotein (HDL) cholesterol. The TOMHS study included an assessment of changes in lipid profile. Doxazosin was associated with a drop in LDL and a small increase in HDL. The HDL/cholesterol ratio increased by 2.6 with doxazosin. This was significantly different from the HDL/cholesterol increases reported with acebutolol (1.2) amlodipine (1.5), chlorthalidone (1.4), or the placebo (1.2), but not significantly different from enalapril (1.9) (25). Oxidized LDL plays a central role in atherogenesis; it has recently been reported that doxazosin decreases oxidized LDL (38).

α_1-blocking drugs have been found to improve insulin sensitivity by 20–25%, which results in increased glucose uptake. Calcium antagonists and ACE inhibitors do not affect insulin resistance; diuretics and β-blockers increase insulin resistance (39). It also has been found that the improvement in insulin sensitivity with doxazosin is greater in hypertensive patients with insulin resistance, with a greater improvement in fibrinolytic activity (40).

XV. HEART FAILURE

Acute studies with prazosin in heart failure have demonstrated hemodynamic improvement with an increase in cardiac output and stroke volume during exercise. Chronic administration is disappointing, however; benefit is lost, which may be reversed by the addition of spironolactone (9). A comparison of prazosin with a placebo failed to show any benefit from prazosin with respect to survival in heart failure (41). The hemodynamic benefit in heart failure patients from metoprolol administration after 3 months treatment was not influenced by the addition of doxazosin (42).

XVI. BENIGN PROSTATIC HYPERPLASIA

About 40% of the prostate tissue in benign prostatic hyperplasia is α-adrenoceptor-possessing smooth muscle. Benefit was first demonstrated with the nonspecific α-inhibiting drug phenoxybenzamine, but side effects limited its use. Better results were obtained initially with prazosin and then subsequently with the longer-acting doxazosin and terazosin, both of which are suitable for once-daily treatment. Improvement in symptoms is rapid, and urine flow is improved; however, postural hypotension may limit the dose and thus the benefit. More recently, uroselective α_1-receptor-blocking drugs (such as tamsulosin or alfuzosin), that is, drugs that are selective for α_{1a} receptors have been described. These drugs have a lower incidence of dizziness and postural hypotension (17).

Finasteride, a 5-α-reductase inhibitor, reduces testosterone levels and after 6 months of treatment also shows benefit in benign prostatic hyperplasia. Although studies over 1 year do not indicate any value in combination therapy, a 4 year study demonstrated greater relief of symptoms with doxazosin and finasteride in combination than with either agent alone (43).

XVII. PHAEOCHROMOCYTOMA

The α-blockers have been used to inhibit the vasoconstrictor effects of circulating adrenaline and noradrenaline in this rare cause of hypertension. A β-blocker is used to control their tachycardiac effect. The noncompetitive agent phenoxybenzamine is the preferred α-blocker for long-term therapy (14).

XVIII. OTHER POSSIBLE APPLICATIONS OF α-BLOCKERS

The use of α-blocking drugs has been reported in a variety of other conditions: in Raynaud's phenomenon, to antagonize the peripheral vasoconstriction; in the case of shock, to improve peripheral blood flow without inhibiting the chromotropic effects of catecholamines; and in bronchoconstriction to antagonize the α-mediated component (14).

XIX. SIDE EFFECTS OF α-BLOCKERS

The most important side effects from α_1-blocking drugs are those associated with too much inhibition of the α receptor, principally postural hypotension (9–13,15,16). If α-receptor inhibition is too great initially, the first-dose phenomenon results, that is, after the first dose, symptoms of severe postural hypotension occur. This side effect was of considerable concern in the early use of prazosin. Loss of consciousness occurred in several instances, and, thus, a specific effect on cerebral blood flow was suggested. However, prazosin does not appear to alter cerebral blood flow. This first-dose phenomenon is dose dependent and related to the speed of onset of α blockade. The use of a low initial dose of 0.5 mg, particularly if it is taken just before bedtime, is likely to result in only minimal if any dizziness and no occurrence of the first-dose phenomenon. The chronic administration of prazosin is probably associated with an increase in systemic blood volume and the initial excessive sensitivity to α blockade declines. There are other factors besides a low initial dose that influence the first-dose phenomenon. The consumption of a low-sodium diet provokes the phenomenon, and a high-sodium diet inhibits it. Previous treatment of a patient with a diuretic or a β-adrenoceptor-blocking drug may increase the drop in blood pressure that is associated with the initial dose of prazosin (9). Although the first-dose phenomenon has been reported with other α_1 drugs, such as doxazosin (16) or terazosin (44), its incidence is less than with prazosin. A slower onset of action for other α-blockers may contribute to this, but an important factor also is that since this first-dose phenomenon was recognized, the starting doses for other α-blockers was relatively lower than had been used with prazosin.

Whatever an α_1-blocking drug is being used, it is always wise to advise that the initial dose be small; this is particularly true when an α_1-blocking drug is being added to a drug regimen because the patient may be more sensitive to α blockade. It is also important that increases in subsequent dosages be carefully made to avoid dizziness that larger increment can produce; the dosage should normally be decreased in small decrements if any dizziness occurs.

The symptoms of orthostatic hypotension from α_1 blockade vary and depend greatly on how carefully dose increments are calculated. The incidence orthostatic hypotension reported from prazosin has been typically 10–20%, but an even higher occurrence has been seen in some studies (9). There is an incidence of dizziness with doxazosin of $\sim$5% at a dose of 1–4 mg/day and 10% at $\geq$8 mg/day (16). Likewise with terazosin, dizziness occurs $\sim$10% more frequently than when the patient is taking a placebo. When results from double-blind trials were pooled, it was reported that 3.2% of patients withdrew from studies because of dizziness with terazosin (10). Dizziness is possibly seen in $\sim$5% of patients treated with urapidil (13), and it has been reported in 4–10% of patients treated with indoramin, although diuretics were used in combination with indoramin (12). The incidence of significant dizziness with the competitive α_1-blocking drugs should be very low and the dose increments kept small, particularly when they are used in combination with other antihypertensive drugs. Very small doses should be used initially because if the patient is already receiving a diuretic and blood volume is reduced, the patient will then be particularly sensitive to an agent that increases vascular capacity which occurs with the administration of an α-blocker.

As is the case with other vasodilators, peripheral edema may occur; an incidence with terazosin 4% greater than that with a placebo has been reported (10). Nasal congestion, which may be troublesome occasionally because of a reduction in vasoconstriction tone in the nasal mucosa, is a further side effect that is attributable to cardiovascular α_1 blockade (9). Exercise tolerance does not appear to be limited by α_1 blockade.

Nausea has been reported to occur in $\sim$3–5% of patients receiving α_1-blocking drugs. Lack of energy, drowsiness, and weakness have an incidence of $\sim$7% with α_1 blockade (9,10). Fatigue has been reported in 1.4% of patients receiving urapidil (13). Indoramin also is a competitive inhibitor at the histamine$_1$ receptor and is associated with much higher incidence of somnolence (20–50%) than other α_1-receptor-blocking agents (12). Also, indoramin is associated with dry mouth overall $\sim$11% of the time; in some studies, up to 25% of patients experience this symptom (12).

Sexual dysfunction is relatively rare (3.2%). For example, impotence occurs less with prazosin than with hydrochlorothiazide (9).

Other side effects are relatively minor, and overall adverse effects in these drugs—with the exception of indoramin, with its high incidence of sedation and dry mouth—compare reasonably with the other classes of antihypertensive drugs. In the TOMHS study, there was no significant difference in the overall score for adverse reactions among the drugs doxazosin, acebutolol, amlodipine, chlorthalidone, and enalapril (25). No withdrawal reaction after discontinuing α_1-receptor-inhibitory drugs would be expected, as has been confirmed after discontinuing terazosin treatment (10).

XX. PLACE OF α_1-RECEPTOR-BLOCKING DRUGS IN ANTIHYPERTENSION TREATMENT AND CONCLUSIONS

Although α_1-blocking agents are no longer regarded as first-choice agents in the treatment of hypertension, they remain useful agents to be used in combination with other drugs (24). There are three possible important advantages in the treatment of hypertension with α_1-receptor-blocking drugs: their hemodynamic profile, the relative ease of patient selection, and the apparent absence of long-term adverse metabolic side effects.

The pathological hemodynamic changes of hypertension are reversed by α-receptor-inhibitory drugs toward conditions seen in normotensive subjects. The reduction in peripheral resistance is the principal effect.

There are no important contraindications to α-adrenoceptor-blocking drugs. They do not worsen asthma; in fact, they may have a modest anti-asthmatic effect. α_1-blocking drugs increase peripheral blood flow and have been used in the treatment of Raynaud's disease. Provided that care is taken to reduce the incidence of first-dose excessive drops in blood pressure, particularly in susceptible subjects such as the elderly, there are no problems in the selection of patients, and there are no co-morbidities that represent an absolute contraindication to their use. Unlike some other first-line antihypertensive drugs, α_1-blockers increase HDL, improve the HDL/LDL cholesterol ratio, have other favorable effects on lipid profile and improve insulin sensitivity.

REFERENCES

1. Guimarães S, Moura D. Vascular adrenoceptors: an update. Pharmacol Rev 2001; 53:319–356.
2. Van Zwieten PA. α Adrenoceptor blocking agents in the treatment of hypertension. In: Laragh JH, Brenner BM, eds. Hypertension; Pathophysiology, Diagnosis, and Management. 2nd ed. New York: Raven Press Ltd., 1995:2917–2935.
3. Langer SZ, Shepperson NB. Recent developments in vascular and smooth muscle pharmacology: The postsynaptic α2-adrenoceptor. Trends Pharmacol Sci. 1982; 3:440.
4. Prichard BNC. Principles and practice of α-antiadrenergic therapy. In: Messerli FH, ed. Cardiovascular Drug Therapy. Philadelphia: W.B. Saunders, 1996:601–616.
5. Prichard BNC, Graham BR. I$_1$ imidazoline agonists: general clinical pharmacology of imidazoline receptors. Drugs Aging 2000; 17:133–159.
6. Guyton AC, Coleman TG, Cowley AW Jr, Manning RD Jr, Norman RA Jr, Ferguson JD. A systems analysis approach to understanding long-range arterial blood pressure control and hypertension. Circ Res 1974; 35:159–176.
7. Di Bona GF. The sympathetic nervous system and hypertension; recent developments. Hypertension 2004; 43:147–150.
8. Julius S. The changing relationship between autonomic control and haemodynamics of hypertension. In: Swales JD, ed. Textbook of Hypertension. London: Blackwell, 1994:77–84.
9. Stanaszek WF, Kellerman D, Brogden RN, Romankiewicz JA. Prazosin update: a review of its pharmacological properties and therapeutic use in hypertension and congestive heart failure. Drugs 1983; 25:339–384.
10. Titmarsh S, Monk JP. Terazosin. A review of its pharmacodynamic and pharmaco-kinetic properties, and therapeutic efficacy in essential hypertension. Drugs 1987; 33:461–477.
11. Young RA, Brogden RN. Doxazosin. A review of its pharmacodynamic and pharmacokinetic properties, and therapeutic efficacy in mild to moderate hypertension. Drugs 1988; 35:525–541.
12. Holmes B, Sorkin EM. Indoramin. A review of its pharmacodynamic and pharmacokinetic properties, and therapeutic efficacy in hypertension and related vascular, cardiovascular and airway diseases. Drugs 1986; 31:467–499.
13. Dooley M, Goa KL. Urapidil. A reappraisal of its use in the management of hypertension. Drugs 1998; 56:929–955.
14. Frishman WH, Kotob F. α-adrenergic blocking drugs in clinical medicine. J Clin Pharmacol 1999; 39:7–16.
15. Brogden RN, Heel RC, Speight TM, Avery GS. Prazosin: a review of its pharmacological properties and therapeutic efficacy in hypertension. Drugs 1977; 14:163–197.
16. Fulton B, Wagstaff AJ, Sorkin EM. Doxazosin. An update of its clinical pharmacology and therapeutic applications in hypertension and benign prostatic hyperplasia. Drugs 1995; 49:295–320.
17. Cooper KL, McKiernan JM, Kaplan SA. α-Adrenoceptor antagonists in the treatment of benign prostatic hyperplasia. Drugs 1999; 57:9–17.
18. Lund-Johansen P. Central haemodynamics in essential hypertension at rest and during exercise. A 20 year follow up study. Hypertension 1989; 7(suppl):s52–s55.
19. Lund-Johansen P, Omvik P, Haugland H. Acute and chronic haemodynamic effects of doxazosin in hypertension at rest and during exercise. Br J Clin Pharmacol 1986; 21(suppl 1):45S–54S.
20. Thompson PD, Cullinane EM, Nugent AM, Sady MA, Sady SP. Effect of atenolol or prazosin on maximal exercise performance in hypertensive joggers. Am J Med 1989; 86(1B):104–109.
21. Izzo JL, Horwitz D, Keiser HR. Physiologic mechanisms opposing the hemodynamic effects of prazosin. Clin Pharmacol Ther 1981; 29:7–11.

22. Dahlof B, Pennert K, Hansson L. Reversal of left ventricular hypertrophy in hypertensive patients. A metaanalysis of 109 treatment studies. Am J Hyperten 1992; 5:95–110.

23. Gottdiener JS, Reda DJ, Massie BM, Materson BJ, Williams DW, Anderson RJ. Effect of single-drug therapy on reduction of left ventricular mass in mild to moderate hypertension. Circulation 1997; 95:2007–2014.

24. ESH/ESC Guidelines Committee. 2003 European Society of Hypertension–European Society of Cardiology guidelines for the management of arterial hypertension. J Hypertens 2003; 21:1011–1053.

25. Neaton JD, Grimm RH Jr, Prineas RJ, Stamler J, Grandits GA, Elmer PJ, Cutler JA, Flack JM, Schoenberger JA, McDonald R. For the Treatment of Mild Hypertension Study Research Group. Treatment of mild hypertension study. Final results. J Am Med Assoc 1993; 270:713–724.

26. Materson BJ, Reda DJ, Cushman WC, Massie BM, Freis ED, Kochar MS, Hamburger RJ, Fye C, Lakshman R, Gottdiener J. Single-drug therapy for hypertension in men. A comparison of six antihypertensive agents with placebo. The Department of Veterans Affairs Cooperative Study Group on Antihypertensive Agents. N Engl J Med 1993; 328(13):914–921.

27. Materson BJ, Reda DJ, Cushman WC. Department of veterans Affairs single-drug therapy of hypertension study. Revised figures and new data. Department of Veterans Affairs Cooperative Study Group on Antihypertensive Agents. Am J Hypertens 1995; 8(2):189–192.

28. ALLHAT Collaborative Research Group. Major cardiovascular events in hypertensive patients randomised to doxazosin vs chlorthalidone: the antihypertensive and lipid-lowering treatment to prevent heart attack trial (ALLHAT). J Am Med Assoc 2000; 283:1967–1975.

29. ALLHAT Collaborative Research Group. Diuretic versus α-blocker as first step anti-hypertensive therapy: Final results from the antihypertensive and lipid-lowering treatment to prevent heart attack trial (ALLHAT). Hypertension 2003; 42:239–246.

30. Wang JG, Staessen JA. Antihypertensive drug therapy in older patients. Curr Opin Nephrol Hypertens 2001; 10:263–269.

31. Williams B. Drug treatment of hypertension: implications of ALLHAT. Heart 2003; 89:589–590.

32. Sever PS. α1 blockers in hypertension. Curr Med Res Opin 1999; 15:95–103.

33. Brown MJ, Cruickshank JK, Dominiczak AF, MacGregor GA, Poulter NR, Russell GI, Thom S, Williams B. Better blood pressure control: how to combine drugs. J Human Hypertens 2003; 17:81–86.

34. Brown MJ, Dickerson JE. α-blockade and calcium antagonism: an effective and well-tolerated combination for the treatment of resistant hypertension. J Hypertens 1995; 13:701–707.

35. Mann SJ, Gerber LM. Low-dose α/β blockade in the treatment of essential hyper-tension. Am J Hypertens 2001; 14:553–558.

36. Langdon CG, Packard RS. Doxazosin in hypertension: result of a general practice study in 4809 patients. Br J Clin Prac 1994; 48:293–298.

37. Houston MC. α1-blocker combination therapy for hypertension. Postgrad Med 1998; 104:167–187.

38. Kinoshita M, Shimazu N, Fujita M, Fujimaki Y, Kojima K, Mikuni Y, Horie E, Teramoto T. Doxazosin, an α1-adrengergic antihypertensive agent, decreases serum oxidised LDL. Am J Hypertens 2001; 14:267–270.

39. Lithell HO. Hyperinsulinemia, insulin resistance, and the treatment of hypertension. Am J Hypertens 1996; 9:150s–154s.

40. Jeng JR, Sheu WH, Jeng CY, Huang SH, Shieh SM. Effect of doxazosin on fibrinolysis in hypertensive patients with and without insulin resistance. Am Heart J 1996; 132(4):783–789.

41. Cohn JN, Archibald DG, Ziesche S, Franciosa JA, Harston WE, Tristani FE, Dunkman WB, Jacobs W, Francis GS, Flohr KH, Goldman S, Cobb FR, Shah PM, Saunders R, Fletcher RD, Loeb HS, Hughes VC, Baker B. Effect of vasodilator therapy on mortality in chronic congestive heart failure: results of a Veterans Administration Cooperative Study (V-Heft) N Engl J Med 1986; 314:1547–1552.

42. Kukin ML, Kalman J, Maninno M, Freudenberger R, Buchholz C, Ocampo O. Combined α-β blockade (doxazosin plus metoprolol) compared with β blockade alone in chronic congestive heart failure. Am J Cardiol 1996; 77:486–491.

43. McConnell JD, Roehrborn CG, Bautista OM, Andriole GL Jr, Dixon CM, Kusek JW, Lepor H, McVary KT, Nyberg LM Jr, Clarke HS, Crawford ED, Diokno A, Foley JP, Foster HE, Jacobs SC, Kaplan SA, Kreder KJ, Lieber MM, Lucia MS, Miller GJ, Menon M, Milam DF, Ramsdell JW, Schenkman NS, Slawin KM, Smith JA; Medical Therapy of Prostatic Symptoms (MTOPS) Research Group. The long-term effect of doxazosin, finasteride, and combination therapy on the clinical progression of benign prostatic hyperplasia. N Engl J Med 2003; 349:2387–2398.

44. Luther RR, Glassman HN, Estep CB, Schmitz PJ, Horton JK, Jordan DC. Terazosin, a new selective α1 adrenergic blocking agent. Results of long-term treatment in patients with essential hypertension. Am J Hypertens 1988; 1(3 Pt 3):237S–240S.

29

Angiotensin-Converting Enzyme Inhibitors

DOMENIC A. SICA

Virginia Commonwealth University, Richmond, Virginia, USA

KEYPOINTS

- ACE inhibitors are compounds commonly used for the treatment of hypertension—either as monotherapy or in combination with a diuretic or a calcium-channel blocker. ACE inhibitors compare favorable with other antihypertensive medication classes as to blood pressure reduction.
- ACE inhibitors are mechanistically diverse in their pathobiologic actions beyond simple reduction in the level of angiotensin-II.
- ACE inhibitors are compounds with positive effects on outcomes in diverse disease states including: heart failure, post-myocardial infarction, chronic proteinuric kidney disease, stroke, and coronary artery disease settings.

- ACE inhibitor side-effects include functional renal insufficiency, cough, angioneurotic edema, hyperkalemia, and anemia.

SUMMARY

ACE inhibitors have enjoyed a lengthy history of use. The first application of ACE inhibitors was in the treatment of hypertension where they were shown to reduce blood pressure in a not insignificant number of individuals with hypertension. Soon these compounds were also being routinely employed in disease states such as heart failure, chronic kidney disease, and coronary artery disease. The results of large carefully conducted studies validated what was as first the empiric use of these compounds in such end-organ disease conditions. Innumerable ACE inhibitors are available and the concept of class effect is now a routine topic of discussion for these compounds. Class effect is an acceptable viewpoint when ACE inhibitor-related blood pressure reduction is being considered; however, it is a somewhat awkward concept when it is applied to the end-organ protection seen with ACE inhibitors. ACE inhibitor side-effects include cough, angioneurotic edema, functional renal insufficiency, and hyperkalemia. Angioneurotic edema is a class effect with all ACE inhibitors and is potentially life-threatening. Other ACE inhibitor-related side-effects are not common causes for discontinuation of these drugs.

I. INTRODUCTION

In the treatment of hypertension and cardiovascular disease, multiple treatment strategies have risen and fallen in popularity over the last half-century. At the forefront of most of these strategies has been the so-called *stepped-care* approach, which relies heavily on diuretic and/or β-blocker therapy. The stepped-care approach, utilizing diuretics as the first treatment option, was strongly evidence-based (1). However, adopting a stepped-care approach *per se* to the treatment of hypertension disregarded the *individualized* pathophysiology of this disease. Its backers valued its harmonizing sameness and therefore the simplicity of the approach, while others took issue with its unbending nature.

The alternative concept of individualized therapy, however attractive, did not gain its current acceptance until two events had come to pass; first, sufficient treatment options (with a minimum of side effects) had been tested, and second, these same treatment options had been submitted to study in diverse disease states with the goal of assessing outcomes. Angiotensin-converting enzyme (ACE) inhibitors—in that they were a targeted therapy intended to interfere with production of angiotensin-II—were the first therapeutic option that was truly individualized in its purpose. Over time, the ACE inhibitor drug class has effectively stood up to the concept of stepped-care; however, it has been less so on the basis of their offering individualized therapy [i.e., by reducing output from the renin–angiotensin–aldosterone system (RAAS)] but more so because of their efficacy, tolerability, and more recently positive outcomes data (2,3).

The ACE inhibitor class has grown to the degree that there are currently 10 ACE inhibitors available in the United States and many more to be had world-wide. In addition to their antihypertensive properties, ACE inhibitors were promptly recognized experimentally for their capacity to slow progressive renal, cardiac, and/or vascular disease (2,3). Thus, it was a rational step in their

Table 29.1 FDA-Approved Indications for ACE Inhibitors

DRUG	HTN	CHF	Diabetic nephropathy	High-risk patients without left ventricular dysfunction
Captopril	•	• (post-MI)[a]	•	
Benazepril	•			
Enalapril	•	•[b]		
Fosinopril	•	•		
Lisinopril	•	• (post-MI)[a]		
Moexipril	•			
Perindopril	•			
Quinapril	•	•		
Ramipril	•	• (post-MI)		•
Trandolapril	•	• (post-MI)		

[a]Captopril and lisinopril are indicated for CHF treatment both post-MI and as adjunctive therapy in general heart failure therapy.
[b]Enalapril is indicated for asymptomatic, left ventricular dysfunction.

development to seek additional usage indications in conditions such as congestive heart failure (CHF), post-myocardial infarction (post-MI), and diabetic nephropathy (Tables 29.1 and 29.2) (2,3). Most recently, a treatment indication has been granted to the ACE inhibitor ramipril for reducing cardiovascular event rates in the high-risk cardiac patient without obvious left ventricular dysfunction (4).

This chapter will by and large address the pharmacokinetic and pharmacodynamic characteristics of ACE inhibitors. In addition, it will describe the end-organ disease outcomes data for ACE inhibitors. The reader will be directed to sources that provide more comprehensive discussion on certain themes that cannot be completely discussed because of space considerations.

II. PHARMACOLOGY

In 1981, the first orally active ACE inhibitor was introduced. This was the sulfhydryl-containing compound captopril. Shortly thereafter, the more long-acting compounds enalapril maleate and lisinopril became available. Enalapril is a prodrug requiring *in vivo* esterolysis (occurring in the liver and intestinal wall) to yield its active diacid enalaprilat. All other ACE inhibitors are also prodrugs with the exception of lisinopril and captopril (3,5). Most ACE inhibitors are given as a prodrug for a specific reason, which is to improve their bioavailability (most of the active diacid ACE inhibitor forms are poorly absorbed). Although it was originally thought that formation of the active diacid metabolite of an ACE inhibitor, such as enalapril, could be inhibited in the presence of hepatic impairment, as

Table 29.2 ACE Inhibitors (Dosage Strengths and Treatment Guidelines)

| Drug | Trade name | Usual total dose and/or range | | Comment | Fixed dose combination[a] |
		Hypertension (Frequency day)	Heart Failure (Frequency day)		
Benazepril	Lotensin®	20–40 (1)	Not FDA approved for heart failure		Lotensin HCT®
Captopril	Capoten®	12.5–100 (2–3)	18.75–150 (3)	Generically available	Capozide®b
Enalapril	Vasotec®	5–40 (1–2)	5–40 (2)	Available generically and intravenously	Vaseretic®
Fosinopril	Monopril®	10–40 (1)	10–40 (1)	Renal and hepatic elimination	Monopril-HCT®
Lisinopril	Prinivil®, Zestril®	2.5–40 (1)	5–20 (1)	Generically available	Prinizide®, Zestoretic®
Moexipril	Univasc®	7.5–30 (1)	Not FDA approved for heart failure		Uniretic®
Perindopril	Aceon®	2–16 (1)	Not FDA approved for heart failure		
Quinapril	Accupril®	5–80 (1)	10–40 (1–2)		Accuretic®
Ramipril	Altace®	2.5–20 (1)	10 (2)	Indicated in high-risk vascular patients	
Trandolapril	Mavik®	1–8 (1)	1–4 (1)	Renal and hepatic elimination	Tarka®

[a]Fixed-dose combinations in this class typically contain a thiazide-like diuretic.
[b]Capozide is indicated for first-step treatment of hypertension.

exists in advanced CHF, this delay in metabolism proves to be of limited clinical consequence (6).

The binding ligand for ACE is the basis for dividing these drugs into three structurally heterogeneous groups: sulfhydryl, phosphinyl, and carboxyl-containing moieties. These structural differences in the ligand for ACE purport to offer pharmacologic advantages, such as a free-radical scavenging ability with the sulfhydryl-containing ACE inhibitor captopril, but to date any such distinctions remain clinically unproven (7). Alternatively, the sulfhydryl group contained within captopril is regarded as the basis for the more frequent skin rashes (usually maculopapular in form) and the dysgeusia observed with this compound (8). The idea that the phosphinyl group (present on the ACE inhibitor fosinopril) might determine its ability to penetrate the myocardium and thereby improve myocardial inotropic and lusitropic responses is likewise unproven (9).

ACE inhibitors can be further distinguished by differences in rate and extent of absorption, plasma protein binding, systemic half-life, and means of systemic clearance; however, any such differences (beyond frequency of dosing) appear to offer no obvious advantage in BP reduction (if comparable doses are given) (Table 29.3) (3,5,10,11); however, two pharmacologic considerations for the ACE inhibitors, mode of systemic elimination

and tissue-binding, have generated recent discussion and deserve additional comment (12,13).

A. Route of Elimination

In the presence of chronic kidney disease (CKD), the ACE inhibitors ramipril, enalapril, fosinopril, trandolapril, and benazepril do not accumulate with repetitive dosing, suggesting that these prodrugs either undergo some intact biliary clearance or their conversion to an active diacid form is independent of renal function (14–16). Each of these ACE inhibitors is marginally active as a prodrug; thus, the absence of accumulation in CKD is a moot point and should not be viewed as a clinically relevant property. ACE inhibitor accumulation in CKD is most germane for the diacid metabolites (which are typically the active form) of these compounds. The diacid metabolites of fosinopril and trandolapril, fosinoprilat and trandolaprilat, are the only ones, which undergo dual renal and hepatic elimination (15,16). For all other ACE inhibitors, their systemic clearance is largely renal (with accumulation commencing early in the course of CKD) occurring by varying degrees of filtration and tubular secretion (12). ACE inhibitor accumulation has yet to be associated with the known idiosyncratic side effects of ACE inhibitors, such as cough or angioneurotic edema.

Table 29.3   Predominant Hemodynamic Effects of ACE Inhibitors

Hemodynamic parameter	Effect	Clinical significance
Cardiovascular		
Total peripheral resistance	Decreased	These parameters contribute to a
Mean arterial pressure	Decreased	general decrease in systemic
Cardiac output	Increased or no change	blood pressure
Stroke volume	Increased	
Preload and afterload	Decreased	
Pulmonary artery pressure	Decreased	
Right atrial pressure	Decreased	
Diastolic dysfunction	Improved	
Renal		
Renal blood flow	Usually increased	Contributes to the renoprotective
Glomerular filtration rate	Variable, usually unchanged but may decrease in renal failure	effect of these agents
Efferent arteriolar resistance	Decreased	
Filtration fraction	Decreased	
Sympathetic nervous system		
Biosynthesis of noradrenaline	Decreased	Enhances blood pressure lowering
Reuptake of adrenaline	Inhibited	effect and resets baroreceptor
Circulating catecholamines	Decreased	function

However, elevations in ACE inhibitor concentrations can be attended by significantly reduced BP values and/or evidence of organ underperfusion (17).

B.   Tissue Binding

The second unresolved pharmacologic feature of ACE inhibitors is that of tissue binding (13,18). The physicochemical differences among ACE inhibitors including binding affinity, potency, lipophilicity, and depot effect allows for the arbitrary classification of ACE inhibitors according to affinity for tissue ACE (13,19). The extent to which tissue ACE is blocked by an ACE inhibitor parallels both the inhibitor's intrinsic binding affinity, as well as the free inhibitor concentration found within that tissue. The tissue-based free inhibitor concentration is in a continuous state of flux and at any one time is determined by the sum of ACE inhibitor delivered to tissues and residual ACE inhibitor released from tissues for re-entry into the bloodstream. The quantity of ACE inhibitor conveyed to tissues is determined by several pharmacologic variables including dose frequency/amount, absolute bioavailability, plasma half-life, and tissue penetration. When blood levels of an ACE inhibitor are high— typically in the first third to half of the dosing interval— tissue retention *per se* of an ACE inhibitor is not needed for an enduring level of ACE inhibition. However, as ACE inhibitor blood levels fall during the second-half of the dosing interval, two factors (inhibitor binding affinity and tissue retention) take on added importance if functional ACE inhibition is to be maintained (13).

The question arises as to whether the degree of tissue ACE inhibition may extend to efficacy differences between the various ACE inhibitors. In this regard, there appears to be little difference among the various ACE inhibitors in their capacity to reduce BP. When relative drug-to-drug BP responses differ among ACE inhibitors, it is generally the result of divergent half-lives of the compounds under study.

An additional consideration is whether ACE inhibitors with a high tissue affinity differ in their ability to provide BP-independent end-organ protection as has been theorized for the ACE inhibitor ramipril in the Heart Outcomes Protection (HOPE) study (20). In this regard, endothelial function is observed to improve more regularly with the higher tissue-ACE affinity compounds such as quinapril and ramipril. If improvement in endothelial dysfunction is accepted as a surrogate for protection from end-events, then relevant intraclass differences may exist among ACE inhibitors. Yet, there have been no direct head-to-head outcomes trials between ACE inhibitors, which possess varying tissue affinity. When such head-to-head comparisons have been undertaken, the results do not convincingly support the claim of overall superiority for lipophilic ACE inhibitors (21,22).

C.   Application of Pharmacologic Differences

As there is little that truly separates one long-acting ACE inhibitor from another in the treatment of hypertension, the cost of an ACE inhibitor has assumed increased importance (23). For pricing to be key in the selection of an

ACE inhibitor is not unreasonable if these drugs were only being used for the control of BP. ACE inhibitors, however, are also extensively used for their cardiorenal outcomes benefits and in that only a limited number of ACE inhibitors have been studied. The term *class effect* has entered into the discussion of both of these aspects of ACE inhibitor use, relevant to one and not the other.

Class effect is a phrase often invoked to legitimatize use of a less costly ACE inhibitor when a higher-priced agent in the class has been the one specifically studied in disease states such as CHF, diabetic nephropathy, or high-risk CAD circumstances (20,24–26). The concept of class effect may be best suited for application to the BP effects of ACE inhibitors where scant difference exists among the numerous ACE inhibitors. Alternatively, the concept of class effect, already vague in its definition, becomes even more ambiguous when "true" dose equivalence for a non-BP end-point, such as rate of progression to end-stage renal disease (ESRD) or survival in the setting of CHF, is being determined for the various ACE inhibitors. Determining ACE inhibitor dose equivalence from outcomes trials is particularly confused by differing dose frequency, titration requirements, and level of renal function in individual disease-state studies (27–32). The latter is particularly relevant to the elderly as senescence-related changes in renal function extend the functional half-life of an ACE inhibitor (if it is renally cleared as most are) and make it nearly impossible to determine "true" dose equivalence between various ACE inhibitors.

A prudent action as regards the concept of ACE inhibitor class effect in outcomes trials is to assume that the benefits derive from the compound being tested, for the outcome being studied, at the *per protocol* dose amount and frequency of dosing; however, despite these caveats about the difficulty in establishing dose equivalence, the clinician can presumably estimate what might represent equivalent doses among the various ACE inhibitors if an ACE inhibitor substitution policy exists.

III. MECHANISM OF ACTION AND HEMODYNAMIC EFFECTS

The site of ACE inhibitor activity (within the RAA axis) can be pinpointed at the pluripotent ACE, an enzyme known to catalyze the conversion of angiotensin-I to angiotensin-II as well as to facilitate the degradation of bradykinin to assorted vasoactive peptides (18,33). However, there are inherent limitation as to how well ACE inhibition can reduce angiotensin-II levels (18). ACE inhibition fails to suppress production of angiotensin-II by alternative enzymatic pathways such as chymase and other tissue-based proteases (18,34). These alternative pathways represent the principal mode of

angiotensin-II generation in several tissues including the myocardium and the vasculature (35,36). With long-term ACE inhibitor administration, these alternative pathways upregulate in the course of a sequence of events, which culminate in a return of angiotensin-II concentrations to pretherapy levels (angiotensin-II escape). Substrate for these alternative pathways, in part, is obtained from the increase in angiotensin-I levels arising from a disinhibition of renin secretion by ACE inhibition (36,37).

Because ACE inhibitors reduce angiotensin-II levels only in the order of weeks, other mechanisms for their persistent BP lowering effect must exist (37,38). One possibility is that an increase in the concentrations of the vasodilator bradykinin, which can be expected to enhance the release of nitric oxide (NO), stimulate the production of endothelium-derived hyperpolarizing factor, and accentuate the release of prostacyclin (PGI_2) (39,40). Moreover, ACE is also responsible for the degradation of angiotensin (1–7), an angiotensin peptide (of an autocrine/paracrine nature) with the capacity to counterbalance a number of the pleitrophic (renal and vascular) effects of angiotensin-II (40). The contribution of angiotensin "fragments" (many of which are physiologically active) and prostaglandins/NO to the antihypertensive effect of ACE inhibitors is still debated (40,41).

Alternatively, it has been recognized for some time that nonsteroidal anti-inflammatory drugs (NSAIDs) and selective cyclooxygenase inhibitors (COXIBs), such as celecoxib and rofecoxib, dampen the BP-lowering effect of a number of antihypertensive compounds including ACE inhibitors (42,43). This occurs more commonly in salt-sensitive hypertensives as in the case of many elderly and African-American patients (43) and may relate to a compound's (COXIB or traditional NSAID) half-life for effect and therefore dosing frequency (44).

A question that remains unresolved is the level of interaction for aspirin with the antihypertensive and/or cardioprotective effects of an ACE inhibitor (45–47). Low-dose aspirin (≤ 100 mg/day) appears to minimally affect the BP reduction observed with ACE inhibition (45,46). For example, in the Hypertension Optimal Treatment (HOT) study long term, low-dose ASA did not interfere with the BP-lowering effect of antihypertensive combinations, which in many cases included ACE inhibitors (46). However, higher doses (generally >236 mg/day) can blunt the antihypertensive response to an ACE inhibitor and possibly neutralize the clinical benefits of ACE inhibitors in patients with heart failure (47).

A reduction in both central and peripheral sympathetic nervous system (SNS) activity accounts for a portion of the antihypertensive effect of an ACE inhibitor (Table 29.3) (48,49). ACE inhibitors also preserve circulatory reflexes and baroreceptor function; thus, they do not reflexly increase heart rate, when BP is reduced (50). This latter property accounts for the low incidence of postural hypotension with this drug class and provides an important safety benefit in elderly subjects, who as a group are typically predisposed to orthostatic hypotension (51). ACE inhibitors also improve endothelial function, facilitate vascular remodeling, and favorably modify the viscoelastic properties of structurally abnormal blood vessels (52,53). Such vascular effects are the probable explanation for the incremental reduction in BP with long-term ACE inhibitor administration.

IV. BLOOD PRESSURE LOWERING EFFECT

All ACE inhibitors available in the United States are FDA-approved for the treatment of hypertension (Table 29.2). The Joint National Committee on the Detection, Evaluation, and Treatment of High Blood Pressure (JNC 7), the World Health Organization/International Society of Hypertension, and European Society of Hypertension/European Society of Cardiology and the Canadian Hypertension Education Program Evidence-based Recommendations Task Force now endorse ACE inhibitors as an alternative for first-line therapy in patients with essential hypertension, especially in those with a high coronary disease risk profile, diabetes with renal disease/proteinuria, CHF, and/or are post-MI (54–56).

ACE inhibitors are viewed as a suitable first-step option in the treatment of hypertension. This includes recreational exercisers and athletes who have hypertension (57–59), which is but one of several areas where ACE inhibitor use is accepted but not extensively studied (59). The enthusiasm for the use of ACE inhibitors extends beyond the issue of effectiveness, because they are comparably efficacious (and not better than) to most other drug classes including diuretics, β-blockers, and calcium-channel blockers (CCBs). Response rates with ACE inhibitors range from 40–70% in Stage I or II hypertension with salt intake and race influencing the observed response rate (60). In the interpretation of clinical trial results with ACE inhibitors, a distinction should be made between the mean reduction in BP (which is typically significant) and the percentage of individuals who are poor, average, and excellent responders (which may vary considerably in the different studies).

There are few predictors of the vasodepressor response to ACE inhibitors. Although ACE gene polymorphism (and specific genotypes) among other genetic determinants have been suggested to predict the antihypertensive response to an ACE inhibitors, such findings have been sufficiently inconsistent to warrant a wait-and-see attitude for genotyping (61). There has also been a limited predictive relationship between the pre and/or post-treatment plasma renin activity (PRA) value (used as a marker of RAA axis activity) and the fall in BP with an ACE inhibitor; however, when hypertension is marked by RAA axis activation such as in renal artery stenosis, the response to an ACE inhibitor can be profound (62).

Certain patient groups are recognized as being responsive [high-renin and young hypertensives (age of 6–16)] and others less responsive to ACE inhibitor monotherapy, including low-renin, salt-sensitive, volume-expanded individuals such as the diabetic and African-American hypertensive (2,3,63). However, the BP response to an ACE inhibitor can be highly variable in the African-American and diabetic patient with some individuals in these groups experiencing significant falls in BP (64,65). The low-renin state characteristic of the elderly hypertensive differs from other low-renin forms of hypertension in that it reflects the consequences of senescence-related changes in the RAA axis and not volume expansion (66). The elderly generally respond well to ACE inhibitors at conventional doses (67), though senescence-related renal failure, which slows the elimination of most ACE inhibitors, complicates interpretation of dose-specific treatment successes.

Results from a number of head-to-head trials support the similar antihypertensive efficacy and tolerability of the various ACE inhibitors if comparable doses of the individual ACE inhibitors are given (Table 29.2). However, there are differences among the ACE inhibitors, as to the time to onset and/or the duration of effect, which may relate to the absorption and tissue distribution characteristics of a compound.

Enalaprilat is the lone ACE inhibitor available in an intravenous form; however, multiple choices exist for the orally available ACE inhibitors (3). ACE inhibitors labeled as "once-daily," vary in their ability to reduce BP for a full day, as defined by a trough: peak ratio >50% (68). Consequently, the dosing frequency for ACE inhibitors should occur with the understanding that response patterns to these drugs are highly individualized with many patients requiring a second daily dose to maintain effect. However, senescence-related changes in renal function (and reduced ACE inhibitor renal clearance) and/or giving a high dose may obviate a second ACE inhibitor dose during the day treatment period (69).

A frequent question asked is what steps to take when an ACE inhibitor fails to normalize BP. This question is best answered in the context of the magnitude of the response. If there is a minimal BP-reducing effect, then a switch to an alternative drug class is justified unless continuation of an ACE inhibitor is warranted on the basis of a high risk profile from cardiac and/or renal disease; however, ACE inhibitor nonresponders fairly regularly "respond" upon addition of a diuretic or a CCB. This latter observation would suppose that very few patients should have an ACE inhibitor discontinued simply on the basis of a failure to initially "respond."

If the BP response is modest, one can increase the daily dose (this can occur by reverting to twice daily administration) understanding that the dose–response curve for ACE inhibitors, like many antihypertensive agents, is fairly steep at the beginning doses and thereafter flattens (70,71). Increasing the dose of an ACE inhibitor does not generally change the peak effect, rather it extends the duration of response. In fact, several of the shorter acting ACE inhibitors, such as enalapril, can behave as once-a-day medications if high-enough doses are given. A final consideration with ACE inhibitor therapy is that of an incremental BP benefit (over several weeks) relating to factors such as vascular remodeling and/or improvement in endothelial function (53).

V. ACE INHIBITORS IN COMBINATION WITH OTHER AGENTS

The BP-lowering ability of an ACE inhibitor is bettered with the concurrent administration of a diuretic, particularly when a salt-sensitive pattern of hypertension exists (72). This type response has encouraged the development of several fixed-dose combination products, comprised an ACE inhibitor and varying doses (as low as 12.5 mg) of a thiazide-type diuretic (72,73). The rationale for combining these two drug classes arises from the observation that diuretic-related sodium depletion activates the RAA axis; therein BP shifts to an angiotensin-II dependent mode, which is a circumstance most conducive to the BP-reducing properties of an ACE inhibitor.

β-Blockers have been administered in conjunction with ACE inhibitors, an approach which was possible *per protocol* in the Antihypertensive and Lipid-lowering Treatment to Prevent Heart Attack Trial (ALLHAT) (58). The β-blocker atenolol was the most commonly added second medication in ALLHAT and was, in part, the basis for the greater use of Step 3 therapy with hydralazine in this trial. If a physiologic basis exists for this combination, it is that of β-blockade blunting the reactive rise in PRA that goes along with ACE inhibitor therapy (72); alternatively, this combination can be considered for use in the setting of coronary artery disease (CAD) with any BP gain being a secondary consideration (74). When a meaningful drop in BP follows from the addition of a β-blocker to an ACE inhibitor, it often occurs in sequence with a reduction in pulse-rate. Alternatively, adding a peripheral α-antagonist, such as doxazosin, to an ACE inhibitor can further reduce BP, albeit without a clear mechanistic basis (75).

Finally, the BP-lowering effect of an ACE inhibitor is reinforced with the addition of a CCB, be it either a dihydropyridine or a nondihydropyridine-type compound. This particular pattern of additivity has been the basis for several fixed-dose combination products comprised both drug classes (76–78); however, the consequence of these two drug classes being combined may go beyond that of additivity for BP reduction. Combined ACE inhibitor and CCB treatment with the compounds benazepril and amlodipine has also been demonstrated to be more effective than high doses of these individual agents in improving arterial compliance and/or reducing left ventricular mass (79). In addition, a verapamil–trandolapril-based treatment strategy was as clinically effective as an atenolol-hydrochlorothiazide regimen in hypertensive CAD patients (80). The addition of an ACE inhibitor to a CCB is also of use in attenuating and/or preventing CCB-related peripheral edema (81). In addition, preliminary evidence exists in support of CCB-therapy attenuating the drop in glomerular filtration rate that can accompany ACE inhibitor therapy (82). This is of particular relevance to the elderly as one reason for underuse of ACE inhibitors in older subjects is fear of a decline in renal function on top of already reduced renal function. This CCB and ACE inhibitor hemodynamic interaction at a renal level may also occasionally result in false positive captopril renography studies.

The efficacy of both ACE inhibitors and angiotensin-receptor blockers (ARBs) as antihypertensive agents is well established. This has fueled the belief that in combination, these two drug classes may provide an incremental benefit in both BP reduction and end-organ protection. However, there is an insufficient evidence to support a general recommendation for the combination of these two drug classes in BP management (83,84).

Finally, studies have established the utility of ACE inhibitors in regressing left ventricular hypertrophy induced by complex medical regimens employing the potent vasodilator minoxidil (85). In addition, if an acute reduction in BP is needed, oral or sublingual captopril—with an onset of action as soon as 15 min after administration—can be administered. An additional option for the management of hypertensive emergencies is intravenous enalaprilat with a dose of 0.625 mg representing a maximum effect dose (higher doses may only extend the duration of action) (86). ACE inhibitors should be administered cautiously in patients suspected of a marked activation of the RAA axis (e.g., prior treatment with diuretics and/or immediately after-MI). In such subjects, sudden and extreme drops in BP (so-called first dose hypotension) have been observed (87).

VI. ACE INHIBITORS IN HYPERTENSION ASSOCIATED WITH OTHER CONDITIONS

A. Cardiac Disorders

ACE inhibitors effectively alter ventricular geometry and thereby regress left ventricular hypertrophy (LVH) (88). This is an important property of ACE inhibitors given that LVH portends a significant future risk of sudden death or MI (89). ACE inhibitors can be safely utilized in patients with CAD (90) and are indicated for secondary prevention after acute MI (2,3). In addition, the ACE inhibitor perindopril has been shown to reduce cardiovascular risk in a low-risk population with stable CAD and no apparent heart failure (91). Although they are not proven coronary vasodilators, ACE inhibitors improve hemodynamic factors such that myocardial oxygen consumption is reduced with no worsening of angina and possibly some attendant benefits on ischemia (Table 29.3). ACE inhibitors do not reflexly increase myocardial sympathetic tone in hypertensive patients with angina, as can take place with other antihypertensives (90,92). However, when studied quinapril, doses as high as 80 mg were not found to favorably improve transient ischemia in a normotensive CAD cohort without left ventricular dysfunction (90). ACE inhibitors can also be cautiously used in two other patient types; first, pediatric cancer survivors previously exposed to anthracyclines (93), and second, symptomatic patients with aortic stenosis (particularly if there is a component of aortic insufficiency); however, patients with aortic stenosis, left ventricular dysfunction and low BP are prone to symptomatic hypotension with their use (94).

B. Systolic Hypertension and Peripheral Arterial Disease

ACE inhibitors are effective in the management of either isolated systolic hypertension or systolic-predominant forms of hypertension (95), which partly relates to their capacity to improve vessel compliance as well as to reduce central aortic pressures (53,96,97). ACE inhibitors are of value in the treatment of patients with cerebrovascular disease, since they maintain cerebral autoregulation in the setting of lowered BP, a property of particular importance to the elderly hypertensive (98).

ACE inhibitors vasodilate various caliber arteries (small and large) without producing a steal phenomenon. This property allows these drugs to be used safely in patients with peripheral arterial disease (PAD) (99). In the Heart Outcomes Prevention Evaluation (HOPE) study, 3099 of the 8986 patients had PAD (defined by an ankle-brachial index <0.90). When the effects of ACE inhibition with ramipril were assessed in this PAD cohort and were compared with those without PAD, the risk of fatal and nonfatal ischemic events was comparably reduced whether PAD patients were symptomatic or subclinical in their disease (100).

C. Diabetes

ACE inhibitors are also considered as preferred agents in the hypertensive diabetic patient for several reasons; first

for BP reduction (101) and second for organ protection, an attribute in all probability independent of BP lowering (102). In the former instance, it is often necessary to co-administer a diuretic (sometimes with the specific intention to diurese the patient) as ACE inhibitor monotherapy only modestly reduces BP in the low-renin, volume expanded hypertensive diabetic (72). Finally, ACE inhibitors have also been shown to influence diabetic retinopathy. In the EURODIAB Controlled Trial of Lisinopril in Insulin-Dependent Diabetes Mellitus (EUCLID) study, the ACE inhibitor lisinopril reduced the risk of progression of retinopathy by ~50% and also significantly reduced the risk of progression to proliferative retinopathy (103). These findings are consistent with the hypothesis that the RAS is expressed in the eye and that adverse effects of angiotensin-II on retinal angiogenesis and function can be inhibited by ACE inhibitors or ARBs (104).

A concluding consideration in the hypertensive diabetic is the effect of ACE inhibition on lipids and/or insulin sensitivity and their utility in the obese hypertensive. As to the latter, ACE inhibitors are useful agents (in combination therapy) in obese hypertensives (105). Alternatively, ACE inhibitors have not yet demonstrated a clear-cut effect on serum lipids (106). However, in the CAPtopril Prevention Project (CAPPP), the HOPE study, and ALLHAT, the ACE inhibitors captopril, ramipril, and lisinopril decreased the incidence of new-onset type 2 diabetes mellitus, respectively (58,107,108). Being that a similar reduction in the rate of new-onset diabetes has been observed with ARB therapy, the suggestion has been made that this phenomenon links to some aspect of angiotensin-II effect on insulin sensitivity; however, the basis for this effect on glucose homeostasis remains uncertain at this time though under active investigation.

VII. END-ORGAN EFFECTS AND RECENT CLINICAL TRIALS RENAL

The JNC 7 recommends the use of ACE inhibitors in patients with hypertension and CKD both to control hypertension and to slow its rate of progression (1,54). However, the renoprotective features of ACE inhibitors should never substitute for tight BP control or smoking cessation, which are of importance in the management of the hypertensive CKD patient. As to the latter, cigarette smoking exacerbates renal injury in type 2 diabetes despite BP control and ACE inhibitor therapy, but its cessation ameliorates the progressive renal injury caused by continued smoking (109).

As regards BP targets in CKD, the JNC 7 suggests a goal BP of <130/80 mmHg in albuminuric patients (>300 mg/day) with or without CKD (54). In hypertensive CKD patients, ACE inhibitor monotherapy (without concomitant diuretic administration) rarely yields a brisk

BP-lowering response—because of the volume dependency of this form of hypertension. For example, in the African-American Study of Kidney Disease and Hypertension (AASK), those hypertensive African-American CKD patients treated with ramipril and randomized to a mean arterial BP of 102–107 mmHg required three additional medications (most times including a diuretic) on average to achieve this goal BP range (110).

Both macroproteinuria and microalbuminuria have come forward as strong indicators of the rate of CKD progression (111). In particular, microalbuminuria warns of the succession of the stages of diabetic nephropathy and now should be routinely determined in all diabetics (111). The choice of risk terms for proteinuria (macroproteinuria or microalbuminuria) has been arbitrarily established at a cut-point above or below 300–500 mg/day; however, these partition values for urine albumin excretion should not be taken to mean that the incremental risk with proteinuria exists solely by progressing from microalbuminuria to macroproteinuria when, in fact, there appears not to be a specific threshold value for the risk associated with microalbuminuria (112). In either case, proteinuria also serves as an independent risk factor for fatal and nonfatal cardiovascular events (112,113). Screening for microalbuminuria is recommended in all diabetics and increasingly in others perceived to be at high risk for renal or cardiovascular disease (114,115). It is now recommended that proteinuria is therapeutically targeted when present in both diabetic and nondiabetic renal disease (116,117). In this regard, ACE inhibitors and ARBs, given separately or together, effectively reduce protein excretion and thereby are important tools in the treatment of micro- or macroalbuminuria patients (with or without hypertension) (117,118). With combination of ACE inhibitor and ARB therapy, the greater antiproteinuric effect most likely relates to favorably renal hemodynamic effects, in addition to glomerular size selectivity amelioration (119).

ACE inhibitors have demonstrated renoprotective effects in various settings including established type 1 insulin-dependent diabetic nephropathy (25), type 2 non-insulin dependent diabetic nephropathy (120,121), normotensive type 1 patients with microalbuminuria (122), and an assortment of nondiabetic renal diseases (116,123–125).

ACE inhibitor therapy (trandolapril), together with ARB therapy (losartan), has also been shown to be renoprotective (more than either drug alone) in nondiabetic glomerular disease (126). In some diabetic patients, ACE inhibitor therapy has resulted in the remission of nephrotic range proteinuria and long-term stabilization of renal function (127,128). However, aggressive BP control (<130/80 mmHg) in elderly patients with type 2 diabetes and preserved renal function stabilizes renal function regardless of whether the initial therapy is with an ACE inhibitor or a CCB (129,130). Moreover, recent experimental data suggests that much more of the renoprotective effects of ACE inhibition are BP dependent and go underappreciated when insensitive measurement techniques are used to determine day BP load (131).

More recently, the benefits of ACE inhibitor therapy in nondiabetic renal diseases have become clear. In the AASK, ramipril was more effective than amlopidine at slowing the rate of decline in glomerular filtration rate (GFR) in patients with hypertensive nephrosclerosis and a urinary protein:creatinine ratio >0.22 (urinary protein excretion of >300 mg/day) (125). Moreover, a recent meta-analysis of ACE inhibitor use in nondiabetic renal disease concluded that ACE inhibitors conferred renal benefit in nondiabetic patients distinguished by having >0.5 gms/day of proteinuria (132). In many of these studies comprising this meta-analysis, the target BP was <140/90 mmHg, which is significant in that the renoprotective effects of ACE inhibitors (compared with other antihypertensive agents) may not be as prominent at lesser BP values.

However, positive renal outcomes with ACE inhibitors in nephropathic states are not guaranteed. In the Ramipril Efficacy in Nephropathy (REIN) study patients with proteinuric chronic nephropathies were assigned randomly to treatment with the ACE inhibitor ramipril or placebo plus conventional antihypertensive therapy. ACE inhibitors significantly reduced the rate of proteinuria, the decline in GFR, and the risk of ESRD in patients with >3 g/day of proteinuria; however, during the study period, those with proteinuria <2 g/day, type 2 diabetes, or polycystic kidney disease did not benefit to an appreciable extent from ACE inhibitor therapy (133).

ACE inhibitor regimens that slow the rate of CKD progression include benazepril 10 mg/day, captopril 25 mg/day, enalapril 5–10 mg/day, and ramipril 2.5–5 mg/day (3). Each of these ACE inhibitors is renally cleared; thus, it can be presumed that reduced renal clearance in the presence of CKD would have prolonged their pharmacologic effect (134). Whereas it is accepted that the beneficial effects of ACE inhibition are greatest when urinary protein excretion is excessive (>3 g/day) (135). The ACE inhibitor dose providing optimal renoprotection is still openly debated. For example, low dose ramipril (1.25 mg/day) in addition to conventional therapy has no effect on cardiovascular and renal outcomes of patients with type 2 diabetes and albuminuria, despite a slight decrease in blood pressure and urinary albumin (136). Conversely, in the HOPE trial ramipril given at a high dose (titrated to 10 mg/day) prevented or delayed progression of microalbuminuria (137).

Dose titration of an ACE inhibitor should be viewed in the context of the sought after therapeutic end-point because targeted reductions in protein excretion, lipid parameters and BP show evidence of differing dose–responses to the upwards titration of an ACE inhibitor (138,139). For example, in chronic proteinuric nondiabetic nephropathies, uptitration of the ACE inhibitor lisinopril to maximum tolerated doses improves hypertriglyceridemia by a direct, dose-dependent effect, and hypercholesterolemia (through increases in serum albumin/total protein concentration and thereby oncotic pressure). These lipid benefits with upward dose titration even with the majority of the BP-lowering effect having occurred at the low-end doses of lisinopril (Fig. 29.1) (139).

Therapies directed at reducing the production or effects of angiotensin-II offer a mixture of potentially beneficial renal effects involving hemodynamic, cellular, and lipid-related pathways; however, the expected positive hemodynamic effects of ACE inhibition can sometimes be misconstrued to represent a "nephrotoxic" process.

ACE inhibitors transiently reduce GFR in tandem with their reducing glomerular capillary pressures (140,141). Such falls in GFR are typically inconsequential and generally in the order of 10–15%; moreover, these changes are reversible and in point of fact predictive of renal protection in the long-term (141). The elderly are more liable to GFR reductions with ACE inhibitors at least, in part, because of their typically more advanced micro- and macrovascular renal disease (Section X) (142). A question commonly put forward with ACE inhibitors, particularly in the elderly, is whether a specific level of renal function exists at which an ACE inhibitor should not be started. In this regard, there is not a specific level of renal function, which prohibits the start of an ACE inhibitor, unless clinically important hyperkalemia is anticipated.

Several factors can be regarded as being able to adjust the renal effects of ACE inhibition. First, a low sodium intake improves both the antiproteinuric and the antihypertensive response to ACE inhibition (143,144). Second, short-term studies show that dietary protein restriction enhances the ACE inhibitor effect on protein excretion in nephrotic patients, suggesting that the combination of dietary protein restriction and ACE inhibition could prove more effective than ACE inhibition alone in slowing the progression of CKD (145). A third adjudicating factor is that of resistance to the antiproteinuric effect of ACE inhibition during the nighttime hours despite a persistent day BP-lowering effect (146).

Finally, ACE activity varies according to inherited variations in its structure. Two common forms of the ACE gene I (insertion) and D (deletion) give rise to three potential genotypes II, ID, and DD. The DD genotype is associated with higher circulating ACE levels and an increased pressor response to infused angiotensin-I when compared with the II genotype and with the ID genotype displaying intermediate characteristics (147). The observation that DD patients were at increased risk for MI and ischemic cardiomyopathy was the earliest sign that an inherited variation in ACE activity could be of clinical significance (148). Recent studies have found that renal function declines more rapidly in CKD patients with the DD genotype. Moreover, when such patients are given ACE inhibitors, the anticipated reduction in urine protein excretion and the slowing in the rate of CKD progression are less apparent (149). Although ACE genotyping seems promising, as a means to pharmacogenetically selecting out those CKD patients likely to be more responsive to ACE inhibition, studies to date do not provide a sufficiently definitive answer to warrant more widespread use of genotyping (150).

VIII. CARDIAC

ACE inhibitor therapy has been shown to provide positive outcome benefits in a number of cardiac scenarios including CHF (24,29,151), post-MI (152–155), and in the hypertensive patient with a definable cardiac risk (20,57,58,91). More recently, these drugs have even been shown to reduce the occurrence of atrial fibrillation in the post-operative period following coronary artery bypass grafting (156). ACE inhibitor benefits have been demonstrated both in normotensive (20) and hypertensive (20,57,58) individuals, in diabetics (157), as well as patients with varying risk profiles (20,57,58,91). This beneficial effect has now been observed with several ACE inhibitors, suggesting that a class effect may be present for the positive cardiac outcomes benefits with these compounds (20,57,58,91).

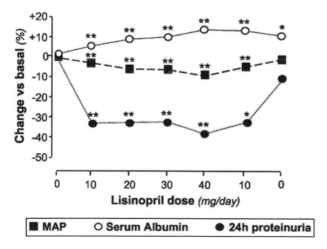

Figure 29.1 Percent changes vs. baseline in MAP, 24 h urinary protein excretion rate, and serum albumin at different lisinopril treatment periods in 22 patients with nondiabetic proteinuric nephropathies (*P < 0.05, **P < 0.01 vs. baseline). [Adapted with permission from Ruggenenti et al. (139).]

The results from both placebo-controlled and open-label trials suggest that ACE inhibitors improve CHF symptomatology and more importantly reduce the risk of death and hospitalization from CHF (24,29,151). These positive results for heart failure outcomes have established ACE inhibitors as first-line therapy in the treatment of CHF (158,159). ACE inhibitors decrease angiotensin-II production (at least in the short-term) (35,36) and thereby readjust the neurohumoral imbalance of CHF (160,161). ACE inhibitor effect in heart failure is at least, in part, related to changes in bradykinin effect (and possibly concentration), which distinguishes these drugs from ARBs (162). Low doses of ACE inhibitors are sufficient to improve exercise tolerance, and CHF symptoms (28,31) as well as more recently being shown to arrest the weight loss otherwise seen with progressive CHF (163); however, improvement in CHF mortality at least, in part, requires high-dose ACE inhibitor therapy (29,32). The optimal frequency of ACE inhibitor dosing in CHF is as of yet undecided. This has proven to be a tricky question to answer, in part, because few studies have even addressed the question. When formally studied (at least for surrogate markers of CHF), twice-daily regimens appear superior to once-daily treatment regimens (164). Until incontrovertible evidence otherwise becomes available, the treatment of CHF should include sequential dose titration to those ACE inhibitor doses proven to favorably affect mortality in randomized clinical trials. The ability to reach these doses in the CHF patient can often prove challenging because systemic hypotension and/or a decline in GFR often arise with high-dose ACE inhibitor therapy (165–167); thus, reaching goal ACE inhibitor doses calls for a well-developed understanding of the relationship between volume status, BP, and the sought after ACE inhibitor dose (165,166).

Several ACE inhibitors—including captopril, fosinopril, lisinopril, quinapril, ramipril, and trandolapril—have demonstrated positive outcomes data in a range of CHF types (151,152,168). Despite the compelling makeup of these outcomes data, physician-prescribing practice has lagged behind. As such, only a modest fraction (50–75%) of those CHF patients eligible for ACE inhibitor therapy actually receives such therapy (143,144). Moreover, the ACE inhibitor dosages commonly employed in "real world practice" are on average less than one-half the dose proven effective in the randomized, controlled mortality trials (169,170). As an example, of a case sample of 767 patients, discharged alive with the diagnosis of acute MI, 274 received an ACE inhibitor. The daily mean doses of the four ACE inhibitors used in this study were captopril 69.8 ± 36.9 mg, enalapril 13.6 ± 8.1 mg, lisinopril 11.0 ± 7.2 mg, and ramipril 8.4 ± 4.5 mg. The doses were unchanged after 6 months except for captopril, which showed a rise in mean daily dose to 84.4 ± 36.7 mg (171).

Factors predicting either the use or optimal dosing of ACE inhibitors include variables relating to the treatment setting (prior hospitalization and/or specialty clinic follow-up), the prescribing physician (cardiology specialty vs. family practitioner/general internist), the patient-status (increased severity of symptoms, male, younger), and the drug (lower frequency of administration) (169). Underdosing of ACE inhibitors has a negative economic impact in heart failure as it is associated with more frequent heart failure hospitalizations (172). Finally, some question has emerged as to the observation that African-Americans with CHF may respond less well to ACE inhibitors. Although, the nuances of the observed differences in the response to ACE inhibitors are not yet clear (this should not deny African-Americans) the benefits of these therapies (173).

Enalapril, captopril, lisinopril, and trandolapril have each been shown to significantly reduce morbidity and mortality in the post-MI patient with a wide range of ventricular dysfunction (152,154,155). In a hemodynamically stable patient (systolic BP >100 mmHg) following a MI, an oral ACE inhibitor should be initiated (generally within the first day of the event), particularly if the MI is accompanied by depressed left ventricular function (174). The hemodynamic effects and overall benefit of ACE inhibition are secured early after a MI with the 30 day survival increasing by 40% in the first day, 45% in 2–7 days, and ~15% thereafter (175). This benefit may be explained by an early effect on infarct expansion, reduced neurohumoral activity, or an increase in collateral coronary flow. Recent trends show a promising increase in ACE inhibitor prescriptions in patients discharged followed an acute MI (153).

At present, captopril, lisinopril, ramipril, and trandolapril are approved specific to post-MI left ventricular dysfunction and enalapril is indicated for use in asymptomatic left ventricular dysfunction (Table 29.1) (3). The uniformity of these positive findings implies a class-effect for this aspect of ACE inhibitor action (155). There are presently very few data to conclude that clinically significant differences exist among the ACE inhibitors in the post MI setting given both the lack of head-to-head trials and the differing trial designs and study circumstances for individually studied ACE inhibitors (154,155).

Several trials have recently been completed that assess the utility of ACE inhibitors in modifying cardiac endpoints (20,57,58,91). These trials have either compared ACE inhibitor therapy with placebo (20,91) or with an active comparator such as a thiazide diuretic (57,58). A number of these trials have served as the basis for the belief that ACE inhibitors are drugs that favorably influence cardiac outcomes; however, in the broader scheme of things, there appear to be insignificant differences in total major cardiovascular events between regimens based on ACE inhibitors, calcium antagonists, diuretics, or β-blockers, as viewed in the context of unequal BP reduction favoring therapies other than ACE inhibitor regimens (176). The ALLHAT trial (58) showed a smaller reduction in total major cardiovascular events—as was the case for stroke and heart failure—with the ACE inhibitor lisinopril than with the diuretic chlorthalidone. This difference in event rate was almost entirely attributable to findings in the African-American cohort in this study and may have related to the smaller reduction in BP with an ACE inhibitor-based regimen in that subgroup.

IX. STROKE

Given the considerable public health impact of stroke and the recognition of important nonmodifiable (age, gender, and race/ethnicity) and modifiable (BP, diabetes, lipid profile, and lifestyle) risk factors, early deterrence strategies are increasingly being implemented. When a patient experiences a stroke, the focus of care becomes the prevention of secondary occurrences. This can be accomplished with anti-platelet and lipid-lowering as well as BP-reduction strategies. Despite the clear risk reduction with effective realization of these preventative strategies, new approaches are needed. One such "new" approach is to determine whether the stroke benefit gained from BP reduction is unique to the agent employed, such as an ACE inhibitor or an ARB, or a simple consequence of upgrading the hemodynamic profile (177–179).

The data and opinions supporting ACE inhibitors in specifically reducing stroke rate have been mixed and in the process some debate has emerged as to whether ARBs are more cerebroprotective than ACE inhibitors (on the basis of AT_2-receptor stimulation) (178–181). In the ALLHAT study, the stroke incidence was 15% greater with the ACE inhibitor lisinopril (primarily in African-Americans) than with the thiazide-type diuretic chlorthalidone, although the BP reduction was less in the lisinopril group than what was observed with chlorthalidone (58). Similar negative data for ACE inhibitors and stroke exists from the Perindopril Protection Against Recurrent Stroke (PROGRESS) trial for the ACE inhibitor perindopril in the context of secondary stroke prevention (177). In this study, 6105 hypertensive and nonhypertensive patients who had sustained a stroke without a major disability within the past 5 years were randomized to a 4 mg dose of perindopril with or without a 2.5 mg dose of indapamide (diuretic therapy was at the discretion of the treating physician).

In the PROGRESS trial, BP was reduced an average of 9/4 mmHg in the active treatment group, resulting in a 28% risk reduction of major stroke in all participants. This reduction of risk extended to all forms of stroke

(major disabling, hemorrhagic, ischemic, or unknown), to patients with and without hypertension and to those with and without diabetes. However, the most beneficial effect was seen in the group receiving perindopril and indapamide in which BP decreased 12/5 mmHg. Surprisingly, patients who received perindopril monotherapy had no reduction in cerebrovascular morbidity and mortality despite a significant 5/3 mmHg fall in BP (177). The PROGRESS data are important, because it has been debated whether the long-term lowering of BP, in patients who have sustained a prior cerebrovascular event, reduces recurrent stroke rate comparably to the benefit observed for primary stroke rate with BP reduction.

The HOPE trial results with the ACE inhibitor ramipril showed that the benefits of lowering BP on the risk of stroke are not confined to patients with hypertension, but they also extend to individuals with BP in the normotensive range. Compared with placebo, ramipril reduced the risk of any stroke by 32% and that of fatal stroke by 61%. Benefits were consistent across baseline BPs, drugs used, and subgroups defined by prior stroke status, PAD, diabetes or hypertension (182). On the basis of the HOPE study, the recently published American Heart Association guidelines for the primary prevention of stroke recommend ramipril to prevent stroke in high-risk patients and in patients with diabetes and hypertension (183).

In choosing an antihypertensive therapy regimen in the post-stroke circumstance, several factors, beyond a proposed cerebroprotective effect of ACE inhibitors, deserve consideration if this drug class is being considered. First, the ability of this drug class to preserve (if not improve) cerebral autoregulatory ability in the face of BP reduction offers the possibility of these drugs being better tolerated, particularly in the elderly. Secondly, the neurotransmitter, substance P, is believed to play a major role in both the cough and swallow sensory pathways. ACE inhibitors prevent the breakdown of substance P and may theoretically be useful in the management of patients (particularly with Asians) with a tendency to develop aspiration pneumonia as may occur in the post-stroke patient (184). Further supporting this substance P theory, a significantly lower rate of pneumonia has been observed in elderly hypertensive patients randomized to an ACE inhibitor compared with an ARB (185). Finally, ACE inhibitors with or without diuretics decrease cognitive decline (PROGRESS, HOPE) and stroke-related dementia (PROGRESS) not dissimilar to what has been observed with CCBs. At this time, the mechanism is unclear behind dementia prevention with ACE inhibitors in the post-stroke patient (182,186).

X. SIDE EFFECTS OF ACE INHIBITORS

Soon after their release, a syndrome of "functional renal insufficiency" was observed as a class effect with ACE inhibitors (187). This phenomenon was initially reported in patients with renal artery stenosis and a solitary kidney or in the presence of bilateral renal artery stenosis. Predisposing conditions to this development include dehydration, CHF, NSAID use, and/or either micro- or macrovascular renal disease (167,188). The mechanistic prompt in these conditions is a fall in afferent arteriolar flow. When this occurs, glomerular filtration temporarily declines. In response to this reduction in glomerular filtration, local production of angiotensin-II increases. In concert with this increase in angiotensin-II, the efferent or post-glomerular arteriole constricts, which re-establishes hydrostatic pressures within the more proximal glomerular capillary bed.

The abrupt removal of angiotensin-II, as occurs with an ACE inhibitor (or an ARB), will abruptly dilate the efferent arteriole in tandem with a reduction in systemic BP. In combination, these hemodynamic changes drop glomerular hydrostatic pressure such that glomerular filtration plummets. This type of "functional renal insufficiency" is best treated by discontinuation of the responsible agent, careful volume expansion (if intravascular volume contraction is a contributing factor), and, if warranted on clinical grounds, evelution for the presence of renal artery stenosis (Fig. 29.2) (165).

A situation comparable to that of "functional renal insufficiency" is exposure to ACE inhibitors after the first trimester of pregnancy. When this occurs *in utero*, acute renal failure can occur and with it oligohydroamnios and specific abnormalities thought to be secondary to reduced amniotic fluid volume (limb deformities, cranial ossification deficits, and lung hypoplasia). This sequence of events is the basis for the ACE inhibitor contraindication in the second and third trimester of pregnancy (189).

Hypotension is not a specific side-effect with ACE inhibitors, rather it is an extension of the physiologic effect of these drugs, which is more common when a patient becomes volume contracted. Unanticipated hypotension with an ACE inhibitor occurs when either recognized (post-exercise) or unanticipated (intercurrent febrile or gastrointestinal illness) forms of dehydration occur. Hyperkalemia is an additional ACE inhibitor-associated side-effect (190). ACE inhibitor-related hyperkalemia occurs infrequently unless a specific predisposition to hyperkalemia exists such as diabetes and CHF with renal failure (receiving K^+-sparing diuretics or K^+ supplements) (191,192). Conversely, ACE inhibitors will cut the potassium loss ordinarily occurring with diuretic therapy.

A dry, irritating, nonproductive cough is a common complication with ACE inhibitors, with an incidence between 0% and 44% (193). Cough is a class phenomenon with ACE inhibitors and has ostensibly been attributed to an increase in bradykinin and/or other vasoactive peptides, such as substance P, which may play a second messenger role in setting off the cough reflex. Although numerous therapies have been tried, few have had any lasting success in eliminating ACE inhibitor-induced cough. The sensible clinical approach for suspected ACE

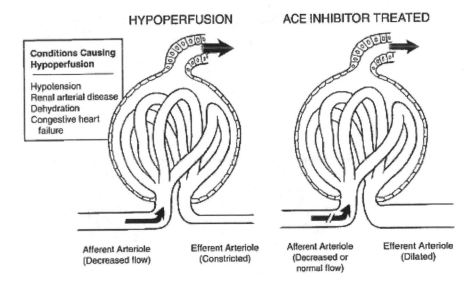

Figure 29.2 Schematic illustration of settings wherein ACE inhibitor therapy may worsen renal function. Conditions causing renal hypoperfusion include systemic hypotension, high-grade renal artery stenosis, extracellular fluid volume contraction (simplified as "dehydration" in the figure), and administration of vasoconstrictor agents (NSAIDs or cyclosporine, not shown), and CHF. These conditions typically increase renin secretion and angiotensin-II production. Angiotensin-II constricts the efferent arteriole to a greater extent than the afferent arteriole such that glomerular hydrostatic pressure and GFR can be maintained despite hypoperfusion. When these conditions occur in ACE-inhibitor treated patients, angiotensin-II formation and effect are diminished, and GFR may decrease. [Adapted with permission from Schoolwerth et al. (165).]

inhibitor-related cough is to reassess the patient several weeks after drug discontinuation. Disappearance of the cough can then be taken as proof of an ACE inhibitor etiology.

Nonspecific side-effects with ACE inhibitors are generally uncommon with the exception of taste disturbances, leucopenia, skin rash, and dysgeusia, which are largely seen in captopril-treated patients (194). Whereas a number of antihypertensives have headache as an accompanying side-effect with their use, this is not so with ACE inhibitors. In fact, ACE inhibitors have been used for migraine prophylaxis (195). Moreover, they have been proven effective in reducing the risk of headache with nitrate therapy (196).

Angioneurotic edema is a potentially life-threatening complication of ACE inhibitors, which is more common in blacks (197). Angioedema can be effectively managed in the long-term with simple discontinuation of the ACE inhibitor at fault (198). Angioedema can occasionally recur with ARB therapy in patients having previously experienced it with an ACE inhibitor, but it is generally mild and not life-threatening in its severity (199). Angioedema of the intestine (more common in women) can also occur with ACE inhibitor, therapy with a typical presentation being one of abdominal pain/diarrhea with or

without facial and/or oropharyngeal swelling (Fig. 29.3) (200). This process can be intermittent in nature developing even several years after ACE inhibitor therapy has been initiated (201). However, the use of ACE inhibitors is not associated with a significantly increased risk of acute pancreatitis (202).

A final side-effect consideration with ACE inhibitors is that of anemia. ACE inhibitors suppress the production of erythropoietin in a dose-dependent manner, which presents a particular problem when ACE inhibitors are administered in the presence of renal failure (203). ACE inhibitor-related anemia is at least, in part, related to *N*-acetyl-seryl-aspartyl-lysyl-proline accumulation. This substance is a potent natural inhibitor of hematopoietic stem cell proliferation as well as an antifibrotic moiety, which is degraded mainly by ACE (204). Because of the increase in *N*-acetyl-seryl-aspartyl-lysyl-proline concentrations with ACE inhibitor therapy, these compounds may possibly be better suited for suppression of red cell production when it is a desired clinical goal (Fig. 29.4) (205). Such settings include post-transplant erythrocytosis (205,206) and high-altitude polycythemia with as much as a 4.5 gm/dL fall in hemoglobin concentration being observed with ACE inhibitor therapy (207).

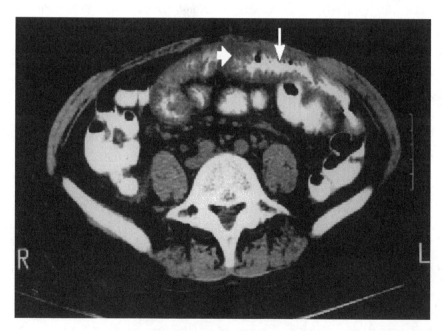

Figure 29.3   Abdominal computed tomography was performed in a 58-year-old woman with acute abdominal pain, nausea, vomiting, and abdominal distention. The patient had had recurrent swelling of the tongue and pharynx during therapy with lisinopril, but the medication had been continued. On the scan, the mucosa of a loop of small intestine is markedly thickened, and the irregularities within the wall are most consistent with the presence of edema (thick arrow). The valvulae conniventes are prominent and widened (thin arrow), resulting in a severely narrowed lumen. All of the patient's symptoms resolved within 24 h after the discontinuation of lisinopril. [Adapted with permission from Gregory and Davis (200).]

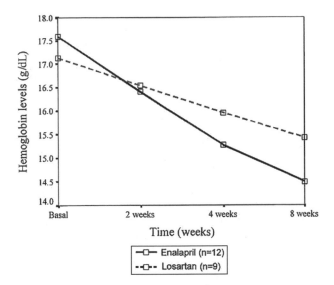

Figure 29.4 The change in mean hemoglobin levels in both study groups with post-renal transplant erythrocytosis among responders. Enalapril was administered in a dose of 10 mg/day and losartan at a dose of 50 mg/day. The decrease in hemoglobin was more prominent with enalapril than with losartan (-3.26 ± 0.65 vs. -1.70 ± 0.39 g/dL, $P = 0.05$). [Adapted with permission from Yildiz et al. (205).]

XI. CONCLUSIONS

ACE inhibitors are commonly used drugs in the elderly patient. These compounds are employed either in their capacity to reduce blood pressure or to take advantage of their cardio- and/or renoprotective effects. ACE inhibitors can be expected to provide the greatest end-organ protection in the elderly having CHF, proteinuric renal disease, or in the post-MI setting. Dosing guidelines exist for each of these scenarios, although such guidelines may not be followed as closely in clinical practice as is advised. ACE inhibitor-related side-effects are for the most part easily recognized and other than functional renal insufficiency, which is occasionally seen with their use, do not occur more commonly in the elderly.

REFERENCES

1. Chobanian AV, Bakris GL, Black HR, Cushman WC, Green LA, Izzo JL Jr, Jones DW, Materson BJ, Oparil S, Wright JT Jr, Roccella EJ; National Heart, Lung, and Blood Institute Joint National Committee on Prevention, Detection, Evaluation, and Treatment of High Blood Pressure; National High Blood Pressure Education Program Coordinating Committee. The Seventh Report of the Joint National Committee on Prevention, Detection, Evaluation, and Treatment of High Blood Pressure: the JNC 7 report. J Am Med Assoc 2003; 289:2560–2572.

2. Sica DA, Gehr TWB. Angiotensin converting enzyme inhibitors. In: Oparil S, Weber M, eds. Hypertension: A Companion to the Kidney. 1st ed. Philadelphia: W.B. Saunders, 2000:599–608.

3. Sica DA, Gehr TWB, Frishman WH. The renin–angiotensin axis: angiotensin converting enzyme inhibitors and angiotensin-receptor blockers. In: Frishman W, Sonnenblick S, Sica DA, eds. Cardiovascular Pharmacotherapeutics. 2nd ed. McGraw-Hill, 2003:131–156.

4. Warner GT, Perry CM. Ramipril: a review of its use in the prevention of cardiovascular outcomes. Drugs 2002; 62:1381–1405.

5. White CM. Pharmacologic, pharmacokinetic, and therapeutic differences among ACE inhibitors. Pharmacotherapy 1998; 18:588–599.

6. Dickstein K, Till AE, Aarsland T, Tjelta K, Abrahamsen AM, Kristianson K, Gomez HJ, Gregg H, Hichens M. The pharmacokinetics of enalapril in hospitalized patients with congestive heart failure. Br J Clin Pharmacol 1987; 23:403–410.

7. Lapenna D, De Gioia S, Ciofani G, Daniele F, Cuccurullo F. Captopril has no significant scavenging antioxidant activity in human plasma in vitro or in vivo. Br J Clin Pharmacol 1996; 42:451–456.

8. Chalmers D, Whitehead A, Lawson DH. Postmarketing surveillance of captopril for hypertension. Br J Clin Pharmacol 1992; 34:215–223.

9. Sica DA. Angiotensin converting enzyme inhibitors: fosinopril. In: Messerli F, ed. Cardiovascular Drug Therapy. 2nd ed. Philadelphia: W.B. Saunders, 1996:801–809.

10. Brockmeier D. Tight binding influencing the future of pharmacokinetics. Meth Find Exp Clin Pharmacol 1998; 20:505–516.

11. Reid JL. From kinetics to dynamics. are there differences between ACE inhibitors? Eur Heart J 1997; 18(suppl E):E14–E18.

12. Hoyer J, Schulte K-L, Lenz T. Clinical pharmacokinetics of angiotensin converting enzyme inhibitors in renal failure. Clin Pharmacokinet 1993; 24:230–254.

13. Dzau VJ, Bernstein K, Celermajer D, Cohen J, Dahlof B, Deanfield J, Diez J, Drexler H, Ferrari R, van Gilst W, Hansson L, Hornig B, Husain A, Johnston C, Lazar H, Lonn E, Luscher T, Mancini J, Mimran A, Pepine C, Rabelink T, Remme W, Ruilope L, Ruzicka M, Schunkert H, Swedberg K, Unger T, Vaughan D, Weber M. Working Group on Tissue Angiotensin-converting enzyme, International Society of Cardiovascular Pharmacotherapy. The relevance of tissue angiotensin-converting enzyme: manifestations in mechanistic and endpoint data. Am J Cardiol 2001; 88(suppl 9):1L–20L.

14. Ebihara A, Fujimura A. Metabolites of antihypertensive drugs. An updated review of their clinical pharmacokinetic and therapeutic implications. Clin Pharmacokinet 1991; 21:331–343.

15. Hui KK, Duchin KL, Kripalani KJ, Chan D, Kramer PK, Yanagawa N. Pharmacokinetics of fosinopril in patients with various degrees of renal function. Clin Pharmacol Ther 1991; 49:457–467.

16. Danielson B, Querin S, LaRochelle P, Sultan E, Mouren M, Bryce T, Stepniewski JP, Lenfant B. Pharmacokinetics and pharmacodynamics of trandolapril after repeated administration of 2 mg to patients with chronic renal failure and healthy control subjects. J Cardiovasc Pharmacol 1994; 23(suppl 4):S50–S59.

17. Brunner-La Rocca HP, Weilenmann D, Kiowski W, Maly FE, Follath F. Plasma levels of enalaprilat in chronic therapy of heart failure: relationship to adverse events. J Pharmacol Exp Ther 1999; 289:565–571.

18. Brown NJ, Vaughn DE. Angiotensin-converting enzyme inhibitors. Circulation 1998; 97:1411–1420.

19. Johnston CI, Fabris B, Yamada H, Mendelsohn FA, Cubela R, Sivell D, Jackson B. Comparative studies of tissue inhibition by angiotensin converting enzyme inhibitors. J Hypertens 1989; 7(suppl):S11–S16.

20. Yusuf S, Sleight P, Pogue J, Bosch J, Davies R, Dagenais G. Effects of an angiotensin-converting enzyme inhibitor, ramipril, on cardiovascular events in high-risk patients. The Heart Outcomes Prevention Evaluation Study Investigators. N Engl J Med 2000; 342:145–153.

21. Leonetti G, Cuspidi C. Choosing the right ACE inhibitor. A guide to selection. Drugs 1995; 49:516–535.

22. Zeitz CJ, Campbell DJ, Horowitz JD. Myocardial uptake and biochemical and hemodynamic effects of ACE inhibitors in humans. Hypertension 2003; 41:482–487.

23. Huskamp HA, Deverka PA, Epstein AM, Epstein RS, McGuigan KA, Frank RG. The effect of incentive-based formularies on prescription-drug utilization and spending. N Engl J Med 2003; 349:2224–2232.

24. The SOLVD investigators. Effect of enalapril on survival in patients with reduced left ventricular ejection fractions and congestive heart failure. N Engl J Med 1991; 325:293–302.

25. Lewis EJ, Hunsicker LG, Bain RP, Rohde RD. The effect of angiotensin converting enzyme inhibition on diabetic nephropathy. The Collaborative Study Group. N Engl J Med 1993; 329:1456–1462.

26. Sica DA. The HOPE Study: ACE inhibitors—are their benefits a class effect or do individual agents differ? Curr Opin Nephrol Hypertens 2001; 10:597–601.

27. Segura J, Christiansen H, Campo C, Ruilope LM. How to titrate ACE inhibitors and angiotensin receptor blockers in renal patients: according to blood pressure or proteinuria? Curr Hypertens Rep 2003; 5:426–429.

28. Tang WH, Vagelos RH, Yee YG, Benedict CR, Willson K, Liss CL, Fowler MB. Neurohormonal and clinical responses to high- versus low-dose enalapril therapy in chronic heart failure. J Am Coll Cardiol 2002; 39:70–78.

29. Packer M, Poole-Wilson PA, Armstrong PW, Cleland JG, Horowitz JD, Massie BM, Ryden L, Thygesen K, Uretsky BF. Comparative effects of low and high doses of the angiotensin-converting enzyme inhibitor, lisinopril, on morbidity and mortality in chronic heart failure. ATLAS Study Group. Circulation 1999; 100:2312–2318.

30. Massie B. Neurohormonal blockade in chronic heart failure. How much is enough? can there be too much? J Am Coll Cardiol 2002; 39:79–82.

31. Tang WH, Vagelos RH, Yee YG, Benedict CR, Willson K, Liss CL, Fowler MB. Neurohormonal and clinical responses to high- versus low-dose enalapril therapy in chronic heart failure. J Am Coll Cardiol 2002; 39:70–78.

32. van Veldhuisen DJ, Genth-Zotz S, Brouwer J, Boomsma F, Netzer T, Man In 'T Veld AJ, Pinto YM, Lie KI, Crijns HJ. High versus low-dose ACE inhibition in chronic heart failure. A double-blind, placebo-controlled study of imidapril. J Am Coll Cardiol 1998; 32:1811–1818.

33. Carretero OA, Scicli AG. The kallikrein–kinin system as a regulator of cardiovascular and renal function. In: Brenner BM, Laragh JH, eds. Hypertension: Pathophysiology, Diagnosis, and Management. 2nd ed. New York: Raven Press Ltd., 1995:983–999.

34. Urata H. Nishimura H, Ganten D. Chymase-dependent angiotensin II forming system in humans. Am J Hypertens 1996; 9:277–284.

35. Petrie MC, Padmanabhan N, McDonald JE, Hillier C, Connell JM, McMurray JJ. Angiotensin converting enzyme and non-ACE dependent angiotensin II generation in resistance arteries from patients with heart failure and coronary heart disease. J Am Coll Cardiol 2001; 37:1056–1061.

36. Ennezat PV, Berlowitz M, Sonnenblick EH, Le Jemtel TH. Therapeutic implications of escape from angiotensin-converting enzyme inhibition in patients with chronic heart failure. Curr Cardiol Rep 2000; 2:258–262.

37. Mooser V, Nussberger J, Juillerat L, Burnier M, Waeber B, Bidiville J, Pauly N, Brunner HR. Reactive hyperreninemia is a major determinant of plasma angiotensin II during ACE inhibition. J Cardiovasc Pharmacol 1990; 15:276–282.

38. Swedberg K, Eneroth P, Kjekshus J, Wilhelmsen L. Hormones regulating cardiovascular function in patients with severe congestive heart failure and their relation to mortality. CONSENSUS Trial Study Group. Circulation 1990; 82:1730–1736.

39. Gainer JV, Morrow JD, Loveland A, King DJ, Brown NJ. Effect of bradykinin-receptor blockade on the response to angiotensin-converting enzyme inhibitor in normotensive and hypertensive subjects. N Engl J Med 1998; 339:1285–1292.

40. Tom B, Dendorfer A, Danser AH. Bradykinin, angiotensin (1–7), and ACE inhibitors: how do they interact? Int J Biochem Cell Biol 2003; 35:792–801.

41. Rodriguez-Garcia JL, Villa E, Serrano M, Gallardo J, Garcia-Robles R. Prostacyclin: its pathogenic role in essential hypertension and the class effect of ACE inhibitors on prostaglandin metabolism. Blood Press 1999; 8:279–284.

42. Johnson AG. NSAIDs and increased blood pressure. What is the clinical significance? Drug Saf 1997; 17:277–289.

43. Morgan T, Anderson A. The effect of nonsteroidal anti-inflammatory drugs on blood pressure in patients treated with different antihypertensive drugs. J Clin Hypertens (Greenwich) 2003; 5:53–57.

44. Izhar M, Alausa T, Folker A, Hung E, Bakris GL. Effects of COX inhibition on blood pressure and kidney function

in ACE inhibitor-treated blacks and Hispanics. Hypertension 2004; 43:573–577.

45. Nawarskas JJ, Townsend RR, Cirigliano MD, Spinler SA. Effect of aspirin on blood pressure in hypertensive patients taking enalapril or losartan. Am J Hypertens 1999; 12:784–789.

46. Zanchetti A, Hansson L, Leonetti G, Rahn KH, Ruilope L, Warnold I, Wedel H. Low-dose aspirin does not interfere with the blood pressure-lowering effects of antihypertensive therapy. J Hypertens 2002; 20:1015–1022.

47. Cleland JG, John J, Houghton T. Does aspirin attenuate the effect of angiotensin-converting enzyme inhibitors in hypertension or heart failure? Curr Opin Nephrol Hypertens 2001; 10:625–631.

48. Lang CC, Stein CM, He HB, Wood AJ. Angiotensin converting enzyme inhibition and sympathetic activity in healthy subjects. Clin Pharmacol Ther 1996; 59:668–674.

49. Ranadive SA, Chen AX, Serajuddin AT. Relative lipophilicities and structural-pharmacological considerations of various angiotensin-converting enzyme (ACE) inhibitors. Pharm Res 1992; 9:1480–1486.

50. Fagard R, Amery A, Reybrouck T, Lijnen P, Billiet L. Acute and chronic systemic and hemodynamic effects of angiotensin converting enzyme inhibition with captopril in hypertensive patients. Am J Cardiol 1980; 46:295–300.

51. Slavachevsky I, Rachmani R, Levi Z, Brosh D, Lidar M, Ravid M. Effect of enalapril and nifedipine on orthostatic hypotension in older hypertensive patients. J Am Geriatr Soc 2000; 48:807–810.

52. Vanhoutte PM. Endothelial dysfunction and inhibition of converting enzyme. Eur Heart J 1998; 19(suppl J):J7–J15.

53. Schiffrin EL. Effects of antihypertensive drugs on vascular remodeling: do they predict outcome in response to antihypertensive therapy? Curr Opin Nephrol Hypertens 2001; 10:617–624.

54. Chobanian AV, Bakris GL, Black HR, Cushman WC, Green LA, Izzo JL Jr, Jones DW, Materson BJ, Oparil S, Wright JT Jr, Roccella EJ; Joint National Committee on Prevention, Detection, Evaluation, and Treatment of High Blood Pressure. National Heart, Lung, and Blood Institute; National High Blood Pressure Education Program Coordinating Committee. Seventh report of the Joint National Committee on Prevention, Detection, Evaluation, and Treatment of High Blood Pressure. Hypertension 2003; 42:1206–1252.

55. Guidelines Committee. 2003 European Society of Hypertension–European Society of Cardiology guidelines for the management of arterial hypertension. J Hypertens 2003; 21:1011–1053.

56. Khan NA, McAlister FA, Campbell NR, Feldman RD, Rabkin S, Mahon J, Lewanczuk R, Zarnke KB, Hemmelgarn B, Lebel M, Levine M, Herbert C. Canadian Hypertension Education Program. The 2004 Canadian recommendations for the management of hypertension: Part II—Therapy. Can J Cardiol 2004; 20:41–54.

57. Wing LM, Brown MA, Beilin LJ, Ryan P, Reid CM. ANBP2 Management Committee and Investigators. Second Autralian National Blood Pressure Study. A comparison of outcomes with angiotensin-converting enzyme

58. inhibitors and diuretics for hypertension in the elderly. N Engl J Med 2002; 348:583–592.

58. The ALLHAT Officers and Co-ordinators for the ALLHAT Collaborative Group. Major outcomes in high-risk hypertensive patients randomized to angiotensin converting enzyme inhibitor or calcium channel blocker vs diuretic. The Antihypertensive and Lipid-Lowering Treatment to Prevent Heart Attack Trial (ALLHAT). J Am Med Assoc 2002; 288:1981–1997.

59. Pescatello LS, Franklin BA, Fagard R, Farquhar WB, Kelley GA, Ray CA; American College of Sports Medicine. Exercise and hypertension. Med Sci Sports Exerc 2004; 36:533–553.

60. Materson BJ, Reda DJ, Cushman WC, Massie BM, Freis ED, Kochar MS, Hamburger RJ, Fye C, Lakshman R, Gottdiener J et al. Single-drug therapy for hypertension in men. A comparison of six antihypertensive agents with placebo. N Engl J Med 1993; 328:914–921.

61. Li X, Du Y, Du Y, Huang X. Correlation of angiotensin-converting enzyme gene polymorphism with effect of antihypertensive therapy by angiotensin-converting enzyme inhibitor. J Cardiovasc Pharmacol Ther 2003; 8:25–30.

62. Smith RD, Franklin SS. Comparison of effects of enalapril plus hydrochlorothiazide versus standard triple therapy on renal function in renovascular hypertension. Am J Med 1985; 79(suppl 3C):14–23.

63. Soffer B, Zhang Z, Miller K, Vogt BA, Shahinfar S. A double-blind, placebo-controlled, dose–response study of the effectiveness and safety of lisinopril for children with hypertension. Am J Hypertens 2003; 16:795–800.

64. Mokwe E, Ohmit SE, Nasser SA, Shafi T, Saunders E, Crook E, Dudley A, Flack JM. Determinants of blood pressure response to quinapril in black and white hypertensive patients. Hypertension 2004; 43:1–6.

65. Seghal AR. Overlap between whites and blacks in response to antihypertensive drugs. Hypertension 2004; 43:566–572.

66. Weidmann P, De Myttenaere-Bursztein S, Maxwell MH. Effect of aging on plasma renin and aldosterone in normal man. Kidney Int 1975; 8:325–333.

67. Israili ZH, Hall WD. ACE Inhibitors: differential use in elderly patients with hypertension. Drugs Aging 1995; 7:355–371.

68. Omboni S, Fogari R, Palatini P, Rappelli A, Mancia G. Reproducibility and clinical value of the trough-to-peak ratio of the antihypertensive effect. Evidence from the sample study. Hypertension 1998; 32:424–429.

69. Morgan TO, Morgan O, Anderson A. Effect of dose on trough peak ratio of antihypertensive drugs in elderly hypertensive males. Clin Exp Pharmacol Physiol 1995; 22:778–780.

70. Sica DA, Gehr TWB. Dose–response relationship and dose adjustments. In: Izzo JL, Black HR, eds. Hypertension Primer. 2nd ed. Baltimore, Maryland: Lippincott Williams & Wilkins, 1999:342–344.

71. Elung-Jensen T, Heisterberg J, Kamper AL, Sonne J, Strandgaard S. Blood pressure response to conventional and low-dose enalapril in chronic renal failure. Br J Clin Pharmacol 2003; 55:139–146.

72. Sica DA. Rationale for fixed-dose combinations in the treatment of hypertension: the cycle repeats. Drugs 2002; 62:443–462.

73. Law MR, Wald NJ, Morris JK, Jordan RE. Value of low dose combination treatment with blood pressure lowering drugs: analysis of 354 randomised trials. Brit Med J 2003; 326:427–434.

74. Docherty A, Dunn FG. Treatment of hypertensive patients with coexisting coronary arterial disease. Curr Opin Cardiol 2003; 18:268–271.

75. Black HR, Sollins JS, Garofalo JL. The addition of doxazosin to the therapeutic regimen of hypertensive patients inadequately controlled with other antihypertensive medications: a randomized, placebo-controlled study. Am J Hypertens 2000; 13:468–474.

76. Gradman AH, Cutler NR, Davis PJ, Robbins JA, Weiss RJ, Wood BC. Combined enalapril and felodipine extended release for systemic hypertension. Enalapril–Felodipine ER Factorial Study Group. Am J Cardiol 1997; 79:431–435.

77. DeQuattro V, Lee D. Fixed-dose combination therapy with trandolapril and verapamil SR is effective in primary hypertension. Am J Hypertens 1997; 10(suppl 2):138S–145S.

78. Pool J, Kaihlanen P, Lewis G, Ginsberg D, Oparil S, Glazer R, Messerli FH. Once-daily treatment of patients with hypertension: a placebo-controlled study of amlodipine and benazepril vs amlodipine or benazepril alone. J Hum Hypertens 2001; 15:495–498.

79. Neutel JM, Smith DH, Weber MA. Effect of antihypertensive monotherapy and combination therapy on arterial distensibility and left ventricular mass. Am J Hypertens 2004; 17:37–42.

80. Pepine CJ, Handberg EM, Cooper-DeHoff RM, Marks RG, Kowey P, Messerli FH, Mancia G, Cangiano JL, Garcia-Barreto D, Keltai M, Erdine S, Bristol HA, Kolb HR, Bakris GL, Cohen JD, Parmley WW; INVEST Investigators. A calcium antagonist vs a non-calcium antagonist hypertension treatment strategy for patients with coronary artery disease. J Am Med Assoc 2003; 290:2805–2816.

81. Sica DA. Calcium-channel blocker edema: can it be resolved? J Clin Hypertens 2003; 5:291–294.

82. Zuccala G, Onder G, Pedone C, Cesari M, Marzetti E, Cocchi A, Carbonin P, Bernabei R. Use of calcium antagonists and worsening renal function in patients receiving angiotensin-converting-enzyme inhibitors. Eur J Clin Pharmacol 2003; 58:695–699.

83. Sica DA. Combination angiotensin-converting enzyme inhibitor and angiotensin receptor blocker therapy: its role in clinical practice. practical aspects of combination therapy with angiotensin-receptor blockers and angiotensin-converting enzyme inhibitors. J Clin Hypertens 2003; 5:414–420.

84. Taylor AA. Is there a place for combining angiotensin-converting enzyme inhibitors and angiotensin-receptor antagonists in the treatment of hypertension, renal disease or congestive heart failure? Curr Opin Nephrol Hypertens 2001; 10:643–648.

85. Pogatsa-Murray G, Varga L, Varga A, Abraham G, Nagy I, Forster T, Csanady M, Sonkodi S. Changes in left ventricular mass during treatment with minoxidil and cilazapril in hypertensive patients with left ventricular hypertrophy. J Hum Hypertens 1997; 11:149–156.

86. Hirschl MM, Binder M, Bur A, Herkner H, Brunner M, Mullner M, Sterz F, Laggner AN. Clinical evaluation of different doses of intravenous enalaprilat in patients with hypertensive crises. Arch Intern Med 1995; 155:2217–2223.

87. Sica DA. Dosage considerations with perindopril for hypertension. Am J Cardiol 2001; 88(suppl 1):13–18.

88. Gottdiener JS, Reda DJ, Massie BM, Materson BJ, Williams DW, Anderson RJ. For the VA Cooperative Study Group on Antihypertensive Agents: Effect of single-drug therapy on reduction of left ventricular mass in mild to moderate hypertension. Comparison of six antihypertensive agents. Circulation 1997; 95:2007–2014.

89. Koren MJ, Devereux RB, Casale PN, Savage DD, Laragh JH. Relation of left ventricular mass and geometry to morbidity and mortality in uncomplicated essential hypertension. Ann Intern Med 1991; 114:345–352.

90. Pepine CJ, Rouleau JL, Annis K, Ducharme A, Ma P, Lenis J, Davies R, Thadani U, Chaitman B, Haber HE, Freedman SB, Pressler ML, Pitt B, QUASAR Study Group. Effects of angiotensin-converting enzyme inhibition on transient ischemia: the Quinapril Anti-Ischemia and Symptoms of Angina Reduction (QUASAR) trial. J Am Coll Cardiol 2003; 42:2049–2059.

91. Fox KM; EURopean trial On reduction of cardiac events with Perindopril in stable coronary Artery disease Investigators. Efficacy of perindopril in reduction of cardiovascular events among patients with stable coronary artery disease: randomised, double-blind, placebo-controlled, multicentre trial (the EUROPA study). Lancet 2003; 362:782–788.

92. Daly P, Mettauer B, Rouleau JL, Cousineau D, Burgess JH. Lack of reflex increase in myocardial sympathetic tone after captopril: potential antianginal mechanism. Circulation 1985; 71:317–325.

93. Silber JH, Cnaan A, Clark BJ, Paridon SM, Chin AJ, Rychik J, Hogarty AN, Cohen MI, Barber G, Rutkowski M, Kimball TR, Delaat C, Steinherz LJ, Zhao H. Enalapril to prevent cardiac function decline in long-term survivors of pediatric cancer exposed to anthracyclines. J Clin Oncol 2004; 22:820–828.

94. Chockalingam A, Venkatesan S, Subramaniam T, Jagannathan V, Elangovan S, Alagesan R, Gnanavelu G, Dorairajan S, Krishna BP, Chockalingam V; Symptomatic Cardiac Obstruction-Pilot Study of Enalapril in Aortic Stenosis. Safety and efficacy of angiotensin-converting enzyme inhibitors in symptomatic severe aortic stenosis: Symptomatic Cardiac Obstruction-Pilot Study of Enalapril in Aortic Stenosis (SCOPE-AS). Am Heart J 2004; 147:E19.

95. Morgan T, Anderson AI, MacInnis RJ. ACE inhibitors, β-blockers, calcium blockers, and diuretics for the control of systolic hypertension. Am J Hypertens 2001; 14:241–247.

96. Morgan T, Lauri J, Bertram D, Anderson A. Effect of different antihypertensive drug classes on central aortic pressure. Am J Hypertens 2004; 17:118–123.

97. Schiffrin EL. Effect of antihypertensive treatment on small artery remodeling in hypertension. Can J Physiol Pharmacol 2003; 81:168–176.

98. Walters MR, Bolster A, Dyker AG, Lees KR. Effect of perindopril on cerebral and renal perfusion in stroke patients with carotid disease. Stroke 2001; 32:473–478.

99. Regensteiner JG, Hiatt WR. Current medical therapies for patients with peripheral arterial disease: a critical review. Am J Med 2002; 112:49–57.

100. Ostergren J, Sleight P, Dagenais G, Danisa K, Bosch J, Qilong Y, Yusuf S; HOPE study investigators. Impact of ramipril in patients with evidence of clinical or subclinical peripheral arterial disease. Eur Heart J 2004; 25:17–24.

101. Vijan S, Hayward RA. Treatment of hypertension in type 2 diabetes mellitus: blood pressure goals, choice of agents, and setting priorities in diabetes care. Ann Int Med 2003; 138:593–602.

102. Position Statement. Hypertension management in adults with diabetes. Diabetes Care 2004; 27:S65–S67.

103. Chaturvedi N, Sjolie AK, Stephenson JM, Abrahamian H, Keipes M, Castellarin A, Rogulja-Pepeonik Z, Fuller JH. Effect of lisinopril on progression of retinopathy in normotensive people with type 1 diabetes. Lancet 1998; 351:28–31.

104. Sjolie AK, Chaturvedi N. The retinal renin–angiotensin system: implications for therapy in diabetic retinopathy. J Hum Hypertens 2002; 16(suppl 3):S42–S46.

105. Douketis JD, Sharma AM. The management of hypertension in the overweight and obese patient: is weight reduction sufficient? Drugs 2004; 64:795–803.

106. Lithell HO, Pollare T, Berne C. Insulin sensitivity in newly detected hypertensive patients: influence of captopril and other antihypertensive agents on insulin sensitivity and related biological parameters. J Cardiovasc Pharmacol 1990; 15(suppl 5):S46–S52.

107. Yusuf S, Gerstein H, Hoogwerf B, Pogue J, Bosch J, Wolffenbuttel BH, Zinman B; HOPE Study Investigators. Ramipril and the development of diabetes. J Am Med Assoc 2001; 286:1882–1885.

108. Hansson L, Lindholm LH, Niskanen L, Lanke J, Hedner T, Niklason A, Luomanmaki K, Dahlof B, de Faire U, Morlin C, Karlberg BE, Wester PO, Bjorck JE. Effect of angiotensin-converting-enzyme inhibition compared with conventional therapy on cardiovascular morbidity and mortality in hypertension: the Captopril Prevention Project (CAPPP) randomised trial. Lancet 1999; 353:611–616.

109. Chuahirun T, Simoni J, Hudson C, Seipel T, Khanna A, Harrist RB, Wesson DE. Cigarette smoking exacerbates and its cessation ameliorates renal injury in type 2 diabetes. Am J Med Sci 2004; 327:57–67.

110. Wright JT Jr, Agodoa L, Contreras G, Greene T, Douglas JG, Lash J, Randall O, Rogers N, Smith MC, Massry S, African American Study of Kidney Disease and Hypertension Study Group. Successful blood pressure control in the African American study of kidney disease and hypertension. Arch Intern Med 2002; 162:1636–1643.

111. Yu HT. Progression of chronic renal failure. Arch Intern Med 2003; 163:1417–1429.

112. Wachtell K, Ibsen H, Olsen MH, Borch-Johnsen K, Lindholm LH, Mogensen CE, Dahlof B, Devereux RB, Beevers G, de Faire U, Fyhrquist F, Julius S, Kjeldsen SE, Kristianson K, Lederballe-Pedersen O, Nieminen MS, Okin PM, Omvik P, Oparil S, Wedel H, Snapinn SM, Aurup P. Albuminuria and cardiovascular risk in hypertensive patients with left ventricular hypertrophy: the LIFE study. Ann Intern Med 2003; 139:901–906.

113. Donnelly R, Yeung JM, Manning G. Microalbuminuria: a common, independent cardiovascular risk factor, especially but not exclusively in type 2 diabetes. J Hypertens 2003; 21(suppl 1):S7–S12.

114. Brown WW, Peters RM, Ohmit SE, Keane WF, Collins A, Chen SC, King K, Klag MJ, Molony DA, Flack JM. Early detection of kidney disease in community settings: the kidney early evaluation program (KEEP). Am J Kidney Dis 2003; 42:22–35.

115. Boulware LE, Jaar BG, Tarver-Carr ME, Brancati FL, Powe NR. Screening for proteinuria in US adults: a cost-effectiveness analysis. J Am Med Assoc 2003; 290:3101–3114.

116. Jafar TH, Stark PC, Schmid CH, Landa M, Maschio G, de Jong PE, de Zeeuw D, Shahinfar S, Toto R, Levey AS; AIPRD Study Group. Progression of chronic kidney disease: the role of blood pressure control, proteinuria, and angiotensin-converting enzyme inhibition: a patient-level meta-analysis. Ann Intern Med 2003; 139:244–252.

117. Laverman GD, Remuzzi G, Ruggenenti P. ACE inhibition versus angiotensin receptor blockade: which is better for renal and cardiovascular protection? J Am Soc Nephrol 2004; 15(suppl 1):S64–S70.

118. Laverman GD, de Zeeuw D, Navis G. Between-patient differences in the renal response to renin–angiotensin system intervention: clue to optimising renoprotective therapy? J Renin Angiotensin Aldosterone Syst 2002; 3:205–213.

119. Campbell R, Sangalli F, Perticucci E, Aros C, Viscarra C, Perna A, Remuzzi A, Bertocchi F, Fagiani L, Remuzzi G, Ruggenenti P. Effects of combined ACE inhibitor and angiotensin II antagonist treatment in human chronic nephropathies. Kidney Int 2003; 63:1094–1103.

120. Ravid M, Lang R, Rachmani R, Lishner M. Long-term renoprotective effect of angiotensin converting enzyme inhibition in non-insulin dependent diabetes mellitus. A 7-year follow-up study. Arch Int Med 1996; 156:286–289.

121. Lebovitz HE, Wiegmann TB, Cnaan A, Shahinfar S, Sica DA, Broadstone V, Schwartz SL, Mengel MC, Segal R, Versaggi JA. Renal protective effects of enalapril in hypertensive NIDDM: role of baseline albuminuria. Kidney Int Suppl 1994; 45:S150–S155.

122. Viberti G, Mogensen CE, Groop LC, Pauls JF. Effect of captopril on progression to clinical proteinuria in patients

with insulin-dependent diabetes mellitus and microalbuminuria: European Microalbuminuria Captopril Study Group. J Am Med Assoc 1994; 271:275–279.

123. Ihle BU, Whitworth JA, Shahinfar S, Cnaan A, Kincaid-Smith PS, Becker GJ. Angiotensin-converting enzyme inhibition in nondiabetic progressive renal insufficiency: a controlled double-blind trial. Am J Kidney Dis 1996; 27:489–495.

124. Giatras I, Lau J, Levey AS. For the Angiotensin-Converting Enzyme Inhibition and Progressive Renal Disease Study Group: Effect of angiotensin-converting enzyme inhibitors on the progression of nondiabetic renal disease: a meta-analysis of randomized trials. Ann Intern Med 1997; 127:337–347.

125. Agodoa LY, Appel L, Bakris GL, Beck G, Bourgoignie J, Briggs JP, Charleston J, Cheek D, Cleveland W, Douglas JG, Douglas M, Dowie D, Faulkner M, Gabriel A, Gassman J, Greene T, Hall Y, Hebert L, Hiremath L, Jamerson K, Johnson CJ, Kopple J, Kusek J, Lash J, Lea J, Lewis JB, Lipkowitz M, Massry S, Middleton J, Miller ER III, Norris K, O'Connor D, Ojo A, Phillips RA, Pogue V, Rahman M, Randall OS, Rostand S, Schulman G, Smith W, Thornley-Brown D, Tisher CC, Toto RD, Wright JT Jr, Xu S; African American Study of Kidney Disease and Hypertension (AASK) Study Group. Effect of ramipril vs amlodipine on renal outcomes in hypertensive nephrosclerosis: a randomized controlled trial. J Am Med Assoc 2001; 285:2719–2728.

126. Nakao N, Yoshimura A, Morita H, Takada M, Kayano T, Ideura T. Combination treatment of angiotensin-II receptor blocker and angiotensin-converting-enzyme inhibitor in non-diabetic renal disease (COOPERATE): a randomised controlled trial. Lancet 2003; 361:117–124.

127. Wilmer WA, Hebert LA, Lewis EJ, Rohde RD, Whittier F, Cattran D, Levey AS, Lewis JB, Spitalewitz S, Blumenthal S, Bain RP. Remission of nephrotic syndrome in type 1 diabetes: long-term follow-up of patients in the captopril study. Am J Kidney Dis 1999; 34:308–314.

128. Lewis JB, Berl T, Bain RP, Rohde RD, Lewis EJ. Effect of intensive blood pressure control on the course of type 1 diabetic nephropathy. Am J Kidney Dis 1999; 34:809–817.

129. Estacio RO, Esler A, Mehler P. Effects of aggressive blood pressure control in normotensive type 2 diabetic patients on albuminuria, retinopathy and strokes. Kidney Int 2002; 61:1086–1097.

130. Estacio R, Jeffers R, Gifford N, Schrier R. Effect of blood pressure control on diabetic microvascular complications in patients with hypertension and type 2 diabetes. Diabetes Care 2000; 23:B54–B64.

131. Griffin KA, Abu-Amarah I, Picken M, Bidani AK. Renoprotection by ACE inhibition or aldosterone blockade is blood pressure-dependent. Hypertension 2003; 41:201–206.

132. Jafar TH, Schmid CH, Landa M, Giatras I, Toto R, Remuzzi G, Maschio G, Brenner BM, Kamper A, Zucchelli P, Becker G, Himmelmann A, Bannister K, Landais P, Shahinfar S, de Jong PE, de Zeeuw D, Lau J, Levey AS. Angiotensin-converting enzyme inhibitors and progression of nondiabetic renal disease. A meta-analysis of patient-level data. Ann Intern Med 2001; 135:73–87.

133. Ruggenenti P, Perna A, Gherardi G, Benini R, Remuzzi G. Chronic proteinuric nephropathies: outcomes and response to treatment in a prospective cohort of 352 patients with different patterns of renal injury. Am J Kidney Dis 2000; 35:1155–1165.

134. Sica DA. Kinetics of angiotensin converting enzyme inhibitors in renal failure. J Cardiovasc Pharmacol 1992; 20(supp 10):S13–S20.

135. Jafar TH, Stark PC, Schmid CH, Landa M, Maschio G, Marcantoni C, de Jong PE, de Zeeuw D, Shahinfar S, Ruggenenti P, Remuzzi G, Levey AS; AIPRD Study Group. Angiotensin-Converting Enzymne Inhibition and Progression of Renal Disease. Proteinuria as a modifiable risk factor for the progression of non-diabetic renal disease. Kidney Int 2001; 60:1131–1140.

136. Marre M, Lievre M, Chatellier G, Mann JF, Passa P, Menard J; DIABHYCAR Study Investigators. Effects of low dose ramipril on cardiovascular and renal outcomes in patients with type 2 diabetes and raised excretion of urinary albumin: randomised, double blind, placebo controlled trial (the DIABHYCAR study). Brit Med J 2004; 328:495.

137. Mann JF, Gerstein HC, Yi QL, Lonn EM, Hoogwerf BJ, Rashkow A, Yusuf S. Development of renal disease in people at high cardiovascular risk: results of the HOPE randomized study. J Am Soc Nephrol 2003; 14:641–647.

138. Laverman G, Ruggenenti P, Remuzzi G. Angiotensin-converting enzyme inhibition or angiotensin receptor blockade in hypertensive diabetics? Curr Hypertens Rep 2003; 5:364–367.

139. Ruggenenti P, Mise N, Pisoni R, Arnoldi F, Pezzotta A, Perna A, Cattaneo D, Remuzzi G. Diverse effects of increasing lisinopril doses on lipid abnormalities in chronic nephropathies. Circulation 2003; 107:586–592.

140. Bakris GL, Weir MR. Angiotensin-converting enzyme inhibitor-associated elevations in serum creatinine: is this a cause for concern? Arch Intern Med 2000; 160:685–693.

141. Apperloo AJ, de Zeeuw D, de Jong PE. A short-term anti-hypertensive-treatment induced drop in glomerular filtration rate predicts long-term stability of renal function. Kidney Int 1997; 51:793–797.

142. Sica DA. Assessment of the role of ACE inhibitors in the elderly. In: Prisant M, ed. Hypertension in the Elderly. Humana Press Inc., 2004. In Press.

143. Heeg JE, de Jong PE, van der Hem GK, de Zeeuw D. Efficacy and variability of the antiproteinuric effect of ACE inhibition by lisinopril Kidney Int 1989; 36:272–279.

144. Buter H, Hemmelder MH, Navis G, de Jong PE, de Zeeuw D. The blunting of the antiproteinuric efficacy of ACE inhibition by high sodium intake can be restored by hydrochlorothiazide. Nephrol Dial Transplant 1998; 13:1682–1685.

145. Gansevoort RT, de Zeeuw D, de Jong PE. Additive antiproteinuric effect of ACE inhibition and a low protein diet in human renal disease. Nephrol Dial Transplant 1995; 10:497–504.

146. Buter H, Hemmelder MH, van Paassen P, Navis G, de Zeeuw D, de Jong PE. Is the antiproteinuric response to inhibition of the renin–angiotensin system less effective during the night? Nephrol Dial Transplant 1997; 12(suppl 2):53–56.

147. Ueda S, Elliott HL, Morton JJ, Connell JM. Enhanced pressor response to angiotensin I in normotensive men with the deletion genotype (DD) for angiotensin-converting enzyme. Hypertension 1995; 25:1266–1269.

148. Cambien F, Poirier O, Lecerf L, Evans A, Cambou JP, Arveiler D, Luc G, Bard JM, Bara L, Ricard S. Deletion polymorphism in the gene for angiotensin-converting enzyme is a potent risk factor for myocardial infarction. Nature 1992; 359:641–644.

149. Parving HH, Jacobsen P, Tarnow L, Rossing P, Lecerf L, Poirier O, Cambien F. Effect of deletion polymorphism of angiotensin converting enzyme gene on progression of diabetic nephropathy during inhibition of angiotensin converting enzyme. Observational follow-up study. Brit Med J 1996; 313:591–594.

150. Rudnicki M, Mayer G. Pharmacogenomics of angiotensin converting enzyme inhibitors in renal disease—pathophysiological considerations. Pharmacogenomics 2003; 4:153–162.

151. Garg R, Yusuf S. For the Collaborative Group on ACE Inhibitor Trials. Overview of randomized trials of angiotensin-converting enzyme inhibitors on mortality and morbidity in patients with heart failure. J Am Med Assoc 1995; 273:1450–1456.

152. Flather MD, Yusuf S, Kober L, Pfeffer M, Hall A, Murray G, Torp-Pedersen C, Ball S, Pogue J, Moye L, Braunwald E. Long-term ACE-inhibitor therapy in patients with heart failure or left-ventricular dysfunction: a systematic overview of data from individual patients. ACE-Inhibitor Myocardial Infarction Collaborative Group. Lancet 2000; 355:1575–1581.

153. Burwen DR, Galusha DH, Lewis JM, Bedinger MR, Radford MJ, Krumholz HM, Foody JM. National and state trends in quality of care for acute myocardial infarction between 1994–1995 and 1998–1999: the medicare health care quality improvement program. Arch Intern Med 2003; 163:1430–1439.

154. Megarry SG, Sapsford R, Hall AS, Ball SG. Do ACE inhibitors provide protection for the heart in the clinical setting of acute myocardial infarction? Drugs 1997; 54(suppl 5):48–58.

155. Indications for ACE inhibitors in the early treatment of acute myocardial infarction: systematic review of individual data from 100,000 patients in randomised trials. Circulation 1998; 97:2202–2212.

156. Mathew JP, Fontes ML, Tudor IC, Ramsay J, Duke P, Mazer CD, Barash PG, Hsu PH, Mangano DT; Investigators of the Ischemia Research and Education Foundation; Multicenter Study of Perioperative Ischemia Research Group. A multicenter risk index for atrial fibrillation after cardiac surgery. J Am Med Assoc 2004; 291:1720–1729.

157. Shekelle PG, Rich MW, Morton SC, Atkinson CS, Tu W, Maglione M, Rhodes S, Barrett M, Fonarow GC, Greenberg B, Heidenreich PA, Knabel T, Konstam MA, Steimle A, Warner Stevenson L. Efficacy of ACE inhibitors and β-blockers in the management of left ventricular systolic dysfunction according to race, gender, and diabetic status: a meta-analysis of major clinical trials. J Am Coll Cardiol 2003; 41:1529–1538.

158. Liu P, Arnold JM, Belenkie I, Demers C, Dorian P, Gianetti N, Haddad H, Howlett J, Ignazewski A, Jong P, McKelvie R, Moe G, Parker JD, Rao V, Rouleau JL, Teo K, Tsuyuki R, White M, Huckel V, Issac D, Johnstone D, LeBlanc MH, Lee H, Newton G, Niznick J, Ross H, Roth S, Roy D, Smith S, Sussex B, Yusuf S; Canadian Cardiovascular Society. The 2002/3 Canadian Cardiovascular Society consensus guideline update for the diagnosis and management of heart failure. Can J Cardiol 2003; 19:347–356.

159. ACC/AHA Guidelines for the Evaluation and Management of Chronic Heart Failure in the Adult: Executive Summary—A Report of the American College of Cardiology/American Heart Association Task Force on Practice Guidelines. Circulation 2001; 104:2996–3007.

160. Massie B. Neurohormonal blockade in chronic heart failure; How much is enough? can there be too much? J Am Coll Cardiol 2002; 39:79–82.

161. Remme WJ. Effect of ACE inhibition on neurohormones. Eur Heart J 1998; 19(suppl J):J16–J23.

162. Cruden NL, Witherow FN, Webb DJ, Fox KA, Newby DE. Bradykinin contributes to the systemic hemodynamic effects of chronic angiotensin-converting enzyme inhibition in patients with heart failure. Arterioscler Thromb Vasc Biol 2004; 24(suppl 6):1043–1048 (Epub 2004 Apr 22).

163. Anker SD, Negassa A, Coats AJ, Afzal R, Poole-Wilson PA, Cohn JN, Yusuf S. Prognostic importance of weight loss in chronic heart failure and the effect of treatment with angiotensin-converting-enzyme inhibitors: an observational study. Lancet 2003; 361:1077–1083.

164. Hirooka K, Koretsune Y, Yoshimoto S, Irino H, Abe H, Yasuoka Y, Yamamoto H, Hashimoto K, Chin W, Kusuoka H. Twice-daily administration of a long-acting angiotensin-converting enzyme inhibitor has greater effects on neurohumoral factors than a once-daily regimen in patients with chronic congestive heart failure. J Cardiovasc Pharmacol 2004; 43:56–60.

165. Schoolwerth AC, Sica DA, Ballermann BJ, Wilcox CS. Renal considerations in angiotensin converting enzyme inhibitor therapy: a statement for healthcare professionals from the Council on the Kidney in Cardiovascular Disease and the Council for High Blood Pressure Research of the American Heart Association. Circulation 2001; 104:1985–1991.

166. Kittleson M, Hurwitz S, Shah MR, Nohria A, Lewis E, Givertz M, Fang J, Jarcho J, Mudge G, Stevenson LW. Development of circulatory-renal limitations to angiotensin-converting enzyme inhibitors identifies patients with severe heart failure and early mortality. J Am Coll Cardiol 2003; 41:2029–2035.

167. Agusti A, Bonet S, Arnau JM, Vidal X, Laporte JR. Adverse effects of ACE inhibitors in patients with chronic heart failure and/or ventricular dysfunction: meta-analysis of randomised clinical trials. Drug Saf 2003; 26:895–908.

168. Valsartan, captopril, or both in myocardial infarction complicated by heart failure, left ventricular dysfunction, or both. N Engl J Med 2003; 349:1893–1906.

169. Bungard TJ, McAlister FA, Johnson JA, Tsuyuki RT. Underutilization of ACE inhibitors in patients with congestive heart failure. Drugs 2001; 61:2021–2033.

170. Chen YT, Wang Y, Radford MJ, Krumholz HM. Angiotensin-converting enzyme inhibitor dosages in elderly patients with heart failure. Am Heart J 2001; 141:410–417.

171. Kvan E, Reikvam A. The problem of underdosing of angiotensin-converting enzyme inhibitors is markedly overrated: results from a study of patients discharged from hospital after an acute myocardial infarction. Eur J Clin Pharmacol 2004; 60:205–210.

172. Schwartz JS, Wang YR, Cleland JG, Gao L, Weiner M, Poole-Wilson PA; ATLAS Study Group. High- versus low-dose angiotensin converting enzyme inhibitor therapy in the treatment of heart failure: an economic analysis of the Assessment of Treatment with Lisinopril and Survival (ATLAS) trial. Am J Manag Care 2003; 9:417–424.

173. Dries DJ, Yancy CW, Strong MA, Drazner MH. Racial response to angiotensin-converting enzyme therapy in systolic heart failure. Cong Heart Fail 2004; 10:30–33.

174. Ryan TJ, Antman EM, Brooks NH, Califf RM, Hillis LD, Hiratzka LF, Rapaport E, Riegel B, Russell RO, Smith EE III, Weaver WD, Gibbons RJ, Alpert JS, Eagle KA, Gardner TJ, Garson A Jr, Gregoratos G, Smith SC Jr. 1999 update: ACC/AHA Guidelines for the Management of Patients with Acute Myocardial Infarction: Executive Summary and Recommendations: A Report of the American College of Cardiology/American Heart Association Task Force on Practice Guidelines (Committee on Management of Acute Myocardial Infarction). Circulation 1999; 100:1016–1030.

175. Naccarella F, Naccarelli GV, Maranga SS, Lepera G, Grippo MC, Melandri F, Gatti M, Pazzaglia S, Spinelli G, Angelini V, Ambrosioni E, Borghi C, Giovagnorio MT, Nisam S. Do ACE inhibitors or angiotensin II antagonists reduce total mortality and arrhythmic mortality? A critical review of controlled clinical trials. Curr Opin Cardiol 2002; 17:6–18.

176. Turnbull F; Blood Pressure Lowering Treatment Trialists' Collaboration. Effects of different blood-pressure-lowering regimens on major cardiovascular events: results of prospectively-designed overviews of randomised trials. Lancet 2003; 362:1527–1535.

177. PROGRESS Collaborative Group. Randomised trial of a perindopril-based blood-pressure-lowering regimen among 6105 individuals with previous stroke or transient ischaemic attack. Lancet 2001; 358:1033–1041.

178. Anderson C. Blood pressure-lowering for secondary prevention of stroke: ACE inhibition is the key. Stroke 2003; 34:1333–1334.

179. Bath P. Blood pressure-lowering for secondary prevention of stroke: ACE inhibition is not the key. Stroke 2003; 34:1334–1335.

180. Davis SM, Donnan GA. Blood pressure reduction and ACE inhibition in secondary stroke prevention: mechanism uncertain. Stroke 2003; 34:1335–1336.

181. Fournier A, Messerli FH, Achard JM, Fernandez L. Cerebroprotection mediated by angiotensin II: a hypothesis supported by recent randomized clinical trials. J Am Coll Cardiol 2004; 43:1343–1347.

182. Bosch J, Yusuf S, Pogue J, Sleight P, Lonn E, Rangoonwala B, Davies R, Ostergren J, Probstfield J; HOPE Investigators. Heart outcomes prevention evaluation. Use of ramipril in preventing stroke: double blind randomised trial. Brit Med J 2002; 324:699–702.

183. Goldstein LB, Adams R, Becker K, Furberg CD, Gorelick PB, Hademenos G, Hill M, Howard G, Howard VJ, Jacobs B, Levine SR, Mosca L, Sacco RL, Sherman DG, Wolf PA, del Zoppo GJ. Primary prevention of ischemic stroke: a statement for healthcare professionals from the Stroke Council of the American Heart Association. Stroke 2001; 32:280–299.

184. Ohkubo T, Chapman N, Neal B, Woodward M, Omae T, Chalmers J; Perindopril Protection Against Recurrent Stroke Sutdy Collaborative Group. Effects of an angiotensin-converting enzyme inhibitor-based regimen on pneumonia risk. Am J Respir Crit Care Med 2004; 169:1041–1045.

185. Arai T, Yasuda Y, Takaya T, Toshima S, Kashiki Y, Shibayama M, Yoshimi N, Fujiwara H. Angiotensin-converting enzyme inhibitors, angiotensin-II receptor antagonists, and pneumonia in elderly hypertensive patients with stroke. Chest 2001; 119:660–661.

186. Tzourio C, Anderson C, Chapman N, Woodward M, Neal B, MacMahon S, Chalmers J; PROGRESS Collaborative Group. Effects of blood pressure lowering with perindopril and indapamide therapy on dementia and cognitive decline in patients with cerebrovascular disease. Arch Intern Med 2003; 163:1069–1075.

187. Textor SC. Renal failure related to angiotensin-converting enzyme inhibitors. Semin Nephrol 1997; 17:67–76.

188. Bouvy ML, Heerdink ER, Hoes AW, Leufkens HG. Effects of NSAIDs on the incidence of hospitalisations for renal dysfunction in users of ACE inhibitors. Drug Saf 2003; 26:983–989.

189. Tabacova S, Little R, Tsong Y, Vega A, Kimmel CA. Adverse pregnancy outcomes associated with maternal enalapril antihypertensive treatment. Pharmacoepidemiol Drug Saf 2003; 12:633–646.

190. Textor SC, Bravo EL, Fouad FM, Tarazi RC. Hyperkalemia in azotemic patients during angiotensin-converting enzyme inhibition and aldosterone reduction with captopril. Am J Med 1982; 73:719–725.

191. Juurlink DN, Mamdani M, Kopp A, Laupacis A, Redelmeier DA. Drug-drug interactions among elderly patients hospitalized for drug toxicity. J Am Med Assoc 2003; 289:1652–1658.

192. Cruz CS, Cruz AA, Marcilio de Souza CA. Hyperkalaemia in congestive heart failure patients using ACE inhibitors and spironolactone. Nephrol Dial Transplant 2003; 18:1814–1819.

193. Israili ZH, Hall WD. Cough and angioneurotic associated with angiotensin-converting enzyme inhibitor therapy: a

review of the literature and pathophysiology. Ann Intern Med 1992; 117:234–242.

194. Chalmers D, Dombey SL, Lawson DH. Post-marketing surveillance of captopril (for hypertension): a preliminary report. Br J Clin Pharmacol 1987; 24:343–349.

195. Rahimtoola H, Buurma H, Tijssen CC, Leufkens HG, Egberts AC. Reduction in the therapeutic intensity of abortive migraine drug use during ACE inhibition therapy—a pilot study. Pharmacoepidemiol Drug Saf 2004; 13:41–47.

196. Onder G, Pahor M, Gambassi G, Federici A, Savo A, Carbonin P, Bernabei R, GIFA Study. Association between ACE inhibitors use and headache caused by nitrates among hypertensive patients: results from the Italian group of pharmacoepidemiology in the elderly. Cephalalgia 2003; 23:901–906.

197. Gibbs CR, Lip GYH, Beevers DG. Angioedema due to ACE inhibitors: increased risk in patients of African origin. Br J Clin Pharmacol 1999; 48:861–865.

198. Cicardi M, Zingale LC, Bergamaschini L, Agostoni A. Angioedema associated with angiotensin-converting enzyme inhibitor use: outcome after switching to a different treatment. Arch Int Med 2004; 164:910–913.

199. Granger CB, McMurray JJ, Yusuf S, Held P, Michelson EL, Olofsson B, Ostergren J, Pfeffer MA, Swedberg K; CHARM Investigators and Committees. Effects of candesartan in patients with chronic heart failure and reduced left ventricular systolic function intolerant to angiotensin-converting enzyme inhibitors: the CHARM-Alternative trial. Lancet 2003; 362:772–776.

200. Gregory KW, Davis RC. Images in clinical medicine. Angioedema of the intestine. N Engl J Med 1996; 334:1641.

201. Orr KK, Myers JR. Intermittent visceral edema induced by long-term enalapril administration. Ann Pharmacother 2004; 38:825–827.

202. Cheng RM, Mamdani M, Jackevicius CA, Tu K. Association between ACE inhibitors and acute pancreatitis in the elderly. Ann Pharmacother 2003; 37:994–998.

203. Sica DA, Gehr TWB. The pharmacokinetics and pharmacodynamics of angiotensin receptor blockers in end-stage renal disease. J Renin–Angio Aldo Sys 2002; 3:247–254.

204. Rasoul S, Carretero OA, Peng H, Cavasin MA, Zhuo J, Sanchez-Mendoza A, Brigstock DR, Rhaleb NE. Antifibrotic effect of Ac-SDKP and angiotensin-converting enzyme inhibition in hypertension. J Hypertens 2004; 22:593–603.

205. Yildiz A, Cine N, Akkaya V, Sahin S, Ismailoglu V, Turk S, Bozfakioglu S, Sever MS. Comparison of the effects of enalapril and losartan on posttransplantation erythrocytosis in renal transplant recipients: prospective randomized study. Transplantation 2001; 72:542–545.

206. Trivedi H, Lal SM. A prospective, randomized, open labeled crossover trial of fosinopril and theophylline in post renal transplant erythrocytosis. Ren Fail 2003; 25:77–86.

207. Plata R, Cornejo A, Arratia C, Anabaya A, Perna A, Dimitrov BD, Remuzzi G, Ruggenenti P, Commission on Global Advancement of Nephrology (COMGAN), Research Subcommittee of the International Society of Nephrology. Angiotensin-converting-enzyme inhibition therapy in altitude polycythaemia: a prospective randomised trial. Lancet 2002; 359:663–666.

30

Angiotensin II Receptor Antagonists

MARC MAILLARD, MICHEL BURNIER

Service of Nephrology, CHUV, Lausanne, Switzerland

KEYPOINTS

- Seven angiotensin II antagonists are currently marketed and used Worldwide to hypertensive patients and patients with congestive heart failure and type 2 diabetes.
- These agents have a common mechanism of action, but pharmacokinetic and pharmacodynamic differences clearly account for clinically significant differences.
- A large number of outcome trials have demonstrated their efficacy in decreasing the cardiovascular morbidity and mortality in hypertensive patients and in retarding progression of diabetic nephropathy in type 2 diabetes.
- Because of their efficacy and tolerability profile, these drugs have the potential to become the

leading compounds for managing hypertensive patients with cardiovascular and renal diseases.

SUMMARY

Ten years after the introduction for clinical use of losartan, the first orally active angiotensin II receptor antagonist, seven compounds—the pharmacological characteristics of which are described in this chapter—are registered by the US Food and Drug Administration and are used in the United States and in various European countries for the treatment of hypertension, heart failure and for the prevention of type-2 diabetic nephropathy. Indeed a large number of clinical studies and the completion of several large outcome trials have demonstrated their efficacy to lower morbidity and mortality in these various groups of patients. All these agents that selectively block the binding of angiotensin II to the subtype 1 receptor have an excellent tolerability profile which is a real advantage as these agents are prescribed most frequently to asymptomatic patients. While pharmacokinetic and pharmacodynamic differences clearly accounted for clinically significant differences at least in term of blood pressure control between antagonists, some unresolved questions still remain such as the right dose to use in order to achieve the optimal target organ protection, the role of the AT2 receptors or the potential benefits of a combination with ACE inhibitors. These questions will probably find their answers in the next few years with the results of the ongoing studies.

I. INTRODUCTION

In the last decades, blockade of the renin–angiotensin–aldosterone cascade (RAS), an important blood pressure-regulating mechanism, has proven to be very effective in treating hypertension and related disorders including heart failure and renal disease. Nonetheless, angiotensin-converting enzyme inhibitors (ACE inhibitors), the first drugs available to inhibit the generation of angiotensin II, are not devoid of side effects that sometimes limit their clinical use. Thus, cough occurs in ~10% of patients treated with an ACE inhibitor, and some individuals may develop angioedema because the ACE enzyme is also involved in the metabolism of bradykinin (42).

Another limitation of these drugs is that during chronic treatment some angiotensin II is still found at measurable levels in the circulation (39). This phenomenon is due to the reactive rise in plasma renin activity and plasma angiotensin I levels, which results in the generation of the angiotensin II as soon as some enzyme becomes available. This so-called "escape" phenomenon is particularly pronounced if the activity of ACE is not fully inhibited around the clock. Angiotensin II can also be produced through non-ACE pathways.

Thus, there was clearly a possibility of improving the ability to block the renin–angiotensin system even more effectively by acting directly at the receptor level. This hypothesis led to the development of the selective angiotensin II type 1 (AT_1) receptor antagonists, one of the latest class of drugs to be introduced for treating hypertension (52). These drugs act at the final step of the renin–angiotensin pathway by selectively inhibiting the AT_1 receptor subtype. In contrast to what is observed with ACE inhibition, there is no possible bypass.

As already discussed in Chapter 10, the AT_1 receptor subtype is responsible for most of the known actions of angiotensin II such as smooth muscle contraction, aldosterone, catecholamine, and arginine vasopressin release and cell proliferation. There is another angiotensin II receptor subtype, the AT_2 receptor, whose role is being increasingly delineated. This receptor appears to be predominantly involved in embryonic development, but it may also play a vasodilatory role in certain situations such as the response to shear stress. Some authors have suggested that this AT_2 activation may contribute to the pharmacological effects of the AT_1 receptor antagonists (13). Indeed, the selective blockade of AT_1 receptors, which reduces the effects of angiotensin II, leads to a compensatory rise in circulating angiotensin II levels that may stimulate the AT_2 receptors, as the latter are not blocked by the AT_1 antagonists. In fact, *in vitro* data effectively suggest that chronic stimulation of the AT_2 receptor may be beneficial in reducing cardiovascular remodeling by inhibiting cardiac and vascular smooth muscle growth and proliferation, stimulating apoptosis, and promoting extracellular matrix synthesis. However, whether these effects are also present clinically is still debated.

Orally active angiotensin II antagonists became available in the early 1990s. The first drug marketed from this group was losartan in 1995. Since then, many antagonists have been synthesized, and several have received approval for the treatment of hypertension by the United States Food and Drug Administration. Seven antagonists are currently marketed and used in the United States and Europe to treat hypertensive patients and patients with congestive heart failure and type 2 diabetes (4) (Fig. 30.1).

II. PHARMACOLOGY OF ANGIOTENSIN II RECEPTOR ANTAGONISTS

All angiotensin II receptor antagonists share a common mechanism of action; they selectively block the angiotensin II subtype-1 (AT_1) receptors. However, these various antagonists differ in their pharmacological profile, and these differences may sometimes affect their clinical efficacy. On the basis of *in vitro* binding studies, AT_1 receptor antagonists have been divided into two groups:

- Surmountable antagonists (losartan and eprosartan);
- Insurmountable antagonists (EXP3174, valsartan, irbesartan, candesartan, telmisartan, and olmesartan).

Although both groups produce a rightward shift of the angiotensin II dose–response curve, the maximal response is unaffected by surmountable antagonists, whereas it is reduced by insurmountable antagonists, leading to a non-parallel displacement of the angiotensin II response curve. Of note, the surmountable vs. insurmountable antagonism describes the ligand–antagonist interaction occurring when cells or tissue preparations are preincubated

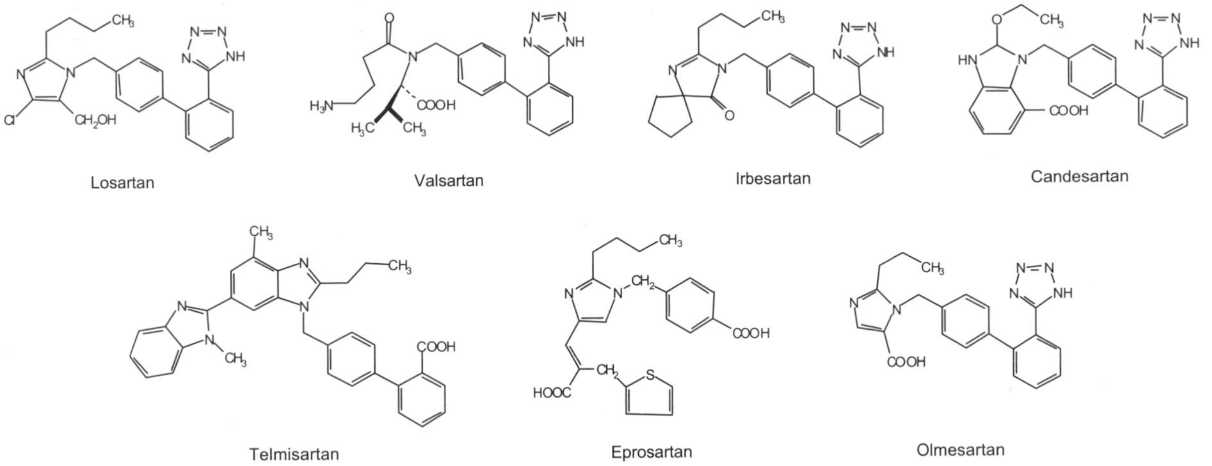

Figure 30.1 Oral angiotensin II receptor antagonists that are currently used in the United States and Europe for the management of hypertension and congestive heart failure.

with the antagonist and thereafter exposed to the agonist. In contrast, the competitive or noncompetitive nature of a drug is related to experimental conditions in which the ligand and the antagonist are added simultaneously. Recent studies have actually demonstrated that even though some AT_1 receptor antagonists are surmountable and others insurmountable, all are competitive antagonists, which means that they compete with angiotensin II at the receptor level according to the law of mass action (16).

The molecular basis for insurmountable antagonism is still a matter of debate. Several different potential mechanisms have been proposed (16,29). Recently, increasing evidence suggests that a slow dissociation from the receptor resulting in increased longevity of the antagonist–receptor complex is one of the leading mechanisms of the insurmountable characteristic of angiotensin II receptor antagonists. Although the specific mode of receptor occupancy has not been clearly linked with the blood pressure response to an angiotensin II antagonist, it is likely that a slow off-rate from the AT_1 receptor may extend the time of occupancy of the receptor protein and lengthen the duration of antagonism (29).

Another common feature of all angiotensin II receptor antagonists is their high binding to plasma proteins (>95%), mainly albumin and α_1-acid glycoprotein. In general, the protein binding of antihypertensive drugs has little, if any, effect on its clinical efficacy. Yet, we have reported that the strength of the binding between proteins and angiotensin II antagonists differs with the various compounds and may actually affect their clinical efficacy. Thus, for example, some AT_1 receptor antagonists are so tightly bound to plasma proteins when administered to humans that they do not exhibit any antagonistic effect, even though they were found to be very effective antagonists when investigated *in vitro* (27). These observations

suggest that the qualitative interaction between AT_1 receptor antagonists and proteins, and not necessarily the quantitative aspect of the binding, is an important pharmacological characteristic of angiotensin II receptor antagonists.

Despite numerous chemical similarities, the angiotensin II receptor antagonists differ from one another in their pharmacokinetic profiles including absorption, bioavailability, tissue distribution, metabolism, and rate of elimination, as shown in Table 30.1. The absorption rate of a compound generally influences the speed with which this latter acts, while the extent of compound absorption is another feature determining the drug effect. Tissue distribution (V_D) is a parameter that in theory characterizes the penetration of drug into deep tissue compartments. It has been suggested that larger V_D correlates with higher and facilitated extravascular AT_1 receptor access. Finally, the pharmacokinetic half-life of a compound roughly approximates its duration of effect. Long-lasting drugs such as irbesartan, candesartan, telmisartan, or olmesartan can effectively be considered as once-a-day compounds.

A. Losartan

Losartan (Cozaar®, Merck), was the first orally bioavailable, nonpeptide AT_1 antagonist to be used in humans. It has been studied extensively in both animals and human volunteers, and its effectiveness as an antihypertensive agent was established in the early 1990s. *In vitro*, losartan selectively competes with the binding of angiotensin II to the AT_1 receptor, with a median inhibitory concentration (IC_{50}) of 17–20 nmol/L. Losartan undergoes first-pass hepatic metabolism via cytochrome P-450 (CYP) isoenzymes 2C9 and 3A4 to its active carboxylic acid metabolic

Table 30.1 Pharmacokinetic Properties of Angiotensin II Receptor Antagonists

Variable	Losartan	Valsartan	Irbesartan	Candesartan	Eprosartan	Telmisartan	Olmesartan
Prodrug	No	No	No	Yes: candesartan cilexetil	No	No	Yes: olmesartan medoxomil
Active metabolite	Yes: EXP3174	No	No	No	No	No	No
AT_1-receptor affinity	(Losartan) IC_{50}: 20 nmol/L (EXP3174) IC_{50}: 3.7 nmol/L	IC_{50}: 2.7 nmol/L	IC_{50}: 1.7 nmol/L	K_i: 0.6 nmol/L	IC_{50}: 1.5 nmol/L	K_i: 3.5 nmol/L	IC_{50}: 8.0 nmol/L
In vitro angiotensin II antagonism	(Losartan) surmountable (EXP3174) insurmountable	Insurmountable	Insurmountable	Insurmountable	Surmountable	Insurmountable	Insurmountable
Bioavailability $F(\%)$	33	25	60–80	40	15	40–60	26
Food interaction	10% decrease in F (clinically NS)	50% decrease in absorption	No	No	Delayed absorption (clinically nonsignificant)	No	No
T_{max} (h)	1 (EXP3174: 2–4)	2–4	1.5–2	2–5	1–2	0.5–1	≈2
Protein binding (%)	98.7 (95.8)	95.0	99	99.5	98	>99	>99
V_d (L)	28–50 (10–12)	17	50–100	8–10	15	500	35
Metabolism	Oxidation, mainly by CYP2C9 and CYP3A4	Unknown	Oxidation and glucuronide conjugation	O-Demethylation	Glucuronide conjugation	Glucuronide conjugation	No
$t_{1/2}$ (h)	2 (6–9)	6–10	11–15	3–11	5–9	24	15
Elimination (renal/biliary)	40/60	30/70	20/80	60/40	37/63	0/100	40/60
Daily dosage (mg)	50–100	80–320	150–300	8–32	400–800	40–80	10–40
Dose adjustment: Renal	None	None	None (starting dose: 75 mg max. in dialysis patient)	None (starting dose: reduced in severe renal disease)	None	None	Reduced dose (max. 20 mg) in severe renal impairment
Hepatic	Reduced dose	None	None (do not give in severe case)	Starting dose: 2 mg (do not give in severe cases)	None	Starting dose: 40 mg in mild to moderate cases	None
Elderly	None	None	Starting dose: 75 mg	Starting dose: 4 mg	None	None	None
Drug interaction	None	None	Fluconazole	None	None	Digoxin; warfarin	None

Note: IC_{50}, concentration that displaces specifically 50% of the binding of angiotensin II; K_i, inhibition constant; T_{max}, time to peak plasma concentration; V_d, apparent volume of distribution; $t_{1/2}$, elimination half-life.

EXP-3174. EXP-3174 is 10–20 times more potent than losartan and has a longer duration of action than that of losartan. In fact, most of the effects observed after drug intake are due to EXP-3174. However, as the oral bioavailability of EXP-3174 is very low, the drug on the market is losartan. On the isolated rabbit aorta, losartan produces a surmountable blockade of the contractile response induced by angiotensin II, whereas EXP-3174 causes an insurmountable blockade. Food tends to slow the absorption of the drug, but this effect has only a minimal clinical impact. Losartan and its metabolite are excreted by the kidney and bile, and neither compound is dialyzed. Finally, in contrast to other angiotensin II receptor antagonists, losartan has been documented to lower plasma uric acid levels after single or multiple doses in healthy subjects as well as in hypertensive subjects (6,57). This effect, which potentially could be an advantage in patients concomitantly treated with a diuretic or with hyperuremia for other reasons, is due to the losartan molecule itself and not to its active metabolite. Losartan increases urinary uric acid excretion by inhibiting the urate/anion exchanger found in the brush-border of the renal proximal tubule (5).

The recommended doses of losartan are 50–100 mg once daily. Most clinical studies have been conducted with the 50 mg dose, but more recent trials have used losartan 100 mg once daily (19). Fixed combinations of losartan (50 and 100 mg) and hydrochlorothiazide (12.5 or 25 mg) are available in many countries. Losartan has received the indication for treating hypertension and, in some countries, also for treating congestive heart failure and prevention of diabetic nephropathy in type 2 diabetes.

B. Valsartan

Valsartan (Diovan®, Tareg®, Nisis®; Novartis) was the second nonpeptide angiotensin II receptor antagonist available for treating hypertension. Valsartan is a nonheterocyclic compound in which the imidazole of losartan has been replaced with an acylated amino acid. *In vitro*, it blocks the AT_1 receptor in an insurmountable fashion. Valsartan inhibits the binding of angiotensin II to rat aorta AT_1 receptors with an IC_{50} of 2.7 nmol/L. In contrast to losartan, valsartan does not require conversion to an active metabolite and ~80–90% of the drug is excreted unchanged in the bile (70%) and by the kidney (30%). Only one metabolite (valeryl-4-hydroxy valsartan), which is not active, accounting for 10% of recovered drug, is also found in the feces. After oral application, valsartan is rapidly absorbed, with a bioavailability of 25%, which is reduced by ~40% if the drug is taken with food (31).

The recommended starting doses of valsartan are 80–160 mg once daily, with possible titration to doses up to 320 mg daily. In heart failure, valsartan has been used safely at a dose of 160 mg bid. As observed for losartan, the safety profile of valsartan is excellent, with adverse reactions such as headache, upper-respiratory-tract infections, diarrhea, fatigue, and cough occurring at rates comparable with placebo. At higher dosages (320 mg/day), dizziness became more prevalent (31).

No clinically important pharmacokinetic interactions were reported when valsartan was given with other drugs such as digoxin, warfarin, glyburide, cimetidine, or hydrochlorothiazide, currently administered in elderly patients. Fixed combinations of valsartan and hydrochlorothiazide are also marketed.

C. Irbesartan

Like losartan, irbesartan (Aprovel®, Avapro®, Karvea®; Bristol-Myers Squibb/Sanofi Synthelabo) is an imidazole-derivative with a biphenyl-tetrazol side chain. The molecule has an imidazolinone ring in which the carbonyl group replaces the hydroxylmethyl group of losartan (or the carboxylic moieties of EXP-3174) as hydrogen bond acceptor. Irbesartan has a high affinity for the AT_1 receptor, with an IC_{50} of 1.7 nmol/L in human vascular smooth muscle cells. *In vitro*, irbesartan induces an insurmountable blockade of AT_1 receptors. Irbesartan has no active metabolite, and food does not affect its bioavailability which, with an average of 60–80%, is higher than that of other angiotensin II receptor antagonists. Irbesartan is longer acting than losartan and valsartan, with an elimination half-life of about 11–15 h.

There are some controversies about the binding of this drug to plasma proteins. This latter was originally claimed to be smaller than those usually observed within other angiotensin II antagonists (90–92%), but in a more recent study, irbesartan was found to have a protein binding (<99%) comparable with other antagonists (40). Irbesartan is mainly excreted (60–80%) in the feces, whereas ~25% appears in urine. As irbesartan is strongly metabolized via hepatic glucuronidation and oxidation (mainly CYP 2C9), only ~1% is excreted as the unchanged molecule. Warfarin and digoxin appear to have negligible effects on CYP 2C9 metabolism of irbesartan, and no potential drug interactions have been reported except with fluconazole (18).

The recommended doses of irbesartan are 150 and 300 mg once daily. Antihypertensive effects are seen within 2 weeks of initiating therapy, with maximum effects occurring between 2 and 6 weeks. In clinical studies, there was no relationship between the dosage and the overall frequency of adverse events, which remained similar to those observed for placebo (18). Irbesartan is also available in fixed combinations with a small dose of hydrochlorothiazide for use in patients who have not achieved the desired blood pressure-lowering effect with irbesartan monotherapy. Irbesartan is indicated for treating hypertension and preventing diabetic nephropathy in type 2 diabetes.

D. Candesartan

Candesartan (Atacand®, Kenzen®, Blopress®; Astra-Zeneca/Takeda) is a potent long-lasting angiotensin II receptor antagonist that is rapidly produced in the gastro-instestinal tract by hydrolysis of an easily orally absorbed ester-prodrug candesartan–cilexetil (TCV-116). Candesartan inhibits the *in vitro* binding of angiotensin II to AT_1 receptors of rabbit aortic membrane, with an inhibition constant (K_i) of 0.64 nmol/L (35). This drug produces an insurmountable antagonism because of a tight binding to and a slow dissociation from the AT_1 receptors. Following oral administration, candesartan–cilexetil is quantitatively converted to candesartan, with an average absolute bioavailability of candesartan of ~40%. Candesartan has an elimination half-life of ~9 h, which might be prolonged in elderly patients. It is mainly eliminated unchanged by the kidneys (30%) and the bile (70%). Of note, candesartan has a rather small apparent volume of distribution (0.1 L/kg), which results in starting and maintenance doses of candesartan (8–16 mg once-a-day) that are smaller than those of other antagonists (35). Titration to 32 mg has been used in some clinical trials and has been shown to provide a greater antihypertensive efficacy. No reports of clinically important interactions between candesartan and other drugs commonly prescribed in hypertensive patients or with oral contraceptives have been noticed. The dosage of candesartan must be individualized, especially in patients with severe renal or hepatic impairments or in the elderly. Candesartan/hydrochlorothiazide fixed combinations are also available with different doses of candesartan (35).

E. Eprosartan

Eprosartan (Teveten®; SmithKline Beecham/Solvay) was the fourth selective nonpeptide angiotensin II receptor antagonist to gain approval for use in treating hypertension in the United States. Eprosartan is the unique representative of a nonbiphenyl, nontetrazole AT_1 antagonist class. This compound is the last development of an imidazole-5-acrylic acid series of nonpeptide angiotensin II receptor antagonists. Introduction of a *p*-carboxylic acid on the *N*-benzyl ring resulted in nanomolar affinity for the AT_1 receptor and good oral activity; the presence of a thienyl ring (sulfur-containing heterocycle) together with two acid groups was important to achieve good potency. Eprosartan does not require any metabolic activation or transformation to produce an effective AT_1 receptor antagonism (34). Eprosartan is a specific antagonist of the AT_1 receptor, which shows a true surmountable competitive antagonism *in vitro*. It inhibits [^{125}I]-angiotensin II binding to rat mesenteric artery membranes with an IC_{50} of 1.5 nmol/L, and it is also a potent inhibitor of labeled-angiotensin binding to human liver membranes (IC_{50} = 1.7 nmol/L). The bioavailability of eprosartan is smaller than those of other antagonists. It is limited by an incomplete oral absorption rather than high first-pass metabolism. In addition, depending on the formulation, eprosartan absorption may be reduced by 25% and retarded by 1.5 h when the drug is administered with food (9). The bile represents the main excretory pathway (90%); 7% of eprosartan is found as unchanged drug in urine.

Several studies have investigated the ability of eprosartan to block presynaptic AT_1 receptors, located at the vascular neuroeffector junction, but with contrasted results (34). The usual maintenance dose of eprosartan is 600 mg daily. Because eprosartan has a half-life of 5–7 h, most initial studies have been conducted using a twice-a-day regimen. However, a double-blind, parallel group, placebo-controlled, and multicenter study comparing the antihypertensive efficacy in 243 patients of one daily dose vs. half-doses given twice a day showed that there was no significant difference in efficacy and tolerability of eprosartan between the two regimens and that both regimens induced significant blood pressure reductions (20). Thus, eprosartan is now rather used in a once-daily regimen with a recommended dose of 400–800 mg/day. Eprosartan does not inhibit CYP450 isoenzymes and is not metabolized via this pathway. Thus, eprosartan would not be expected to be at risk of drug interactions.

F. Telmisartan

Telmisartan (Micardis®, Pritor®, Kinzal®; Boehringer Ingelheim/Glaxo Wellcome/Bayer) is a long-acting angiotensin II receptor antagonist that gained approval for use in treating hypertension in 1998. Chemically, telmisartan lacks the tetrazole unit and has a common benzimidazole group with candesartan. The substitution of this benzimidazole moiety with a basic heterocycle results in potent AT_1 antagonism and good absorption after oral application. Telmisartan is an insurmountable antagonist of the AT_1 receptor that does not affect other receptor systems involved in cardiovascular regulation. It inhibits the binding of labeled angiotensin II to AT_1 receptors in rat lungs with a K_i of 3.7 nmol/L. The absolute bioavailability of telmisartan is dose-dependent and varies from 30% to 60%. Telmisartan is more lipophilic than other antagonists; this feature, coupled with a high volume of distribution, could result in good tissue penetration.

Telmisartan is not a prodrug and has a long terminal elimination half-life (~24 h), making it suitable for once-a-day dosing. The compound, which is not metabolized by cytochrome P450 isoenzymes, undergoes minimal glucuro-transformation and is almost completely excreted in the feces (98%) (56). In contrast to other angiotensin II receptor antagonists, some drug interactions with telmisartan have been described. In particular, telmisartan causes an increase in serum digoxin, and it may also decrease warfarin plasma levels during coadministration (50).

The overall frequency of adverse events with telmisartan 20–160 mg/day was reported to be similar to that with placebo. Telmisartan is used at the recommended starting dose of 40 mg once daily; this dose may be increased to 80 mg in case of insufficient blood pressure-lowering effect. The fixed dose combination of telmisartan and hydrochlorothiazide is now available in some countries.

G. Olmesartan

Olmesartan medoxomil (Benikar®; Sankyo) is a new orally active angiotensin II receptor antagonist that recently (2002) gained FDA approval for use in treating hypertension. It is also now on the market in Europe. This compound is a prodrug containing, like candesartan–cilexetil, an ester-moiety that after oral administration is rapidly converted *in vivo* to the active metabolite olmesartan. *In vitro*, the affinity of olmesartan for AT_1 bovine adrenal cortical receptors is comparable to other angiotensin II receptor antagonists (IC_{50} 8.0 nmol/L). Olmesartan produces selective insurmountable inhibition of all-induced contractions of the guinea-pig aorta.

Following oral administration, olmesartan has a faster onset but similar elimination half-life when compared with candesartan cilexetil. The absolute biovailabilty of olmesartan after a single oral dose of olmesartan medoxomil is 26% in healthy volunteers. The remaining unabsorbed drug is excreted without further metabolism. Feces is the major route of excretion of olmesartan, with urinary excretion accounting for 5–12% of the administered dose. Because olmesartan is not metabolized by the CYT P450 system, drugs that induce, inhibit, or are metabolized by these enzymes do not appear to interact with it. In addition, dosing adjustments do not appear necessary for elderly patients or for patients with moderate to mild renal dysfunction or with hepatic disease (3).

Olmesartan exhibited a pronounced dosage-related efficacy across the entire dosage range evaluated, with a tolerability profile similar to that of placebo. The usual recommended doses of olmesartan are 10–40 mg once daily. Twice-daily dosing offers no advantage over the same total dose given once daily (55).

III. TOLERABILITY AND SAFETY PROFILE OF ANGIOTENSIN II RECEPTOR ANTAGONISTS

Despite the wide choice of antihypertensive agents at the disposition of practitioners, only low hypertension control rates (25–30%) are generally reported in the literature. These disappointing results have multiple causes: one of them is undoubtedly the occurrence of side effects and a low tolerability profile, which in turn may result in poor long-term adherence to therapy. In this regard, angiotensin II receptor antagonists are unique, as they have an excellent safety and tolerability profile with an incidence of side effects that is not different from placebo (32). None of the seven drugs reviewed here has a specific, dose-dependent adverse effect that can be attributed to the drug itself. For example, unlike ACE inhibitors, angiotensin II receptor antagonists do not cause cough. Although some cases of angioedema, another side effect of ACE inhibitors, were associated with the consumption of losartan (7), it is difficult to ascertain whether these published cases of angioedema are really linked to the administration of losartan or simply a coincidence, because angioedema may occur with many substances including other drugs and some food products.

No consistent adverse effects on routine hematological parameters were noted with the use of angiotensin II receptor antagonists. Only minor clinically nonsignificant decreases in hemoglobin levels have been reported in hypertensive patients. Some cases of anemia have been reported in dialyzed patients or inpatients with chronic renal failure treated with losartan (49). However, AT_1 receptor blockade has been found to lower hemoglobin in posttransplant erythrocytosis (22). Occasional elevations of liver enzymes (particularly ALAT) have been reported and usually resolved with or without discontinuation of therapy (32). Increases in serum potassium levels have been observed during angiotensin II receptor blockade. Of note, hyperkalemia is more likely to develop in patients with renal insufficiency, or with diabetes mellitus, or in those patients taking potassium-sparing diuretics or potassium supplementation.

The safety and tolerability of angiotensin II receptor antagonists as well as their efficacy were carefully evaluated with regard to patient gender, age, and race. None of these factors was found to influence the incidence of side effects. In particular, angiotensin II receptor antagonists are equally well tolerated by elderly (>65 years), younger (<65 years), and very old (>75 years) patients. Because all antagonists are cleared through the bile, no dosage adjustment is recommended in patients with moderate to marked renal impairment (creatinine clearance <40 mL/min) or with moderate hepatic dysfunction (32). In case of severe hepatic dysfunction, the antihypertensive efficacy may be prolonged. For patients with possible depletion of intravascular volume (e.g., patients treated with diuretics, particularly those with impaired renal function), blockade of the renin–angiotensin system should be initiated carefully and consideration should be given to the use of a lower starting dose. In studies evaluating the use of ACE inhibitors in patients with unilateral or bilateral renal artery stenosis, increases in serum creatinine or blood urea nitrogen, together with oliguria and/or progressive azotemia and (rarely) with acute renal failure and/or death, have been reported (15). So far, few studies have evaluated the safety of angiotensin II receptor antagonists in patients with renal artery stenosis, but preliminary reports suggest that similar results may be expected (32).

IV. USE OF ANGIOTENSIN II RECEPTOR ANTAGONISTS IN HYPERTENSION

Numerous clinical studies have evaluated the antihypertensive efficacy of angiotensin II receptor antagonists in patients with mild to moderate or severe hypertension. In these studies, angiotensin II receptor antagonists were compared with other first-line antihypertensive agents such as ACE inhibitors, calcium-channel blockers, β-blockers, and diuretics (4). Approximately half of the hypertensive patients treated with a monotherapy of angiotensin II receptor blockers were considered as responders to treatment. This percentage is similar to that obtained with other monotherapies. In studies evaluating their efficacy in various populations and age groups when administered either alone or in combination with diuretics, angiotensin II receptor antagonists were as effective as other antihypertensive drugs. They also lowered blood pressure in hypertensive patients without affecting heart rate, regardless of gender and age (18,19,31,34,35,50,55). In monotherapy, angiotensin II receptor antagonists, like ACE inhibitors, were less effective in reducing blood pressure in black patients, but this was not the case when angiotensin II antagonists were combined with a diuretic.

V. DIFFERENCES BETWEEN ANGIOTENSIN II RECEPTOR ANTAGONISTS

As discussed previously, the antihypertensive activity of marketed angiotensin II receptor antagonists has been evaluated extensively, and it was found to be comparable to that of other blood pressure-lowering drugs. A meta-analysis also compared the antihypertensive efficacy of four AT_1 receptor antagonists (losartan, valsartan, irbesartan, and candesartan) on the basis of the results of the

clinical trials submitted for their registration (11). In this analysis, no significant difference in terms of antihypertensive efficacy was found among the four compounds, despite their pharmacological differences. However, specially designed head-to-head comparisons among these antagonists have revealed some significant differences; the biggest being observed when losartan was compared with longer acting drugs such as candesartan, irbesartan, telmisartan, or olmesartan. In fact, in all these studies, losartan was found to produce a smaller decrease in blood pressure, less at trough, suggesting a less effective 24 h control of blood pressure. Yet, one has to stress that head-to-head comparison studies have generally concluded that the new compound is better than the older, an observation that may be true but might also be the subject of bias.

Another important issue in this type of studies is the choice of doses. Thus, the results of the CLAIM study II (54) and the Losartan trial (30) illustrate how drug comparisons can be misleading if the doses are not adequately defined. Indeed, in the first trial comparing candesartan and losartan, the doses of candesartan and losartan were 16/32 mg vs. 50/100 mg, respectively (the CLAIM II study), and the results showed a significantly greater antihypertensive effect for candesartan. In contrast, in the Losartan trial, losartan was found to be as effective as candesartan, but the doses of candesartan were twice as small.

When differences in antihypertensive efficacy are observed between two angiotensin II receptor antagonists acting through the same mechanism of action, one reasonable question is "does this difference persist when the doses of the comparators are increased?" To answer these questions, we have evaluated the blockade of the renin–angiotensin system produced by a series of angiotensin receptor antagonists using two different techniques (Fig. 30.2):

- The inhibition of blood pressure increase to exogenous angiotensin I or II (8).
- An *ex vivo in vitro* binding assay that quantifies the displacement of angiotensin II by the blocking agents (28).

With these techniques, we found that the recommended starting doses of the marketed drugs are generally able to achieve a significant blockade of the angiotensin II receptor during the first hours after drug intake.

However, that is not always the case at trough. Significant differences between the antagonists were found, which suggests that some antagonists do not block the system around the clock (17,28,33). As observed with valsartan, increasing the dose from 80 to 320 mg had a small additional effect at peak, but it clearly enhanced the receptor blockade at trough and prolonged the duration of action of the compound.

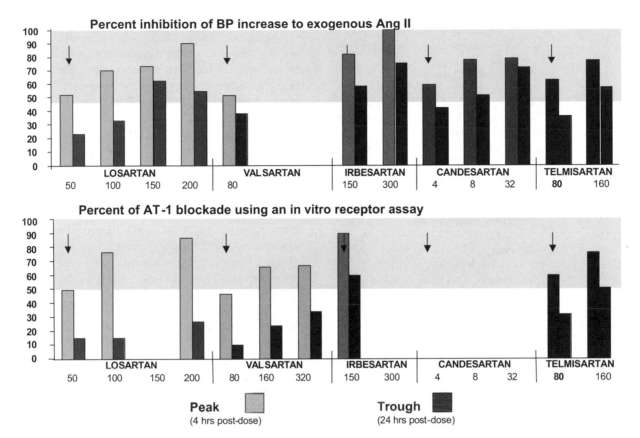

Figure 30.2 Assessment of angiotensin II receptor blockade induced by a series of angiotensin II receptor antagonists in normotensive volunteers by using two different techniques.

The clinical importance of a 24 h blockade of the renin–angiotensin system can be discussed. Indeed, because some ACE inhibitors have been shown to decrease blood pressure around the clock despite a relatively short duration of action, it may not be absolutely necessary to continuously block this system at least in term of blood pressure control. Nevertheless, a more complete blockade of the renin–angiotensin system may be of greater importance when considering the ability of these agents to provide end-organ target protection. This assumption was recently corroborated by the results of several morbidity and mortality trials that have clearly shown that higher doses were more effective to achieve target organ protection.

Thus, as will be discussed subsequently, the LIFE and RENAAL studies have demonstrated the clear benefit of 100 mg of losartan in reducing the primary end-points in hypertensive patients (12) and inpatients with type 2 diabetes (2), whereas 50 mg of losartan in the ELITE II (47) and in the OPTIMAAL (14) trials failed to demonstrate an advantage for losartan when compared with an adequate dose of captopril (50 mg tid) in patients with congestive heart failure or myocardial infarction. In IRMA-2, irbesartan 300 mg was found to be superior to irbesartan 150 mg in preventing the development of overt proteinuria

in type 2 diabetes (43). Finally, in VALHeFT, valsartan was found to provide clear benefits in patients with heart failure, but at an average dose of 240 mg per day (10).

These clinical results on the basis of large groups of patients therefore suggest that a complete 24 h blockade of the renin–angiotensin system with an AT_1 receptor blocker is probably more beneficial than a lower dose that blocks the system only transiently.

VI. COMBINING ANGIOTENSIN II RECEPTOR ANTAGONISTS WITH ACE INHIBITORS

Another approach to achieve a more complete blockade of the renin–angiotensin system would be to act at two levels of the cascade—for example, to combine an angiotensin II antagonist and an ACE inhibitor (1). Several small clinical studies have suggested that combining an ACE inhibitor with an AT_1 receptor antagonist provides an additional benefit, mainly in urinary protein excretion in diabetics (the Candesartan and Lisinopril Microalbuminuria (CALM) study) (38) and in nondiabetic patients (the COOPERATE study) (41). However, most of these studies combined a relatively low dose of an AT_1 receptor

Table 30.2   Medical Trial Names and Acronyms

ACCESS	Acute Candesartan CilExetil therapy in Stroke Survivors
CALM	CAndesartan and Lisinopril Microalbuminuria
CHARM	Candesartan in Heart failure-Assessment of Reduction in Mortality and morbidity
ELITE	Evaluation of Losartan In The Elderly
IDNT	Irbesartan Diabetic Nephropathy Trial
I-PRESERVE	Irbesartan in heart failure with PRESERVEd systolic sunction
IRMA-2	IRbesartan MicroAlbuminuria study
LIFE	Losartan Intervention For Endpoint reduction in hypertension
MARVAL	MicroAlbuminuria Reduction with VALsartan
ONTARGET	ONgoing Telmisartan Alone and in combination with Ramipril Global Endpoint Trial
OPTIMAAL	OPtimal Therapy In Myocardial infarction with the Angiotensin II Antagonist Losartan
RENAAL	Reduction in End points in NIDDM with the Angiotensin II Antagonist Losartan
RESOLVD	Randomized Evaluation Strategies fOr Left Ventricular Dysfunction
SCOPE	Study on COgnition and Prognosis in the Elderly
TRANSCEND	Telmisartan Randomized AssessmeNt Study in aCE iNtolerant subjects with cardiovascular Disease
VALHeFT	VALsartan Heart Failure Trial
VALIANT	VALsartan In Acute myocardial iNfarction Trial
VALUE	Valsartan Antihypertensive Long-term Use Evaluation

blocker, usually losartan 50 or 100 mg od, with various doses of ACE inhibitors. Again, the main issue is to demonstrate that the same effect could not be obtained with a higher dose of the receptor antagonist alone. To test this hypothesis, we have recently quantified the degree of blockade obtainable in normotensive subjects with increasing doses of losartan and telmisartan given once or twice a day alone or in combination with lisinopril (17). When both drugs were administered at their maximum recommended doses, 100 mg for losartan and 80 mg for telmisartan, the addition of lisinopril 20 mg provided a clear additional blockade of the receptor at trough. However, with the use of higher doses of antagonist (upto 200 mg for losartan and 160 mg for telmisartan), as much blockade of the renin–angiotensin system could be obtained with the receptor antagonist as with the ACE inhibitor/angiotensin II receptor blocker combination.

This suggests that combining an ACE inhibitor with an AT_1 receptor blocker may indeed provide additional benefits if the dose of the receptor antagonist is relatively low and does not block the system for 24 h. However, with the use of higher doses of the antagonists, the combination may not be necessary. In line with this idea, the newly published VALIANT trial did not convincingly demonstrate the benefits of combining an ACE inhibitor and an AT_1 receptor antagonist following an acute myocardial infarction (45); nor did the CHARM (44) and VALHeft (10) studies demonstrate a clear advantage of combining these drugs in heart failure.

Thus, whether combining two drugs interfering with the renin–angiotensin system is really beneficial remains to be demonstrated. Additional information will be generated by two large ongoing trials conducted in patients with a high cardiovascular risk—the ONTARGET trial and the TRANSCEND substudy. These studies will provide important information on the efficacy and safety of this combined therapy.

VII.   CLINICAL TRIALS WITH ANGIOTENSIN II RECEPTOR ANTAGONISTS

Several large trials have been designed to assess the effects of angiotensin II receptor antagonists on morbidity and mortality in hypertensive patients (Tables 30.2 and 30.3). The first trial demonstrating the clinical efficacy of an antagonist on morbidity and mortality was the LIFE trial (12). This study compared two regimens—losartan-based and atenolol-based—in 9193 hypertensive patients with ECG-documented left-ventricular hypertrophy. Patients were followed for an average of 4.7 years. Although blood pressure was comparably reduced in both the losartan-based and the atenolol-based treatments, the losartan-based treatment was associated with a significantly lower relative risk of primary cardiovascular event (i.e., death, myocardial infarction, or stroke) and with significantly less fatal and nonfatal strokes (−25%, $P < 0.001$). In a subgroup of 1195 diabetic patients, the protection was even more marked, with a highly significant 24% reduction of the combined risk and a 39% decrease in mortality (26). In addition, losartan also diminished new-onset diabetes and was more effective than atenolol in reversing left-ventricular hypertrophy. Thus, this study effectively suggests that angiotensin II receptor blockade presents additional cardiac and metabolic benefits beyond the reduction of blood pressure when compared with a β-blocker (12).

A second study, SCOPE, has been designed to evaluate the effects of candesartan cilexetil compared with placebo on cardiovascular mortality and morbidity and on cognitive performances in a population of 4500 elderly hypertensive patients (70–89 years old) over 4 years (21). Unfortunately, because of ethical considerations, many of the placebo-allocated patients went on to treatment and only 16% received placebo alone as defined per protocol. Thus, the power of the trial was reduced, and there was only a nonsignificant 11% decrease in the primary endpoint (cardiovascular mortality/nonfatal myocardial infarction/stroke) but a 28% reduction in nonfatal stroke ($P = 0.04$). When considering only those patients who had no "add-on" drugs other than hydrochlorothiazide, candesartan reduced the relative risk of a primary end-point event by 32%. Also in this study, angiotensin II receptor blockade significantly diminished new-onset diabetes compared with controls. In addition, candesartan has no deleterious effect on cognition, despite strict control of blood pressure.

Recently, the result of a third study, the VALUE trial has been published (23). This trial compared a valsartan-based regimen (80–160 mg od) and the long-acting calcium channel blocker amlodipine (5 to 10 mg od) in more than 15,000 hypertensive patients older than 50 years who are at high risk for a cardiovascular event. The hypothesis that for a same level of blood-pressure control ($<140/90$ mmHg), angiotensin II receptor blockade will be more effective than amlodipine to decrease cardiovascular mortality (acute MI, heart failure, and cardiac death) was not verified. Indeed, a significant difference in blood pressure control in favor of amlodipine, partly due to the relatively low dose of valsartan used in the beginning of the study, precluded valid comparison of drug effects on outcomes. However, despite poorer blood pressure control, valsartan-treated patients did as well as those prescribed amlodipine for the primary composite outcome.

ONTARGET is an ongoing trial, which compares the efficacy of the angiotensin II receptor blocker telmisartan with that of the ACE inhibitor ramipril, either drug given alone or in association with telmisartan in about 30,000 patients at high risk of cardiovascular disease with or without hypertension for an observation period of up to 5.5 years (58). This study is the first large trial directly comparing an ACE inhibitor and an angiotensin II receptor antagonist in reducing stroke, myocardial infarction, cardiovascular death, and hospitalization for congestive heart failure. It should also provide important information on the potential benefits of combining an ACE inhibitor and an antagonist, particularly in diabetic patients.

As part of the ONTARGET trial program, the TRANSCEND trial will be the largest cardiovascular protection trial ever conducted in patients intolerant to ACE inhibitors (58). The TRANSCEND trial is specially set up because there is increasing awareness of treatment discontinuations in patients on ACE inhibitors because of their specific side effects. Approximately 5000 patients will be enrolled worldwide in this double-blind, parallel-group study. The primary objective of the study is the effect of angiotensin II blockade on the composite endpoint of cardiovascular mortality, stroke, acute myocardial infarction, and hospitalization for congestive heart failure. The secondary objective is the impact of angiotensin II receptor blockade on the incidence of re-vascularization procedures, newly diagnosed diabetes, dementia, new-onset atrial fibrillation, and microvascular complications of diabetes.

VIII. CARDIAC AND RENAL EFFECTS OF ANGIOTENSIN II RECEPTOR ANTAGONISTS

Besides their antihypertensive properties, the angiotensin II receptor antagonists may also be active in other clinical indications. Indeed, it is well established from ACE inhibitor trials that inhibition of RAS:

- prolongs the survival of patients after acute myocardial infarction or of patients with congestive heart failure;
- retards or even inhibits left-ventricular hypertrophy progression in hypertensive patients;
- slows progression of renal disease in patients with diabetes;
- reduces morbidity associated with atherosclerotic disease.

Because angiotensin II receptor antagonists share most of the pharmacological actions of ACE inhibitors but with a better tolerability profile, they were of course considered as an ideal alternative to this therapeutic approach. Table 30.3 presents a summary of the major clinical trials conducted so far with AT_1 receptor antagonists in various clinical indications.

Several randomized trials have been designed to assess the efficacy and safety of angiotensin II receptor antagonists in chronic heart failure and acute myocardial infarction. These latter were triggered by the results of the ELITE I trial, which compared the renal safety of losartan 50 mg qd and captopril 50 mg tid in elderly patients with heart failure. In this study, a secondary end-point (combined mortality from and hospital admission for heart failure) was astonishingly lower in the losartan group (46). Unfortunately, these results were not confirmed by the larger ELITE II follow-up trial (47). Although there was no significant difference in all-cause mortality or sudden death between the two treatment groups, because of the statistical and regulatory definitions due to the special design of the study, the investigators were obliged to conclude that losartan was not superior to the ACE inhibitor captopril in reducing the primary

Table 30.3 Ongoing and Completed Trials for Angiotensin II Receptor Antagonists

	Trial	Patient population	Number of subjects	Endpoints	Year study completed	Treatment group	Results
Hypertension	LIFE	Hypertensive with LVH	9124	CV morbidity and mortality	2001	Losartan vs. atenolol	Losartan 100 mg is better than atenolol to reduce the risk of primary CV events.
	SCOPE	Elderly hypertensive 70–90 years	4964	CV mortality, MI, stroke, prevention of cognitive impairment	2002	Candesartan vs. placebo	Candesartan reduces CV mortality, especially in stroke. No deleterious effect on cognition.
	VALUE	Hypertensive (>50 years) with high CV risks	15,000	CV mortality	2004	Valsartan vs. amlodipine	Valsartan is not superior to amlodipine to reduce CV mortality and morbidity
	ONTARGET	High CV risk patients	~30,000	CV morbidity and mortality (stroke, MI, CHF, and cardiac deaths)	2007	Telmisartan vs. ramipril or combined therapy	—
	TRANSCEND	High CV risk patients intolerant to ACE-I	~5000	CV morbidity and mortality (stroke, MI, CHF, and cardiac deaths)	2007	Telmisartan vs. placebo	—
Heart failure	ELITE I	Elderly patients (>60 years) with CHF	722	Renal safety	1997	Losartan vs. captopril	Losartan is safe and effective in the treatment of CHF.
	ELITE II	Elderly patients (>60 years) with CHF	3121	All cause mortality	1999	Losartan vs. captopril	Losartan 50 mg is not better than captopril in the treatment of CHF.
	RESOLVD	Patients with HF due to systolic dysfunction	768	Improvement of the physical capacity, remodeling	Stopped 1999	Candesartan vs. enalapril or combined therapy	Combination was more effective than either therapy alone. Increase, though not significant in HF hospitalization, in candesartan groups.
	Val-HeFT	Patients with HF and LVEF <40%	5010	All cause mortality	2001	Valsartan vs. placebo (ACE-I background)	Valsartan is better than placebo to reduce morbidity and mortality in CHF patients.
	CHARM-alternative	Patients with HF and LVEF <40% (ACE-I intolerant)	2028	All cause mortality	2003	Candesartan vs. placebo (no ACE-I background)	Candesartan reduces CV deaths or hospitalization for CHF.
	CHARM-added	Patients with HF and LVEF <40%	2548	All cause mortality	2003	Candesartan vs. placebo (ACE-I background)	Candesartan reduces CV deaths and hospitalization for CHF.
	CHARM-preserved	Patients with HF and LVEF >40%	3025	All cause mortality	2003	Candesartan vs. placebo (ACE-I background)	No significant effect of candesartan.
	I-PRESERVE	Patients with HF (>60 years) and LVEF >45%	~3600	CV morbidity and mortality	2005	Irbesartan vs. placebo (no ACE-I background)	—

	Trial	Patients	N	Endpoint	Year	Comparison	Conclusion
Post-MI	OPTIMAAL	High-risk patients post-MI with LV dysfunction	5477	All cause mortality	2002	Losartan vs. captopril	Losartan 50 mg is not better than captopril in post-MI follow-up.
	VALIANT	High-risk patients post-MI with LVEF <35%	14,500	All cause mortality	2003	Valsartan vs. captopril or combined therapy	Valsartan is not inferior to captopril or combined therapy to reduce morbidity and mortality in CHF patients post-MI.
Stroke	ACCESS	Patients with acute cerebral ischemia	339	Safety	2003	Candesartan vs. placebo within 7 days post-stroke, candesartan background afterwards	Candesartan is safe, and significantly reduces 1-year mortality.
Renal	IDNT	NIDDM patients with nephropathy	1650	Renal protection, composite of ESRD, doubling of creatinine, and mortality	2000	Irbesartan vs. amlodipine vs. placebo (no ACE-I background)	Irbesartan provides better renal protection and disease-retarding effect than amlodipine or placebo.
	RENAAL	NIDDM patients with nephropathy	1520	Renal protection, composite of ESRD, doubling of creatinine, and mortality	2000	Losartan vs. placebo (no ACE-I background)	Losartan provides renal protection and has disease-retarding effect.
	IRMA-2	NIDDM patients with hypertension	611	Microalbuminuria	2000	Irbesartan vs. placebo (no ACE-I background)	Irbesartan 300 mg decreases microalbuminuria and retard the progression towards proteinuria.
	CALM	NIDDM patients with hypertension	197	Proteinuria	2000	Candesartan vs. lisinopril or combined therapy	Reduction of proteinuria is greater after combined therapy than after candesartan alone but not lisinopril alone.
	MARVAL	NIDDM patients with hypertension	332	Microalbuminuria	2001	Valsartan vs. placebo (ACE-I background)	Valsartan has antiproteinuric effect in type 2 diabetes.

end-point. Hence, after this study, ACE remained the standard of therapy in patients with heart failure due to systolic dysfunction (47).

The RESOLVD pilot study comparing candesartan, enalapril, and a combination of both drugs in patients with heart failure also failed to find a significant difference between treatments in term of improvement of the physical capacity, quality of life, and tolerability. In addition, this study was discontinued earlier than expected because of an increase, albeit nonsignificant, of heart-failure-related hospitalizations and deaths in the candesartan and combination group compared with the enalapril group (36).

The relatively negative findings of both the ELITE II and RESOLVD trials have yet to be interpreted carefully. Thus, in the ELITE II study, the chosen dose of losartan (50 mg qd) was probably too small to achieve effective 24 h AT_1 blockade (32). In the RESOLVD study, although it was terminated early because of the increase in heart failure-induced hospitalization after angiotensin II receptor blockade, the number of patients in the ACE inhibitor group was small and the mortality rate was considerably lower than that reported in SOLVD, an earlier, larger trial of ACE inhibition (51). Thus, conclusions regarding mortality differences cannot really be drawn from these trials.

The VALHeFT trial was designed to evaluate the long-term effects of the addition of valsartan 160 mg or a placebo twice daily on top of standard therapy for heart failure (10). In addition to mortality, a combined end-point of mortality and morbidity (cardiac arrest, hospitalization for heart failure, or receipt of intravenous inotropic or vasodilator therapy) was the primary outcome measure. After a mean follow-up of 23 months, no difference was observed in all-cause mortality, but valsartan significantly lowered the incidence of the combined end-point, mainly because of a high reduction rate in hospitalizations for worsening heart failure. The favorable impact of valsartan was particularly impressive in patients who were not being treated with an ACE inhibitor, with a 42% reduction of the relative risk.

The emergence of a new class of drug for RAS inhibition has also presented the opportunity to investigate additional questions not formally tested in previous trials with ACE inhibitors. This is the case with studies of patients with chronic heart failure with preserved left-ventricular systolic function. The series of CHARM trials (45) evaluated the potential benefits of candesartan in 7600 patients divided into three groups with different cardiac function and concomitant therapies. The results of this large study showed that the long-acting candesartan reduces both cardiovascular mortality and hospitalization for heart failure, whatever the concomitant therapies, with the greatest benefits in ACE-intolerant patients. Of note, patients with preserved left-ventricular function did not gain significant further benefit from candesartan in this study. Moreover, no interaction was found in patients treated with a β-blocker. Another trial, the I-PRESERVE study, is currently ongoing. This trial is enrolling subjects with heart failure, left-ventricular ejection fraction >45%, and raised plasma brain natriuretic peptide. It will determine whether irbesartan is effective in decreasing mortality and decreasing cardiovascular hospitalization. Results are expected in mid-2006.

The use of angiotensin II receptor antagonists in managing patients with acute myocardial infarction has been studied in the OPTIMAAL and VALIANT trials.

The OPTIMAL trial hypothesized that the addition of losartan 50 mg daily to standard care would reduce mortality in patients with left-ventricular dysfunction following myocardial infarction compared with captopril three times 50 mg daily (14). Unfortunately, this study did not show any significant difference between the two treatment groups. But, as in the ELITE II trial, suboptimal dosing and relatively slow uptitration of losartan may have accounted for these apparently negative results.

The results of the second study, VALIANT, have recently been published (45). This study demonstrates that valsartan 160 mg bid is equally as effective as ACE inhibition with captopril 50 mg tid in reducing death and cardiovascular events in patients at high risk after acute myocardial infarction. A combination of both drugs did not improve survival over the effect of single-agent treatment, but it did increase the rate of adverse events in these patients. In addition, it also showed that in contrast to VALHeFT, there is no particular interaction in patients receiving a β-blocker (44).

Finally, angiotensin II receptor antagonists have also been evaluated in managing stroke survivors. Although mechanisms by which these drugs affect cardiovascular morbidity and mortality are still unclear, the phenomenal results of the ACCESS study represent a major breakthrough in the treatment of ischemic stroke, because they show that a modest blood pressure reduction by candesartan in the early moment of stroke (reduction by 10–15% of the blood pressure within 24 h during the first 7 days after stroke) significantly affects the cumulative 12 month mortality (odds ratio, 0.475; 95%; 0.252–0.985) (48).

Numerous experimental and small clinical studies have demonstrated that angiotensin II receptor antagonists have effects on kidney function similar to those of ACE inhibitors. They have no influence on glomerular filtration rate, but they increase renal blood flow, resulting in a decrease of filtration fraction (6). Because ACE inhibitors were known to have a favorable impact on long-term renal function in diabetic and nondiabetic proteinuric or microalbuminuric patients (2,24,37), the role of angiotensin II receptor antagonists has been the subject of several large clinical studies, particularly in type 2 diabetes. Recent trials with losartan (RENAAL), irbesartan (IRMA-2 and IDNT), and valsartan (MARVAL) have provided strong evidence that this drug class has renoprotective effects in patients with type 2 diabetes, macro- or micro-albuminuria, and varying levels of renal dysfunction. These favorable renal effects seemed to be, at least in part, independent of blood-pressure control (2,25,43,53).

IX. CONCLUSIONS

Angiotensin II receptor antagonists represent an effective new therapeutic approach to block the renin–angiotensin system and to lower blood pressure in hypertensive patients. Because of their high selectivity for the AT$_1$ receptor, angiotensin II receptor antagonists have an excellent tolerability profile, which in large placebo-controlled studies is comparable to placebo. Within a decade, several large clinical trials have demonstrated their usefulness in decreasing the cardiovascular morbidity of patients with essential hypertension, in reducing mortality and morbidity in patients suffering from congestive heart failure, and in retarding the progression of diabetic nephropathy in type 2 diabetes. Thus, because of their efficacy and tolerability profile, angiotensin II receptor antagonists could become the leading compounds for managing patients with cardiovascular and renal diseases.

REFERENCES

1. Azizi M, Chatellier G, Guyene TT, Murieta-Geoffroy D, Ménard J. Additive effects of combined angiotensin-converting enzyme inhibition and angiotensin II antagonism on blood pressure and renin release in sodium-depleted normotensives. Circulation 1995; 92:825–834.
2. Brenner BM, Cooper ME, de Zeeuw D, Keane WF, Mitch WE, Parving HH, Remuzzi G, Snapinn SM, Zhang Z, Shahinfar S. Effects of losartan on renal and cardiovascular outcomes in patients with type 2 diabetes and nephropathy. N Engl J Med 2001; 345:861–869.
3. Brunner HR. The new oral angiotensin II antagonist olmesartan medoxomil: a concise overview. J Hum Hypertens 2002; 16:S13–S16.
4. Burnier M, Brunner HR. Angiotensin II receptor antagonists. Lancet 2000; 355:637–645.
5. Burnier M, Roch-Ramel F, Brunner HR. Renal effects of angiotensin II receptor blockade in normotensive subjects. Kidney Int 1996; 49:1787–1790.
6. Burnier M, Rutschmann B, Nussberger J, Versaggi J, Shahinfar S, Waeber B, Brunner HR. Salt-dependent renal effects of an angiotensin II antagonist in healthy subjects. Hypertension 1993; 22:339–347.
7. Chiu AG, Krowiak EJ, Deeb ZE. Angioedema associated with angiotensin II receptor antagonists: challenging our knowledge of angioedema and its etiology. Laryngoscope 2001; 111:1729–1731.
8. Christen Y, Waeber B, Nussberger J, Porchet M, Borland RM, Lee RJ, Maggon K, Shum LY, Timmermans PB, Brunner HR. Oral administration of DuP 753, a specific angiotensin II receptor antagonist, to normal volunteers. Circ Res 1991; 83:1333–1342.
9. Chung O, Unger T. Pharmacology of angiotensin receptors and AT$_1$ receptor blockers. Basic Res Cardiol 1999; 93:15–23.
10. Cohn JN, Tognoni G. A randomized trial of the angiotensin-receptor blocker valsartan in chronic heart failure. N Engl J Med 2001; 345:1667–1675.
11. Conlin PR, Spence JD, Williams B, Ribeiro AB, Saito I, Benedict C, Bunt AMG. Angiotensin II antagonists for hypertension: are there differences in efficacy? Am J Hypertens 2000; 13:418–426.
12. Dahlöf B, Devereux RB, Kjeldsen SE, Julius S, Beevers G, Faire U, Fyhrquist F, Ibsen H, Kristiansson K, Lederballe-Pedersen O, Lindholm LH, Nieminen MS, Omvik P, Oparil S, Wedel H. Cardiovascular morbidity and mortality in the Losartan Intervention For Endpoint reduction in hypertension study (LIFE): a randomized trial against atenolol. Lancet 2002; 359:995–1003.
13. De Gasparo M, Siragy HM. The AT$_2$ receptor: fact, fancy, and fantasy. Regul Pept 1999; 81(1–3):11–24.
14. Dickstein K, Kjekshus J. Effects of losartan and captopril on mortality and morbidity in high-risk patients after acute myocardial infarction: the OPTIMAAL randomised trial. Optimal Trial in Myocardial Infarction with Angiotensin II Antagonist Losartan. Lancet 2002; 360:752–760.
15. Dominiczak A, Isles C, Gillen G, Brown JJ. Angiotensin converting enzyme inhibition and renal insufficiency in patients with bilateral renovascular disease. J Hum Hypertens 1988; 2:53–56.
16. Fierens FLP, Vanderheyden PML, de Backer JP, Vauquelin G. Insurmountable angiotensin AT$_1$ receptor antagonists: the role of tight antagonist binding. Eur J Pharmacol 1999; 372:199–206.
17. Forclaz A, Maillard M, Nussberger J, Brunner HR, Burnier M. Angiotensin II receptor blockade: is there truly a benefit of adding an ACE inhibitor? Hypertension 2003; 41:1–36.
18. Gillis JC, Markham A. Irbesartan: a review of its pharmacodynamic and pharmacokinetic properties and therapeutic use in the management of hypertension. Drugs 1997; 54:885–902.
19. Goa KL, Wagstaff AJ. Losartan potassium: a review of its pharmacology, clinical efficacy and tolerability in the management of hypertension. Drugs 1996; 51:820–845.
20. Hedner T. The clinical profile of the angiotensin II receptor blocker eprosartan. J Hypertens 2002; 20:S33–S38.
21. Innocenti AD, Elmfeldt D, Hansson L, Breteler M, James O, Lithell H, Olofsson B, Skoog I, Trenkwalder P, Zanchetti A, Wiklund I. Cognitive function and health-related quality of life in elderly patients with hypertension—baseline data from the study on cognition and prognosis in the elderly (SCOPE). Blood Press 2002; 11:157–163.
22. Julian BA, Brantley RR Jr, Barker CV, Stopka T, Gaston RS, Curtis JJ, Lee JY, Prchal JT. Losartan, an angiotensin II type 1 receptor antagonist, lowers hematocrit in

posttransplant erythrocytosis. J Am Soc Nephrol 1998; 9:1104–1108.

23. Julius S, Kjeldsen SE, Weber M, Brunner HR, Eckman S, Hansson L, Hua T, Laragh J, McInnes GT, Mitchell L, Plat F, Smith B, Zanchetti A. Value trial group. Outcomes in hypertensive patients at high cardiovascular risk treated with regimens based on valsartan or amlodipine: The VALUE randomised trial. Lancet 2004; 363:2022–2031.

24. Lewis EJ, Hunsicker LG, Bain RP, Rohde RD. The effect of angiotensin-converting-enzyme inhibition on diabetic nephropathy. The collaborative study group. N Engl J Med 1993; 329:1456–1462.

25. Lewis EJ, Hunsicker LG, Clarke WR, Berl T, Pohl MA, Lewis JB, Ritz E, Atkins RC, Rohde R, Raz I. Renoprotective effect of the angiotensin-receptor antagonist irbesartan in patients with nephropathy due to type 2 diabetes. N Engl J Med 2001; 345:851–860.

26. Lindholm LH, Ibsen H, Dahlof B, Devereux RB, Beevers G, de Faire U, Fyhrquist F, Julius S, Kjeldsen SE, Kristiansson K, Lederballe-Pedersen O, Nieminen M, Omvik P, Oparil S, Wedel H, Aurup P, Edelman J, Snapinn S, for the LIFE study group. Cardiovascular morbidity and mortality in patients with diabetes in the Losartan Intervention For Endpoint reduction in hypertension study (LIFE): a randomised trial against atenolol. Lancet 2002; 359:1004–1010.

27. Maillard M, Centeno C, Frostell-Karlsson A, Brunner HR, Burnier M. Does protein binding modulate the effect of angiotensin II receptor antagonists. JRAAS 2001; 2:S54–S58.

28. Maillard M, Mazzolai L, Daven C, Centeno C, Nussberger J, Brunner HR, Burnier M. Assessment of angiotensin II-receptor blockade in humans using a standardized angiotensin II-receptor binding assay. Am J Hypertens 1999; 12:1201–1208.

29. Maillard M, Perregaux C, Centeno C, Stangier J, Wienen W, Brunner HR, Burnier M. *In vitro* and *in vivo* characterization of telmisartan: an insurmountable angiotensin II receptor antagonist. J Pharmacol Exp Ther 2002b; 302:1089–1095.

30. Manolis AJ, Grossman E, Jelakovic B, Jacovides A, Bernhardi DC, Cabrera WJ, Watanabe LA, Barragan J, Matadamas N, Mendiola A, Woo KS, Zhu JR, Mejia AD, Bunt T, Dumortier T, Smith RD. Effects of losartan and candesartan monotherapy and losartan/hydro-chlorothiazide combination therapy in patients with mild to moderate hypertension. Losartan Trial Investigators. Clin Ther 2000; 22:1186–1203.

31. Markham A, Goa KL. Valsartan: a review of its pharmacology and therapeutic use in essential hypertension. Drugs 1997; 54:299–311.

32. Mazzolai L, Burnier M. Comparative safety and tolerability of angiotensin II receptor antagonists. Drug Safety 1999; 21:23–33.

33. Mazzolai L, Maillard M, Rossat J, Nussberger J, Brunner HR, Burnier M. Angiotensin II receptor blockade in normotensive subjects: a direct comparison of three AT_1 receptor antagonists. Hypertension 1999; 33:850–855.

34. McClellan KJ, Balfour JA. Eprosartan. Drugs 1998; 55:713–718.

35. McClellan KJ, Goa KL. Candesartan cilexetil: a review of its use in essential hypertension. Drugs 1998; 56:847–869.

36. McKelvie RS, Yusuf S, Pericak D, Avezum A, Burns RJ, Probstfield J, Tsuyuki RT, White M, Rouleau J, Latini R, Maggioni A, Young J, Pogue J. Comparison of candesartan, enalapril, and their combination in congestive heart failure: randomized evaluation of strategies for left ventricular dysfunction (RESOLVD) pilot study. The RESOLVD Pilot Study Investigators. Circulation 1999; 100:1056–1064.

37. McKenzie HS, Brenner BM. Current strategies for retarding the progression of renal disease. Am J Kidney Dis 1998; 31:161–170.

38. Mogensen CE, Neldam S, Tikkanen I, Oren S, Viskoper R, Watts RW, Cooper ME. Randomised controlled trial of dual blockade of renin–angiotensin system in patients with hypertension, microalbuminuria, and non-insulin dependent diabetes: the Candesartan and Lisinopril Microalbuminuria (CALM) study. Br Med J 2000; 321:1440–1444.

39. Mooser V, Nussberger J, Juillerat L, Burnier M, Waeber B, Bidiville J, Pauly N, Brunner HR. Reactive hyperreninemia is a major determinant of plasma angiotensin II during ACE inhibition. J Cardiovasc Pharmacol 1990; 15:276–282.

40. Morsing P, Adler G, Brandt-Eliasson U, Karp L, Ohlson K, Renberg L, Sjöquist P-O, Abrahamsson T. Mechanistic differences of various AT-1 receptor blockers in isolated vessels of different origin. Hypertension 1999; 33:1406–1413.

41. Nakao N, Yoshimura A, Morita H, Takada M, Kayano T, Ideura T. Combination treatment of angiotensin II receptor blocker and angiotensin-converting-enzyme inhibitor in non-diabetic renal disease (COOPERATE): a randomised controlled trial. Lancet 2003; 361:117–124.

42. Nussberger J, Cugno M, Amstutz C, Cicardi M, Pellacani A, Agostoni A. Plasma bradykinin in angioedema. Lancet 1998; 351:1693–1697.

43. Parving HH, Lehnert H, Brochner-Mortensen J, Gomis R, Andersen S, Arner P. The effect of irbesartan on the development of diabetic nephropathy in patients with type 2 diabetes. N Engl J Med 2001; 345:870–878.

44. Pfeffer MA, Swedberg K, Granger CB, Held P, McMurray JJV, Michelson EL, Olofsson B, Ostergren J, Yusuf S. Effects of candesartan on mortality and morbidity in patients with chronic heart failure: the CHARM-Overall programme. Lancet 2003a; 362:759–766.

45. Pfeffer MA, McMurray JJ, Velazquez EJ, Rouleau JL, Kober L, Maggioni AP, Solomon SD, Swedberg K, Van de Werf F, White H, Leimberger JD, Henis M, Edwards S, Zelenkofske S, Sellers MA, Califf RM. Valsartan in Acute Myocardial Infarction Trial Investigators. Valsartan, captopril, or both in myocardial infarction complicated by heart failure, left ventricular dysfunction, or both. N Engl J Med 2003b; 349:1893–1906.

46. Pitt B, Segal R, Martinez FA, Meurers G, Cowley AJ, Thomas I, Deedwania PC, Ney DE, Snavely DB, Chang PI. Randomised trial of losartan versus captopril in patients over 65 with heart failure (Evaluation of Losartan In The Elderly study, ELITE). Lancet 1997; 349:747–752.

47. Pitt B, Poole-Wilson PA, Segal R, Martinez FA, Dickstein K, Camm AJ, Konstam MA, Riegger G, Klinger GH, Neaton J, Sharma D, Thiyagarajan B. Effect of losartan compared with captopril on mortality in patients with symptomatic heart failure: randomised trial—the Losartan Heart Failure Survival Study ELITE II. Lancet 2000; 355:1582–1587.

48. Schrader J, Lüders S, Kulschewski A, Berger J, Zidek W, Treib J, Einnhäupl K, Diener HC, Dominiak P. On behalf of the ACCESS Study Group. The ACCESS Study: evaluation of acute candesartan cilexetil therapy in stroke survivors. Stroke 2003; 34:1699–1703.

49. Schwarzberg A, Wittenmeier KW, Hallfritzsch U. Anemia in dialysis patients as a side-effects of sartans. Lancet 1998; 352:286.

50. Sharpe M, Jarvis B, Goa KL. Telmisartan: a review of its use in hypertension. Drugs 2001; 61:1501–1529.

51. The SOLVD investigators. Effects of enalapril on survival in patients with reduced left ventricular ejection fractions and congestive heart failure. N Engl J Med 1991; 325:293–302.

52. Timmermans PB, Wong PC, Chiu AT, Herblin WF, Benfield P, Carini DJ, Lee RJ, Wexler RR, Saye JA, Smith RD. Angiotensin II receptors and angiotensin II receptor antagonists. Pharmacol Rev 1993; 45:205–251.

53. Viberti G, Wheeldon NM. Microalbuminuria reduction with valsartan in patients with type 2 diabetes mellitus: a blood pressure-independent effect. Circulation 2002; 106:672–678.

54. Vidt DG, White WB, Ridley E, Rahman M, Harris S, Vendetti J, Michelson EL, Wang R. A forced titration study of antihypertensive efficacy of candesartan cilexetil in comparison to losartan: CLAIM Study II. J Hum Hypertens 2001; 15:475–480.

55. Warner GT, Jarvis B. Olmesartan medoxomil. Drugs 2002; 62:1345–1353.

56. Wienen W, Hauel N, Busch U, Ebner T. Characterization of the PK/PD profile of BIBR-277 1-O-acylglucuronide, the metabolite of telmisartan [abstr]. J Hum Hypertens 1999; 13:S11.

57. Wuerzner G, Gerster JC, Chioléro A, Maillard M, FalLab-Stubi CL, Brunner HR, Burnier M. Comparative effects of losartan and irbesartan on serum uric acid in hypertensive patients with hyperuricemia and gout. J Hypertens 2001; 19:1855–1860.

58. Yusuf S. From the HOPE Study to ONTARGET and the TRANSCEND studies: challenges in improving prognosis. Am J Cardiol 2002; 89:18A–26A.

31

Calcium Antagonists

DONNA S. HANES, MATTHEW R. WEIR
University of Maryland Medical System, Baltimore, Maryland, USA

KEYPOINTS

- Calcium antagonists dilate arterioles and thus reduce peripheral resistance.
- Calcium antagonists reduce cardiovascular morbidity and mortality.
- Calcium antagonists are metabolically neutral.

SUMMARY

Calcium antagonists are primarily arteriolar vasodilators that reduce peripheral resistance. They are safe and effective antihypertensive drugs in their recommended dosage range and have been shown to reduce cardiovascular morbidity and mortality. The antihypertensive properties of calcium antagonists are dependable in a variety of patients regardless of race, age, gender, salt-intake, or the use of concomitant drugs (such as NSAIDS). Calcium antagonists can be used safely in combination with other antihypertensive drugs and have uniquely neutral metabolic interactions. Calcium antagonists help delay the progression of renal disease when used in combination with drugs that block the renin–angiotensin system.

I. INTRODUCTION

Over the past 30 years, calcium antagonists have emerged as an essential therapeutic class of medications for a wide variety of cardiovascular indications. Initially, in 1962, they were observed to significantly lower blood pressure and improve renal blood flow; subsequently, in the 1970s, they were introduced as antianginal agents. But it was not until the 1980s that the administration of calcium antagonists for the long-term treatment of hypertension became widespread. Multiple clinical trials have convincingly demonstrated the efficacy and safety of calcium antagonists and have lead to widespread recommendations that they be used as "first-line" monotherapy for hypertension (1,2). In general, calcium antagonists are potent antihypertensive drugs that are particularly effective in the elderly, in African-Americans, and in patients with low renin hypertension. Recently, interest has focused on the protective effects of calcium antagonists on target organs, both independent of and in addition to their ability to lower blood pressure; these other protective effects include antioxidant activity, potentiation of nitric oxide, and their ability to reduce atherosclerosis.

II. MECHANISM OF ACTION

The pharmacologic and clinical effects of calcium antagonists are related to their ability to attenuate calcium transport in a variety of tissues. Cells normally maintain a low resting intracellular concentration of ionized calcium in the setting of a large, inwardly directed extracellular calcium concentration. Upon entering the cell, calcium binds to calcium-binding proteins, including calmodulin, which causes stimulation of a number of second messenger systems within the cell. Calcium entry is then coupled to cellular responses in physiologic and pathologic states. Excessive calcium influx after cell injury is toxic and may lead to irreversible cell death (3). Control of calcium mobilization by pharmacologic agents provides a therapeutic means to manipulate cellular communication and regulatory functions and prevent cellular injury.

Calcium antagonists inhibit the entry of calcium into the cytosolic space from both extracellular and intracellular stores. They do not antagonize the effects of calcium directly.

Among the various calcium channels that have been described, the L-type calcium channels dominate the majority of functions in the cardiovascular system. This voltage-gated channel is a multimeric complex with binding sites for both activators and antagonists. Despite the ubiquitous distribution of voltage-gated calcium channels, calcium antagonists are highly selective for the cardiovascular system. Each class of calcium antagonist is quantitatively and qualitatively unique, possessing differential sensitivity and selectivity for binding pharmacologic receptors in various vascular beds. Nondihydropyridines typically exhibit significant cardiac depressant activities, whereas the dihydropyridines are vasodilators. Even among subclasses, minor structural changes impart considerable pharmacologic variability and specificity for the vascular system. For example, lacidipine has a 60-fold greater vascular selectivity than nitrendipine (4). This differential selectivity of action has important clinical implications for the use of these drugs. It explains why the different calcium antagonists vary considerably in their

effects on regional circulatory beds, sinus and atrioventricular nodal function, and myocardial contractility, as well as in the diversity of clinical indications and side effects.

III. PHARMACOLOGY

Despite their shared mechanism of action, the calcium antagonists represent a very heterogeneous group of compounds and cannot be used interchangeably. As stated previously, they differ with respect to their receptor binding, chemical structure, and pharmacokinetic profiles. Two primary categories are distinguished on the basis of their behavior: 1,4-dihydropyridines and nondihydropyridines. The nondihydropyridines are further divided into the papaverine-like diphenylalkylamines (verapamil) and the benzothiazepines (diltiazem). All calcium antagonists vasodilate coronary and peripheral arteries (Table 31.1).

The dihydropyridines, a membrane-active group, exert their most potent effects on the peripheral vessels, with very little effect on myocardial cells, which depend less heavily on external calcium influx. This vasodilatory action stimulates baroreceptor reflexes, eliciting a prompt compensatory increase in sympathetic nervous activity and activation of the renin–angiotensin system. This positive inotropic stimulus appears to be important for the first-generation, short-acting dihydropyridines (nifedipine), but clinically unimportant for the long-acting drugs (5). This is an important distinction because short-acting drugs are no longer recommended for the treatment of hypertension and may predispose patients to

Table 31.1   Hemodynamic Effects of Calcium Antagonists

	Calcium antagonist		
	Dihydropyridines	Diltiazem	Verapamil
Arteriolar dilation	↑↑↑	↑↑	↑↑
Coronary dilation	↑↑↑	↑↑↑	↑↑
Cardiac afterload	↓↓	↓	↓
Cardiac contractility	↔	↓	↓↓
Myocardial oxygen demand	↓	↓	↓
Cardiac output	↑ ↔	↔	↔
Avioventricular conduction	↔	↓	↓↓
Sinoatrial automaticity	↔	↓↓	↓
Heart rate			
Acute	↑	↓	↓
Chronic	↑	↓ ↔	↓ ↔
Activation of baroreceptor reflexes	↑ ↔	↔	↔

stroke, angina, and myocardial infarction as a result of their rapid blood pressure lowering effects (6).

Second-generation and third-generation drugs have been modified so that they have a slower onset of action and longer half-lives and only require once daily dosing. They have no significant effect on cardiac output except in patients with severely impaired systolic ventricular function (Table 31.1). In fact, because of the increased vasoselectivity, these drugs have lesser effects on cardiac rate, contractility, and sympathetic activity. Third-generation dihydropyridines have been found to improve the exercise capacity in patients with mild to moderate heart failure (7).

Conversely, the nondihydropyridines have only moderate arterial vasodilatory effects, but they have significantly slow atrioventricular nodal conduction and possess negative inotropic and chronotropic effects (Table 31.1). Because of their negative inotropic action, they are more useful for inhibiting stress-induced cardiovascular responses and tachyarrhythmias, but they are contraindicated in patients with systolic heart failure.

IV. ANTIHYPERTENSIVE MODE OF ACTION

Calcium antagonists have attracted a great deal of interest as antihypertensive agents because they reduce peripheral vascular resistance uniformly. They have reliable clinical effects in patients regardless of race, age, gender, or co-morbid conditions. They reduce blood pressure through inhibition of calcium influx into the cell through the L-type calcium channel. In hypertensive patients, there is an abnormal influx of calcium into the cytosol, where it binds with calmodulin. This initiates a sequence of cellular events that promotes the interaction between actin and myosin, which results in smooth muscle contraction. Therefore, blockade of the channel interferes with contraction and basal vascular tone.

There are several other properties of calcium antagonists that facilitate blood pressure reduction (8). First, there is considerable evidence that calcium antagonists interfere with α_2 (and possibly α_1) adrenergic receptor-mediated vasoconstriction. They also dampen the vascular responses to angiotensin II and reduce the synthesis of aldosterone. Interestingly, patients with low renin and angiotensin II activity exhibit the greatest vasodilatory responses to calcium antagonists, which suggests a more important role for calcium-mediated vasoconstriction in these patients. Alternatively, amlodipine and others may partially inhibit local angiotensin-converting enzyme (ACE) activity that results in increased activity of the vasodilatory kinins and nitric oxide (9). An equally important property of calcium antagonists is that they facilitate natriuresis by several mechanisms. They cause increases in atrial natriuretic peptide, and the dihydropyridines, in particular, cause preferential dilation of the afferent arteriole, resulting in

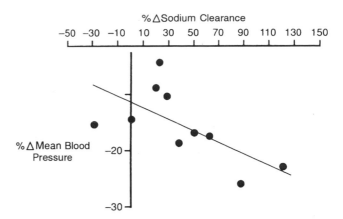

Figure 31.1 Relationship between change in the mean arterial pressure to the percent change in sodium clearance induced by calcium antagonists.

reduced tubular sodium re-absorption and improved renal blood flow (10). The sodium excretion rate has been shown to correlate with blood pressure reduction (Fig. 31.1) (11).

V. PHARMACOKINETICS AND UNIQUE PROPERTIES

Despite the wide range of pharmacodynamic effects, the original calcium antagonists have remarkably similar pharmacokinetic profiles (Table 31.2).

Overall, the drugs are well absorbed, but they undergo extensive first-pass hepatic metabolism and biotransformation. With the exception of diltiazem, verapamil, and possibly nifedipine, the metabolites are inactive. Dose adjustments are necessary in hepatic failure, but not with renal disease. Many studies have demonstrated a consistent–concentration effect relationship of the calcium antagonist, which allows prediction of the long-term effectiveness of the therapy from the first dose response. The recommended daily doses are outlined in Table 31.3.

The most important goal of hypertension treatment is to reduce total peripheral resistance without interfering with cardiac output. Patients with hypertension frequently have normal or slightly reduced cardiac output and blunted baroreceptor-mediated responses to exercise as a result of inadequate compensatory increases in stroke volume. Many patients, particularly those with isolated systolic hypertension, also have reduced arterial compliance that contributes to the increased blood pressure, and these patients may be susceptible to exaggerated hemodynamic fluctuations with antihypertensive therapy. Similarly, older patients frequently lack the appropriate compensatory sympathetic vasoconstrictor responses and may experience more acute drops in blood pressure. Therefore, the best approach to management of these patients is to begin with a low dose of calcium antagonist and titrate the dose as needed over several weeks.

Table 31.2 Pharmacokinetic Properties of Calcium Antagonists

Drug	Oral absorption (%)	First-pass effect	Bioavailability (%)	Peak blood level (hours except as noted)	Elimination half-life (h)	Metabolism excretion	Protein binding (%)	Active metabolites
Diltiazem	98	50%	40	2–3	4–6	Liver/feces and urine	77–93	Yes
Diltiazem SR	>80	50%	35	6–11	5–7	Liver/feces and urine	77–93	Yes
Diltiazem CD	95	Extensive	35	10–14	5–8	Liver/feces and urine	77–93	Yes
Diltiazem XR	95	Extensive	41	4–6	5–10	Liver/feces and urine	95	Yes
Diltiazem ER	93	Extensive	40–60	4–6	10	Liver/feces and urine	95	Yes
Amlodipine	>90	Minimal	88	6–12	30–50	Liver/urine	>95	Yes
Felodipine	>90	Extensive	13–18	2.5–5	11–16	Liver/urine	>95	No
Isradipine	>90	Extensive	15–25	1–2	8	Liver/feces and urine	>95	No
Isradipine CR	>90	Extensive	15–25	7–18	—	Liver/feces and urine	>95	No
Nicardipine	>90	Extensive	35	0.5–2	8.6	Liver/feces and urine	>95	No
Nicardipine SR	>90	Extensive	30	1–4	—	Liver/feces and urine	>95	No
Nifedipine	>90	20–30%	60	<30 min	2	Liver/urine	98	Yes
Nifedepine GITS	>90	25–35%	86	6	—	Liver/urine	98	Yes
Nifedipine ER	>90	25–35%	89	2.5–5; 6–12	7	Liver/urine	98	Yes
Nisoldipine	>85	Extensive	4–8	6–12	10–22	Liver/feces and urine	98	No
Verapamil	>90	70–80%	20–35	1–2	2.8–7.4	Liver/feces and urine	99	Yes
Verapamil SR	>90	70–80%	20–35	5–6	4–12	Liver/feces and urine	85–95	Yes
Verapamil SR pellet	>90	70–80%	20–35	7–9	12	Liver/feces and urine	85–95	Yes
Verapamil COER-24/CODAS	>90	70–80%	20–35	11	—	Liver/feces and urine	85–95	Yes

Note: SR, sustained release; CD, controlled-diffusion; XR and ER, extended release; GITS, gastrointestinal therapeutic system; COER, controlled-onset extended release.

Table 31.3 Pharmacodynamic Properties of Calcium Antagonists

Drug generic name (trade name)	First dose (mg)	Usual daily dose (mg)	Maximum daily dose (mg)	Maximal hypotensive response (h)	Duration of hypotensive response (h)
Diltiazem (Cardizem)	60	60–120 tid/qid	480	2.5–4	8
Diltiazem SR (Cardizem SR)	180	120–240 bid	480	6	12
Diltiazem CD (Cardizem CD)	180	240–280 qd	480	—	24
Diltiazem XR (Dilacor XR)	180	180–480 qd	480	3–6	24
Diltiazem ER (Tiazac)	180	180–480 qd	480	6–10	24
Amlodipine (Norvasc)	5	5–10 qd	10	—	24
Felodipine (Plendil ER)	5	5–10 qd	20	2.5	24
Isradipine (DynaCirc)	2.5	2.5–5 bid	20	2–3	12
Isradipine CR (DynaCirc CR)	5	5–20 qid	20	2	7–18
Nicardipine (Cardene)	20	20–40 tid	120	1–2	8
Nicardipine SR (Cardene SR)	30	30–60 bid	120	2–6	12
Nifedipine (Procardia, Adalat)	10	10–30 tid/qid	6,120	0.5–1	12
Nifedipine GITS (Procardia XL)	30	30–90 qd	120	4–6	24
Nifedipine ER (Adalat CC)	30	30–90 qd	120	2–4	24
Nisoldipine (Sular)	20	20–40 qd	60	—	24
Verapamil (Calan, Isoptin)	80	80–120 tid	480	6–8	8
Verapamil SR (Calan SR, Isoptin SR)	90	90–240 bid	480	—	12–24
Verapamil SR pellet (Veralan)	120	240–480 qd	480	—	24
Verapamil COER-24 (Covera-HS)	180	180–480 qHS	480	>4–5	24
Mibefradil (Posicor)	50	50–100 qd	100	2–4	17–25

Note: SR, sustained release; CD, controlled-diffusion; XR and ER, extended release; GITS, gastrointestinal therapeutic system; COER, controlled-onset extended release.

VI. CLASSIFICATION

With the development of novel formulations and newer drugs, the most practical clinical approach is to divide drugs into classes according to their onset and offset of action (Table 31.4). With this method, the first-generation calcium antagonists consist of immediate-release nifedipine, verapamil, and diltiazem. The second-generation compounds were modified to improve the pharmacokinetic profile and improve vascular selectivity and are subdivided into slow-release formulations or novel agents. The third-generation compounds, typified by amlodipine, possess increased lipophilicity and a much longer onset and duration of action, providing more consistent peak-to-trough levels and steadier blood pressure control.

A. First-Generation Drugs

Diltiazem hydrochloride is almost completely absorbed following oral administration, but due to extensive first pass metabolism, the bioavailability is only 40%.

Table 31.4 Clinical Pharmacologic Classification of Calcium Antagonists

Group (tissue selectivity)	First generation	Second generation Novel formulations (IIa)	Second generation New chemical entities (IIb)	Third generation
Dihydropyridine	Nifedipine Nicardipine Nicardipine	Nifedipine SR/GITS Felodipine ER Nicardipine SR	Isradipine Manidipine Nimoldipine Nisolidpine Nitrendipine	Amlodipine Lacidipine Lercanidipine
Benzothiazepine	Diltiazem	Diltiazem SR		
Phenylalkylamine	Verapamil	Verapamil SR		

Note: ER, extended release; SR, sustained release; GITS, gastrointestinal therapeutic system.

Diltiazem is metabolized in the liver into metabolites that possess only 25–50% of the original biologic activity. This pathway is responsible for metabolism of numerous other drugs, accounting for the substantial number of interactions that occur with diltiazem. Diltiazem is highly protein bound and widely distributed. Renal excretion accounts for 35%, with the remainder eliminated in the feces. Rates of elimination are slower with repeated oral dosing in the elderly and in patients with liver disease and are unaffected by renal function. Newer formulations include tablets, sustained-release (SR) capsules, controlled-diffusion (CD) capsules, and Geo-matrix extended release capsules. Buccoadhesive formulations that bypass the effects of hepatic metabolism are under investigation. The usual daily doses are outlined in Table 31.3. Peak responses occur in 4–6 h, and the half-life averages 10 h.

Verapamil hydrochloride is also well absorbed (>90%) from the gastrointestinal tract but undergoes extensive first-pass metabolism, resulting in only 10–30% bioavailability. Consequently, there is significant variation in plasma levels between patients from dose to dose. Verapamil consists of a racemic mixture of the two optically active isomers, D and L, which have different pharmacologic properties and, therefore, contribute to further variability. Verapamil is metabolized in the liver into 13 known metabolites. Of these, norverapamil is the only one with cardiovascular activity, and it has ∼20% of the potency of the parent compound.

The bioavailability increases from twofold to threefold with chronic administration, relative to single-dose administration, as a result of saturated hepatic elimination pathways. This prolongs the half-life from 4–5 h with a single dose to 8–12 h with chronic administration. The onset of action is achieved in 6–8 h, and the maximal therapeutic effect occurs in 1–4 weeks.

Sustained release caplets have an onset of action of 5–6 h, but this is delayed by concurrent food ingestion. The usual daily dose is equal to that of the immediate release preparation, but twice-daily dosing improves the antihypertensive effect of this formulation. The sustained-release, pellet-filled verapamil capsules are gel-coated, which renders the medication immune to the effects of food on absorption. The onset of action is 7–9 h, and the peak concentration is ∼65% that of the immediate-release tablet, but with 30% higher trough concentrations. The controlled-onset, extended release (COER) and chronotherapeutic oral drug absorption system (CODAS) formulations are uniquely designed to deliver verapamil 4–5 h after ingestion, making it ideal for nighttime dosing. Blood levels are low during the nighttime hours (minimizing diurnal blood pressure variations), but they increase during the early morning from 6:00 a.m. to 12:00 noon and remain sustained through the course of the day.

Nifedipine is the prototype dihydropyridine calcium antagonist that causes reduced peripheral resistance with no significant depression of atrioventricular conduction, sinus node recovery, or sinus rate. Administration of the immediate-release preparation results in vasodilation, with a reflex increase in sympathetic tone that prompts slight increases in cardiac index and heart rate. In general, it causes a modest antihypertensive effect that is well tolerated. However, in the elderly and others, the effect is profound and has been associated with a threefold increase in mortality from myocardial infarction, stroke, and death when compared with other antihypertensive drugs, including other calcium antagonists. Therefore, the immediate release form should be used only for short periods, if at all, and certainly not in the setting of acute coronary syndromes. There is no clinical advantage to the bite-and-swallow route or sublingual route of administration.

Nifedipine is rapidly absorbed with a 60% bioavailability and can be detected in the serum within 10 min. Peak drug levels are achieved within 30 min, with a half-life of 2 h. Nifedipine is extensively metabolized in the liver into at least two inactive metabolites that are excreted into the urine. Doses should be adjusted in patients with liver disease.

Several creative modifications to the delivery vehicle allow a more extended release and sustained absorption of nifedipine. The gastrointestinal therapeutic system formulation consists of an inner, active drug core that is surrounded by an osmotically active inert layer; this outer layer swells within the gastrointestinal tract and dissolves the inner core. The drug is then slowly released over 16–18 h. Peak concentration is reached in 6 h and remains steady for 24 h, with a bioavailability of 86%. Dosage conversion from the immediate-release form is done on an equi-milligram basis. The gastrointestinal therapeutic system tablet should not be divided or crushed.

The core-coat form of nifedipine is composed of an outer layer that contains slow-release nifedipine, surrounding an inner layer of immediate release drug. The peak serum concentrations occur within 3–5 h, followed by a second peak 6–12 h later when the inner core is exposed. However, the peak serum level may be variable and unreliable. Ingestion of three 30 mg tablets results in a 29% higher peak plasma concentration when compared with the 90 mg tablet. Therefore, substitution of 30 mg for 90 mg tablets is not recommended. The bioavailability of the core-coat form is 89%, and its half-life is prolonged to 7 h.

B. Second-Generation Drugs

Felodipine is a dihydropyridine calcium antagonist that is almost completely absorbed from the gastrointestinal tract.

Because of extensive first-pass hepatic metabolism, the bioavailability is only ~18%, but it increases to 50% with concomitant ingestion of grapefruit juice or large meals. The elimination half-life of felodipine extended release (ER) is 11–16 h and is triphasic. Felodipine is solubilized into a matrix-embedded tablet, with a release rate that is determined by the amount of gel coat swelling generated by contact with gastrointestinal secretions. Felodipine is metabolized into inactive metabolites that are excreted primarily in the urine. The peak clinical response occurs within four weeks, and doses can be titrated at 2 week intervals. Felodipine has a higher affinity for peripheral vascular smooth muscle cells than for cardiac tissue, which results in reduced peripheral vascular resistance.

Isradipine is a dihydropyridine calcium antagonist that has a high affinity for the peripheral vessels, lowering peripheral vascular resistance by 37% and increasing arterial compliance. *In vitro* studies show SA node depression. The clinical effect appears to be insignificant. Isradipine is rapidly and almost completely absorbed following oral administration, with a bioavailability of 25%. Isradipine drug delivery is formulated upon the gastrointestinal therapeutic system principle. The peak anti hypertensive activity can be seen as early as 2–3 h after ingestion, but the full clinical response may take up to 2 weeks. The terminal half-life of isradipine is 8 h, and the metabolites are inactive.

Manidipine is a dihydropyridine that structurally resembles nifedipine. Up to 60% is absorbed after oral administration. Manidipine undergoes extensive hepatic metabolism into metabolites that are excreted primarily in the feces. The elimination half-life is 5–8 h. Doses should be adjusted at 2 week intervals for maximum clinical effect.

Nicardipine is a dihydropyridine calcium antagonist that is well absorbed, with 35% systemic bioavailability. The long-acting sustained-release form activates in 1–4 h, with a half-life of 8.6 h. Nicardipine also selectively inhibits vascular smooth muscle contraction and can elicit a compensatory increase in heart rate that usually disappears after several weeks of therapy.

Nisoldipine is available in a core-coat formulation that allows drug delivery in variable amounts throughout the gastrointestinal tract. Eighty percent of the dose is contained in the outer layer, and is absorbed slowly in the stomach and upper intestine. In the lower intestine, where, in general, absorption is slow, the remaining 20% of the drug is released rapidly. This core-coat formulation results in a true once-daily dosing with continuous 24 h drug delivery. The pharmacokinetic profile is variable because of fluctuations in hepatic blood flow. The drug is metabolized in the liver and small intestine into primarily inactive metabolites. The elimination half-life is 10–22 h. Recently available in the United States,

nisoldipine has demonstrated efficacy comparable to the third-generation drug, amlodipine (12).

C. Third-Generation Drugs

Newer dihydropyridine medications with intrinsically longer half-lives do not require unique delivery systems for maximum drug effect. They offer a more sustained onset of action and fewer peak-trough variations in blood levels and therapeutic response, and they may enhance compliance. In addition, because of the long half-lives of these drugs, the therapeutic effects persist for several days, even if a patient misses a dose.

Amlodipine possesses a distinctly unique pharmacologic profile when compared with other dihydropyridines. Absorption is slower and more complete after oral administration. It does not undergo significant first-pass metabolism, which results in a bioavailability of up to 88%. The peak plasma concentrations occur 6 h after dosing and reach their maximal effect after 7 days. The serum levels are linear with increasing doses and do not appear to be affected by the age of the patient. Amlodipine is metabolized extensively in the liver into inactive fragments. The elimination half-life is 30–50 h, which provides a clinical therapeutic response for several days beyond the last dose that was administered. Amlodipine also is unique among the dihydropyridines in that it appears also to bind to nondihydropyridine calcium channels, which results in peripheral arterial vasodilation without the compensatory activation of the sympathetic nervous system (8).

Recently, significant interest has focused on ancillary properties of amlodipine that are attributable to the effects on nondihydropyridine binding sites. Amlodipine has been demonstrated to depress smooth muscle cell proliferation and matrix formation modulate nitric oxide production. It also improves arterial compliance when it is combined with HMGCoA reductase inhibitors (13). In addition, amlodipine shows antioxidant activity *in vivo*, reduces LDL cholesterol uptake by the vessel wall, and can cause a dose-dependent regression of atherosclerotic lesion formation in the aorta, possibly by inhibiting monocyte-endothelial adhesion (14).

Lacidipine is an unusually potent dihydropyridine calcium antagonist, with a great degree of vascular selectivity. Lacidipine has an intrinsically slow onset of action, resulting in no significant reflex tachycardia. It has a long duration of action, in part due to unique membrane binding properties and greater diffusion into lipid bilayers. Lacidipine is absorbed rapidly after oral administration. However, it undergoes extensive first-pass metabolism and has a bioavailability of only 2–9%. The duration of action is 12–24 h, with an elimination half-life ranging of 3–19 h. Hepatic metabolism into inactive compounds is complete. Although lacidipine is not currently available in the United States, it is attractive as an antihypertensive drug because it is as effective as other drugs and causes less peripheral edema. In addition to its increasing vasodilation of peripheral vascular beds, lacidipine has greater antioxidant activity in comparison with other dihydropyridines, and it has been shown in clinical trials to significantly reduce atherosclerotic disease progression and plaque formation when compared with the effects of β-blockers (15).

Lercandipine is similar to lacidipine, but it demonstrates an even greater solubility within the arterial cellular membrane, which results in a 10-fold increase in vasoselectivity when compared with amlodipine. After oral administration, the time to peak dose is 2–3 h, and bioavailability is limited by extensive first-pass hepatic metabolism. The terminal half-life of lercandipine is only 8–10 h, although there is a long-lasting effect at the receptor level and membrane level that corresponds to extended clinical effects. It causes less peripheral edema and flushing than other third-generation calcium antagonists and has no cardiodepressant or reflex stimulatory properties (16). Dosage reductions in cases of severe hepatic and renal impairment are necessary to prevent drug accumulation.

Although lercandipine is not widely available in the United States, it is an important therapeutic agent in much of Europe, Asia, South America, and Australia. It has considerable efficacy in the management of hypertension and may be particularly effective in severe or resistant hypertension. Like other third-generation calcium antagonists, lercandipine possesses antiatherogenic activity that is independent of its blood pressure-lowering effect. In both diabetic and nondiabetic patients, lercandipine reduces LDL oxidation and promotes vascular protection.

In animal models, lercandipine also has been reported to dilate the efferent renal arteriole in contrast to other drugs in this class, which results in a 10% increase in creatinine clearance (17). The clinical consequences of these findings are currently under investigation.

VII. CARDIOVASCULAR EFFECTS OF CALCIUM ANTAGONISTS

The widespread availability of calcium channel antagonists has been an important advance for a variety of cardiovascular disorders. They are now indicated for first-line treatment of arterial hypertension and ischemic heart disease and for the treatment and prevention of supraventricular arrhythmias. They are beneficial as second-line therapy in hypertrophic cardiomyopathy, primary pulmonary hypertension, migraine, and other vasculospastic disorders.

A. Hemodynamic Effects

Most patients with primary hypertension have an increased peripheral vascular resistance. This is in large part due to an abnormal influx of calcium into the cytosol. This influx is blunted by calcium antagonists. The result is a reduction in peripheral vascular resistance and a lowering of systemic blood pressure. Thus, the primary hemodynamic effect is vasodilation. Interestingly, calcium antagonists are the most potent in constricted vascular beds, and the greatest vasodepressor responses occur in patients with the highest pretreatment blood pressures. There is little, if any, change observed in normotensive patients. Calcium antagonists preferentially dilate the arterial vasculature over the venous system. This may contribute to fewer orthostatic responses in comparison to the effects of conventional vasodilators, but it also may contribute to the development of peripheral edema. Multiple studies have demonstrated that total peripheral vascular resistance and regional vascular resistance are reduced in the short term and with chronic therapy. There is no significant affect on cardiac function unless the patient has an ejection fraction <30%. In these patients, the dihydropyridines (particularly amlodipine and felodipine) are the least likely to depress cardiac output and are safe. To variable degrees, all of the drugs dilate coronary arteries and improve cardiac perfusion (Table 31.1). They are effective for the treatment of hypertension-induced diastolic dysfunction, and because they act as coronary vasodilators and reduce afterload, the negative inotrophic effects (of verapamil and diltiazem) are rarely of clinical consequence.

The effects on heart rate vary but are clinically negligible. Diltiazem reduces sinoatrial node conduction and has more potent effects on the atrioventricular node. This makes it, along with verapamil, very useful for the treatment of supraventricular arrhythmias. Conversely, dihydropyridines may acutely induce a reflex increase in heart rate, which normalizes with long-term therapy. Although higher doses may be expected to increase the pulse rate, the doses commonly recommended for the treatment of hypertension have no effect on heart rate. A few patients may experience a 10% heart rate reduction with the nondihydropyridines, but this effect is only one-half to one-third the effect observed in treatment with β-blocker therapy. In addition, calcium antagonists do not interfere with exercise performance, and they do not inhibit stress-related increases in blood pressure.

B. Renal Effects

The beneficial effects of calcium antagonist therapy in hypertensive patients with renal disease is well described. Calcium antagonists exert natriuretic effects that can facilitate antihypertensive activity and protect existing renal function, probably by direct inhibition of sodium reabsorption at the distal tubule sodium channels, by inhibition of aldosterone synthesis, and by augmentation of atrial natriuretic peptide action (8). In hypertensive patients, calcium antagonists acutely increase sodium excretion onefold to threefold, often unrelated to any reduction in blood pressure. Natriuresis occurs after the first 6 h of dosing, then plateaus after 2–3 days and persists for the duration of therapy. Although there are no significant changes in body weight, the effects of natriuresis are most pronounced on a high-salt diet and are reversible after cessation of calcium antagonist treatment. In general, calcium antagonists increase glomerular filtration rate by preferentially dilating the afferent renal arteriole. Chronic administration causes no significant change in glomerular filtration rate, and calcium antagonists may help slow progression of chronic kidney disease when they are used in conjunction with drugs that block the renin–angiotensin system, in large part due to better blood pressure reduction (18). However, when calcium antagonists are used without a renin–angiotensin system blocker, they may increase glomerular hyperfiltration and are not as renoprotective as ACE inhibitors or angiotensin II receptor blockers (19).

There is clinical evidence that nondihydropyridines, such as diltiazem and verapamil, can reduce proteinuria when they are used as monotherapy (20,21). This is a unique effect that is not seen with dihydropyridines unless there is a substantial reduction in blood pressure. The mechanism of this differential effect is not known for certain, but it may reflect an alteration in glomerular basement membrane permselectivity to proteins (20,22). The clinical significance of this difference is unknown because most patients will already be treated with an ACE inhibitor or an angiotensin receptor blocker.

C. Clinical Use

All calcium antagonists have been shown to be equally efficacious in reducing systolic and diastolic blood pressure. Overall response rates for monotherapy are ~50% in all patients, but the response rates approach 85% in patients with mild to moderate hypertension alone. However, the initial calcium antagonist that is selected for a particular patient should take into account concomitant conditions (Table 31.1) and, where possible, be selected from the longer-acting preparations to facilitate more reliable blood pressure control and compliance. Initial doses should be started at the lowest recommended range and then titrated upward over 1–2 weeks as needed. The higher the patient's initial blood pressure, the more effective the therapy will be. It was thought initially that the dosages required to achieve satisfactory blood pressure reduction were lower than those required to control

angina, but clinical experience and more recent trials do not support this theory. Dosages do not need to be adjusted for high dietary salt intake. Sustained systolic and diastolic blood pressure reductions of 16–28 and 14–17 mmHg, respectively, can be expected, particularly with the dihydropyridines. There is a moderately steep dose-response relationship. The development of tolerance to the clinical effects has not been reported.

Several factors may help predict the response to calcium antagonists. The drugs have been demonstrated to be effective in young, middle aged, and elderly patients, with blood pressure levels that range from white coat and mild hypertension to severe hypertension. Moreover, calcium antagonists tend to be more effective than β-blockers and ACE inhibitors in older patients, particularly at preventing strokes. The response may be inversely related to plasma renin, comparable to diuretic responses. Specifically, they normalize blood pressure in ~20% of patients under the age of 40 or with high renin, compared with 80% of patients over the age of 60 or with low plasma renin (8). Gender does not determine the effectiveness of calcium antagonists, although women may be more likely to report side effects. In contrast to other antihypertensive classes, calcium antagonists are reliably effective in African-American hypertensive patients and may be the most potent drugs for this subgroup of patients. Moreover, the responses do not depend on underlying renal function; therefore, patients with end-stage renal disease can be treated effectively. Calcium antagonists maintain a robust ability to lower blood pressure regardless of dietary salt consumption or NSAID use (23–25). However, modest dietary salt restriction can facilitate better blood pressure reduction (24).

Long-acting calcium antagonists, in general, improve myocardial oxygen demand, improve ventricular filling, conserve contractility, and decrease ventricular arrhythmias. They are equally as effective as β-blockers for reducing angina symptoms, cardiac events, variant angina, and hypertrophic cardiomyopathy in patients with coronary artery disease. Acutely, calcium antagonists facilitate diastolic relaxation, and, chronically, they can prevent or reverse left ventricular hypertrophy better than a β-blocker or a thiazide can (26) (Fig. 31.2). This may be particularly important because left ventricular hypertrophy is a powerful risk factor for cardiovascular endpoints. When treatment with calcium antagonists is initiated early in the course of hypertension, they can normalize altered-resistance arteriolar structure and endothelial dysfunction and, thus, prevent progression to higher stages of hypertension (27).

Only diltiazem and verapamil have been shown to be effective for secondary prevention of cardiac events after myocardial infarction. Verapamil may be preferred in those patients who cannot tolerate a β-blocker, when treatment is initiated 1–2 weeks after a myocardial infarction.

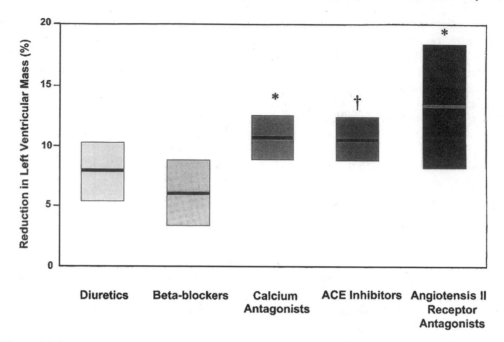

Figure 31.2 Percent reduction in left ventricular mass with various classes of antihypertensive drugs.

It should be emphasized that abrupt cessation of nondihydropyridines in patients with variant angina or diastolic dysfunction may precipitate anginal events. Calcium antagonists offer a particularly important therapeutic strategy for patients with peripheral vascular disease or bronchospastic disorders, such as asthma, who may be unable to tolerate β-blocker therapy. High-risk patients, such as those with dysmetabolic syndrome or diabetes, may benefit especially from the reduction of atherogenesis induced by calcium antagonists.

The dihydropyridine amlodipine was as effective as chlorthalidone or lisinopril, either alone or with other antihypertensive therapy, in preventing fatal or nonfatal myocardial infarction in the Antihypertensive and Lipid-Lowering Treatment to Prevent Heart Attack Trial (ALLHAT) study (28). Additionally, nitrendipine was demonstrated to be as effective in reducing stroke-related morbidity and mortality in the Systolic Hypertension in Europe (Sys-Eur) study (29).

There are relatively few contraindications for calcium antagonists. However, they should not be used in patients with ejection fractions <30% (with the exception of amlodipine or felodipine), sick sinus syndrome (unless the patient has a functional pacemaker), or second-degree or third-degree heart block. Verapamil and diltiazem are preferred in patients with acute and chronic supraventricular arrhythmias unless these arrhythmias are associated with an accessory pathway. Patients with pre-excitation syndromes associated with a rapid ventricular response should not be treated with verapamil because it may accentuate conduction through the accessory pathway.

D. Combination Therapy

Numerous recent clinical trials have proven that the most effective way to achieve the desired blood pressure level is with the use of multiple classes of medications. The calcium antagonists are an attractive class of drugs to use in combination with other drugs because of their efficacy and relatively neutral side-effect profile. Overall, the greatest antihypertensive efficacy is achieved with the combination of calcium antagonist with a β-blocker, ACE inhibitor, or angiotensin receptor blocker. There is less of an anithypertensive effect when a calcium antagonist is combined with a diuretic, which reflects the fact that calcium antagonists possess inherent diuretic activity. Treatment response rates approach 70% when dihydropyridines are added to ACE-inhibitor or angiotensin receptor blocker therapy. The combination of these classes takes advantage of simultaneous precapillary and postcapillary vasodilation to lower peripheral resistance. This approach may cause synergistic blood pressure lowering, more complete renal protection, and result in less peripheral edema. In fact, the addition of verapamil to chronic ACE inhibitor therapy has been shown to reverse the decrease in glomerular filtration rate that is associated with the ACE inhibitor, without further lowering blood pressure (30).

In the recently published International Verapamil–Trandolapril Study (INVEST), hypertensive patients with coronary artery disease were randomized to receive either verapamil, alone or in combination with the ACE inhibitor trandolapril, and hydrochlorothiazide (HCTZ) as needed; or atenolol, with or without hydrochlorothiazide, and the ACE inhibitor as needed. After 2.7 years of follow-up, there were no significant differences between treatment strategies with respect to the primary endpoints of death, fatal or nonfatal myocardial infarction, stroke, angina, hospitalizations, or adverse events (31). Blood pressure control over the 2 year period was similar between groups, and the calcium antagonist-based therapy was associated with significantly fewer new diagnoses of diabetes. This important trial provides convincing evidence that verapamil, alone or in combination with an ACE inhibitor, is as effective as a β-blocker and thiazide combination for the treatment of hypertensive patients with coronary artery disease (31).

Because β-blockers and diuretics decrease insulin sensitivity and impair glucose tolerance, there is some concern with using these drugs in diabetics. Holzgrove et al. (32) recently demonstrated in diabetics that the same calcium antagonist strategy used in the INVEST trial was associated with no short-term or long-term change in HbA1c levels (7.9%), whereas the β-blocker group had significant impairment of glycemic control (HgA1c increased from 7.8% to 8.6%).

Another attractive approach combines the use of a dihydropyridine with a β-blocker to maximize protection against adverse effects that are caused by either drug alone. Calcium antagonists can inhibit potential vasoconstriction that is induced by the β-blocker; the β-blockers can attenuate the reflex activation that is induced by dihydropyridines. The use of nondihydropyridines with β-blockers can accentuate conduction delays, contractility, and heart rate and should only be used with extreme caution and close monitoring.

Combining dihydropyridines with other calcium antagonists has been effective for blood pressure control, but data supporting the safety and rationale for this approach is limited, and the incidence of pedal edema is increased (33). Routine use of calcium antagonists with even three or four additional antihypertensive classes, however, is safe and frequently necessary to control blood pressure.

VIII. PITFALLS, DANGERS, AND SIDE EFFECTS

Calcium antagonists as a group are well tolerated. Unlike conventional antihypertensive drugs, calcium antagonists are not associated with significant alterations in sexual function, depression, or masking of hypoglycemic awareness. Orthostatic blood pressure changes are uncommon because the mechanisms for venoconstriction remain intact. However, because calcium antagonists are primarily vasodilators, hypotension can occur. Hypotension is less frequent with oral dosing than with intravenous treatment and is more common, as expected, with the more potent dihydropyridines. Hypotension is more common with

initiation of drug therapy or in patients who are receiving multiple antihypertensive drugs, particularly β-blockers (34). The vasodilatory action also is directly associated with flushing, dizziness, nausea, and headaches. These side effects are more pronounced with the shorter acting drugs and are often dose related and transient. Perhaps the most common and bothersome side effect of the dihydropyridines is peripheral (and occasionally periorbital) edema. The edema is likely the result of uncompensated precapillary vasodilation, which increases intracapillary hydrostatic pressure and results in a transudative shift of fluid into the extravascular space. Because this edema is neither gravitational nor associated with increased sodium retention, it does not respond well to diuretics (35). In contrast, preferential postcapillary vasodilation with ACE inhibitors or angiotensin receptor blockers reduces intracapillary hydrostatic pressure and reverses the hydrostatic forces favoring extravascular fluid shifts (35,36).

Another common side effect of the dihydropyridines is gingival hyperplasia. Nifedipine, in particular, enhances the ability of oral bacterial plaques to stimulate an inflammatory B-cell infiltration in the gingiva that results in growth of the bacteria. This effect is exaggerated in the presence of cyclosporine (37). Gingival hypertrophy is reversible with cessation of drug therapy. Side effects of the nondihydropyridines, particularly verapamil, are more likely to result from direct inhibition of calcium-dependent smooth muscle contraction. In the gastrointestinal tract, they cause relaxation of the lower esophageal sphincter and a reduction in peristaltic contractions in the bowel wall. Clinically, patients experience nausea and constipation. The effects of diltiazem and verapamil on cardiac conduction may be more troublesome. Because they inhibit conduction at the sinus and atrioventicular node, they can cause conduction delays and atrioventicular block (8). These effects are seldom associated with any clinical symptoms and, indeed, form the basis for the use of these drugs in tachycardia syndromes.

As stated previously, calcium antagonists are unique among antihypertensive drugs with regard to their neutral metabolic side effect profile. They do not impair glucose or insulin homeostatis, do not reduce HDL cholesterol or increase oxidized LDL cholesterol or triglycerides, and are not associated with changes in serum sodium, potassium, or uric acid. On the contrary, they have been shown to have additive vasculoprotective metabolic effects when they are used in combination with statins (38). Therefore, they may be one of the preferred drugs for patients with the dysmetabolic syndrome or diabetes.

A. Safety and Drug Interactions

A number of questions about the long-term safety of calcium antagonists have been raised over the last 10 years, and there has been considerable debate about their cardiovascular safety. The use of short-acting drugs, particularly nifedipine, has been associated with a small increased risk of cardiovascular events due to compensatory activation of the renin–angiotensin and sympathetic nervous system activity (6). For this reason, the indications for short-acting drugs have been modified to exclude their use from the treatment of hypertension. Similar concerns have been raised about the clinical safety of dihydropyridines in diabetics, which are based on the results of several clinical trials in which dihydropyridines were compared to ACE inhibitors (39,40). In these studies, diabetic patients treated with the ACE inhibitors experienced fewer cardiovascular events. However, these data need to be interpreted with caution, as there were no placebo groups with which to compare the calcium antagonists. Recent, well-controlled trials demonstrate unequivocally the beneficial effects of calcium antagonists in diabetics and nondiabetics (28,29,41–45). Concerns about possible increased risks of gastrointestinal bleeding or cancers have not been substantiated (46). The large number of patients currently being treated with calcium antagonists and the ongoing trials and observational studies in which there is more aggressive blood pressure reduction are expected to allay many of these concerns (28).

Perhaps more clinically relevant are the multiple potential drug interactions that occur with calcium antagonists. Table 31.5 outlines the more frequent drug interactions that are encountered in clinical practice. Simultaneous use of the combinations are not contraindicated; they merely warrant closer clinical observation.

IX. CONCLUSIONS

Since their introduction >30 years ago, calcium antagonists have generated both significant debates as well as ongoing excitement. Calcium antagonists reduce peripheral vascular resistance by inhibiting the intracellular influx of calcium, a process that is abnormal in a majority of hypertensive patients. As a result, they interfere with excitation–contraction coupling in vascular and, to some extent, in cardiac smooth muscle. As a class, they have considerably more variable effects on the vasculature, heart, and target organs, such as the kidney, than most antihypertensive drugs. However, their pharmacokinetic profiles are remarkably similar.

Numerous studies have demonstrated the efficacy of calcium antagonists in treating hypertension. They are reliably effective in patients regardless of age, gender, race, salt intake, or even NSAID use. Calcium antagonists are as effective as all other antihypertensive drugs in reducing blood pressure and cardiovascular events and may be better for stroke reduction. Because of their neutral or favorable metabolic profile, ease of dosing, and low incidence of side effects, they are ideal drugs for a variety of patients, both as monotherapy and in combination therapy with other drugs.

In general, doses should be started at the lowest recommended range, and a slow-release or long-acting form should be selected to improve compliance and reduce blood pressure variability and reflex stimulation of the sympathetic nervous system. Side effects are infrequent

Table 31.5   Drug–Drug Interactions with Calcium Antagonists

Calcium antagonist	Interacting drug	Result
Verapamil	Digoxin	Increases digoxin levels by 50–90%
Diltiazem	Digozin	Increases digoxin level by 40%
Verapamil	β-blockers	Increases AV nodal blockade, hypotension, bradycardiaasystole
Verapamil, diltiazem	Cyclosporine/tacrolimus and sirolimus	Increases cyclosporine levels by 25–100%
Verapamil, diltiazem	Cimetidine	Increases verapamil and diltiazem levels by decreasing metabolism
Verapamil	Rifampin/phenytoin	Decreases verapamil levels by enzyme induction
Dihydropyridines	Amiodarone	Exacerbates sick sinus syndrome and AV nodal blockade
Dihydropyridines	β-blockers	Results in excessive hypotension
Dihydropyridines	Propanolol	Increases propanolol levels
Dihydropyridines	Cimetidine	Increases area under the blood pressure curve and plasma levels of calcium antagonist
Nicardipine	Cyclosporine	Increases cyclosporine levels (nicardipine 40–50%; amlodipine 10%)
Amlodipine		
Felodipine	Flavonoids	Increases bioavailability by 50%
Diltiazem	Methylprednisone	Increases methylprednisone 0.5-fold
Nifedipine	Diltiazem	Increases nifedipine levels 100–200%

and can be managed easily. The choice of a particular calcium antagonist should take into account other co-morbidities as discussed previously in this chapter.

Emerging data indicates that calcium antagonists also may have protective effects that are independent of their blood pressure-lowering properties. Many have intrinsic antioxidant activity, improve endothelial function and arterial compliance, and reduce atherogenesis. The clinical importance of these findings has not yet been established, but in addition to the clinical efficacy and safety of calcium antagonists, they provide compelling reasons to support the widespread use of drugs from this class for the treatment of hypertension.

REFERENCES

1. Chobanian AV, Bakris GL, Black HR, Cushman WC, Green LA, Izzo JL Jr et al. The Seventh Report of the Joint National Committee on Prevention, Detection, Evaluation, and Treatment of High Blood Pressure: the JNC 7 Report. JAMA 2003; 289(19):2560–2572.
2. 1999 World Health Organization-International Society of Hypertension Guidelines for the Management of Hypertension. Guidelines Subcommittee. J Hypertens 1999; 17(2):151–183.
3. Triggle. Mechanisms of action of calcium antagonists. In: Epstein M, ed. Calcium Antagonists in Clinical Medicine. Philadelphia, PA: Hanley & Belfus, Inc., 2002:1–32.
4. Angelico P, Guarneri L, Leonardi A, Testa R. Vascular-selective effect of lercanidipine and other 1,4-dihydropyridines in isolated rabbit tissues. J Pharm Pharmacol 1999; 51(6):709–714.
5. Lefrandt JD, Heitmann J, Sevre K, Castellano M, Hausberg M, Fallon M et al. The effects of dihydropyridine and phenylalkylamine calcium antagonist classes on autonomic function in hypertension: the VAMPHYRE study. Am J Hypertens 2001; 14(11 Pt 1):1083–1089.
6. Pahor M, Psaty BM, Alderman MH, Applegate WB, Williamson JD, Cavazzini C et al. Health outcomes associated with calcium antagonists compared with other first-line antihypertensive therapies: a meta-analysis of randomised controlled trials. Lancet 2000; 356(9246):1949–1954.
7. Dunselman PH, van der Mark TW, Kuntze CE, van Bruggen A, Hamer JP, Scaf AH et al. Different results in cardiopulmonary exercise tests after long-term treatment with felodipine and enalapril in patients with congestive heart failure due to ischaemic heart disease. Eur Heart J 1990; 11(3):200–206.
8. Weir MR, Klaussen DR, Hanes Ds. Antihypertensive drugs. In: Brenner BM, ed. The Kidney. Philadelphia: W.B. Saunders Company, 2003:2381–2451.
9. Xu B, Xiao-hong L, Lin G, Queen L, Ferro A. Amlodipine, but not verapamil or nifedipine, dilates rabbit femoral artery largely through a nitric oxide- and kinin-dependent mechanism. Br J Pharmacol 2002; 136(3):375–382.
10. Papadopoulos CL, Kokkas BA. Atrial natriuretic peptide contributes to the antihypertensive action of many drugs. Eur J Drug Metab Pharmacokinet 2003; 28(1):55–57.
11. Buhler FR. Antihypertensive care with calcium antagonists. In: Laragh JH, Brenner BM, eds. Hypertension: Pathophysiology, Diagnosis and Management. New York: Raven Press, 1995:2801–2814.
12. White WB, Saunders E, Noveck RJ, Ferdinand K. Comparative efficacy and safety of nisoldipine extended-release (ER) and amlodipine (CESNA-III study) in African American patients with hypertension. Am J Hypertens 2003; 16(9 Pt 1):739–745.
13. Mason RP, Marche P, Hintze TH. Novel vascular biology of third-generation L-type calcium channel antagonists: ancillary actions of amlodipine. Arterioscler Thromb Vasc Biol 2003; 23(12):2155–2163.
14. Yu T, Morita I, Shimokado K, Iwai T, Yoshida M. Amlodipine modulates THP-1 cell adhesion to vascular endothelium via inhibition of protein kinase C signal transduction. Hypertension 2003; 42(3):329–334.
15. McCormack PL, Wagstaff AJ. Lacidipine: a review of its use in the management of hypertension. Drugs 2003; 63(21):2327–2356.
16. Fogari R, Mugellini A, Zoppi A, Corradi L, Rinaldi A, Derosa G et al. Differential effects of lercanidipine and nifedipine GITS on plasma norepinephrine in chronic treatment of hypertension. Am J Hypertens 2003; 16(7):596–599.
17. Bang LM, Chapman TM, Goa KL. Lercanidipine: a review of its efficacy in the management of hypertension. Drugs 2003; 63(22):2449–2472.
18. Lewis EJ, Hunsicker LG, Clarke WR, Berl T, Pohl MA, Lewis JB et al. Renoprotective effect of the angiotensin-receptor antagonist irbesartan in patients with nephropathy due to type 2 diabetes. N Engl J Med 2001; 345(12):851–860.
19. Delles C, Klingbeil AU, Schneider MP, Handrock R, Weidinger G, Schmieder RE. Direct comparison of the effects of valsartan and amlodipine on renal hemodynamics in human essential hypertension. Am J Hypertens 2003; 16(12):1030–1035.
20. Tarif N, Bakris GL. Preservation of renal function: the spectrum of effects by calcium-channel blockers. Nephrol Dial Transplant 1997; 12(11):2244–2250.
21. Kloke HJ, Branten AJ, Huysmans FT, Wetzels JF. Antihypertensive treatment of patients with proteinuric renal diseases: risks or benefits of calcium channel blockers? Kidney Int 1998; 53(6):1559–1573.
22. Smith AC, Toto R, Bakris GL. Differential effects of calcium channel blockers on size selectivity of proteinuria in diabetic glomerulopathy. Kidney Int 1998; 54(3):889–896.
23. Houston MC, Weir M, Gray J, Ginsberg D, Szeto C, Kaihlenen PM et al. The effects of nonsteroidal anti-inflammatory drugs on blood pressures of patients with hypertension controlled by verapamil. Arch Intern Med 1995; 155(10):1049–1054.
24. Weir MR, Chrysant SG, McCarron DA, Canossa-Terris M, Cohen JD, Gunter PA et al. Influence of race and dietary

salt on the antihypertensive efficacy of an angiotensin-converting enzyme inhibitor or a calcium channel antagonist in salt-sensitive hypertensives. Hypertension 1998; 31(5):1088–1096.

25. Weir MR, Hall PS, Behrens MT, Flack JM. Salt and blood pressure responses to calcium antagonism in hypertensive patients. Hypertension 1997; 30(3 Pt 1):422–427.

26. Klingbeil AU, Schneider M, Martus P, Messerli FH, Schmieder RE. A meta-analysis of the effects of treatment on left ventricular mass in essential hypertension. Am J Med 2003; 115(1):41–46.

27. Schiffrin EL, Pu Q, Park JB. Effect of amlodipine compared to atenolol on small arteries of previously untreated essential hypertensive patients. Am J Hypertens 2002; 15(2 Pt 1):105–110.

28. ALLHAT Collaborative Research Group. Major cardiovascular events in hypertensive patients randomized to doxazosin vs chlorthalidone: the antihypertensive and lipid-lowering treatment to prevent heart attack trial (ALLHAT). JAMA 2000; 283(15):1967–1975.

29. Staessen JA, Fagard R, Thijs L, Celis H, Arabidze GG, Birkenhager WH et al. Randomised double-blind comparison of placebo and active treatment for older patients with isolated systolic hypertension. The Systolic Hypertension in Europe (Syst-Eur) Trial Investigators. Lancet 1997; 350(9080):757–764.

30. Bitar R, Flores O, Reverte M, Lopez-Novoa JM, Macias JF. Beneficial effect of verapamil added to chronic ACE inhibitor treatment on renal function in hypertensive elderly patients. Int Urol Nephrol 2000; 32(2):165–169.

31. Pepine CJ, Handberg EM, Cooper-DeHoff RM, Marks RG, Kowey P, Messerli FH et al. A calcium antagonist vs a non-calcium antagonist hypertension treatment strategy for patients with coronary artery disease. The International Verapamil–Trandolapril Study (INVEST): a Randomized Controlled Trial. JAMA 2003; 290(21):2805–2816.

32. Holzgreve H, Nakov R, Beck K, Janka HU. Antihypertensive therapy with verapamil SR plus trandolapril versus atenolol plus chlorthalidone on glycemic control. Am J Hypertens 2003; 16(5 Pt 1):381–386.

33. Kiowski W, Erne P, Linder L, Buhler FR. Arterial vasodilator effects of the dihydropyridine calcium antagonist amlodipine alone and in combination with verapamil in systemic hypertension. Am J Cardiol 1990; 66(20):1469–1472.

34. Epstein M. Calcium antagonists in the management of hypertension. In: Epstein M, ed. Calcium Antagonists in Clinical Medicine. Philadelphia: Hanley and Belfus Inc., 2002:293–313.

35. Weir MR, Rosenberger C, Fink JC. Pilot study to evaluate a water displacement technique to compare effects of diuretics and ACE inhibitors to alleviate lower extremity edema due to dihydropyridine calcium antagonists. Am J Hypertens 2001; 14(9 Pt 1):963–968.

36. Messerli FH, Weir MR, Neutel JM. Combination therapy of amlodipine/benazepril versus monotherapy of amlodipine in a practice-based setting. Am J Hypertens 2002; 15(6):550–556.

37. Bullon P, Machuca G, Armas JR, Rojas JL, Jimenez G. The gingival inflammatory infiltrate in cardiac patients treated with calcium antagonists. J Clin Periodontol 2001; 28(10):897–903.

38. Leibovitz E, Beniashvili M, Zimlichman R, Freiman A, Shargorodsky M, Gavish D. Treatment with amlodipine and atorvastatin have additive effect in improvement of arterial compliance in hypertensive hyperlipidemic patients. Am J Hypertens 2003; 16(9 Pt 1):715–718.

39. Estacio RO, Jeffers BW, Hiatt WR, Biggerstaff SL, Gifford N, Schrier RW. The effect of nisoldipine as compared with enalapril on cardiovascular outcomes in patients with non-insulin-dependent diabetes and hypertension. N Engl J Med 1998; 338(10):645–652.

40. Tatti P, Pahor M, Byington RP, Di Mauro P, Guarisco R, Strollo G et al. Outcome results of the Fosinopril Versus Amlodipine Cardiovascular Events Randomized Trial (FACET) in patients with hypertension and NIDDM. Diabetes Care 1998; 21(4):597–603.

41. Tuomilehto J, Rastenyte D, Birkenhager WH, Thijs L, Antikainen R, Bulpitt CJ et al. Effects of calcium-channel blockade in older patients with diabetes and systolic hypertension. Systolic Hypertension in Europe Trial Investigators. N Engl J Med 1999; 340(9):677–684.

42. Hansson L, Zanchetti A, Carruthers SG, Dahlof B, Elmfeldt D, Julius S et al. Effects of intensive blood-pressure lowering and low-dose aspirin in patients with hypertension: principal results of the hypertension optimal treatment (HOT) randomised trial. HOT Study Group. Lancet 1998; 351(9118):1755–1762.

43. Bakris GL, Weir MR, Shanifar S, Zhang Z, Douglas J, van Dijk DJ et al. Effects of blood pressure level on progression of diabetic nephropathy: results from the RENAAL study. Arch Intern Med 2003; 163(13):1555–1565.

44. Epstein M. Safety of calcium antagonists as antihypertensive agents: an update. In: Epstein M, ed. Calcium Antagonists in Clinical Medicine. Philadelphia: Hanley and Belfus Inc., 2002:807–832.

45. Turnbull F. Effects of different blood-pressure-lowering regimens on major cardiovascular events: results of prospectively-designed overviews of randomised trials. Lancet 2003; 362(9395):1527–1535.

46. *Ad Hoc* Subcommittee of the Liaison Committee of the World Health Organisation and the International Society of Hypertension. Effects of calcium antagonists on the risks of coronary heart disease, cancer and bleeding. J Hypertens 1997; 15(2):105–115.

32

Direct Vasodilators

BANSARI SHAH
University of Illinois/Christ Hospital, Chicago, Illinois, USA

GEORGE L. BAKRIS
Rush University Medical Center, Chicago, Illinois, USA

KEYPOINTS

- Direct vasodilators are useful in the treatment of specific types of hypertension characterized by a failure to achieve goal if BP is >140 systolic and on maximum doses of 4 drugs. Also conditions such as heart failure.
- Direct vasodilators generally are not recommended as first-line agents except in the case of preeclampsia.

SUMMARY

Direct vasodilators can be used alone or in conjunction with other drugs to achieve blood pressure goals or to address situations of hypertensive emergency or urgency. There are currently four drugs in this class of medications: hydralazine, minoxidil, nitroprusside, and fenoldopam.

I. INTRODUCTION

Direct vasodilators are antihypertensive medications, which produce direct relaxation of the arteriolar smooth muscles and, hence, result in vasodilation. Medications in this class include hydralazine, minoxidil, nitroprusside, and fenoldopam. The first two drugs are recommended as adjunct agents to be used with more established therapy to achieve blood pressure goals (1); the latter two drugs are recommended for cases of hypertensive urgency (2).

A summary of these drugs is presented in Table 32.1, including clinical, dosing, and side-effect profiles.

The specific mechanism of vascular relaxation and the reason for the selectivity of resistance vessels for hydralazine are not known. Minoxidil is known to open potassium channels and, hence, result in smooth muscle relaxation. Nitroprusside is a direct acting intravenous vasodilater that disrupts cerebral autoregulation and has limited usefulness in people with advance nephropathy due to increase in this cynate concentration. Fenoldopam is a selective dopamine-1 (D1) receptor agonist, which results in a dose-dependent relaxation of vascular smooth muscle, but it can only be administered intravenously.

II. HYDRALAZINE (APRESOLINE)

Hydralazine is the prototype direct vasodilator. It was one of the first orally active antihypertensive agents on the market. However, it is generally not used as a single agent to achieve blood pressure goals and requires some other agents such as a β-blocker that blocks sympathetic tone secondary to development of tachycardia and tachyphylaxis (3). Its recommended use is as a fourth-line agent in concert with diuretics and sympatholytic agents so that it can be better tolerated.

A. Mechanism of Action

Hydralazine causes direct relaxation of the arteriolar smooth muscle by a mechanism, which is currently unknown. However, a number of mechanisms have been proposed for the vasodilating action of hydralazine. One is the inhibition of calcium influx into the smooth muscle; another is the inhibition of phosphorylation of myosin light chain kinases (4).

Hydralazine has a greater effect on the precapillary resistance than on the postcapillary resistance vessels. It also causes a preferential decrease in the vascular resistance in coronary, cerebral, and renal vascular beds when compared with skin and muscular beds (5). Because of its preferential dilation of arterioles over veins, postural hypotension is not a common problem. Although, theoretically hydralazine may be useful for treating pulmonary hypertension, the vasodilation this drug produces in the pulmonary vasculature is offset by the relatively greater increase in cardiac output, which, in turn results in mild pulmonary hypertension. It is difficult to predict what patients will respond to hydralazine in this manner, but the increase in cardiac output can be attenuated by the concurrent use of a β-adrenergic blocking agent (6,7).

Although most of hydralazine's effect in increasing heart rate and cardiac output is due to baroreceptor-mediated responses, hydralazine also may stimulate the release of norepinephrine from the sympathetic nerve terminals and augment myocardial contractility directly (8). In addition, fluid retention results from a decrease in blood pressure, which stimulates the renin–angiotensin–aldosterone system, and an increase mechanism to also increase sodium reabsorption from the proximal tubule of the nephron (9).

Table 32.1 Oral and Intravenous Vasodilating Agents

Vasodilator	Mechanism	Dose	Onset of action	Side effects
Hydralazine	Opens potassium channels	Intravenously, 10–50 mg IV/IM q 4–6 h for 15–30 min. Orally, 50 mg bid up to 150 mg bid[a]	Within 2 h	Hypotension, reflex sympathetic stimulation, exacerbate angina, myocardial infarction
Minoxidil	Opens potassium channels	Start oral dose 2 mg bid, and increase up to 40 mg/day in divided doses[a]	Within 2 h	Reflex sympathetic stimulation, exacerbate angina, myocardial infarction, pericardial effusion
Sodium nitroprusside	Increases cyclic GMP; blocks cell calcium	0.25–10 μg/kg per min	Immediate	Nausea, severe hypotension, thiocyanate toxicity. (Check thiocyanate levels every 48 h, especially in cases of renal failure.)
Fenoldopam	D1 receptor agonist	0.1–0.3 μg/kg per min	<5 min	Tachycardia, headache, nausea, flushing

[a]bid, to be ingested twice daily.

B. Pharmacokinetics and Pharmacodynamics

The peak serum concentration of hydralazine and the peak hypotensive effect of the drug occur within 30–120 min of ingestion. However, when hydralazine is given intravenously, the peak blood level of the drug and the time of maximal effect differ from those observed with oral administration. This is because hydralazine is extensively metabolized in the gastrointestinal mucosa and the liver, which results in the inactivation of 75–90% of an orally administered dose.

Hydralazine is N-acetylated in the liver and the bowel. The rate of acetylation is genetically determined. About half of the hypertensive patients in the United States are fast acetylators, and the other half are slow acetylators (10,11). Because the acetylated compound is inactive, the oral dose that is required to produce a systemic effect is larger in fast acetylators. No difference exists in dose effect between fast and slow acetylators when hydralazine is administered intravenously (12,13).

The half-life of hydralazine is 1 h, and the systemic clearance of the drug is ~50 mL/kg per min. Because systemic clearance exceeds hepatic blood flow, extrahepatic metabolism must occur; hydralazine combines with circulating α keto acids to form hydrazones. The major metabolite recovered from the plasma is hydralazine pyruvic acid hydrazone (14). However, although hydralazine's half-life is only ~1 h, the duration of the hypotensive effect can last ~12 h. The reason for this discrepancy is not understood clearly. One explanation is the persistence of the active metabolites in the plasma. Another possible explanation is the tissue binding of hydralazine that occurs in the walls of arteries in the muscles, which might allow hydralazine to persist much longer and exert a prolonged pharmacologic effect. It has also been postulated that its prolonged pharmacologic effect is due to a sustained effect on endothelium-derived relaxing factor (15).

C. Adverse Effects

The most common adverse effects of hydralazine are related to its direct reflex-mediated hemodynamic actions including flushing, headache, palpitations, hypotension, and angina. It can cause electrocardiographic changes of myocardial ischemia that are a result of an increased oxygen demand that is imposed by the baroreflex-mediated stimulation of the sympathetic nervous system. Moreover, because hydralazine does not dilate the epicardial coronary arteries, the arteriolar dilation it produces results in the blood flowing away from the ischemic region. For this reason, parenteral administration to patients with coronary artery disease is contraindicated.

The salt and fluid retention that result from using hydralazine also may precipitate heart failure. Therefore, as previously mentioned, hydralazine is better tolerated with the concomitant use of a β-blocker and a diuretic.

Repeated administration of hydralazine can cause a drug-induced, lupus-like syndrome. This syndrome is frequently dose dependant and rarely occurs in patients who receive <200 mg/day of hydralazine. The occurrence of this syndrome is also related to the age, gender, and acetylator phenotype of the patient (16). The syndrome is four times more common in women than in men. Its clinical features are similar to most other drug-induced lupus syndromes and include arthralgias, arthritis, fever, and, occasionally, pleuritis, and pericarditis. The symptoms disappear when the drug is discontinued. The majority of patients who develop a positive antinuclear antibody titer do not develop the drug-induced lupus syndrome, and the drug need not be discontinued unless clinical symptoms develop.

The use of hydralazine also can result in an antineutrophil cytoplasmic antibody-positive vasculitis or in a rapidly proliferative glomerulonephritis (17). Note that these conditions are extremely uncommon. The mechanism for the genesis of these conditions is unknown; however, hydralazine is known to inhibit the methylation of DNA, and it induces self-reactivity in T-cells (18). Hydralazine also can produce a pyridoxine-responsive polyneuropathy, although this side effect is encountered very seldom.

D. Clinical Uses

Hydralazine has several clinical uses in the treatment of hypertension and cardiac failure:

- Preeclamptic conditions in pregnant women.
- Hypertensive emergencies.
- Perioperative hypertension.
- Management of refractory hypertension.
- Management of hypertension during pregnancy.
- Heart failure.

However, hydralazine has no role as a first-line agent except in one circumstance: in preeclamptic pregnant women, where this drug should be considered as one of several other possible agents. A systolic blood pressure of >169 mmHg and a diastolic blood pressure of 109 mmHg are considered an emergency in a pregnant woman. Eclampsia poses a great risk to both maternal and fetal well-being. Poor maternal outcomes are related to complications, such as cerebral hemorrhage and seizures, if eclampsia develops. The recommended dose is 5–10 mg administered intravenously every 20–30 min (19).

Parenteral antihypertensive therapy with hydralazine is indicated in patients with symptomatic stage 2 hypertension as defined by the Joint National Committee 7th Report classification (1). This is the class of patients who have severe hypertension with evidence of progressive target organ damage to the central nervous system, retina, cardiovascular system, or the kidney as evidenced by severe headache, mental status changes, seizures, loss or blurring of vision, chest pain, shortness of breath, or edema, with the physical findings of focal or diffuse neurological deficits, papilledema, gallop rhythm, or pulmonary crackles. In this setting, an initial dose of 10–20 mg should be administered intravenously and repeated as needed.

Perioperative hypertension is one of the most common settings for episodic severe hypertension. Hydralazine can be used both intraoperatively and postoperatively. Improved blood pressure control may decrease surgical bleeding and protect vascular anastomotic suture lines.

As mentioned previously in this chapter, hydralazine is very useful in the management of refractory hypertension as an adjunct to other drugs to help achieve blood pressure goal (20).

Hydralazine also is used in the management of hypertension during pregnancy, which helps to prevent maternal and perinatal morbidity and mortality (21).

In addition, hydralazine is used in conjunction with nitrates for the treatment of chronic heart failure, which is a result of systolic dysfunction in patients who cannot tolerate angiotensin-converting enzyme inhibitors or angiotensin receptor blockers. Hydralazine confers a favorable effect on left ventricular function and on decreasing the mortality rate (22).

III. MINOXIDIL (LONITEN)

Minoxidil was discovered in 1965. It has been proven to be efficacious in the treatment of patients with very severe hypertension and drug-resistant hypertension (20).

A. Mechanism of Action

Minoxidil is inactive *in vitro*. It is metabolized by hepatic sulfotransferase to the active molecule minoxidil N–O sulfate. Minoxidil sulfate relaxes vascular smooth muscle by activating adenosine triphosphate (ATP)-modulated potassium channels in smooth muscle, which results in a potassium efflux and the hyperpolarization of smooth muscle (23).

Minoxidil produces arteriolar vasodilation with no effect on the capacitance vessels, in which regard it resembles hydralazine. It increases blood flow to the heart, skin, skeletal muscle, and gastrointestinal tract more than it affects blood flow to the central nervous system. Hence, the administration of minoxidil causes an increase in myocardial contractility and cardiac output (24). However, long-term use can result in the development of pericardial effusions and, rarely, cardiac tamponade.

Minoxidil is a renal vasodilator, but the systemic hypotension produced by the drug can decrease renal blood flow. It is a potent stimulator of renin secretion and leads to profound sodium retention and the development of substantial edema.

B. Pharmacokinetics and Pharmacodynamics

Minoxidil is absorbed well from the gastrointestinal tract. Peak concentrations of the drug occur 1 h after oral administration, but the maximum hypotensive effect occurs later because the formation of the active metabolite is delayed. Twenty percent of the drug is excreted unchanged in the urine, and the main route of elimination is through hepatic metabolism.

C. Adverse Effects

Minoxidil causes the retention of salt and water secondary to increased proximal tubular absorption, which is, in turn, secondary to reduced renal perfusion pressure and reflex stimulation of renal tubular α adrenergic receptors. Fluid retention can be controlled with a diuretic.

Minoxidil can cause direct reflex-mediated hemodynamic actions that include flushing, headache, palpitations, and hypotension and also angina and electrocardiogram changes of myocardial ischemia that are a result of an increased oxygen demand, which is imposed by the baroreflex-mediated stimulation of the sympathetic nervous system. These effects are similar to the effects of hydralazine. They can be attenuated by the concomitant use of a β-blocker.

The increased cardiac output that is caused by minoxidil can adversely affect patients who have left ventricular hypertrophy and diastolic dysfunction. The poorly compliant ventricles do not respond optimally to an increased volume load, which results in an increase in left ventricular filling pressure. This is the major contributor to the increase in pulmonary artery pressure that is observed with minoxidil therapy. Heart failure can occur in this patient population secondary to minoxidil therapy.

Pericardial effusion also can occur in rare cases. In most instances, it is reversible when administration of the drug is discontinued (25).

Hypertrichosis occurs in all patients who use minoxidil for an extended period of time. It is secondary to the potassium channel activation. Growth of hair is seen on the face, arms, legs, and back. Topical minoxidil is now marketed commercially for the treatment of male pattern baldness.

Other rare side effects include Stevens–Johnson syndrome, antinuclear antibody formation, and glucose intolerance.

D. Clinical Uses

Because of its side-effect profile, minoxidil is used only as a last resort to help achieve the blood pressure goal. Minoxidil is used in both adults and children in the management of severe refractory hypertension and is always used in conjunction with a diuretic and a β-adrenergic blocking agent. It is administered once or twice a day. The initial dose is 2.5–5 mg/day. The maximum dose is 100 mg/day.

Minoxidil is also used in the treatment of alopecia. It modifies the hair cycle by prolonging the anagen phase and has been used for treatment of both androgenetic alopecia and alopecia areata. Its use is being studied in the treatment of chemotherapy-induced alopecia (26).

In addition, minoxidil is being investigated as a combination drug with tamoxifen in the treatment of breast cancer (27).

IV. NITROPRUSSIDE

Nitroprusside is a direct-acting vasodilator, which is used for hypertensive emergencies.

A. Mechanism of Action and Pharmacology

Nitroprusside increases cyclic guanosine monophosphate (GMP) and partially blocks calcium fluxes in the cell. In this way, nitroprusside catalyzes events that lead to vasodilation (2,28). It has a half-life of minutes and, thus, can be titrated easily when it is used to lower blood pressure. An intravenous dose of 0.25–10 µg/kg per min usually reduces arterial pressure.

B. Adverse Effects

A number of adverse effects have been reported with nitroprusside, including nausea, severe hypotension, and thiocyanate toxicity. Thiocyanate toxicity is especially prominent in people with renal insufficiency. Therefore, levels of thiocyanate should be checked every 48 h, especially in patients with renal failure (2,28).

C. Clinical Uses

This agent is used in hypertensive crisis when parenteral therapy is required should be used with caution in people with kidney disease due to increases in thiocynate

and potential cynaide toxicity if levels are not monitored. Most commonly used in conditions where patients have decreased mental status with very high blood pressure ($>$190–200 mmHg systolic) already receiving oral therapy.

V. FENOLDOPAM

Fenoldopam is a direct-acting vasodilator that is used for hypertensive crisis.

A. Mechanism of Action and Pharmacology

Fenoldopam is a selective dopamine agonist that causes peripheral vasodilation via the stimulation of D1 receptors. The half-life of fenoldopam is on the order of minutes (2,29).

B. Adverse Effects

Because fenoldopam is indicated only for hypertensive urgencies or emergencies, the only untoward effects are hypotension that may result from too large a dose. Given the fenoldopam's short half-life, this hypotension is corrected easily by reducing the dose of the drug (2,29).

C. Clinical Uses

The efficacy of an intravenous infusion of fenoldopam for decreasing blood pressure in patients with hypertensive urgency (including patients who develop hypertension after coronary artery bypass graft surgery and in a small number of patients with hypertensive emergency) is similar to the efficacy of treatment with sodium nitroprusside. However, unlike sodium nitroprusside, fenoldopam also increases renal blood flow and causes diuresis and natriuresis (29). There is no evidence of rebound hypertension after stopping the infusion. Because the tolerability profile of fenoldopam is generally similar to that of sodium nitroprusside, fenoldopam appears to be an effective alternative to sodium nitroprusside in the immediate treatment of patients who develop severe hypertension and for whom oral treatment is not practical. Fenoldopam may be particularly useful in patients who develop hypertension after coronary artery bypass graft surgery, but further studies are required to confirm its role in hypertensive emergency.

REFERENCES

1. Chobanian AV, Bakris GL, Black HR, Cushman WC, Green LA, Izzo JL Jr, Jones DW, Materson BJ, Oparil S, Wright JT Jr, Roccella EJ. The Seventh Report of the

Joint National Committee on Prevention, Detection, Evaluation, and Treatment of High Blood Pressure: the JNC 7 report. JAMA 2003; 289:2560–2572.

2. Black HR, Bakris GL, Elliott WJ. Hypertension: epidemiology, pathophysiology, diagnosis and treatment. In: Fuster V, Alexander W, O'Rourke R et al., eds. Hurst's: The Heart. New York: McGraw-Hill, 2001:1553–1604.

3. John O, Nancy B. Antihypertensive Agents and the Drug Therapy of Hypertension. In: Hardman JG, Limbird LE, eds. Goodman and Gilman's the Pharmacological Basis of Therapeutics. Chapter 33. 10th ed. McGraw-Hill Companies, 2001:784–796.

4. Kirsten R, Nelson K, Kirsten D, Heintz B. Clinical pharmacokinetics of vasodilators, part I. Clin Pharmacokinet 1998; 34(6):457–482.

5. Ebeige AB, Aloamaka CP. Mechanisms of hydralazine induced relaxation of arterial smooth muscle. Cardiovasc Res 1985; 19:400–405.

6. Powers D, Papadakos P, Wallin J. Parenteral hydralazine revisited. J Emerg Med 1998; 16(2):191–196.

7. Jacobs M. Mechanism of action of hydralazine on vascular smooth muscle. Biochem Pharmacol 1984; 33:2915–2919.

8. Azuma J, Sawamura A, Awata N, Kishimoto S, Sperelakis N. Mechanism of direct cardiostimulating effects of hydralazine. Eur J Pharmacol 1987; 135:137–144.

9. Direct acting vasodilators. In: Brenner BM, Rector F, eds. The Kidney. 6th ed. 2265–2267.

10. Lesser JM, Israili ZH, Davis DC, Dayton PG. Metabolism and disposition of hydralazine in man and dog. Drug Metab Dispos 1974; 2:351–360.

11. Ludden TM, McNay JL, Shepard AMM. Clinical pharmacokinetics of hydralazine. Clin Pharmacokinetics 1982; 7:185–205.

12. Ludden TM, Shepard AMM, McNay JL, Lin MS. Hydralazine kinetics in hypertensive patients after intravenous administration. Clin Pharmacol Ther 1980; 28:736–742.

13. Reece PA, Cozamanis I, Zacest R. Hydralazine kinetics after single and repeated oral doses. Clin Pharmacol Ther 1980; 28:769–778.

14. Reece PA, Stafford I, Prager RH, Walker GJ, Zacest R. Synthesis formulation and clinical pharmacologic evaluation of hydralazine pyruvic acid hydrazone in two healthy volunteers. J Pharm Sci 1985; 74:193–196.

15. Wei S, Kasayu Y, Yanagisawa M, Kimura S, Masaki T, Goto K. Studies on endothelium dependant vasorelaxation by hydralazine in porcine coronary artery. Eur J Pharmacol 1997; 321(3):307–314.

16. Cameron HA, Ramsey LE. The lupus syndrome induced by hydralazine. Br Med J 1984; 289:410–412.

17. Merkel PA. Drug associated vasculitis. Curr Opin Rheumatol 1998; 10:45–50.

18. Cornacchia E, Globus J, Maybum J, Strahler J, Hanash S, Richardson B. Hydralazine and procainamide inhibit T cell DNA methylation and induce auto reactivity. J Immunol 1988; 140:2197–2200.

19. Rey E, Le Lorier J, Burgess E, Lange I, Leduc L. Pharmacologic treatment of hypertensive disorders in pregnancy. Can Med Assoc J 1997; 157:1245–1254.

20. Ram CV. Management of refractory hypertension. Am J Ther 2003; 10:122–126.

21. Hibbard JU. Hypertensive disease and pregnancy. J Hypertension 2002; 20(suppl 2):S29–S33.

22. Cohn JN, Archibald DG, Ziesche S, Franciosa JA, Harston WE, Tristani FE, Dunkman WB, Jacobs W, Francis GS, Flohr KH et al. Effect of vasodilator therapy on mortality in chronic congestive heart failure. Results of a Veterans Administration Cooperative Study. NEJM 1986; 240:1547–1552.

23. Leblanc N, Wilde DW, Keef KD, Hume JR. Electrophysiological mechanisms of minoxidil sulfate induced vasodilation of rabbit portal vein. Circ Res 1989; 65:1102–1111.

24. Ogilvie RI. Comparative effects of vasodilator drugs on flow distribution and venous return. Can J Physiol Pharmacol 1985; 63:1345–1355.

25. Reichgott MJ. Minoxidil and pericardial effusion. An idiosyncratic reaction. Clin Pharmacol Ther 1981; 30:64–70.

26. Duvic M, Lemak NA, Valero V, Hymes SR, Farmer KL, Hortobagyi GN, Trancik RJ, Bandstra BA, Compton LD. A randomized trial of minoxidil in chemotherapy-induced alopecia. J Am Acad Dermatol 1996; 35(1):74–78.

27. Abdul M, Santo A, Hoosein N. Activity of potassium channel-blockers in breast cancer. Anticancer Res 2003; 23(4):3347–3351.

28. Leeuwenkamp OR, van Bennekom WP, van der Mark EJ, Bult A. Nitroprusside, antihypertensive drug and analytical reagent. Review of (photo)stability, pharmacology and analytical properties. Pharm Weekbl Sci 1984; 6(4):129–140.

29. Brogden RN, Markham A. Fenoldopam: a review of its pharmacodynamic and pharmacokinetic properties and intravenous clinical potential in the management of hypertensive urgencies and emergencies. Drugs 1997; 54(4):634–650.

33

Investigational Drugs for the Treatment of Hypertension

ALEXANDER M. M. SHEPHERD

University of Texas Health Sciences Center at San Antonio, San Antonio, Texas, USA

KEYPOINTS

- Aldosterone antagonists may prevent the development of cardiac fibrosis.
- Dopamine 1 agonists cause arterial vasodilation in the renal, mesenteric, cerebral, and coronary arterial beds.
- Peripheral dopamine 2 receptor agonists reduce norepinephrine and aldosterone release.
- Endothclin antagonists may reduce blood pressure, prevent left ventricular hypertrophy, and preserve myocardial function.
- Central imidazoline agonists and 5HT1A antagonists reduce central sympathetic outflow.
- Neutral endopeptidase inhibitors prevent ANP breakdown and angiotensin II generation.
- Potassium channel openers are of limited use because of reflex tachycardia and headache.
- Renin inhibitors prevent angiotensin II formation.

SUMMARY

Several groups of drugs are in development for treatment of hypertension. While some may come to fruition,

difficulties with the development of each has limited their potential. The most promising at present appears to be the metalloprotease inhibitors, if the problem of the angioedema can be solved.

I. INTRODUCTION

Several groups of drugs are in development for treatment of hypertension. Although some may come to fruition, difficulties with the development of each have limited their potential. The most promising, at present, appears to be the metalloprotease inhibitors, if the problem of the angioedema can be solved. Several other groups look as though they may not add to our useful armamentarium for treating hypertension for the reason that they lower blood pressure, but not with fewer adverse effects or with more efficacy than the drugs that we have available already. Part of their dilemma is that with some exceptions, the risk of hypertension appears to fall largely as a function of the extent of the blood pressure reduction, rather than as a function of the form of therapy used to reduce it. This means that it is much more difficult for a new form of therapy to distinguish itself from currently available therapy.

Several classes of drugs are under investigation as therapy of hypertension. These include the following:

- *Aldosterone antagonists* may prevent the development of cardiac fibrosis.
- *Dopamine 1 agonists* cause arterial vasodilation in the renal, mesenteric, cerebral, and coronary arterial beds.
- *Peripheral dopamine 2 receptor agonists* reduce norepinephrine and aldosterone release.
- *Endothelin antagonists* mixed endothelin ETA/ ETB receptor antagonists may reduce blood pressure, prevent left ventricular hypertrophy, and preserve myocardial function.
- *Central imidazoline agonists* reduce central sympathetic outflow without the sedation.
- *5HT1A antagonists* reduce central sympathetic outflow.
- *Neutral endopeptidase inhibitors* prevent ANP breakdown and angiotensin II generation.
- *Potassium channel openers* are of limited use because of reflex tachycardia and headache.
- *Renin inhibitors* are a specific way to prevent angiotensin II formation.

II. ALDOSTERONE ANTAGONISTS

It is no longer considered sufficient to lower blood pressure to normal or near-normal in essential hypertension. Clinicians now also have a duty to try to reverse the pathophysiologic changes which have occurred in the cardiovascular system as a result of the hypertension. It has been shown that aldosterone plays a central role in inducing fibrosis of the heart muscle and of the large arteries. It probably does this by acting directly on the heart through cardiac mineralocorticoid receptors (1). Administration of the aldosterone antagonist spironolactone prevents the development of cardiac fibrosis in rats with experimentally induced left ventricular hypertrophy at doses which do not alter blood pressure. It does so without reducing the left ventricular hypertrophy itself. This finding supports the idea of a direct effect of aldosterone on generation of cardiac fibrosis and on the ability of aldosterone antagonists to oppose the formation of this fibrous tissue.

Two aldosterone antagonists, eplerenone and spironolactone, have been used clinically in the therapy of hypertension. They cause a greater increase in left ventricular diastolic indices compared with a control group, without changing blood pressure, and with a similar decrease in left ventricular mass index. In essential hypertension patients, left ventricular diastolic function was improved when a low dose of aldosterone antagonist was added to other hypertensive therapy.

Eplerenone has recently been approved for use in hypertension in doses of 50–100 mg daily. Peak blood levels are seen ~2 h after oral dosing. The plasma protein binding is 50%, and the apparent distribution volume is ~1 L/kg. The drug is broken down by cytochrome P450 3A4, principally in the liver. The plasma half-life is ~5 h. Side effects are few in number and include gynecomastia and hyperkalemia. These adverse effects appear to occur with lower frequency than with spironolactone. They occur in <1% of patients receiving eplerenone. Eplerenone appears to have greater selectivity for aldosterone receptors compared with other receptors. There has been no direct comparison between eplerenone and spironolactone with regard to efficacy and safety. These two drugs are approximately equi-effective in reducing blood pressure in hypertension, but their ability to reverse target organ damage has not been compared.

Spironolactone is extensively metabolized to several breakdown products including canrenone and 7 α-thiomethylspirolactone. Both these metabolites are pharmacologically active. Canrenone is the dethioacetylated (i.e., nonsulfur-containing) breakdown product. It is canrenone which is thought to account for much of spironolactone's therapeutic effect. Canrenone and canrenoate exist in equilibrium in plasma. Canrenoate does not contribute much antagonism of mineralocorticoid activity (2–5).

Canrenone acts by competing with aldosterone for intracellular mineralocorticoid receptors. Canrenoate potassium has one major advantage over spironolactone in that it is soluble in water. This permits intravenous administration when rapid effect is required.

Blood pressure lowering is seen in hypertensive patients within ~1 week after administration of canrenoate potassium. Oral absorption of both canrenone and canrenoate potassium is good (>80%) after oral administration (6). The drugs are highly protein-bound, 85–90% in plasma, volume of distribution is 0.5 L/kg for canrenoate potassium, and 1.8 L/kg for canrenone (2,7). Total body clearance of canrenoate potassium is ~1 L/h and of canrenone is ~0.3 L/h (8,9). Elimination half-life varies from 4 to 22 h depending on which study is reviewed.

III. DOPAMINE 1 RECEPTOR AGONISTS

Dopamine 1 (DA1) receptors cause arterial vasodilation in the renal, mesenteric, cerebral, and coronary arterial beds when stimulated. Dopamine 2 (DA2) receptors, when stimulated, prevent norepinephrine release in presynaptic areas.

Dopamine is used in the emergency treatment of hypertension, but its use in essential hypertension is limited by its failure to be absorbed when it is given by mouth. Several agents which are absorbed from the gastrointestinal tract are being investigated for use in hypertension. One of these is the drug ibopamine. This drug is an agonist at DA1, DA2, β and α receptors. It is a pro-drug and is de-esterified by esterase hydrolysis in the gastrointestinal tract, in the liver, and in the blood, to form N-methyl dopamine (epinine), which is the active component. It is rapidly absorbed when given by mouth and has an elimination half-life of $\sim$2.5 h. Approximately 60% of the drug is excreted through the kidneys (10–12). Because of its multiple actions, its main use will probably be in heart failure and possible in acites, caused by hepatic cirrhosis, rather than in the treatment of essential hypertension.

The dopamine agonist presently available for use in hypertension in the United States is fenoldopam. It has selective postsynaptic DA1 receptor agonist properties (13). It is effective after being given by mouth but at present is used only after administration by the parental route, as there have been problems with the formulation of an oral preparation. This drug lowers blood pressure by vasodilation, particularly in the renal and splanchnic vascular beds. Oral administration is followed $\sim$1 h later by an anti-hypertensive response (14). The oral preparation is quite well absorbed, but there is extensive pre-systemic extraction, which results in low blood levels of the compound. The volume of distribution is $\sim$0.5 L/kg (15), and the drug is broken down in the liver by Phase I and Phase II metabolism to sulfate, glucuronide, and methoxy metabolites (14). Half-life is extremely short, between 5 and 10 min, which is a problem for a drug proposed to be used by mouth in the treatment of essential hypertension (16). The oral bioavailability is <6%, which is also a problem.

Dopexamine is being investigated in heart failure. It stimulates vascular DA1 receptors, resulting in arterial vasodilation, and also stimulates β-2-adrenergic receptors, which adds to the degree of peripheral vasodilation (17).

IV. PERIPHERAL DA2 RECEPTOR AGONISTS

Peripheral DA2 receptor agonists are found presynaptically on adrenergic nerve terminals and on the ganglia of the sympathetic nervous system. Activation of these receptors reduces norepinephrine release. In theory, selective stimulation of DA2 receptors provides a desirable therapy for hypertension with reduction of norepinephrine-induced vasoconstriction and also reduction of aldosterone release. The aldosterone reduction would prevent the adverse restructuring effects caused by

aldosterone in the vasculature, and inhibition of norepinephrine release causes arterial vasodilation with reduction in peripheral resistance.

V. ENDOTHELIN ANTAGONISTS

The endothelins are a group of vasoconstrictor peptides, which are important in the control of blood pressure. They are produced in many tissues, including in the vascular endothelium. Stimulation of the ETA receptors causes arterial vasoconstriction, myocardial hypertrophy, and fibrosis. Stimulation of the ETB receptors, on the other hand, causes differing effects depending on where the stimulation is seen. In vascular smooth muscle, there is vasoconstriction, and the vascular endothelial cells release nitric oxide and prostacyclin, which results in vasodilation. It may be seen, therefore, that antagonism of endothelin A and B receptors in the vascular smooth muscle, and the myocardium, may be of use in treating both hypertension and some of the end-organ damage (18). It is not clear whether it would be better to develop specific ETA receptor antagonists or mixed ETA/ETB receptor antagonists for the treatment of hypertension.

We know at least three different endothelins, which have significance with regard to the cardiovascular system in hypertension. The main endothelin produced by the endothelium is endothelin-1 (ET-1). This substance interacts with ETA or ETB receptors in the vascular smooth muscle to cause vasoconstriction and with ETB receptors in the endothelial cells to cause vasodilation.

Bosentan is the first orally administered endothelin antagonist. Oral bioavailability is 50%. Plasma protein binding is >98%, mainly to plasma albumen. Distribution volume is 0.5 L/kg (19). Bosentan is broken down in the liver by the hepatic isoenzymes cytochrome P450 2C9 and 3A4. It induces the activity of these enzymes and may induce the rate of its own metabolism, making dosing adjustment difficult when the drug is given chronically. The blood concentrations of bosentan on multiple dosing are $\sim$50% of those seen after single dose administration, possibly caused by this auto-induction. The elimination half-life in adults is between 5 and 8 h. This means that multiple daily doses may have to be taken (20,21). The most common adverse effect is mild-to-moderate headache occurring in about one-quarter of patients. Elevations in liver enzyme levels to more than three times the upper limits of normal are seen in $\sim$11% of patients. They tend to be asymptomatic and be reversible after reduction or cessation of dosing with bosentan. Drug interactions with other drugs metabolized by the same liver isoenzymes will be expected. These drugs will include warfarin and ketoconazole.

In one study, the mixed ETA/ETB receptor antagonist bosentan was given to adult hypertensive patients and was found to reduce blood pressures to approximately the same extent as was seen with 20 mg/day of the angiotensin converting inhibitor, enalapril (22). It did this without altering plasma levels of norepinephrine, angiotensin II, and plasma–renin activity. Unfortunately, bosentan is classified as being a pregnancy category X, indicating that it is expected to cause fetal harm if it is administered to pregnant women.

Tezosentan is also an ETA/ETB antagonist. However, it must be administered by intravenous infusion and is, therefore, not likely to be of use in the chronic treatment of hypertension. Most studies have been in the treatment of acute heart failure, where it has been shown to be effective at infusion rates of 20–50 mg/h for up to 48 h (23).

Enrasentan is a mixed endothelin ETA/ETB receptor antagonist, which reduces blood pressure, prevents left ventricular hypertrophy, and preserves myocardial function in an animal model of hypertension. Further studies are needed to determine whether it will be of clinical use in the treatment of hypertension (24).

The selective ETA receptor antagonist darusentan has been studied in patients with severe heart failure, being added to standard therapy, including angiotensin-converting enzyme inhibitors and β adergernic receptor antagonists. The drug produced some beneficial effects on hemodynamic parameters, together with reduction of neurohormonal levels in the blood (25).

VI. CENTRAL IMIDAZOLINE AGONISTS

Clonidine is an anti-hypertensive agent, which has been used for many years in the treatment of essential hypertension, with considerable success. It is quite effective at lowering blood pressure and the main limitation to its use is the high incidence of side effects. These side effects are symptomatic and troublesome to patients, thereby limiting its use. They include sedation and dry mouth, which occur in up to 30% of patients taking the drug. In addition, with doses approximately >0.8 mg/day, there is a risk of significant rebound hypertension, if the drug is stopped abruptly. This could readily occur in patients who forget to take their medications or who run out of tablets without ready access to a further prescription.

Clonidine acts in the brain by stimulating both α-2-adrenergic receptors and imidazoline receptors. The anti-hypertensive action is by reduction in central sympathetic outflow. This lowers blood pressure, principally by peripheral vasodilation, thus lowering peripheral resistance. It does so without stimulating the heart and without causing sodium retention. Thus, the hemodynamic profile is desirable but the side effects are a problem. Most, not all of these side effects, have been shown to occur by its action on the central α 2 adrenergic receptors. However, drugs have been developed, which act preferentially on imidazoline (Ii) receptors. Thus far, the two which are furthest along in development are moxonidine and rilmenidine. Figure 33.1 shows the central action of this group of drugs.

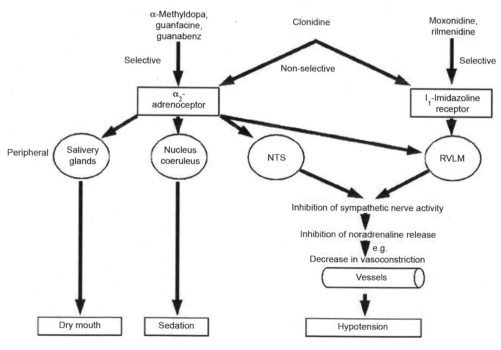

Figure 33.1   Targets of [α]2-adrenoceptor and imidazoline (I1)-receptor stimulants in the central nervous system. [With permission from van Zwieten. J Hypertens 1999; 17(12):1787–1797.]

Moxonidine acts centrally at imidazoline (Ii) receptors and has up to a 600-fold selectivity at these sites than at $\alpha 2$ receptors. It reduces serum norepinephrine and epinephrine levels by about one-third and also reduces plasma renin activity. After oral administration, plasma levels peak within 2 h. Oral bioavailability is $\sim$90% (26). Plasma protein binding is low at $\sim$7% (27). Distribution volume is between 2 and 3 L/kg. A 10–20% of the drug is broken down in the liver to metabolites, which have little activity. Plasma half-life is relatively short, 2–3 h, but duration of effect is quite long, permitting once daily dosing. The usual initial dose is 200 μg daily, which may be increased to a maximum of 600 μg daily in two divided doses. Because of the renal excretion, the plasma half-life increases with severe renal impairment, and thus, dose should be reduced.

Rilmenidine acts in the same way but does not appear to be quite so specific for imidazoline receptors as is moxonidine. Rilmenidine is well absorbed after oral administration with oral bioavailability of $\sim$100%. Food ingestion does not appear to change bioavailability. Peak blood levels occur within $\sim$2 h after oral dosing. Like moxonidine, rilmenidine is little bound to plasma proteins ($\sim$11%) and has a distribution volume between 4 and 5 L/kg. Most of the drug excreted is unchanged in the urine and the elimination half-life is between 8 and 10 h. The usual dose is 1–2 mg once daily.

It appears likely that even more selective agonists of I1 receptors will become available, thus reducing further the likelihood of adverse effects and reducing the potential for hypertensive rebound with sudden cessation of the drug.

VII. SEROTONIN 5HT1A AGONISTS

Stimulation of $5HT_{1A}$ receptors in the rostral ventrolateral medulla in the brain stem (28) will cause peripheral sympathetic inhibition and a reduction in heart rate (29,30).

Urapidil is a non stereoisomer drug with at least two clinically significant actions. The first is peripheral postsynaptic alpa 1 adrenoceptor antagonism, and the second is probably stimulation of the 5HT1A receptors in the brain stem. In animal experiments, the central action has been shown to be inhibited by the 5HT1A receptor antagonist, spiroxatrine (29,30). Because of ethical concerns, it is not possible at present to determine whether the same agonism occurs in humans with hypertension. There are, however, some suggestions that this is clinically relevant. It is known from animal experiments that reduced sympathetic outflow caused by agonism at 5HT1A receptors will reduce heart rate. Culbertson et al. (32) found that with increasing doses of urapidil, the heart rate did not increase as would be expected if the sole anti-hypertensive action was peripheral postsynaptic α-1 adrenoceptor antagonism.

The pharmacokinetics of urapidil are simple. It is rapidly and well absorbed with oral bioavailability of 78%. Terminal half-life is $\sim$3 h, and plasma clearance is 12 L/h. Approximately 17% of the drug appears in the urine as parent compound within 24 h of dosing. There is extensive hepatic metabolism to the para-hydroxylated (34% in urine), N-demethylated (4% in urine), and O-demethylated (3% in urine) products. Elimination is linear at usual clinical doses. This drug is not yet approved for use in the United States, but it has been in use in many European and other countries for some time. The drug is administered as a sustained-release capsule on a once or twice daily basis. Initial dose is usually 30 mg once daily in the morning, ranging up to a total of 180 mg daily in some patients. Dizziness occurs in $\sim$10% of patients, headache in 3%, and fatigue in 2%. Orthostatic hypotension and palpitations are seen in 1–2% of patients. As would be expected from knowledge of its mechanism of action, there are no alterations in biochemical parameters including cholesterol, triglycerides, and fasting blood sugar (33).

Several other 5HT1A agonists have also been investigated, but at this time it is not clear whether they will prove to be useful in treating systemic hypertension.

VIII. NEUTRAL ENDOPEPTIDASE INHIBITORS

The natriuretic peptides are substances secreted in the body, which possess the three properties of being diuretics, natriuretics, and vasodilators. Three different groups have been identified. Atrial natriuretic peptide (ANP) is produced mainly in the atria of the heart. Brain natriuretic peptide (BNP) is produced in the ventricles of the heart and of the brain. C-type natriuretic peptide (CNP) is produced in the vascular endothelium. The site and mechanism of action of the natriuretic peptides is shown in Fig. 33.2.

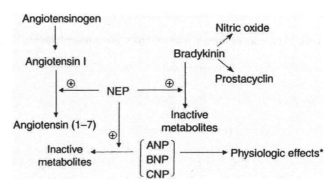

Figure 33.2 Description of the natriuretic peptide system. [With permission from Burnett JC Jr. Vasopeptidase inhibition: a new concept in blood pressure management. J Hypertens 1999; 17(suppl 1):S37–S43.]

ANP is a 28 residue peptide, which has diuretic, natriuretic, and vasodilator properties. It also inhibits vasopressin, aldosterone, and renin release. Other potentially beneficial effects in hypertension and heart failure include increase in glomerular filtration rate and reduction in cardiac pre- and after-load. Because blood levels of ANP are elevated in hypertension (34), it was initially felt that giving exogenous ANP might be of benefit in treating systemic hypertension. However, this largely failed to be of benefit, because the drug is poorly absorbed when given by mouth, and in addition, is rapidly cleared from the circulation.

Efforts then turned to prevent the breakdown of endogenous ANP. These efforts were met with much more success. This is done by inhibiting the zinc-dependent membrane-bound endopeptidase known as neutral endopeptidase (NEP). This endopeptidase is very similar to angiotensin-converting enzyme. At present, three classes of compounds are identified. These groups are well described in the article by Nawarskas et al. (35).

1. The first is the carboxyl inhibitors. Compounds identified are SCH 39370 (36) and UK 69578 (37).
2. The second is the thiol inhibitors, of which thiorphan was the first (38,39).
3. The third group is the phosphoryl and hydroxamic acid inhibitors represented by kelatorphan (40).

By inhibiting the degradation of ANP, its half-life is prolonged and its clinical effect is increased. In addition to its direct effect of diuresis and natriuresis, these compounds may increase the level of bradykinin in the kidney (41). This may increase the levels of bradykinin in the heart, which would be expected to have a cardioprotective effect. In addition, these compounds decrease circulating endothelin levels. Endothelin is a potent vasoconstrictor substance.

There is no doubt that inhibiting neutral endopeptidase in healthy volunteers can cause increases in plasma ANP levels and can cause a natriuresis. The drugs which have been used are UK 69578 (37) and acetorphan (42). Neither of these drugs has demonstrated a reduction in blood pressure in healthy volunteers. Hypertensive subjects have, in some instances, had lowering of blood pressure, and in other instances, failed to have any anti-hypertensive effects. Patients on a high salt diet failed to have a reduction in blood pressure, and the blood pressure in patients on a normal salt diet was minimally reduced. It appears, therefore, that selective NEP inhibition by itself is not likely to provide useful anti-hypertensive effects in hypertensive patients. Their effect in heart failure is more likely to be of clinical benefit.

When an NEP inhibitor was combined with an angiotensin-converting enzyme inhibitor, the blood pressure reduction was enhanced in rats (39) and in hypertensives (43). Because of this finding, molecules have been synthesized, which will inhibit both NEP and angiotensin-converting enzyme. The first of these to come close to being on the market is omapatrilat, being developed by Bristol Myers Squibb. This drug has the appearance of being almost ideal because the angiotensin-converting enzyme inhibitors are more likely to be efficacious in high renin hypertension and the NEP inhibitors to be more effective in low renin hypertension. Thus, this drug should be effective in both high and low renin hypertension. Omapatrilat is a dual vasopeptidase (metalloprotease) inhibitor.

Omapatrilat has 20–30% systemic bioavailability when given by mouth and this is not altered by concomitant food ingestion. Protein binding is 80% in plasma, and the volume of distribution is ~21 L/kg. The drug is extensively metabolized in the liver, and there dots not appear to be significant accumulation of active metabolites in blood. The plasma half-life in healthy subjects is between 14 and 19 h, probably permitting once daily dosing. The clinical efficacy is good. Blood pressure is reduced by 26/17 mmHg at peak effect (44). The safety profile appeared to be what one would expect, that is, very few, symptomatic adverse effects. However, the drug was found to cause a threefold higher incidence of angioedema in hypertensive patients than enalapril (2.2% vs. 0.7%). In heart failure, the likelihood of angioedema was not different between the two agents. The risk of angioedema from omapatrilat has been well reviewed by Floras (45). It was found that ~2.2% of all patients, 5.5% of blacks, 3.9% of smokers, and 1.8% of nonsmokers had symptomatic angioedema when given omapatrilat. In congestive heart failure, the likelihood is much lower, with only 0.8% of patients having symptomatic angioedema. Further work on defining the risk in the different groups is being undertaken.

IX. POTASSIUM CHANNEL OPENERS

The ability to open potassium channels resides in a broad range of endogenous and synthetic substances. Adenosine $5'$-triphosphate (ATP)-sensitive K+ channels have been identified in vascular smooth muscle (46). They are activated by ATP-dependent K+ channel openers (47,48). This results in hyperpolarization of the plasma membrane and vasodilation of the smooth muscle, possibly by preventing the opening of voltage-activated calcium channels in the smooth muscle. These ATP-sensitive K+ channel openers have been investigated for the treatment of hypertension and angina (49,50).

Several potassium channel openers have been investigated, including SKP-450, aprikalim, cromakalim, lemakalim, and nicorandil. Other potassium channel openers, including diazoxide, pinacidil, and minoxidil, have been in clinical use for some time. None is used a great deal for the treatment of hypertension, although each has a niche in our armamentarium. The main reason for their limited use is that the vasodilation induced causes a reflex increase in heart rate and a longer term induction of edema to limit the fall in blood pressure. This means that they cannot be used as monotherapy. In addition, a migraine-like head-ache is an expected adverse effect caused by cerebral vasodilation.

KR-30450 is orally absorbed in humans and 200–300 μg causes arterial vasodilation. Concurrent food intake does not affect the extent of absorption. Aprikalim may have utility in cardioplegic arrest and dilates human coronary arteries. Cromokalim has been investigated for treating hypertension and asthma (51,52).

Although this group of substances may have utility in treating other forms of human disease, the hemodynamic profile and the symptomatic adverse effects will signifi-cantly limit their use in the maintenance therapy of hypertension.

X. RENIN INHIBITORS

The development and utilization of angiotensin-converting enzyme inhibitors in the treatment of systemic hypertension was a major advance. Their use has permitted clinicians to effectively treat hypertension with a lower likelihood of symptomatic adverse effects than was seen with older medications. However, their nonspe-cificity may well be the basis for the adverse effects seen. These adverse effects may be due to accumulation of bradykinin and consist of a dry, irritating cough, seen in approximately one patient in 10, and angioedema, which is usually mild but may result in the necessity for emergency tracheostomy in a few patients.

Renin and pro-renin are found in the juxtaglomerular apparatus in the tubules of the kidneys. They are released in response to several stimuli and cause cleavage of angio-tensinogen, resulting in liberation of angiotensin I. Angiotensin I interacts with angiotensin-converting enzyme, resulting in angiotensin II, a potent vasoconstric-tor. Unfortunately, angiotensin-converting enzyme not only interacts with angiotensin I but also with bradykinin, encephalon, and other hormones. This nonspecificity results in accumulation of bradykinin, which not only contributes to the anti-hypertensive effect but also probably to the adverse effects described earlier. An alternative, and more specific, way to prevent angiotensin II formation would be to inhibit the action of renin. Renin is highly specific for angiotensinogen.

A diagram of the renin–angiotensin system, with the site of action of the renin inhibitors is shown in Fig. 33.3.

Development of clinically useful renin inhibitors has been difficult for several reasons. The first group to be

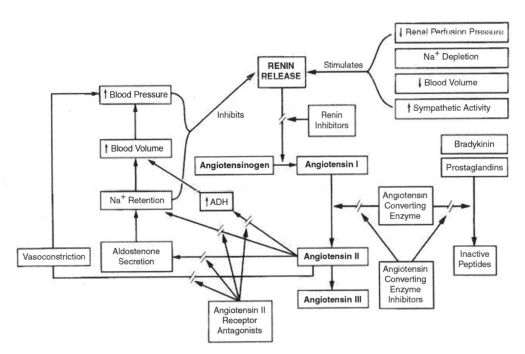

Figure 33.3 Diagram of renin–angiotensin aldosterone system. [With permission from Foote EF, Halstenson CE. New therapeutic agents in the management of hypertension: angiotensin II-receptor antagonists and renin inhibitors. Ann Pharmacother 1993; 27(12):1495–1503.]

developed were antibodies to renin. Initially, these were nonspecific, being prepared from crude kidney extracts. Because these are antibodies, they must be given parenterally, and in addition, when given over a period of time, they are likely to be significantly antigenic.

Subsequently, molecules based on angiotensinogen were developed which bound tightly to renin and prevented its action. The next step was the development of pepstatin analogs which resulted, unfortunately, in a low level of renin inhibition with poor specificity. More recently, an angiotensinogen analog substrate was found to compete for renin activity and resulted in an inactive compound being formed. This development process has been advanced by the synthesis of lower molecular weight peptides, with substances as small as dipeptides (53,54) being developed. Most recently, nonpeptide compounds have been found to have high potency and specificity as substrate renin inhibitors (55–57). This development has been well described in the excellent review article by Lin and Frishman (58). The development of this latter group of renin inhibitors has not been without its problems. Their systemic bioavailability after oral administration has generally been poor because of poor absorption from the gastrointestinal tract and high first-pass uptake by the liver. In addition, they have tended to have small volumes of distribution, with most of the drug being found in the central compartment. This makes it available for elimination by the liver and also results in them penetrating less well into the tissues, which is their site of action. Remikiren has a longer plasma half-life than prior drugs of the same class, probably because it is distributed more peripherally to the tissues rather than because it is broken down by the liver more slowly (59). Their potency in inhibiting renin activity has been significantly lower *in vivo* than *in vitro*, probably because of extensive plasma protein binding. This results in a much lower free, active, drug concentration in the blood. For example, the potency of remikiren, enalkiren, and CGP 38560 was up to 35-fold lower in human plasma than against pure renin in solution (60).

When these drugs are given to salt replete healthy volunteers, there is no change in blood pressure or in heart rate, as is seen also with the angiotensin-converting enzyme inhibitors (55,59,61). Their efficacy in hypertensive patients appears to improve with salt depletion. Remikiren was given to hypertensive patients for 1 week, and over that week, the anti-hypertensive effect diminished (62,63). One of the most recently developed and investigated renin inhibitors is aliskiren, an octanamide which is a nonpeptidic orally active renin inhibitor (64). Aliskiren seems to be closer to a clinically useful drug, from a pharmacokinetic point of view, as it has dose-dependent drug levels in the plasma. Angiotensin 2 levels were also reduced in a dose-dependent fashion,

indicating the potential for clinically useful effect in humans. Maximal reduction of angiotensin II was achieved within 1 h of aliskiren administration. The plasma half-life is ~24 h, indicating that once-a-day dosing would be possible.

The incidence of adverse effects has generally been low with this group of drugs, as would be expected from their high specificity for inhibition of renin.

REFERENCES

1. Lombes M, Farman N, Bonvalet JP, Zennaro MC. Identification and role of aldosterone receptors in the cardiovascular system. Ann Endocrinol (Paris) 2000; 61(1):41–46.
2. Overdiek HW, Merkus FW. The metabolism and biopharmaceutics of spironolactone in man. Rev Drug Metab Drug Interact 1987; 5(4):273–302.
3. LaCagnin LB, Lutsie P, Colby HD. Conversion of spironolactone to 7 α-thiomethylspironolactone by hepatic and renal microsomes. Biochem Pharmacol 1987; 36(20):3439–3444.
4. Merkus FW. Is canrenone the major metabolite of spironolactone? Clin Pharm 1983; 2(3):209–210.
5. Ramsay L, Shelton J, Harrison I, Tidd M, Asbury M. Spironolactone and potassium canrenoate in normal man. Clin Pharmacol Ther 1976; 20(2):167–177.
6. Sadee W, Dagcioglu M, Schroder R. Pharmacokinetics of spironolactone, canrenone and canrenoate-K in humans. J Pharmacol Exp Ther 1973; 185(3):686–695.
7. Dahlof CG, Lundborg P, Persson BA, Regardh CG. Re-evaluation of the antimineralocorticoid effect of the spironolactone metabolite, canrenone, from plasma concentrations determined by a new high-pressure liquid-chromatographic method. Drug Metab Dispos 1979; 7(2):103–107.
8. Karim A, Ranney RE, Maibach HI. Pharmacokinetic and metabolic fate of potassium canrenoate (SC-14266) in man. J Pharm Sci 1971; 60(5):708–715.
9. Krause W, Karras J, Seifert W. Pharmacokinetics of canrenone after oral administration of spironolactone and intravenous injection of canrenoate-K in healthy man. Eur J Clin Pharmacol 1983; 25(4):449–453.
10. Azzollini F, de Caro L, Longo A, Pelosi G, Rolandi E, Ventresca GP, Lodola E. Ibopamine kinetics after single and multiple dosing in patients with congestive heart failure. Int J Clin Pharmacol Ther Toxicol 1988; 26(11):544–551.
11. Lodola E, Borgia M, Longo A, Pocchiari F, Pataccini R, Sher D. Ibopamine kinetics after a single oral dose in healthy volunteers. Arzneimittelforschung 1986; 36(2A):345–348.
12. Leier CV, Ren JH, Huss P, Unverferth DV. The hemodynamic effects of ibopamine, a dopamine congener, in patients with congestive heart failure. Pharmacotherapy 1986; 6(1):35–40.
13. Lokhandwala MF, Hegde SS. Cardiovascular pharmacology of adrenergic and dopaminergic receptors:

therapeutic significance in congestive heart failure. Am J Med 1991; 90(5B):2S–9S.

14. Boppana VK, Dolce KM, Cyronak MJ, Ziemniak JA. Simplified procedures for the determination of fenoldopam and its metabolites in human plasma by high-performance liquid chromatography with electrochemical detection: comparison of manual and robotic sample preparation methods. J Chromatogr 1989; 487(2):385–399.

15. Allison NL, Dubb JW, Ziemniak JA, Alexander F, Stote RM. The effect of fenoldopam, a dopaminergic agonist, on renal hemodynamics. Clin Pharmacol Ther 1987; 41(3):282–288.

16. Weber RR, McCoy CE, Ziemniak JA, Frederickson ED, Goldberg LI, Murphy MB. Pharmacokinetic and pharmacodynamic properties of intravenous fenoldopam, a dopamine1-receptor agonist, in hypertensive patients. Br J Clin Pharmacol 1988; 25(1):17–21.

17. Brown RA, Dixon J, Farmer JB, Hall JC, Humphries RG, Ince F, O'Connor SE, Simpson WT, Smith GW. Dopexamine: a novel agonist at peripheral dopamine receptors and β 2-adrenoceptors. Br J Pharmacol 1985; 85(3):599–608.

18. Ram CV. Possible therapeutic role of endothelin antagonists in cardiovascular disease. Am J Ther 2003; 10(6):396–400.

19. Dingemanse J, Bodin F, Weidekamm E, Kutz K, van Giersbergen P. Influence of food intake and formulation on the pharmacokinetics and metabolism of bosentan, a dual endothelin receptor antagonist. J Clin Pharmacol 2002; 42(3):283–289.

20. van Giersbergen PL, Halabi A, Dingemanse J. Single- and multiple-dose pharmacokinetics of bosentan and its interaction with ketoconazole. Br J Clin Pharmacol 2002; 53(6):589–595.

21. Weber C, Schmitt R, Birnboeck H, Hopfgartner G, van Marle SP, Peeters PA, Jonkman JH, Jones CR. Pharmacokinetics and pharmacodynamics of the endothelin-receptor antagonist bosentan in healthy human subjects. Clin Pharmacol Ther 1996; 60(2):124–137.

22. Krum H, Viskoper RJ, Lacourciere Y, Budde M, Charlon V. The effect of an endothelin-receptor antagonist, bosentan, on blood pressure in patients with essential hypertension. Bosentan Hypertension Investigators [see comment]. N Engl J Med 1998; 338(12):784–790.

23. Dingemanse J, Clozel M, van Giersbergen PL. Pharmacokinetics and pharmacodynamics of tezosentan, an intravenous dual endothelin receptor antagonist, following chronic infusion in healthy subjects. Br J Clin Pharmacol 2002; 53(4):355–362.

24. Cosenzi A. Enrasentan, an antagonist of endothelin receptors. Cardiovasc Drug Rev 2003; 21(1):1–16.

25. Nakov R, Pfarr E, Eberle S, HEAT Investigators. Darusentan: an effective endothelin A receptor antagonist for treatment of hypertension. Am J Hypertens 2002; 15(7):583–589.

26. Theodor RA et al. Influence of food on the oral bioavailability of moxonidine. Eur J Drug Metab & Pharmaco 1992; 17(1):61–66.

27. Kirch W, Hutt HJ, Planitz V. The influence of renal function on clinical pharmacokinetics of moxonidine. Clin Pharmaco 1988; 15(4):245–253.

28. Dreteler GH, Wouters W, Saxena PR. Comparison of the cardiovascular effects of the 5-HT1A receptor agonist flesinoxan with that of 8-OH-DPAT in the rat. Eur J Pharmacol 1990; 180(2–3):339–349.

29. Kolassa N, Beller KD, Sanders KH. Involvement of brain 5-HT1A receptors in the hypotensive response to urapidil. Review Am J Cardiol 1989; 64(7):7D–10D.

30. Ramage AG. The mechanism of the sympathoinhibitory action of urapidil: role of 5-HT1A receptors. Br J Pharmacol 1991; 102(4):998–1002.

31. Dabire H, Cherqui C, Fournier B, Schmitt H. Vascular postsynaptic effects of some 5-HT1-like receptor agonists in the pithed rat. Eur J Pharmacol 1988; 150(1–2):143–148.

32. Culbertson VL, Bryant PJ, Cady WJ, Rubison RM, Piepho RW, Nies AS, Byyny RL. Acute effects of increasing doses of urapidil in patients with hypertension. Clin Pharmacol Ther 1986; 39(6):690–696.

33. Prichard BN, Tomlinson B, Renondin JC. Urapidil, a multiple-action α-blocking drug. Am J Cardiol 1989; 64(7):11D–15D.

34. Sagnella GA, Markandu ND, Shore AC, MacGregor GA. Raised circulating levels of atrial natriuretic peptides in essential hypertension. Lancet 1986; 1(8474):179–181.

35. Nawarskas J, Rajan V, Frishman WH. Vasopeptidase inhibitors, neutral endopeptidase inhibitors, and dual inhibitors of angiotensin-converting enzyme and neutral endopeptidase. Heart Dis 2001; 3(6):378–385.

36. Sybertz EJ, Chiu PJ, Vemulapalli S, Pitts B, Foster CJ, Watkins RW, Barnett A, Haslanger MF. SCH 39370, a neutral metalloendopeptidase inhibitor, potentiates biological responses to atrial natriuretic factor and lowers blood pressure in desoxycorticosterone acetate-sodium hypertensive rats. J Pharmacol Exp Ther 1989; 250(2):624–631.

37. Northridge DB, Jardine AG, Alabaster CT, Barclay PL, Connell JM, Dargie HJ, Dilly SG, Findlay IN, Lever AF, Samuels GM. Effects of UK 69 578: a novel atriopeptidase inhibitor. Lancet 1989; 2(8663):591–593.

38. Trapani AJ, Smits GJ, McGraw DE, Spear KL, Koepke JP, Olins GM, Blaine EH. Thiorphan, an inhibitor of endopeptidase 24.11, potentiates the natriuretic activity of atrial natriuretic peptide. J Cardiovasc Pharmacol 1989; 14(3):419–424.

39. Seymour AA, Sheldon JH, Smith PL, Asaad M, Rogers WL. Potentiation of the renal responses to bradykinin by inhibition of neutral endopeptidase 3.4.24.11 and angiotensin-converting enzyme in anesthetized dogs. J Pharmacol Exp Ther 1994; 269(1):263–270.

40. Roques BP. New approach in the research of analgesics and antihypertensive agents. Ann Pharm Fr 1991; 49(6):317–326.

41. Granger JP. Inhibitors of ANF metabolism. Potential therapeutic agents in cardiovascular disease [comment]. Circulation 1990; 82(1):313–315.

42. Gros C, Souque A, Schwartz JC, Duchier J, Cournot A, Baumer P, Lecomte JM. Protection of atrial natriuretic factor against degradation: diuretic and natriuretic responses after in vivo inhibition of enkephalinase (EC 3.4.24.11) by acetorphan. Proc Natl Acad Sci USA 1989; 86(19):7580–7584.

43. Favrat B, Burnier M, Nussberger J, Lecomte JM, Brouard R, Waeber B, Brunner HR. Neutral endopeptidase versus angiotensin converting enzyme inhibition in essential hypertension. J Hypertens 1995; 13(7):797–804.

44. Waeber B. Vasopeptidase inhibition: a new mechanism of action—a new antihypertensive drug. Schweiz Rundsch Med Prax 2000; 89(16):649–653.

45. Floras JS. Vasopeptidase inhibition: a novel approach to cardiovascular therapy. Can J Cardiol 2002; 18(2):177–182.

46. Standen NB, Quayle JM, Davies NW, Brayden JE, Huang Y, Nelson MT. Hyperpolarizing vasodilators activate ATP-sensitive K+ channels in arterial smooth muscle. Science 1989; 245(4914):177–180.

47. Hiraoka M, Fan Z. Activation of ATP-sensitive outward K+ current by nicorandil (2-nicotinamidoethyl nitrate) in isolated ventricular myocytes. J Pharmacol Exp Ther 1989; 250(1):278–285.

48. Arena JP, Kass RS. Activation of ATP-sensitive K channels in heart cells by pinacidil: dependence on ATP. Am J Physiol 1989; 257(6 Pt 2):H2092–H2096.

49. Quast U. Potassium channel openers: pharmacological and clinical aspects. Fundam Clin Pharmacol 1992; 6(7):279–293.

50. Di Somma S, Liguori V, Petitto M, Carotenuto A, Bokor D, de Divitiis O, de Divitiis M. A double-blind comparison of nicorandil and metoprolol in stable effort angina pectoris. Cardiovasc Drugs Ther 1993; 7(1):119–123.

51. Williams AJ, Lee TH, Cochrane GM, Hopkirk A, Vyse T, Chiew F, Lavender E, Richards DH, Owen S, Stone P. Attenuation of nocturnal asthma by cromakalim. Lancet 1990; 336(8711):334–336.

52. Suzuki S, Yano K, Kusano S, Hashimoto T. Antihypertensive effect of levcromakalim in patients with essential hypertension. Study by 24-h ambulatory blood pressure monitoring. Arzneimittelforschung 1995; 45(8):859–864.

53. Kokubu T, Hiwada K, Murakami E, Imamura Y, Matsueda R, Yabe Y, Koike H, Iijima Y. Highly potent and specific inhibitors of human renin. Hypertension 1985; 7(3): 8–11.

54. Glassman HN, Kleinert HD, Boger RS, Moyse DM, Griffiths AN, Luther RR. Clinical pharmacology of enalkiren, a novel, dipeptide renin inhibitor. J Cardiovasc Pharmacol 1990; 16:S76–S81.

55. de Gasparo M, Cumin F, Nussberger J, Guyenne TT, Wood JM, Menard J. Pharmacological investigations of a new renin inhibitor in normal sodium-unrestricted volunteers. Br J Clin Pharmacol 1989; 27(5):587–596.

56. Boyd SA, Fung AK, Baker WR, Mantei RA, Armiger YL, Stein HH, Cohen J, Egan DA, Barlow JL, Klinghofer V. C-terminal modifications of nonpeptide renin inhibitors: improved oral bioavailability via modification of physico-chemical properties. J Med Chem 1992; 35:1735–1746.

57. Sham HL, Bolis G, Stein HH, Fesik SW, Marcotte PA, Plattner JJ, Rempel CA, Greer J. Renin inhibitors. Design and synthesis of a new class of conformationally restricted analogues of angiotensinogen. J Med Chem 1988; 31:284–295.

58. Lin C, Frishman WH. Renin inhibition: a novel therapy for cardiovascular disease. Am Heart J 1996; 131(5):1024–1034.

59. Kleinbloesem CH, Weber C, Fahrner E, Dellenbach M, Welker H, Schroter V, Belz GG. Hemodynamics, biochemical effects, and pharmacokinetics of the renin inhibitor remikiren in healthy human subjects. Clin Pharmacol Ther 1993; 53(5):585–592.

60. Clozel JP, Fischli W. Comparative effects of three different potent renin inhibitors in primates. Hypertension 1993; 22(1):9–17.

61. Nussberger J, Delabays A, de Gasparo M, Cumin F, Waeber B, Brunner HR, Menard J. Hemodynamic and biochemical consequences of renin inhibition by infusion of CGP 38560A in normal volunteers. Hypertension 1989; 13(6):948–953.

62. Rongen GA, Lenders JW, Smits P, Thien T. Clinical pharmacokinetics and efficacy of renin inhibitors. Clin Pharmacokinet 1995; 29:6–14.

63. Kobrin I, Viskoper RJ, Laszt A, Bock J, Weber C, Charlon V. Effects of an orally active renin inhibitor, Ro 42–5892, in patients with essential hypertension. Am J Hypertension 1993; 6(5):349–356.

64. Nussberger J, Wuerzner G, Jensen C, Brunner HR. Angiotensin II suppression in humans by the orally active renin inhibitor Aliskiren (SPP100): comparison with enalapril. Hypertension 2002; 39(1):E1–E8.

34

Combination Therapy in the Treatment of Hypertension

BARRY J. MATERSON, RICHARD A. PRESTON

University of Miami School of Medicine, Miami, Florida, USA

KEYPOINTS

- Worldwide, far less than one-third of all hypertensive patients are treated to goal blood pressure of $<140/90$ mmHg or to $130/80$ mmHg if they have concomitant diabetes mellitus or chronic renal disease.
- Achieving these goal blood pressures usually requires more than one antihypertensive drug.
- Commercially available combination drugs can be substituted for individual drugs in order to improve patient compliance with therapy and often reduce cost.
- Combination drugs can be used as initial antihypertensive therapy when the baseline blood pressure is

$>20/10$ mmHg above goal blood pressure or when goal is unlikely to be achieved with a single agent.
- Ideal combination products last at least 24 h, have at least additive components, and have minimal adverse effects.

SUMMARY

Evidence supports the concept that therapeutic reduction of intra-arterial pressure (blood pressure) well into the biologically normal range confers substantial protection against death and target organ damage associated with arterial hypertension. This is especially true for patients who also have diabetes mellitus, chronic renal disease, isolated systolic hypertension, or other cardiovascular risk factors. There is also evidence that most patients will require more than one drug in order to achieve these more aggressive therapeutic goals. Therefore, it has become appropriate to use more than one drug as initial therapy for such patients (1). Many commercially available combination products are now recommended for initial antihypertensive therapy.

I. INTRODUCTION

Although one always hopes for a "magic bullet" that will target a specific problem when used alone, many diseases have been treated more effectively with combination chemotherapy. Examples include combination chemotherapy for tuberculosis, cancer, certain diseases of the kidney, and Human Immunodeficiency Virus (HIV). Combination therapy for the treatment of hypertension is not new. Dr. Edward D. Freis designed his landmark trial of antihypertensive therapy to use the combination of reserpine 0.1 mg and hydrochlorothiazide 50 mg in a single tablet to be given twice daily. Hydralazine 25 mg given three times daily was added to that combination (2). The triple combination was later marketed as Ser-Ap-Es, which contained 0.1 mg reserpine, 25 mg hydrochlorothiazide, and 15 mg hydralazine in the same tablet. This combination continues to be marketed worldwide under many trade names (see Table 34.1). Simply put, the majority of hypertensive patients are going to require two or more drugs in order to achieve their goal blood pressure.

Much has been written about what the clinician can do or should do when confronted by failure of the initially selected antihypertensive drug. We have recently reviewed the basic concepts (3). If the practitioner has carefully matched the patient to the drug selected, the odds of success are considerably increased. Should the drug fail to achieve goal, the practitioner should consider possible causes for that failure such as unidentified secondary hypertension, unrecognized sleep apnea, countereffects by drugs such as nonsteroidal anti-inflammatory drugs or pressor agents, office or clinic (white coat) hypertension, psychological problems, or failure of the patient to take the drug as prescribed. If these factors are ruled out, the practitioner has four basic choices:

1. Stop the first drug and select a drug better matched to the patient's age-by-race profile (sequential therapy).
2. Titrate the first drug to maximum dose or toxicity and then add a second drug (stepped care). If the first drug was not a diuretic, a diuretic should be strongly considered as the second drug.
3. Add a second drug without reaching the maximum or toxic dose of the first drug (combination therapy).

4. By-pass this entire sequence by recognizing those patients who are likely to benefit from at least two drugs (4) and treat with two drugs initially (initial combination therapy).

II. MONOTHERAPY

Before we consider combination therapy in detail, it is important to address single-drug therapy in that population of hypertensive patients who are most likely to benefit from only one drug.

A. Veterans Administration Cooperative Study on Single-Drug Therapy

The Veterans Administration Cooperative Study Group on Antihypertensive Agents (5) performed a prospective, double-masked clinical trial on the monotherapy of hypertension (6–8). In this trial, 1292 hypertensive men were randomly assigned to placebo or one of the following drugs: the diuretic hydrochlorothiazide (12.5–50 mg/d), the β-blocker atenolol (25–100 mg/d), the calcium antagonist diltiazem (120–360 mg/d, sustained-release preparation), the α_1-blocker prazosin (4–20 mg/d), or the centrally acting sympatholytic, clonidine (0.2–0.6 mg/d). The study started with a 4–8 week titration period and continued for 1 year. Good responders were defined as patients with diastolic blood pressure <90 mmHg at the end of the titration phase and <95 mmHg at 1 year.

Together, the six classes of agents controlled diastolic blood pressure in ~62% of the patients. However, when the patients were divided into four groups, two by age (<60 or ≥60 years) and two by race (white Euro-American, or black African-American), substantial differences in the response to the six drugs became evident. Blacks responded best to the calcium antagonist and older blacks also responded well to the diuretic but poorly to the angiotensin-converting enzyme (ACE) inhibitor. Younger whites responded well to the β-blocker and ACE inhibitor as well as the calcium antagonist, but poorly to the diuretic. Older whites responded similarly to all of the drug classes. Therefore, the overall 62% response underestimates some drugs and overestimates others in the age-by-race categories.

The age-by-race paradigm was tested against the Laragh–Sealey method of plasma renin profiling (9). Logistic regression analysis determined that the most important predictor of response to a single drug was the baseline diastolic blood pressure. This is one of the reasons that we suggest limitation of the age-by-race paradigm to patients with stage 1 hypertension. The other is that we expect the majority of patients with stage 2 hypertension will require combination therapy. Nevertheless, the

Table 34.1 Combination Antihypertensive Medications

Chemical name	Trade name(s)
ACE inhibitors in combination with calcium antagonists	
Amlodipine–benazepril (2.5/10, 5/10/5/20, 10/20)	Lotrel (Novartis)
Enalapril–felodipine (5/5)	Lexxel (Astra-Zeneca)
Enalapril–diltiazem	Teczem[a]
Ramipril–felodipine (2.5/2.5, 5/5)	Triapin Mite, Triapin (Aventis, UK)
Trandolapril–verapamil (2/180, 1/240, 2/240, 4/240)	Tarka (Abbott)
ACE inhibitors and diruretics	
Benazepril–HCT (5/6.25, 10/12.5, 20/12.5, 20/25)	Lotensin–HCT (Novartis)
	Cibadrex (Novartis)
Captopril–HCT (25/15, 25/25, 50/15, 50/25)	Acezide, Capozide (Bristol–Myers–Squibb, Apothecon);
	Capozide, Capozide LS (Squibb, UK); Captozide (Par);
	Tensobon (Schwarz); Generic (Geneva, Mylan)
Enalapril–HCT (5/12.5,10/25)	Vaseretic (Biovail, Merck); Co-Renitic (Merck);
	Neotensin-Diu (Schwarz, Spain); Innozide (Merck, UK);
	Renacor, Renidur (Merck); Generic (Mylan, Par, Taro)
Fosinopril–HCT (10/12.5, 20/12.5)	Monopril–HCT (Bristol–Myers–Squibb)
Lisinopril–HCT (10/12.5, 20/12.5, 20/25)	Prinzide, Vivazid, Novazyd (Merck);
	Zestoretic (AstraZeneca); Carace Plus (Squibb, UK);
	Generic (Geneva, Mylan)
Moexipril–HCT (7.5/12.5, 15/25)	Uniretic (Schwartz)
Perindopril–indapamide (4/1.25)	Coversyl Plus (Servier)
Quinapril–HCT (10/12.5, 20/12.5, 20/25)	Accuretic (Parke–Davis)
Angiotensin receptor blockers and diuretics	
Candesartan–HCT (16/12.5, 32/12.5)	Atacand–HCT (AstraZeneca)
Eprosartan–HCT (600/12.5, 600/25)	Teveten–HCT (Biovail)
Irbesartan–HCT (150/12.5, 300/12.5)	Avalide (Bristol–Myers–Squibb); CoAprovel (Sanofi/BMS,
	France); Karvezide (BMS, France); CoAprovel
	(Sanofi Synthelabo, UK)
Losartan–HCT (50/12.5, 100/25)	Hyzaar (Merck); Cozaar–Comp (Merck, UK)
Olmesartan–HCT (20/12.5, 40/12.5, 40/25)	Benicar–HCT (Forest, Sankyo)
Telmisartan–HCT (40/12.5, 80/12.5)	Micardis–HCT (Boehringer, Ingelheim); BolusacPlus,
	Kinzelcomb (Bayer); MicardisPlus (B–I, UK & Germany);
	Pritor Plus (Glaxo, Germany)
Valsartan–HCT (80/12.5, 160/12.5)	Diovan–HCT, Co-Diovan (Novartis); Miten Plus
	(Schwarz, Spain)
β-blockers and diuretics	
Atenolol–chlorthalidone (50/12.5, 50/25, 100/25)	Tenoret 50, Tenoretic (AstraZeneca); Generic (Mylan, Watson)
Bisoprolol–HCT (2.5/6.25, 5/6.25, 10/6.25)	Ziac (Wyeth); Generic (Geneva, Mylan, Watson)
Metoprolol–chlorthalidone (100/12.5, 200/25)	Legroton Retard (Novartis); Co-Betaloc, Co-Betaloc LA
	(Pharmacia, UK)
Nadolol–bendrofluazide (40/5)	Corgaretic (Sanofi Synthelabo)
Oxprenolol–chlorthalidone	Trasitensin
Oxprenolol–cyclopenthiazide (160/0.25)	Trasidrex (Novartis)
Pindolol–clopamide (10/5)	Viskaldix (Novartis)
Pindolol–HCT (10/25, 10/50)	Viskazide
Propranolol–bendrofluazide (80/2.5, 160/5)	Inderetic, Inderex (AstraZeneca, UK)
Propranolol LA–HCT (40/25.80/25)	Inderide LA (Wyeth); Generic (Mylan)
Metoprolol–HCT (50/25, 100/25)	Lopressor HCT (Novartis)
Nadolol–bendroflumethiazide (40/5, 80/5)	Corzide (Monarch)
Timolol–bendrofluazide (10/2.5)	Prestim (ICN Pharmaceuticals, UK)
Timolol–HCT (10/25)	Timolide (Merck)

(continued)

Table 34.1 *Continued*

Chemical name	Trade name(s)
Centrally acting drugs and diuretics	
Clonidine–chlorthalidone	Clorpres
Clonidine–chlorthalidone	Combipres
	Generic (Mylan)
Deserpidine–methychlothiazide	Enduronyl
Methyldopa–chlorothiazide (250/250)	Aldoclor (Merck)
Methyldopa–HCT (250/15, 250/25, 500/30, 500/50)	Aldoril (Merck);
	Generic (Mylan)
Rauwolfia serpentina–bendroflumethiazide	Rauzide
Reserpine–chlorthalidone	Demi-Regroton, Regroton
Reserpine–chlorothiazide (0.125/250, 0.25/500)	Diupress
Reserpine–HCT (0.125/15, 0.125/25, 0.125/50)	Hydropres, Hydro-Reserp (Camall); Hydro-Serp,
	Hydroserpine; Hydrotensin (Mayrand Pharmaceutical);
	Mallopres (Mallard, Inc.)
Reserpine–hydroflumethiazide (0.125/25–50)	Salutensin (Apothecon)
	Hydropine, Hydropine H.P. (Rugby Laboratories)
Reserpine–methyclothiazide (0.125/2.5)	Wallace Laboratories
Reserpine–polythiazide	Renese-R
Reserpine–methyclothiazide	Diutensen-R
Reserpine–trichlormethiazide (0.125/2)	Metatensin;
	Naquival (Schering)
Diuretics and diuretics	
Amiloride–HCT (2.5/25, 5/50)	Moduretic (Merck; BMS, UK), Moduret 25 (BMS, UK);
	Moduret (DuPont Merck) Diuzine (Schwarz, Spain)
	Generic (Mylan, Par)
Amiloride–cyclopenthiazide (2.5/0.25)	Navispare (Novartis)
Spironolactone–furosemide (50/20)	Lasilactone (Borg Medicare, UK)
Spironolactone–HCT (25/25, 50/50)	Aldactazide (Searle);
	Generic (Geneva, Mylan, Schein)
Tiamterene–chlorthalidone (50/50)	Kalspare (Pliva, UK)
Triamterene–HCT (37.5/25, 75/50)	Dyazide (GlazoSmithKlein);
	Maxzide (Bertek); Apo-Triazide (Arlington Scientific);
	Generic (Barr, Geneva, Mylan, Schein, Watson)
Other drug combinations	
Guanethidine–HCT	Esimil
Hydralazine–HCT (25/25,50/50, 100/50)	Apresazide (Par)
Nifedipine–atenolol (20/50)	β-Adalat (Bayer); Tenif (AstraZeneca)
Prazosin–polythiazide	Minizide
Multiple-drug combinations	
Atenolol–HCT–amiloride (50/25/2.5)	Kalten (AstraZeneca)
Oxprenolol–hydralazine-chlorthalidone	Trepress
Reserpine, dihydroergocristine, clopamide	Brinerdina (Giofil, Italy)
Reserpine, dihydroergocristine, clopamide, Hydralazine	Brinerdin (Novartis)
Reserpine, hydralazine–HCT (0.1/25/15)	Ser-Ap-Es (Novartis); Cam-Ap-Es (Camall);
	Cherapas (Key); Hydrap-Es, Marpres, Ser-A-Gen,
	Seralazide, Serpazide, Tri-Hydroserpine, Unipres,
	Uni-Serp, Marpres
Timolol–HCT–amiloride (10/25/2.5)	Moducren (Merck, UK)

[a]Discontinued by original supplier.

Note: Drug combinations are listed alphabetically with known dose combinations expressed as milligrams in parentheses. Not all doses are available in all countries or in all brands. Brand names are listed with the original or last-known supplier in parentheses. The suppliers may not be current or the same in each country. HCT, Hydrochlorothiazide; BMS, Bristol–Myers–Squibb; B–I, Boehringer–Ingelheim.

age-by-race paradigm not only compared well to the plasma renin profiling method, but also was actually somewhat superior to it.

On the basis of these data, we believe that the results of single-drug therapy of stage 1 hypertension in a racially diverse population may be misleading if not considered by the age-by-race paradigm.

The Veterans Administration Cooperative Study Group on Antihypertensive Agents also had an opportunity to look at sequential therapy in their single-drug therapy of hypertension trial. In brief, of the 410 men (of the original 1292) who did not achieve goal blood pressure with the initial drug to which they were randomized, 352 qualified for random allocation to a second single drug. The double mask was maintained. Forty-nine percent of these patients achieved the goal with the second single drug. Keep in mind that, as patients had already failed to respond to one drug, it is not surprising that a drug given as the second choice was less effective as when it was given as the first choice. What was surprising is how close the initial and sequential response rates were for all of the drugs except atenolol (60% initial response vs. 41% second response), and captopril (50% vs. 37%). The age-by-race subgroups also were similar. For example, captopril and clonidine had the highest rates and hydrochlorothiazide had the lowest rates for younger whites. Diltiazem, hydrochlorothiazide, and clonidine had the highest rates for older blacks, whereas captopril had the lowest response rate. If a patient failed initial hydrochlorothiazide therapy, they achieved the best response when the second drug was diltiazem. Similar pairs were clonidine best after atenolol failure, prazosin after captopril failure, diltiazem after clonidine, captopril after diltiazem, and clonidine after prazosin failure. This study supported the concept of sequential therapy for patients with stage 1 hypertension.

B. Role of Single-Drug Therapy

Approximately two-thirds of all hypertensive patients have stage 1 hypertension, which means that their systolic blood pressure is between 140 and 159 mmHg and diastolic pressure is between 90 and 99 mmHg (10). If a single drug is selected carefully according to the patient's individual characteristics, including age and race, the success rate in this group should be ~60–80% (6–8). If the initial drug fails to control the blood pressure adequately, one strategy is to substitute another single drug from a class with different pharmacological properties (*sequential therapy*) (5). Alternatively, a second drug, preferably a diuretic if the first drug is not a diuretic, can be added.

But in the majority of hypertensive patients it is unlikely that a single drug will control blood pressure to target levels (1). Clinical trials demonstrate that combination therapy is required in approximately two-thirds of hypertensive individuals. For example, in the Hypertension Optimal Treatment (HOT) trial (11), 33% of patients reached their blood pressure target with one drug, 45% required two drugs, and 22% needed three or more agents. In a recent meta-analysis of studies involving renal disease of various etiologies, Bakris et al. (12) reported that an average of more than three drugs per patient was required.

C. Issues Related to Monotherapy

There are several possible reasons for the inability of single-drug therapy (*monotherapy*) to adequately control blood pressure in a large number of patients (Table 34.2).

First, recommended blood pressure goals are being reduced for many high-risk hypertensive subgroups including isolated systolic hypertension (140 mmHg), diabetes (130/80 mmHg), and renal impairment (130/80 mmHg). The added benefit of the new lower goals is paid for by the cost of adding antihypertensive drugs to reach the new lower target. There is growing evidence that systolic blood pressure is more important than elevated diastolic blood pressure as a cardiovascular risk factor (1), and thus controlling systolic blood pressure provides significant protection against major cardiovascular complications. This has been demonstrated in large trials involving elder patients with isolated systolic hypertension (1).

This recent emphasis on the control of systolic as well as diastolic blood pressure has probably further increased the number of patients requiring multi-drug therapy. Systolic blood pressure is often less responsive to treatment than diastolic blood pressure. Over 50% of patients with isolated systolic hypertension participating in the Systolic Hypertension in the Elderly (SHEP) study (13) needed more than one drug despite the fact that the target systolic

Table 34.2 Potential Reasons for Failure of a Single Drug

Lower blood pressure goals
  Isolated systolic hypertension (140 mmHg)
  Diabetes mellitus (130/80 mmHg)
  Renal impairment (130/80 mmHg)
Higher prevalence of factors that produce resistance to
  antihypertensives
  Obesity
  Renal disease
Counter regulatory mechanisms
Unpredictability of blood pressure response
Volume overload
Nonadherence

blood pressure was much higher than the currently rec-ommended goal of 140 mmHg. In the Losartan Inter-vention for Endpoint reduction (LIFE) trial (14), where treatment to goal (<140/90 mmHg) was aggressively pursued for both systolic and diastolic blood pressure in >9000 patients with an average baseline blood pressure of 175/98 mmHg, >90% of patients required multiple agents.

A second reason monotherapy is not effective is that a variety of factors that coexist with hypertension, such as obesity, renal impairment, and the concomitant use of nonsteroidal anti-inflammatory drugs (NSAIDS), can attenuate and complicate hypertension management by producing or exacerbating resistance to antihypertensives. Therefore, goals are decreasing while clinical conditions that make blood pressure control more difficult are becom-ing more prevalent.

A third reason is that some counter-regulatory mechan-isms are activated in response to blood pressure lowering and can attenuate the antihypertensive effects of a given agent. For example, reducing intravascular volume with diuretics activates the renin–angiotensin–aldosterone system, leading to renal sodium retention and vasocon-striction. In addition, vasodilators stimulate the sympath-etic nervous system, increasing both cardiac output and vascular resistance, further leading to renal sodium retention.

A fourth reason for the failure of monotherapy in many patients is the unpredictability of blood pressure response to a given drug in a given patient. There has been a large body of data gathered to allow prediction of which patient will respond to which drug, but on an individual basis the physician must still resort to trial and error. This process can lead to frustration both for the physician and for the patient. The multifactorial nature of primary hypertension is also reflected by the unpredictability of individual blood pressure responses to antihypertensive agents belonging to various classes. This is apparent when each patient receives sequentially all test agents in studies performed according to a cross-over design. As shown repeatedly, a patient may respond favorably to one given agent only, two or more drugs, or possibly not to any drug (5–8). This is important conceptually because any antihyperten-sive drug, whatever its mechanism of action, may be the best one for one patient but unsatisfactory for another. The only way to ascertain whether a medication is appro-priate is to administer it empirically for several weeks.

Volume overload is a common underlying cause for failure to respond to a single drug in many patients, and often aggravates hypertension in patients receiving mono-therapy with nondiuretic agents. It is especially important in many salt-sensitive patients whose blood pressure is very responsive to small variations in sodium intake. It is also a factor in patients with hypertension and renal disease, heart failure, primary aldosteronism, or those with renal artery stenosis as the etiology of their hyperten-sion. Concomitant medications, in particular nonsteroidal anti-inflammatory agents (which are available over-the-counter and are commonly used or abused), may also contribute significantly to undesired volume overload.

Nonadherence to prescribed therapy is altogether too often an underlying cause of the failure of monotherapy. Several surveys found a large number of patients begun on antihypertensive drug treatment were no longer taking their medication a year later. Side effects related to drug therapy are a common reason for patient discon-tinuation of treatment.

Primary hypertension is not only highly heterogeneous in terms of response to treatment, but also various patho-physiologic mechanisms might be involved to a greater or lesser degree in the abnormal blood pressure elevation in a given patient. There is also reciprocal reinforcement among pressor systems. For example, angiotensin II facili-tates the presynaptic release of norepinephrine and epi-nephrine which stimulates renin secretion by activating β-adrenoceptors. These two vasoconstrictors also have a sodium retaining effect. Further, renin secretion depends on the state of sodium balance; sodium depletion leads to hyper-reninemia, so that controlling high blood pressure becomes angiotensin II-dependent. The pathogenesis of primary hypertension might involve many abnormalities other than excessive sodium reten-tion and/or hyperactivity of the renin–angiotensin–aldosterone and sympathetic nervous systems. On the other hand, medications are available to decrease total body sodium (diuretics), or interfere with the renin–angiotensin–aldosterone system (ACE inhibitors, angio-tensin II antagonists), or the sympathetic nervous system (β- and α_1-blockers, and centrally acting sympatholytics). Therefore, one advantage of combinations of antihyperten-sive drugs is that selection can be tailored to offset the each drug's counter-regulatory effects.

III.   PROFILE OF COMBINATION DRUG THERAPY

Combining drugs with additive properties makes good pharmacological sense. This is especially true of combi-nations with a diuretic drug. When two or more drugs are combined, any age-by-race interaction attributable to a single drug is abolished and need not be considered further (Fig. 34.1).

A summary of the characteristics of an ideal drug com-bination is presented in Table 34.3. The combination should contain components that have an approximately equal duration of action and should control blood pressure over 24 h. They should have at least an additive effect and

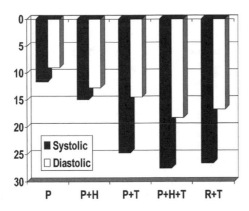

Figure 34.1 An example of racial difference in response to antihypertensive medication that is abolished by combination therapy. These data are from 130 white and 178 African-American patients who were treated with bendroflumethiazide alone (*n* = 68), nadolol alone (*n* = 104), or the combination of the two drugs (*n* = 136). [From Veterans Administration Cooperative Study Group on Antihypertensive Agents (15).]

should mutually reduce their adverse drug reactions. For example, the ACE inhibitor benezepril has been shown to reduce the frequency of edema associated with the dihydropyridine amlodipine (16). The adverse drug effects should be distinguishable. The preceding two drugs have very different side effect profiles, so a clinician who is confronted with a new onset, unexplained chronic cough might want to substitute an angiotensin receptor blocker for the ACE inhibitor.

When prescriptions are filled individually, there is a cost for the pharmacist who is doing the work that may be passed on to the patient. In some healthcare delivery models such as Health Maintenance Organizations (HMOs), the patient may be required to pay a fee for each prescription filled. A combination drug would incur only one such fee. Finally, although we are not aware of such a product on the market at the time of this writing, delivery of combination products transdermally may be

Table 34.3 Characteristics of Ideal Antihypertensive Drug Combinations

Long-acting components for once-daily administration
Equal duration of action of component drugs
At least an additive effect of the component drugs
Few or no adverse drug effects for each component drug
Component drugs mutually reduce adverse drug effects
Component drugs should have distinguishable adverse effects
Combination should cost less than the sum of the components purchased separately (includes cost of dispensing and co-payments by patient)
Possible application by long-lasting transdermal patch

technically feasible and would increase both convenience and patient compliance.

IV. VETERANS ADMINISTRATION COOPERATIVE STUDY GROUP ON ANTIHYPERTENSIVE AGENTS

The 1993 Veterans Administration Cooperative Study Group on Antihypertensive Agents tested the concept of sequential therapy as described earlier and also tested the concept of combination therapy (17). This preplanned phase of the study was conducted on a small subset of 102 patients who had failed to achieve goal blood pressure both during the initial trial and with the randomly allocated alternate drug in the second trial. They were given a combination of the first and second drug which they had previously received. This part of the study could not be masked for either the patient or the staff because both drugs were known to be active, and placebos were not permitted.

Of the 102 patients, 59 (57.8%) responded to the combination of the two drugs. If one of the two drugs was the diuretic hydrochlorothiazide, the response rate was higher: 69% for diastolic and 77% for systolic blood pressure compared with 51% and 46%, respectively, if neither drug was a diuretic (Fig. 34.2). Eight patients were discontinued from the trial because of adverse effects. Of these, six were taking prazosin as one of the two drugs.

Although the numbers are small, ranging from 2 to 14 in each group, it is interesting to observe how each available combination fared in achieving diastolic goal blood pressure of <90 mmHg. This is displayed in Table 34.4.

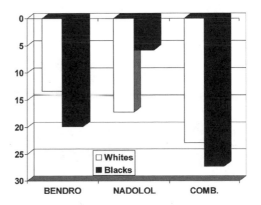

Figure 34.2 In combinations of two drugs, blood pressure control was greater if one of the two drugs was hydrochlorothiazide (HCTZ) (solid bars), as compared to the combination of two nondiuretic drugs (shaded bars). The combinations were of drugs that had each had failed to achieve blood pressure control when used alone. [From Materson et al. (17); data reconstructed from source information.]

Table 34.4   Goal Blood Pressure (<90 mmHg) Achieved with Various Combinations of Antihypertensive Drugs

Drug combination	N	% at goal
Hydrochlorothiazide + atenolol	9	77.8
Hydrochlorothiazide + captopril	14	71.4
Hydrochlorothiazide + clonidine	5	80.0
Hydrochlorothiazide + diltiazem	5	60.0
Hydrochlorothiazide + prazosin	6	50.0
Atenolol + captopril	11	36.4
Atenolol + clonidine	2	50.0
Atenolol + diltiazem	6	50.0
Atenolol + prazosin	6	66.7
Captopril + clonidine	6	33.3
Captopril + diltiazem	7	57.1
Captopril + prazosin	10	60.0
Clonidine + diltiazem	3	100.0
Clonidine + prazosin	8	50.0
Diltiazem + prazosin	4	25.0

Note: This is not an original untreated population. Each patient had failed to achieve goal blood pressure when exposed to the component drugs as single-drug therapy.
Source: Materson et al. (5)

As noted earlier combinations with hydrochlorothiazide fared best, from 50% to 77.8%.

All three of the patients who received the combination of clonidine plus diltiazem achieved goal. Figure 34.3 compares the response to combinations containing each of the six drugs with combinations that did not contain each of the drugs.

The Group posed the question of whether it mattered which drug the patient received first, and two types of "order effect" were found (18). The first was the case in which there were different results for each of the components, but the combination result was the same. An

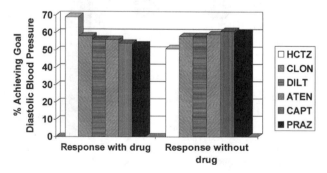

Figure 34.3   There were 15 possible pairings of each of the six drugs used in the third phase (Combination) of the Veterans Administration Cooperative Study on Antihypertensive Agents. This illustration shows the response of combinations that did or did not contain each drug. HCTZ (hydrochlorothiazide), CLON (clonidine), DILT (diltiazem-SR), ATEN (atenolol), CAPT (captopril), PRAZ (prazosin). [From Materson et al. (17).]

example is that when a patient failed on diltiazem, only 6% of patients responded to prazosin, but 86% responded to the combination. For patients who had failed on prazosin, diltiazem had a 22% response rate and the combination rate was 84%, similar to the other order.

The second type of response was one in which the order of drug administration yielded a different combination result. For patients who had failed atenolol, 30% responded to clonidine, but the combination added only 2% for a total of 97% response rate. For patients who received clonidine first and failed, only 9% responded to atenolol and the combination added 13% for a total of 87% response rate. If captopril was followed by the addition of diltiazem, the combination was 88% effective, but reversing the order yielded 97%. These results included some effects of age and race, but the numbers were quite small in each subgroup.

V.   SPECIFIC COMBINATIONS OF ANTIHYPERTENSIVE DRUGS

There are several possible drug class combinations that potentially could be effective for a particular patient.

A.   Drug Combinations that Include a Thiazide Diuretic

Thiazide diuretics are often included in antihypertensive drug combinations. These agents combine the advantages of low cost with proven efficacy in reducing the long-term target organ complications of hypertension. Low-dose diuretics are recommended by the seventh report of the Joint National Committee on the Detection, Evaluation, and Treatment of High Blood Pressure (JNC7) as first-line therapy. At the low doses generally prescribed in current practice, diuretics are well tolerated and their side effect profile is often improved when other agents are added. Many fixed-dose combinations are available that include a diuretic in combination with other diuretics, β-blockers, ACE inhibitors, and angiotensin receptor blockers. In all of these combinations, additive effects on blood pressure are observed.

Figure 34.4 shows the results of various combinations. In every case, the addition of hydrochlorothiazide enhanced the result of the single drug and was superior to the combination of two nondiuretic drugs.

Figure 34.5 further supports this point and gives some insight to triple-combination therapy. Propranolol alone was not as effective as propranolol plus hydralazine. Propranolol plus hydrochlorothiazide was even more effective. Reserpine, although not widely used now, was quite effective when combined with a diuretic.

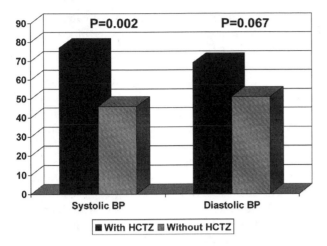

Figure 34.4 Percent achievement of goal blood pressure by one-, two-, or three-drug therapy in a variety of Department of Veterans Affairs Cooperative studies. These studies were done at different times, with different protocols, and on different patient populations. Nevertheless, the results are remarkably similar. TZ, hydrochlorothiazide; Bendro-TZ, bendroflumethiazide. [From Veterans Administration Cooperative Study Group on Antihypertensive Agents (15,23) and Materson et al. (24).]

Diuretic combinations that include potassium-sparing agents such as triamterene, spironolactone, or amiloride lower the risk of serious hypokalemia and appear to improve the long-term outcome of diuretic treatment.

Selected Combination Data

Drug(s)	1	2	3
Propranolol	52		
Nadolol	49		
Reserpine + TZ		88	
Propranolol + TZ		81	
Propranolol + TZ		86	
Nadolol + Bendro-TZ		85	
Enalapril + TZ		87	
Propranolol + Hydralazine		72	
Nadolol + Hydralazine		75	
Propran. + Hydralazine + TZ			92
Nadolol + Hydral. + Bendro-TZ			93

Figure 34.5 Reduction of systolic and diastolic blood pressure (mmHg) by propranolol (P) alone, combined with hydralazine (H), hydrochlorothiazide (T), both hydralazine and hydrochlorothiazide, and the combination of reserpine (R) with hydrochlorothiazide. The combinations with hydrochlorothiazide were more effective than the combination of propranolol plus hydralazine. Triple therapy was most effective. Note the high efficacy of the reserpine plus hydrochlorothiazide combination. [From Veterans Administration Cooperative Study Group on Antihypertensive Agents (23).]

Current recommendations emphasize the use of low-dose diuretics.

The combination of either an ACE inhibitor or an angiotensin receptor blocker with a low-dose diuretic, in addition to lowering blood pressure, may confer additional long-term benefits in cardiovascular endpoint reduction via blockade of the renin–angiotensin–aldosterone system. In the Heart Outcomes Prevention Evaluation (HOPE) study (19), for example, the ACE inhibitor ramipril reduced the subsequent risk of death, myocardial infarction, and stroke. The effect could not be accounted for on the basis of blood pressure reduction alone. In the Irbesartan Diabetic Nephropathy Trial (IDNT) (20), Reduction of Endpoints in Non-Insulin Dependent Diabetes Mellitus (NIDDM) with the Angiotensin II Antagonist Losartan (RENAAL) (21), Irbesartan Microalbuminuria Study (IRMA)-2 (22), and LIFE in hypertension study (14), antihypertensive regimens that included an angiotensin receptor blocker (irbesartan and losartan) were associated with more effective endpoint reduction compared with regimens based on standard therapy (placebo), dihydropyridine calcium channel blocker, or β-blocker. In fact, these trials were studies of combination therapy. In RENAAL, approximately three additional drugs were administered to each patient. In LIFE, >90% of patients in the losartan group also received a diuretic.

B. Combination of an ACE Inhibitor and a Calcium Channel Antagonist

Calcium channel blockers are very effective antihypertensive agents that remain an essential component of therapy for many hypertensive patients in whom blood pressure control cannot be achieved control with a single drug. In the RENAAL study, 78% received calcium channel blockers even though calcium channel blockers were not given as first-line treatment.

Calcium channel blockers are effective in combination with ACE inhibitors, and the combination of low doses of a calcium antagonist and an ACE inhibitor is associated with reduced edema compared with titration of the calcium antagonist to higher doses (25–28). The ACE inhibitor partially neutralizes the dependent edema that is the most frequent dose-limiting side effect seen with calcium antagonists. The edema is believed to be a result of the selective reduction in precapillary resistance produced by calcium channel blockers. ACE inhibitors lower postcapillary resistance, decreasing the hydrostatic pressure gradient across capillary membranes and the tendency for fluid extravasation.

Messerli et al. (28) studied 1079 patients whose diastolic blood pressure remained between 95 and 115 mmHg after treatment with either nifedipine or amlodipine randomized to 8 weeks of amlodipine 5 mg/benazepril 10 mg, amlodipine 5 mg/benazepril 20 mg, nifedipine 30 mg or nifedipine 60 mg and amlodipine 5 mg/benazepril 10 mg, amlodipine 5 mg/benazepril 20 mg, amlodipine 5 mg, or amlodipine 10 mg. Both doses of the calcium antagonist/ ACE inhibitor combination therapy lowered diastolic pressure as much as the high dose of the calcium antagonist and more than the lower dose. This finding was the same for both nifedipine and amlodipine. In addition, there was a reduced rate of edema with the combination treatment compared with the highest dose of the calcium antagonist.

Gradman et al. (26) studied 707 patients with diastolic blood pressures in the range of 95–110 mmHg who were randomized to receive enalapril, felodipine extended release, or the combination of the two drugs. Following 8 weeks of treatment, the combination had a significant additive effect on blood pressure. The combination produced a reduction of 15.4 mmHg compared with the highest dose of felodipine extended release monotherapy (10 mg/d) which reduced blood pressure by an average of 11.7 mmHg. Peripheral edema was reduced from 10.8% with felodipine single drug therapy to only 4.1% in patients receiving the combination of felodipine and enalapril.

Given the success of these combinations, it would appear logical to combine an angiotensin receptor blocker with a calcium channel antagonist. We are aware of two products that are under development: telmisartan plus amlodipine and telmisartan plus lacidipine. We would expect to see many similar products to be studied and eventually marketed.

C. Combination of an ACE Inhibitor and an Angiotensin Receptor Blocker

There has been recent investigative interest in the combination of ACE inhibitors and angiotensin receptor blockers both for lowering blood pressure and for reducing hypertensive target organ injury. ACE inhibitors and angiotensin receptor blockers inhibit the renin–angiotensin–aldosterone system via different mechanisms and several studies have suggested that they may produce additive antihypertensive effects when used in combination. ACE inhibitors reduce the production of angiotensin II, whereas angiotensin receptor blockers block its effects directly at the AT_1 receptor site. In the Candesartan and Lisinopril Microalbuminuria (CALM) study (29), the combination of candesartan (16 mg) and lisinopril (20 mg) appeared to have additive effects in reducing diastolic blood pressure. The study also reported greater reduction in proteinuria with the combination. Maximum doses of each agent were not tested, which leaves the question open of whether there is a true additive effect in the drug classes when both are given at maximum dosages. It is

also unclear from this study whether the greater reduction of proteinuria is the result of the greater blood pressure reduction with the combination vs. a selective effect upon the renal microvasculature.

Nakao et al. (30) assessed the efficacy and safety of combined treatment of ACE inhibitor and angiotensin-II receptor blocker, and monotherapy of each drug at its maximum dose, in 263 patients with nondiabetic renal disease randomly assigned angiotensin-II receptor blocker (losartan, 100 mg daily), ACE inhibitor (trandolapril, 3 mg daily), or a combination of both drugs at equivalent doses (COOPERATE trial). Survival analysis compared the effects of each regimen on the combined primary endpoint of time to doubling of serum creatinine concentration or end-stage renal disease.

Ten of eighty five patients (11%) on combination treatment reached the combined primary endpoint compared with 20 of 85 (23%) on trandolapril alone ($P = 0.018$) and 20 of 86 (23%) on losartan alone ($P = 0.016$). Frequency of side effects with combination treatment was the same as with trandolapril alone. This trial suggests that the combination of an ACE inhibitor and an angiotensin receptor blocker has a synergistic effect on progression of nondiabetic renal disease.

Song et al. (31) attempted to avoid the confounding effects of blood pressure reduction and of disease heterogeneity by treating a group of patients with either IgA or diabetic nephropathy who had their blood pressure controlled long-term with the ACE inhibitor ramipril. They added 4–8 mg of candesartan or placebo once daily and measured urinary protein excretion and urinary transforming growth factor β_1 levels as surrogate indicators of renal injury. There was no change in 24 h mean blood pressure by the addition of candesartan in either group. In the IgA nephropathy group, but not the diabetics, the combination of ramipril and candesartan significantly reduced both urinary protein excretion (−12.3%) and transforming growth factor β_1 levels (−28.9%) compared with the addition of a placebo. There were no such significant changes in the patients with diabetic nephropathy although there was a nonsignificant (−14.3%) decrease in transforming growth factor β_1 urinary excretion. This study is important in that it used 24 h ambulatory blood pressure monitoring, it selected patients whose blood pressure was already controlled before the addition of the angiotensin receptor blocker, it was double-blind and placebo controlled, and the renal disease was proven by biopsy.

The African American Study of Kidney Disease and Hypertension (AASK) trial (32) found ramipril-based therapy to be superior to amlodipine-based treatment in reducing the progression of hypertensive renal disease. This landmark study also demonstrated that blood pressure levels in patients with renal impairment, a documented cause of resistance to antihypertensive therapy, could be controlled to below the newer recommendations of 130/80 mmHg for renal patients. Thus, the work of the AASK investigators demonstrated that patients with significant levels of hypertension and coexisting renal impairment can reach lower target blood pressure.

Further, the addition of a low-dose diuretic significantly enhances the effectiveness of ACE inhibitors or angiotensin receptor blockers in African-American patients. For example, Flack et al. (33) studied 433 African-Americans with a diastolic blood pressure of 95–109 mmHg randomized to either placebo, high-dose losartan (150 mg/d), or the combination of losartan 100 mg/HCTZ 25 mg. A diastolic blood pressure goal of <90 mmHg was reached in 56% of patients treated with the combination compared with 36% of patients receiving losartan alone.

D. Fixed Low-Dose Combinations of Drugs

According to the stepped-care approach, the initial step in treating hypertension is selecting a single drug and increasing its dosage to reach treatment goals. A second drug is added to the regimen only if blood pressure control cannot be obtained with a single agent at the maximum dosage. A disadvantage of this approach is that upward dose titration of antihypertensive agents may result in a significant increase in side effects with little additional blood pressure reduction. Addition of a low dose of a second agent may be a more successful strategy for achieving blood pressure control without side effects in some patients. This alternative approach to antihypertensive therapy is recognized in JNC 7. Low-dose combinations may also be used as first-step therapy, particularly in patients with initial diastolic blood pressures >100 mmHg or systolic pressures >160 mmHg.

Numerous trials have suggested that fixed-dose combinations are as or more effective in lowering blood pressure than the single components given alone. This enhanced efficacy can be regarded as an important condition for approval of a fixed-dose combination. Fixed-dose combinations are very attractive because of their high efficacy and their excellent tolerability (34–36). They offer a good chance of success whether used as first- or second-line therapy compared with sequential therapy which requires changing or withdrawing drugs in order to find the most appropriate regimen for an individual patient. The latter has a tangible cost in terms of medications, number of visits, and aggravation for both physician and patient. The fact that fixed-dose combinations reduce the number of tablets to be taken every day is an additional factor facilitating the adherence to antihypertensive treatment (37). As a result, the use of fixed-dose combinations may yield a better cost-effectiveness and long-term compliance than monotherapy (38). Beyond the protection afforded by their blood pressure-lowering

action, fixed-dose combinations might confer prognostic advantages. For instance, the untoward metabolic effects associated with thiazide diuretics (hyperglycemia, hypercholesterolemia, hyperuricemia, and hypokalemia) are reduced when the diuretic is co-administered with a blocker of the renin–angiotensin system (39,40), primarily because minimal doses of diuretics are required when the renin–angiotensin system is blocked. Another example is the synergy of ACE inhibition and calcium entry blockade with verapamil in reducing proteinuria (41). Further studies are needed to establish whether some drugs protect better against target organ damage when they are combined than when they are administered as single agents.

Current recommendations propose that fixed low-dose combinations may be appropriate for initiating antihypertensive therapy (1). There is general consensus that hypertension should be more consistently treated to target goals than it has in the past, and that the treatment should be individualized not only to achieve the target blood pressures but also to preserve as much as possible the patients' quality of life. Fixed low-dose combinations are useful in everyday practice, whether prescribed as first- or second-line therapy, because they can increase the probability of rapidly finding an effective and well-tolerated treatment. This is key because the achievement of sustained blood pressure normalization represents the over-riding aim of antihypertensive therapy today.

E. Combinations of Calcium Antagonists

Dihydropyridine (DHP), diltiazem-like (D-type), and verapamil-like (V-type) calcium antagonists bind at different sites on the α_1 subunit of the calcium channel (42). If a DHP (N-type) or a D-type drug binds to the receptor, the other receptor is up-regulated, at least in vitro. Receptor blockade with a V-type drug appears to down-regulate the N- and D-type receptors. On the basis of this information that was originally obtained in a conference in 1991, Materson (43) later proposed a pharmacological separation of calcium antagonists with the idea that it would then be logical to combine an N-type with a D-type drug for clinical purposes. Clinical trials of these combinations are difficult to perform. Nevertheless, there is evidence to support this powerful interaction. In contrast to the in vitro studies, clinical trials suggest that verampamil potentiates and is also potentiated by DHP calcium antagonists (44,45). There is a suggestion that verapamil must be used in much higher doses than comparable doses of diltiazem and that the incidence of lower extremity edema is much higher. One study (44) demonstrated that diltiazem increased the area under the curve for nifedipine levels and imputed a pharmacokinetic mechanism to the positive interaction. This potent combination may avert the need for the use of minoxidil in patients with very severe hypertension. Adverse effects include the risk of hypotension, lower extremity edema (as much as 30%), and gingival hypertrophy. The combination must be titrated carefully to the desired effect.

F. Dual or Multiple Purpose Combinations

A new trend in therapeutics is emerging: combination of two or more drugs for the treatment of separate but related conditions. Pfizer has marketed Caduet®, a combination of the antihypertensive dihydropyridine, amlodipine, with the lipid-lowering "statin," atorvastatin. The concept is to attack two components of the metabolic syndrome simultaneously. Possible future combinations include an antihypertensive with one or more drugs to improve glucose metabolism.

In the United Kingdom, Law and colleagues (46) performed a meta-analysis of 354 randomized, double-blind, placebo-controlled trials of five classes of antihypertensive medication. This robust database of 40,000 actively treated patients and 16,000 subjects who received placebo permitted them to develop a mathematical model for treatment effect. They estimated that the use of a combination of three antihypertensive drugs at half-dose would lower blood pressure by 20/11 mmHg and effect a dramatic reduction in the risk of stroke (63%) and ischemic heart disease events (46%) for patients aged 60–69 years. Wald and Law (47) have proposed a 6-drug combination in one delivery system. They have coined the term "Polypill" for a pill that would target elevated LDL cholesterol, hypertension, elevated homocysteine, and increased clotting tendency. The tentative drugs would be: atorvastatin 10 mg or simvastatin 40 mg; half-doses of hydrochlorothiazide, atenolol and enalapril; folic acid 0.8 mg; and 75 mg aspirin. They estimated that if such a polypill were used as a preventive strategy, especially in people aged 55 years or over with known cardiovascular disease, ischemic heart disease could be reduced by 88% and stroke by 80%. Whether it will be possible to manufacture, gain regulatory approval for and market such a product remains to be seen.

VI. COMPILATION OF COMBINATION PRODUCTS

We reviewed the *2003 Physicians Desk Reference*, wrote to pharmaceutical companies, queried contacts within the pharmaceutical industry, and reviewed multiple Web sites in order to identify combination antihypertensive products that are marketed worldwide. This effort will always be a work in progress because of the frequent mergers and spin-offs of pharmaceutical companies and their divisions,

a wide variety of world-wide licensing agreements executed by the companies (all subject to rapid change), the evolution of brand name drugs to generic as they lose patent protection, the sale or licensing of drugs to other companies, and the laws and marketing needs of different countries. We have made an effort to be as complete as possible; however, some material available on the Internet reflects companies that no longer exist as independent entities, and there are many other errors. Corporate Web sites generally promote their branded name drugs that remain under patent. It is therefore difficult, if not impossible, to determine what company in at any given time actually markets a given drug. The information on manufacturers is a best effort but by no means should it be considered authoritative. For example, the combination of clonidine and chlorthalidone has been discontinued by its original supplier but is marketed by other companies as a generic. In contrast, the combination of enalapril and diltiazem (Teczem) was discontinued by its original supplier but has not, to our knowledge, been picked up by any other company. Nevertheless, we have elected to list it as an example in the hope that it may have a future market.

As with other products, pharmaceuticals that are approaching the end of their marketing life cycle must either be reinvented or fall into decline. Some smaller pharmaceutical companies have carved a niche by identifying these drugs, acquiring the rights to them and selling them in a more defined market. As a consequence, relatively few drugs simply just disappear. Interest in marketing combination antihypertensive drugs is not yet a worldwide phenomenon. Nevertheless, with the increased emphasis on achieving goal blood pressure, the lowering of some target blood pressures, which makes them difficult to achieve, and the legitimization of combination therapy by organizations that write treatment guidelines, we expect that the market for antihypertensive drug combinations will blossom the world over.

The following Web sites were used in the compiling information about combination drugs currently on the market. You can use these as a starting point for researching available drugs for specific conditions.

1. MEDLINEplus Drug Information (http://www.nlm.nih.gov/medlineplus/druginfo)
2. Prentice Hall Health—Drug Guides. Wilson BA, Shannon MT, Stang CL. Drug Guide 2003: (http://wps.prenhall.com/chet_wilson_drugguides_1/0%2C5513%2C403550-%2C00.html)
3. Mythos Pharmacy (http://www.mythos.com/pharmacy)
4. HYPERTENSION MEDICATIONS (http://www.hypertensionmeds.com)

Note that Web sites are subject to change. These were accurate and functional as of October 2003.

VII. CONCLUSIONS

The many millions of people whose blood pressure averages between 140 and 149 mmHg systolic are likely to respond to a carefully selected single drug. Those whose systolic pressure averages between 150 and 159 mmHg are more likely to require two drugs in order to achieve goal blood pressure. Those whose systolic blood pressure is 20 or more mmHg or diastolic 10 or more mmHg above goal will most likely require two or even more drugs in order to achieve goal.

The growing availability of combinations of two or more drugs should facilitate adherence for the patient as well as possible cost savings. Numerous combinations already exist. Many more will be marketed in the future. Expect to see combinations of antihypertensive medications with other medications directed at cardiovascular risk factors in addition to hypertension.

REFERENCES

1. Chobanian AV, Bakris GL, Black HR, Cushman WC, Green LA, Izzo JI Jr, Jones DW, Materson BJ, Oparil S, Wright JT Jr, Roccella EJ, and the National High Blood Pressure Coordinating Committee. The seventh report of the Joint National Committee on Prevention, Detection, Evaluation, and Treatment of High Blood Pressure: the JNC 7 report. JAMA 2003; 289:2560–2572.

2. Veterans Administration Co-operative Study Group on Antihypertensive Agents. Effects of treatment on morbidity in hypertension. I. Results in patients with diastolic blood pressure averaging 115 through 129 mmHg. JAMA 1967; 202:1028–1034.

3. Materson BJ. Remedies for Single-Dose therapy Failure. In: Egan BM, Basile JN, Lackland DT, eds. Hot Topics: Hypertension. Philadelphia: Hanley & Belfus, 2003:237–242.

4. Materson BJ. Combination therapy as the Initial Drug Treatment for Hypertension: When is it appropriate? Am J Hypertens 2001; 14:293–295.

5. Materson BJ, Reda DJ, Preston RA, Cushman WC, Massie BM, Freis ED, Kochar MS, Hamburger RJ, Fye C, Lakshman R, Gottdiener J, Ramirez EA, Henderson WG. For the Department of Veterans Affairs Co-operative Study Group on Antihypertensive Agents: Response to a second single antihypertensive agent used as monotherapy for hypertension after failure of the initial drug. Arch Intern Med 1995; 155:1757–1762.

6. Materson BJ, Reda DJ, Cushman WC, Massie BM, Freis ED, Kochar MS, Hamburger RJ, Fye C, Lakshman R, Gottdiener J, Ramirez EA, Henderson WG. Single-drug therapy for hypertension in men. A comparison of six antihypertensive agents with placebo. N Engl J Med 1993; 328:914–921.

7. Materson BJ, Reda DJ. Correction: single-drug therapy for hypertension in men (letter). N Engl J Med 1994; 330:1689.

8. Materson BJ, Reda DJ, Cushman WC. For the Department of Veterans Affairs Cooperative Study Group on Antihypertensive Agents: Department of Veterans Affairs Single-Drug therapy of hypertension study: revised figures and new data. Am J Hypertens 1995; 8:189–192.

9. Preston RA, Materson BJ, Reda DJ, Williams DW, Hamburger RJ, Cushman WC, Anderson RJ. For the Department of Veterans Affairs Cooperative Study Group on Antihypertensive Agents. Age-race subgroup compared with renin profile as predictors of blood pressure response to antihypertensive therapy. JAMA 1998; 280:1168–1172.

10. Hypertension Detection and Follow-up Program Co-operative Group. The Hypertension Detection and Follow-up Program. A progress report. Circ Res 1977; 40(suppl 1):I106–I109.

11. Hansson L, Zanchetti A, Carruthers SG, Dahlof B, Elmfeldt D, Julius S, Menard J, Rahn KH, Wedel H, Westerling S. Effects of intensive blood-pressure lowering and low-dose aspirin in patients with hypertension: principal results of the Hypertension Optimal Treatment (HOT) randomised trial. HOT Study Group. Lancet 1998; 351:1755–1762.

12. Bakris GL, Williams M, Dworkin L, Elliott WJ, Epstein M, Toto R, Tuttle K, Douglas J, Hsueh W, Sowers J. Preserving renal function in adults with hypertension and diabetes: a consensus approach. National Kidney Foundation Hypertension and Diabetes Executive Committees Working Group. Am J Kidney Dis 2000; 36:646–661.

13. Systolic Hypertension in the Elderly Program (SHEP) Co-operative Research Group. Prevention of stroke by antihypertensive drug treatment in older persons with isolated systolic hypertension: final results of SHEP. JAMA 1991; 265:3255–3264.

14. Lindholm LH, Ibsen H, Dahlof B, Devereux RB, Beevers G, de Faire U, Fyhrquist F, Julius S, Kjeldsen SE, Kristiansson K, Lederballe-Pedersen O, Nieminen MS, Omvik P, Oparil S, Wedel H, Aurup P, Edelman J, Snapinn S. The LIFE Study Group. Cardiovascular morbidity and mortality in patients with diabetes in the Losartan Intervention For Endpoint reduction in hypertension study (LIFE): a randomised trial against Atenolol. Lancet 2002; 359:1004–1010.

15. Veterans Administration Co-operative Study Group on Antihypertensive Agents. Efficacy of Nadolol alone combined with bendroflumethiazide and hydralazine. Am J Cardiol 1983; 52:1230–1237.

16. Messerli FH, Weir MR, Neutel JM. Combination therapy of amlodipine/benazepril versus monotherapy of amlodipine in a practice-based setting. Am J Hypertens 2002; 15:550–556.

17. Materson BJ, Reda DJ, Cushman WC, Henderson WG. For the Department of Veterans Affairs Co-operative Study Group on Anti-hypertensive Agents: Results of combination anti-hypertensive therapy after failure of each of the components. J Human Hypertens 1995; 9:791–796.

18. Materson BJ, Reda DJ, Williams D. Lessons from combination therapy in Veterans Affairs studies. Am J Hypertens 1996; 9:187S–191S.

19. Yusuf S, Sleight P, Pogue J, Bosch J, Davies R, Dagenais G. Effects of an angiotensin-converting-enzyme inhibitor, ramipril, on cardiovascular events in high-risk patients. The Heart Outcomes Prevention Evaluation Study Investigators. N Engl J Med 2000; 342:145–153.

20. Lewis EJ, Hunsicker LG, Clarke WR, Berl T, Pohl MA, Lewis JB, Ritz E, Atkins RC, Rohde R, Raz I. Collaborative Study Group. Renoprotective effect of the angiotensin-receptor antagonist irbesartan in patients with nephropathy due to type 2 diabetes. N Engl J Med 2001; 345:851–860.

21. Brenner BM, Cooper ME, de Zeeuw D, Keane WF, Mitch WE, Parving HH, Remuzzi G, Snapinn SM, Zhang Z, Shahinfar S. RENAAL Study Investigators. Effects of losartan on renal and cardiovascular outcomes in patients with type 2 diabetes and nephropathy. N Engl J Med 2001; 345:861–869.

22. Parving HH, Lehnert H, Brochner-Mortensen J, Gomis R, Andersen S, Arner P. Irbesartan in Patients with Type 2 Diabetes and Microalbuminuria Study Group. The effect of irbesartan on the development of diabetic nephropathy in patients with type 2 diabetes. N Engl J Med 345:870–878.

23. Veterans Administration Co-operative Study Group on Antihypertensive Agents. Propranolol in the treatment of essential hypertension. JAMA 1977; 237:2303–2310.

24. Materson BJ, Eidelson BA, Nash DT, Michelson EL, Zager PG, McCall MM III, Rush JE, Lengerich RA Langendörfer: Enalapril/hydrochlorothiazide vs. propranolol/hydrochlorothiazide in patients with mild to moderate hypertension. J Drug Development 1988; 1:40–49.

25. Gradman AH, Acevedo C. Evolving strategies for the use of combination therapy in hypertension. Current Hypertension Reports 2002; 4:343–349.

26. Gradman AH, Cutler NR, Davis PJ, Robbins JA, Weiss RJ, Wood BC. Combined enalapril and felodipine extended release (ER) for systemic hypertension. Enalapril-Felodipine ER Factorial Study Group. Am J Cardiol 1997; 79:431–435.

27. Elliott WJ. Is fixed combination therapy appropriate for initial hypertension treatment? Current Hypertension Reports 2002; 4:278–285.

28. Messerli FH, Oparil S, Feng Z. Comparison of efficacy and side effects of combination therapy of angiotensin-converting enzyme inhibitor (benazepril) with calcium antagonist (either nifedipine or amlodipine) versus high-dose calcium antagonist monotherapy for systemic hypertension. Am J Cardiol 2000; 86:1182–1187.

29. Mogensen CE, Neldam S, Tikkanen I, Oren S, Viskoper R, Watts RW, Cooper ME. Randomized controlled trial of dual blockade of renin–angiotensin system in patients with hypertension, microalbuminuria, and non-insulin dependent diabetes: the candesartan and lisinopril microalbuminuria (CALM) study. BMJ 2000; 321:1440–1444.

30. Nakao N, Yoshimura A, Morita H, Takada M, Kayano T, Ideura T. Combination treatment of angiotensin-II receptor blocker and angiotensin-converting-enzyme inhibitor in non-diabetic renal disease (COOPERATE): a randomised controlled trial. Lancet 2003; 361:117–124.

31. Song JH, Lee SW, Suh JH, Kim ES, Hong SB, Kim KA, Kim MJ. The effects of dual blockade of the renin–angiotensin system on urinary protein and transforming growth factor-β; excretion in 2 groups of patients with IgA and diabetic nephropathy. Clin Nephrology 2003; 60:318–326.

32. Wright JT Jr, Agodoa L, Contreras G, Greene T, Douglas JG, Lash J, Randall O, Rogers N, Smith MC, Massry S. African American Study of Kidney Disease and Hypertension Study Group. Successful blood pressure control in the African American Study of Kidney Disease and Hypertension. Arch Intern Med 2002; 162:1636–1643.

33. Flack JM, Saunders E, Gradman A, Kraus WE, Lester FM, Pratt JH, Alderman M, Green S, Vargas R, Espenshade M, Ceesay P, Alexander J Jr, Goldberg A. Antihypertensive efficacy and safety of losartan alone and in combination with hydrochlorothiazide in adult African Amerians with mild to moderate hypertension. Clin Ther 2001; 23:1193–1208.

34. Waeber B. Fixed low-dose combinations for hypertension. Current hypertension Reports 2002; 4:298–306.

35. Waeber B, Brunner HR. Low-dose combinations versus monotherapies in the treatment of hypertension. J Hypertens 1997; 5(suppl 2):17–20.

36. Neutel JM, Smith DH, Weber MA. Low-dose combination therapy: an important first-line treatment in the management of hypertension. Am J Hypertens 2001; 14:286–292.

37. Waeber B, Burnier M, Brunner HR. Compliance with antihypertensive therapy. Clin Exp Hypertens 1999; 21:5–6.

38. Ambrosioni E. Pharmacoeconomics of hypertension management: the place of combination therapy. Pharmacoeconomics 2001; 19:337–347.

39. Weinberger MH. Blood pressure and metabolic responses to hydrochlorothiazide, captopril, and the combination in black and white mild-to-moderate hypertensive patients. J Cardiovasc Pharmacol 1985; 7:S52–S55.

40. MacKay JH, Arcuri KE, Goldberg AI, Snapinn SM, Sweet CS. Losartan and low-dose hydrochlorothiazide in patients with essential hypertension. A double-blind, placebo-controlled trial of concomitant administration compared with individual components. Arch Intern Med 1996; 156:278–285.

41. Bakris GL, Williams B. Angiotensin converting enzyme inhibitors and calcium antagonists alone or combined: does the progression of diabetic renal disease differ? J Hypertens 1995; 13:S95–S101.

42. Triggle DJ. Mechansim of action of calcium channel antagonists. In: Epstein M, 2nd ed. Calcium Antagonists in Clinical Medicine. Philadelphia: Hanley & Belfus, 1997:1–26.

43. Materson BJ. Calcium channel blockers: is it time to split the lump? Am J Hypertens 1995; 8:325–329.

44. Saseen JJ, Carter BL, Brown TE, Elliott WJ, Black HR. Comparison of nifedipine alone and with diltiazem or verapamil in hypertension. Hypertension 1996; 28:109–114.

45. Kaesemeyer WH, Carr AA, Bottini PB, Prisant LM. Verapamil and nifedipine in combination for the treatment of hypertension. J Clin Pharmacol 1994; 34:48–51.

46. Law MR, Wald NJ, Morris JK, Jordan RE. Value of low dose combination treatment with blood pressure lowering drugs: analysis of 354 randomised trials. BMJ 2003; 326:1427–1434.

47. Wald NJ, Law MR. A strategy to reduce cardiovascular disease by more than 80%. BMJ 2003; 326:1419–1424.

35

Compliance with Antihypertensive Medication

ANDREAS ZELLER, EDOUARD J. BATTEGAY
University Hospital Basel, Basel, Switzerland

KEYPOINTS

- Compliance is the extent to which patient's behavior in terms of taking medication corresponds with agreed recommendations from a health care provider.
- Compliance with antihypertensives is affected by the interplay of patient-related, condition-related, therapy-related, health care system-related, and socio-economic factors.
- Measuring compliance is difficult, a gold standard does not exist.
- Medical event monitoring system improves the assessment of compliance substantially.

- Hearing patients' thoughts about taking drugs (e.g., antihypertensives) and patients' disease model is essential.
- An open and trusting partnership between patient and physician is crucial for optimal compliance.
- Side effects, complex treatment regimen, and therapy failure of antihypertensives substantially lower compliance.
- An effective, simple, and side effects free antihypertensive therapy for an optimal compliance is mandatory.
- Non- or mal-compliance as the single cause not achieving target blood pressure is overestimated.

SUMMARY

Compliance is a multidimensional phenomenon that is affected by the interplay of many dynamic issues: social and economic factors, condition-related-factors, therapy-related factors, patient-related factors, health care team, and system-related factors. In hypertension, a chronic and frequently asymptomatic condition, the handling of noncompliance with antihypertensive medication remains a difficult task. However, compliance rates in patients resistant to antihypertensive drugs is better than often assumed and corresponds to compliance rates for many drugs in many conditions and diseases.

The measuring of compliance is difficult and a golden standard does not exist. Medical event monitoring system (MEMS®) improved the assessment of compliance substantially. However, electronic monitoring is expensive and not readily available in busy clinical practice.

There is no single intervention that has been shown to be effective in all patients or settings. Poor compliance to long-term therapies, such as hypertension, severely worsens the clinical outcome regarding hypertension-related morbidity and mortality.

The most important element in determining compliance is the relationship between physician and patient. Patients need to be supported and not blamed. Open and trusting partnerships concerning the management of hypertension improve compliance. Similarly, sufficient information in the patient's own language and taking account of the patients' disease model increase compliance. Unpleasant aspects, such as forgotten doses of antihypertensive drugs, side effects, the difficulty in attaining an effect, and other impediments, to therapy have to be discussed openly. Both partners have to evaluate the success and failure of therapy in regularly fixed consultations and to find individually tailored solutions.

The aim of an antihypertensive therapy is to make it an effective and simple therapy that is free of side effects. Achieving this aim provides the basis for optimal compliance. Obviously, the patient needs to know that this can be difficult and may require time or be impossible all together.

I. INTRODUCTION

Effective and usually well-tolerated drugs are available for the treatment of arterial hypertension. Nevertheless, normal blood pressures are not achieved, even after prolonged treatment, in a substantial number of patients (1,2). Poor compliance might be one explanation for unsatisfactory blood pressure control with antihypertensive therapy (3).

Compliance of the patient with the physician's prescriptions and adherence to medication is a much-debated problem in hypertension. Often, physicians would like to believe that a lack of compliance is the main reason for therapy-resistant hypertension, and that resistance to therapy is therefore the patient's problem. In line with this, efforts to understand poor blood pressure control have focused especially on patient's compliance with antihypertensive medication and patient characteristics associated with non- or poor-adherence. On the other hand, more and more evidence is emerging that physicians may not be aggressive enough with the management of hypertension (4). Although physicians seem to be familiar with guidelines for treating hypertension, this knowledge is not fully implemented into daily clinical practice. Nevertheless, lack of adherence by the patient has been identified as one reason that antihypertensive therapy is not successful (5,6).

Nonadherence to medication is believed to be especially common when complex antihypertensive drug regimens have to be established. The complexity of regimens includes multiple drugs and dosages. Reducing the number of daily doses seems to be effective in increasing compliance with blood pressure-lowering medication (5,7). Furthermore, if the patient's knowledge, understanding (5,8), and perception (5,9) of hypertension is insufficient, an optimal compliance to antihypertensive therapy is unlikely (5,10).

The nature and determinants of noncompliant behavior is multifaceted, and despite of intense research efforts not fully understood. Incompliant behavior is a problem with self-administered treatments for all disorders. Additionally, patients tend to miss appointments and drop out of care when there are, for instance, long waiting times at clinics or long time lapses between appointments. These factors are definitely not patient-related.

Obviously, adherence to pharmacological therapy is a critical factor for the success of any therapy. Nonadherence to prescribed medication increases the economic burden of disease and also precludes beneficial effects, especially of antihypertensive treatments. In clinical practice, the differentiation between nonresponse to prescribed medication and noncompliance to medication is crucial for the treating physician and the quality of the interaction between the patient and physician.

II. DEFINITIONS

Most research has focused on compliance with medication. However, compliance also includes several health-related behaviors that extent beyond taking prescribed pharmaceuticals. The definition of compliance as "the extend to which the patient follows medical instructions" is assumed to be insufficient in describing the range of intervention used to treat chronic diseases such as arterial hypertension. Furthermore, the term "instructions" implies that the patient is a passive, acquiescent recipient of expert advice as opposed to an active partner and collaborator in the treatment process and decisions about it (5,11).

Two different terms are used to describe compliance. However, in our view, the terms compliance and adherence should be used as synonyms. The point to be stressed is that both terms are intended to be nonjudgmental, a statement of fact rather than of blame of the prescribing physician, patient, or treatment (5,12).

A. Persistence

Persistence is the continued taking of the initially prescribed medication over the long-term. The duration of time, a patient remains on a prescribed treatment, is based on the physician's willingness to continue prescribing a medication and the patient's willingness to continue taking it. Persistence is thus a reflection of both efficacy and tolerability (Fig. 35.1). It depends on adverse effects, comorbidity, and costs. Especially, patients with chronic and asymptomatic conditions are at risk to discontinue treatment due to real or falsely attributed adverse effects or because they perceive the medication to be ineffective. Hypertension is a prime example for a chronic condition without typical symptoms and therefore a particular challenge in terms of persistence. Persistence with antihypertensive therapy decreased in the first 6 months after treatment was started and continued to decline over the next 4 years (5,13). At the end of 1 year only 78% of the patients with newly diagnosed hypertension persisted with therapy. These results have been confirmed and reproduced (5,14,15). Among those with newly diagnosed hypertension, older patients were more likely than younger ones to persist, and women were more likely than men to persist ($p < 0.001$) (Fig. 35.1).

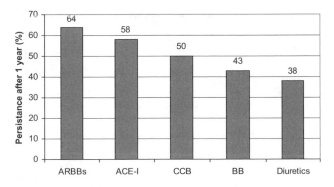

Figure 35.1 Compliance medication regimens after 1 year according to drug class initially prescribed to patients. [From Bloom (14).]

B. Compliance

Compliance (or "adherence") is the extent to which the patient's actual dosing history conforms to the prescribed regimen or the extent to which the patient's behavior in terms of taking medications, following diets, or making other lifestyle changes corresponds with recommendations from a health care provider to which the patient has agreed (16).

Compliance affects persistence, but it explains only a minor part of low persistence rates on antihypertensive drugs (8). Moreover, a patient may still persist on a prescribed drug while being partially noncompliant. Compliance is a mainly patient-centered variable that is affected by physician–patient interactions. The definition of persistence and compliance shows the difficulties that many medical regimens present for the patient. For example, the regimen described for a patient with metabolic syndrome includes a special diet, increased physical activity, smoking cessation, antidiabetic drugs and/or injection of insulin, antihypertensive treatment, antilipidemic medication, and possibly additional drugs. Such a therapy fulfills theoretical, physiological, and empirical considerations about optimal care of patients with metabolic syndrome. At the same time, practical patient-centered concerns, such as the nature, culture, and personal attitudes of the patient or costs, and adverse effects of the treatment are ignored. As a result the patient may get confused with the complex treatment and become (partially) incompliant to the therapy regimen.

Definitions of compliance using pill counting data can complicate the interpretation of knowledge achieved from clinical trials. To address this problem, Eisen et al. (17) compared two definition of compliance in patients based on counting the prescribed daily doses. A first definition represents the percentage of prescribed doses that the patient removed during the interval of observation (no. of doses removed/no. of doses prescribed). This definition corresponds to pill counting during a consultation or in clinical trials. It is independent of information about timing of dose removal and suggests perfect compliance (100%) even if the patient forgets doses and removes all doses briefly before the consultation. A second definition equals the percentage of days during which less than the prescribed number of doses or greater than the prescribed number of doses were removed. This definition suggests a worse than real compliance in patients who do not remove the prescribed number of doses of a multiple dose regimen each day. Using the first definition, patient compliance was higher on a once- (96%) or twice- (93%) daily dose regimen compared with a three times (84%) daily regimen ($p < 0.05$) (17) (Fig. 35.2).

Examining mean daily compliance according to the second definition revealed that the percentage of days on

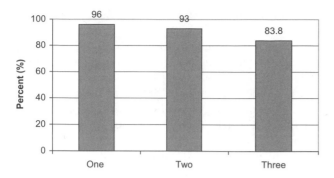

Figure 35.2 Compliance defined as the percentage of prescribed doses that the patient removed during the interval of observation. One, once daily; two, twice daily; three, three times daily. [From Eisen et al. (17).]

which the prescribed were removed correctly, decreased significantly with dose frequency (once-daily 83.6%, twice-daily 75%, three times daily 59%) (17) (Fig. 35.3). This example shows how compliance can vary depending on the definition used. Both definitions can be used to measure compliance and provide substantially different compliance rates. This complicates the interpretation of findings from clinical trials enormously. It also demonstrates the degree to which compliance may be overestimated with the simple pill count method or underestimated with other methods.

If one uses the MEMS the definition of compliance has to be very precise in order to correct compare findings from various studies.

Timing compliance is the strictest of the definitions of adherence. It can be defined as the percentage of the prescribed number of doses taken within a correct interval. The correct interval between two doses is determined by the prescribed drug regimen. For a regimen with one dose per day the correct inter-dose interval is 24 h, for

two doses per day it is 12 h, and for three doses per day it is 8 h. Allowing for a tolerance of $\pm 25\%$, for a regimen of one dose per day the correct inter-dose interval is between 18 and 32 h. The percentage of doses taken within a correct interval is the number of correct inter-dose intervals divided by the total number of doses taken less one, because there is one less interval between doses than the total number of doses taken.

"Correct dosing" is the percentage of days on which the correct number of doses was taken. *Taking compliance* is the number of doses taken divided by the number of doses prescribed during a monitored interval. The number of doses prescribed corresponds with the number of monitored days multiplied by the number of doses prescribed per day and provides the equivalent data to a "pill count." This adherence measure is the least strict of the three described.

III. THE FIVE INTERACTING DIMENSIONS AFFECTING COMPLIANCE

Recently, the World Health Organization described the issue of compliance as a multidimensional phenomenon determined by the interplay of five sets of factors (Fig. 35.4) (18): (1) social/economic factors; (2) health care team and system-related factors; (3) condition-related factors; (4) therapy-related factors; and (5) patient-related factors. The authors of this document point out that patient-related factors are just one determinant affecting compliance (19). They also stress that the common belief patients are solely responsible for taking their medication is obviously misleading (19).

The socio-economic status of a patient has been reported to have an effect on adherence (18). Notably, poverty, illiteracy (20), low level of education, and

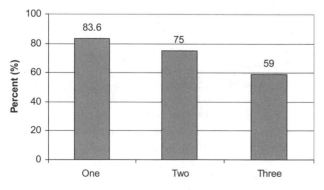

Figure 35.3 Compliance defined as the percentage of days with 100% of the doses removed from the monitor. One, once daily; two, twice daily; three, three times daily. [From Eisen et al. (17).]

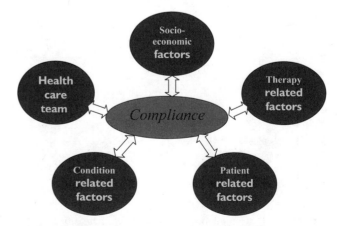

Figure 35.4 The five dimensions that affect compliance according to the World Health Organization. [From Sabate (18).]

unemployment seem to lower adherence to medication (21,22). For example, in a case–control study examining an inner-city minority population (low income or no employment, black or Hispanic, drug addiction, or unskilled employee), severe, uncontrolled hypertension was found to be more common among patients who had no primary care physician [adjusted odds ratio, 3.5; 95% confidence interval (CI) 1.6–7.7] or lack of health insurance compared with a hypertensive control group (23).

In developing countries, factors, such as unstable living conditions (24), long distance from treatment centers or nonaffordable costs of medication (25), also influence the level of adherence. In a cross-sectional study of hypertensive patients in eastern Sudan, inability to buy drugs was negatively and significantly associated with noncompliance (26). Poorly developed health services, poor medication distribution systems, and lack of knowledge and training for health care workers on managing chronic diseases are important factors, which have negative effects on adherence independent of the patient's performance (18).

Condition-related factors refer to disease-specific demands faced by the patient. Hypertensive patients are at risk to become incompliant, because the condition is asymptomatic for a long time. Other strong determinants of adherence with respect to condition-related factors are rate of progression or severity of disease, and the availability of treatments.

Therapy-related factors affecting adherence are manifold. Side effects and complexity of the medical regimen substantially affect compliance. Also, frequent changes in treatment lowers adherence. Availability of accurate information for the patient concerning the prescribed medication improves compliance.

Patient-related factors include patient's knowledge and beliefs about their illness and the motivation to manage it. Patients seem to be concerned about the necessity of their prescribed medication and are interested in information about the necessity of their medication weighed against the potential adverse effects of taking it (27). Patients also seem to have a fairly negative view of drugs. They attribute generally harmful effects of drugs that are over-used by doctors in other situations (27). In a qualitative study in two urban general practices, the thoughts of taking antihypertensive drugs were analyzed by interviewing hypertensive patients in a primary care setting (28). Results showed that four in every five people (80%) had reservations about taking antihypertensives and two-thirds preferred to lower blood pressure without taking drugs. Nearly, 40% of patients were concerned of having side effects in the near future or in the long run (28). About half of these patients (17%) stated feeling unwelcome side effects from the actually taken antihypertensive medication.

IV. MEASURING COMPLIANCE

These are the factors to consider in measuring compliance.

- Patient interview
- Keeping arranged appointments
- Prescription refills
- Pill counts
- Standardized patient-administered questionnaires
- Drug concentration in urine or serum
- Concentrations of marker substances in urine or serum
- Electronic medication monitoring

Accurate assessment of compliance is necessary for effective and efficient treatment planning, and for ensuring that changes in health outcomes can be attributed to the recommended regimens. One of the most important problem is the lack of entirely satisfactory methods to measure compliance. This has made research into compliance difficult. Most methods are indirect and fault-prone. Indisputably, a commonly accepted gold standard does not exist (29,30). Although no clinical measurement of compliance approaches perfection, clinical information can be used to find situations in which the patient may be incompliant to medication. Generally, patients should be informed about the assessment of compliance and asked for consent, because possibly the patient's privacy could be invaded against patient's will. Patients usually agree to have their compliance measured or measure it themselves if the physician explains the purpose of the assessments. The patient should be informed that the aim is to better understand how effective the taken medicine is or why a therapy does not work as expected (31).

Pill boxes that electronically record every opening, such as MEMS (Fig. 35.5), have substantially improved the assessment of compliance and have been successfully used in several clinical trials in arterial hypertension and in other conditions (32–34).

This electronic monitor consists of a container similar to traditional drug bottles and a large lid, which holds a microchip and a pressure release system. Closure and opening of the bottles activates the system and is called a medication event. The monitor stores the exact time and date of each opening sequence, and summary data can be downloaded onto a personal computer (Fig. 35.6). The medication event is defined as the electronically detected, time-stamped maneuver made by the electronic monitor, which is a necessary condition for removing a dose of a drug. In practice, this is assumed to designate the taking of a prescribed drug dose. There is no assurance that patients actually consume their medications, but they have to open and close the bottle at prescribed intervals on a daily basis to create a false pattern of adherence. This is very unlikely. Results based on electronic monitoring have

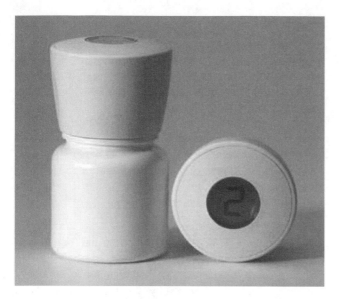

Figure 35.5 MEMS. Pill box that measures compliance by recording openings.

been reported in over 350 publications, including over 50 peer-reviewed original research papers. Electronic monitoring is now considered as a "gold standard" for the measurement of adherence (35,36). MEMS is reliable with a failure rate (dysfunction of the electronic chip or problems of downloading data) of <1% (37).

Keeping arranged appointments or prescription refills can give a crude estimate of patients compliance. Patient interviews seem to be more accurate despite their potential for inaccuracy. Obviously, it is very helpful when patients admit noncompliance upon appropriate questions, but denial of noncompliance is common. Patients who reveal that they have not followed treatment advice in general terms tend to describe details of their behavior accurately (11,38), whereas patients who deny their failure to follow

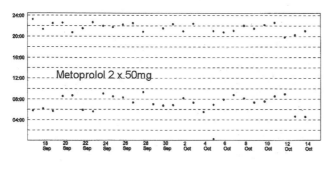

% days correct number of doses taken   96.43 %
% prescribed doses taken on schedule   62.50 %
Taking compliance   98.21 %

Figure 35.6 Example of optimal compliance with antihypertensive therapy. Once-daily drug regimen measured by MEMS.

recommendations in general terms report details of their behavior inaccurately (39). Generally, when health care providers have to rate the degree to which patients follow their recommendations they overestimate compliance (40). In one study, primary care physicians were asked to estimate compliance of patients they felt to know well (41). The sensitivity of clinical judgment was only 10%. This value is very low and physicians should not trust their unaided judgment regarding the compliance of individual patients.

Pill counts have been widely used in various studies. However, pill counts may not adequately describe true compliance because unused pills can be discarded by patients. Furthermore, timing of dosage and patterns of missed doses are not detected. Still, weekly pill counts provide better information than long-term average pill counts (42).

The use of brief medication questionnaires to screen for adherence and barriers to adherence have been validated and been made available to physicians in busy clinical practice. Ogedegbe et al. (43) recently developed and evaluated a 26-item medication self-efficacy scale. The authors aimed to identify situations in which patients have low self-efficacy, which is a known predictor for a wide range of health behaviors. This scale showed good internal consistency and stable scores, and it was easy to use and understand for patients. However, it has only been evaluated among African-Americans in the United States and it seems to be too extensive for a busy primary care practice. Furthermore, the scale did not quantify prediction of adherence to prescribed antihypertensive medication. A much shorter questionnaire to assess patient's compliance to antihypertensive medication was developed recently (44). The tool includes a five-item Regimen Screen, which asks patients about they took their medication during in the past week, a two-item Belief Screen asking about drug effects and bothersome features of drugs, and a two-item Recall Screen about potential difficulties of memory. The validity of this instrument was assessed in 20 patients who were prescribed ACE inhibitors by using MEMS as a comparator. This questionnaire showed an 80–100% sensitivity for different types of adherence, suggesting that this tool is more sensitive than existing tools. This study was the first to demonstrate that sensitivity levels vary by type of nonadherence and by type of screening tool.

Another method to gage medication compliance is measurements of drug concentrations in serum or urine (45) or of low dose chemical markers added to the drugs in plasma and urine. However, in most clinical settings, these methods are not readily available for any of the antihypertensive drugs and may strain the relationship and mutual trust between physician and patient. Furthermore, satisfactory serum or urine levels of drugs can usually be attained if the patient takes the drugs for a few days before the consultation, that is, patients with white coat compliance or a "*tooth brush effect*" are not identified. In other words, in patients with toothbrush effect drug levels may be high or even toxic and compliance still very poor (Fig. 35.7).

A few drugs induce typical clinical effects that can be assessed as a measure of compliance, such as pulse rate reduction with beta-blocking agents, increased urinary frequency with the initiation of diuretics, dry mouth with anticholinergics, or dark stool with oral iron.

Independent of the technique used to gage compliance threshold of good and poor compliance are widely used, despite the lack of evidence to support such thresholds. In practice, good and poor compliance might be grossly inadequate terms because a poor compliance of 50% may be sufficient in a patient that responds well to the therapy, whereas a good compliance of 80% may be insufficient because of a poor response. A demonstrative example that compliance should not be treated as a dichotomous variable (e.g., taking >80% compliance is good, taking <80% compliance is poor) is adherence to oral anticontraceptive therapy. A taking compliance of 80% in this condition may not suffice for contraception and lead to pregnancy. Similarly, for highly active antiretroviral therapy to suppress emergence of viral mutations in HIV, compliance should exceed even 95% (46). In sinusitis, compliance with a specific antibiotic treatment during the first 3 days of treatment may be sufficient (47).

Measurement of compliance gives useful information that monitoring of outcome alone cannot provide. However, available methods can only estimate the patient's actual behavior. No single measurement is optimal. An approach using multiple methods that combines self-reporting and objective measurements is currently the best way to assess compliance.

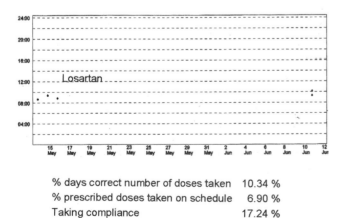

% days correct number of doses taken	10.34 %
% prescribed doses taken on schedule	6.90 %
Taking compliance	17.24 %

Figure 35.7 Example of partial compliance with antihypertensive therapy (toothbrush effect). Once-daily drug regimen measured by MEMS.

V. TYPES OF NONCOMPLIANCE

Noncompliance can be described as falling into one or more of several categories.

- Total
- Nondeclared
- Partial
- Drug holiday
- Over-compliance
- Toothbrush effect or white coat compliance

Degrees of noncompliance with drug regimens vary from total, nondeclared noncompliance (taking no drug at all and not telling the treating physician) to over-compliance which means taking more drugs than prescribed and agreed. The most common form of poor compliance in hypertension, and almost all other conditions, is partial compliance. An example of partial compliance is a "drug holiday"; patients intentionally omit or unintentionally forget their medication for a few days, for example on a business trip or on weekends. Another form of partial compliance is termed as the toothbrush effect or white coat compliance, that is, an increase of compliance before and after a consultation at the doctor's office. In general, patients frequently change their degree and pattern of noncompliance. Compliance is therefore a dynamic process and any measurement of compliance only looks at a selected phase of the patients variegated lives.

VI. COMPLIANCE IN HOME BLOOD PRESSURE MEASUREMENTS

Measuring blood pressure at home is recommended to distinguish sustained from white coat hypertension and to monitor treatment (48,49). Furthermore, home blood pressure measurement can improve compliance with medication and empower patients in the management of their condition (50,51).

An analysis of 1350 consecutive patients in a representative sample of the hypertensive population showed that home blood pressure measurement is widely performed by hypertensive patients managed in a hypertension hospital clinic (52). This practice was associated with a significantly higher rate of clinic blood pressure control (52). In addition, age, male gender, and educational level were associated with the use of home blood pressure measurement (52). Home blood pressure measurement also lead to less intensive drug treatment and lowered costs marginally (53). On the other hand, patients measuring their home blood pressure more often stopped their antihypertensive therapy (25.6% vs. 11.3%; $P < 0.001$). Furthermore, patients monitoring their therapy with office blood

Table 35.1 Types of Mistakes in Incorrectly Reported Measurements of Blood Pressure ($n = 794$) Taken at Home (27% of All Performed Measurements) (54)

Mistake	No. of mistakes (%)	No. of patients ($n = 54$)
Timing	270 (34)	27
Averaging	231 (29)	25
Single measurements	209 (26)	23
False high systolic values	50 (6)	14
False high diastolic values	51 (6)	18
False low systolic values	48 (6)	13
False low diastolic values	60 (8)	16
Invented measurements	57 (7)	9
Measurements not reported	13 (2)	7
Miscellaneous	14 (2)	7

pressure and ambulatory blood pressure had significantly lower blood pressure values after a mean of 350 days of follow-up (53).

We, recently, examined whether patients with hypertension or suspected hypertension, who had been referred for 24 h ambulatory blood pressure monitoring, accurately reported their home blood pressure measurements (54) (Table 35.1) and whether reporting accuracy affected the assessment of the patients' condition (55). Reporting accuracy of blood pressure measurements taken at home was acceptable in most patients (73%). Patients of lower educational level tended to report less accurately (relative risk 3.39 for reporting <80% correct measurements). Inadequate conclusions regarding the assessment of a hypertensive patient owing to poor reporting were possible but rarely clinically relevant (55).

VII. COMPLIANCE WITH DRUG TREATMENT

Obviously, individuals with hypertension need to stay on therapy with antihypertensive medication to obtain the full benefits of blood pressure reduction. The complex pathophysiology of hypertension is an important factor influencing the success of pharmacological treatment (56). Thus, the antihypertensive agent prescribed may not be effective because its mechanism of action is inappropriate for the underlying condition. Unfortunately, the response to a particular agent can seldom be predicted on clinical grounds alone.

The initial choice of an antihypertensive agent may influence the extent to which patients stay on therapy. In a retrospective study, drug persistence over nearly 5 years was significantly associated with the initial choice of drug class (57). Angiotensin receptor blockers had the highest persistence followed by ACE inhibitors, calcium

channel blockers, beta-blocker, and diuretics (57). Generally, persistence decreased with time.

Compliance to antihypertensive medication is also affected by the frequency of daily dosage. A meta-analysis of eight studies involving >10,000 observations demonstrated that once-daily dosing is associated with higher rates of adherence than either twice-daily or multiple-daily regimens (58). In elderly outpatients aged between 65 and 99 years, good compliance (≥80%) was associated with the use of newer agents such as angiotensin-converting enzyme inhibitors (OR 1.9, 95% CI 1.6–2.2) and calcium channel blockers (OR 1.7, 95% CI 1.5–2.1) (59). In addition, adverse drug reactions to antihypertensive medication, especially in older patients, correlate with noncompliance (60). Avoiding side effects can, therefore, be an important consideration when prescribing antihypertensive drugs. However, perceived side effects are more likely to occur at the beginning of therapy and tend to decrease over time (61). In general, younger patients tend to quit their medication because blood pressure has improved, whereas older patients tend to discontinue treatment because adverse effects have occurred (62). Women are more likely to adhere to antihypertensive therapy and to achieve better blood pressure control than men (62). Furthermore, discontinuation of antihypertensive medication is associated with younger age, lower prevalence of previous hospitalizations for cardiovascular disease, and less concurrent chronic pharmacotherapies (62). Depressive symptoms may be an underrecognized but modifiable risk factor for poor compliance with antihypertensive medications (63).

VIII. COMPLIANCE IN THERAPY-RESISTANT HYPERTENSION

Patients in whom a prespecified blood pressure cannot be achieved are commonly referred to as having therapy-resistant hypertension (2,49). Therapy-resistant hypertension is described in details in Chapter 37. Noncompliance with antihypertensive therapy can be a limiting factor in achieving the therapeutic goals in hypertensive patients. To obtain reliable prevalence data is difficult because therapy resistance strongly depends on the setting. For example, therapy-resistant hypertension in a primary care setting (64) or among New York employees (65) is ~3%. In referred patients (66) and hypertension clinics (67), the prevalence of therapy-resistant hypertension is much higher and can exceed 20% of all patients.

Earlier studies had shown relatively poor compliance in patients with arterial hypertension (68,69). However, many recent hypertension trials have shown compliance rates ~80% with antihypertensive drugs (70,71). We, recently, performed a prospective study in which medication compliance was >80% in patients with an adequate response to treatment and also in patients with resistance to treatment in hypertension (34). In the study, 103 consecutive patients were analyzed on stable treatment with at least two antihypertensive agents, that is, 49 nonresponders were compared with 54 responders (34). Compliance, measured by using MEMS during 1 month for two drugs, did not significantly differ between the two groups (82% in nonresponders, 85% in responders) (34). Furthermore, the compliance rate in most patients was >80% (Fig. 35.8). Patients with compliance rate <50% were an exception (8.7%).

Another recent study investigated whether monitoring compliance with MEMS affected therapy resistance in 41 patients without controls (32). Although similar rates of compliance were obtained in comparison to our study, blood pressure levels improved significantly upon MEMS monitoring, suggesting that increasing compliance can ameliorate blood pressure control in therapy-resistant patients. However, even with almost perfect compliance rates achieved through MEMS monitoring, most blood pressures remained in the range that would commonly be described as therapy resistant and further improvements of blood pressures occurred upon modifications of the drug regimen (32). Similarly, MEMS monitoring improved blood pressure control significantly in those patients categorized as nonresponders in our study, but not in those categorized as responders to therapy (Edouard Battegay et al., unpublished data). Nevertheless, the majority of patients with therapy resistance remained poorly controlled upon compliance monitoring in spite of high compliance rates in both studies. Compliance, therefore, turns out to be only one of the many variables in explaining resistance in the majority of patients. Indeed, the lack of a perceived effect of an antihypertensive drug, that is, therapy resistance itself, may hypothetically induce patients assessing their own blood pressure to become noncompliant.

IX. IMPROVING COMPLIANCE

Compliance with treatment recommendations by physicians has a major impact on health outcomes and costs of care for patients with arterial hypertension. The process aims at achieving normal blood pressure values by an individually tailored, well-tolerated treatment regimen. Physicians must be aware of several important factors that influence patients' compliance with antihypertensive therapy. Factors that might affect compliance should be systematically evaluated and discussed with the patient. If possible, measurement of compliance should be done by appropriate methods.

A recent systematic review of randomized controlled trials that assessed, which types of intervention to increase adherence. Simplification of dosing regimens increased adherence (measured by MEMS) by 8–19.8% (7) and was the most effective measure to be taken. The effects of motivational (e.g., nurse telephone calls, written educational material, group education) or complex health and organizational interventions (work-side management by nurse/physician, intervention by clinical pharmacist, combined postcard/telephone/nurse-led educational appointments reminders) were mixed, that is, partly successful or inconclusive. These results add evidence in the field of adherence to antihypertensive medication; however, included trials were heterogeneous and often of poor methodological quality, and more evidence from carefully designed randomized trials is needed. With respect to the following points, adherence to antihypertensive drugs may be improved in clinical practice.

A. Side Effects

Patient surveys, which attempted to determine risk factors for poor compliance, have repeatedly shown that side effects of antihypertensive drugs are strongly associated with reduced compliance rates (8,60). Furthermore, the fear of dose-dependent side effects are probably one of the important reasons that physicians accept inadequate blood pressure control and do not titrate the dose upward. Low-dose combination therapy may provide an effective alternative to titrating upward with monotherapy regimen. In fact, guidelines suggest the use of low-dose combination therapy as antihypertensive first-step treatment (49), and this may be a more efficient way to achieve blood pressure targets with acceptable side effects (72).

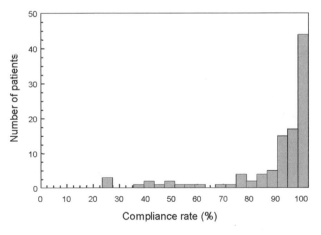

Figure 35.8 Compliance rates in 103 patients taking antihypertensive medication measured by MEMS. [From Nuesch et al. (34).]

B. Dosing Interval

Antihypertensive agents that are dosed once-daily are taken more regularly than drugs that have to be taken more than twice-daily (7,73). Indeed, there is no evidence for improved blood pressure control or better outcomes when drugs are taken or must be taken three times a day in a hypertensive patient. Therefore, it is important to choose a drug that provides adequate blood pressure control over an entire 24 h interval. Duration of action can be best assessed by instructing patients to omit dosing on the morning of their clinical visit.

C. Avoidance of Polypharmacy

The number of drugs that a patient has to take and their compliance with a drug regimen correlates inversely (74). Patients may become confused by complex multiple drug regimen and might therefore take them incorrectly.

D. Exploration of Patients' Thoughts About Antihypertensive Medication

For the treating physician, it is crucial to explore patients' ideas and concerns when planning an antihypertensive treatment. Patients balance their reservations about antihypertensives and drugs, in general, with reasons to take them. Generally, patients felt medicines were best avoided and seen unnatural or unsafe. Some patients spoke with doctors prescribing medicine too readily, and taking tablets were seen as an unwelcome sign of ill health (75). Regarding antihypertensive medication, in particular, patients were worried about taking drugs for the rest of their lives (75) and long-term or hidden risks. On the other hand, patients' reasons for taking antihypertensive medication were advice from physicians, achieving a good outcome, and improved blood pressure reading (75).

E. Patient Involvement in Treatment

Patients need advice, support, and information from the physician in order to better understand the importance of maintaining blood pressure control, to use their drugs rationally, to learn how to deal with missed doses, how to identify side effects and what to do when they occur (18). Sharing this responsibility with the physician is a must. The patient does not need to cope alone with his condition. Compliance to long-term medication regimen requires behavioral change, which involves learning, adopting, and sustaining a medication-taking behavior. Getting patients involved in their antihypertensive treatment influences compliance.

Use of home blood pressure monitors might empower patients to take control of their blood pressure treatment. Adequate patient education in this situation is crucial. Patients should understand the disease to a degree that lets them adequately judge the consequences of poor compliance. Patients should be instructed to use a validated monitor and to correctly measure blood pressure.

F. Other Interventions

A telephone-linked-computer system was tested as an aid to staying on therapy (76). Subjects reported self-measured blood pressures, knowledge and adherence to antihypertensive medication regimens, and medication side effects weekly. Mean antihypertensive medication adherence moderately improved by 17.7% for telephone system users and 11.7% for controls ($P = 0.03$).

Incorporating family members (77), office assistants, or technical aids such as MEMS-devices can help to improve compliance (32). For that, simple communication and negotiation skills are necessary.

Various interventions to remind the patient taking antihypertensive medication were tested in terms of improving adherence. Postal reminders (78), and e-mail reminders (79) or educational newsletter (79) may improve adherence. Furthermore, avoiding too many changes from one clinic to the other may substantially improve persistence on specific antihypertensive drugs (80). However, these studies used less reliable methods of measuring adherence, such as pill counts, direct questioning, and prescription refill reports.

X. CONCLUSIONS

Compliance with antihypertensive medication is a multi-dimensional phenomenon which is affected by the interplay of several dynamic issues such as social and economic factors, therapy-related factors, patient-related factors, interaction with the health care team, and system-related factors. Many clinicians find it difficult to differentiate between non- or poor compliance and non-response to antihypertensive drug treatment if a patient does not improve despite being prescribed effective drugs. Particularly in chronic medical conditions such as arterial hypertension, knowing the reasons why a patient's blood pressure isn't getting better is important, since the management strategies will be different.

Compliance rates in patients resistant to antihypertensive drugs is better than often assumed and corresponds to compliance rates for many drugs in many conditions and diseases. Efforts should be made to improve compliance such as simplifying dosing interval and choosing the most effective drug with least side effects.

The most important element in determining compliance is the relationship between physician and patient. Open and trusting partnerships concerning the management of hypertension improve compliance. Patients need to be supported and not blamed. Sufficient information in the patient's own language and taking account of the patient's disease model increases compliance. Provided an optimal compliance with antihypertensive medication as the result of a substantial effort by patients and physicians cardiovascular damage can be prevented.

REFERENCES

1. Graves JW. Management of difficult-to-control hypertension. Mayo Clin Proc 2000; 75:278–284.
2. Setaro JF, Black HR. Refractory hypertension. N Engl J Med 1992; 327:543–547.
3. Rudd P. Clinicians and patients with hypertension: unsettled issues about compliance. Am Heart J 1995; 130:572–579.
4. Oliveria SA, Lapuerta P, McCarthy BD, L'Italien GJ, Berlowitz DR, Asch SM. Physician-related barriers to the effective management of uncontrolled hypertension. Arch Intern Med 2002; 162:413–420.
5. The sixth report of the Joint National Committee on prevention, detection, evaluation, and treatment of high blood pressure. Arch Intern Med 1997; 157:2413–2446.
6. Miller NH, Hill M, Kottke T, Ockene IS. The multilevel compliance challenge: recommendations for a call to action. A statement for healthcare professionals. Circulation 1997; 95:1085–1090.
7. Schroeder K, Fahey T, Ebrahim S. How can we improve adherence to blood pressure-lowering medication in ambulatory care? Systematic review of randomized controlled trials. Arch Intern Med 2004; 164:722–732.
8. Dusing R, Weisser B, Mengden T, Vetter H. Changes in antihypertensive therapy—the role of adverse effects and compliance. Blood Press 1998; 7:313–315.
9. Wright EC. Non-compliance—or how many aunts has Matilda? Lancet 1993; 342:909–913.
10. Kjellgren KI, Ahlner J, Saljo R. Taking antihypertensive medication—controlling or co-operating with patients? Int J Cardiol 1995; 47:257–268.
11. Sabate E. Adherence Meeting Report. Geneva, World Health Organization, 2001.
12. McDonald HP, Garg AX, Haynes RB. Interventions to enhance patient adherence to medication prescriptions: scientific review. JAMA 2002; 288:2868–2879.
13. Caro JJ, Salas M, Speckman JL, Raggio G, Jackson JD. Persistence with treatment for hypertension in actual practice. CMAJ 1999; 160:31–37.
14. Bloom BS. Continuation of initial antihypertensive medication after 1 year of therapy. Clin Ther 1998; 20:671–681.
15. Hasford J, Mimran A, Simons WR. A population-based European cohort study of persistence in newly diagnosed hypertensive patients. J Hum Hypertens 2002; 16:569–575.
16. Sabate E. Defining adherence. In: World Health Organization, ed. Adherence to Long-term Therapies—Evidence for Action. Geneva: World Health Organization, 2003:3.
17. Eisen SA, Miller DK, Woodward RS, Spitznagel E, Przybeck TR. The effect of prescribed daily dose frequency on patient medication compliance. Arch Intern Med 1990; 150:1881–1884.
18. Sabate E. Adherence to long-term therapy—Evidence of action. Geneva: World Health Organization, 2003.
19. Towards the solution. In: Sabate E, ed. Adherence to Long-Term Therapies—Evidence for Action. Geneva: World Health Organization, 2003:27–38.
20. Hungerbuhler P, Bovet P, Shamlaye C, Burnand B, Waeber B. Compliance with medication among outpatients with uncontrolled hypertension in the Seychelles. Bull World Health Organ 1995; 73:437–442.
21. Khalil SA, Elzubier AG. Drug compliance among hypertensive patients in Tabuk, Saudi Arabia. J Hypertens 1997; 15:561–565.
22. Francis CK. Hypertension, cardiac disease, and compliance in minority patients. Am J Med 1991; 91:29S–36S.
23. Shea S, Misra D, Ehrlich MH, Field L, Francis CK. Predisposing factors for severe, uncontrolled hypertension in an inner-city minority population. N Engl J Med 1992; 327:776–781.
24. Joshi PP, Salkar RG, Heller RF. Determinants of poor blood pressure control in urban hypertensives of central India. J Hum Hypertens 1996; 10:299–303.
25. van der Sande MA, Milligan PJ, Nyan OA, Rowley JT, Banya WA, Ceesay SM, Dolmans WM, Thien T, McAdam KP, Walraven GE. Blood pressure patterns and cardiovascular risk factors in rural and urban gambian communities. J Hum Hypertens 2000; 14:489–496.
26. Elzubier AG, Husain AA, Suleiman IA, Hamid ZA. Drug compliance among hypertensive patients in Kassala, eastern Sudan. East Mediterr Health J 2000; 6:100–105.
27. Horne R. Patients' beliefs about treatment: the hidden determinant of treatment outcome? J Psychosom Res 1999; 47:491–495.
28. Benson J, Britten N. Patients' views about taking antihypertensive drugs: questionnaire study. BMJ 2003; 326:1314–1315.
29. Melnikow J, Kiefe C. Patient compliance and medical research: issues in methodology. J Gen Intern Med 1994; 9:96–105.
30. Urquhart J. Patient non-compliance with drug regimens: measurement, clinical correlates, economic impact. Eur Heart J 1996; 17(suppl A):8–15.
31. Stephenson BJ, Rowe BH, Haynes RB, Macharia WM, Leon G. The rational clinical examination. Is this patient taking the treatment as prescribed? JAMA 1993; 269:2779–2781.
32. Burnier M, Schneider MP, Chiolero A, Stubi CL, Brunner HR. Electronic compliance monitoring in resistant hypertension: the basis for rational therapeutic decisions. J Hypertens 2001; 19:335–341.
33. Mallion JM, Dutrey-Dupagne C, Vaur L, Genes N, Renault M, Elkik F, Baguet P, Boutelant S. Benefits of

electronic pillboxes in evaluating treatment compliance of patients with mild to moderate hypertension. J Hypertens 1996; 14:137–144.

34. Nuesch R, Schroeder K, Dieterle T, Martina B, Battegay E. Relation between insufficient response to antihypertensive treatment and poor compliance with treatment: a prospective case-control study. BMJ 2001; 323:142–146.

35. Cramer JA, Mattson RH, Prevey ML, Scheyer RD, Ouellette VL. How often is medication taken as prescribed? A novel assessment technique. JAMA 1989; 261:3273–3277.

36. Rudd P, Ahmed S, Zachary V, Barton C, Bonduelle D. Improved compliance measures: applications in an ambulatory hypertensive drug trial. Clin Pharmacol Ther 1990; 48:676–685.

37. Metry J. Measuring compliance in clinical trials and ambulatory care. In: Metry J, Meyer U, eds. Drug Regimen Compliance—Issue in Clinical Trails and Patient management. Chichester: Wiley & Sons, 1999.

38. Cramer JA, Mattson RH, Spilker B. Patient Compliance. In: Raven Press, ed. Patient Compliance in Medical Practice and Clinical Trials. New York, 1991:123–137.

39. Spector SL, Kinsman R, Mawhinney H, Siegel SC, Rachelefsky GS, Katz RM, Rohr AS. Compliance of patients with asthma with an experimental aerosolized medication: implications for controlled clinical trials. J Allergy Clin Immunol 1986; 77:65–70.

40. Norell SE. Accuracy of patient interviews and estimates by clinical staff in determining medication compliance. Soc Sci Med [E] 1981; 15:57–61.

41. Gilbert JR, Evans CE, Haynes RB, Tugwell P. Predicting compliance with a regimen of digoxin therapy in family practice. Can Med Assoc J 1980; 123:119–122.

42. Rudd P, Byyny RL, Zachary V, LoVerde ME, Titus C, Mitchell WD, Marshall G. The natural history of medication compliance in a drug trial: limitations of pill counts. Clin Pharmacol Ther 1989; 46:169–176.

43. Ogedegbe G, Mancuso CA, Allegrante JP, Charlson ME. Development and evaluation of a medication adherence self-efficacy scale in hypertensive African-American patients. J Clin Epidemiol 2003; 56:520–529.

44. Svarstad BL, Chewning BA, Sleath BL, Claesson C. The brief medication questionnaire: a tool for screening patient adherence and barriers to adherence. Patient Educ Couns 1999; 37:113–124.

45. Urquhart J. Role of patient compliance in clinical pharmacokinetics. A review of recent research. Clin Pharmacokinet 1994; 27:202–215.

46. Paterson DL, Swindells S, Mohr J, Brester M, Vergis EN, Squier C, Wagener MM, Singh N. Adherence to protease inhibitor therapy and outcomes in patients with HIV infection. Ann Intern Med 2000; 133:21–30.

47. Williams JW Jr, Holleman DR Jr, Samsa GP, Simel DL. Randomized controlled trial of 3 vs 10 days of trimethoprim/sulfamethoxazole for acute maxillary sinusitis. JAMA 1995; 273:1015–1021.

48. 2003 European Society of Hypertension-European Society of Cardiology guidelines for the management of arterial hypertension. J Hypertens 2003; 21:1011–1053.

49. Chobanian AV, Bakris GL, Black HR, Cushman WC, Green LA, Izzo JL Jr, Jones DW, Materson BJ, Oparil S, Wright JT Jr, Roccella EJ. Joint National Committee on Prevention, Detection, Evaluation, and Treatment of High Blood Pressure. National Heart, Lung, and Blood Institute; National High Blood Pressure Education Program Coordinating Committee. Seventh report of the Joint National Committee on Prevention, Detection, Evaluation, and Treatment of High Blood Pressure. Hypertension 2003; 42:1206–1252.

50. Vetter W, Hess L, Brignoli R. Influence of self-measurement of blood pressure on the responder rate in hypertensive patients treated with losartan: results of the SVATCH Study. Standard vs Automatic Treatment Control of COSAAR in Hypertension. J Hum Hypertens 2000; 14:235–241.

51. Zarnke KB, Feagan BG, Mahon JL, Feldman RD. A randomized study comparing a patient-directed hypertension management strategy with usual office-based care. Am J Hypertens 1997; 10:58–67.

52. Cuspidi C, Meani S, Fusi V, Salerno M, Valerio C, Severgnini B, Catini E, Leonetti G, Magrini F, Zanchetti A. Home blood pressure measurement and its relationship with blood pressure control in a large selected hypertensive population. J Hum Hypertens 2004; 18(10):725–731.

53. Staessen JA, Den Hond E, Celis H, Fagard R, Keary L, Vandenhoven G, O'Brien ET; Treatment of Hypertension Based on Home or Office Blood Pressure (THOP) Trial Investigators. Antihypertensive treatment based on blood pressure measurement at home or in the physician's office: a randomized controlled trial. JAMA 2004; 291:955–964.

54. Nordmann A, Frach B, Walker T, Martina B, Battegay E. Reliability of patients measuring blood pressure at home: prospective observational study. BMJ 1999; 319:1172.

55. Nordmann A, Frach B, Walker T, Martina B, Battegay E. Comparison of self-reported home blood pressure measurements with automatically stored values and ambulatory blood pressure. Blood Press 2000; 9:200–205.

56. Sever P. The heterogeneity of hypertension: why doesn't every patient respond to every antihypertensive drug? J Hum Hypertens 1995; 9(suppl 2):S33–S36.

57. Marentette MA, Gerth WC, Billings DK, Zarnke KB. Antihypertensive persistence and drug class. Can J Cardiol 2002; 18:649–656.

58. Iskedjian M, Einarson TR, MacKeigan LD, Shear N, Addis A, Mittmann N, Ilersich AL. Relationship between daily dose frequency and adherence to antihypertensive pharmacotherapy: evidence from a meta-analysis. Clin Ther 2002; 24:302–316.

59. Monane M, Bohn RL, Gurwitz JH, Glynn RJ, Levin R, Avorn J. The effects of initial drug choice and comorbidity on antihypertensive therapy compliance: results from a population-based study in the elderly. Am J Hypertens 1997; 10:697–704.

60. Nelson EC, Stason WB, Neutra RR, Solomon HS. Identification of the noncompliant hypertensive patient. Prev Med 1980; 9:504–517.

61. Edmonds D, Greminger P, Vetter W, Baumgart P, Vetter H. The neglected time factor and antihypertensive therapy. A pitfall in evaluating side effects in a cross-over study. Postgrad Med 1988; Spec No:40–45.

62. Degli Esposti L, Degli Esposti E, Valpiani G, Di Martin M, Saragoni S, Buda S, Baio G, Capone A, Sturani A. A retrospective, population-based analysis of persistence with antihypertensive drug therapy in primary care practice in Italy. Clin Ther 2002; 24:1347–1357.

63. Wang PS, Bohn RL, Knight E, Glynn RJ, Mogun H, Avorn J. Noncompliance with antihypertensive medications: the impact of depressive symptoms and psychosocial factors. J Gen Intern Med 2002; 17:504–511.

64. Andersson O. Management of hypertension. Clinical and hemodynamic studies with special reference to patients refractory to treatment. Acta Med Scand Suppl 1977; 617:1–62.

65. Alderman MH, Budner N, Cohen H, Lamport B, Ooi WL. Prevalence of drug resistant hypertension. Hypertension 1988; 11:II71–II75.

66. Yakovlevitch M, Black HR. Resistant hypertension in a tertiary care clinic. Arch Intern Med 1991; 151:1786–1792.

67. Swales JD, Bing RF, Heagerty A, Pohl JE, Russell GI, Thurston H. Treatment of refractory hypertension. Lancet 1982; 1:894–896.

68. Caldwell JR. Drug regimens for long-term therapy of hypertension. Geriatrics 1976; 31:115–119.

69. Eraker SA, Kirscht JP, Becker MH. Understanding and improving patient compliance. Ann Intern Med 1984; 100:258–268.

70. Andrejak M, Genes N, Vaur L, Poncelet P, Clerson P, Carre A. Electronic pill-boxes in the evaluation of antihypertensive treatment compliance: comparison of once daily versus twice daily regimen. Am J Hypertens 2000; 13:184–190.

71. Waeber B, Leonetti G, Kolloch R, McInnes GT. Compliance with aspirin or placebo in the Hypertension Optimal Treatment (HOT) study. J Hypertens 1999; 17:1041–1045.

72. Law MR, Wald NJ, Morris JK, Jordan RE. Value of low dose combination treatment with blood pressure lowering drugs: analysis of 354 randomised trials. BMJ 2003; 326:1427.

73. Sica DA. Fixed-dose combination antihypertensive drugs. Do they have a role in rational therapy? Drugs 1994; 48:16–24.

74. Neutel JM, Smith DH. Improving patient compliance: a major goal in the management of hypertension. J Clin Hypertens (Greenwich) 2003; 5:127–132.

75. Benson J, Britten N. Patients' decisions about whether or not to take antihypertensive drugs: qualitative study. BMJ 2002; 325:873.

76. Friedman RH, Kazis LE, Jette A, Smith MB, Stollerman J, Torgerson J et al. A telecommunications system for monitoring and counseling patients with hypertension. Impact on medication adherence and blood pressure control. Am J Hypertens 1996; 9:285–292.

77. Morisky DE, DeMuth NM, Field-Fass M, Green LW, Levine DM. Evaluation of family health education to build social support for long-term control of high blood pressure. Health Educ Q 1985; 12:35–50.

78. Skaer TL, Sclar DA, Markowski DJ, Won JK. Effect of value-added utilities on prescription refill compliance and health care expenditures for hypertension. J Hum Hypertens 1993;7:515–518.

79. Sclar DA, Skaer TL, Chin A, Okamoto MP, Gill MA. Utility of a transdermal delivery system for antihypertensive therapy. Part 1. Am J Med 1991; 91:50S–56S.

80. Chou CC, Lee MS, Ke CH, Chuang MH. Factors influencing the switch in the use of antihypertensive medications. Int J Clin Pract 2005; 59:85–91.

36

Management of Patients with Refractory Hypertension

SANDRA J. TALER

Mayo Clinic College of Medicine, Rochester, Minnesota, USA

KEYPOINTS

- Resistant hypertension is the failure to control blood pressure to goal levels using at least three antihypertensive agents, including a diuretic.
- Causes for resistance include errors in drug selection and dosing, secondary causes, and the interaction of other medications and lifestyle practices.
- The key to management of resistant hypertension lies in recognition by the practitioner and the patient that blood pressure readings are above goal levels.
- A detailed review of historical features, physical findings, basic laboratory test results, and an inventory of all medications and lifestyle factors will often provide clues to the cause of drug resistance.
- Decisions on the extent of testing indicated require careful examination of the patient's health status, balancing the risks of intervention against the risks of missing a contributing cause.
- Although a number of theoretic methods have been proposed, systematic approaches to treatment have demonstrated some success in trial settings, including supervised regular nurse intervention and follow-up, and use of serial measurement of hemodynamic parameters or volume indicators.

SUMMARY

Resistant hypertension is increasing in prevalence related in part to lower blood pressure goals in an aging population. Costs of this condition are high including target organ damage and the financial burden and emotional frustration of using increasing numbers of medications at higher dosages yet without achieving normal blood pressure levels. The key to managing this condition lies in recognition by the treating practitioner that first, the blood pressure is not controlled and requires a change in treatment and second, that further historical information, examination and laboratory testing may reveal the cause for resistance and the pathway to successful control. Causes for resistant hypertension include flaws in medication selections and dosing, secondary hypertension (most commonly due to renal parenchymal disease, renovascular hypertension, primary aldosteronism, or obstructive sleep apnea), lifestyle factors, and drug interactions. Decisions on the extent of testing or intervention appropriate for an individual patient require careful review to balance the risks of intervention against the risks of leaving a secondary cause unrecognized. A single treatment approach has not been proven superior, but several systematic approaches show demonstrated success in study settings, including protocol-based nurse intervention and follow-up, or use of serial physiologic measurements (systemic hemodynamic measurements, plasma renin activity, plasma volume) to adjust treatment.

I. INTRODUCTION

Resistant hypertension is increasing in prevalence, fueled by an aging population and stepwise lowering of blood pressure targets. Within our tertiary hypertension practice, resistant hypertension is now the most common reason for referral. The patient may be aware of the importance of blood pressure control but frustrated by the large number of medications prescribed and their failure to achieve blood pressure targets. Laboratory testing may be minimal, or may harbor clues to a secondary cause that has been missed. Many patients with resistant hypertension carry a high cardiovascular risk burden, significant co-morbidity, and sub-clinical or symptomatic target organ damage. Evaluation of these patients provides an opportunity to treat or definitively exclude a reversible cause, adjust and simplify often complex medication regimens, educate the patient on the effects of lifestyle practices and achieve blood pressure goals. Particularly for those with multiple co-morbidities, blood pressure control may slow further injury and improve quality of life.

Although awareness and treatment rates have improved over the past 20 years, hypertension control rates remain disappointingly low. On the basis of the most recent National Health and Nutrition Examination Survey (NHANES), 34% of hypertensive Americans achieve blood pressure levels <140/90 mmHg using antihypertensive therapy (1). With the implementation of lower targets for those at high cardiovascular risk or with target organ damage, control rates are even lower. Surveys of two nephrology practices reported control rates of 15% for <125/75 mmHg in a population of 201 patients with proteinuric renal disease (2) and 5% for <130/85 of 107 patients requiring initiation of dialysis support (3). Even with focused efforts and expertise, hypertension control may be difficult to achieve, particularly in the setting of renal disease.

II. DEFINITIONS

Resistant hypertension is the failure to control blood pressure <140 mmHg systolic and 90 mmHg diastolic, using a rational combination of at least three antihypertensive agents, including a diuretic (4). Refractory hypertension is a more inclusive term designating treatment failure using two or more agents; the terms are sometimes used interchangeably. With recent trends to lower diuretic prescription rates (5), some patients present taking three or more agents without a diuretic. Although outside the classic definition, these patients may be considered to have resistant hypertension as well. On the basis of target blood pressure levels <140/90 mmHg, reported prevalence rates for resistant hypertension vary from <1% at a hypertension job site clinic to 11–13% in hypertension referral clinics (6,7). Prevalence rates are likely much higher for those with cardiac or renal compromise where goal blood pressure levels are <130/80 mmHg. These patients with evident target organ damage carry a disproportionately high risk of cardiovascular events (8).

Blood pressure measurement is classically defined by American Heart Association (AHA) standards on the basis of carefully standardized office technique (9). Advances in technology now provide convenient affordable electronic units for home or out of office measurement. Because some patients do show stereotypic blood pressure elevations at physician visits, termed "office" or "white-coat hypertension," out of office measurements are essential to the identification of truly resistant hypertension (10). We utilize multiple approaches to blood pressure measurement including standardized AHA measurements by trained nurses, shortened versions of ambulatory blood pressure monitoring, and patient home measurements with physician review (9,11,12). Accurate measurement may be challenging in the obese patient where cuff size may be inadequate. As specified by AHA guidelines, the bladder of the blood pressure cuff must be wide enough to cover at least two-thirds the distance from axilla to antecubital space and long enough to encircle at least 80% of the arm (9). The use of a cuff that is too short or too narrow may lead to erroneously high readings; a cuff that is too large may produce false low or normal values. For accurate measurement, it is vital to keep four cuff sizes easily available, including pediatric, standard adult arm, large adult arm, and thigh versions. With the increasing prevalence of obesity in the Western world, the large adult arm cuff is appropriate for most patients. Cuff sizes for home blood pressure equipment are limited to standard and large, and are not adequate for the morbidly obese arm. Electronic wrist measurement devices are becoming more reliable and may be a better choice in this setting.

III. PATHOPHYSIOLOGY

Causes for resistant hypertension are listed in Table 36.1. Despite the introduction of several new classes of antihypertensive agents over the past two decades, suboptimal selection of drug therapy remains among the most common causes for treatment failures. In a series of 91 patients referred to a tertiary care center with resistant hypertension, 43% were felt to be resistant due to suboptimal therapy, another 10% due to noncompliance, and 14% from adverse effects (13). Results from randomized clinical trials indicate that 19–47% of enrolled hypertensive subjects require two or more antihypertensive agents to achieve treatment goals (14–17). For patients with manifest target organ damage, diabetes mellitus or renal disease where treatment goals are lower (<130/80 mmHg), 78–93% require two or more medications (18,19). Current guidelines advise initiation of treatment with combination agents if starting pressures are 20 mmHg systolic or 10 mmHg diastolic above targets to improve early response and compliance (1). Although diuretics potentiate the effectiveness of angiotensin-converting enzyme inhibitors, angiotensin receptor blockers and other agents, the effects of other combinations are less clear. Combination therapy agents are limited to those brought forth from the pharmaceutical industry and may not concur with patterns of combination tested to be effective in rigorous trials. For treatment with more than two agents, there are few data evaluating added efficacy of the third and fourth agents or the risks for drug interactions or side effects.

Several reports implicate physician inattention as a cause for inadequate blood pressure treatment. Hyman and Pavlik (20) analyzed data from the NHANES to elucidate patient characteristics and health care practices that contribute to poor blood pressure control. Among those receiving treatment, hypertension control rates fell with increasing patient age. The predominant elevation was in systolic pressure and the extent of elevation above target blood pressure was mild. Inadequate control was concentrated in older individuals with access and contact with health care providers. Berlowitz et al. (21) examined practice patterns within the Veterans Administration system to elucidate clinical factors that led to intensified therapy. Even though blood pressure was poorly controlled in many, there was a clear link between more intensive treatment and improved control. Oliveria et al. (22) queried physicians 10–90 days after a patient visit regarding reasons they changed or did not change treatment. The most frequently cited reason for no change was satisfaction with blood pressure control even though blood pressure remained above national targets. To evaluate the impact of patient adherence, Nuesch et al. (23) compared blood pressure control by 12 h ambulatory blood pressure monitoring to medication usage as recorded by electronic medication containers. Adherence to treatment, defined as taking at least 80% of prescribed doses, was similar in those responsive to medication (85%) and those with treatment resistant hypertension (82%). The traditional profile of the resistant hypertension patient as a young man, often African-American, with poor adherence may be changing, with increasing prevalence of this condition in an older, but compliant population manifest primarily as systolic pressure elevation.

Secondary hypertension is the presence of a specific condition known to cause hypertension. Major secondary causes of hypertension are listed in Table 36.2. This condition may be the primary cause for hypertension in an individual, or may be a contributing factor in a patient who already has essential hypertension. Secondary hypertension may contribute to drug resistance related to increased severity and underlying hormonal abnormalities. Although the Yakovlevitch and Black (13) series reported a prevalence of 11%, our own experience suggests it may occur more commonly, as noted in 31% of a group of 104 patients enrolled in a resistant hypertension treatment trial (Fig. 36.1) (24).

Table 36.1 Causes of Resistant Hypertension

Improper blood pressure measurement
Excess sodium intake
Inadequate diuretic therapy
Medication related causes
  Inadequate doses
  Drug actions and interactions (oral contraceptives, NSAIDs, illicit drugs)
  Over-the-counter drugs; herbal supplements
Excess alcohol intake
Identifiable (secondary) causes of hypertension
Obesity

Note: NSAIDs, Nonsteroidal anti-inflammatory drugs.
Source: Adapted from Chobanian et al. (1).

Table 36.2 Causes of Secondary Hypertension

Category of condition	Specific cause
Renal	Renal parenchymal disease
	Ureteral or bladder outlet obstruction
Renovascular	Renovascular hypertension
	Aortic coarctation
Endocrine	Primary aldosteronism
	Hypothyroidism or hyperthyroidism
	Pheochromocytoma
	Cushing's disease
	Hyperparathyroidism
Other causes	Obstructive sleep apnea

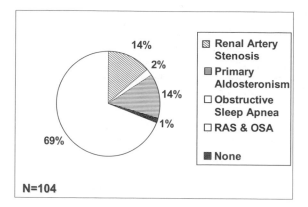

Figure 36.1 Causes of resitant hypertension in a hypertension treatment trial. Thirty-one percent of 104 patients referred for an intensive treatment program had one or more secondary causes as shown.

In some situations, correction of the secondary cause even if feasible, does not resolve the resistant hypertension. Although 13% of the patients in our series received treatment directed specifically at the secondary cause, they remained resistant to therapy. This underscores the challenge of distinguishing between the presence of an exacerbating condition and defining its contribution to resistance. Rates of secondary hypertension reported in other series range from 6% to 18% (25,26). Prevalence rates vary widely depending on whether patients are screened prior to the diagnosis of resistant hypertension and the extent of screening or exclusions. Some individuals with secondary hypertension can be treated to achieve goal blood pressure levels using medical therapy. Decisions regarding the extent of evaluation appropriate must consider the patient's age, long-term prognosis, and the adequacy of medical therapy, then balance the risks of leaving the condition undetected against the risks of intervention. If the risks are prohibitive, one should consider forgoing complex diagnostic procedures. Patient response to medical treatment and tolerance of that treatment must be reviewed. If medical therapy fails, one may need to go back then and address the secondary cause. In fact, a key role for the hypertension specialist is to determine the extent of testing and indications for treatment appropriate for the individual patient.

Recent trends in hypertension management emphasize lifestyle changes and initiation of drug treatment with limited laboratory investigation. Thus many hypertensive patients receive treatment over years, without extensive testing to exclude secondary causes. The most common indication for secondary evaluation is the failure to achieve blood pressure targets on escalating numbers and doses of medication. Secondary hypertension is more likely when the clinical picture departs from

expected patterns with atypical features in the patient's history, clues on physical exam, or unexpected laboratory findings. Decisions on extent of testing and indications for intervention are often complex. The over-riding goal is to address the causative mechanisms for resistance as a means to improve responsiveness to prescribed antihypertensive medications. It is appropriate to evaluate for curable forms of hypertension although they are rare. Efforts to detect and treat secondary causes should focus on younger and more severely afflicted hypertensives to achieve maximum benefit. In older individuals, it is commonly the failure to achieve blood pressure targets or a progressive decline in renal function that merit reconsideration of a secondary cause. Renal parenchymal disease is the most common secondary cause, but urinary outlet obstruction should be considered. Renovascular disease occurs in young and old hypertensive patients, although from different causes. There are a number of endocrine disorders that cause hypertension including primary aldosteronism, pheochromocytoma, and cortisol or thyroid abnormalities. Obstructive sleep apnea is an increasing problem with the current obesity epidemic and may mediate a relative aldosterone excess state (27,28).

Clues to secondary hypertension can be historical, physical, or biochemical. Historical clues include early age of onset (i.e., under the age of 30), severe or accelerated hypertension (29–31), and absence of a family history of hypertension. The diagnosis of hypertension in a young person merits more aggressive evaluation, as the long-term economic and medical costs of drug treatment over a lifetime are substantial, even if the blood pressure is well controlled. In this setting, early diagnosis may provide an opportunity for cure that will be lost later if hypertension persists over a longer time. Drug intolerance can be a clue to secondary hypertension. Development of hypokalemia disproportionate in severity to that anticipated or the need for large amounts of potassium supplementation to maintain normokalemia suggests excessive aldosterone or other mineralocorticoid production, whether primary or secondary, or corticosteroid excess. It is important to distinguish renal parenchymal disease from renovascular hypertension or renal outflow obstruction. The development of acute renal failure with introduction of an angiotensin-converting enzyme inhibitor or angiotensin receptor blocker or the rapid onset of pulmonary edema ("flash pulmonary edema") suggest bilateral renovascular disease. Specific symptom constellations merit further investigation. These include hypertensive spells and lability suggesting pheochromocytoma, urinary obstructive symptoms suggesting obstructive uropathy, and snoring with daytime hypersomnolence suggesting obstructive sleep apnea. Although multiple drug intolerance is not related to secondary hypertension directly, the inability to tolerate multiple agents may result in inadequate control and greater risk of target organ damage. In this setting, it is appropriate to search more extensively for a reversible cause that if treated could reduce the need for multiple medications.

Physical findings are infrequent and require additional studies to confirm a diagnosis. Specific features include café au lait spots or neurofibroma (pheochromocytoma, paraganglioma), posterior pharyngeal soft tissue crowding and large shirt collar size (obstructive sleep apnea), moon facies, cervical fat pad and pigmented striae (Cushing's disease), reduced thigh blood pressure (coarctation), carotid or femoral bruits or abdominal bruit (renovascular disease), and enlarged palpable kidneys (polycystic kidney disease). Abdominal systolic bruits are not specific for renovascular disease, but the detection of an abdominal bruit increases the possibility of renal artery disease fivefold (32). Laboratory abnormalities relate primarily to serum potassium, higher or lower than normal or detection of reduced renal function. Secondary hypertension is associated with disturbances in circadian blood pressure rhythm and increased risk for target organ damage. The presence of target organ damage out of proportion to office blood pressure levels provides a clue to nocturnal hypertension and may reflect a secondary cause.

An extensive discussion of the work-up of secondary hypertension is beyond the scope of this chapter and the reader is referred to more in-depth reviews in Part E of this book. A classification of testing procedures by diagnosis is presented in Table 36.3.

For the patient with resistant hypertension, one must begin with a general consideration of multiple secondary causes then focus in on contributing mechanisms based on preliminary test results (Fig. 36.2). Beyond the basic laboratory tests advised by JNC 7, preliminary testing should include a noninvasive imaging study of the kidneys and renal arteries and hormonal screening for excess aldosterone or catecholamine states. It is important to distinguish renal parenchymal disease from renovascular hypertension. Parenchymal renal disease is

Table 36.3 Laboratory Evaluation for Secondary Causes

Secondary cause	Tests
Renal parenchymal disease	Renal ultrasound
	Vasculitis serologies
	Renal biopsy
Renovascular disease or co-arctation	Renal artery imaging
	Renal artery duplex ultrasound
	Renogram
	MR angiography
	CT angiography
	Angiography
Primary aldosteronism	Aldosterone/renin ratio
	Nonsuppressible aldosterone after sodium load
	Adrenal imaging by CT or MR
	Adrenal vein sampling
	Aldosterone antagonist treatment trial
Pheochromocytoma	Plasma metanephrines
	24 h urine metanephrines and fractionated catecholamines
	Adrenal CT
	MIBG scanning
Cushing's disease	24 h urine cortisol
	1 mg overnight dexamethasone suppression test
	Adrenal CT
Hyperthyroidism or hypothyroidism	Thyroid stimulating hormone
	Total and free thyroxine, tri-iodothyronine
	Thyroid ultrasound
Hyperparathyroidism	Serum calcium, phosphorous, parathyroid hormone
Obstructive sleep apnea	Overnight oximetry
	Polysomnography with CPAP trial
Coarctation	Simultaneous arm and thigh blood pressure measurement;
	Aortogram/MR angiography/ultrasound

Note: MR, Magnetic resonance; CT, Computed tomography; MIBG, Iodine 123 meta-iodobenzylguanidine scintigraphy; CPAP, Continuous positive airway pressure.

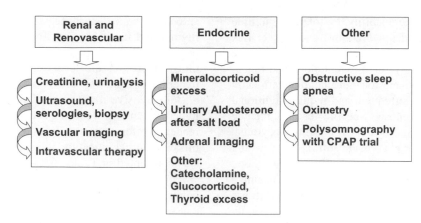

Figure 36.2 Outline of the laboratory evaluation for secondary causes of resistant hypertension, highlighting the more common contributing causes.

characterized by an elevated serum creatinine and in some settings, an active urinary sediment. Renal biopsy may be necessary for definitive diagnosis. Renal outflow tract obstruction due to prostatic obstruction, mass lesion or complications of prior surgery, should be excluded before moving to invasive vascular testing. Normal renal imaging and a bland urinary sediment suggest renal vascular disease and coupled with drug resistant hypertension merit further vascular imaging. Duplex ultrasonography provides images of the renal arteries and blood-flow velocity and pressure waveforms, but with failure rates of 10–20% related to operator inexperience, obese body habitus or intestinal gas (36). Current techniques for gadolinium-enhanced magnetic resonance angiography and computed tomographic angiography offer excellent views of the renal circulation and aorta, but are less reliable for visualizing distal segments and small accessory arteries (37,38). Gadolinium is safe for patients with renal insufficiency, without evident nephrotoxicity. Significant renal vascular disease causing resistant hypertension or progressive renal dysfunction may respond well to renal revascularization and for selected individuals, percutaneous or surgical intervention may salvage critical renal function.

Clinical features should guide the investigation of hormonal secondary causes. Hypokalemia may occur due to mineralocorticoid or glucocorticoid excess. Hyperaldosteronism is increasingly recognized as a correctable cause for resistant hypertension, thus screening should be considered early in the evaluation. The obese patient with resistant hypertension may have a relative aldosterone excess but fall short of the classic criteria for primary aldosteronism. Chemokines in visceral fat may stimulate the renin–angiotensin–aldosterone system, particularly in patients with concurrent sympathetic activation from untreated sleep apnea (27). The initial evaluation is

directed to demonstration of inappropriate aldosterone production, using the aldosterone/renin ratio for screening and confirmed by demonstration of inappropriate aldosterone production after salt loading. After the diagnosis of primary hyperaldosteronism is confirmed, imaging studies are indicated to discriminate adenomatous disease from adrenal hyperplasia. Invasive adrenal vein sampling may be necessary to predict the success of adrenalectomy in individual cases (35).

Less common secondary causes may present with subtle findings and screening is appropriate even without florid clinical manifestations. The pursuit of secondary causes is intended to ensure treatment of all potential contributing mechanisms so that blood pressure control is achieved. At each step in the pathway, the clinician must decide whether the condition has been sufficiently excluded in the individual patient or whether more definitive testing is indicated. Such decisions should consider patient age, long-term prognosis, risks of leaving the condition undetected, risks of intervention, and adequacy of medical therapy.

IV. PITFALLS, DANGERS, AND SIDE EFFECTS

Although secondary hypertension must be considered and excluded, resistant hypertension more commonly results from effects of concurrent drug use or drug interactions that interfere with antihypertensive treatment efficacy. Although there are numerous drugs causing potential interference, the most common and most significant today is the nearly universal use of nonsteroidal antiinflammatory agents (NSAIDS) and COX II inhibitors, causing sodium retention and reduced drug efficacy of many antihypertensive agents. These agents reduce vasodilatory prostaglandins, particularly within the kidney and produce a rise in

Table 36.4 Drugs that Cause Resistant Hypertension

Prescription drugs	Nonprescription drugs
NSAIDS	NSAIDS
Sympathomimetic agents	Sympathomimetic agents
Exogenous corticosteroids	Licorice
Immunosuppressive agents	Illicit drugs (cocaine,
Erythropoietin	amphetamines)
Antidepressants	Herbal preparations
Oral contraceptives	(ephedra)

systemic resistance and impaired sodium excretion. Epidemiologic studies indicate that NSAID exposure causes enough blood pressure elevation to trigger the initial diagnosis of hypertension in some individuals (39). Use of NSAIDs during antihypertensive therapy can blunt the effectiveness of several classes of drugs and allow blood pressures to rise substantially (40,41). COX II inhibitors appear to have similar class effects, although product differences have been emphasized by marketers (42).

A variety of vasoconstrictive sympathomimetic agents may cause hypertension or exacerbate control (Table 36.4). Among the most common of these are cold remedies containing agents such as phenylephrine, pseudoephedrine and until recently, phenylpropanolamine. Numerous herbal preparations containing ephedra, Ma Hwong, St. John's wort or ginseng have been associated with worsened hypertension (43). Confectioners' black licorice and chewing tobacco contain glycyrrhizic acid causing a clinical picture suggestive of primary aldosteronism. Other prescription medications may also aggravate hypertension. Specific offending agents include the immunosuppressive calcineurin inhibitors cyclosporine and tacrolimus, and erythropoietin. Some of the medications used for treatment of mood disorders or depression

(e.g., methylphenidate, modafinil, venlafaxine) can produce labile and sometimes severe rises in blood pressure. Sibutramine, an anorexiant/stimulant used for weight reduction, may cause or exacerbate hypertension by inhibiting catecholamine reuptake.

Equally important to drug interactions are lifestyle factors including obesity, high sodium intake, and excessive alcohol use that may cause hypertension and drive resistance. In the setting of a high sodium diet so common in our society, most patients show no outward signs of excess cardiopulmonary volume. Recent trends to use of micro-dose diuretic therapy or avoidance of diuretics (5) are based on marketing strategies that emphasize potential metabolic interactions, and sometimes weaken the practitioner's resolve to advance diuretic therapy. Ethanol abuse may be easily overlooked yet contributes to drug resistance and poor adherence to treatment.

V. TREATMENT APPROACHES

An algorithm for approaching resistant hypertension is shown in Fig. 36.3, highlighting potential measurement, lifestyle and treatment factors. Nonadherence is more likely with increasing complexity of treatment, numbers of agents and dosing frequency. Drug intolerance, financial constraints or other causes contribute to missed or reduced doses of medication and may result in inadequately treated hypertension and acceleration to more severe levels (29). Nonadherence with prescribed medications can at times be addressed by simplifying the regimen or changing to agents better tolerated by the individual patient. Some individuals label themselves intolerant to agents that were ineffective in past trials, but perhaps this was with their use as monotherapy. Use of these agents in combination

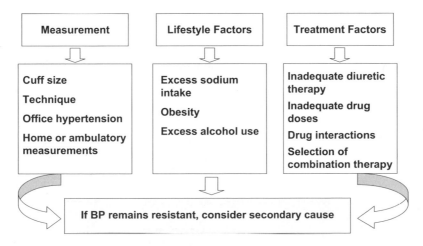

Figure 36.3 Considerations in the evaluation of resistant hypertension: addressing measurement errors, contributing lifestyle factors, drug selection, and dosage.

or at different dosage may be effective and well tolerated. In examining the pre-existing drug regimen, the use of agents with overlapping mechanisms of action, or at inadequate doses, should be considered. Blood pressure lability or loss of blood pressure control may occur with the use of short acting agents or rapid drug metabolism.

Previous resistant hypertension treatment trials in the 1980s utilized standardized multi-drug regimens with agents added in stepwise fashion starting with a diuretic or β-adrenergic blocker then adding peripheral vasodilatory agents. These trials were not randomized, with the more potent agents reserved for those most refractory. (7,44). More intensive treatment was limited by an increase in side effects. More recently, Yakovlevitch and Black (13) controlled blood pressure in 34 and improved blood pressure in another 8 of 46 patients with resistant hypertension attributed to a suboptimal treatment regimen. For half of these patients, diuretic therapy was started or intensified. In another 17, the addition of a newer agent or the reduction of sympatholytic medications led to improved blood pressure. There were no specific guidelines or clinical features used to guide treatment changes. Studies by Calhoun and coworkers and others (45,46) report additive blood pressure reduction from the addition of low dose spironolactone to multiple agent regimens in subjects with and without primary aldosteronism. Extent of the blood pressure reduction was similar in those with and without demonstrated aldosterone excess.

When considering actual medication options for treatment of resistant hypertension, there are several choices. One can add a fourth agent, use higher than recommended doses of those agents already prescribed, or substitute another agent from the same drug class to see if there is a better individual response. New medications should be introduced individually to simplify the interpretation of drug reactions or side effects should they occur. Beyond these adjustments, most experts utilize a systematic approach with examples listed in Table 36.5.

Decisions regarding treatment changes are based on algorithms for drug selection. The Birmingham Hypertension Square is designed to optimize the choice of add-in drugs in the management of resistant hypertension (47). One can choose any of four agent classes on the corners of a square on the basis of clinical characteristics of the patient or compelling indications as specified in JNC VI. If a single agent is not effective, one would select a second agent using one of the drug classes adjacent on the square to the initial selection, but avoid the selection at the corner opposite to that initial choice. Variations to this schematic have also been published (48). The evidence for this approach is based on a few small trials using limited agents and small patient numbers then extrapolated to generalizations about entire drug classes and the resistant hypertension population. The authors note that third drug selection is speculative, anecdotal, and based on less reliable trial evidence. Other approaches to treatment focus on system changes for intervention (49,50) and follow-up (12). Stroebel et al. reported use of a team approach with a nurse safety net using nurse measurements and an algorithm for repeat measurements to maintain focus on the blood pressure until control was achieved. During a pilot study, control rates improved from 33% to 50% during the intervention period and remained at 56% 1 year later. Corresponding rates for the control group were 25% at entry, 31% at the end of the intervention, and 24% 1 year later. Denver et al. (50) reported threefold greater hypertension control rates using a nurse-led hypertension clinic compared with

Table 36.5 Treatment Approaches to Resistant Hypertension

Type of treatment change	Examples of treatment
System change approach	Nurse–physician team with nurse follow-up (49)
	Nurse-based follow-up and drug titration (50)
	Rapid titration followed by home measurement reports to a nurse (12)
Add-on treatment	Not randomized; usually a single add-on agent
	Fourth agent
	Higher than recommended doses
	Substitution of another agent from same drug class
Treatment algorithms	Birmingham Hypertension Square (47)
	Round 1, Round 2 (48)
Treatment using serial measurements	Laragh method of sodium-volume and renin vasoconstrictor drugs (51)
	Hemodynamic measurements by thoracic bioimpedance (24)
Attention to volume	Plasma volume measurements (65)
	Volume assessment by thoracic bioimpedance (24)
	Empiric use of combination diuretic treatment

conventional primary care. Patients were seen monthly for blood pressure measurement, review of medication adherence and recommendations for lifestyle interventions and initiation of physician supervised medication adjustments. Canzanello et al. demonstrated the long-term efficacy of rapid initiation of physician directed medication titration over days followed by interval home blood pressure measurements and medication adjustments over 1 year to achieve and maintain extended control. These approaches may be effective, but most of the patients in these treatment trials did not have resistant hypertension but less severe forms of hypertension.

Beyond these system change approaches, some experts utilize spot or serial measurements to adjust complex drug therapy. The Laragh method classifies antihypertensive agents according to their effects on sodium-volume and renin vasoconstrictor determinants of blood pressure. Using a standardized measurement of plasma renin, medications are selected to correct the primary pathologic mechanism behind the blood pressure elevation, either a high sodium and volume state or a renin–angiotensin mediated vasoconstricted state (51). Serial measurements are utilized to guide treatment decisions and titrate or alter treatment for patients already taking medications who remain hypertensive (Laragh Protocol II). We use noninvasive hemodynamic measurements obtained by thoracic bioimpedance to adjust and change complex antihypertensive treatment. The premise of this approach is to control the compensatory responses to initial treatment by use of antihypertensive agents with different hemodynamic actions. It is recognized that effective blood pressure control requires a reduction in vascular resistance; however, the effects of specific drugs can be heterogeneous and can lead to both volume retention and reflex changes that offset the desired result (52–54). Use of hemodynamic measurements to characterize blood pressure disorders is not new (55–57); application to guide therapy has been limited by a lack of methods to obtain reproducible measurements noninvasively. Recent developments have improved consistency and reliability of systemic hemodynamic measurements using thoracic bioimpedance in normal and disease states (58–61). This technique detects changes in thoracic fluid volume during electrical systole using skin electrodes and a low voltage current to derive stroke volume. Coupled with heart rate and blood pressure measurements, thoracic impedance offers real-time measurement of cardiac output and systemic vascular resistance. Absolute impedance measurements and changes in impedance with posture change from a supine to a standing position serve as markers of cardiopulmonary volume on the basis of data from normal subjects studied on controlled sodium intakes. Application of this method in a randomized clinical trial demonstrated improved control rates and lower blood pressure levels in resistant hypertensive patients using serial hemodynamic measurements compared to standard drug adjustment made by hypertension experts. Improved blood pressure control correlated with an incremental reduction in systemic vascular resistance in those treated according to hemodynamic values. Nearly all subjects were taking a diuretic at entry (91%), but more intensive diuretic therapy was prescribed in the hemodynamic treatment group than in the specialist care group. Our results indicate that therapy based on hemodynamic measurements with an emphasis on targeted control of volume using diuretic therapy achieved blood pressure control superior to that attained by empiric selection of drugs.

Volume expansion is well recognized as a cause for resistance to antihypertensive therapy (54,62). The mechanism of resistance is an insensitivity to standard diuretic therapy, perhaps mediated by obesity and the sodium retaining properties of certain antihypertensive agents, regardless of renal function. Plasma volume is normal in untreated essential hypertensives but increased in patients with renal parenchymal disease (63). Studies in resistant hypertensives support a positive correlation between measured blood volume and systolic and diastolic blood pressure in patients treated with sympatholytic agents or vasodilators (54). Intensified diuretic treatment effects improve blood pressure control by a reduction in plasma volume (54,62,64,65). Practical assessment of effective cardiopulmonary volume may be difficult in the setting of arterial vasodilating agents, such as calcium channel blocking agents, where edema formation may not reflect accurately total body sodium (66). Other markers of volume status, such as plasma renin activity, can be affected by numerous drugs and other conditions. Hence, titration of diuretic dose in a specific patient can be difficult. An alternative explanation for resistance may relate to the effects of antihypertensive agents in combination, a consequence of the use of multiple agents leading to secondary volume retention, activation of the sympathetic nervous system or the RAA system. Increased fluid volume occurs commonly as a compensatory response to antihypertensive therapy and may manifest as fluid retention (weight gain, edema) or a poor response to increased amounts of medication. Graves et al. (65) used measurements of plasma volume to adjust therapy in a sample of nine patients with resistant hypertension. Plasma volume was increased in eight of the nine, all of whom responded to aggressive diuretic therapy allowing simplification of their regimens. For the one patient with contracted plasma volume, vasodilation was effective in controlling blood pressure. None of the patients had clinical evidence of volume overload and those with expanded plasma volume were already taking diuretic agents, either thiazide or loop diuretics at conventional dosages.

VI. REFERING PATIENTS FOR MORE SPECIALIZED CONSULTATION

Decisions on when to refer a patient depend largely on the comfort and experience of the treating practitioner. The discussion in this chapter is directed to the level of the internist or sub-specialist physician with expertise in the selection and use of multiple agents for the treatment of hypertension. After a patient has been diagnosed with resistant hypertension, it is appropriate to consider the causes discussed here, with a focus on potential secondary causes. Decisions regarding the extent of evaluation require consideration of the likelihood of diagnosis, the patient's overall health status and prognosis, and balancing the risks of intervention against the risks of missing a diagnosis. Referral is indicated when these risks appear prohibitive, there are questions regarding selection of optimal studies or extent of intervention and blood pressure remains uncontrolled. Referral patterns vary with regional expertise and the question at hand. Resources include Nephrologists (renal parenchymal disease, renovascular hypertension, volume overload), Pharmacists and Pharmacologists (drug interactions, regimen simplification, adherence), and Endocrinologists (endocrine secondary causes, referral and interpretation of adrenal imaging, and adrenal vein sampling).

VII. CONCLUSIONS

The availability of multiple effective antihypertensive medications in recent years offers greater choice in antihypertensive therapy than ever before. Yet hypertension resistant to treatment with three or more agents continues to present complex challenges to the clinician. Although suboptimal treatment is most common, other causes include secondary hypertension, lifestyle practices, and drug interactions. Careful evaluation provides the opportunity to treat or definitively exclude a reversible cause, adjust and simplify complex medication regimens, educate the patient on the effects of lifestyle practices and achieve blood pressure goals. A variety of treatment strategies are reviewed including systems approaches that often depend on nonphysician pathways.

REFERENCES

1. Chobanian AV, Bakris GL, Black HR, Cushman WC, Green LA, Izzo JL Jr, Jones DW, Materson BJ, Oparil S, Wright JT Jr, Roccella EJ. Joint National Committee on Prevention, Detection, Evaluation, and Treatment of High Blood Pressure. National Heart, Lung, and Blood Institute; National High Blood Pressure Education Program Coordinating Committee. The Seventh Report of the Joint National Committee on Prevention, Detection, Evaluation and Treatment of High Blood Pressure: The JNC 7 Report. J Am Med Assoc 2003; 289:2560–2572.
2. Schwenger V, Ritz E. Audit of antihypertensive treatment in patients with renal failure. Nephrol Dial Transplant 1998; 13:3091–3095.
3. Dasgupta I, Madeley RJ, Pringle MAL, Savill J, Burden RP. Management of hypertension in patients developing end-stage renal failure. Q J Med 1999; 92:519–525.
4. Gifford RW Jr. Resistant hypertension: introduction and definitions. Hypertension 1988; 11(suppl II):II-65–II-66.
5. Psaty BM, Manolio TA, Smith NL, Heckbert SR, Gottdiener JS, Burke GL, Weissfeld J, Enright P, Lumley T, Powe N, Furberg CD. Cardiovascular Health Study. Time trends in high blood pressure control and the use of antihypertensive medications in older adults: The Cardiovascular Health Study. Arch Intern Med 2002; 162:2325–2332.
6. Alderman MH, Budner N, Cohen H, Lamport B, Ooi WL. Prevalence of drug resistant hypertension. Hypertension 1988; 11(3, suppl II):II-71–II-75.
7. Swales JD, Bing RF, Heagerty AM, Pohl JE, Russell GI, Thurston H. Treatment of refractory hypertension. Lancet 1982; 1:894–896.
8. McAlister FA, Lewanczuk RZ, Teo KK. Resistant hypertension: an overview. Can J Cardiol 1996; 12:822–828.
9. Pickering TG, Hall JE, Appel LJ, Falkner BE, Graves J, Hill MN, Jones DW, Kurtz T, Sheps SG, Roccella EJ. Recommendations for blood pressure measurement in humans and experimental animals: Part 1 : Blood pressure measurement in humans: A statement for professionals from the subcommittee of professional and public education of the American Heart Association Council on High Blood Pressure Research. Hypertension 2005; 45(1):142–161.
10. Brown MA, Buddle ML, Martin A. Is resistant hypertension really resistant? Am J Hypertens 2001; 14:1263–1269.
11. Zachariah PK, Schwartz GL, Sheps SG, Schirger A, Smith RL. Ambulatory blood pressure for better diagnosis of hypertension: correlation between office and automatic blood pressure recording. Am J Hypertens 1988; 1:81A.
12. Canzanello VJ, Jensen PL, Hunder I. Rapid adjustment of antihypertensive drugs produces a durable improvement in blood pressure. Am J Hypertens 2001; 14:345–350.
13. Yakovlevitch M, Black HR. Resistant hypertension in a tertiary care clinic. Arch Intern Med 1991; 151:1786–1792.
14. Staessen JA, Fagard R, Thijs L, Celis H, Arabidze GG, Birkenhager WH, Bulpitt CJ, de Leeuw PW, Dollery CT, Fletcher AE, Forette F, Leonetti G, Nachev C, O'Brien ET, Rosenfeld J, Rodicio JL, Tuomilehto J, Zanchetti A. Randomised double-blind comparison of placebo and active treatment for older patients with isolated systolic hypertension. Lancet 1997; 350:757–764.
15. Wang J, Staessen JA, Gong L, Liu L. Chinese trial on isolated systolic hypertension in the elderly. Arch Intern Med 2000; 160:211–220.
16. Hansson L, Lindholm LH, Ekbom T, Dahlof B, Lanke J, Schersten B, Wester PO, Hedner T, de Faire U. Randomised trial of old and new antihypertensive drugs in elderly patients: cardiovascular mortality and morbidity

in the Swedish Trial in Old Patients with Hypertension-2 study. Lancet 1999; 354:1751–1756.

17. ALLHAT. Major cardiovascular events in hypertensive patients randomized to doxazosin vs. chlorthalidone. J Am Med Assoc 2000; 283:1967–1975.

18. Estacio R, Jeffers BW, Hiatt WR, Biggerstaff SL, Gifford N, Schrier RW. The effect of nisoldipine as compared with enalapril on cardiovascular outcomes in patients with non-insulin dependent diabetes and hypertension. N Engl J Med 1998; 338:645–652.

19. Wright JT Jr, Bakris G, Greene T, Agodoa LY, Appel LJ, Charleston J, Cheek D, Douglas-Baltimore JG, Gassman J, Glassock R, Hebert L, Jamerson K, Lewis J, Phillips RA, Toto RD, Middleton JP, Rostand SG; African-American study of kidney disease and hypertension study group. Effect of blood pressure lowering and antihypertensive drug class on progression of hypertensive kidney disease. J Am Med Assoc 2002; 288:2421–2431.

20. Hyman DJ, Pavlik VN. Characteristics of patients with uncontrolled hypertension in the United States. N Engl J Med 2001; 345:479–486.

21. Berlowitz DR, Ash AS, Hickey EC, Friedman RH, Glickman M, Kader B, Moskowitz MA. Inadequate management of blood pressure in a hypertensive population. N Engl J Med 1998; 339:1957–1963.

22. Oliveria SA, Lapuerta P, McCarthy BD, L'Italien GJ, Berlowitz DR, Asch SM. Physician-related barriers to the effective management of uncontrolled hypertension. Arch Intern Med 2002; 162:413–420.

23. Nuesch R, Schroeder K, Dieterle T, Martina B, Battegay E. Relation between insufficient response to antihypertensive treatment and poor compliance with treatment: a prospective case-control study. Br Med J 2001; 323:142–146.

24. Taler SJ, Textor SC, Augustine JE. Resistant hypertension: comparing hemodynamic management to specialist care. Hypertension 2002; 39:982–988.

25. Garg JP, Folker AC, Munavvar I, Elliott WJ, Black H. Resistant hypertension revisited. Am J Hypertens 2002 15(4), [Part 2 of 2]:25A.

26. Martell N, Rodriguez-Cerrillo M, Grobbee DE, Lopez-Eady MD, Fernandez-Pinilla C, Avila M et al. High prevalence of secondary hypertension and insulin resistance in patients with refractory hypertension. Blood Press 2003; 12:149–154.

27. Goodfriend TL, Calhoun DA. Resistant hypertension, obesity, sleep apnea, and aldosterone: theory and therapy. Hypertension 2004; 43:518–524.

28. Calhoun DA, Nishizaka MK, Zaman MA, Harding SM. Aldosterone excretion among subjects with resistant hypertension and symptoms of sleep apnea. Chest 2004; 125:112–117.

29. Shea S, Misra D, Ehrlich MH, Field L, Francis CK. Predisposing factors for severe, uncontrolled hypertension in an inner-city minority population. N Engl J Med 1992; 327:776–781.

30. Davis BA, Crook JE, Vestal RE, Oates JA. Prevalence of renovascular hypertension in patients with grade III or IV hypertensive retinopathy. N Engl J Med 1979; 301:1273–1276.

31. Vaughan CJ, Delanty N. Hypertensive emergencies. Lancet 2000; 356:411–417.

32. Krijnen P, van Jaarsveld BC, Steyerberg EW, Man in't Veld AJ, Schalekamp MADH, Habbema JKF. A Clinical Prediction Rule for renal artery stenosis. Ann Intern Med 1998; 129:705–711.

33. Safian RD, Textor SC. Medical progress: renal artery stenosis. N Engl J Med 2001; 344:431–442.

34. Young WF. Pheochromocytoma and primary aldosteronism: Diagnostic approaches. Endocrinol Metab Clin North Am 1997; 26(4):801–827.

35. Young WF. Primary aldosteronism: a common and curable form of hypertension. Cardiol Rev 1999; 7(4):207–214.

36. Hansen KJ, Tribble RW, Reavis SW, Canzanello VJ, Craven TE, Plonk GW Jr, Dean RH. Renal duplex sonography: evaluation of clinical utility. J Vasc Surg 1990; 12:227–236.

37. Gedroyc WM, Neerhut P, Negus R, Palmer A, al Kutoubi A, Taube D, Hulme B. Magnetic resonance angiography of renal artery stenosis. Clin Radiol 1995; 50:436–439.

38. Elkohen M, Beregi JP, Deklunder G, Artaud D, Mounier-Vehier C, Carre A. Evaluation of the spiral computed tomography alone and combined with color doppler ultrasonography in the detection of renal artery stenosis: a prospective study of 114 renal arteries. Arch Mal Coeur Vaiss 1995; 88:1159–1164.

39. Gurwitz JH, Avorn J, Bohn RL, Glynn RJ, Monane M, Mogun H. Initiation of antihypertensive treatment during nonsteroidal anti-inflammatory drug therapy. J Am Med Assoc 1994; 272:781–786.

40. Pope JE, Anderson JJ, Felson DT. A meta-analysis of the effects of nonsteroidal and anti-inflammatory drugs on blood pressure. Arch Intern Med 1993; 153:477–484.

41. Johnson AG, Nguyen TV, Day RO. Do nonsteroidal anti-inflammatory drugs affect blood pressure? A meta-analysis. Ann Intern Med 1994; 121:289–300.

42. Frishman WH. Effects of nonsteroidal anti-inflammatory drug therapy on blood pressure and peripheral edema. Am J Cardiol 2002; 89(suppl):18D–25D.

43. Ernst E. The risk-benefit profile of commonly used herbal therapies: Ginkgo, St. John's wort, ginseng, echinacea, saw palmetto, and kava. Ann Intern Med 2002; 136:42–53.

44. Vandenburg MJ, Sharman VL, Drew P, Barnes J, Wright P. Quadruple therapy for resistant hypertension. Br J Clin Pract 1985; 39:17–19.

45. Nishizaka MK, Zaman MA, Calhoun DA. Efficacy of low-dose spironolactone in subjects with resistant hypertension. Am J Hypertens 2003; 16:925–930.

46. Ouzan J, Perault C, Lincoff AM, Carre E, Mertes M. The role of spironolactone in the treatment of patients with refractory hypertension. Am J Hypertens 2002; 15:333–339.

47. Lip GYH, Beevers M, Beevers DG. The 'Birmingham Hypertension Square' for the optimum choice of add-in drugs in the management of resistant hypertension. J Hum Hypertens 1998; 12(11):761–763.

48. Giles TD, Sander GE. Beyond the usual strategies for blood pressure reduction: Therapeutic considerations and combination therapies. J Clin Hypertens 2001; 3(6):346–353.

49. Stroebel RJ, Broers JK, Houle SK, Scott CG, Naessens JM. Improving hypertension control: a team approach in a primary care setting. J Qual Improv 2000; 26(11):623–632.

50. Denver EA, Barnard M, Woolfson RG, Earle KA. Management of uncontrolled hypertension in a nurse-led clinic compared with conventional care for patients with type 2 diabetes. Diab Care 2003; 26:2256–2260.

51. Laragh JH. Lesson XVI. How to choose the correct drug treatment for each hypertensive patient using a plasma renin-based method and the volume-vasoconstriction analysis. Am J Hypertens 2001; 14:491–503.

52. Lund-Johansen P. Hemodynamic effects of antihypertensive agents. In: Doyle AE, ed. Handbook of Hypertension. Elsevier Science Publishers B.V., 1988: 41–72.

53. Johns DW, Peach MJ. Factors that contribute to resistant forms of hypertension: pharmacological considerations. Hypertension 1988; 11(suppl II):II-88–II-95.

54. Dustan HP, Tarazi RC, Bravo EL. Dependence of arterial pressure on intravascular volume in treated hypertensive patients. N Engl J Med 1972; 286(16):861–866.

55. Tarazi RC. The hemodynamics of hypertension. In: Genest J, Kuchel O, Hamet P, Cantin M, ed. Hypertension: Physiopathology and Treatment. New York: McGraw-Hill Book Company, 1983:15–42.

56. Franciosa JA. Application of noninvasive techniques for measuring cardiac output in hypertensive patients. Am Heart J 1988; 116:650–656.

57. Messerli FH, DeCarvalho JGR, Christie B, Frohlich ED. Systemic and regional hemodynamics in low, normal and high cardiac output borderline hypertension. Circulation 1978; 3:441–448.

58. De Maria AN, Raisinghani A. Comparative overview of cardiac output measurement methods: has impedance cardiography come of age? Congest Heart Fail 2000; 6:60–73.

59. Van De Water JM, Miller TW, Vogel RL, Mount BE, Dalton ML. Impedance cardiography: the next vital sign technology? Chest 2003; 123:2028–2033.

60. Greenberg BH, Hermann DD, Pranulis MF, Lazio L, Cloutier D. Reproducibility of impedance cardiography hemodynamic measures in clinically stable heart failure patients. Congest Heart Fail 2000; 6:74–80.

61. Pickett BR, Buell JC. Validity of cardiac output measurement by computer-averaged impedance cardiography, and comparison with simultaneous thermodilution determinations. Am J Cardiol 1992; 69:1354–1358.

62. Finnerty Jr FA, Davidov M, Mroczek WJ, Gavrilovich L. Influence of extracellular fluid volume on response to antihypertensive drugs. Circ Res 1970; 26–27(suppl I): I-71–I-82.

63. Tarazi RC, Dustan HP, Frohlich ED, Gifford RW Jr, Hoffman GC. Plasma volume and chronic hypertension: relationship to arterial pressure levels in different hypertensive diseases. Arch Intern Med 1970; 125: 835–842.

64. Ramsay LE, Silas JH, Freestone S. Diuretic treatment of resistant hypertension. Br Med J 1980; 281:1101–1103.

65. Graves JW, Bloomfield RL, Buckalew VM. Plasma volume in resistant hypertension: guide to pathophysiology and therapy. Am J Med Sci 1989; 298(6):361–365.

66. Gustafsson D. Microvascular mechanisms involved in calcium antagonist edema formation. J Cardiovasc Pharmacol 1987; 10(suppl 1):S121–S131.

37

The Role of Nurses and Nurse Practitioners in Hypertension Management

CHERYL R. DENNISON, MARTHA N. HILL

The Johns Hopkins University School of Nursing, Baltimore, Maryland, USA

KEYPOINTS

- Incorporating nurses in the care of patients has consistently produced more effective control of hypertension.
- Nurses and nurse practitioners can contribute to many aspects of the every day management of hypertension.

SUMMARY

The management of hypertension requires longterm, effective collaboration among healthcare professionals and patients. The benefits of nurses participating in or leading hypertension care has been demonstrated in a wide variety of studies from uncontrolled community-based and clinic based surveys to randomized multi-site clinical trials, and in studies in developing as well as developed countries. An interdisciplinary team approach to hypertension care that includes nurses has consistently produced effective control of hypertension in clinical trials and many practice settings. The roles of the nurse and nurse practitioner in hypertension management include all aspects of hypertension management: detection, referral, and follow-up; medication management; patient education, counseling, and skill building; coordination of care; and clinic or office management.

I. INTRODUCTION

Since the late 1960s, when the detection, evaluation, and treatment of hypertension became a public health, as well as a medical mandate, nurses have contributed to improved care and outcomes for patients with hypertension. The benefits of nurses participating in or leading hypertension care have been demonstrated in a wide variety of studies from uncontrolled community-based and clinic-based surveys to randomized, multisite clinical trials, and in studies in developing as well as developed countries (1–17). Moreover, a multidisciplinary team approach, including nurses, has consistently produced effective control of hypertension in clinical trials and many practice settings (14,18–22). The proactive involvement of nurses, and other providers, such as pharmacists, nutritionists, social workers, and community health workers, allows flexibility in matching patient needs with the competencies of providers and staff members who have different but complementary skills and interests.

Nurses are the largest group of health professionals; they practice in all settings where patients are seen, including specialty clinics, private practice offices, worksite settings, primary care clinics, hospitals, and community centers. Patients with hypertension are identified, evaluated, and treated in all of these settings as well as in hypertension specialty clinics. As the health care environment is challenged across the world by increasing rates of chronic illness, aging populations, and concerns about escalating healthcare costs, awareness is increasing that a team approach to hypertension management is needed. Physicians, working in collaboration with nurses, pharmacists, nutritionists, social workers, and community health workers, can help patients develop the knowledge and skills they need to control their hypertension and to optimize their health. This chapter will describe the roles of the nurse and nurse practitioner (see Table 37.1) in hypertension management in outpatient or ambulatory settings and provide examples of their effectiveness.

Table 37.1 Roles of Nurses and Nurse Practitioners in Hypertension Management

- Detection, referral, and follow-up
- Medication management
- Patient education, counseling, and skill building
- Coordination of care
- Management of clinic or office

II. ROLE OF THE NURSE

Nurses have demonstrated the necessary critical clinical judgment in the management of patients with hypertension. The role of nurses in the care of patients with hypertension includes all aspects of hypertension management, although the role of any individual nurse may vary by education, motivation, the staffing needs of the practice site, and the needs of the patients. For example, in a physician's private practice office, the nurse's involvement may be limited to the measurement of vital signs prior to the patient being seen by the physician. Alternatively, in another setting, the nurse may not only measure blood pressure when assessing vital signs but also assess patient adherence to the prescribed treatment regimen and any barriers to optimal adherence to that regimen. They may provide counseling regarding risk factor modification, for example, smoking cessation or dietary sodium reduction. As the patient visit concludes, the nurse may assess the need for prescription renewals and reinforce the recommended treatment plan. Nurse involvement in hypertension management provides an ideal example of nurse specialty practice with a variety of potential roles.

In managing a cohort of patients in a hypertension clinic, the nurse is responsible for taking a thorough medical history and for ordering appropriate diagnostic tests, such as sodium, potassium, creatinine, blood urea nitrogen, cholesterol, a complete blood cell count, a urinalysis, and an electrocardiogram. This allows physicians to devote their efforts during a subsequent visit to perform the physical examination and to formulate an appropriate treatment plan that is based on extensive medical social history and laboratory data provided by the nurse. In settings in which the nurses do not have advanced practice credentials, physicians are responsible for making the diagnosis of hypertension and for determining secondary causes that may influence decisions about appropriate treatment. Physicians help formulate a treatment plan and provide consultation to nurses in the management of complex cases.

III. ROLE OF THE NURSE PRACTITIONER/ ADVANCED PRACTICE NURSE

Nurse practitioners are registered nurses who have acquired the expert knowledge base, complex decision-making skills, and clinical competencies for expanded practice, characteristics which are shaped by the context or country in which he or she has credentials to practice (23). The nurse practitioner role was developed in response to the need for creative ways to improve health care by providing competent, approachable, and accessible health care services. This role was first developed in the

United States in the early 1970s when pediatricians and nurses began to practice collaboratively, with the nurses assuming greater responsibility for the continuous primary care of well children. The role was developed to improve the care of well children and children with common, self-limiting, problems such as otitis media, and chronic illness, such as diabetes mellitus, by complementing and supplementing the role of the physician. Initially designed as certificate programs, the preparation has been integrated into masters-level preparation or into a level following masters certificate programs. In addition to advanced training, the functional role that distinguishes a nurse practitioner from other nurses is the legal authority to write prescriptions. The legal aspects of practice, which include continuing education requirements, credentialing, and scope of practice (including prescribing medication) are regulated by the government and depend on local custom and requirements.

With the increasing emphasis on health promotion and disease prevention and the recognition of the benefits of an interdisciplinary approach to care, nurse practitioners are part of the solution to care. It has been established in developed countries that 60–80% of primary and preventive services traditionally performed by physicians can be provided by nurses with similar or better clinical outcomes, and high levels of patient and provider satisfaction, and for less money (24,25). This cost effectiveness is explained by a variety of factors that relate to lower salaries, lower cost of liability insurance, and lower cost of educating nurse practitioners compared with physicians (24). Furthermore, in a randomized trial that compared physician primary care ($n = 510$) with nurse practitioner primary care ($n = 806$), Mundinger et al. (26) found that at 6 months, there were no differences in patients' health status, health care utilization, or satisfaction. For patients with hypertension, diastolic blood pressure was significantly lower for patients of nurse practitioners than for patients of primary care physicians (82 vs. 85 mmHg, $P = 0.04$).

Depending on local practice regulations, nurse practitioners who are caring for patients with hypertension can practice independently, using protocols developed jointly with they collaborating physician with whom they collaborate. Nurse practitioners follow the same hypertension treatment consensus guidelines as physicians do. (See Chapter 23 for an overview of treatment and management guidelines.) Implementation of treatment guidelines in a practice setting decreases variation in practice and improves appropriateness and efficacy of care. The effective implementation of guidelines requires not only dissemination and awareness but also a commitment by all providers and staff to set expectations for the standards, encourage implementation, create and explain incentives for adoption, build skills, and provide resources (i.e., tools). Nurses and nurse practitioners play an important role in enforcing the use of hypertension treatment guidelines.

IV. ROLE OF INTERDISCIPLINARY TEAM APPROACH IN HYPERTENSION MANAGEMENT

To achieve effective management of hypertension, in addition to engaging the patient as an active partner in care it is important that all health professionals must understand the value of their own contribution, the roles and skills of other professionals, as well as the importance of interdisciplinary collaboration. When pharmacists, nutritionists, social workers, community health workers, and others join nurses and physicians the expertise of each discipline supplements and complements that of the others. Case conferences, chart review sessions, and journal clubs are effective strategies to bring together other health professionals who are involved in hypertension management. Team case conferences are an ideal forum for discussion of guidelines and the extent to which they need to be modified, if at all, for implementation at the individual patient level. Selecting a case with particularly complex and challenging issues for the conference can be an effective method to gain input from the interdisciplinary team in revising the plan of care to assist the patient in achieving blood pressure control. Sample questions to guide a Hypertension Team Management Case Conference are provided in Table 37.2. Journal clubs can provide a forum to increase team awareness of new or revised treatment guidelines as well as newly published research findings that may lead

Table 37.2 Questions for a Hypertension Team Management Case Conference

- Have blood pressure goals been set, clearly communicated to the patient and all members of the care team, and achieved?
- What type of care does the patient require?
- What is the ideal approach (e.g., individual or group basis) to providing the needed care?
- Which team members are skilled and licensed to provide the various elements of care?
- Which team members provide the various elements of care in the most effective and efficient manner?
- Does this patient need to be referred to specialty medical care, a social worker, a nutritionist, or others?
- What are the barriers to hypertension control? What is the plan for overcoming barriers to blood pressure control?
- Does the patient have the resources to pay for the needed care, including prescription medications?
- Does the patient have family or others who offer social support and assist the patient with blood pressure control behaviors? How can this support be engaged?
- How can quality care be delivered at a reasonable cost?

to changes in practice patterns and improved patient outcomes.

An interdisciplinary team approach to hypertension care and control permits flexibility in matching patients' needs with the competencies of staff with different, yet complementary skills and interests. Nonphysician health professionals, particularly nurses, nurse practitioners, nurse case-managers, pharmacists, health educators, and nurse-supervised community health workers, working in collaboration with physicians in a variety of settings have demonstrated effective, safe, and well-received interventions to effectively improve adherence and blood pressure control among patients with hypertension (13,14,18–22). In addition, involving family, friends, community resources, as well as other health professionals can assist patients in modifying lifestyle and home blood pressure care behaviors and maintaining these changes over time.

Classic hypertension care and control clinical trials, such as HDFP, MRFIT, SHEP, and TOMHS, demonstrated that extensive and continuous interventions provided by interdisciplinary teams improved adherence and outcomes (3,6,27,28). These and other studies designed to meet patient, provider, and organizational needs and minimize barriers to blood pressure control have been effective in a variety of clinical and community settings. One innovative program in which a nurse practitioner-led, interdisciplinary team addressed patient's beliefs and concerns in a multifaceted manner, providing outreach, follow-up, feedback, and free medication, if needed, has been highly successful (14). In this randomized clinical trial with 309 hypertensive, urban black men 21–54 years old, Hill et al. (14) evaluated the effectiveness of a more intensive comprehensive educational–behavioral–pharmacological intervention by a nurse practitioner–community health worker–physician team and a less intensive education and referral intervention in controlling blood pressure and minimizing progression of left ventricular hypertrophy and renal insufficiency. At 36 months, the mean systolic blood pressure/diastolic blood pressure change from baseline was $-7.5/-10.1$ mmHg for the more intensive group and $+3.4/-3.7$ mmHg for the less intensive group ($P = 0.001$ and 0.005 for between-group differences in systolic blood pressure and diastolic blood pressure, respectively). The proportion of men with controlled blood pressure ($<140/90$ mmHg) was 44% in the more intensive group and 31% in the less intensive group ($P = 0.045$). Left ventricular mass was significantly lower in the more intensive group than in the less intensive group (274 g, more intensive; 311 g, less intensive; $P = 0.004$). There was a trend towards slowing of the progression of renal insufficiency (incidence of 50% increase in serum creatinine) in the more intensive group compared with the less intensive group (5.2%, more intensive; 8.0%, less intensive; $P = 0.08$). Most important, the clinical and

cost effectiveness of an interdisciplinary team approach to care compared with physician care alone for chronic illness has been demonstrated (21).

V. SPECIFIC ROLES

Specific roles of the nurse and nurse practitioner in hypertension care reported in the literature have been reviewed (29–31). In addition to clinical care, a significant amount of work has been carried out by nurses in the field of hypertension research, including research focused on blood pressure measurement techniques, hypertension knowledge, blood pressure measurement training, sphygmomanometer validation, and various aspects of clinical care (29). The roles of the nurse and nurse practitioner in hypertension management, which will be further delineated in this section, involve all aspects of hypertension management, including detection, referral, and follow-up; medication management; patient education, counseling, and skill building; coordination of care; management of the clinic or office.

A. Detection, Referral, and Follow-Up

Nurses routinely measure blood pressure in most health care settings as part of the initial and ongoing assessments of each patient. In addition, nurses lead many blood pressure screening and verification initiatives in community, work site, church, school, and other settings. After blood pressure is measured and recorded, the nurse analyzes the data to determine whether the readings are in the normal, pre-hypertensive, or hypertensive range per site protocol. A system to flag charts can help to ensure that uncontrolled hypertension is recognized and treated. In addition, the nurse often assesses the patient's level of cardiovascular risk. There are a number of tools, such as the interactive tool found on the National Heart, Lung, and Blood Institute Web site, that are helpful in guiding healthcare providers as they assess cardiovascular risk; these tools can also be utilized in patient education efforts (32). It may be necessary to refer the patient for specialist evaluation as needed when blood pressure remains uncontrolled despite intervention or for abnormal renal or vascular findings. The nurse often plays an important role in implementing referrals and in educating patients regarding the purpose and importance of the referral.

Follow-up between visits via telephone or mail can be an effective method to reinforce goals and enhance provider–patient relationship. Moreover, it is essential to follow-up on all missed appointments to maintain contact with the patient and to reinforce the importance of achieving blood pressure targets. Nurses are often the first health professionals to detect hypertension and therefore have a key role in communicating with patients and other health professionals to enforce treatment guidelines through development and appropriate revision of the patient's treatment plan.

B. Medication Management

Nurses or nurse practitioners may also be responsible for the pharmacological aspects of hypertension management. Using well-defined protocols based on national treatment guidelines such as the Seventh Report of the Joint National Committee on Prevention, Detection, Evaluation, and Treatment of High Blood Pressure (JNC7), nurse practitioners can prescribe and titrate medications to achieve blood pressure control (33). Nurse management of antihypertensive medication has been demonstrated to result in greater rates of blood pressure control than those achieved with standard care (2,14,18,26,34). These improved outcomes have resulted from nurses placing a greater number of patients on medications, altering drug regimens more frequently in response to inadequate blood pressure control, and placing a higher proportion of patients on multiple drug regimens in order to achieve greater control (2,14,18,26,34). Greater use of antihypertensive medications may produce higher costs initially, as noted by Logan (35). However, if the goals of a clinic are to keep patients in treatment and achieve greater adherence and blood pressure control rates, then obtaining the best regimen for the patient must be paramount (36). In addition to management of hypertension, nurses have been shown to effectively manage other cardiovascular risk factors, such as diabetes (12,13,15) and dyslipidemia (37).

C. Patient Education, Counseling, and Skill Building

In the majority of hypertension clinics as well as in other settings, nurses provide the education, counseling, and skill building necessary to ensure that patients are undertaking lifestyle changes that may favorably influence blood pressure (36). A combination of strategies is required to maximize long-term adherence and blood pressure control by engaging patients and maintaining them in care and preventing, recognizing, and responding to adherence problems. Effective, evidence-based strategies to promote blood pressure control are identified in Table 37.3 and are clustered under the following general approaches (36,38):

- identify patient knowledge, attitudes, beliefs, and experiences;
- educate the patient about conditions and treatment;

- individualize the treatment regimen;
- provide reinforcement;
- promote social support;
- collaborate with other professionals.

It is important to consider that patient education is a means to an end. That is, knowledge is necessary but insufficient to bring about the desired behaviors without the development of skills and other multiple reinforcing factors. The ultimate goal is for the patient to have the skills and resources, in addition to the knowledge, to follow treatment recommendations, and to achieve and sustain blood pressure control.

1. Identifying Patient Knowledge, Attitudes, Beliefs, and Experience

A classic framework to guide healthcare professionals in assessing four critical patient behaviors with concomitant knowledge, attitudes, and skills necessary to achieve and sustain long-term blood pressure control has been adapted and is presented in Table 37.4 (39). This presentation is most useful in guiding nurses and other professionals as they provide patient education, counseling, and skill building to facilitate patients' attainment of the following four critical behaviors:

1. make the decision to control blood pressure;
2. take the medication as prescribed;
3. monitor progress towards the target blood pressure;
4. resolve barriers that prevent reaching the target blood pressure.

The premise of this evidence-based framework is that active participation by the patient as the decision-maker and problem-solver with the nurse or other health professional functioning as advisor and guide favors successful management of hypertension (39).

2. Educating the Patient About Conditions and Treatment

Adequate knowledge of hypertension, including consequences of uncontrolled hypertension and treatment regimen is essential to achieve blood pressure control. It has been shown that patients who receive education and counseling on hypertension management exhibit increased adherence (40). The nurse must practice patient centered care, engaging the patient in shared decision making and establishing mutually agreed upon blood pressure targets. The patient must always be informed of blood pressure and related diagnostic testing values. This provides an ideal opportunity to assess patient knowledge, educate, and establish clear goals with the patient as well as to follow-up regularly to assess and discuss progress towards goals. The nurse must emphasize the need

Table 37.3 Strategies to Promote Blood Pressure Control

Identify knowledge, attitudes, beliefs, and experience:
- Assess patient's understanding and acceptance of the diagnosis and expectations of being in care
- Discuss patient's concerns, and clarify misunderstandings

Educate about conditions and treatment:
- Inform patient of blood pressure level
- Agree with patients on a target blood pressure
- Inform patient about recommended treatment, providing specific oral and written information
- Elicit concerns and questions and provide opportunities for patient to state specific behaviors to carry out treatment recommendations
- Emphasize need to continue treatment, that patient cannot tell if blood pressure is elevated, and that control does not mean cure
- Teach self-monitoring skills

Individualize the regimen:
- Include patient in decision-making
- Simplify the regimen
- Incorporate treatment into patient's daily lifestyle
- Set (with the patient) realistic short-term objectives for specific components of the treatment plan
- Encourage discussion of side effects and concerns
- Encourage self-monitoring of blood pressure
- Prioritize critical aspects of the regimen
- Implement treatment plan in steps
- Modify dosages or change medications to reduce side effects
- Minimize cost of therapy
- Indicate that you will ask about adherence at next visit
- When weight loss is established as a treatment goal, discourage quick weight-loss regimens, fasting, or unscientific methods because these methods are associated with weight cycling, which may increase cardiovascular morbidity and mortality

Provide reinforcement:
- Provide feedback regarding blood pressure level
- Ask about behaviors to achieve blood pressure control
- Give positive feedback for behavioral and blood pressure improvement
- Hold exit interviews to clarify regimen
- Make appointment for next visit before patient leaves the office
- Use appointment reminders, and contact patients to confirm appointments
- Schedule more frequent visits to counsel patients who do not adhere to program
- Contact and follow-up patients who missed appointments
- Consider clinician-patient contracts
- Consider home visits

Promote social support:
- Educate family members to be part of the blood pressure control process and to provide daily reinforcement
- Suggest small group activities to enhance mutual support and motivation

Collaborate with other professionals:
- Draw upon complementary skills and knowledge of nurses, pharmacists, dietitians, optometrists, dentists, and physician assistants
- Recognize shared practice goals
- Refer patients for more intensive counseling

Source: Adapted from the U.S. Department of Health and Human Services (38) and Miller and Hill (36).

to continue treatment even when blood pressure control has been achieved, that is, control does not mean cure. The nurse also plays a key role in educating patients regarding the necessary self-monitoring skills (e.g., home blood pressure monitoring). Patient knowledge is necessary but insufficient if appropriate action does not follow. In addition to patient education, effective communication and a trustful relationship between the patient and the nurse along with patient skill building are of paramount importance to sustained blood pressure control.

3. Individualizing the Treatment Regimen

Successful education and counseling to promote adherence to treatment regimen and blood pressure control requires that nurses and other health professionals individualize care to maximize the patient's motivation to control their hypertension by remaining in care, maintaining a healthy lifestyle, taking prescribed medication, and monitoring progress towards goals. Nurse efforts to individualize the regimen should focus on patient response to the treatment regimen as well as self-care behaviors and skills necessary to hypertension control. The nurse can assist the patient to incorporate the treatment regimen into the patient's daily lifestyle which is required for long-term sustainability. The nurse works with the patient to mutually develop realistic, outcome-oriented goals and strategies for attaining the goals. Equally important, the nurse follows up with the patient frequently to assess progress towards goal and if necessary to revise strategies for attaining goals.

Table 37.4 Four Critical Patient Behaviors with Concomitant Knowledge, Attitudes, and Skills

Knowledge (The patient is able to state:)	Attitude (The patient believes that:)	Skill (The patient is able to:)
Make Decision to Control Blood Pressure		
Current blood pressure and normal limits	His/her blood pressure exceeds normal	Differentiate between normal and abnormal
That high blood pressure can be asymptomatic	His/her blood pressure is high even if there are no symptoms	
That untreated high blood pressure can lead to stroke, kidney failure, or heart disease	Although consequences may not occur for years, they are nevertheless real and serious	
That drug therapy can control high blood pressure and reduce risk of these complications	Drug therapy and high blood pressure control lessen risk of stroke, kidney failure, or heart disease	Explain the benefits of high blood pressure control, e.g., increased length and quality of life
The necessity of lifelong therapy for control of high blood pressure	Potential problems can be resolved	Differentiate between control and cure
	The benefits of control outweigh the costs	Identify potential problems related to medication regimen, fear of medication, time, and money
Take Medication as Prescribed		
Medical regimen: which pill to take, when to take it, what to do if doses are missed	Prescribed medicine will lower blood pressure, is needed every day for blood pressure control, should not be stopped without medical advice	Develop habit of taking medicine by tailoring plan to fit personal schedule
	Folk remedies are not substitutes for prescribed medication	Cue medication taking (if necessary) by associating with daily activities, storing in a prominent place, marking medication calendar
		Select accessible source to obtain medications
		Make financial plan and arrangements to obtain medications
		Renew prescription before supply exhaustion
Monitor Progress toward Blood Pressure Goal		
Individualized blood pressure target	As a partner with provider(s), he has the right to understand what is expected of him, follow own progress, interact with advisor concerning progress	Identify and communicate progress toward goal: state of health, problems encountered with therapy
That blood pressure readings vary and the trend during time is the basis for therapeutic decisions	Accepts daily blood pressure fluctuations (within range provider defines) without undue concern	Keep track of blood pressure trend (if the provider recommends self-monitoring of blood pressure, then additional skills need to be developed)
That medication may need to be changed		
Date and time for next appointment	Continuous therapy is important, including appointment keeping	Reschedule appointment
Resolve Barriers that Prevent Achieving Blood Pressure Control		
A. Communication		
That blood pressure control requires a combined effort by both provider and patient	Provider is interested in his concerns	State concerns; ask questions
	As a partner, he has responsibility to know what is expected, state what he expects of provider	With the provider: identify possible solutions, select and try out solutions, evaluate progress
That other health professionals can help solve problems	Others can assist him to solve problems	Select appropriate health professionals
	Aforementioned attitudes apply here as well	Aforementioned skills apply here as well

(continued)

Table 37.4 *Continued*

Knowledge (The patient is able to state:)	Attitude (The patient believes that:)	Skill (The patient is able to:)
That blood pressure control requires emotional support from friends and relatives	He/she can ask and will gain empathy, support, and assistance with high blood pressure therapy from friends and relatives	State when and how family members can help and ask for that assistance Request instruction for friends and relatives about blood pressure control and its management Accept and use reinforcement and support
B. Medication regimen		
Important side effects of his blood pressure drugs	Side effects occur	Recognize symptoms as possibly being drug-induced
Action to be taken if symptoms occur	Provider will correct problems that pose danger to health	Consult provider about bothersome symptoms
Methods of minimizing side effects, e.g., dosage scheduling, dietary supplements, activity precautions		Utilize methods when necessary
That other medications are available if side effects are intolerable	Living with minor side effects is more acceptable than consequences of uncontrolled blood pressure	Request that other medication be prescribed if side effects are intolerable
That other drugs can interfere with blood pressure target, e.g., over-the-counter medications such as decongestants	Drug interactions can interfere with blood pressure goals	Inform all providers of current regimen Seek advice before taking nonprescription medications
C. Costs		Inform provider of special time constraints
Time required for follow-up visits, getting medication	Time commitment to high blood pressure therapy is as important as conflicting time demands	Request advice on how to minimize time spent on treatment of high blood pressure
How this time will be built into his life		Inform provider of special financial problems
Dollar costs of medicine and follow-up visits	Treatment of high blood pressure has high priority in budget	Request advice on resources to assist with cost

Source: Adapted from Working Group to Define Critical Patient Behaviors in High Blood Pressure Control (39).

Nurses are trained to provide counseling regarding lifestyle modification, which is recommended for all hypertensive patients with lifestyle risk factors, for example, obesity, excessive alcohol consumption, and a high-sodium diet (33). Weight loss, which may be the most successful nonpharmacological technique for lowering blood pressure, requires behavior change in both diet and physical activity patterns (33). Such nonpharmacological approaches include helping patients to initiate or maintain an aerobic exercise program and to limit sodium intake and alcohol consumption to one to two drinks per day (33). In addition, many hypertensive patients present with multiple risk factors for cardiovascular disease. The nurse can also provide education and counseling for smoking cessation and lipid reduction to help patients further lower their risk of cardiovascular disease. Modifying lifestyle behaviors requires many clinical interventions: assessment of an individual's baseline behaviors; education about how to make the appropriate changes; counseling to develop strategies such as setting short-term goals and self-monitoring that will ensure the achievement and maintenance of the changes; constant follow-up with the patient to determine whether adherence is a problem; working with patient to identify and resolve barriers to blood pressure control; reinforcement of progress toward the goal of change in behavior (39).

The extent to which patients are able to adhere to or comply with treatment recommendations is a major issue in blood pressure control and depends on many factors. A review of adherence in randomized controlled trials on cardiovascular disease prevention strategies identified the following successful approaches: signed agreements; behavioral skill training; self-monitoring; telephone/mail contact; spouse support; self-efficacy enhancement; contingency contracting; exercise prescriptions; external cognitive aids; persuasive communication; nurse–managed clinics; work- or school-based programs (40). Patients, nurses, and other health care professionals and health care organizations can prevent, monitor, and address adherence problems by utilizing effective strategies. Improving adherence to evidence-based guidelines is a multilevel challenge and multiple strategies are required beginning with patient education, counseling, and skill building (18).

Another important aspect of individualizing the regimen to promote blood pressure control involves assessing potential barriers to blood pressure control. Nurses are motivated and trained to assess common barriers to blood pressure control. Barriers may include: knowledge deficits, lack of health care or pharmacy insurance, inadequate communication with clinicians, cost of medication, complexity of the regimen, adverse effects of medication, transportation to and from the visit, work schedule, inconvenient clinic or office location or difficulty in scheduling appointments, child or elder care, or other competing life demands (41,42). Following identification of barriers, the nurse works with the patient and collaborating health professionals to minimize or eliminate the barriers, thereby promoting blood pressure control.

4. Providing Reinforcement

It is important to work with individual patients to assure that they understand what is necessary to achieve treatment goals and that they participate in treatment decisions. Nurse responsiveness to patient concerns with joint problem solving to prevent or minimize barriers to care and treatment as well as reinforcement and support are crucial. Provision of reminders, outreach, and follow-up services are beneficial. Follow-up between visits via telephone and/or mail can be an effective method to reinforce goals and enhance provider–patient relationship. It is essential to follow-up on all missed appointments to maintain contact with the patient and to reinforce the importance of achieving blood pressure goals. Success in implementing the treatment regimen to achieve blood pressure control requires frequent monitoring of blood pressure, modification of treatment regimen, and interaction with the patient. These roles are most appropriate for a health professional, such as a nurse, who has requisite training and dedicated time to provide the education and counseling necessary to build skills for and reinforce successful behavior change.

5. Promoting Social Support

The nurse can also be effective in educating family members and/or friends to participate in the blood pressure control process. Family members can play a fundamental role providing daily reinforcement of the patient's efforts to achieve blood pressure control. If the patient desires greater family participation, the nurse should encourage the patient to invite family members to attend and participate in clinic visits. In addition, some patients may benefit from small group activities, for example, clinic support groups or group visits, to enhance social support and motivation.

6. Collaborating with Other Professionals

In planning care, the nurse works in conjunction with the patient, physician, and other members of the care team. The nurse functions as a co-interventionist with any or all of the following roles: detection, referral, and follow-up; medication management; patient education, counseling, and skill building; coordination of care; managing the clinic or office. Ongoing collaboration with other professionals with complementary skills and shared practice goals is in the best interest of the patient. It may be necessary to refer the patient for specialist evaluation as needed when managing complex cases with uncontrolled hypertension despite intervention. Nurse-supervised community health workers, nurse case-managers, and nurse practitioners, in collaboration with physicians and other health professionals, in a variety of settings have effectively improved the outcomes of patients with hypertension (13,14,16–20). Involving family, friends, community resources, and other health professionals can help patients to achieve and sustain blood pressure control.

Achieving and sustaining target blood pressure levels over time requires continuous educational and behavioral strategies, an individualized regimen, and reinforcement so that patients have the knowledge, skills, motivation, and resources to carry out treatment recommendations. Successful blood pressure control requires that patients know what steps to take and develop skills in problem identification and problem solving to address barriers. Strategies to help patients develop these skills need to be adapted so that they are culturally salient and feasible for staff to implement.

D. Coordination of Care

Long-term maintenance of hypertension control requires continual monitoring of blood pressure, refilling of prescriptions, providing counseling and reinforcement of behavior change efforts, and titrating therapy as indicated. Each patient's plan of care must be individualized. It is also important that costs incurred by patients be minimized. Patients often see different providers at several settings for various health problems, fill prescriptions in more than one pharmacy, receive inconsistent messages, and experience interruption of therapy and inadequate communication among providers. Nurses are skilled at building and maintaining both informal and formal collaborative linkages among providers, resources, and services within and outside their practice setting. Nurse can assist patients in understanding complex treatment regimen

(45) and navigating through the complex, challenging, and commonly confusing health care structure.

E. Managing the Clinic or Office

A nurse may be in the position of managing or planning for the initiation of a hypertension clinic. A simple checklist for use in developing a hypertension clinic is shown in Table 37.5 (46). Nurses frequently direct and/or coordinate the efforts of other team members who are working within the clinic or providing direct consultation. Collaborative teams may include physicians, nurses, nutritionists, pharmacists, and community health care workers. To enhance consistency and quality of care and to facilitate adherence to treatment guidelines, in collaboration with other team members the nurse may develop decision support systems (electronic and paper) such as flow sheets and feedback reminders. In addition, it may be the responsibility of the nurse to hire, supervise, and train the community health workers to deliver appropriate intervention strategies and other staff, such as office assistants and receptionists, to take blood pressures, schedule appointments, make reminder telephone calls, obtain laboratory results, and enter data to support evaluation of clinical outcomes, which can be

helpful and can also decrease costs (36). Nurses influence utilization of resources including appropriate length of visit and caseload size as well as reimbursement for services in the hypertension clinic setting.

It is imperative that all health professionals who measure blood pressure use correct measurement technique following guidelines developed and promulgated by professional societies such as the World Hypertension League (47,48). In addition to ensuring proper blood pressure measurement technique among staff, nurses often are responsible for ensuring that blood pressure measurement equipment is properly calibrated and functioning (47).

Documentation of clinical outcomes is becoming increasingly important and necessary. Often it is the nurse in the hypertension care setting who has responsibility for tracking process and outcome measures. Integrated systems with continuous quality improvement approaches enhance provider's delivery of care and patient outcomes. Tracking the blood pressures, frequency of visits, medications, patient adherence, hospitalizations, and emergency room visits, through a computer program enables timely evaluation of clinical outcomes and the costs incurred in providing antihypertensive treatment.

Table 37.5   Outpatient Hypertension Clinic Start-Up Checklist

1. Establish need and cost benefits	7. Determine sequence and pathway of patient visit flow
2. Assess and establish staff support and qualifications	Schedule for new and return visit
3. Designate physician medical director and coordinator	Physician consultation schedule with new patients
4. Ensure efficient assessment and educational physical space	8. Develop patient data tracking system
5. Develop written policies and procedures	Assess existing patient tracking software packages
Entry and referral criteria	Determine protocol for monitoring clinical events and associated costs
Treatment Algorithms	9. Acquire and maintain patient education materials
Exit criteria	Pharmacological information
Laboratory standards	Lifestyle information
Pricing	Other resources
Fee-for-service schedule	10. Marketing and promotion plan
Compute capitation rate or contribution to global rate for managed care contracts	Internal marketing and promotion: Medical and ancillary staff
Billing and corrections policy	Patients
Operational budget and pro forma outcome measures (JNC7 goals)	Referring physicians, PPOs and HMOs
6. Develop standard forms	Business and industry
Patient information (medical history, lifestyle)	Alliances with hospitals, PPOs and drug companies to form organized and efficient disease-management programs
Initial assessment and treatment plan	11. Develop continuing education schedule for clinic staff
Return visit and progress report	New research funding
Drug descriptions and patient administration instructions	New reimbursement guidelines and legislation
Individual lifestyle counseling prescription (dietary, exercise, stress management)	12. Develop link and network with national hypertension organizations
Dietary and body fat assessment (BMI)	

Note: BMI, body mass index; PPOs, preferred provider organizations; HMOs, health maintenance organizations.
Source: Adapted from La Forge and Thomas (46).

VI. ADVANTAGES AND BARRIERS TO NURSE INVOLVEMENT

The advantages of involving nurses in the management of hypertension are numerous. Nurses provide effective care by adhering to treatment guidelines and protocols resulting in improved outcomes, including patient satisfaction and retention in care, and physician satisfaction. They function as essential hypertension care team members in the following roles: providing detection, referral and follow-up; medication management; patient education, counseling, and skill building; coordination of care; managing the clinic or office.

The barriers to optimal participation of nurses in the management of hypertension are similar to the barriers that limit the most effective involvement of physicians and other health professionals in the care of patients with any chronic illness. These include inadequate awareness of the role, lack of time and resources, and lack of incentives and reimbursement. The reporting of hypertension clinical trial methods has historically limited our understanding of the role of nurses in hypertension care (29). For example, the American Hypertension Detection and Follow-up Program (HDFP) was a randomized trial of efficient and organized stepped care vs. routine clinical practice or referred care. Both heart attacks and strokes were prevented in the stepped care group. These patients were largely managed by well trained and highly motivated nurses. However, in most of the publications from this study, information about who provided the care to the stepped care group was not well described (3,29). In some settings the barriers also include lack of practical implementation tools, such as decision support systems, and local social norms and ethics that preclude nurses from assuming greater responsibility for patient care and outcomes. A major barrier to nurse practitioners' practice in some provinces or states involves practice regulations.

VII. CONCLUSIONS

The prevalence and asymptomatic nature of hypertension and the need for life-long treatment to prevent complications pose challenges that require professional expertise beyond that of physicians. Nurses, who are the largest group of nonphysician providers, participate importantly in the care of patients with hypertension, especially in the care of patients with uncomplicated essential hypertension. The care of patients with hypertension is commonly provided by physician–nurse teams, even in settings where the team approach is not clearly recognized. Advanced practice nurses are trained and licensed to provide management of acute and chronic conditions including the diagnosis, treatment, and management of hypertension.

Collaborative partnerships, based upon recognition of nurses' roles and a supportive environment, are essential to the successful involvement of nurses in the management of hypertension. The meaningful involvement of nurses in the management of hypertension involves bringing nurses, physicians, and other health professionals together to improve patient care, to advance nurses and nursing, and to influence health policy.

REFERENCES

1. Alderman MH, Schoenbaum EE. Detection and treatment of hypertension at the work site. N Engl J Med 1975; 293:65–68.
2. Logan AG, Milne BJ, Achber C, Campbell WP, Haynes RB. Work-site treatment of hypertension by specially trained nurses. Lancet 1979; 2:1175–1178.
3. Hypertension Detection and Follow-up Program Co-operative Group. Five-year findings of the Hypertension Detection and Follow-up program. I. Reduction in mortality of persons with hypertension, including mild hypertension. J Am Med Assoc 1979; 242:2562–2571.
4. Viskoper RJ, Silverberg DS. Community control in Israel: cardiovascular risk factor control. In: Bulpitt CJ, ed. Handbook of Hypertension: Epidemiology of Hypertension. Vol. 2. Amsterdam: Elsevier Science Publishers, 1985.
5. Curzio JL, Rubin PC, Kennedy SS, Reid JL. A comparison of the management of hypertensive patients by nurse practitioners compared with conventional hospital care. J Hum Hypertens 1990; 4:665–670.
6. SHEP Co-operative Research Group. Prevention of stroke by antihypertensive drug treatment in older persons with isolated systolic hypertension. J Am Med Assoc 1991; 265:3255–3264.
7. Medical Research Council Working Party. Medical Research Council trial of treatment of hypertension in older adults: principal results. Br Med J 1992; 304:405–412.
8. Becker DM, Yook RM, Moy TF, Blumenthal RS, Becker LC. Markedly high prevalence of coronary risk factors in apparently healthy African-American and white siblings of persons with premature coronary heart disease. Am J Cardiol 1998; 82:1045–1051.
9. Montgomery A, Fahey T, Peters T, MacIntosh C, Sharp D. Evaluation of computer based clinical decision support system and risk chart for management of hypertension in primary care: randomized controlled trial. Br Med J 2000; 320:686–690.
10. Rice VH, Stead LF. Nursing Interventions for Smoking Cessation (Cochrane Review). Oxford: The Cochrane Library, 2002.
11. McPherson CP, Swenson KK, Pine DA, Leimer L. A nurse-based pilot program to reduce cardiovascular risk factors in a primary care setting. Am J Manag Care 2002; 8:543–555.

12. Denver EA, Barnard M, Woolfson RG, Earle KA. Management of uncontrolled hypertension in a nurse-led clinic compared with conventional care for patients with type 2 diabetes. Diabetes Care 2003; 26:2256–2260.

13. Gary TL, Bone LR, Hill MN, Levine DM, McGuire M, Saudek C, Brancati FL. Randomized controlled trial of the effects of nurse case manager and community health worker interventions on risk factors for diabetes-related complications in urban African-Americans. Prev Med 2003; 37:23–32.

14. Hill MN, Han HR, Dennison CR, Kim MT, Roary MC, Blumenthal RS, Bone LR, Levine DM, Post WS. Hypertension care and control in underserved urban African American men: behavioral and physiologic outcomes at 36 months. Am J Hypertens 2003; 16:906–913.

15. New JP, Mason JM, Freemantle N, Teasdale S, Wong LM, Bruce NJ, Burns JA, Gibson JM. Specialist nurse-led intervention to treat and control hypertension and hyperlipidemia in diabetes (SPLINT). A randomized controlled trial. Diabetes Care 2003; 26:2250–2255.

16. Canzanello VJ, Jensen PL, Schwartz LL, Worra JB, Klein LK. Improved blood pressure control with a physician-nurse team and home blood pressure measurement. Mayo Clin Proc 2005; 80(1):31–36.

17. Bosworth HB, Olsen MK, Gentry P, Orr M, Dudley T, McCant F, Oddone EZ. Nurse administered telephone intervention for blood pressure control: a patient-tailored multifactorial intervention. Patient Educ Couns 2005; 57(1):5–14.

18. Reichgott MJ, Pearson S, Hill MN. The nurse practitioner's role in complex patient management: hypertension. J Natl Med Assoc 1983; 75:1197–1204.

19. Ginsberg GM, Viskoper JR, Fuchs Z, Drexler I, Lubin F, Berlin S, Nitza H, Zulty L, Chetrit A, Bregman L. Partial cost-benefit analysis of two different modes of nonpharmacological control of hypertension in the community. J Hum Hypertens 1993; 7:593–597.

20. Miller NM, Hill MN, Kottke T, Ockene IS. The multilevel compliance challenge: recommendations for a call to action: a statement for health care professionals. Circulation 1997; 95:1085–1090.

21. Litaker D, Mion L, Planavsky L, Kippes C, Mehta N, Frolkis J. Physician-nurse practitioner teams in chronic disease management: the impact on costs, clinical effectiveness, and patients' perception of care. J Interprof Care 2003; 17:223–237.

22. Norby SM, Stroebel RJ, Canzanello VJ. Physician-Nurse Team Approaches to Improve Blood Pressure Control. J Clin Hypertens 2003; 5:386–392.

23. International Council of Nurses. Available at: http://www.icn.ch (accessed May 14, 2004).

24. American Nurses Association. Advanced Practice Nursing: A New Age in Health Care. Washington, DC: American Nurses Association, 1993.

25. Horrocks S, Anderson E, Salisbury C. Systematic review of whether nurse practitioners working in primary care can provide equivalent care to doctors. Br Med J 2002; 324:819–823.

26. Mundinger MO, Kane RL, Lenz ER, Totten AM, Tsai W, Cleary PD, Friedewald WT, Siu AL, Shelanski ML. Primary care outcomes in patients treated by nurse practitioners or physicians. A randomized trial. J Am Med Assoc 2000; 283:59–68.

27. Grimm RH, Cohen JD, Smith WM, Falvo-Gerard L, Neaton JD. Hypertension management in the Multiple Risk Factor Intervention Trial (MRFIT). Six-year intervention results for men in special intervention and usual care groups. Arch Intern Med 1985; 145:1191–1199.

28. Treatment of Mild Hypertension Study Research Group. Treatment of mild hypertension study: final results. J Am Med Assoc 1993; 270:713–724.

29. Curzio JL, Beevers M. The role of nurses in hypertension care and research. J Hum Hypertens 1997; 11:541–550.

30. Bengtson A, Drevenhorn E. The Nurse's Role and Skills in Hypertension Care. Clin Nurse Spec 2003; 17:260–268.

31. Oakeshott P, Kerry S, Austin A, Cappuccio F. Is there a role for nurse-led blood pressure management in primary care? Fam Pract 2003; 20:469–473.

32. National Cholesterol Education Program. Third Report of the expert panel on Detection, Evaluation, and Treatment of High Blood Cholesterol in Adults (Adult Treatment Panel III). Risk assessment tool for estimating 10-year risk of developing hard CHD (Myocardial Infarction and coronary death). Available at: http://hin.nhlbi.nih.gov/atpiii/calculator.asp?usertype = prof (acccessed May 14, 2004).

33. The Seventh Report of the Joint National Committee on Prevention, Detection, Evaluation, and Treatment of High Blood Pressure (JNC VII). National High Blood Pressure Education Program. Bethesda, MD: National Institutes of Health, National Heart, Lung and Blood Institute, 2003: NIH publication 03-5233.

34. Runyan KW Jr. The Memphis Chronic Disease Program. Comparisons in outcome and the nurse's extended role. J Am Med Assoc 1975; 231:264–267.

35. Logan AC, Milne BJ, Flanagan PT, Haynes RB. Clinical effectiveness and cost-effectiveness of monitoring blood pressure of hypertensive employees at work. Hypertension 1983; 5:828–836.

36. Miller NM, Hill MN. Nursing clinics in the management of hypertension. In: Oparil, Weber, eds. Hypertension. 2nd ed. Philadelphia: WB Saunders, 2004.

37. Debusk RF, Miller NH, Superko HR, Dennis CA, Thomas RJ, Lew HT, Berger WE, Heller RS, Rompf J, Gee D, Kraemer HC, Bandura A, Ghandour G, Clark M, Shah RV, Fisher L, Taylor CB. A case-management system for coronary risk factor modification after acute myocardial infarction. Ann Intern Med 1994; 120:721–729.

38. The Fifth Report of the Joint National Committee on Prevention, Detection, Evaluation, and Treatment of High Blood Pressure (JNC V). National High Blood Pressure Education Program. Bethesda, MD: National Institutes of Health, National Heart, Lung and Blood Institute, 1993: NIH publication 98-98-4080.

39. Working Group to Define Critical Patient Behaviors in High Blood Pressure Control. Patient behavior for blood pressure control. Guidelines for professionals. J Am Med Assoc 1979; 241:2534–2537.

40. Levine DM, Green LW, Deeds SG, Chwalow J, Russell RP, Finlay J. Health Education for hypertensive patients. J Am Med Assoc 1979; 241:1700–1703.

41. Miller NH, Taylor CB. Lifestyle Management for Patients With Coronary Heart Disease. Current Issues in Cardiac Rehabilitation, Monograph No. 2. Champaign, IL: Human Kinetics, 1995.

42. Haynes RB. Improving patient adherence: state of the art, with a special focus on medication taking for cardiovascular disorders. In: Burke LE, Ockene IS, eds. Compliance in Healthcare and Research. Armonk, NY: Futura Publishing Company, Inc, 2001.

43. Eaton LE, Buck EA, Catanzaro JE. The nurse's role in facilitating compliance in clients with hypertension. Med Surg Nursing 1996; 5:339–364.

44. Hill MN, Bone LR, Kim MT, Miller DJ, Dennison CR, Levine DM. Barriers to hypertension care and control in young urban black men. Am J Hypertens 1999; 12:951–958.

45. Aminoff UB, Kjellgren KI. The nurse—a resource in hypertension care. J Adv Nurs 2001; 35:582–589.

46. La Forge R, Thomas T. Outpatient management of lipid disorders. J Cardiovasc Nurs 1996; 11:39–53.

47. Beevers G, Lip GY, O'Brien E. ABC of hypertension. Blood pressure measurement. Part I-sphygmomanometry: factors common to all techniques. Br Med J 2001; 322:981–985.

48. World Hypertension League. Measuring your blood pressure. Available at: http:www.mco.edu/org/whl/bloodpre.html. (accessed May 14, 2004).

38

Orthostatic Disorders in Hypertension

WANPEN VONGPATANASIN, RONALD G. VICTOR

University of Texas Southwestern Medical Center, Dallas, Texas, USA

KEYPOINTS

- Postural changes in blood pressure (BP) are common in patients with hypertension.
- To avoid overtreatment or undertreatment of hypertension, BP, and heart rate should be measured in the supine, sitting, and standing positions in all hypertensive patients.
- Orthostatic hypotension could be due to excessive reduction in effective intravascular volume despite appropriate autonomic reflex compensation (hyperadrenergic) or primary abnormalities in the autonomic reflex adjustments to postural fall in venous return (hypoadrenergic).

- Treatment of orthostatic hypotension is depending on the cause and the presence or absence of intact autonomic nervous system function. However, diuretics should be avoided in patients with hypoadrenergic orthostatic hypotension.

SUMMARY

Orthostatic hypotension is commonly found in hypertensive patients with the prevalence between 10–30%. Orthostatic hypotension can be classified as either (a) "hyperadrenergic" indicating that the autonomic nervous system is responding appropriately to an excessive postural fall in venous return, or (b) "hypoadrenergic," indicating a defective reflex compensation to a normal fall in venous return. Patients with hyperadrenergic states should be treated according to the cause of intravascular volume depletion. Patients with hypoadrenergic orthostatic hypotension require both nonpharmacologic and pharmacologic intervention to reduce the postural symptoms. Although diuretics are first-line antihypertensive therapy for most patients with hypertension, they should be avoided in patients with hypoadrenergic orthostatic hypotension. Supine hypertension in the setting of autonomic failure is a rare indication for short-acting vasodilator therapy at bedtime. Orthostatic hypertension (elevated blood pressure only when standing) is less common than orthostatic hypotension and often goes undetected. The pathophysiology is not well understood but overactivity of sympathetic nervous system may play a major role. Alpha-adrenergic receptor blockade should be considered.

I. INTRODUCTION

When a normal subject assumes upright posture, ~500–800 cc of blood pools in the leg and splanchnic veins, reducing central blood volume, cardiac output, and blood pressure. The adequate circulatory adjustment to upright posture requires the activation of several autonomic reflexes shown in Fig. 38.1. First, reduced central blood volume unloads cardiopulmonary ("low pressure") baroreceptors located in the left atrium, left ventricle, and pulmonary veins. The deactivation of these receptors trigger a reflex increase in sympathetic outflow to the peripheral circulation, increasing peripheral vascular resistance to

maintain blood pressure with little effect on the heart rate or cardiac output. Secondly, reduction in systemic blood pressure decreases the stretch of the carotid sinus and aortic arch ("high pressure") baroreceptors, which project centrally via the glossopharyngeal or vagus nerve to the nucleus tractus solitarius into the brainstem. The reflex response is to increase sympathetic efferent discharge to the blood vessels to increase vascular resistance and to the sinus node to increase heart rate and cardiac output. Withdrawal of cardiac vagal activity also contributes to immediate rise in heart rate within the first 30 s of standing, resembling the abrupt increase in the heart rate observed in normal subjects at the onset of exercise. The more gradual increase in the heart rate 1–2 min after standing is due to baroreflex-mediated further decrease in cardiac vagal activity and increase in sympathetic tone to the sinus node. In addition to the autonomic reflex adjustments, skeletal muscle contraction in the legs plays a critical role in emptying the vein and increasing the venous driving pressure back toward the heart to maintain cardiac output. For this muscle pump to be effective, venous valves must be competent.

Therefore, in normal subjects, postural reduction in blood pressure is usually 20/10 mmHg and increase in heart rate is 30 beats/min. Any abnormalities in the arterial or cardiopulmonary baroreceptors, afferent nerves, the nucleus tractus solitarius where the afferent nerves terminate, and the efferent nerve output in the sympathetic nervous system to increase norepinephrine release to the heart and blood vessels can lead to OH. On the other hand, patients with severe reduction in intravascular volume may experience OH or tachycardia despite intact autonomic nervous system function.

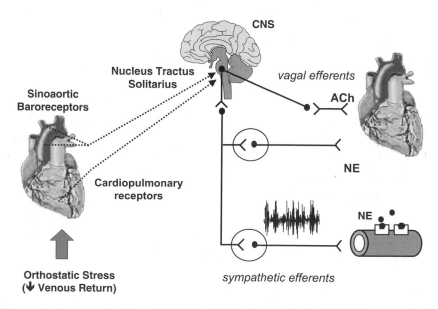

Figure 38.1 Diagram showing neural pathway that is involved in the regulation of blood pressure during orthostatic stress.

II. PATHOPHYSIOLOGY OF ORTHOSTATIC HYPOTENSION

OH is defined by the Consensus Committee of the American Autonomic Society and the American Academy of Neurology as a reduction of systolic blood pressure of at least 20 mmHg or diastolic blood pressure of at least 10 mmHg within 3 min of standing (1). The prevalence of OH in individuals with hypertension varied between 10% and 30% (2–5).

OH can occur in hypertensive patients in the presence or absence of intact autonomic function (Fig. 38.2). Patients with intact autonomic function usually have features of hyperadrenergic state, such as reflex tachycardia and elevated plasma catecholamines, indicating an appropriate compensation to excessive intravascular volume reduction or vasodilation from variety of causes. Patients with autonomic dysfunction have hypoadrenergic features with fixed or blunted heart rate and plasma catecholamine responses to postural changes, indicating an impaired reflex compensation.

A. Hyperadrenergic OH

Volume depletion from gastrointestinal or renal loss is the common cause of hyperadrenergic type of OH. Severe venous insufficiency reduces ability of muscle pump to prevent pooling of blood in the legs. Patients with pheochromocytoma frequently have both hypertension and OH from reduced intravascular volume and vasodilation effects of epinephrine. Phenylpropanolamine, a nonprescription sympathomimetic drug used for weight reduction, can lead to OH probably by a mechanism similar to pheochromocytoma (6). Mastocytosis and carcinoid syndrome are potential causes of episodic OH, flushing, and palpitation related to massive intermittent release of histamine from the mast cells and serotonin from carcinoid tumors, leading to excessive peripheral vasodilation. Antihypertensive medications can also lead to OH. α-Adrenergic receptor blocker (7), dihydropyridine calcium channel blockers (8), and diuretics (7) appeared to cause this problem more than angiotensin-converting enzyme (ACE) inhibitors. However, the use of slow-release forms or drugs with longer half-life reduced this difference in the incidence of postural hypotension among different classes of antihypertensive drugs (9).

B. Hypoadrenergic OH

The lesions producing hypoadrenergic OH could be at the level of postganglionic efferent sympathetic fibers, central nervous system, or afferent baroreceptor input.

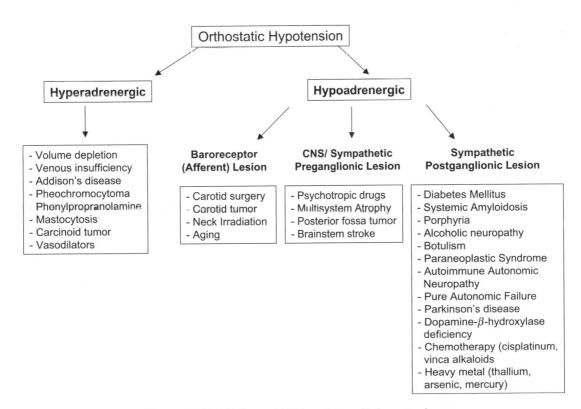

Figure 38.2 Etiology of OH in patients with hypertension.

1. Lesions in Afferent Baroreceptor Input (Baroreflex Failure)

Abnormalities in the baroreceptors, the glossopharyngeal or vagus nerve, or their brainstem connections can lead to baroreflex failure. Carotid surgery, such as carotid endarterctomy or carotid body tumor resection, either unilaterally or bilaterally can lead to acute increases in blood pressure immediately after surgery (10). A smaller subset of patients develop persistent reduction in baroreflex sensitivity and episodic labile hypertension and tachycardia, resembling clinical picture of pheochromocytoma (11). Patients with baroreflex failure have exaggerated pressor response to cold pressor test but may or may not present with OH (11). The same clinical presentation have been reported as a late complication of neck irradiation (12).

Aging is commonly associated with increased prevalence of OH, possibly related to age-related decline in baroreflex function and/or attenuated vasoconstrictor responses to norepinephrine ~30% of noninstitutionalized subjects >65 years of age have OH (3,13), most of whom are asymptomatic (14). However, aging alone should not cause symptomatic OH unless patients have concomitant volume depletion, venous insufficiency, or postprandial hypotension (15).

2. Lesions in the Central Nervous System/Sympathetic Preganglionic Site

Multisystem atrophy (MSA) (Shy–Drager syndrome) is a neurodegenerative disorder characterized by the loss of sympathetic preganglionic neurons in the intermediolateral cell column (16). The disease usually begins in middle age around the fifth decade of life and affects more men than women. In addition to OH, MSA patients also suffer from genitourinary dysfunction and other neurological involvement due to subcortical white matter disease. Movement disorders similar to Parkinson's disease, such as bradykinesia, inexpressive facies, hypertonia, truncal ataxia, are also present. Patients with MSA have limited survival of approximately only 9 years from the symptom onset (17). Unlike Parkinson's disease, MSA is generally unresponsive to levodopa. Indeed, the clinical response of the movement disorder to levodopa often is used to distinguish MSA from Parkinson's disease. MSA patients have a large reduction in supine blood pressure with ganglionic blocker trimethaphan and a large pressor response to α2 antagonist yohimbine, indicating residual sympathetic activity (18).

Tricyclic antidepressant and psychotropic drugs are common causes of central hypoadrenergic OH (6). Orthostatic symptoms can persistent even months after discontinuation of medication. Brainstem stroke is an obvious cause of OH. Posterior fossa tumors are important to consider as a reversible cause and should be excluded with neuroimaging studies including posterior fossa cut.

3. Lesions in the Postganglionic Sympathetic Efferents

Pure autonomic failure (PAF) (Bradbury–Eggleston syndrome) is the classic idiopathic form of postganglionic efferent cause of OH. Patients with PAF have diminished postganglionic sympathetic neuron in the sympathetic ganglia, resulting in denervation supersensitivity. Patients have both OH and supine hypertension, beginning in the sixth decade of life. Autonomic involvement of other organs is also present leading to impotence, decreased sweating, papillary dysfunction, neurogenic bladder, and gastrointestinal dysmotility. The consequence of supine hypertension is pressure diuresis, particularly at nighttime, which leads to intravascular volume depletion and exacerbation of OH in the morning hours (19). In marked contrast to MSA, PAF patients usually do not have neurologic abnormalities other than involvement of autonomic nervous system. Mechanism of supine hypertension in PAF is not well understood. Unlike MSA, PAF is characterized by little or no residual SNA as evidenced by minimal reduction in blood pressure with ganglionic blocker trimethaphan (18).

Parkinson's disease is frequently accompanied by symptoms of autonomic failure such as OH, constipation, urinary incontinence, erectile dysfunction. Despite similarity in clinical presentation to MSA, recent data suggest an important component of peripheral denervation in Parkinson's disease with OH (20). Most patients with Parkinson's disease and OH have low baroreflex gain, low levels of plasma norepinephrine both in supine and in upright position, and reduced cardiac sympathetic innervation as evidenced by reduced myocardial concentration of 6-[^{18}F]fluorodopamine-derived radioactivity by PET scanning (20–22). Patients with Parkinson's disease with autonomic involvement, OH often becomes symptomatic when the neurologists titrate the dose of levodopa, a potent peripheral vasodilator through activation of the dopamine 1 receptor in the vascular smooth muscle or stimulation presynaptic dopamine 2 receptor to inhibit norepinephrine release from sympathetic nerve endings.

Deficiency of the enzyme dopamine-β-hydroxylase (DβH) is a very rare congenital disorder resulting in defective conversion of dopamine to norepinephrine in the adrenal medulla and in the sympathetic nerve terminals at the central and peripheral sites. DβH deficiency is characterized by isolated failure of noradrenergic neurotransmission with normal sympathetic cholinergic and parasympathetic function. Therefore, patients with DβH deficiency suffer from OH and ptosis, but have normal sweating and respiratory variation of the heart rate.

Patients have undetectable levels of epinephrine and norepinephrine with elevated dopamine levels. Patients have normal postganglionic sympathetic nerve traffic as evidenced by direct microneurographic studies with appropriate increase in response to handgrip exercise and cold pressor test and normal baroreflex-mediated suppression in SNA with phenylephrine, indicating an intact central sympathetic outflow with defective catecholamine synthesis (23).

Diabetes mellitus is a frequent cause of secondary autonomic failure, accounting up to 15% of patients referred for evaluation of symptomatic OH (6). Prevalence of postural hypotension in patients with diabetes mellitus is between 17% and 43%, but only one-third of diabetic patients with postural hypotension have postural dizziness (24,25). Patients usually have had diabetes for 15–20 years prior to symptom onset. Involvement of vagal efferent fibers, resulting in loss of respiratory sinus arrhythmia, usually precedes involvement of postganglionic sympathetic efferent fibers leading to OH. Autonomic neuropathy involving other organ systems, causing erectile dysfunction, diarrhea, constipation, sudomotor dysfunction, urinary retention or incontinence, and diabetic nephropathy are commonly present. Patients with asymptomatic autonomic neuropathy have much poorer prognosis than those with normal autonomic function (26). Patients with symptomatic OH have highest mortality rate, ranging from 25% to 50% >5 years of follow-up (27,28). By contrast, the 5 year mortality rate is <5%, if autonomic function tests are normal. The most common cause of death is renal failure followed by sudden cardiac death, which could be related to cardiac vagal denervation.

Amyloid neuropathy can present as autonomic failure and OH. Patients develop clinical signs of widespread sympathetic and parasympathetic failure, such as anhidrosis, constipation alternating with diarrhea due to involvement of myenteric and submucosal plexus, and dysphagia due to esophageal involvement. Distal sensory loss, macroglossia, weight loss, and impotence may also develop.

Porphyrias are rare cause of autonomic dysfunction, characterized by acute or subacute onset of tachycardia, peripheral motor neuropathy, skin manifestation, and central nervous system involvement. Constipation, bladder distention, abdominal pain, nausea, and vomiting may also occur.

Botulism should be suspected when patients develop acute onset of ptosis, blurred vision, dysphagia, extraocular muscle weakness, generalized muscle weakness, and OH after ingestion of food contaminated by *Clostridium botulinum* for 12–36 h. Patients may have severe cholinergic failure, resulting in anhidrosis, dry eyes, dry mouth, ileus, and urinary retention.

Autoimmune autonomic neuropathy, or acute pandysautonomia, has a classic triad of OH, anhidrosis, and gastrointestinal dysmotility involving previously healthy individuals. Patients develop acute or subacute onset of generalized autonomic failure involving both sympathetic and parasympathetic nervous system with relative sparing of somatic nerves. The pathogenesis of autoimmune autonomic neuropathy is not completely understood, but is thought to be immune-mediated because of frequent history of preceding viral illness and detectable levels of ganglionic nicotinic acetylcholine receptor antibodies. Clinical pictures of autoimmune autonomic neuropathy can be separated from those of Guillain–Barré syndrome (GBS) by the absence of somatic nerve involvement that leads to generalized muscle weakness and areflexia seen with GBS.

Patients with malignancy may develop subacute or acute onset of paraneoplastic autonomic neuropathy. Small-cell carcinoma of the lung is the most common cause (25), and is thought to be related to antineuronal nuclear antibody type-1. Gastrointestinal motility problems are also common in this setting. Some chemotherapeutic agents, such as cisplatinum and vinca alkaloids, can result in autonomic neuropathy.

III. DIAGNOSIS OF OH

Clinical recognition of OH requires measurement of blood pressure and heart rate both in the standing and in the supine positions. Blood pressure and heart rate measurements should then be repeated immediately upon standing and after 3 min of standing. Measurement of blood pressure in the sitting and then in the standing position may be more convenient, but could miss OH up to two-thirds of the patients (29). Therefore, both supine and standing blood pressure should be part of routine assessment in all hypertensive patients with postural dizziness, diabetes mellitus, or those over the age of 50.

Once OH is detected, careful history taking and physical examination should be obtained to determine the temporal pattern of symptoms and the associated neurological and autonomic abnormalities. If the onset of disease is acute or subacute, the main differential diagnosis should be autonomic neuropathy due to autoimmune disease, paraneoplastic syndrome, drugs, toxins, botulism, or porphyria. For chronic progressive onset, one should consider diabetes mellitus, amyloidosis, neurodegenerative disorders such as PAF, MSA, and Parkinson's disease.

Initial laboratory evaluation should begin with routine chemistry and complete blood count to exclude systemic disease that may cause autonomic failure such as diabetes mellitus or uremia. Twenty-four hour ambulatory blood pressure monitoring may be helpful in determining severity and frequency of symptomatic OH and labile hypertension. Patients with large orthostatic drop in clinic blood pressure are more like to have blunted nocturnal blood pressure dipping or even reversed dipping during 24 h ambulatory blood pressure monitoring (4,30).

Other laboratory studies such as immunoelectrophoresis of blood or urine, fat aspirate for amyloid, paraneoplastic autoantibody panel, and urinary porphyrins should be considered depending on the history and index of suspicion. Autonomic function testing should be performed. The normal range of commonly used autonomic testing is shown subsequently in Table 38.1.

Autonomic function tests can be separated into two major categories, bedside tests and specialized tests.

A. Bedside Tests

Respiratory sinus arrhythmia can be assessed during controlled breathing at the rate of six deep breaths per minute at the bedside. The sinus arrhythmia ratio is calculated by dividing the longest to shortest RR interval and is considered to be abnormal, if the ratio is <1.2. Heart rate response to standing provides similar information to heart rate response during Valsava maneuver (see subsequently). Subject is asked to lie quietly in bed, then stand up, and remain standing quietly for 3 min, while ECG is constantly monitored. In normal subject, reduction in blood pressure upon standing is accompanied by baroreflex-mediated increase in the heart rate (or shortening of the RR interval), reaching the nadir at about the 15th beat. The increase in sympathetic outflow to the heart and peripheral circulation cause recovery of blood pressure and relative prolongation of the RR interval at about the 30th beat. The ratio of RR interval at 30th beat of standing to the RR interval at 15th beat (30:15 ratio) should be >1.04 (31). Cold pressor test is another simple and noninvasive test of autonomic function. The test is accomplished by immersing patients' hands in the cold water

of 4°C for 2 min. In normal subjects, muscle sympathetic nerve increased by more than twofold (32) and mean arterial pressure increases by >20 mmHg. Such responses exclude presence of autonomic failure, but subnormal blood pressure response is not definitive for because 10–15% of normal subjects show negative response.

B. Specialized Autonomic Function Tests

More specialized autonomic function test include Valsava's maneuver, which can be performed by having the subject blow against a 40 mmHg for at least 12 s, while a continuous beat-to-beat measurement of blood pressure is monitored. Blood pressure monitoring can be done noninvasively by using finger plethysmography device or radial artery tonometry. Typically, the Valsava response is divided into four phases (Fig. 38.3).

In the first phase, there is brief increase in blood pressure due to direct compression of aorta form elevated intrathoracic pressure. Blood pressure is then reduced in the early part of second phase when venous return is reduced during continued straining. The reduction in blood pressure is accompanied by baroreflex-mediated increase in heart rate and peripheral vascular resistance. Thus, there is a partial recovery of blood pressure during the late part of second phase. In the third phase, there is a further reduction in blood pressure immediately after Valsava release due to sudden reduction in intrathoracic pressure that compresses the aorta. In the fourth phase, blood pressure overshoots above baseline values because there is increase in venous return and cardiac output, whereas the peripheral resistance remains elevated. The increase in blood pressure during this phase is accompanied by baroreflex-mediated increase in cardiac vagal tone causing reduction in the heart rate. For patients with autonomic failure, blood pressure will decrease progressively throughout the early and late part of second phase without reflex increase in sympathetic outflow to the sinus node and peripheral circulation. In addition, blood pressure of patients with autonomic failure fail to overshoot in phase IV and heart rate also remains constant. The Valsava ratio can be calculated by dividing the fastest heart rate during phase II by the slowest heart rate during phase IV. The ratio of <1.2 was considered to be abnormal (31,33).

Blood pressure responses to isometric handgrip provide similar information to cold pressor tests. During this test, subject is asked to maintain handgrip at 30% of maximal voluntary contraction, using a handgrip dynamometer, for 5 min. The increase in systolic or diastolic blood pressure just before release of the handgrip in normal subjects is >15 mmHg compared with baseline (18,31).

Plasma catecholamines and metanephrines should be obtained at rest in the supine position for 15–30 min,

Table 38.1   Autonomic Function Tests

Test	Normal values
Bedside tests	
Sinus arrhythmia ratio	>1.2
30:15 ratio	>1.04
ΔSBP or DBP during cold pressor test	>20 mmHg
Specialized tests	
Valsava HR ratio	>1.2
ΔSBP in Valsava phase II	<20 mmHg
ΔSBP in Valsava phase IV	>20 mmHg
ΔSBP during isometric handgrip	>15 mmHg
Percent increase in plasma norepinephrine with standing	>60%
PHE_{BP25}	204 ± 28 μg
NTP_{BP25}	1.2 ± 0.2 μg/kg

Note: SBP, systolic blood pressure; DBP, diastolic blood pressure.

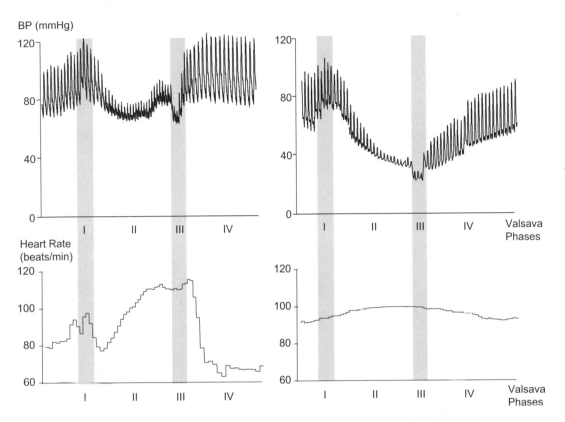

Figure 38.3 Changes in blood pressure (top panel) and heart rate (bottom panel) during phase I–IV Valsava maneuver in a normal subject (left panel) and an 18-year-old patient with baroreflex failure from brainstem tumor.

and after 15–30 min of standing. In normal subjects, the concentration of norepinephrine in the plasma doubles within 5 min of standing from the supine position. Failure of plasma norepinephrine to increase >60% while standing suggests impaired baroreflex-mediated increase in sympathetic activity (34). Thus, patients with PAF, MSA, and Parkinson's disease with OH have subnormal increase of plasma norepinephrine in the upright posture. However, plasma levels of catecholamines in the supine position may help separate these three groups of patients. Patients with PAF have low supine plasma levels of norepinephrine, epinephrine, normetanephrine, and metanephrine. Patients with PD and OH have normal supine plasma levels of norepinephrine, epinephrine, and metanephrine, but low plasma normetanephrine (35). The mechanism responsible for low plasma normetanephrine in PD patients are not known, but is thought to be because of decreased uptake of NE by extraneuronal cells, the main site of conversion of norepinephrine into normetanephrine (35). MSA patients with OH have normal supine plasma levels of catecholamines and metanephrines. Patients with DβH deficiency have low plasma levels of norepinephrine, but high plasma dopamine levels with the ratio of dopamine to norepinephrine greater than 10:1 (23).

Other specialized autonomic function tests include responses to bolus infusion of phenylephrine and nitroprusside. In normal subjects, the dose of phenylephrine that increases systolic blood pressure by 25 mmHg (PHE_{BP25}) and nitroprusside dose that decreases systolic blood pressure by 25 mmHg (NTP_{BP25}) is 204 ± 28 µg and 1.2 ± 0.2 µg/kg, respectively. Patients with autonomic failure have augmented pressor responses to phenylephrine and depressor response to nitroprusside; therefore, PHE_{BP25} and NTP_{BP25} are much lower. Furthermore, at this dose of phenylephrine or nitroprusside, there will be minimal or no change in the heart rate due to impaired baroreflex control of heart rate.

Other autonomic testing can also be considered are thermoregulatory sweat test and bladder function test. The detail of these tests has been described elsewhere (36) and beyond the scope of this book chapter. Heart rate variability has also been advocated to test influence of sympathetic and parasympathetic nervous system on the sinus node. The low frequency power of the spectral analysis of heart rate was proposed to reflect both sympathetic and parasympathetic influences, whereas the high frequency (HF) power is accepted as a reliable, valid, and rather specific index of cardiac vagal activity (37). However, our recent study indicates that the HF component of heart rate variability can also be influenced by sympathetic activity and nonneural mechanism and, thus, cannot be used to substitute other autonomic testing as a specific measure of vagal control of sinus node function (38). Direct intraneural recording of post-ganglionic sympathetic action potentials using micro-neurographic technique may be useful in some patients with OH whom are not suspected to have autonomic failure but are treated with medications that interfere with accurate interpretation of heart rate responses to Valsava maneuver such as β-blockers or vagolytic drug. The presence of normal sympathetic traffic responses with normal increase during nitroprusside infusion and decrease during phenylephrine infusion excludes diagnosis of autonomic failure. However, the technique is cumbersome, operator-dependent, and may not be successful in detecting sympathetic nerve activity in 10–20% of subjects even in the presence of intact autonomic function. Neurochemical assessment to detect norepinephrine spillover from a specific organ can be used to determine sympathetic outflow in humans, but the technique is more invasive. Sympathoneural imaging studies using [^{18}F]fluorodopamine or [^{123}I]metaiodobenzylguanidine of the heart has been used to determine presence or absence of cardiac sympathetic denervation. However, experiences are still limited in a few centers and the clinical applicability of the tests are unclear as cardiac denervation may be present even in subjects without OH (20).

IV. TREATMENT OF OH AND SIDE EFFECTS

Patients with hyperadrenergic OH with intact autonomic function should be treated according to etiology of reduced intravascular volume or excessive vasodilation. Hypoadrenergic OH is very challenging to treat for both OH and supine hypertension. Rarely is there an exception to the rules for antihypertensive therapy such as high-salt diet, no diuretics, and short-acting vasodilators. The goal of treatment for patients with hypoadrenergic features is to achieve functional capacity and avoid falls during the daytime, while minimizing target-organ damage from supine hypertension.

A. Nonpharmacological Therapy

Patients with no history of heart failure should be encouraged to increase fluid and salt intake. To minimize OH, patients should also be instructed to avoid hot environments, limit early morning and postmeal activities, and have frequent small meals with caffeinated beverages to minimize postprandial hypotension (39). Compression garments encompassing abdomen (Jobst stocking) may be useful in patients with venous insufficiency to prevent venous pooling in the lower extremities and pelvis. At nighttime, patients should be instructed to sleep in the head-up tilt position with the head of the bed elevated by 6–9 in. to minimize nocturnal diuresis and sodium loss (40). Drinking water rapidly was reported to be effective in some patients.

B. Pharmacological Therapy for OH

Pharmacologic treatment of postural hypotension may exacerbate supine hypertension, and thus, it should be reserved only for patients with symptoms of postural-related cerebral hypoperfusion or underperfusion of other organs such as visual disturbance or angina. Patients with asymptomatic postural hypotension should not be treated as reduction in blood pressure may not be accompanied by reduction in cerebral blood flow until systolic blood pressure was <80 mmHg in some patients (41). Antihypertensive medication should be given mainly at nighttime (as indicated in Section C of treatment of supine hypertension) and titrated according to standing blood pressure during the day.

1. Fludrocortisone

Fludrocortisone reduces OH primarily by plasma volume expansion. Therefore, it should not be used in patients with congestive heart failure. The therapeutic dose is between 0.05 and 0.4 mg/day. Fludrocortisone is a potent mineralocorticoid with little, if any, glucocorticoid effect at this dose range. Orthostatic symptoms may not improve until several weeks after drug administration or until adequate volume expansion has occurred. Hypokalemia and hypomagnesemia are frequent side effects and are needed to be monitored and replaced.

2. Sympathomimietic Drugs

Sympathomimetic drugs are another class of pharmacotherapy used to reduce OH. These drugs should be given early in the days to improve symptoms and minimize supine hypertension. Because of the vasoconstricting properties, the use of these drugs should be avoided in patients with coronary artery disease or peripheral vascular disease.

Midodrine is a prodrug that is converted to desglymidodrine after absorption. Midodrine increases blood pressure by α1-adrenergic-mediated constriction of arterioles and veins. It has high (>90%) oral bioavailability with the half-life of active metabolites of 2–3 h. Because of the hypersensitivity of α1-adrenergic receptor in patients with autonomic failure, midodrine should be titrated from low dose of 5 mg/day until symptoms improve or the dose of 30 mg/day is reached. To minimize nocturnal hypertension, midodrine should not be given after 6 p.m.

Midodrine does not cross the blood-brain barrier and, therefore, has no central nervous system side effects. In a large multicenter randomized trial, midodrine has been shown to be safe and effective in improving standing blood pressure and symptoms of lightheadedness (42). However, patients with supine blood pressure >180/110 mmHg was excluded from the study and the safety of midodrine in this group of patients remains unknown. Side effects of midodrine are sensation of gooseflesh from piloerection, prutitus, and paresthesia of the scalp were reported in ~10% of patients (42,43).

Ergot alkaloids have long been used for treatment of hypoadrenergic OH because of their predominant venoconstricting effects (44,45), which can reduce orthostasis without exacerbation of supine hypertension. The bioavailability of oral ergotamine is variable. Inhaled ergotamine may have higher bioavailability, but experience is still limited (46). Caffeine may increase absorption of ergotamine and we found that combination of ergotamine and caffeine are effective in reducing OH in 90% of patients with MSA or Parkinson's disease with autonomic failure (45). The main side effect of ergot alkaloids is vasospasm in the peripheral, cerebral, or even retinal arteries. Valvular heart disease, resembling carcinoid or methysergide-induced heart disease, has been reported with long term use in patients receiving ergot alkaloids for migraine headache, but has not been reported in patients with OH from autonomic failure (47).

Clonidine administration has been shown to reduce frequency and severity of episodic hypertension in patients with baroreflex failure from lesions in the afferent input. However, when it is used in patients with autonomic failure from damage in the postganglionic sympathetic efferents, it can increase both standing and supine blood pressure by its postjunctional $\alpha2$-adrenergic-mediated arterial vasoconstriction without venoconstrictor effect (44). Compared with ergotamine, clonidine was not shown to prolong standing time in patients with neurogenic OH and even exacerbate supine hypertension (44). Thus, its use should be avoided in these patients.

Yohimbine can increase blood pressure in patients with PAF or MSA, presumably by increasing the residual central sympathetic outflow through its central $\alpha2$ antagonistic property (48,49). It has been shown to be as effective as midodrine in increasing blood pressure in PAF and MSA patients in one study (49). It is ineffective in patients with DβH enzyme deficiency.

Dihydroxyphenylserine (DOPS) is a synthetic precursor of norepinephrine and is a treatment of choice for patients with DβH enzyme deficiency. DOPS is converted to norepinephrine by aromatic acid decarboxylase (AADC) enzyme and can reverse norepinephrine deficiency even in the absence of DβH enzyme. Recent studies have indicated that it is also effective in other forms of primary autonomic failure such as PAF and MSA (50). However, concomitant use of carbidopa in patients with Parkinson's disease inhibits peripheral L-AADC enzyme and blunt the increase in plasma norepinephrine and the pressor response, thereby limiting its usefulness (51).

3. Erythropoietin

Up to 40% of patients with primary autonomic failure have anemia, which is unrelated to iron deficiency, megaloblastic disease, or inflammatory states (52). In these patients, plasma upright norepinephrine levels directly correlates with hemoglobin levels, suggesting an important role of sympathetic nervous system in stimulating erythropoiesis in humans (52). Erythropoietin has been shown to reduce OH in patients with primary autonomic failure and anemia. Mechanism by which erythropoietin increases blood pressure is not known, but may be related to increased blood viscosity and/or vasoconstriction (43). Although erythropoietin has a clear role in treatment of patients with anemia and primary autonomic failure, its role in patients without anemia is not known.

C. Pharmacological Therapy for Supine Hypertension

The goal of treatment for supine hypertension is to minimize hypertensive target-organ damage and the consequent nocturnal diuresis, which further promotes OH. Although the use of long-acting antihypertensive medication is recommended for treatment of essential hypertension in general, the use of short-acting medication at bedtime is preferable in treatment of supine hypertension to avoid exacerbation of OH during the daytime. Hypertensive diabetic patients with OH should be given short-acting ACE inhibitor, such as captopril, because of benefit of this class of drugs in preventing adverse cardiovascular outcomes. Transdermal nitrates should be used before bedtime and removed in the morning in patients with primary autonomic failure because it is effective in lowering supine blood pressure without augmenting nocturnal diuresis or fall in standing blood pressure (53). In contrast, bedtime nifedipine reduced supine blood pressure by a similar magnitude, but caused a more prolonged reduction in standing blood pressure by augmenting nocturnal sodium excretion (53). Thus, nifedipine should be avoided in these patients. ACE inhibitor and angiotensin receptor blocker have been shown to reduce intraglomerular hypertension and reduce the rate of decline in renal function in patients with chronic renal insufficiency and diabetes mellitus. It is unknown whether an ACE inhibitor may reduce both supine blood pressure and nocturnal diuresis in patients with primary autonomic failure.

V. ORTHOSTATIC HYPERTENSION

Although described for over 50 years, there is still no consensus on the definition of orthostatic hypertension. Some studies have advocated the definition of "increase in blood pressure from normal values in the supine position to hypertensive range upon standing (diastolic blood pressure from <90 to ≥90 mmHg and/or increase in systolic blood pressure form <140 to ≥140 mmHg)" (54,55). Others have defined orthostatic hypertension as an increase in systolic blood pressure ≥10 (56) or ≥20 mmHg (5) upon assuming an upright position from a supine position. Although very few studies so far have focused attention on this clinical condition, it is not a rare clinical condition. Approximately 10–15% of hypertensive subjects were reported to have orthostatic hypertension (54,55). Patients with diabetes mellitus (54), patients with nephroptosis (abnormal mobility of kidney) (57), and patients with excessive dipping (≥20% decrease in nocturnal blood pressure from awake blood pressure) during 24 h ambulatory blood pressure monitoring (56) are more likely to have orthostatic hypertension. One large epidemiological study in both normotensive and hypertensive subjects indicated that blacks and people who are obese were also associated independently with increased systolic blood pressure upon standing (58). Therefore, it is essential to obtain both sitting and standing blood pressure because failure to recognize orthostatic hypertension can lead to undertreatment of hypertension, particularly during the daytime.

The precise mechanism mediating orthostatic hypertension is unknown, but sympathetic overactivity may play an important role. Patients with orthostatic hypertension were reported to have normal plasma catecholamines in supine position but have excessive increase in plasma norepinephrine and vasopressin levels, decrease in cardiac output, and increase in peripheral vascular resistance upon standing (5,55). Such an increase in sympathetic activity could be due to excessive gravitational pool of blood in the legs, increase vascular adrenergic sensitivity, or augmented cardiopulmonary baroreflex gain (55,59). In observational studies, patients with orthostatic hypertension were reported to have increased carotid intimal thickness (60) and elevated risks of silent cerebrovascular disease (5). In one study, α-adrenergic receptor blockers have been shown to abolish increase in orthostatic blood pressure without affecting supine blood pressure (5).

VI. POSTURAL TACHYCARDIA SYNDROME OR ORTHOSTATIC INTOLERANCE

Postural tachycardia syndrome (POTS) is a clinical syndrome characterized by excessive tachycardia (increased heart rate by ≥30 beats/min or heart rate ≥110 beats/min) and symptoms of cerebral hypoperfusion upon standing without OH. Although POTS is thought to be one of the most common disorders of autonomic regulation, most patients with this condition do not have hypertension. Patients affected by this syndrome are generally young women between the age of 20 and 50 (61). Pathogenesis of POTS is not completely understood. Patients with POTS have high-normal or elevated levels of plasma norepinephrine in supine position with exaggerated increase upon standing than normal subjects (62). The ratio of dihydroxyphenylglycol, a product of intraneuronal metabolite of norepinephrine, to plasma norepinephrine is usually low, resembling biochemical changes seen in normal subjects receiving norepinephrine reuptake inhibitors such as desipramine (62). As a result, impairment in norepinephrine transporter function is thought to be the main mechanism of orthostatic intolerance (63). Indeed, this syndrome has been identified in one patient and her identical twin with loss-of-function mutation in norepinephrine transporter gene encoding a change from guanine to cytosine at position 237 of exon 9 (G237C) (63). However, more recent studies indicated that this mutation is absent in most patients with POTS and elevated heart rate in these patients is explained by elevated cardiac sympathetic activity as measured by cardiac norepinephrine spillover technique, causing increased norepinephrine release rather than impairment of norepinephrine reuptake (64). The mechanisms underlying increased cardiac sympathetic outflow are also not known, but could be related to hypovolemia (65) or excessive venous pooling in the lower extremities from partial sympathetic denervation in the legs (66), resulting baroreflex-mediated increase in cardiac SNA. The mechanism underlying dizziness or symptoms of cerebral hypoperfusion, despite absence of OH, is also unknown but may be related to impaired regulation of cerebrovascular tone upon standing in POTS patients (67).

Therapy for POTS includes volume expansion with salt and hydrocortisone, because it has been shown to decrease both supine and upright heart rate at least in the acute setting (68). Treatment with α-1 agonist, such as phenylephrine and midodrine, but not α-2 agonist clonidine, have also been shown to be effective in reducing orthostatic symptoms and heart rate (68,69). However, both fludrocortisone and midodrine should not be used in patients with uncontrolled hypertension. β-adrenergic receptor blockers were reported to be efficacious in some (61,70), but not all studies (69). Patients with POTS have favorable prognosis. A cross-sectional study reported 80% patients are improved, 60% are functionally normal, and 90% are able to return to work over a 5.5 year follow-up period (61).

VII. CONCLUSIONS

Our approach to orthostatic abnormalities in hypertensive patients is shown in Fig. 38.4.

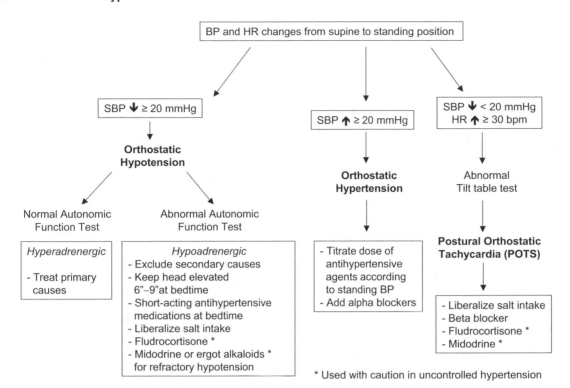

Figure 38.4 Algorithm in management of patients with hypertension and orthostatic abnormalities.

Patients with OH and supine hypertension should undergo formal autonomic function tests. Patients with suspected hyperadrenergic OH, the purpose of the autonomic function test is to confirm that autonomic reflexes are intact and respond appropriately to hypovolemia. Blood pressure and heart rate are normalized by volume repletion. The treatment is to remove primary cause of intravascular volume depletion and/or inappropriate vasodilation. Patients with suspected hypoadrenergic OH, the goal is to establish impaired autonomic adjustments to standard stimuli. Most of conditions are not reversible, but it is important to exclude underlying carcinoma, offending drugs, or posterior fossa tumor. Once excluded, patients with primary autonomic failure should be given short-acting antihypertensive medication mainly at bedtime to avoid postural hypotension in the morning. They should sleep on an incline with head of bed elevated 6–9 in. to minimize supine hypertension. Patients with orthostatic symptoms should liberalize salt intake. Patients who remain symptomatic should be treated with fludrocortisone to further expand blood volume. Sympathomimetics can exacerbate supine hypertension should be reserved for refractory cases of OH. Sympathomimetic drug, which has more venoconstrictor property such as ergotamine, is preferable to arterial vasoconstrictor, such as midodrine, because it is less likely to cause such side effects.

REFERENCES

1. The Consensus Committee of the American Autonomic Society and the American Academy of Neurology. Consensus statement on the definition of orthostatic hypotension, pure autonomic failure, and multiple system atrophy. Neurology 1996; 46:1470.

2. Beckett NS, Connor M, Sadler JD, Fletcher AE, Bulpitt CJ. Orthostatic fall in blood pressure in the very elderly hypertensive: results from the Hypertension in the Very Elderly Trial (HYVET)—pilot. J Hum Hypertens 1999; 13:839–840.

3. Luukinen H, Koski K, Laippala P, Kivela S-L. Prognosis of diastolic and systolic orthostatic hypotension in older persons. Arch Intern Med 1999; 159:273–280.

4. Fotherby MD, Robinson TG, Potter JF. Clinic and 24 h blood pressure in elderly treated hypertensives with postural hypotension. J Hum Hypertens 1994; 8:711–716.

5. Kario K, Eguchi K, Hoshide S, Hoshide Y, Umeda Y, Mitsuhashi T, Shimada K. U-curve relationship between orthostatic blood pressure change and silent cerebrovascular disease in elderly hypertensives orthostatic hypertension as a new cardiovascular risk factor. J Am Coll Cardiol 2002; 40:133–141.

6. Robertson D, Robertson RM. Causes of chronic orthostatic hypotension. Arch Intern Med 1994; 154:1620–1624.

7. Masuo K, Mikami H, Ogihara T, Tuck ML. Changes in frequency of orthostatic hypotension in elderly

hypertensive patients under medications. Am J Hypertens 1996; 9:263–268.

8. Slavachevsky I, Rachmani R, Levi Z, Brosh D, Lidar M, Ravid M. Effect of enalapril and nifedipine on orthostatic hypotension in older hypertensive patients. J Am Geriatr Soc 2000; 48:807–810.

9. Meredith PA. Is postural hypotension a real problem with antihypertensive medication? Cardiology 2001; 96:19–24.

10. Timmers HJ, Wieling W, Karemaker JM, Lenders JW. Denervation of carotid baro- and chemoreceptors in humans. J Physiol 2003; 553:3–11.

11. Robertson D, Hollister AS, Biaggioni I, Netterville JL, Mosqueda-Garcia R, Robertson RM. The diagnosis and treatment of baroreflex failure. N Engl J Med 1993; 329:1449–1455.

12. Sharabi Y, Dendi R, Holmes C, Goldstein DS. Baroreflex failure as a late sequela of neck irradiation. Hypertension 2003; 42:110–116.

13. Raiha I, Luutonen S, Piha J, Seppanen A, Toikka T, Sourander L. Prevalence, predisposing factors, and prognostic importance of postural hypotension. Arch Intern Med 1995; 155:930–935.

14. Tilvis RS, Hakala SM, Valvanne J, Erkinjuntti T. Postural hypotension and dizziness in a general aged population: a four-year follow-up of the Helsinki Aging Study. J Am Geriatr Soc 1996; 44:809–814.

15. Maurer MS, Karmally W, Rivadeneira H, Parides MK, Bloomfield DM. Upright posture and postprandial hypotension in elderly persons. Ann Intern Med 2000; 133:533–536.

16. Parikh SM, Diedrich A, Biaggioni I, Robertson D. The nature of the autonomic dysfunction in multiple system atrophy. J Neurol Sci 2002; 200:1–10.

17. Gilman S, Low PA, Quinn N, Albanese A, Ben-Shlomo Y, Fowler CJ, Kaufmann H, Klockgether T, Lang AE, Lantos PL, Litvan I, Mathias CJ, Oliver E, Robertson D, Schatz I, Wenning GK. Consensus statement on the diagnosis of multiple system atrophy. J Neurol Sci 1999; 163:94–98.

18. Shannon JR, Jordan J, Diedrich A, Pohar B, Black BK, Robertson D, Biaggioni I. Sympathetically mediated hypertension in autonomic failure. Circulation 2000; 101:2710–2715.

19. Biaggioni I, Robertson RM. Hypertension in orthostatic hypotension and autnomic dysfunction. Cardiol Clin 2002; 20:291–301.

20. Goldstein DS, Holmes CS, Dendi R, Bruce SR, Li ST. Orthostatic hypotension from sympathetic denervation in Parkinson's disease. Neurology 2002; 58:1247–1255.

21. Goldstein DS, Holmes C, Li ST, Bruce S, Metman LV, Cannon ROr. Cardiac sympathetic denervation in Parkinson disease. Ann Intern Med 2000; 133:338–347.

22. Goldstein DS. Dysautonomia in Parkinson's disease: neurocardiological abnormalities. Lancet Neurol 2003; 2:669–676.

23. Rea RF, Biaggioni I, Robertson RM, Haile V, Robertson D. Reflex control of sympathetic nerve activity in dopamine β-hydroxylase deficiency. Hypertension 1990; 15:107.

24. Wu J-S, Lu F-H, Yang Y-C, Chang C-J. Postural hypotension and postural dizziness in patients with non-

insulin-dependent diabetes. Arch Intern Med 1999; 159:1350–1356.

25. Low PA, Vernino S, Suarez G. Autonomic dysfunction in peripheral nerve disease. Muscle Nerve 2003; 27:646–661.

26. O'Brien IA, McFadden JP, Corrall RJ. Influence of autonomic neuropathy on mortality of insulin-dependent diabetes. Q J Med 1991; 79:495–502.

27. Ewing DJ, Campbell IW, Clarke BF. The natural history of diabetic autonomic neuropathy. Q J Med 1980; 49:95–108.

28. O'Brien IA, McFadden JP, Corrall RJ. The influence of autonomic neuropathy on mortality in insulin-dependent diabetes. Q J Med 1991; 79:495–502.

29. Carlson JE. Assessment of orthostatic blood pressure: measurement technique and clinical applications. South Med J 1999; 92:167–173.

30. Lagi A, Rossi A, Comelli A, Rosati E, Cencetti S. Postural hypotension in hypertensive patients. Blood Press 2003; 12:340–344.

31. Hohnloser SH, Klingenheben T. Basic autonomic tests. In: Malik M, ed. Clinical Guide to Cardiac Autonomic Tests. Dordrecht: Kluwer Academic Publishers, 1998:51–66.

32. Victor RG, Leimbach WN, Seals DR, Wallin BG, Mark AL. Effects of the cold pressor test on muscle sympathetic nerve activity in humans. Hypertension 1987; 9:429–436.

33. Campbell IW, Ewing DJ, Clarke BF. Tests of cardio-vascular reflex function in diabetic autonomic neuropathy. Horm Metab Res Suppl 1980; 9:61–67.

34. Lake CR, Ziegler MG, Kopin IJ. Use of plasma norepi-nephrine for evaluation of sympathetic neuronal function in man. Life Sci 1976; 18:1315–1325.

35. Goldstein DS, Holmes C, Sharabi Y, Brentzel S, Eisenhofer G. Plasma levels of catechols and metane-phrines in neurogenic orthostatic hypotension. Neurology 2003; 60:1327–1332.

36. Bannister R, Mathias C. Testing autonomic reflexes. In: Bannister R, ed. Autonomic Failure: A Textbook of Clinical Disorders of the Autonomic Nervous System. New York: Oxford University Press, 1988:289–307.

37. Task Force of the European Society of Cardiology and the North American Society of Pacing and Electrophysiology. Heart rate variability: Standard of measurement, physio-logical interpretation, and clinical use. Circulation 1996; 93:1043–1065.

38. Vongpatanasin W, Taylor JA, Victor RG. Effects of cocaine on heart rate variability in healthy subjects. Am J Cardiol 2004; 93:385–388.

39. Onrot J, Goldberg MR, Biaggioni I, Hollister AS, Kingaid D, Robertson D. Hemodynamic and humoral effects of caffeine in autonomic failure. Therapeutic impli-cations for postprandial hypotension. N Engl J Med 1985; 313:549–554.

40. Bannister R, Ardill L, Fentem P. An assessment of various methods of treatment of idiopathic orthostatic hypotension. Quart J Med 1969; 38:377–395.

41. Thomas DJ, Bannister R. Preservation of autoregulation of cerebral blood flow in autonomic failure. J Neurol Sci 1980; 44:205–212.

42. Low PA, Gilden JL, Freeman R, Sheng KN, McEllingott MA. Efficacy of midodrine vs placebo in neurogenic orthostatic hypotension. A randomized, double-blind multicenter study. Midodrine Study Group. JAMA 1997; 277:1046–1051.

43. Robertson D, Davis TL. Recent advances in the treatment of orthostatic hypotension. Neurology 1995; 45:S26–S32.

44. Victor RG, Tallman WT. Comparative effects of clonidine and dihydroergotamine on venomotor tone and orthostatic tolerance in patients with severe hypoadrenergic orthostatic hypotension. Am J Med 2002; 112:361–368.

45. Dewey RB Jr, Rao SD, Holmberg SL, Victor RG. Ergotamine/caffeine treatment of orthostatic hypotension in parkinsonism with autonomic failure. Eur J Neurol 1998; 5:593–599.

46. Biaggioni I, Zygmunt D, Haile V, Robertson D. Pressor effects of inhaled ergotamine in orthostatic hypotension. Am J Cardiol 1990; 65:89–92.

47. Redfield MM, Nicholson WJ, Edwards WD, Tajik AJ. Valve disease associated with ergot alkaloid use: echocardiographic and pathologic correlations. Ann Intern Med 1992; 117:50–52.

48. Onrot J, Goldberg MR, Biaggioni I, Wiley RG, Hollister AS, Robertson D. Oral yohimbine in human autonomic failure. Neurology 1987; 37:215–220.

49. Jordan J, Shannon JR, Biaggioni I, Norman R, Black BK, Robertson D. Contrasting actions of pressor agents in severe autonomic failure. Am J Med 1998; 105:116–124.

50. Mathias CJ, Senard JM, Braune S, Watson L, Aragishi A, Keeling JE, Taylor MD. L-threo-dihydroxyphenylserine (L threo-DOPS; droxidopa) in the management of neurogenic orthostatic hypotension: a multi-national, multicenter, dose-ranging study in multiple system atrophy and pure autonomic failure. Clin Auton Res 2001; 11:235–242.

51. Kaufmann H, Saadia D, Voustianiouk A, Goldstein DS, Holmes C, Yahr MD, Nardin R, Freeman R. Norepinephrine precursor therapy in neurogenic orthostatic hypotension. Circulation 2003; 108:724–728.

52. Biaggioni I, Robertson D, Krantz S, Jones M, Haile V. The anemia of primary autonomic failure and its reversal with recombinant erythropoietin. Ann Intern Med 1994; 121:181–186.

53. Jordan J, Shannon JR, Pohar B, Paranjape SY, Robertson D, Robertson RM, Biaggioni I. Contrasting effects of vasodilators on blood pressure and sodium balance in the hypertension of autonomic failure. J Am Soc Nephrol 1999; 10:35–42.

54. Yoshinari M, Wakisaka M, Nakamura U, Yoshioka M, Uchizono Y, Iwase M. Orthostatic hypertension in patients with type 2 diabetes. Diabetes Care 2001; 24:1783–1786.

55. Streeten DH, Auchincloss JHJ, Anderson GHJ, Richardson RL, Thomas FD, Miller JW. Orthostatic hypertension: pathogenic studies. Hypertension 1985; 7:196–203.

56. Kario K, Eguchi K, Nakagawa Y, Motai K, Shimada K. Relationship between extreme dippers and orthostatic hypertension in eldery hypertensive patients. Hypertension 1998; 31:77–82.

57. Takada Y, Shimizu H, Kazatani Y, Azechi H, Hiwada K, Kokubu T. Orthostatic hypertension with nephroptosis and aortic disease. Arch Intern Med 1984; 144:152–154.

58. Nardo CJ, Chambless LE, Light KC, Rosamond WD, Sharrett AR, Tell GS, Heiss G. Descriptive epidemiology of blood pressure response to change in body position: the ARIC study. Hypertension 1999; 33:1123–1129.

59. Benowitz NL, Zevin S, Carlsen S, Wright J, Schambelan M, Cheitlin M. Orthostatic hypertension due to vascular adrenergic hypersensitivity. Hypertension 1996; 28:42–46.

60. Kohara K, Tabara Y, Yamamoto Y, Miki T. Orthostatic hypertension: another orthostatic disorder to be aware of. J Am Geriatr Soc 2000; 48:1538–1539.

61. Sandroni P, Opfer-Gehrking TL, McPhee BR, Low PA. Postural tachycardia syndrome: clinical features and follow-up study. Mayo Clin Proc 1999; 74:1106–1110.

62. Jordan J, Shannon JR, Diedrich A, Black BK, Robertson D. Increased sympathetic activation in idiopathic orthostatic intolerance: role of systemic adrenoreceptor sensitivity. Hypertension 2002; 39:173–178.

63. Shannon JR, Flattem NL, Jordan J, Jacob G, Black BK, Biaggioni I, Blakely RD, Robertson D. Orthostatic intolerance and tachycardia associated with norepinephrine-transporter deficiency. N Engl J Med 2000; 342:541–549.

64. Goldstein DS, Holmes C, Frank SM, Dendi R, Cannon ROr, Sharabi Y, Esler MD, Eisenhofer G. Cardiac sympathetic dysautonomia in chronic orthostatic inteolerance syndromes. Circulation 2002; 106:2358–2365.

65. Jacob G, Robertson D, Mosqueda Garcia R, Ertl AC, Robertson RM, Biaggioni I. Hypovolemia in syncope and orthostatic intolerance role of the renin–angiotensin system. Am J Med 1997; 103:128–133.

66. Jacob G, Costa F, Shannon JR, Robertson RM, Wathen M, Stein M, Biaggioni I, Ertl A, Black B, Robertson D. The neuropathic postural tachycardia syndrome. N Engl J Med 2000; 343:1008–1014.

67. Jacob G, Atkinson D, Jordan J, Shannon JR, Furlan R, Black BK, Robertson D. Effects of standing on cerebrovascular resistance in patients with idiopathic orthostatic intolerance. Am J Med 1999; 106:59–64.

68. Jacob G, Shannon JR, Black B, Biaggioni I, Mosqueda-Garcia R, Robertson RM, Robertson D. Effects of volume loading and pressor agents in idiopathic orthostatic tachycardia. Circulation 1997; 96:575–580.

69. Stewart JM, Munoz J, Weldon A. Clinical and physiological effects of an acute α-1 adrenergic agonist and a β-1 adrenergic antagonist in chronic orthostatic intolerance. Circulation 2002; 106:2946–2954.

70. Freitas J, Santos R, Azevedo E, Costa O, Carvalho M, de Freitas AF. Clinical improvement in patients with orthostatic intolerance treatment with bisoprolol and fludrocortisone. Clin Auton Res 2000; 10:293–299.

39

Anaesthesia and Surgery in Hypertension

JONATHAN HULME, KIN-L. KONG
University of Birmingham, Birmingham, UK

KEYPOINTS

- Hypertension is a common disease in patients presenting for surgery.
- End organ damage is caused to cardiovascular, cerebrovascular, and renal systems.
- Poorly controlled hypertension and end organ damage indicates high risk patients.
- Drugs used to treat hypertension can affect responses to anaesthesia and surgery.
- Cardiovascular stability during anaesthesia reduces risk of increased morbidity and mortality in the hypertensive patient.
- Cardiovascular stability is more difficult to achieve in hypertensive patients.
- Good knowledge is required of agents which are used to treat acutely high blood pressure.
- Some diseases in which hypertension is present require expert management.

SUMMARY

Hypertension is a common disease and its prevalence is increasing. It is associated with end organ disease which increases peri-operative morbidity and mortality predominantly due to cardiovascular complications.

Anaesthetic management of the hypertensive patient should include assessment to identify end organ damage, treatment to ameliorate hypertensive responses to surgery, and maintenance of cardiovascular stability. Appropriate monitoring to detect adverse occurrences and provide correct treatment is mandatory. The extent of monitoring depends on the severity of the disease and its effects.

There are a variety of agents used to treat acute hypertensive episodes, of which some are better than others. β-Blockade and nitroglycerin are most appropriate. A thorough knowledge of agents used in hypertension is required due to the deleterious effects some popular treatments have and the potential for interaction with anaesthesia.

Hypertension does occur as part of more complex conditions and experienced assistance should be sought for appropriate management.

I. INTRODUCTION

In the first half of the 20th century, hypertension and ischaemic heart disease were considered to be contraindications to anaesthesia because of high perioperative morbidity and mortality rates. In the beginning of the 21st century, hypertension is a common problem, with 10–25% of the population affected, including >50% of

people over the age of 65. With an aging population, its prevalence is likely to increase (1).

Initially, the introduction of treatments for hypertension caused further concern, with reports of severe hypotension and bradycardia attributed to the preoperative administration of these agents. The benefits of treatment have now been established and there are fewer cardiovascular deaths and complications in treated patients in the nonsurgical setting.

The outcome of hypertensive subjects undergoing anaesthesia and surgery has also been extensively studied. Uncontrolled systemic hypertension alone may pose a minor risk for perioperative cardiovascular complications when compared with major risk factors such as unstable coronary syndromes and decompensated heart failure (2).

However, chronic hypertension is a marker for numerous potential predictors of perioperative complications, as well as being a risk itself.

The range of problems encountered in hypertensive patients during the perioperative period can be due to one or more of the following:

- Pathophysiological changes in the cardiovascular system, that cause an exaggerated pressor response.
- End-organ damage, especially to the heart and kidneys, and cerebrovascular disease.
- Co-morbid problems commonly associated with hypertension, for example, diabetes.
- Drug therapy for the treatment of hypertension or sequelae.

Management of the hypertensive patient is based on:

- Increased understanding of the pathophysiology of hypertension.
- Problems associated with hypertension.
- Preoperative assessment requirements.
- Intra-operative anaesthetic management.
- Postoperative care, and
- Treatment and prevention of acute hypertensive episodes.

This chapter will consider the potential problems caused by hypertension and its treatment with respect to anaesthesia and surgery and present an approach to these patients as dictated by current best evidence and expert consensus opinion.

A number of still widely quoted studies were completed >20 years ago (3–5), but subsequent changes in anaesthesia, monitoring and treatment may change their relevance to current practice. Conclusions and recommendations in this chapter are based on numerous studies of the peri-operative hypertensive patient. Major complications in the hypertensive patient are relatively uncommon and consequently, difficult to study. Large randomised controlled trials into best practice are lacking.

II. PATHOPHYSIOLOGY OF HYPERTENSION

The pathophysiology of essential hypertension is uncertain, but the derangement of several interrelated factors controlling blood pressure is probably responsible. A discussion of these factors can be found elsewhere in this book.

Features associated with essential hypertension include arteriolar changes, ventricular hypertrophy, altered autoregulation, and accelerated atheromatous plaque formation.

A. Arteriolar Changes

Cardiac output and systemic vascular resistance determine arterial blood pressure. Arterioles determine the systemic vascular resistance. Arteriolar changes lead to pathological increases in resistance; most patients with essential hypertension have a normal cardiac output and raised peripheral arteriolar resistance.

The changes that occur in arterioles are increased wall thickness to lumen ratio and reduction in arteriolar density to particular tissues.

1. Increased Wall Thickness to Lumen Ratio

At equal external diameters, the internal diameter of these vessels is less than those of the normotensive patient as a result of medial smooth muscle hypertrophy and deposition of mucopolysaccharides, fibrin, and elastin into the media and intima. Because of the smaller internal diameter, there is a greater change in resistance with changes in intra-luminal diameter in the hypertensive patient. This is expected from Poiseuille's equation and is the basis of the exaggerated responses to constriction and dilatation that are observed in the hypertensive patient.

2. Reduction in Arteriolar Density of Particular Tissues

Reduction in arteriolar density of particular tissues (*arteriolar rarefaction*) can be considered as compensatory effects to prevent raised arterial pressure from being transmitted to a capillary bed, where it may have deleterious results. Loss of elastin and deposition of collagen, glycosaminoglycans, and calcium as an individual ages results in a more rigid vascular tree. This leads to systolic hypertension with a relatively normal diastolic pressure.

B. Ventricular Hypertrophy

The greater workload required to maintain cardiac output with longstanding increased after-load leads to left ventricular hypertrophy. Diastolic compliance also decreases as a result of impaired muscle distensability, and filling is compromised. Cardiac output becomes more dependent on the Frank–Starling mechanism, that is, if preload decreases, filling is reduced more than in a normal heart and may lead to an exaggerated decrease in stroke volume. Volume overload is more likely to result in pulmonary oedema that is caused by high pulmonary venous pressures.

C. Altered Autoregulation

Chronic hypertension leads to a shift of the autoregulation curve to the right. Decreasing the mean arterial pressure by 25% in normotensive and hypertensive patients reaches the lower limit of autoregulation (6). That is, autoregulation is lost at a higher mean arterial pressure in hypertensive patients.

D. Accelerated Atheromatous Plaque Formation

Hypertension is associated with endothelial dysfunction and abnormalities of blood constituents and flow (cf. Virchow's triad), resulting in a hypercoagualable state. Atheroma development is promoted in the presence of high plasma lipoprotein levels.

III. POTENTIAL PROBLEMS ASSOCIATED WITH HYPERTENSION

Chronic hypertension leads to pathological changes, and compensatory mechanisms that are present during normal activity may not be sufficient during anaesthesia. The types of complications that can occur as a result of these compensatory mechanisms failing to perform adequately during anaesthesia are cardiovascular complications, cerebrovascular complications, renal complications, and surgery-specific complications.

A. Cardiovascular Complications

Perioperative cardiac morbidity is a leading cause of death after surgery. In England and Wales, ~18,000 deaths occur within 30 days of anaesthesia and surgery, with ~8000 attributable to cardiovascular causes. Hypertension is associated with an increased risk (7).

Up to 20 major cardiovascular complications, such as myocardial infarction, new or unstable angina, acute left ventricular failure, or life-threatening arrhythmias occur for each cardiovascular death. These are high-risk events; for example, postoperative myocardial infarction and unstable angina reduce 2 year survival from 95% to 23% (8).

Myocardial ischaemia is a risk factor for these complications (9). It is often not painful ("silent"). Why it is silent is unclear, but the effects are the same as when pain is present. Silent myocardial ischaemia is common in hypertensive patients, especially in the presence of left ventricular hypertrophy, previous myocardial infarction [per history or electrocardiogram (ECG) evidence] and in patients presenting for coronary artery bypass grafting (10). Patients with more acute cardiovascular abnormalities (hypertensive episodes, dysrhythmias, infarction, left ventricular dilatation, and pump failure) also have significantly more episodes of ischaemia than those do not have these abnormalities (9).

Silent myocardial ischaemia is clinically important whenever it occurs because the prognosis of patients who have it is worse than those who do not have it. Adverse events are temporally associated with its presence and support current consensus that preventing silent myocardial ischaemia is important (11). Whether it occurs pre-operatively or perioperatively, it predicts immediate postoperative complications. In one study, >90% of major postoperative cardiac events occurred in patients with silent myocardial ischaemia (12).

Silent myocardial ischaemia may be a marker of patients with more severe cardiovascular disease, or its occurrence may lead to adverse events that increase the long-term risk. Silent perioperative myocardial ischaemia has been associated with increased mortality at 2 years. (Mortality rate without silent myocardial ischaemia is 5%; mortality rate with silent myocardial ischaemia is 9%.) (8). Because hypertension causes silent myocardial ischaemia, and silent myocardial ischaemia is associated with an increased number of adverse cardiac events, it is not surprising that preoperative hypertension is a significant predictor of postoperative morbidity. A 36% incidence of perioperative silent myocardial ischaemia in uncontrolled or poorly controlled hypertensive patients falls to 16% in controlled hypertensive or normotensive patients (13,14). This indicates that appropriate preoperative treatment of hypertension may reduce the number of adverse cardiac events.

Major cardiovascular complications are uncommon. Adequately powered trials to detect the link between well controlled hypertension and a reduction in cardiovascular morbidity and mortality have not been performed. Still, there are important studies that have added significantly to our knowledge of the hypertensive patient under anaesthesia and surgery.

Prys-Roberts et al. (5) demonstrated the haemodynamic problems of anaesthetizing untreated patients and suggested that preoperative blood pressure control reduced problems. However, at least four out of seven untreated hypertensive patients were less healthy than those who were treated, which created bias for the preoperative treatment. Blood pressure levels did not differ between treated and untreated groups, and the overall number of patients studied were not large. Therefore, the efficacy of preoperative treatment cannot be stated confidently from these results, but these results do reveal the haemodynamic problems of inadequate treatment.

The findings of Goldman and Caldera (4) were different, concluding that treatment does not affect outcomes, but there were flaws in the data gathering methods. In this study, for example, groups were not randomized; the patients who were more sick were allocated to the treatment group, and this adversely affected the results of treatment vs. nontreatment. Only 34 of 117 "hypertensive" patients had a diastolic blood pressure ≥ 100 mmHg, and no patients had severe hypertension (diastolic blood pressure >120 mmHg). The total number of patients included makes it unlikely that a difference would have been detected, and the authors noted that adverse effects number were too small to analyze meaningfully.

Despite deficiencies in these and other studies, it is an important, well-demonstrated fact that hypertension remains a marker of cardiovascular, renal, and neurological risks (3,15–17). Poor preoperative control can lead to haemodynamic instability though to date we do not know the true efficacy of treatment in the mild, moderate, and severe hypertensive patient.

B. Cerebrovascular Complications

There is a strong association between cerebrovascular disease and hypertension. Chronic hypertension causes two problems that put the brain at risk perioperatively. They are vascular dysfunction and altered autoregulation.

1. Vascular Dysfunction

Vascular degeneration and accelerated atheroma formation predispose subjects to cerebrovascular incidents. These are usually thrombotic rather than haemorrhagic, despite the blood vessels being exposed to high pressure (the so-called "Birmingham Paradox") (1). The same is true for the myocardium and is due to plaque rupture, and the resultant thrombosis and infarction.

2. Altered Autoregulation

In altered autoregulation, the autoregulatory curve is shifted to the right, which means the ischaemic threshold is at a higher mean arterial pressure. A decrease of 25% in mean arterial pressure reaches the lower limit of autoregulation. A decrease of 50% in nonanaesthetized patients causes reversible cerebral ischaemia (18). Hypertensive patients are at risk at the same mean arterial pressures that adequately perfuse the brain in normotensive subjects. Increases in mean arterial pressure of similar degrees exceed the upper limit of autoregulation.

In animal studies, chronic treatment may restore the lower limit of autoregulation to normal (19). Similar results occur in humans, especially with the use of ACE inhibitors, but it may take 12 months to happen and then may still be incomplete (20).

Anaesthesia affects autoregulation. Intravenous agents have no effect, but all volatile agents (with the possible exception of sevoflurane) impair control as a consequence of direct cerebral vasodilatation. With impaired autoregulation, increases and decreases in the mean arterial pressure have greater effects on cerebral perfusion than they do in the nonanaesthetized patient.

Acute hypertensive episodes increase the risk of atheromatous plaque and vessel wall rupture. Hypotension causes global ischaemia or "watershed infarction" in areas of prior critical perfusion.

C. Renal Complications

Chronic hypertension is associated with renal impairment that is a result of nephrosclerosis. This is associated with pathological changes in the preglomerular vasculature (e.g., arteriolar intimal thickening and atheroma) and secondary changes that involve the glomeruli and interstitium.

The reduction in renal blood flow may be further compromised during hypotensive episodes perioperatively, which increases the risk of pre-renal renal failure (i.e., renal failure due to inadequate perfusion of the kidneys).

Impaired renal clearance has implications for the elimination of the drugs that are administered during the perioperative period.

D. Surgery-Specific Complications

Two examples of surgery-specific complications are

- *Haemorrhage*. High intra-luminal pressure increases the risk of bleeding. This may make haemostasis more difficult intra-operatively and increase the risk of ocular bleeding and haematoma formation postoperatively.
- *Increased intra-ocular pressure*. Intra-ocular pressure is raised by an increase in choroidal blood volume. Transient changes in intra-ocular pressure have no significant effect within the intact globe. During surgery, or following a penetrating eye injury, when the globe is open, high intra-ocular pressure can cause further damage, including lens prolapse, vitreous extrusion, and haemorrhage with potential loss of vision.

IV. PREOPERATIVE ASSESSMENT

The goal of preoperative assessment is the detection of poorly controlled hypertension and end-organ damage, which is relevant to how anaesthesia will be administered.

If these tasks have not already been performed, a sufficient medical history, examination, and investigation are necessary to exclude secondary hypertension.

Not all of the investigations described subsequently are required for all hypertensive patients. This would be impractical. The type of surgery required and the identification of higher risk patients through evaluation of their medical history and examination determine the need for further tests. Attempts have been made to stratify risk and provide the rationale for subsequent investigation (2).

The treatable problems that are identified should be corrected to optimize the patient's condition. This might include treatment of hypertension and might necessitate postponing surgery and referring the patient to another specialty. Problems range from diuretic-induced hypokalemia, requiring potassium supplements, to reversible ischaemia generally considered an indication for coronary angiography and revascularization prior to major surgery.

Preoperative hypertension is a predictor of post operative morbidity and mortality. Untreated and poorly controlled hypertensive patients have more intra-operative haemodynamic instability, and this may cause adverse cardiovascular events. It has been suggested that patients with mild and moderate hypertension (blood pressure <180/110 mmHg) are at no more risk than normotensive patients and may proceed with surgery if they are carefully monitored and treated to prevent hypotensive or hypertensive episodes (4). Owing to the original patient selection on which this conclusion is based, this cut-off point may not prevent putting the hypertensive patient at risk of myocardial ischaemia. More recent work reveals ischaemia also occurs perioperatively in patients with mild and moderate hypertension (15). If the patient is otherwise fit for surgery but the blood pressure is $\geq 180/\geq 110$ advice based on Prys-Robert's original studies recommended postponing surgery. This is probably not necessary but care should be taken to maintain cardiovascular stability (21).

Optimal preoperative treatment of blood pressure leads to fewer haemodynamic fluctuations and is widely recommended before elective surgery. The evidence for this is clearest in those with the most severe hypertension. For patients with mild or moderate untreated or poorly controlled hypertension, it may be wise to delay elective surgery in the presence of end-organ damage. This allows further assessment of the degree of damage and treatment of the blood pressure and end-organ decompensation.

Untreated or poorly controlled mild to moderate hypertension without end-organ damage is a more controversial area but relevant to for greater numbers of patients. Careful monitoring and treatment of cardiovascular instability is necessary. Additional treatments, such as acute perioperative β-blockade, also may prove to be beneficial. The true value of such additional interventions is still to be determined.

The availability of monitoring for physiological factors (i.e., electrocardiography including ST segment analysis, blood pressure, oxygen saturation, and end tidal carbon dioxide), the availability and quality of perioperative care facilities, and the experience of the anaesthetist may be more important than any specific cut-off points (9).

A. History

Problems including angina and its precipitants, dyspnaea, orthopnaea, and paroxysmal nocturnal dyspnaea should be sought. Evidence of heart failure is a major predictive risk factor (22), and exercise tolerance (functional capacity) is very informative (2).

History alone may not be very reliable for the detection of coronary artery disease. Ischaemia may be silent or absent during usual activity if the activity is limited by other co-morbidities, for example, osteoarthrosis.

Other important factors are smoking history, age, other relevant illnesses (e.g., diabetes), previous arteriopathic diseases (e.g., end-organ damage), myocardial infarction (especially if recent) (22), heart failure, stroke, retinopathy, claudication, and renal failure.

A current list of medications and any recent changes in medication that are indicative of a progressive disease should be established. The use of various antihypertensive agents during anaesthesia is discussed later in this chapter.

B. Examination

Clinical examination may reveal important evidence of arrhythmias, raised venous pressure, cardiomegaly, additional heart sounds, or pulmonary oedema (22). Other signs of end-organ damage may include impaired vision, haemiplegia, and evidence of renal disease, for example, arterio-venous fistulae.

C. Investigations

Investigations performed pre-operatively include those considered to be baseline for any hypertensive patient and those performed in patients considered to be higher risk as judged by their history, clinical examination or type of surgery for which they have presented. Guidance has been issued in the United Kingdom for this purpose (23).

Some investigations used to guide therapy associated with better peri-operative outcomes are not feasible on a large scale at this time due to economic constraints (24).

1. Blood Pressure

Poorly controlled hypertension is a significant predictor of postoperative morbidity (17). Several individual readings are recommended for assessment of blood pressure

though this may not be possible between admission and surgery. Cooperation with primary care physicians can help. Arterial pressures measurements made at the time of admission to the hospital may be useful to identify patients at risk of perioperative ischaemia (9,13) although findings are not consistent (25).

2. 12-Lead Electrocardiograph

The resting 12-lead ECG does not identify increased perioperative risk in patients undergoing low-risk surgery (26) and is often normal despite the presence of heart disease. It is important as a comparison in case a perioperative event occurs. Some abnormalities are predictors of adverse events in intermediate-risk and high-risk patients. These include evidence of ischaemia, previous myocardial infarction, left ventricular hypertrophy, conduction defects, and a rhythm other than sinus (10,22).

Ambulatory (Holter) monitoring has shown that silent myocardial ischaemia is common in hypertensive patients and that it is an important risk factor (17). Holter monitoring is relatively inexpensive and simple to use except when there are significant ECG abnormalities (such as left bundle branch block, pacemaker, left ventricular hypertrophy with significant strain, and digitalis effect) that prevent analysis. It should be used in those patients who have been identified as being at risk on the basis of their past medical history and current physical state. It is a tool for determining which patients require further evaluation but by itself is not the definitive end investigation.

3. Chest Radiograph

The chest radiograph may reveal signs of pulmonary congestion and increased cardiothoracic ratio. Rarely, coarctation of the aorta may be identified.

4. Blood and Urine Tests

Full blood count. Anaemia decreases oxygen delivery to an ischaemic myocardium.

Urea and electrolytes. Evidence of renal dysfunction or electrolyte abnormalities associated with drug therapy. Rarely, hypokalaemia may be associated with hyperaldosteronism, causing hypertension.

Glucose. Many diabetics are currently undiagnosed.

Urine. Proteinuria and glycosuria are associated with renal impairment and diabetes.

Other discretionary blood tests may be performed.

5. Echocardiography

Echocardiography is noninvasive and relatively inexpensive; it is not routinely required, but it is useful to confirm or refute the presence of left ventricular hypertrophy suggested by ECG changes (27). Low ejection fractions are associated with silent myocardial ischaemia, but objective measurement by transthoracic echocardiography is often inaccurate. Patients with an ejection fraction of >55% are 10 times less likely to suffer an adverse outcome than those in whom it is <35% (28).

Cardiovascular risk is better determined when echocardiography is used in combination with pharmacological stressing agents (29). This technique has been used to identify at-risk patients who then received perioperative β-blockade. Subsequent improvements in outcome were reported (24).

6. Exercise Stress Testing

Approximately 20–50% of patients without a cardiac history and with a normal resting ECG will have an abnormal exercise ECG. In known at-risk patients (e.g., those with previous myocardial infarction, abnormal resting ECG, or peripheral vascular disease), the exercise ECG is higher; when an abnormal exercise ECG occurs at low workloads, it identifies significantly increased risk (30). However, in a general population, routine preoperative exercise stress testing did not predict cardiac risk (31).

7. Dipyridamole Thallium Scanning

Dipyridamole thallium scanning is a noninvasive test for detecting reversible myocardial ischaemia that can be used when baseline ECG abnormalities preclude Holter monitoring. When it is used rationally (32), it may be regarded as a screening test for coronary angiography. It is a widely used tool for risk stratification in high-risk patients. Its use in lower risk patients may be limited by a lack of equipment, time, and skilled personnel to perform the test.

D. Antihypertensive Drugs

Numerous agents are now used for treatment of hypertension in the presence of concurrent disease and end-organ damage and to reduce the side effects associated with high-dose monotherapy. The relevance of commonly used antihypertensive drugs to anaesthesia and surgery should be considered (Table 39.1).

V. MANAGEMENT OF ANAESTHESIA

The practical conduct of anaesthesia for the hypertensive patient requires appropriate monitoring and modification of standard techniques to prevent excessive pressor responses. Up to 50% of intra-operative ischaemic episodes may be preceded by acute hypertension (33). Patient management goals are to maintain safe preoperative levels of blood pressure and heart rate and to avoid the damage that is associated with periods of haemodynamic instability.

A. Monitoring

Adequate intra-operative monitoring is one of the foundations of modern anaesthetic management. Appropriate monitoring should start in the anaesthetic room and continue until recovery (34).

The following are considered essential during induction and maintenance of anaesthesia: pulse oximeter, electrocardiograph, noninvasive blood pressure monitor, and capnograph.

The use or measurement of the following can be considered: invasive blood pressure, central venous pressure, pulmonary artery occlusion pressure, and trans-oesophageal echocardiograph.

B. Pulse Oximeter

Hypoxaemia should be avoided in anaesthetic practice regardless of pre-existing diseases and use of a pulse oximeter is considered by most anaesthetists to be mandatory.

C. Electrocardiograph

CM_5, a modified bipolar lead of V_5, demonstrates the greatest magnitude of ST change, with good P-wave visualization, and it is inexpensive to implement (35). Computerized ST analysis is a significant advance in perioperative monitoring. Both are recommended.

Ischaemic changes are difficult to detect in the presence of right bundle branch block, left ventricular hypertrophy with strain, and atrial fibrillation. They cannot be detected with left bundle branch block and pacemaker dependency.

D. Blood Pressure Monitor

For minor surgery in a well-controlled patient, noninvasive monitoring should suffice. For major surgery and poorly controlled patients, invasive monitoring offers potential benefits:

- Beat-to-beat monitoring that allows early detection and treatment of problems.
- Detection and monitoring of change due to vasoactive drugs.
- Arterial blood gas sampling.
- Supplementary clues from waveform (not validated in subjects with rapidly changing arterial tone, which may include poorly controlled hypertensive patients).

E. Capnograph

Hypocapnia causes decreased cardiac output and hypotension, and may cause dysrhythmias by exacerbating diuretic-associated hypokalaemia.

Table 39.1   Commonly Used Antihypertensive Drugs During Anaesthesia and Surgery

Drug type	Actions	Relevance to anaesthesia and surgery
Diuretics	Vasodilatation and volume contraction (vasodilatation predominates chronically). May lower potassium level.	Not necessary to fluid load pre-op [most patients on diuretic not dehydrated (55)]. Hypocapnia also causes hypokalaemia. This may precipitate tachyarrhythmias.
Calcium channel antagonists	Negative chronotropy and inotropy. Vasodilatation.	Moderate effects additive to those caused by anaesthetic agents.
β-Adrenoreceptor blockers (56)	Sympatholytic effect causing negative chronotropy and inotropy.	Excess sympathetic activity worsens myocardial supply-demand balance and is associated with atheromatous plaque rupture causing coronary artery occlusion. Some studies report lower major cardiovascular complications (e.g., MI/death) in high risk patients treated peri-operatively with β-blockers. Timing of treatment or who best to treat is not known. Chronic β-blockade is not protective. Withdrawal can cause rebound effects. Evidence base does not currently support routine peri-operative, short-term β-blockade.
Angiotensin-converting enzyme (ACE) inhibitors (57)	Inhibits conversion of angiotensin I to angiotensin II. Reduced activity of renin-angiotensin system (RAS) causes vasodilatation.	RAS integrity required during physiological stress to maintain cardiovascular stability and organ perfusion. Blockade by ACE inhibitors may be deleterious. Pre-op administration makes vasopressor use more likely. Stopping drug prior to surgical procedures where large fluid losses or shifts are expected should be considered.
Angiotensin II antagonists (58)	Specific antagonism at angiotensin II receptors. Reduced activity of renin-angiotensin system (RAS) causes vasodilatation.	Effects during anaesthesia are still being elucidated. Similarities to ACE inhibitors are expected.
α-Adrenoreceptor blockers	Vasodilatation.	Moderate effects additive to those caused by anaesthetic agents.
Centrally acting drugs (methyldopa and clonidine)	Variety of mechanisms, including α2 receptor agonism.	Moderate effects additive to those caused by anaesthetic agents. Withdrawal of clonidine can cause rebound effects. Can reduce pressor response to intubation. No effect on peri-operative cardiovascular complication rate (59).

Source: Roberts (55), Howell et al. (56), Mirenda and Grissom (57), Bertrand et al. (58), and Oliver et al. (59).

F.   Central Venous Pressure Monitor

The Central Venous Pressure Monitor is poorly validated in determining the adequacy of circulating blood volume and right ventricular preload. There is little direct evidence of clinical benefits of invasive monitoring, but it may guide treatment if used in combination with other clinical details (36). It is probably no more useful in the hypertensive patient than in others having similar types of surgery.

G.   Pulmonary Artery Occlusion Pressure Monitor

Providing potentially more reliable left heart data by overcoming intrinsic inaccuracies caused by hypertensive heart disease, although clinical outcome studies do not support its use (37). Detection of ischaemia with a pulmonary artery occlusion pressure (PAOP) catheter is possible but not feasible because of the constant or frequent balloon inflation required. Other less invasive methods are likely to supersede it.

H. *Trans*-oesophageal Echocardiograph

Two-dimensional *trans*-oesophageal echocardiography provides a good, real-time view from an ultrasound probe placed in the oesophagus looking forward at the heart. It is one of the most sensitive monitors of cardiac function and is able to detect wall motion abnormalities associated with myocardial ischaemia before ECG changes occur (38). Limitations exist due to training, equipment cost, and poor tolerance during regional anaesthesia and postoperative periods.

VI. INDUCTION

There is insufficient evidence to favor regional or general anaesthetic techniques (39).

A. General Anaesthesia

A major problem with this is sympathetically mediated hypertension and tachycardia caused by laryngoscopy and intubation. The former is the most stimulating. In healthy patients, this transient effect is not a problem, but can be a problem in the presence of cardiovascular and cerebrovascular disease (40).

Hypotension may occur due to venous dilatation, impaired baroreceptor reflexes, and decreased arousal.

In treated and untreated hypertensive patients, induction and laryngoscopy is associated with pronounced cardiovascular instability. Increases in blood pressure and heart rate are more pronounced than in normotensive subjects. Well-controlled hypertensive patients have a smaller pressor response than untreated patients. The latter also have the greatest fall in blood pressure and the highest percentage of arrhythmias and ischaemia (41).

Various factors can limit cardiovascular responses:

- Hypertensive patients should be well controlled on medication
- Several drugs may be effective in attenuating or obliterating the sympathetic pressor response. These include
  - β-blockers,
  - induction agents, and
  - peripheral vasodilators
- Local anaesthetics (topical and intravenous)
- Narcotics
- Centrally acting adrenergic agonists
- Calcium channel blockers

The results of a Cochrane review to substantiate the efficacy and adverse effects of one agent against another will be published in 2005 (42). Currently favored agents are short acting β-blockers (esmolol or labetalol) and high doses of fentanyl.

- Avoidance of laryngoscopy
- Blind nasal intubation (41)
- Laryngeal mask airway (standard and intubating) (43)
- Regional anaesthetic technique
- Avoidance of ketamine in hypertensive patients
- Avoidance of large doses of traditional induction agents, and slowly titrating administration to effect reduction in hypotension.

B. Regional Anaesthesia

There are advantages for using a regional technique but significantly decreased cardiac morbidity has not been demonstrated (39). Well-controlled hypertensive patients tolerate epidural blockade favorably (44). Combining general and regional techniques is well-tolerated and may have significant benefits postoperatively.

In comparison, untreated hypertensive patients frequently develop unacceptable hypotension during extradural blockade requiring vasopressors (44).

VII. MAINTENANCE

There is sufficient evidence to establish if one method for maintenance of general anaesthesia (i.e., volatile or total intravenous anaesthesia) is superior. There may be advantages to avoiding volatile anaesthetics associated with tachyarrythmias or hypertension (e.g., halothane, isoflurane, and desflurane) or using an anaesthetic technique that requires low concentrations (less than 1 minimum alveolar concentration) at which these effects are unlikely to occur.

Either controlled or spontaneous ventilation can be used, although excess hypo- or hypercapnia should be avoided due to effects on vascular tone and serum potassium levels.

Unacceptable hypertension (mean arterial pressure >25% of preoperative pressure) occurring intra-operatively can cause end-organ damage (e.g., ventricular failure, cerebral haemorrhage) and should be treated. Treatment should take into account the likely underlying cause (Table 39.2).

Preoperative blood pressure is determined by taking several readings to ascertain normal values for a particular patient. Pressures at which no evidence exists of increased end-organ compromise may be considered normal. Blood pressure readings that fall outside this range can be considered unacceptable.

VIII. POSTOPERATIVE CARE

There is no significant pressor response associated with extubation if the patient does not cough on the endotracheal tube (5). However, predicting which patients will not cough is unreliable. Extubation can therefore be performed either during deep anaesthesia or following

Table 39.2 Causes of Intra-Operative Hypertension

General category	Specific type
Pre-existing condition	Essential hypertension
	Secondary hypertension
	Pregnancy-related hypertension
Increased sympathetic tone	Inadequate anaesthesia
	Inadequate analgesia
	Hypoxaemia
	Hypercapnia
Drugs	Adrenaline
	Ephedrine
	Ketamine
	Ergometrine
Other	Hypervolaemia
	Aortic cross-clamping
	Phaeochromocytoma
	Malignant hyperthermia

treatment with those agents that are used acutely at laryngoscopy to prevent hypertension.

Common causes of postoperative hypertension are pain, hypoxaemia, anxiety (e.g., associated with residual neuromuscular blockade), full bladder, hypercapnia, and preoperative hypertension.

Rare causes include drug interactions [e.g., pethidine and monoamine oxidase inhibitor (MAOI)], phaeochromocytoma, and malignant hyperthermia.

Treatment of postoperative hypertension includes provision of adequate analgesia, continued adequate monitoring, exclusion of urinary retention, exclusion of residual neuromuscular blockade, and titration of antihypertensive drug of choice to effect.

Most episodes of postoperative hypertension are not long lasting.

When the usual oral medication cannot be administered postoperatively (e.g., for a patient who is not to be fed after bowel resection, prolonged ventilation, nausea, and vomiting), the situation must be addressed. Consider alternative agents or routes of administration.

Patients who have suffered a hypertensive crisis may require transfer to a level-two or level-three area (high-dependency unit or critical care unit) for further treatment or observation.

IX. ACUTE TREATMENT OF HYPERTENSION

Although the ideal agent for the acute treatment of hypertension does not currently exist, the desirable properties of such an agent have been described by several authors (45–47).

Features of the ideal agent are:

- It is short acting.
- It is intravenously administered.

- It prevents reflex tachycardia (maintains subendocardial perfusion).
- It does not cause respiratory depression (avoiding hypoxaemia/hypercapnia).
- It is non-sedating.
- It is non-toxic.

There are several commonly used drugs available for acute hypertension control.

A. Labetalol (IV)

- Competitive blocker for α_1-adrenergic and β-adrenergic receptors.
- Hypotensive effect within 5 min and persists for $\sim$2–4 h.
- Heart rate slightly reduced, cardiac output maintained (unlike pure β-blockers).
- Reduces peripheral vascular resistance without reducing peripheral blood flow; cerebral, renal, and coronary blood flows are maintained.
- Incremental boluses of 20–80 mg cause a rapid, smooth reduction in blood pressure without reflex tachycardia. Injections of 1–2 mg/kg have been reported to produce precipitous falls in blood pressure and should be avoided.
- Used intravenously in hypertensive women in the last trimester of pregnancy, has been shown to not change uteroplacental blood flow or fetal heart rate, despite a significant reduction in maternal blood pressure and heart rate.
- Intravenous use is effective without causing significant hypotension, bradycardia, bronchospasm, or electrocardiographic changes in patients with acute postoperative hypertension and during general anaesthesia. Responses are similar with or without prior treatment with a β-blocker.
- Can cause nausea, vomiting, paraesthesia and sweating, and rarely hepatotoxicity, which can be fatal.

B. Esmolol (IV)

- Very-short-acting cardioselective β_1-adrenergic blocker metabolized by blood esterase to inactive compounds.
- Onset of action is within 60 s with a duration of 10–20 min.
- The recommended initial dose is 0.5 mg/kg followed by an infusion of 25–300 μg/kg per min.
- Safe in patients with acute myocardial infarction, even those who have relative contraindications to β-blockers, and is valuable perioperatively.

- Does not produce excessive reduction in diastolic blood pressure and reflex tachycardia sometimes seen with other agents.

C. Nitroglycerin (IV)

- Interacts with nitrate receptors on vascular smooth muscle with a rapid onset and short half-life (1–4 min).
- Not an effective vasodilator, but a potent venodilator. Affects arterial tone only at high doses.
- Reduced preload or after-load decreases left ventricular myocardial wall tension, reducing oxygen consumption and favoring redistribution of blood flow to the subendocardium.
- May dilate coronary vessels and increase blood supply to ischaemic regions.
- Other drugs are also frequently needed in conjunction to control hypertension.
- Relatively safe when used correctly. May cause headache, nausea and vomiting, hypotension, and rarely bradycardia. A rare but potentially serious complication is methemoglobinaemia, particularly in infants.
- Care needed in patients with left ventricular outflow limitations in order not to precipitate cardiovascular collapse.
- More data needed in humans regarding the safety of such treatment during pregnancy.

D. Sodium Nitroprusside (IV)

- A rapid onset, short-acting vasodilator given as a constant intravenous infusion, effective in decreasing blood pressure in all patients irrespective of severity or etiology.
- Arterial and venous vasodilatation decreases afterload and preload.
- Can cause coronary steal in patients with coronary artery disease, may worsen myocardial ischaemia, increase intracranial pressure, and interfere with hypoxic pulmonary vasoconstriction.
- Contains cyanide. Malnutrition, renal or hepatic disease, and high doses for prolonged periods of time are risk factors for the development of toxicity. Current monitoring methods for cyanide toxicity are inadequate, and toxicity has been seen after short periods of treatment. Metabolic acidosis is usually a preterminal event.
- Even recommended doses can result in cyanide formation at a greater rate than can be detoxified.
- Not as effective or safe as several other agents. Should be used only when other agents are not available, and then only in patients with normal renal and hepatic function. Duration of treatment should be as short as possible.

E. Hydralazine (IV)

- Following a dose of hydralazine (IV), there is an initial latent period of 5–15 min followed by a progressive fall in blood pressure lasting for up to 12 h. Although the circulating half-life is about 3 h, the half-time effect on blood pressure is ~100 h and may cause cerebral, myocardial, and renal ischaemia or infarction.
- Not recommended for treatment of hypertensive episodes in the perioperative period but widely used in pre-eclampsia.

F. Nifedipine (Oral/Sublingual)

- Causes vasodilatation of arterioles, reducing peripheral vascular resistance.
- A significant decrease in blood pressure is observed after 5 min, peak effect at 30–60 min, and duration of action is ~6 h.
- Hypotensive effects cannot be closely regulated following oral or sublingual administration. Serious adverse affects have been reported and there is a lack of evidence of benefit.
- Not approved for the treatment of hypertensive emergencies; the American Food and Drug Administration's 1996 advisory recommended "great caution" in its use for this indication (46).
- Should not be used in the treatment of acute hypertension.

G. Phentolamine (IV)

- An α-adrenergic blocking agent used for management of catecholamine-induced hypertensive crises (i.e., phaeochromocytoma).
- Given in 1–5 mg boluses, the effect is immediate and may last up to 15 min.
- May cause tachydysrhythmias or angina.

Several other group IV drugs, such as nicardipine, fenoldopam, and enaliprat, are increasingly used. The agents described have largely replaced reserpine, methyldopa, and guanethidine.

X. SPECIAL CIRCUMSTANCES

Hypertension may be present in various conditions requiring expert anaesthetic management. These conditions cause hypertension as part of their pathophysiological processes, e.g., pre-eclampsia or phaeochromocytoma, or may depend on a higher than normal blood pressure to perfuse end organs adequately e.g., carotid artery stenoses.

A. Pre-eclampsia

Pre-eclampsia is a multi-system disorder of unknown etiology occurring after the 20th week of pregnancy causing a state of endothelial dysfunction, generalized vasoconstriction, and hypoperfusion. It is one of the leading causes of pregnancy related death, most often occurring after delivery.

Hypertension (diastolic blood pressure ≥ 110 mmHg on one occasion or diastolic blood pressure ≥ 90 mmHg on two occasions >4 h apart) and proteinuria are associated with other variable features (49,50). Severe symptoms include:

- Oliguria due to a reduced glomerular filtration rate.
- Cerebral irritability (visual disturbance, hyper-reflexia, and headache) the cause of which may be due to vasospasm, hypertensive encephalopathy, or cerebral oedema. Seizures (eclampsia) can occur.
- Epigastric/right upper quadrant pain due to liver capsule distension. This is associated with haemo-lysis, elevated liver enzymes, low platelets (HELLP) syndrome.
- Pulmonary oedema, especially with concomitant medical problems (diabetes, chronic hypertension) and older maternal age. It is a common cause of death.
- Severe hypertension (systolic blood pressure >160 mmHg or diastolic blood pressure >110 mmHg).

Early diagnosis, prevention of complications and blood pressure control are management aims. Delivery of the baby is the cure.

An assessment must be made to identify disease manifestations. Haemodynamic monitoring should be established. Good intravenous access is important to administer fluids and drugs especially because haemorrhage and fitting are major complications. Monitoring central venous pressure may be useful. A low central venous pressure is helpful to determine intravascular volume status, but at higher values correlation with pulmonary capillary wedge pressure is poor. Mean arterial pressure should be controlled to 100–140 mmHg.

Labetalol, hydralazine, and methyldopa are commonly used to treat hypertension. The first two are the intravenous agents of choice.

Effective analgesia reduces maternal catecholamines and blood pressure changes. Epidural analgesia is the preferred choice and can be used for labor and Caesarean section, performed as a combined spinal–epidural if necessary. Epinephrine should not be used in the epidural mixture. Hypotension may occur as the block reveals the relative intravascular depletion. It is treated with fluids judiciously because of the risk of pulmonary and cerebral oedema, and vasopressors to which the pre-eclamptic patient is particularly sensitive. Despite previous concerns, mild hypotension may be associated with increased utero-placental perfusion.

Patient refusal or coagulation abnormalities may preclude epidural use. A concern associated with the use of general anaesthesia is the possibility of airway oedema complicating intubation, and exaggerated hypertension during laryngoscopy and intubation.

Awake intubation may be considered if upper body or facial oedema is present. Because oedema may worsen intra-operatively, the cuff should be deflated and an air leak confirmed prior to extubation.

Agents that are used to attenuate the pressor responses to laryngoscopy and extubation are described elsewhere.

Because pre-eclampsia can worsen after delivery and most deaths occur postpartum, close monitoring and treatment must continue during this time in a critical care facility. Particular attention to fluid balance and blood pressure control is essential, and one must be aware that patients with underlying chronic hypertension or diabetes are at the greatest risk for developing pulmonary oedema. Anti-hypertensive drugs and analgesia remain important and may be required for several days before the disease state resolves. Uterine bleeding may be worsened by uterine atony caused by magnesium sulphate.

B. Carotid Endarterectomy

Patients presenting for carotid endarterectomy are at risk from both surgical and anaesthetic technique, although most neurological complications are related to the former. Hypertension is a common comorbidity.

The cohort of patients that presents for all types of vascular surgery there is a high incidence of hypertension and coronary artery disease (51,52). They are at risk from surgical and anaesthetic technique, although most neurological complications are related to the former.

Many consider regional and local techniques the gold standard. There are no differences in the incidence of death, stroke, transient ischaemic attack, or myocardial infarction between general and regional techniques but there are advantages to the latter. They are:

- Continuous assessment of the awake patient without cerebral monitoring.
- Blood pressure that is more stable.
- Reduced vasopressor requirements.
- Reduced luminal shunting requirement (i.e., less intimal dissection, air, and thromboembolism).

Higher catecholamine levels than with general anaesthesia may cause tachycardia, this would require treatment.

Intra-operatively, carotid sinus manipulation can cause bradycardia and hypotension due to baroreceptor reflexes. Infiltration of the carotid bifurcation with lidocaine usually prevents recurrence, but it may increase the likelihood of postoperative hypertension.

Emergence and extubation may cause hypertension and tachycardia requiring intervention. Good control can be more challenging than at induction. Hypertension is common postoperatively, is associated with cerebral and cardiac complications, and must be aggressively controlled. Appropriate drugs to do this are the same as those listed earlier.

Surgical denervation of the baroreceptors has been implicated, although the common causes of postoperative hypertension should be sought and treated if present.

C. Phaeochromocytoma

Anaesthesia can precipitate a hypertensive crisis associated with appreciable morbidity and mortality. Phaeochromocytomata may be known about pre-operatively and be the reason for surgery or may be discovered incidentally. Severe hypertension is a risk in both cases. Management should be at a specialist center; up to 50% of hospital deaths occur during induction of anaesthesia or during surgery for other causes (53,54).

Preoperative assessment should include full investigations for hypertensive end-organ damage. Catecholamine induced cardiomyopathy causing heart failure has a high mortality and is diagnosed in about one-third of patients.

Blockade of vasopressor activity is usually with phenoxybenzamine, a long-acting drug with a high affinity for α_1 receptors. Persistent arrhythmias or tachycardia are treated with a β-blocker. α-adrenoreceptor blockade precedes β-blockade to prevent unopposed α activity. This avoids the risk of unopposed vasoconstriction causing a crisis, although many patients have been on β-blockers before a diagnosis has been made with no problems.

The optimal duration of treatment before resection is performed is not known. Objective tests of pharmacological sympathectomy can be made. Resolving vasoconstriction requires titrated fluid replacement.

Various other antihypertensive agents have been used successfully for control before surgery. These include prazosin, doxazosin, calcium channel-blocking drugs, clonidine, and magnesium.

Premedication should be considered because stress and anxiety can provoke a crisis. Perioperative cardiovascular monitoring is mandatory and allows detection of extremes of blood pressure and their response to anaesthetic intervention.

Many anaesthetic agents and techniques have been used successfully. An epidural may be used for analgesic purposes but will not block receptor-mediated effects of circulating catecholamines and cannot be relied upon to prevent hypertension. The latter is common during manipulation of the tumor.

Phentolamine, labetalol, sodium nitroprusside, and esmolol are commonly used for acute control of intra-operative hypertension. In this setting, cyanide toxicity is not a problem because only small amounts are typically used. Effects are rapid but brief and more effective than nitrates or phentolamine.

Postoperatively, patients should be managed in a critical care unit. Common causes of hypertension should be addressed and blood pressure controlled. Hypertension that is a result of circulating catecholamines is unusual, and it resolves if resection has been successful. Hypotension is a more common problem and has been suggested to be due to the use of phenoxybenzamine and the persistent α-adrenoceptor blockade.

XI. CONCLUSIONS

Hypertension is a common condition and is likely to become more prevalent. Chronically, it causes end organ damage involving the heart, brain, and kidneys. This is due to various pathological changes. These include increased resistance to blood flow through organs, hypertrophy of the heart pumping against a higher pressure, increasing its need for oxygen and making an oxygen deficit more likely, and occlusion, or rupture, of a vessel with resultant stroke or organ infarction.

Treatment of hypertension is associated with a wide range of drug therapy.

The presence of the disease and related sequelae are risk factors for increased morbidity and mortality in patients who require anaesthesia and surgery. Adequate preoperative control, identification, and careful management of high-risk subjects and their appropriate monitoring, perioperative care facilities, and anaesthetic experience can reduce adverse events.

REFERENCES

1. Beevers G, Lip Y, O'Brien E. ABC of Hypertension. 4th ed. BMJ Books.
2. Eagle KA, Berger PB, Calkins H, Chaitman BR, Ewy GA, Fleischmann KE, Fleisher LA, Froehlich JB, Gusberg RJ, Leppo JA, Ryan T, Schlant RC, Winters WL Jr, Gibbons RJ, Antman EM, Alpert JS, Faxon DP, Fuster V, Gregoratos G, Jacobs AK, Hiratzka LF, Russell RO, Smith SC Jr, American College of Cardiology, American

Heart Association. ACC/AHA guideline update for perioperative cardiovascular evaluation for noncardiac surgery—executive summary: a report of the American College of Cardiology/American Heart Association Task Force on Practice Guidelines (Committee to Update the 1996 Guidelines on Perioperative Cardiovascular Evaluation for Noncardiac Surgery). J Am Coll Cardiol 2002; 39(3):542–553.

3. Asiddao CB, Donegan JH, Whitesell RC, Kalbfleisch JH. Factors associated with perioperative complications during carotid endarterectomy. Anesth Analg 1982; 61(8):631–637.

4. Goldman L, Caldera DL. Risks of general anaesthesia and elective operation in the hypertensive patient. Anesthesiology 1979; 50(4):285–292.

5. Prys-Roberts C, Greene LT, Meloche R, Foex P. Studies of anaesthesia in relation to hypertension. I. Cardiovascular responses of treated and untreated patients. Br J Anaesth 1971; 43(2):122–137.

6. Strandgaard S. Autoregulation of cerebral blood flow in hypertensive patients. The modifying influence of prolonged antihypertensive treatment on the tolerance to acute, drug-induced hypotension. Circulation 1976; 53(4):720–727.

7. NCEPOD. The report of the National Confidential Enquiry into Perioperative Deaths. Campling E, ed. London, 1992.

8. Mangano DT, Browner WS, Hollenberg M, Li J, Tateo IM. Long-term cardiac prognosis following noncardiac surgery. The Study of Perioperative Ischaemia Research Group. JAMA 1992; 268(2):233–239.

9. Slogoff S, Keats AS. Does perioperative myocardial ischaemia lead to postoperative myocardial infarction? Anesthesiology 1985; 62(2):107–114.

10. Hollenberg M, Mangano DT, Browner WS, London MJ, Tubau JF, Tateo IM. Predictors of postoperative myocardial ischaemia in patients undergoing noncardiac surgery. The Study of Perioperative Ischaemia Research Group. JAMA 1992; 268(2):205–209.

11. Raby KE, Barry J, Creager MA, Cook EF, Weisberg MC, Goldman L. Detection and significance of intraoperative and postoperative myocardial ischaemia in peripheral vascular surgery. JAMA 1992; 268(2):222–227.

12. Raby KE, Barry J, Treasure CB, Hirsowitz G, Fantasia G, Selwyn AP. Usefulness of Holter monitoring for detecting myocardial ischaemia in patients with nondiagnostic exercise treadmill test. Am J Cardiol 1993; 72(12):889–893.

13. Allman KG, Muir A, Howell SJ, Hemming AE, Sear JW, Foex P. Resistant hypertension and preoperative silent myocardial ischaemia in surgical patients. Br J Anaesth 1994; 73(5):574–578.

14. Howell SJ, Hemming AE, Allman KG, Glover L, Sear JW, Foex P. Predictors of postoperative myocardial ischaemia. The role of intercurrent arterial hypertension and other cardiovascular risk factors. Anaesthesia 1997; 52(2):107–111.

15. Stone JG et al. Myocardial ischaemia in untreated hypertensive patients: effect of a single small oral dose of a β-adrenergic blocking agent. Anesthesiology 1988; 68(4):495–500.

16. Stone JG, Foex P, Sear JW, Johnson LL, Khambatta HJ, Triner L. Risk of myocardial ischaemia during anaesthesia in treated and untreated hypertensive patients. Br J Anaesth 1988; 61(6):675–679.

17. Mangano DT, Browner WS, Hollenberg M, London MJ, Tubau JF, Tateo IM. Association of perioperative myocardial ischaemia with cardiac morbidity and mortality in men undergoing noncardiac surgery. The Study of Perioperative Ischaemia Research Group. N Engl J Med 1990; 323(26):1781–1788.

18. Njemanze PC. Critical limits of pressure-flow relation in the human brain. Stroke 1992; 23(12):1743–1747.

19. Toyoda K, Fujii K, Ibayashi S, Kitazono T, Nagao T, Takaba H, Fujishima M. Attenuation and recovery of brain stem autoregulation in spontaneously hypertensive rats. J Cereb Blood Flow Metab 1998; 18(3):305–310.

20. Waldemar G, Vorstrup S, Andersen AR, Pedersen H, Paulson OB. Angiotensin converting enzyme inhibition and the upper limit of cerebral blood flow autoregulation: effect of sympathetic stimulation. Circ Res 1989; 64(6):1197–1204.

21. Howell SJ, Sear JW, Foex P. Hypertension, hypertensive heart disease and perioperative cardiac risk. BJA 2004; 92(4):570–583.

22. Goldman L, Caldera DL, Nussbaum SR, Southwick FS, Krogstad D, Murray B, Burke DS, O'Malley TA, Goroll AH, Caplan CH, Nolan J, Carabello B, Slater EE. Multifactorial index of cardiac risk in noncardiac surgical procedures. N Engl J Med 1977; 297(16):845–850.

23. National Institute for Clinical Excellence and National Collaborating Centre for Acute Care. CG3—Preoperative testing, the use of routine preoperative tests for elective surgery. www.nice.org.uk 2003.

24. Poldermans D, Boersma E, Bax JJ, Thomson IR, van de Ven LL, Blankensteijn JD, Baars HF, Yo TI, Trocino G, Vigna C, Roelandt JR, van Urk H. The effect of bisoprolol on perioperative mortality and myocardial infarction in high-risk patients undergoing vascular surgery. Dutch Echocardiographic Cardiac Risk Evaluation Applying Stress Echocardiography Study Group. N Engl J Med 1999; 341(24):1789–1794.

25. Howell SJ, Sear YM, Yeates D, Goldacre M, Sear JW, Foex P. Hypertension, admission blood pressure and perioperative cardiovascular risk. Anaesthesia 1996; 51(11):1000–1004.

26. Schein OD, Katz J, Bass EB, Tielsch JM, Lubomski LH, Feldman MA, Petty BG, Steinberg EP. The value of routine preoperative medical testing before cataract surgery. Study of Medical Testing for Cataract Surgery. N Engl J Med 2000; 342(3):168–175.

27. Ramsay L, Williams B, Johnston G, MacGregor G, Poston L, Potter J, Poulter N, Russell G. Guidelines for management of hypertension: report of the third working party of the British Hypertension Society. J Hum Hypertens 1999; 13(9):569–592.

28. Lazor L, Russell JC, DaSilva J, Radford M. Use of the multiple uptake gated acquisition scan for the preoperative

assessment of cardiac risk. Surg Gynecol Obstet 1988; 167(3):234–248.

29. Eichelberger JP, Schwarz KQ, Black ER, Green RM, Ouriel K. Predictive value of dobutamine echocardiography just before noncardiac vascular surgery. Am J Cardiol 1993; 72(7):602–607.

30. McPhail N, Calvin JE, Shariatmadar A, Barber GG, Scobie TK. The use of preoperative exercise testing to predict cardiac complications after arterial reconstruction. J Vasc Surg 1988; 7(1):60–68.

31. Carliner NH, Fisher ML, Plotnick GD, Garbart H, Rapoport A, Kelemen MH, Moran GW, Gadacz T, Peters RW. Routine preoperative exercise testing in patients undergoing major noncardiac surgery. Am J Cardiol 1985; 56(1):51–58.

32. Eagle KA, Coley CM, Newell JB, Brewster DC, Darling RC, Strauss HW, Guiney TE, Boucher CA. Combining clinical and thallium data optimizes preoperative assessment of cardiac risk before major vascular surgery. Ann Intern Med 1989; 110(11):859–866.

33. Roy WL, Edelist G, Gilbert B. Myocardial ischaemia during non-cardiac surgical procedures in patients with coronary-artery disease. Anesthesiology 1979; 51(5):393–397.

34. Recommendations for standards of monitoring during anaesthesia and recovery. 3rd ed. The Association of Anaesthetists of Great Britain and Ireland, 2000.

35. Quyyumi AA, Crake T, Mockus LJ, Wright CA, Rickards AF, Fox KM. Value of the bipolar lead CM5 in electrocardiography. Br Heart J 1986; 56(4):372–376.

36. Pinsky MR. Rationale for cardiovascular monitoring. Curr Opin Crit Care 2003; 9(3):222–224.

37. Sandham JD, Hull RD, Brant RF, Knox L, Pineo GF, Doig CJ, Laporta DP, Viner S, Passerini L, Devitt H, Kirby A, Jacka M; Canadian Critical Care Clinical Trials Group. A randomized, controlled trial of the use of pulmonary-artery catheters in high-risk surgical patients. N Engl J Med 2003; 348(1):5–14.

38. Smith JS, Cahalan MK, Benefiel DJ, Byrd BF, Lurz FW, Shapiro WA, Roizen MF, Bouchard A, Schiller NB. Intraoperative detection of myocardial ischaemia in high-risk patients: electrocardiography versus two-dimensional transesophageal echocardiography. Circulation 1985; 72(5):1015–1021.

39. Go AS, Browner WS. Cardiac outcomes after regional or general anaesthesia. Do we have the answer? Anesthesiology 1996; 84(1):1–2.

40. Low JM, Harvey JT, Prys-Roberts C, Dagnino J. Studies of anaesthesia in relation to hypertension. VII: Adrenergic responses to laryngoscopy. Br J Anaesth 1986; 58(5): 471–477.

41. Prys-Roberts C, Greene LT, Meloche R, Foex P. Studies of anaesthesia in relation to hypertension. II: Hemodynamic consequences of induction and endotracheal intubation. 1971. Br J Anaesth 1998; 80(1):106–122; discussion 104–105.

42. Khan F, Kantor G, Saleemullah H. Pharmacological agents for preventing morbidity associated with the haemodynamic response to tracheal intubation (Protocol for a Cochrane Review). The Cochrane Library, 2003(4).

43. Kihara S, Brimacombe J, Yaguchi Y, Watanabe S, Taguchi N, Komatsuzaki T. Hemodynamic responses among three tracheal intubation devices in normotensive and hypertensive patients. Anesth Analg 2003; 96(3): 890–895; table of contents.

44. Dagnino J, Prys-Roberts C. Studies of anaesthesia in relation to hypertension. VI: Cardiovascular responses to extradural blockade of treated and untreated hypertensive patients. Br J Anaesth 1984; 56(10):1065–1073.

45. British National Formulary. 43rd ed. London: British Medical Association and the Royal Pharmaceutical Society of Great Britain, 2003.

46. Mansoor G. Comprehensive management of hypertensive emergencies and urgencies. Heart Dis 2002; 4(6):358–371.

47. Varon J, Marik P. The diagnosis and management of hypertensive crises. Chest 2000; 118:214–227.

48. Grossman E, Messerli FH, Grodzicki T, Kowey P. Should a moratorium be placed on sublingual nifedipine capsules given for hypertensive emergencies and pseudoemergencies? JAMA 1996; 276(16):1328–1331.

49. Hart E, Coley S. The diagnosis and management of pre-eclampsia. Br J Anaesth CEPD Rev 2003; 3(2):38–42.

50. Miller R. Pre-eclampsia and eclampsia. In: Anaesthesia. Churchill Livingstone, 2000.

51. Miller R. Carotid endartectomy. In: Anaesthesia. Churchill Livingstone, 2000.

52. Rockman CB, Riles TS, Gold M, Lamparello PJ, Giangola G, Adelman MA, Landis R, Imparato AM. A comparison of regional and general anaesthesia in patients undergoing carotid endarterectomy. J Vasc Surg 1996; 24(6):946–953; discussion 953–956.

53. Pace N, Buttigieg M. Phaechromocytoma. Br J Anaesth CEPD Rev 2003; 3(1):20–23.

54. Prys-Roberts C. Phaeochromocytoma—recent progress in its management. Br J Anaesth 2000; 85(1):44–57.

55. Roberts C. Diuretics, in The Hypertensive Patient. In: Marshall A, Barritt D, eds. Tunbridge Wells: Pitman Medical, 1980:389.

56. Howell SJ, Sear JW, Foex P. Peri-operative β-blockade: a useful treatment that should be greeted with cautious enthusiasm. Br J Anaesth 2001; 86(2):161–164.

57. Mirenda JV, Grissom TE. Anesthetic implications of the renin–angiotensin system and angiotensin-converting enzyme inhibitors. Anesth Analg 1991; 72(5):667–683.

58. Bertrand M, Godet G, Meersschaert K, Brun L, Salcedo E, Coriat P. Should the angiotensin II antagonists be discontinued before surgery? Anesth Analg 2001; 92(1):26–30.

59. Oliver MF, Goldman L, Julian DG, Holme I. Effect of mivazerol on perioperative cardiac complications during non-cardiac surgery in patients with coronary heart disease: the European Mivazerol Trial (EMIT). Anesthesiology 1999; 91(4):951–961.

40

Management of Hypertension in Cardiometabolic Syndrome and Diabetes with Associated Nephropathy

SAMEER N. STAS, SAMY I. McFARLANE
SUNY Downstate and Kings County Hospital Center, Brooklyn, New York, USA

JAMES R. SOWERS
University of Missouri and VA Medical Center, Columbia, Missouri, USA

KEYPOINTS

- Hypertension, diabetes and other components of the metabolic syndrome are frequent concomitant conditions.

- Hypertension accounts for substantial excess morbidity and mortality in patients with diabetes.
- Management of hypertension in diabetes or the metabolic syndrome mandates insistent lifestyle measures, blood pressure and lipid lowering.

- Angiotensin-converting enzyme (ACE) inhibitors and angiotensin receptor blockers are often the drugs of choice, but thiazide-type diuretics have also been shown to reduce cardiovascular disease risk in diabetic patients. The latter are usually required as a part of multidrug therapy to control blood pressure.

SUMMARY

Hypertension is twice as common in people with diabetes compared with nondiabetics and accounts for up to 85% excess cardiovascular disease risk; patients with hypertension also are more prone to diabetes compared with normotensive individuals. In type 2 diabetes, hypertension tends to cluster with other components of the metabolic syndrome such as microalbuminuria, central obesity, dyslipidemia increased inflammatory, and procoagulant state. Hypertension in people with diabetes is usually associated with increased salt sensitivity, volume expansion, isolated systolic hypertension, loss of nocturnal dipping of the blood pressure and pulse, orthostatic hypotension, and microalbuminuria. Management of hypertension in this high cardiovascular disease risk population mandates the weight reduction and exercise together with the use of aspirin, lowering of low-density lipoprotein (LDL) cholesterol to 100 mg/dL (2.6 mmol/L), and blood pressure lowering to 130/80 mmHg with agents that afford cardiovascular disease and renal protection such as angiotensin-converting enzyme (ACE) inhibitors and angiotensin receptor blockers. The use of thiazide-type diuretics also has been shown to reduce cardiovascular disease risk in the diabetic patients and is usually required as a part of the multidrug therapy necessary to control blood pressure in this patient population.

I. INTRODUCTION

Cardiovascular disease is the main cause of mortality in diabetic patients (1,2). Hypertension is a frequent co-morbid condition with diabetes and is as up to three times as frequent in diabetic patients when compared with nondiabetics (3). Hypertension markedly increases the risk for cardiovascular disease and accounts for up to 80% of excess morbidity and mortality in these patients. Diabetes mellitus is dramatically increasing throughout the world (4). Among people who are ≥60 years, approximately one-third of them have either diabetes or impaired fasting glucose (5). Furthermore, diabetes is the leading cause of end-stage renal disease, nontraumatic amputation, and blindness in western countries (6). Hypertension also greatly increases the risk for microvascular disease in diabetic patients, that is, blindness and end stage nephropathy (7–9).

In type 1 diabetes, there is a close relation between hypertension and diabetic nephropathy (7). However, hypertension in type 2 diabetes has more complex etiology and is part of a constellation of other cardiovascular risk factors: that is, other components of the cardiometabolic syndrome such as central obesity, insulin resistance, dyslipidemia, hypercoagulation, increased inflammatory status, microalbuminuria, and left ventricular hypertrophy (8,9). Rigorous hypertension control should be an integral part of a comprehensive approach involving management of other cardiovascular risk factors. During the last two decades, our understanding of the mechanisms of hypertension, insulin resistance, and diabetic nephropathy has substantially improved and has lead to development of improved therapeutic strategies.

II. EPIDEMIOLOGY OF HYPERTENSION IN THE METABOLIC SYNDROME

As a component of the metabolic syndrome, hypertension is much more prevalent than diabetes. In a recent analysis of data from the Third National Health and Nutrition Examination Survey (NHANES III) (10), involving a representative sample of 8814 adult United States population and using the National Cholesterol Education Panel (NCEP) Adult Treatment Panel III (ATPIII) definition (11) (Table 40.1), the prevalence of hypertension (as defined by blood pressure >130/85 mmHg or the use of antihypertensive medications) was 34.0% compared with only 12.6% of those with hyperglycemia. In this analysis, hypertension was the second most prevalent component of the metabolic syndrome, compared with central obesity, which was the most prevalent component (38.6%). Hypertension was followed in prevalence by low HDL-cholesterol (37.6%), hypertriglyceridemia (30.0%) and diabetes (12.6%) (10). However, it is important to emphasize that although most patients with the metabolic syndrome do not have diabetes, the prevalence of this syndrome in the diabetic population is very high (86%) (12,13). Furthermore, the prevalence of the metabolic syndrome in patients with impaired glucose tolerance (IGT) was 31% and 71% in those with impaired fasting glucose (>110 mmHg) (12,13).

The overall prevalence of the NCEP-defined metabolic syndrome (11) among adults >20 years of age was 24% and was >40% in those >40 years of age (10,12,13). The prevalence among women was 23.4% when compared with 24% for men. However, there were significant racial differences where Mexican-American women had the highest prevalence of 35.6% compared with 22.8% for white women (10). African-American men in this analysis had the lowest prevalence of the metabolic syndrome (16.4%) (10). This could be explained by the use of separate lipid criteria as defined by NCEP (high triglycerides and

Table 40.1 Definitions of the Cardiometabolic Syndrome

WHO	NCEP
Hyperinsulinemia (upper quartile fasting INS of the nondiabetic population) or FPG ≥110 mg/dL (6.1 mmol/L) or 2 h postglucose load of >200 mg/dL (11.1 mmol/L) plus at least two of the following	At least three of the following
(1) Abdominal obesity: waist-to-hip ratio >0.9, BMI ≥30 kg/m^2, or a waist girth ≥94 cm (37 in.)	(1) FPG ≥110 mg/dL(6.1 mmol/L)
(2) Dyslipidemia: serum TG ≥150 mg/dL (1.7 mmol/L) or HDL-C <35 mg/dL (0.9 mmol/L)	(2) Abdominal obesity: waist girth in men >102 cm and in women >88 cm
(3) Hypertension: ≥140/90 mmHg or on medications	(3) Serum TG >150 mg/dL (1.7 mmol/L)
(4) Microalbuminuria: urinary albuminexcretion rate >20 μg/min or albumin to creatinine ratio >30 mg/g	(4) HDL-C: in men <40 m/dL (1 mmol/L) in women <50 mg/dL (1.3 mmol/L)
	(5) Blood pressure ≥130/85 mmHg or on medications

Note: NCEP, The National Cholesterol Education Program: Adult Treatment Panel III (ATPIII); WHO, World Health Organization; FPG, fasting plasma glucose; BMI, body mass index; INS, insulin; TG, triglyceride; HDL-C, high density lipoprotein cholesterol.
Source: Adapted from The National Cholesterol Education Program (NCEP) Adult Treatment Panel III (ATPIII) (11) and Alberti and Zimmet (16).

low HDL-cholesterol), which likely offset the high prevalence of hypertension and hyperglycemia in this ethnic population (10,12). In fact, African-American men had highest prevalence of hypertension, as a component of the metabolic syndrome, of 49.9%, followed by African-American women (43.3%) and Mexican men (40.2%) (10).

Another analysis of NHANES data aiming to evaluate the risk of coronary heart disease, among people >50 years of age with the metabolic syndrome with and without diabetes showed that the overall prevalence of this syndrome is 44% (14). In this analysis, which also used the NCEP definition (Table 40.1) (11), the prevalence of diabetes was 17% for the entire population and 86% for those with the metabolic syndrome (14). Hypertension was almost as twice as common in the diabetic patients with the metabolic syndrome (82.7%), compared with diabetic patients without the syndrome (43%) (14). These data underscores the common occurrence of diabetes and hypertension as components of the metabolic syndrome particularly in older population.

Hypertension was the strongest predictor for the presence of coronary heart disease in patients >50 years of age, followed by low HDL-cholesterol, and diabetes. The odds ratio, 95% confidence interval (95% CI) was 1.87 (1.37–2.56), 1.74 (1.18–2.58) and 1.55 (1.07–2.25) for hypertension, low HDL cholesterol, and diabetes, respectively (14).

A third analysis, from Europe (15), using the World Heath Organization (WHO) definition (16) (Table 40.1), was conducted to evaluate the prevalence and cardiovascular disease risk associated with the metabolic syndrome. In this analysis, a total of 4483 patients, aged 35–70 participating in a large family study of type 2 diabetes in Finland and Sweden [the Botnia study (17)] were

examined. The metabolic syndrome, as defined by the WHO, was present in 10% of those without diabetes compared with 50% of those with IFG/IGT, and 80% of those with diabetes (15). The prevalence of the metabolic syndrome in diabetic patients in this European population, using the WHO definition, was close to that of the United States population using the NCEP criteria (80% vs. 86%, respectively) (14,15). Furthermore, hypertension occurred frequently in those with diabetes (59%), this prevalence increased with age and was 67% in those 60–69 years of age (15). In this study, hypertension was only second to microalbuminuria as the most predictor for cardiovascular disease mortality with relative risk (RR) = 1.78 (1.06–2.91) (95% CI) (15). These data from United States and Europe across different ethnic population using the NCEP or WHO consistently demonstrate the high prevalence of the metabolic syndrome, which is approaching epidemic proportions in the United States and worldwide. These data also demonstrate the frequent occurrence of hypertension and diabetes mellitus as components of the metabolic syndrome conferring high risk for cardiovascular disease in this patient population (10,14,15).

III. METABOLIC AND HEMODYNAMIC CHARACTERISTICS OF HYPERTENSION IN PATIENTS WITH DIABETES AND THE METABOLIC SYNDROME

Hypertensive patients with diabetes, compared with those without diabetes, have unique features such as increased salt sensitivity, volume expansion, loss of nocturnal dipping of blood pressure and pulse, increased propensity to proetinuria and orthostatic hypotension, and isolated systolic hypertension (6). Most of these features are considered risk factors for cardiovascular disease (9) and are particularly important for selecting the appropriate antihypertensive medication, for example, low dose diuretics for treatment volume expansion and ACE inhibitors or angiotensin receptor blockers for proteinuria.

A. Salt Sensitivity and Volume Expansion

Alterations in sodium balance and extracellular fluid volume have heterogeneous effects on blood pressure in both normotensive and hypertensive subjects (18). Increased salt intake does not raise blood pressure in all hypertensive subjects and sensitivity to dietary salt intake is greatest in the elderly, those with diabetes, obesity, renal insufficiency, low renin status, and African-Americans (19,20). Studies demonstrated that salt sensitivity in normotensive subjects is associated with a greater age-related increase in blood pressure (21). This is particularly important to consider in management of hypertension in patients with diabetes, especially elderly persons, because the prevalence of both diabetes and salt sensitivity increases with age. Thus, a decreased salt intake along with other aspects of diet, such as reduced fat and increased potassium, are important to institute in these patients (6).

B. Loss of Nocturnal Decline of Blood Pressure

In normotensive individuals and in most patients with hypertension, there is a reproducible circadian pattern to blood pressure and heart rate during 24 h ambulatory monitoring (22). Typically, the blood pressure is highest, while the patient is awake and lowest during sleep, a pattern called "dipping", in which blood pressure decreases by 10–15%. Patients with loss of nocturnal decline in blood pressure "nondippers" have <10% decline of blood pressure during the night compared with daytime blood pressure values (23). In patients with diabetes, and many of those with the cardiometabolic syndrome, there is a loss of nocturnal dipping as demonstrated by 24 h ambulatory monitoring of blood pressure. This is particularly important since the loss of nocturnal dipping conveys excessive risk for stroke and myocardial infarction. In fact, ambulatory blood pressure has been reported to be superior to office blood pressure in predicting target organ involvement such as left ventricular hypertrophy (24,25). About 30% of myocardial infarctions and 50% of strokes occur between 6:00 a.m. and noon. This is particularly important in deciding the optimal dosing strategies of antihypertensive medications, where drugs that provide consistent and sustained 24 h blood pressure control will be advantageous (26).

C. Microalbuminuria

There is considerable evidence that hypertension in type 1 diabetes is a consequence, rather than a cause of renal disease, and that nephropathy precedes the rise in blood pressure (27). Persistent hypertension in patients with type 1 diabetes is often a manifestation of diabetic nephropathy as indicated by an elevation of the urinary albumin at diagnosis of the disease (27). Both hypertension and nephropathy appear to exacerbate each other. In type 2 diabetes, microalbuminuria is associated with insulin resistance (9), salt sensitivity, loss of nocturnal dipping, and left ventricular hypertrophy (28). Elevated systolic blood pressure is a significant determining factor in the progression of microalbuminuria (29,30). Indeed, there is an increasing evidence that microalbuminuria is an integral component of the metabolic syndrome associated with hypertension (9,28). This concept is important to consider in selecting the pharmacologic therapy for hypertension in patients with diabetes where medications that decrease both proteinuria and blood pressure, such as ACE inhibitors and angiotensin receptor blockers, have evolved as increasingly important tools in reducing the progression of nephropathy in such patients. Further, aggressive blood pressure lowering, often requiring several drugs, is very important in controlling the progressive diabetic renal disease.

D. Isolated Systolic Hypertension

With the progression of atherosclerosis in patients with diabetes, the larger arteries lose elasticity and become rigid and the systolic blood pressure increases disproportionately because the arterial system is incapable of expansion for any given volume of blood ejected from the left ventricle leading to isolated systolic hypertension, which is more common and occurs at a relatively younger age in patients with diabetes (6,31).

E. Orthostatic Hypotension

Pooling of blood in dependent veins during rising from a recumbent position, normally leads to decrease in stroke volume and systolic blood pressure with concomitant increase in systemic vascular resistance, diastolic blood pressure, and heart rate. In patients with diabetes and autonomic dysfunction, excessive venous pooling can cause immediate or delayed orthostatic hypotension, which might cause reduction in cerebral blood flow leading to intermittent lightheadedness, fatigue, unsteady gait, and syncope (32–34). This is important to recognize in patients with diabetes and concomitant hypertension as it has several diagnostic and therapeutic implications, for example, discontinuation of diuretic therapy and volume repletion might be necessary for the treatment of chronic orthostasis. In addition, in the subset of patients with "hyperadrenergic" orthostatic hypertension as manifested by excessive sweating and palpitation, the use of low dose clonidine might be necessary to blunt excess sympathetic response (35). Furthermore, increased propensity for orthostatic hypertension in patients with diabetes renders α adrenergic receptor blockers less desirable and a second-line agents for these patients. In addition, doses of all antihypertensive agents must be titrated more carefully in patients with diabetes who have greater propensity for orthostatic hypertension, while having high supine blood pressures.

IV. PATHOGENESIS OF HYPERTENSION IN DIABETES AND METABOLIC SYNDROME

The relation among hypertension, obesity, insulin resistance, and diabetes is complex. For example, hypertension is considerably more prevalent in diabetic patients than nondiabetics (7,9). Hypertensive patients are 2.5 times more likely to develop in type 2 diabetes than in normotensive counterparts when matched to age, sex, ethnicity, adiposity, level of physical activity, and family history (9,36). The possible reasons for the increased propensity to develop diabetes in persons with essential hypertension have been extensively reviewed (9,36,37). These included an altered skeletal muscle tissue composition (i.e., more fat and less insulin sensitive slow twitch fibers) and decreased blood flow to skeletal muscle tissue, due to vascular hypertrophy, rarefaction, and vasoconstriction (9).

In type 1 diabetes, hypertension is uncommon in the absence of diabetic renal disease. Blood pressure readings start to rise $\sim$3 years after the onset of microalbuminuria (9). In contrast, in Hypertension in Diabetes Study (HDS), 3648 patients recruited for the UKPDS were examined; hypertension has already existed in 39% of newly diagnosed type 2 diabetes cases (38). In these patients, hypertension was associated with other components of the metabolic syndrome such as obesity, elevated triglycerides, and hyperinsulinemia. The prevalence microalbuminuria in this hypertensive group was 24% (38). These findings highlight differences in the pathophysiology of type 1 and type 2 diabetes.

Microalbuminuria is the first clinical sign of diabetic nephropathy. It is not only a risk factor for diabetic nephropathy, but also a risk factor for cardiovascular disease morbidity and mortality in both diabetic and nondiabetic patients (39). Microalbuminuria reflects generalized endothelial cell dysfunction including renal glomeruli (9). Hypertension and diabetic nephropathy

exacerbate each other and contribute to a cycle of progressive hypertension, nephropathy, and cardiovascular disease. Several factors contribute to the increased propensity to develop hypertension and subsequent complications in diabetic patients. Diabetic patients have an increased propensity to sodium retention and volume expansion (40). Increased salt sensitivity in these patients involve multiple mechanisms including hyperglycemia-induced renal sodium reabsorption in the proximal renal tubule (41), hyperinsulinemia, and renal abnormalities in renin–angiotensin–aldosterone system (42). Thus, restriction of salt in the diet of these patients is important in the management of their hypertension.

Essential hypertension, unlike secondary hypertension, is often associated with hyperinsulinemia. For example, in a cross-sectional study, patients with essential hypertension exhibited significantly higher fasting insulin and C-peptide levels and significantly lower glucose/insulin ratios when compared with normotensive subjects. In contrast, no differences were observed between secondary hypertensive and control subjects (43).

Insulin resistance and hyperinsulinemia increase sympathetic activity and associated with renal sodium retention, and predispose to increased vascular resistance (9). Insulin normally enhances vasodilatation and increases muscle blood flow, which facilitates glucose utilization (42–46). This effect is mediated, in part, by nitric oxide (45), as insulin increases endothelial nitric oxide production. Insulin fails to enhance muscle blood flow in both obese and diabetic patients due to decreased ability to stimulate nitric oxide (46). Hyperinsulinemia and insulin resistance do not consistently lead to hypertension. Pima Indians have an increased incidence of obesity, insulin resistance, and hyperinsulinemia, but have a relatively low incidence of hypertension (2). These observations indicate that the relationship between insulin resistance and hypertension is complex and ethnically dependant.

Obesity, especially central obesity, is a risk factor for both hypertension and diabetes (47,48). Central obesity, insulin resistance, hypertension, and diabetic dyslipidemia are parts of the cardiometabolic syndrome (8,9,49–61). There are other abnormalities found in the cardiometabolic syndrome such as microalbuminuria, increased coagulability, impaired fibrinolysis, and active inflammatory status (9). Several definitions of the cardiometabolic syndrome have been recently published (Table 40.1): one by the World Health Organization (WHO) (16) and other by the National Cholesterol Education Program (NCEP)– Third Adult Treatment Panel (ATP III) in the United States (11). Metabolic syndrome is a common disorder, the prevalence in the United States, using NCEP criteria, is 22% (14). The prevalence of this syndrome, as well as that of type 2 diabetes, increases progressively with advancing age (8,9,41).

The etiology of the cardiometabolic syndrome is complex involving genetic and acquired abnormalities (9). Central obesity is a key element in the pathogenesis of this syndrome (Table 40.2). It is characterized by a greater deposition of fat in the upper or central part of the body (visceral fat). Visceral adipocytes are more metabolically active, and insulin-resistant, than peripheral adipocytes (47). They release several cytokines, such as tumor necrosis factor-α (TNF-α) and interleukin-6 (IL-6), that promotes inflammation, dyslipidemia, hypertension, microalbuminuria, abnormal coagulability, and impaired fibrinolysis (47,48).

Lipolysis of the abdominal fat releases free fatty acids, which are substrates for triglycerides production in the liver (46,53,54). The renin–angiotensin system is very active in the central adipocytes (42,54). Furthermore, adipocytes derived peptide hormones have a role in promoting the cardiometabolic syndrome. Leptin levels are high in obese patients, and elevated leptin levels may stimulate the sympathetic nervous system and may contribute to the pathogenesis of hypertension associated with obesity (42,48,55). Adiponectin has anti-inflammatory effects and its levels are low in insulin resistance conditions (48,56,57). Decreased adiponectin levels may be particularly important, given the role of adiponectin in enhancement of insulin mediated vasodilatation and glucose transport activities (48,58). Finally, high concentrations of resistin (an adipocytes-derived peptide) in visceral fat are correlated to both insulin resistances and obesity (59). This peptide in contradistinction to adiponectin inhibits insulin metabolic actions (47,48,58,60).

Table 40.2 Cardiovascular Risk Factors Associated with Visceral Obesity

Essential hypertension
INS resistance/Hyperinsulinemia
Low serum HDL-C levels
High serum triglyceride levels
Increased serum apolipoprotein B levels
Small, dense LDL-C particles
Increased PAI/PA ratio
Increased serum fibrinogen levels
Increased serum C-reactive protein levels
Increased production of TNF-α
Increased production of interleukin-6
Microalbuminuria
Increased blood viscosity
Increased systolic and pulse pressure
Left ventricular hypertrophy
Premature atherosclerosis

Note: HDL-C, High-density lipoprotein cholesterol; LDL-C, low-density lipoprotein cholesterol; INS, insulin; PAI/PA, plasminogen activator inhibitor/plasminogen activator; TNF-α, tumor necrosis factor α.

A. Cardiovascular Effects of Insulin and IGF-1

Insulin is produced only in the pancreas (61). On the other hand, insulin-like growth factor-1 (IGF-1) is an autocrine/paracrine peptide (61–68) produced by endothelial cells (EC) and vascular smooth muscle cells following stimulation by insulin (62,63), angiotensin 2 (62,64), and mechanical stress (66,67). Furthermore, IGF-1 receptors are expressed to a greater extent than insulin receptors in vascular smooth muscle cells (61,62). IGF-1 has many important biological effects on vascular tissue, including maintenance of the normal differentiated vascular smooth muscle cell phenotype (68), glucose transport (69,70), and modulation of vascular tone (62,65,69–82). IGF-1 and insulin attenuate vasoconstriction/enhance relaxation through a phosphatidylinositol 3-kinase (PI3-K) dependent stimulation of vascular nitric oxide synthase (NOS) enzyme (62,69,70,79,81,82) and Na$^+$, K$^+$-ATPase pump activity (62,65,75,81,83,84). In animal models of obesity, insulin resistance, and hypertension, there is accumulating evidence that resistance to PI3-K-signaling by IGF-1 and insulin plays an important role in the pathogenesis of hypertension (62,76,79,85), impaired myocardial function (62,81,85–94), and attenuated glucose transport (68,84,87). Thus, alterations of cardiovascular and skeletal muscle signaling responses may explain the common coexistence of hypertension, insulin resistance, and type 2 diabetes (62,66,71).

Insulin and IGF-1 induce vasorelaxation, in part, by lowering vascular smooth muscle cell intracellular calcium ($[Ca^{2+}]_i$) levels (68,73,75,84) and myosin light chain (MLC) phosphorylation/Ca^{2+} sensitization (73,84). These actions involve activation of both vascular NOS and Na$^+$, K$^+$-ATPase pump activity (65,69–75,78–84). Upon stimulation, the β subunit of the insulin and IGF-1 receptor not only become phosphorylated on various tyrosine sites but also induces phosphorylation of a number of accessory molecules (61), such as insulin receptor substrate-1 (IRS-1), which serves as an important docking site for many kinases and phosphatases. Many insulin and IGF-1 metabolic effects are mediated by PI3-K upon binding to IRS-1 through its regulatory subunit (p85) SH2 domain (61). An important downstream target of IGF-1/insulin-stimulated PI3-K is the serine–threonine kinase, Akt (protein kinase B) (61,74,95,96). Akt interacts through its pleckstrin homology domain with the phospholipids produced by PI3-K. Phosphorylation of Thr^{308} and Ser^{473} of Akt is important for its activation (95,96). Akt is involved in insulin and IGF-1 regulated glucose transport and other cell functions (95–101). A number of studies have demonstrated a critical role for Akt signaling in mediating the vascular actions of IGF-1/insulin (72,78,98–104). Further, we have observed that Ang II inhibits IGF-1 signaling through the PI3-K/Akt pathway result in less NOS/Na$^+$, K$^+$-ATPase activation in vascular smooth muscle cells (80).

We (9,37,41,42,65,72) and others (74,78,82,98,99) have demonstrated that vascular relaxation in response to insulin and IGF-1 signaling is dependent, in part, on EC and vascular smooth muscle cell production of nitric oxide and reductions in vascular smooth muscle cells [Ca^{2+}]$_i$. The nitric oxide/cGMP increase in response to insulin and IGF-1 stimulation results in inhibition of MLC phosphorylation/activation (105) by increasing the activity of the myosin-bound serine/threonine specific phosphatase (MBP) (105–108). This effect of insulin and IGF-1 thus counterbalances the increase in [Ca^{2+}]$_i$ and the Ca^{2+}-MLC sensitization effects mediated by vasoconstrictor agonists such as Ang II (109–112). Accumulating evidence suggests that Ang II may antagonize the vasodilatory actions of insulin/IGF-1 through a Rho A signaling mechanism (109–111). Rho A inactivates MBP (113,114) and directly increases phosphorylation and activation of MLC (110,111). Thus, there appears to be counterbalancing actions between insulin/IGF-1 and Ang II in the modulation of MLC-Ca^{2+} sensitization/vascular tone.

Insulin and IGF-1 also regulates vascular tone by increasing the vascular smooth muscle cell Na$^+$, K$^+$-ATPase pump activity in vascular smooth muscle cells (65,73,75,78), consequently elevating the transmembrane Na$^+$ gradient that drives Ca^{2+} efflux via Na$^+$/Ca^{2+} exchange (65,73,75,83,84). Insulin (83) and IGF-1 (78) increase α catalytic pump subunit messenger RNA levels. However, the extent of catalytic subunit message expression is inadequate to explain the level of increased pump activity (65,75,78,83), suggesting post-translational modifications such as mobilization of α catalytic subunits to the plasma membrane (75,78), increased β docking subunits (75,78,115), and/or alteration of the phosphorylation state of the catalytic subunits (75,78,115). Furthermore, insulin/IGF-1 may indirectly activate the Na$^+$, K$^+$-ATPase pump, as well as MBP, in vascular smooth muscle cells by stimulating vascular smooth muscle cell nitric oxide/cGMP (78,116). Studies from our laboratory (80), as well as others (75), have shown that the PI3-K/Akt signaling pathway is crucial for insulin and IGF-1 stimulation of the Na$^+$, K$^+$-ATPase pump.

B. Rho A and the Vascular Renin–Angiotensin System

An autocrine/paracrine cardiovascular renin–angiotensin system plays a major role in modulating vascular smooth muscle cell contractility (85,117) growth and remodeling (117,118). Ang II inhibits IGF-1/insulin PI3-K signaling (80,91,119–122) and induces vasoconstriction through an AT$_1$ receptor mediated increase in vascular smooth muscle cells [Ca^{2+}]$_i$ and Ca^{2+}-MLC sensitization (111,112). An important mechanism by which insulin and IGF-1 mediate vasodilation is via EC and vascular smooth muscle cell-NOS activation and consequent increases in vascular production of nitric oxide. Insulin induces vascular smooth muscle cell relaxation by activating MBP and by inhibiting Rho A (106,116). GTP-bound Rho A specifically interacts with the 130 kDa subunit of MBP (MBS), which binds to myosin and regulates the catalytic activity of MBP. Pretreatment with insulin prevented vasoconstrictor agonist-mediated increases in activated/membrane-associated Rho A, site-specific phosphorylation of Thr^{695} of MBS, and thus activates MBP (106,122). Pretreatment with an NOS inhibitor or a cGMP antagonist markedly attenuates insulin's inhibitory effect on Rho translocation and restored Rho-kinase activation and site-specific MBS phosphorylation resulting in MBP inactivation (106,122). It has also been reported that a cGMP agonist mimicked insulin's inhibitory effects of insulin via abrogation of vasoagonist-mediated Rho signaling/phosphorylation of MBS, resulting in MBP activation. Lastly, expression of a dominant-negative construct of Rho A decreases basal as well as agonist-induced MBS Thr^{695} phosphorylation and permits insulin activation of MBP (106).

Given the critical role of nitric oxide in mediating IGF-1 (62,73–80,104), insulin (72,78,82–84,106), and induced vasorelaxation, a major mechanism by which IGF-1 promotes relaxation is via inhibition of Rho A membrane translocation/activation via nitric oxide/cGMP signaling. Nitric oxide promotes MBP activation via site-specific dephosphorylation of its regulatory subunit MBS (108,109). In contrast, Ang II activates Rho A in vascular smooth muscle cells through the coupling of the AT$_1$ receptor to heterotrimeric G proteins (123). These observations are in concert with data indicating that Ang II reduces IGF-1 mediated NOS activation in EC (75,84) and vascular smooth muscle cells (78) through inhibition of PI3-KK/Akt signaling (78). As activation of Rho A is also associated with decreased NOS/nitric oxide in vascular smooth muscle cells (124), Ang II may attenuate IGF-1 induced nitric oxide production via its activation of Rho A (110,113,123). This would result in less nitric oxide/cGMP suppression of post-translational Rho A activation (108,130,132) and a consequent feedback loop accentuating the negative impact of Ang II on IGF-1-induced vasorelaxation. Finally, recent observations that Ang II interferes with IGF-1 stimulation of Na$^+$, K$^+$-ATPase pump activity, via effects on the PI3-KK/Akt signaling pathway (78), suggest another mechanism by which Ang II antagonizes the vasorelaxing effects of IGF-1 (Fig. 40.1).

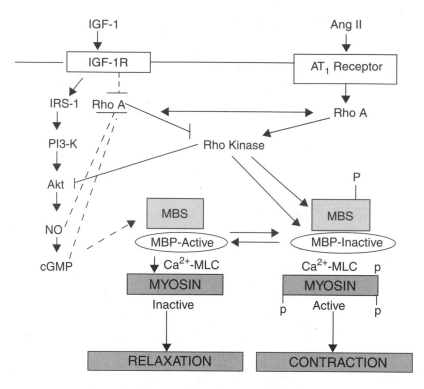

Figure 40.1 Counterregulatory actions of IGF-1 and Ang II in modulation of calcium myosin light chain (MLC) sensitivity. IGF-1 stimulated receptor tyrosine kinase phosphorylates IRS-I, promoting association/activation of PI-3K/Akt and the NO/cGMP pathway, which inactivates Rho A and Rho kinase. This results in enhanced MBP activity and a consequent reduction of Rho-kinase mediated phosphorylation of myosin bound substrate (MBS) is the subunit that binds to myosin and regulates the catalytic activation of MBP. Vascular IGF-1 resistance and/or Ang II overexpression/action is accompanied by enhanced Rho A/Rho-kinase pathway due to impaired activation of Akt and NO/cGMP signaling resulting in reduced MBP activity and higher phosphorylated MBS levels which leads to increased vascular sensitization and contraction.

C. Vascular IGF-1 Resistance and Renin–Angiotensin System Overexpression Impairing of Insulin and IGF-1 Vasorelaxation

Insulin-resistant animal models of hypertension also manifest resistance to the cardiovascular actions of INS/IGF-1 (76–81,87–95,125–131,133). Primary cultured EC (78), and vascular smooth muscle cells (96,97) from insulin/IGF-1 resistant hypertensive rats have decreased insulin and IGF-1 stimulation of NOS related to decreased PI3-K activation. Reduced vascular smooth muscle cells (78,125) and cardiomyocyte (88) glucose transport and associated attenuated PI3-K responses to insulin/IGF-1 have been observed in hypertensive insulin/IGF-1 resistant Zucker obese (ZO) rats. Our laboratory has also reported reduced IGF-1/PI3-K stimulation and reduced NOS expression/activity and glucose transport in vasculature from ZO rats (78,125).

Ang II, like IGF-1, is a pleiotropic autocrine/paracrine peptide, synthesized by vascular smooth muscle cells (117,118) and cardiomyocytes (117). There is increasing

evidence that Ang II is overexpressed in cardiovascular tissue from rodent models of insulin resistant hypertension (91,134–136). Indeed, hyperinsulinemia, as exists in insulin/IGF-1 resistant rodent models (86–88,94,125–127), appears to enhance the renin–angiotensin system in vascular smooth muscle cells (135). In insulin/IGF-1 resistant ZO rats, hypertension is characterized by markedly elevated contractile responses to Ang II (78,86,87,104,136). Collectively, these data suggest that excessive Ang II action in vascular tissue impairs IGF-1 mediated vasorelaxation through Rho A mediated interference with Akt signaling in EC and vascular smooth muscle cells (77,79,103,116,119,120,122).

Like IGF-1 and insulin (107,116,120–123), Ang II modulates vascular smooth muscle cell contraction and relaxation by the phosphorylation/dephosphorylation of MBS, but via a G protein-dependent mechanism (106–113). Vascular smooth muscle cell $[Ca^{2+}]_i$ (regulated by Na^+, K^+-ATPase activity) (78) dynamically controls the relative activity of MBP and MLC and the counterregulatory effects of IGF-I and Ang II (80, 106–125). Further, the Ca^{2+} sensitivity of MLC is also dynamically regulated by insulin/

IGF-1 and Ang II interactions (106–113). Ang II has been shown to interfere with insulin/IGF-1 signaling through the PI3-K pathway (80,98,108,122) resulting in reduced nitric oxide (78–80) and Na^+, K^+-ATPase activity (80–133). Whereas insulin/IGF-1 reduce MBP activity via nitric oxide/cGMP mechanisms (99–108,124), Ang II appears to have opposite effects indirectly via inhibition of IGF-1 stimulation of nitric oxide and directly by activating Rho A (110–113, 123,124). In vasculature in insulin/IGF-1 resistant hypertensive states, there is attenuated insulin and IGF-1 signaling via Akt resulting in reduced NOS/Na^+, K^+-ATPase activation/reduced MBP and impaired relaxation (Fig. 40.1).

V. MANAGEMENT OF HYPERTENSION IN PATIENTS WITH DIABETES

Treatment of hypertension in diabetic patients has two important goals: to decrease the risk of cardiovascular disease morbidity and mortality and to delay, or preferably prevent, the progression of diabetic nephropathy and retinopathy (8). The benefits of tight blood pressure control in diabetic patients are well established (8,48,134,135). However, the two important questions that arise in management of hypertension in diabetic patients are "What level of blood pressure should be the goal of treatment"? And "Which medications should be used, especially in the initial management of these patients?" In recent years, accumulating evidence from large randomized controlled trials provided some answers to these important questions.

The United Kingdom Prospective Diabetes Study (UKPDS) (134) included 1148 hypertensive patients who were followed-up for ~8.4 years. Tight blood pressure control (<140/82 mmHg) compared with less tight control (<180/105 mmHg) was associated with a 24% reduction in diabetic-related end-points, 32% in death related to diabetes, 44% in stroke, and a 37% reduction in microvascular complications (134). Interestingly, the relative benefits of strict blood pressure control outweighed the benefits of tight blood glucose control.

Another major study, the Hypertension Optimal Trial (HOT) demonstrated a 51% reduction in major cardiovascular events in the diabetic subgroup who were randomized to a diastolic blood pressure goal of <80 mmHg compared with a goal of <90 mmHg (135). Other studies reported significant advantages of hypertension treatment in special categories of diabetic patients like the elderly and those with isolated systolic hypertension (136,137). On the basis of the results of these clinical trials and on the data from epidemiological studies which suggested an increase in cardiovascular disease events and mortality with blood pressures >115/75 mmHg (134–139), the currently recommended blood

pressure goal in diabetic patients is now <130/80 mmHg (Fig. 40.2) (139,140).

A. Lifestyle Modifications to Manage Hypertension

Adaptation of a healthy lifestyle is an essential component for managing hypertension in patients with diabetes or the cardiometabolic syndrome (8,40). These interventions include weight loss, dietary sodium reduction, increased aerobic physical activity, cigarette smoking cessation, and moderation of alcohol intake (Table 40.3) (141). The Dietary Approach to Stop Hypertension (DASH) diet when combined with sodium reduction (2300 mg/day) is effective in lowering blood pressure (141). The DASH diet is rich in fiber, potassium, and calcium, low in cholesterol (150 mg/day), and low in total and saturated fat (20% and 6% of daily calories, respectively), with 55% of daily calories comes from carbohydrates.

In addition to lowering blood pressure, weight reduction and increased physical activity improve insulin resistance, serum glucose levels, and lipid profiles (142), Exercise and weight reduction have also been shown to reduce the development of type 2 diabetes in patients with impaired glucose tolerance (143). The protective effects of physical activity have been demonstrated in two prospective cohort studies (144,145) where the development of type 2 diabetes was significantly lower in patients who exercise regularly even after adjustment for obesity, hypertension, and family history of diabetes. In these studies, the reduction in the development of type 2 diabetes was strongest among patients with hypertension, and those with the

Table 40.3 Lifestyle Modification in Management of Hypertension

Modification	Recommendation
Weight reduction	Maintain normal body weight (body mass index $18.5–24.9 kg/m^2$.
Dietary sodium reduction	Not more than 11 mmol/day (2.4 g sodium or 6 g sodium chloride).
Adoption of DASH diet	Foods high in fiber, fruits, vegetables, and low-fat dairy products, with reduced saturated and total fat.
Physical activity	Regular aerobic exercise such as walking 30–45 min at least three times a week.
Reduced alcohol intake	<1 oz. or 30 mL of ethanol (e.g., 24 oz. of beer per day).
Cessation of smoking	Recommended for all smokers.

Note: DASH, Dietary Approaches to Stop Hypertension.
Source: Sowers et al. (41).

highest risk for the development of diabetes (144,145). More recently, the Finnish study and the United States Diabetes Prevention Program (DPP) (146,147) have shown that diet and exercise reduce the risk of development of type 2 diabetes by >50% in high risk patients with glucose intolerance. Therefore, these interventions are highly recommended in patients with hypertension who are at risk for the development of type 2 diabetes.

B. Pharmacological Therapy for Hypertension in Patients with Diabetes

Diet and lifestyle modifications are usually the first step in the management of hypertension, but most patients will also require pharmacological treatment (Fig. 40.2). In fact, most diabetic patients need more than one medication

to maintain their blood pressure within the target range of <130/80 (140). Initiation of therapy with two drugs should be considered if blood pressure is >20/10 mmHg above the goal (i.e., ≥150/90) (140). The optimal goal blood pressure in patients with the cardiometabolic syndrome (without overt diabetes) is not known. However, because these patients are at high risk for cardiovascular disease, it currently appears prudent to treat blood pressure more aggressively than in the general population (i.e., same goal as in type 2 diabetic patients <130/80) (7,9).

1. Thiazide Diuretics

Thiazides are important component of hypertension treatment in almost all hypertension cases. They are

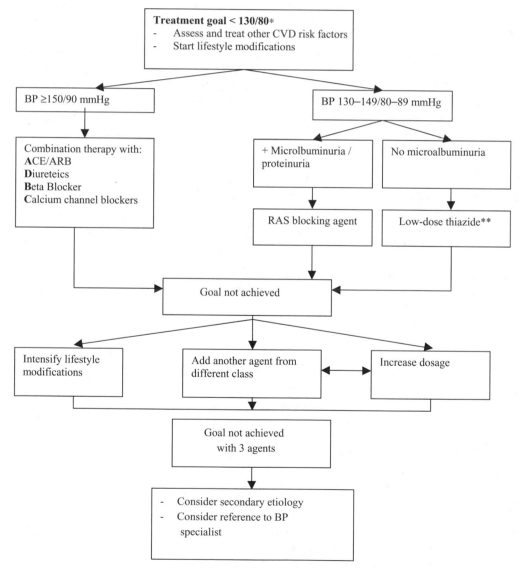

Figure 40.2   Clinical algorithm for hypertension treatment in diabetics. BP, Blood pressure; ARB, Angiotensin receptor blocker. *Goal is 125/75 mmHg in renal insufficiency or proteinuria <1 g/24 h urine. **Not to be used if creatinine is ≥1.8 mg/dL.

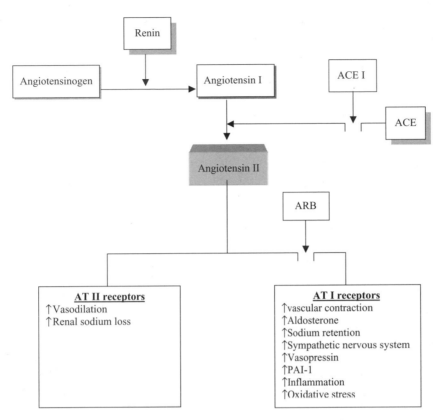

Figure 40.3 Sites of actions of ACE inhibitors and angiotensin receptor blockers. ARB, Angiotensin receptor blocker; PAI-1, Plasminogen activator inhibitor.

inexpensive and effective, especially in treating systolic hypertension (8,148). The Antihypertensive and Lipid Lowering treatment to prevent Heart Attack Trial (ALLHAT) included more than 33000 patients aged ≥ 55 with at least one other coronary heart disease risk factor who were followed up for a mean period of 4.9 years (148). The study showed that there was no difference between chlorthalidone (a thiazide), lisinopril (an ACE inhibitor), and amlodipine (a calcium channel blocker) in preventing major coronary events or in their effects on overall survival. Chlorthalidone was associated with less combined cardiovascular disease, stroke, and better blood pressure control than lisinopril, especially in African-Americans. In addition, Chlorthalidone, however, was associated with less heart failure incidence rate than both lisinopril and amlodipine (148).

The ALLHAT study, the largest hypertension trial to-date, was not designed to prospectively assess the treatment effect in the diabetic patients. However, the diabetic cohort was predesigned for subgroup analysis. About 36% of ALLHAT participants had diabetes (149); the benefits of chlorthalidone were noticed in both diabetic and non-diabetic population, however, for the diabetic patients, several points need to be made in order for the results of the ALLHAT trial to be viewed in the proper context.

First, optimal control of blood pressure in people with diabetes is difficult to achieve and requires multiple medications. Data from our group showed that in a large diabetic cohort with a mean age of 64.5 years (close to ALLHAT 66.6 mean age in the diabetic subgroup), a blood pressure goal of 130/80 was achieved in only 25% of the patients. Furthermore, an average of 3.1 medications was required to achieve such a goal (150). The fact that diabetic patients require multiple antihypertensive medications for blood pressure control is documented in all the major hypertension trials. This fact makes the issue of the initial antihypertensive therapy in people with diabetes less relevant.

Secondly, the study clearly illustrates the importance of lowering blood pressure in order to improve the cardiovascular disease outcome. Therefore, efforts should be directed towards improving blood pressure control that is currently suboptimal (148).

Thirdly, although blood pressure reduction was in favor of the diuretic group, the study did not offer the lack of difference in the primary outcome (fatal coronary heart disease or nonfatal myocardial infarction) among treatment groups. Although ACE inhibitors have been shown to be beneficial in reducing mortality in heart failure patients (149), the observation that diuretic treatment is associated with less incidence of heart failure than ACE inhibitor treatment was largely unexpected and, in this study, the ACE inhibitor group was at disadvantage compared with the diuretic group. This may be explained by the higher blood pressure in the ACE inhibitor group, and in particular African-American subjects who may not respond to ACE inhibitors compared with whites. The efficacy of ACE inhibitors in diabetic nephropathy is well documented. Therefore, it would be of major importance to know the results of the drug comparisons in the diabetic subjects involved in the study.

Fourthly, the ALLHAT with its simple office-based design did not offer information that is particularly relevant for the diabetic population such as the use of antidiabetic agents, glucose control, or microalbuminuria.

Fifthly, it is important to note that thiazide diuretics have been shown to increase insulin resistance (9) and have some adverse metabolic side effects, such as a small increase in serum blood sugar, increased serum triglycerides, increased total cholesterol, increased serum uric acid, hyponatremia, hypokalemia, and hypomagnesaemia. However, all these adverse effects can be minimized by using low doses of thiazides such as 12.5 mg of chlorthalidone or 25 mg of hydrochlorothiazide.

In using diuretics, it is important to avoid volume depletion and orthostatic hypotension. Diabetic patients with autonomic neuropathy, especially elderly people, are more prone to orthostatic hypotension with subsequent risk of falls (9). This is particularly important in elderly diabetic patients who are often on multiple hypertensive medications (32–34).

2. Angiotensin-Converting Enzyme Inhibitors and Angiotensin Receptors Blockers

The renin–angiotensin–aldosterone system is linked to the pathophysiology of various conditions such as hypertension, dyslipidemia, insulin resistance, and inflammation. Angiotensin (Ang) II mainly has two types of receptors. AT I and AT II. AT I receptors are responsible for most of the effects of Ang II including vasoconstriction and aldosterone release (151,152). ACE inhibitors block the conversion of Ang I to Ang II. Angiotensin receptor blockers selectively block the binding of Ang II to (AT1) receptors (Fig. 40.3). ACE is also a kininase, degrading bradykinin to nonactive products, thus ACE inhibitors treatment increases kinins levels (151). Bradykinin is a vasodilator, which might be beneficial for hypertension, as it promotes endothelial production of nitric oxide (9). However, it might be also responsible for the cough that some patients develop while taking ACE inhibitors.

Multiple clinical trials have provided cumulative evidence that using antihypertensive agent that interrupt with the renin–angiotensin system results in beneficial cardiovascular disease and renal outcomes in hypertensive diabetic patients (151,152). For example, the Heart Outcomes Prevention Evaluation (HOPE) study included 3577 diabetic patients who had also at least one other cardiovascular disease risk factor. The participants were randomized to get either ramipril (an ACE inhibitor) or placebo and were followed-up for ~4.5 years. When compared with placebo, ramipril lowered the rates of myocardial infarction, stroke, and all-cause mortality in diabetic patients by 22%, 33%, and 24%, respectively (153). The cardiovascular benefits of an angiotensin receptor blocker (losartan) were compared with a β blocker (atenolol), in the Losartan Intervention For Endpoint reduction (LIFE) study. Losartan in diabetic hypertensive patients with left ventricular hypertrophy lowered the cardiovascular disease mortality and total mortality by 37% and 39%, respectively (154). In the HOPE trial, new onset diabetes was decreased by 35%, and in the LIFE study, new onset diabetes was decreased by 25% of those that began the study without evidence of clinical diabetes (153,154).

Renin–angiotensin–aldosterone system blockade has also been shown to reduce the risk for renal disease and renal disease progression in diabetes (7). In a study conducted in patients with type 1 diabetes and proteinuria, captopril reduced the risk of the combined endpoints of death, dialysis, and renal transplantation by 50% (155). The benefits of ACE inhibitors in renal disease in type 2 appear promising, but there is a need for more investigation (156). On the other hand, several major clinical trials—the Reduction of Endpoints in NIDDM with Angiotensin II Antagonist Losartan (RENAAL) trial (157), the IRbesartan MicroAlbuminuria type II diabetes in hypertension patients (IRMA II) trial (158), the Irbesartan in Diabatic Nephropathy Trial (IDNT) (159), and the Microalbuminuria Reduction with VALsartan (MARVAL) (160) demonstrated the renal protection effects of the angiotensin receptor blockers. Indeed, the mean blood pressure was similar in the placebo and valsaratan treated groups, indicating that angiotensin receptor blockers renal protection effects are independent of blood pressure reduction. In the RENAAL trial, which was done on diabetic patients with impaired renal function (creatinine 1.3–3 mg/dl) and proteinuria, losartan reduced the risk of the primary endpoint [a composite of doubling of serum creatinine, end stage renal disease (ESRD), and death from any cause] by 16%. The risk of doubling of serum creatinine and ESRD was reduced by 25% and 28%, respectively (157). Furthermore, the risk of the first hospitalization for congestive heart failure was reduced by 32%. Treatment with 300 mg irbesartan in IRMA II trial increased regression of microalbuminuria back to values within the normal range by 37% (158). The combination of an ACE inhibitor and an angiotensin receptor blocker in the Candesartan and Lisinopril Microalbuminuria (CALM) trial was associated with significantly more reduction in urinary albumin-to-creatinine ratio (50%) than with either agent alone (24% for candesartan and 39% for lisinopril) (161).

ACE inhibitors are generally well tolerated by patients; they have no adverse effects on lipids or cation metabolism. Clinically, important side effects are cough (up to 15%), hyperkalemia, and rarely angioedema. In patients with underlying renal disease or long standing hypertension, initiation of ACE inhibitor therapy might cause a small increase in scrum creatinine levels, which does not necessitate discontinuation of the agents. If creatinine levels rise to >30% or show progressive increase on repeated measurements, treatment should be stopped and volume status examined carefully (162). Many of these patients will be hypovolumic due to diuretics overtreatment, and with the resumption of more normal volume status, the ACE inhibitors can be safely reinitiated. ACE inhibitors are relatively contraindicated in patients with bilateral renal artery stenosis or unilateral renal stenosis if they have one kidney due to a greater risk of these patients to develope acute renal failure. Angiotensin receptor blockers are very well tolerated, and the incidence rates of cough and angioedema are much lower than those of ACE inhibitor treatment (163,164). Both hyperkalemia and azotemia may be associated with angiotensin receptor blocker, as well as ACE inhibitory therapy. The combination of ACE inhibitors/angiotensin receptor blockers with thiazides helps to minimize the adverse effect on serum potassium levels. The interesting finding from HOPE and LIFE trials suggests that both ACE inhibitors and angiotensin receptor blockers decrease the incidence of new onset diabetes (153,154). Ongoing prospective studies are more definitely evaluating the potential of these agents to lessen the development of clinical diabetes in patients with essential hypertension and others with high risk for developing diabetes.

3. β-Blockers

β-blockers are useful in the treatment of hypertensive diabetic patients with ischemic heart disease. There are some concerns regarding their metabolic adverse effects. In the Atherosclerosis Risk In Communities (ARIC) study, β blockers treatment was associated with 28% increased risk of developing diabetes compared with no-medication group (165). β blockers are a heterogeneous class of medications, having disparate metabolic and hemodynamic properties (165). Both selective β-1 blockers and nonselective β blockers increase insulin resistance. In contrast, vasodilating β blockers may improve insulin action (166). In a study of 45 hypertensive diabetic patients who were treated with either carvedilol or atenolol,

carvedilol was associated with 20% increase in glucose disposal (vs.10% decrease with atenolol), a 20% reduction in serum triglyceride levels (vs. 12% elevation), and an 8% increase in serum HDL cholesterol (vs. 12% decrease with atenolol) (167). Further trials are needed to investigate the potential benefits of vasodilator β blockers in diabetic patients. On the other hand, results from large clinical trials demonstrated the benefits of β-1 selective blockers in diabetic population, particularly in those with coronary heart disease. In the UKPDS study, atenolol was as effective as captopril in reducing microvascular and macrovascular events (168).

4. Calcium Channel Blockers

Calcium channel blockers (CCBs) are generally classified into two classes, dihydropyridines (DHP-CCBs) (e.g., nifedipine and newer agents like amlodipine) and nondihydropyridines (NDHP-CCBs) (e.g., verapamil and diltiazem). Long-acting DHP-CCBs and NDHP-CCBs are safe, effective, and have no adverse effects on serum lipids. They can be added to ACE inhibitors and diuretics in diabetic patients to achieve the blood pressure target of 130/80 mmHg (31). In ALLHAT study, amlodipine had comparable effects to chlorthalidone on coronary heart disease, stroke, and all-cause mortality rate. Interestingly, noncardiovascular mortality rate was significantly lower and renal function was better preserved in amlodipine group (148). The ALLHAT study underscores the value of DHP-CCBs, as one of the antihypertensive drugs that are useful in treating the patients with diabetes and hypertension (31,148).

C. Other Pharmacological Interventions to Treat Cardiovascular Disease Risk Factors

In addition to lifestyle modifications and antihypertensive medications, it is very important to address the other cardiovascular disease risk factors, which are commonly found in hypertensive diabetic population. For example, the degree of hyperglycemia is associated epidemiologically with the incidence of microvascular and macrovascular disease. Controlling blood sugar significantly improves microvascular complications, but effects on macrovascular complications have not been proved (168). On the other hand, statin therapy is highly beneficial for diabetic patients (169,170). The beneficial effects of statins are independent of their classical actions on lipoproteins (171). These effects include reductions in inflammation in the vasculature, kidney, and bone. Potential beneficial effects of these agents also include enhancement of nitric oxide production in vasculature and the kidney. These agents may improve insulin sensitivity and reduce the likelihood of persons progressing from impaired glucose tolerance to type 2 diabetes (171).

The low-density lipoprotein cholesterol (LDL-C) goal in diabetic patient, as generally recognized, is <100 mg/dL (11) or lower. Further, a non-HDL cholesterol of <130 mg/dL, in those with serum triglyceride levels >200 mg/dL is increasingly recognized as an important target goal, as well (11). Diabetes and hypertension associated with high risk for stroke. Using aspirin along with hypertension and lipid treatment significantly reduces the risk (172).

VI. CONCLUSIONS

Diabetes and the cardiometabolic syndrome are rapidly growing public health problems, partly because of increasing obesity and aging in our population. Hypertension is common in diabetic patients and is usually a component of the cardiometabolic syndrome. Treatment of hypertension in those patients is based on therapeutic strategies that have been shown to reduce cardiovascular disease. An effective approach should includes lipid lowering therapy (LDL-C <100 mg/dL), strict blood pressure control (<130/80 mmHg), daily aspirin, and good glycemic control along with adaptation of a healthy diet and lifestyle. Smoking cessation in these patients is a very important lifestyle modification for reducing renal and cardiovascular disease risk. Treatment with antihypertensive medications in patients with diabetes usually requires multiple medications, which should include an agent that modulate renin–angiotensin–aldosterone system. These agents have been shown to reduce cardiovascular disease, and renal disease as well as to improve insulin resistance.

REFERENCES

1. Haffner SM, Lehto S, Ronnemaa T, Pyorala K, Laakso M. Mortality from coronary heart disease in subjects with type 2 diabetes and in nondiabetic subjects with and without prior myocardial infarction. N Engl J Med 1998; 339:229–234.
2. Sowers JR, Lester MA. Diabetes and cardiovascular disease. Diabetes Care 1999; 3:C14–C20.
3. Lehto S, Ronnemaa T, Pyorala K, Laakso M. Predictors of stroke in middle-aged patients with non-INS-dependent diabetes. Stroke 1996; 27:63–68.
4. King H, Aubert RE, Herman WH. Global burden of diabetes, 1995–2025: prevalence, numerical estimates, and projections. Diabetes Care 1998; 21:1414–1431.
5. Harris MI, Flegal KM, Cowie CC, Eberhardt MS, Goldstein DE, Little RR, Wiedmeyer HM, Byrd-Holt DD. Prevalence of diabetes, impaired fasting glucose, and impaired glucose tolerance in U.S. adults. The Third National Health and Nutrition Examination Survey, 1988–1994. Diabetes Care 1998; 21:518–524.
6. Sowers JR, Epstein M, Frohlich ED. Diabetes, hypertension, and cardiovascular disease: an update. Hypertension 2001; 37:1053–1059.
7. Bakris GL, Williams M, Dworkin L, Elliott WJ, Epstein M, Toto R, Tuttle K, Douglas J, Hsueh W, Sowers J. Preserving renal function in adults with hypertension and diabetes: a consensus approach. National Kidney Foundation Hypertension and Diabetes Executive Committees Working Group. Am J Kidney Dis 2000; 36:646–661.
8. Sowers JR, Haffner S. Treatment of cardiovascular and renal risk factors in the diabetic hypertensive. Hypertension 2002; 40:781–788.
9. McFarlane SI, Banerji M, Sowers JR. INS resistance and cardiovascular disease. J Clin Endocrinol Metab 2001; 86:713–718.
10. Ford ES, Giles WH, Dietz WH. Prevalence of the metabolic syndrome among US adults: findings from the Third National Health and Nutrition Examination Survey. J Am Med Assoc 2002; 287:356–359.
11. Third Report of the National Cholesterol Education Program (NCEP) Expert Panel on Detection, Evaluation, and Treatment of High Blood Cholesterol in Adults (Adult Treatment Panel III) final report. National Cholesterol Education Program (NCEP) Expert Panel on Detection, Evaluation, and Treatment of High Blood Cholesterol in Adults (Adult Treatment Panel III). Circulation 2002; 106:3143–3421.
12. Haffner S, Taegtmeyer H. Epidemic obesity and the metabolic syndrome. Circulation 2003; 108:1541–1545.
13. Kereiakes DJ, Willerson JT. Metabolic syndrome epidemic. Circulation 2003; 108:1552–1553.
14. Alexander CM, Landsman PB, Teutsch SM, Haffner SM. NCEP-defined metabolic syndrome, diabetes, and prevalence of coronary heart disease among NHANES III participants age 50 years and older. Diabetes 2003; 52:1210–1214.
15. Isomaa B, Almgren P, Tuomi T, Forsen B, Lahti K, Nissen M, Taskinen MR, Groop L. Cardiovascular morbidity and mortality associated with the metabolic syndrome. Diabetes Care 2001; 24:683–689.
16. Alberti KG, Zimmet PZ. Definition, diagnosis and classification of diabetes mellitus and its complications. Part 1: diagnosis and classification of diabetes mellitus provisional report of a WHO consultation. Diabet Med 1998; 15:539–553.
17. Groop L, Forsblom C, Lehtovirta M, Tuomi T, Karanko S, Nissen M, Ehrnstrom BO, Forsen B, Isomaa B, Snickars B, Taskinen MR. Metabolic consequences of a family history of NIDDM (the Botnia study): evidence for sex-specific parental effects. Diabetes 1996; 45:1585–1593.
18. Semplicini A, Ceolotto G, Massimino M, Valle R, Serena L, De Toni R, Pessina AC, Dal Palu C. Interactions between INS and sodium homeostasis in essential hypertension. Am J Med Sci 1994; 307:S43–S46.

19. Weinberger MH. Salt sensitive human hypertension. Endocr Res 1991; 17:43–51.

20. Luft FC, Miller JZ, Grim CE, Fineberg NS, Christian JC, Daugherty SA, Weinberger MH. Salt sensitivity and resistance of blood pressure. Age and race as factors in physiological responses. Hypertension 1991; 17:I102–I108.

21. Weinberger MH, Fineberg NS. Sodium and volume sensitivity of blood pressure. Age and pressure change over time. Hypertension 1991; 18:67–71.

22. Verdecchia P, Porcellati C, Schillaci G, Borgioni C, Ciucci A, Battistelli M, Guerrieri M, Gatteschi C, Zampi I, Santucci A. Ambulatory blood pressure. An independent predictor of prognosis in essential hypertension. Hypertension 1994; 24:793–801.

23. Nakano S, Kitazawa M, Tsuda S, Himeno M, Makiishi H, Nakagawa A, Kigoshi T, Uchida K. INS resistance is associated with reduced nocturnal falls of blood pressure in normotensive, nonobese type 2 diabetic subjects. Clin Exp Hypertens 2002; 24:65–73.

24. Nielsen FS, Hansen HP, Jacobsen P, Rossing P, Smidt UM, Christensen NJ, Pevet P, Vivien-Roels B, Parving HH. Increased sympathetic activity during sleep and nocturnal hypertension in type 2 diabetic patients with diabetic nephropathy. Diabet Med 1999; 16:555–562.

25. Ohkubo T, Hozawa A, Yamaguchi J, Kikuya M, Ohmori K, Michimata M, Matsubara M, Hashimoto J, Hoshi H, Araki T, Tsuji I, Satoh H, Hisamichi S, Imai Y. Prognostic significance of the nocturnal decline in blood pressure in individuals with and without high 24-h blood pressure: the Ohasama Study. J Hypertens 2002; 20:2183–2189.

26. White WB. A chronotherapeutic approach to the management of hypertension. Am J Hypertens 1996; 9:29S-33S.

27. Arun CS, Stoddart J, Mackin P, MacLeod JM, New JP, Marshall SM. Significance of microalbuminuria in long-duration type 1 diabetes. Diabetes Care 2003; 26:2144–2149.

28. Mitchell TH, Nolan B, Henry M, Cronin C, Baker H, Greely G. Microalbuminuria in patients with non-INS-dependent diabetes mellitus relates to nocturnal systolic blood pressure. Am J Med 1997; 102:531–535.

29. Mogensen CE. Microalbuminuria and hypertension with focus on type 1 and type 2 diabetes. J Intern Med 2003; 254:45–66.

30. Tagle R, Acevedo M, Vidt DG. Microalbuminuria: Is it a valid predictor of cardiovascular risk? Cleve Clin J Med 2003; 70:255–261.

31. McFarlane SI, Farag A, Sowers J. Calcium antagonists in patients with type 2 diabetes and hypertension. Cardiovasc Drug Rev 2003; 21:105–118.

32. Streeten DH, Anderson GH Jr. The role of delayed orthostatic hypotension in the pathogenesis of chronic fatigue. Clin Auton Res 1998; 8:119–124.

33. Streeten DH, Auchincloss JH Jr, Anderson GH Jr, Richardson RL, Thomas FD, Miller JW. Orthostatic hypertension. Pathogenetic studies. Hypertension 1985; 7:196–203.

34. Jacob G, Costa F, Biaggioni I. Spectrum of autonomic cardiovascular neuropathy in diabetes. Diabetes Care 2003; 26:2174–2180.

35. Streeten DH. Pathogenesis of hyperadrenergic orthostatic hypotension. Evidence of disordered venous innervation exclusively in the lower limbs. J Clin Invest 1990; 86:1582–1588.

36. Gress TW, Nieto FJ, Shahar E, Wofford MR, Brancati FL. Hypertension and antihypertensive therapy as risk factors for type 2 diabetes mellitus. Atherosclerosis Risk in Communities Study. N Engl J Med 2000; 342:905–912.

37. Sowers JR, Bakris GL. Antihypertensive therapy and the risk of type 2 diabetes mellitus. N Engl J Med 2000; 342:969–970.

38. Hypertension in Diabetes Study (HDS): I. Prevalence of hypertension in newly presenting type 2 diabetic patients and the association with risk factors for cardiovascular and diabetic complications. J Hypertens 1993; 11:309–317.

39. Mattock MB, Morrish NJ, Viberti G, Keen H, Fitzgerald AP, Jackson G. Prospective study of microalbuminuria as predictor of mortality in NIDDM. Diabetes 1992; 41:736–741.

40. Feldt-Rasmussen B, Mathiesen ER, Deckert T, Giese J, Christensen NJ, Bent-Hansen L, Nielsen MD. Central role for sodium in the pathogenesis of blood pressure changes independent of angiotensin, aldosterone and catecholamines in type 1 (INS-dependent) diabetes mellitus. Diabetologia 1987; 30:610–617.

41. Sowers JR, Sowers PS, Peuler JD. Role of INS resistance and hyperinsulinemia in development of hypertension and atherosclerosis. J Lab Clin Med 1994; 123:647–652.

42. Sowers JR. Effects of INS and IGF-I on vascular smooth muscle glucose and cation metabolism. Diabetes1996; 45:S47–S51.

43. Sechi LA, Melis A, Tedde R. INS hypersecretion: a distinctive feature between essential and secondary hypertension. Metabolism 1992; 41:1261–1266.

44. Frohlich ED. INS and INS resistance: impact on blood pressure and cardiovascular disease. Med Clin North Am 2004; 88:63–82.

45. Steinberg HO, Brechtel G, Johnson A, Fineberg N, Baron AD. INS-mediated skeletal muscle vasodilation is nitric oxide dependent. A novel action of INS to increase nitric oxide release. J Clin Invest 1994; 94:1172–1179.

46. Steinberg HO, Chaker H, Leaming R, Johnson A, Brechtel G, Baron AD. Obesity/INS resistance is associated with endothelial dysfunction. Implications for the syndrome of INS resistance. J Clin Invest 1996; 97:2601–2610.

47. Sowers JR. Obesity and cardiovascular disease. Clin Chem 1998; 44:1821–1825.

48. Sowers JR. Obesity as a cardiovascular risk factor. Am J Med 2003; 115:375–415.

49. El-Atat F, Aneja A, McFarlane S, Sowers JR. Obesity and hypertension. Endocrinol Metab Clin North Amer 2003; 32:823–854.

50. Jensen MD, Haymond MW, Rizza RA, Cryer PE, Miles JM. Influence of body fat distribution on free fatty acid metabolism in obesity. J Clin Invest 1989; 83:1168–1173.

51. Janke J, Engeli S, Gorzelniak K, Luft FC, Sharma AM. Mature adipocytes inhibit *in vitro* differentiation of human preadipocytes via angiotensin type 1 receptors. Diabetes 2002; 51:1699–1707.

52. Hall JE, Hildebrandt DA, Kuo J. Obesity hypertension: role of leptin and sympathetic nervous system. Am J Hypertens 2001; 14:103S–115S.

53. Weyer C, Funahashi T, Tanaka S, Hotta K, Matsuzawa Y, Pratley RE, Tataranni PA. Hypoadiponectinemia in obesity and type 2 diabetes: close association with INS resistance and hyperinsulinemia. J Clin Endocrinol Metab 2001; 86:1930–1935.

54. Ouchi N, Kihara S, Funahashi T, Nakamura T, Nishida M, Kumada M, Okamoto Y, Ohashi K, Nagaretani H, Kishida K, Nishizawa H, Maeda N, Kobayashi H, Hiraoka H, Matsuzawa Y. Reciprocal association of C-reactive protein with adiponectin in blood stream and adipose tissue. Circulation 2003; 107:671–674.

55. Shuldiner AR, Yang R, Gong DW. Resistin, obesity and INS resistance—the emerging role of the adipocyte as an endocrine organ. N Engl J Med 2001; 345:1345–1346.

56. Sowers JR, Ferdinand KC, Bakris GL, Douglas JG. Hypertension-related disease in African Americans. Factors underlying disparities in illness and its outcome. Postgrad Med 2002; 112:24–26.

57. Sowers JR. Diabetic nephropathy and concomitant hypertension: a review of recent ADA recommendations. Am J Clin Proc 2002; 3:27–33.

58. LeRoith D. INS-like growth factors. N Engl J Med 1998; 336:633–640.

59. Sowers J. INS and INS-like growth factor in normal and pathological cardiovascular physiology. Hypertension 1997; 29:691–699.

60. Standley PR, Zhang F, Sowers JR. IGF-1 regulation of Na + -K + -ATPase in rat arterial smooth muscle. Am J Physiol 1997; 273:E113–E121.

61. Standley PR, Obards TJ, Martina CL. Cyclic stretch regulates autocrine IGF-1 in vascular smooth muscle cells: implications in vascular hyperplasia. Am J Physiol 1999; 276:E697–E705.

62. Hayashi K, Saga H, Chimori Y, Kimura K, Yamanaka Y, Sobue K. Differentiated phenotype of smooth muscle cells depends on signaling pathways through INS-like growth factor and phosphatidylinositol 3-kinase. J Biol Chem 1998; 273:28860–28867.

63. Sowers J. Effects of INS and IGF-1 on vascular smooth muscle glucose and cation metabolism. Diabetes 1996; 45:S47-S51.

64. Walsh MF, Barazi M, Sowers JR. IGF-1 diminishes *in vivo* and *in vitro* vascular contractility: role of vascular nitric oxide. Endocrinology 1996; 137:1798–1803.

65. Muniyappa R, Walsh MF, Sowers JR. INS-like growth factor-1 increases vascular smooth muscle nitric oxide production. Life Sci 1997; 61:925–933.

66. Wu HY, Jeng YY, Hsueh WA. Endothelial-dependent vascular effects of INS and INS-like growth factor I in the perfused rat mesenteric artery and aortic ring. Diabetes 1994; 43:1027–1032.

67. Zeng G, Nystrom FH, Quon MJ. Roles for INS receptor, PI3-kinase and Akt in INS-signaling pathways related to production of nitric oxide in human vascular endothelialc cells. Circulation 2000; 101:1539–1545.

68. Sowers J. INS and INS-like growth factor-1 effects on CA2+ and nitric oxide in diabetes. In: Levin ER, Nadler JL, eds. Endocrinology of Cardiovascular Function Boston, MA: Kluwer Academic Publishers, 1998:139–158.

69. Hasdai D, Rizza RA, Holmes DR Jr, Richardson DM, Cohen P, Lerman A. INS and INS-like growth factor-1 cause coronary vasorelaxation *in vitro*. Hypertension 1998; 32:228–234.

70. Li D, Sweeney G, Wang Q, Klip A. Participation of PI3K and atypical PKC in Na+, K+-pump stimulation by IGF-1 in VSMC. Am J Physiol 1999; 276:H2109–H2116.

71. Inishi Y, Katoh T, Okada T. Modulation of renal hemodynamics by IGF-1 is absent in spontaneously hypertensive rats. Kidney Int 1997; 52:165–170.

72. Isenovic ER, Muniyappa R, Sowers JR. Role of PI3-kinase in isoproterenol and IGF-1 induced ecNOS activity. Biochem Biophys Res Commun 2001; 285:954–958.

73. Walsh MF, Ali S. Sowers JR. Vascular INS/INS-like growth factor-1 resistance in female obese Zucker rats. Metabolism 2001; 50:607–612.

74. Vecchione C, Colella S, Fratta L, Gentile MT, Selvetella G, Frati G, Trimarco B, Lembo G. Impaired INS-like growth factor-1 vasorelaxant effects in hypertension. Hypertension 2001; 37:1480–1485.

75. Isenovic ER, Jacobs DB, Kedees MH, Sha Q, Milivojevic N, Kawakami K, Gick G, Sowers JR. Angiotensin II regulation of the Na+ pump involves the phosphatidylinositol-3 kinase and p42/44 mitogen-activated protein kinase signaling pathways in vascular smooth muscle cells. Endocrinology 2004; 145:1151–1160.

76. Sowers JR. INS resistance and hypertension. Am J Physiol Heart Circ Physiol 2004; 286:H1597–H1602.

77. Zeng G, Quon MJ. INS-stimulated production of nitric oxide is inhibited by wortmannin. Direct measurement in vascular endothelial cells. J Clin Invest 1996; 98:894–898.

78. Tirupattur PR, Ram JL, Standley PR, Sowers JR. Regulation of Na +,K(+)-ATPase gene expression by INS in vascular smooth muscle cells. Am J Hypertens 1993; 6:626–629.

79. Sowers JR, Draznin B. INS, cation metabolism and INS resistance. J Basic Clin Physiol Pharmacol 1998; 9:223–233.

80. Sowers JR. Recommendations for special populations: diabetes mellitus and the metabolic syndrome. Am J Hypertens 2003; 16:41S–45S.

81. Zemel MB, Peuler JD, Sowers JR. Hypertension in INS-resistant Zucker obese rats is independent of neural support. Am J Physiol 1992; 262:E368–E371.

82. Henriksen EJ, Jacob S, Kinnick TR, Teachey MK, Krekler M. Selective angiotensin II receptor antagonism reduces INS resistance in obese Zucker rats. Hypertension 2001; 38:884–890.

83. Ouchi Y, Han SZ, Kim S, Akishita M, Kozaki K, Toba K, Orimo H. Augmented contractile function and abnormal Ca^{2+} handling in the aorta of Zucker obese rats with INS resistance. Diabetes 1996; 45:S55–S58.

84. Kolter T, Uphues I, Eckel J. Molecular analysis of INS-resistance in isolated ventricular cardiomyocytes of obese Zucker rats. Am J Physiol 1997; 36:E59–E67.

85. Ren J, Walsh MF, Sowers JR. Altered inotrophic response to IGF-1 in diabetic rat heart: influence of intracellular Ca^{2+} and NO. Am J Physiol 1998; 275:H823–H830.

86. Leri A, Liu Y, Wang X, Kajstura J, Malhotra A, Meggs LG, Anversa P. Overexpression of INS-like growth factor-1 attenuates the myocyte renin-angiotensin system in transgenic mice. Circ Res 1999; 84:752–762.

87. Ren J, Jefferson L, Sowers JR. Influence of age on contractile response to INS-like growth factor 1 in ventricular myocytes from spontaneously hypertensive rats. Hypertension 1999; 34:1215–1222.

88. Ren J, Samson WK, Sowers JR. INS-like growth factor I as a cardiac hormone: physiological and pathophysiological implications in heart disease. J Mol Cell Cardiol 1999; 31:2049–2061.

89. Ren J, Sowers JR, Walsh MF, Brown RA. Reduced contractile response to INS and IGF-I in ventricular myocytes from genetically obese Zucker rats. Am J Physiol 2000; 279:H1708–H1714.

90. Hemmings BA. Akt signaling: linking membrane events to life and death situations. Science 1997; 275:628–630.

91. Somwar R, Srimlani S, Klip A. Temporal activation of p70 S6 kinase and Akt1 by INS: PI3-kinase dependent and −independent mechanisms. Am J Physiol 1998; 38:E618–E625.

92. Begum N, Ragolia L, Rienzie J, McCarthy M, Duddy N. Regulation of mitogen-activated protein kinase phosphatase-1 induction by INS in vascular smooth muscle cells. J Biol Chem 1998; 273:25164–25170.

93. Kaliman P, Canicio J, Testar X, Palacin M, Zorzano A. INS-like growth factor II, phosphatidylinositol 3-kinase, nuclear factor-KB and inducible nitric oxide synthase define a common myogenic signaling pathway. J Biol Chem 1999; 274:17437–17444.

94. Dimmeler S, Fleming I, Fisslthaler B, Hermann C, Busse R, Zeiher AM. Activation of nitric oxide synthase in endothelial cells by Akt-dependent phosphorylation. Nature 1999; 399:601–605.

95. Luo Z, Fujio Y, Kureishi Y, Rudic RD, Daumerie G, Fulton D, Sessa WC, Walsh K. Acute modulation of endothelial Akt/PKB activity alters nitric oxide-dependent vasomotor activity in vivo. J Clin Invest 2000; 106:493–499.

96. Hermann C, Assmus B, Urbich C, Zeiher AM, Dimmeler S. INS-mediated stimulation of protein kinase Akt: a potent survival signaling cascade for endothelial cells. Arterioscler Thromb Vasc Biol 2000; 20:402–409.

97. Begum N, Song Y, Rienzie J, Ragolia L. Vascular smooth muscle cell growth and INS regulation of mitogen-activated protein kinase in hypertension. Am J Physiol 1998; 275:C42-C49.

98. Velloso LA, Folli F, Sun XJ, White MF, Saad MJ, Kahn CR. Cross-talk between the INS and angiotensin signaling systems. Proc Natl Acad Sci USA 1996; 93:12490–12495.

99. Isenovic ER, Divald A, Milivojevic N, Grgurevic T, Fisher SE, Sowers JR. Interactive effects of insulin-like growth factor-1 and beta-estradiol on endothelial nitric oxide synthase activity in rat aortic endothelial cells. Metabolism 2003; 52:482–487.

100. Lee MR, Li L, Kitazawa T. cGMP causes Ca^{2+} desensitization in vascular smooth muscle cells by activating the myosin light chain phosphatase. J Biol Chem 1997; 272:5063–5068.

101. Begum N, Duddy N, Sandu O, Reinzie J, Ragolia L. Regulation of myosin bound protein phosphatase by INS in vascular smooth muscle cells. Evaluation of the role of Rho kinase and PI3-kinase dependent signaling pathways. Mol Endocrinol 2000; 14:1365–1376.

102. Surks HK, Mochizuki N, Kasai Y, Georgescu SP, Tang KM, Ito M, Lincoln TM, Mendelsohn ME. Regulation of myosin phosphatase by a specific interaction with cGMP-dependent protein kinase 1α. Science 1999; 286:1583–1587.

103. Sauzeau V, Le Jeune H, Cario-Toumaniantz C, Smolenski A, Lohmann SM, Bertoglio J, Chardin P, Pacaud P, Loirand G. Cyclic GMP-dependent protein kinase signaling pathway inhibits RhoA-induced Ca2+ sensitization of contraction in vascular smooth muscle. J Biol Chem 2000; 275:21722–21729.

104. Kimura K, Ito M, Amano M, Chihara K, Fukata Y, Nakafuku M, Yamamori B, Feng J, Nakano T, Okawa K, Iwamatsu A, Kaibuchi K. Regulation of myosin phosphatase by Rho and Rho-associated kinase (Rho-kinase). Science 1996; 273:245–248.

105. Uehata M, Ishizaki T, Satoh H, Ono T, Kawahara T, Morishita T, Tamakawa H, Yamagami K, Inui J, Maekawa M, Narumiya S. Calcium sensitization of smooth muscle mediated by a Rho-associated protein kinase in hypertension. Nature 1997; 389:990–994.

106. Yamakawa T, Tanaka A, Inagami T. Involvement of Rho-kinase in angiotensin II-induced hypertrophy of vascular smooth muscle cells. Hypertension 2000; 35:313–318.

107. Kitazawa T, Eto M, Woodsome TP, Brautigan DL. Agonists trigger G protein-mediated activation of the CPI-17 inhibitor phosphoprotein of myosin light chain phosphatase to enhance vascular smooth muscle contractility. J Biol Chem 2000; 275:9897–9900.

108. Kawano Y, Fukata Y, Oshiro N, Amano M, Nakamura T, Ito M, Matsumura F, Inagaki M, Kaibuchi K. Phosphorylation of myosin-binding subunit (MBS) of myosin phosphatase by Rho-kinase in vivo. J Cell Biol 1999; 147:1023–1038.

109. Feng J, Ito M, Ichikawa K, Isaka N, Nishikawa M, Hartshorne DJ, Nakano T. Inhibitory phosphorylation site for Rho-associated kinase on smooth

muscle myosin phosphatase. J Biol Chem 1999; 274:37385–37390.

110. Chibalin AV, Kovalenko MV, Ryder JW, Feraille E, Wallberg-Henriksson H, Zierath JR. INS- and glucose-induced phosphorylation of the Na(+), K(+)-adenosine triphosphatase α-subunits in rat skeletal muscle. Endocrinology 2001; 42:3474–3482.

111. Sandu OA, Ito M, Begum N. Selected Contribution: INS utilizes NO/cGMP pathway to activate myosin phosphatase via Rho inhibition in vascular smooth muscle. J Appl Physiol 2001; 91:1475–1482.

112. Berk B, Duff J, Marrero M. Angiotensin II signal transduction in vascular smooth muscle. In: Sowers JR, ed. Endocrinology of the Vasculature, NJ: Humana press, 1996:187–204.

113. Dzau VJ. Tissue angiotensin and pathobiology of vascular disease: a unifying hypothesis. Hypertension 2001; 37:1047–1052.

114. Kureishi Y, Kobayashi S, Amano M, Kimura K, Kanaide H, Nakano T, Kaibuchi K, Ito M. Rho-associated kinase directly induces smooth muscle contraction through myosin light chain phosphorylation. J Biol Chem 1997; 272:1257–1260.

115. Folli F, Kahn CR, Hansen H, Bouchie JL, Feener EP. Angiotensin II inhibits INS signaling in aortic smooth muscle cells at multiple levels. J Clin Invest 1997; 100:2158–2169.

116. Clark EA, King WG, Brugge JS, Symons M, Hynes RO. Integrin-mediated signals regulated by members of the Rho family of GTPases. J Cell Biol 1998; 142:573–586.

117. Sandu O, Ragolia L, Begum N. Diabetes in the Goto–Kakizaki rat is accompanied by impaired INS-mediated myosin-bound phosphatase activation and vascular smooth muscle cell relaxation. Diabetes 2000; 49:2178–2189.

118. Gohla, A Schultz G, Offermanns S. Role for G12/G13 in agonist-induced vascular smooth muscle cell contraction. Circ Res 2000; 87:221–227.

119. Muniyappa R, Ram JL, Sowers JR. Inhibition of Rho protein stimulates iNOS expression in rat vascular smooth muscle cells. Am J Physiol 2000; 278:H1762-H1768.

120. Standley PR, Rose K, Sowers JR. Increased basal arterial smooth muscle glucose transport in the Zucker rat. Am J Hypertens 1995; 8:48–52.

121. Jacob RJ, Sherwin RS, Greenawalt K, Shulman GI. Simultaneous insulinlike growth factor I and insulin resistance in obese Zucker rats. Diabetes 1992; 41:691–697.

122. Jiang ZY, Lin YW, Clemont A, Feener EP, Hein KD, Igarashi M, Yamauchi T, White MF, King GL. Characterization of selective resistance to INS signaling in the vasculature of obese Zucker (fa/fa) rats. J Clin Invest 1999; 104:447–457.

123. Muniyappa R, Ram J, Walsh MF, Sowers JR. Calcium and protein kinase C mediate high glucose-induced inhibition of inducible nitric oxide synthase in vascular smooth muscle cells. Hypertension 1998; 31:289–295.

124. Bermann MA, Walsh MF, Sowers JR. Angiotensin-II biochemistry and physiology: update on angiotensin-II receptor blockers. Cardiovas Drug Rev 1997; 15:75–100.

125. Goalstone ML, Nadler J, Sowers JR, Draznin B. INS potentiates platelet derived growth factor action in vascular smooth muscle cells. Endocrinology 1998; 139:4067–4072.

126. Draznin B, Olefsky J, Accili D, McClain D. Effects of INS on prenylation as a mechanism of potentially detrimental influence of hyperinsulinemia. Endocrinology 2000; 141:1310–1316.

127. Finder JD, Litz JL. Sebte SM. Inhibition of protein geranylgeranylation causes a superinduction of nitric oxide synthase-2 by interleukin-1 β in vascular smooth muscle cells. J Biol Chem 1997; 272:13484–13488.

128. Ferrer-Martinez A, Felipe A, Casado E. Differential regulation of the Na(+)-K(+)-ATPase in the obese Zucker rat. Am J Physiol 1996; 271:R1123–R1129.

129. Matsubara H, Kanasaki M, Murasawa S, Tsukaguchi Y, Nio Y, Inada M. Differential gene expression and regulation of angiotensin II receptor subtypes in rat fibroblasts and cardiomyocytes. J Clin Invest 1994; 93:1592–1601.

130. Kamide K, Hori MT, Tuck ML. INS-mediated growth in aortic smooth muscle and the vascular renin angiotensin system. Hypertension 1998; 32:482–487.

131. Alonso-Garcia M, Brands MN, Hall J. Hypertension in obese Zucker rats: role of angiotensin II and adrenergic activity. Hypertension 1996; 28:1047–1054.

132. Peuler JD, Johnson BA, Sowers JR. Sex-specific effects of an INS secretagogue in stroke-prone hypertensive rats. Hypertension 1993; 22:214–220.

133. Vesely DL, Gower WR, Farese RV. Elevated atrial natriuretic peptides and early renal failure in type 2 diabetic Goto–Kakizaki rats. Metabolism 1999; 48:771–778.

134. UK Prospective DiabetesStudy Group. Tight blood pressure control and risk of macrovascular and microvascular complications in type 2 diabetes: UKPDS 38. Brit Med J 1998; 317:703–713.

135. Hansson L, Zanchetti A, Carruthers SG, Dahlof B, Elmfeldt D, Julius S, Menard J, Rahn KH, Wedel H, Westerling S. Effects of intensive blood-pressure lowering and low-dose aspirin in patients with hypertension: principal results of the Hypertension Optimal Treatment (HOT) randomised trial. HOT Study Group. Lancet 1998; 351:1755–1762.

136. Tuomilehto J, Rastenyte D, Birkenhager WH, Thijs L, Antikainen R, Bulpitt CJ,Fletcher AE, Forette F, Goldhaber A, Palatini P, Sarti C, Fagard R. Effects of calcium-channel blockade in older patients with diabetes and systolic hypertension. Systolic Hypertension in Europe Trial Investigators. N Engl J Med 1999; 340:677–684.

137. Curb JD, Pressel SL, Cutler JA, Savage PJ, Applegate WB, Black H, Camel G, Davis BR, Frost PH, Gonzalez N, Guthrie G, Oberman A, Rutan GH, Stamler J. Effect of diuretic-based antihypertensive treatment on cardiovascular disease risk in older diabetic patients with isolated systolic hypertension. Systolic Hypertension in

the Elderly Program Cooperative Research Group. J Am Med Assoc 1996; 276:1886–1892.

138. Lewington S, Clarke R, Qizilbash N, Peto R, Collins R. Prospective Studies Collaboration. Age-specific relevance of usual blood pressure to vascular mortality: a meta-analysis of individual data for one million adults in 61 prospective studies. Lancet 2002; 360:1903–1913.

139. Arauz-Pacheco C, Parrott MA, Raskin P. American Diabetes Association. Treatment of hypertension in adults with diabetes. Diabetes Care 2003; 26:S80–S82.

140. Chobanian AV, Bakris GL, Black HR, Cushman WC, Green LA, Izzo JL Jr, Jones DW, Materson BJ, Oparil S, Wright JT Jr, Roccella EJ. National Heart, Lung, and Blood Institute Joint National Committee on Prevention, Detection, Evaluation, and Treatment of High Blood Pressure; National High Blood Pressure Education Program Coordinating Committee. The Seventh Report of the Joint National Committee on Prevention, Detection, Evaluation, and Treatment of High Blood Pressure: the JNC 7 report. J Am Med Assoc 2003; 289:2560–2572.

141. Sacks FM, Svetkey LP, Vollmer WM, Appel LJ, Bray GA, Harsha D, Obarzanek E, Conlin PR, Miller ER III, Simons-Morton DG, Karanja N, Lin PH. DASH-Sodium Collaborative Research Group. Effects on blood pressure of reduced dietary sodium and the Dietary Approaches to Stop Hypertension (DASH) diet. DASH-Sodium Collaborative Research Group. N Engl J Med 2001; 344:3–10.

142. Clinical Guidelines on the Identification, Evaluation, and Treatment of Overweight and Obesity in Adults—The Evidence Report. National Institutes of Health. Obes Res 1998; 6:51S–209S.

143. McFarlane SI, Shin JJ, Rundek T, Bigger JT. Prevention of type 2 diabetes. Curr Diab Rep 2003; 3:235–241.

144. Eriksson KF, Lindgarde F. Prevention of type 2 (non-INS-dependent) diabetes mellitus by diet and physical exercise. The 6-year Malmo feasibility study. Diabetologia 1991; 34:891–898.

145. Helmrich SP, Ragland DR, Leung RW, Paffenbarger RS Jr. Physical activity and reduced occurrence of non-INS-dependent diabetes mellitus. N Engl J Med 1991; 325:147–152.

146. Tuomilehto J, Lindstrom J, Eriksson JG, Valle TT, Hamalainen H, Ilanne-Parikka P, Keinanen-Kiukaanniemi S, Laakso M, Louheranta A, Rastas M, Salminen V, Uusitupa M; Finnish Diabetes Prevention Study Group. Prevention of type 2 diabetes mellitus by changes in lifestyle among subjects with impaired glucose tolerance. N Engl J Med 2001; 344:1343–1350.

147. Knowler WC, Barrett-Connor E, Fowler SE, Hamman RF, Lachin JM, Walker EA, Nathan DM; Diabetes Prevention Program Research Group. Reduction in the incidence of type 2 diabetes with lifestyle intervention or metformin. N Engl J Med 2002; 346:393–403.

148. ALLHAT Officers and Coordinators for the ALLHAT Collaborative Research Group. The Antihypertensive and Lipid-Lowering Treatment to Prevent Heart Attack Trial. Major outcomes in high-risk hypertensive patients randomized to angiotensin-converting enzyme inhibitor or calcium channel blocker vs diuretic: The Antihypertensive and Lipid-Lowering Treatment to Prevent Heart Attack Trial (ALLHAT). J Am Med Assoc 2002; 288:2981–2997.

149. Barzilay JI, Jones CL, Davis BR, Basile JN, Goff DC Jr, Ciocon JO, Sweeney ME, Randall OS; Antihypertensive and Lipid-Lowering Treatment to Prevent Heart Attack Trial (ALLHAT). ALLHAT Collaborative Research Group. Baseline characteristics of the diabetic participants in the Antihypertensive and Lipid-Lowering Treatment to Prevent Heart Attack Trial (ALLHAT). Diabetes Care 2001; 24:654–658.

150. McFarlane SI, Jacober SJ, Winer N, Kaur J, Castro JP, Wui MA, Gliwa A, Von Gizycki H, Sowers JR. Control of cardiovascular risk factors in patients with diabetes and hypertension at urban academic medical centers. Diabetes Care 2002; 25:718–723.

151. McFarlane SI, Kumar A, Sowers JR. Mechanisms by which angiotensin-converting enzyme inhibitors prevent diabetes and cardiovascular disease. Am J Cardiol 2003; 91:30H-37H.

152. Privratsky JR, Wold LE, Sowers JR, Quinn MT, Ren J. AT1 blockade prevents glucose-induced cardiac dysfunction in ventricular myocytes: role of the AT1 receptor and NADPH oxidase. Hypertension 2003; 42:206–212.

153. Heart Outcomes Prevention Evaluation Study Investigators. Effects of ramipril on cardiovascular and microvascular outcomes in people with diabetes mellitus: results of the HOPE study and MICRO-HOPE substudy. Lancet 2000; 355:253–259.

154. Lindholm LH, Ibsen H, Dahlof B, Devereux RB, Beevers G, de Faire U, Fyhrquist F, Julius S, Kjeldsen SE, Kristiansson K, Lederballe-Pedersen O, Nieminen MS, Omvik P, Oparil S, Wedel H, Aurup P, Edelman J, Snapinn S. LIFE Study Group. Cardiovascular morbidity and mortality in patients with diabetes in the Losartan Intervention For Endpoint reduction in hypertension study (LIFE): a randomised trial against atenolol. Lancet 2002; 359:1004–1010.

155. Lewis EJ, Hunsicker LG, Bain RP, Rohde RD. The effect of angiotensin-converting-enzyme inhibition on diabetic nephropathy. The Collaborative Study Group. N Engl J Med 1993; 329:1456–1462.

156. Bakris GL, Weir M. ACE inhibitors and protection against kidney disease progression in patients with type 2 diabetes: what's the evidence. J Clin Hypertens (Greenwich) 2002; 4:420–423.

157. Brenner BM, Cooper ME, de Zeeuw D, Keane WF, Mitch WE, Parving HH, Remuzzi G, Snapinn SM, Zhang Z, Shahinfar S. RENAAL Study Investigators. Effects of losartan on renal and cardiovascular outcomes in patients with type 2 diabetes and nephropathy. N Engl J Med 2001; 345:861–869.

158. Parving HH, Lehnert H, Brochner-Mortensen J, Gomis R, Andersen S, Arner P. Irbesartan in Patients with Type 2 Diabetes and Microalbuminuria Study Group. The effect of irbesartan on the development of diabetic nephropathy in patients with type 2 diabetes. N Engl J Med 2001; 345:870–878.

159. Lewis EJ, Hunsicker LG, Clarke WR, Berl T, Pohl MA, Lewis JB, Ritz E, Atkins RC, Rohde R, Raz I. Collaborative Study Group. effect of the angiotensin-receptor antagonist irbesartan in patients with nephropathy due to type 2 diabetes. N Engl J Med 2001; 345:851–860.

160. Viberti G, Wheeldon NM. MicroAlbuminuria Reduction with VALsartan (MARVAL) Study Investigators. Microalbuminuria reduction with valsartan in patients with type 2 diabetes mellitus: a blood pressure-independent effect. Circulation 2002; 106:672–678.

161. Mogensen CE, Neldam S, Tikkanen I, Oren S, Viskoper R, Watts RW, Cooper ME. Randomized controlled trial of dual blockade of renin–angiotensin system in patients with hypertension, microalbuminuria, and non-INS dependent diabetes: the candesartan and lisinopril microalbuminuria (CALM) study. Brit Med J 2000; 321:1440–1444.

162. Palmer BF. Renal dysfunction complicating the treatment of hypertension. N Engl J Med 2002; 347:1256–1261.

163. Rake EC, Breeze E, Fletcher AE. Quality of life and cough on antihypertensive treatment: a randomized trial of eprosartan, enalapril and placebo. J Hum Hypertens 2001; 15:863–867.

164. Gavras I, Gavras H. Are patients who develop angioedema with ACE inhibition at risk of the same problem with AT1 receptor blockers? Arch Intern Med 2003; 163:240–241.

165. Kirpichnikov D, McFarlane SI, Sowers JR. Heart failure in diabetic patients: utility of β-blockade. J Card Fail 2003; 9:333–344.

166. Jacob S, Rett K, Wicklmayr M, Agrawal B, Augustin HJ, Dietze GJ. Differential effect of chronic treatment with two β-blocking agents on INS sensitivity: the carvedilol–metoprolol study. J Hypertens 1996; 14:489–494.

167. Giugliano D, Acampora R, Marfella R, De Rosa N, Ziccardi P, Ragone R, de Angelis L, D'Onofrio F. Metabolic and cardiovascular effects of carvedilol and atenolol in non-INS-dependent diabetes mellitus and hypertension. A randomized, controlled trial. Ann Intern Med 1997; 126:955–959.

168. Intensive blood-glucose control with sulphonylureas or INS compared with conventional treatment and risk of complications in patients with type 2 diabetes (UKPDS 33). UK Prospective Diabetes Study (UKPDS) Group. Lancet 1998; 352:837–853.

169. Heart Protection Study Collaborative Group. MRC/BHF Heart Protection Study of cholesterol lowering with simvastatin in 20,536 high-risk individuals: a randomised placebo-controlled trial. Lancet 2002; 360:7–22.

170. Goldberg RB, Mellies MJ, Sacks FM, Moye LA, Howard BV, Howard WJ, Davis BR, Cole TG, Pfeiffer MA, Braunwald E. Cardiovascular events and their reduction with pravastatin in diabetic and glucose-intolerant myocardial infarction survivors with average cholesterol levels: subgroup analyses in the cholesterol and recurrent events (CARE) trial. The Care Investigators. Circulation 1998; 98:2513–2519.

171. McFarlane SI, Muniyappa R, Francisco R, Sowers JR. Clinical review 145: pleiotropic effects of statins: lipid reduction and beyond. J Clin Endocrinol Metab 2002; 87:1451–1458.

172. Rolka DB, Fagot-Campagna A, Narayan KM. Aspirin use among adults with diabetes: estimates from the Third National Health and Nutrition Examination Survey. Diabetes Care 2001; 24:197–201.

41

Hypertensive Emergencies and Urgencies: Uncontrolled Severe Hypertension

JOHN KEVIN HIX, DONALD G. VIDT

The Cleveland Clinic Foundation, Cleveland, Ohio, USA

KEYPOINTS

- Most hypertensive emergencies occur in the patients with longstanding untreated or poorly controlled hypertension.
- Hypertensive emergencies are defined as severe uncontrolled hypertension causing ongoing or imminent acute end-organ damage; Reduction of blood pressure in a monitored setting is crucial to patient outcome.
- Hypertensive urgencies are defined as severe uncontrolled hypertension not associated with ongoing or imminent acute organ dysfunction; in these cases, effective oral therapy, brief observation, and appropriate follow-up medical care are indicated.

SUMMARY

Hypertensive emergencies usually start with an abrupt rise in blood pressure to a level which significantly exceeds the normal resting blood pressure of the patient. In normotensive and hypertensive subjects blood flow in critical organ beds is maintained across a wide range of blood pressures by autoregulatory mechanisms. Adaptation of these mechanisms allows a constant blood flow to be maintained even in the setting of chronic hypertension, albeit across a new, higher range of pressures. However, in hypertensive emergencies hyperperfusion overwhelms normal autoregulatory mechanisms and results in target organ damage. Still, the pathophysiology of hypertensive emergencies is poorly understood, but perhaps also involves damage to the endothelium and generation of a prothrombotic state.

The term "hypertensive emergency" is used when severe uncontrolled hypertension is a causative factor in demonstrable ongoing or imminent acute end-organ damage. This represents situations in which immediate reductions of blood pressure in a monitored setting are crucial to patient outcome. Rapid triage followed by immediate attempts to reduce blood pressure to lower, but not necessarily normal, values with appropriate parenteral antihypertensives are the critical, lifesaving steps in the care of patients with hypertensive emergency. Multiple effective parenteral agents are available to the clinician. Certain agents, such as nitroprusside and fenoldopam, are effective for multiple causes of hypertensive emergencies. Others, such as hydralazine or phentolamine, have limited utility. Matching the appropriate agent to the suspected pathophysiology improves the therapeutic utility when treating hypertensive emergencies.

The term "hypertensive urgency" is used in situations in which severe uncontrolled hypertension is observed, but is not associated with ongoing acute organ dysfunction. In these cases, a coordinated approach to management using effective oral therapy, brief observation, and ensuring appropriate follow-up medical care is a cost effective and advisable approach to care.

I. INTRODUCTION

This chapter will discuss the pathogenesis, diagnosis, and management involved in conditions of severe uncontrolled high blood pressure, namely, hypertensive emergencies and urgencies. Hypertension itself is among the most common diseases in the developed countries, over 50 million patients diagnosed in North America alone (1). In the vast majority of patients, hypertension is a chronic condition; morbidity and mortality are typically not prominent until after several years of disease. Similarly, the treatment of chronic hypertension requires an extended period of controlled blood pressure before improvement in outcomes

becomes significant or measurable. However, uncontrolled severe hypertension can cause accelerated damage to patients over a much shorter timeframe. This is seen most commonly in two settings: in patients with longstanding untreated or undertreated hypertension, which progresses to severe levels, or in situations in which severe hypertension occurs rapidly, most often in association with another condition. These crises may affect up to 500,000 Americans each year and represent situations in which extreme elevations in blood pressure can result in adverse outcomes over a much shorter time period than that observed in chronic hypertension (1). Because hypertensive emergencies and urgencies differ in the acuity of the situation as well as the optimal management, a clarification of terminology is both instructive and clinically relevant. In some sense, the two conditions represent points along a continuum of severity of blood pressure elevation which is divided by the presence of acute end-organ damage.

II. DEFINITIONS

The hypertensive emergency represents a situation in which severe uncontrolled high blood pressure is a causative factor in demonstrable ongoing end-organ damage (2,3). This represents a process which, if left untreated, results in morbidity and mortality over a time frame of minutes to hours owing to end-organ dysfunction, most commonly observed in the organ systems outlined in Table 41.1. The hypertensive emergency requires urgent attention and an immediate reduction of blood pressure, if organ damage is to be avoided or minimized.

The hypertensive urgency is a less clearly defined condition in which severe uncontrolled high blood pressure is observed in a patient who may have evidence of previous end-organ damage related to hypertension, but in whom there exists no evidence of ongoing or imminent target-organ dysfunction related to the current episode of hypertension. Most often this occurs in patients with previously diagnosed chronic hypertension (1). In this scenario, there is considerably less benefit associated with an immediate

Table 41.1 End-Organ Damage Seen in Hypertensive Emergencies (4)

Organ system	Pathophysiology
Neurologic	Hypertensive encephalopathy, stroke/intracranial hemorrhage
Cardiac	Acute myocardial infarction, acute left ventricular failure with pulmonary edema
Vascular	Acute aortic dissection, other vascular dissection, arteritis/thrombosis
Endocrine/obstetrical	Eclampsia
Renal	Acute renal failure

reduction in the level of blood pressure; rather, the blood pressure can be treated over a period of time, from several hours to 24 h. These patients are typically at low risk for adverse outcomes related to the present hypertension and can usually be managed outside of the hospital setting.

Hypertensive crises (urgencies and emergencies) represent a clear danger to patients, as well as a significant burden on the health-care system. Although they affect only ~1% of all hypertensive patients, together these diagnoses may account for up to 3–4.9% of all emergency room visits and >27% of all patients presenting to the emergency room with a medical emergency (1,4–7).

III. PATHOPHYSIOLOGY OF HYPERTENSIVE EMERGENCIES

Hypertensive emergencies result when blood pressure is present at a level which overwhelms compensatory mechanisms present in the body, exposing target-organs to the full force of the elevated blood pressure with resultant vascular compromise, arteritis, or ischemia (5,8). The etiology of the high blood pressure itself is not necessarily unique; hypertension of any origin can progress in severity and culminate in a hypertensive emergency or urgency. However, there are specific conditions in which either the rapidity of the development of hypertension or the underlying pathophysiology lowers the threshold for the development of hypertensive urgency or emergency. Often, these are situations in which accelerated hypertension occurs in a previously normotensive patient, overcomes the body's ability to adapt to the rising blood pressure, and overwhelms autoregulatory measures designed to prevent end-organ damage. Situations commonly associated with the development of hypertensive urgencies and emergencies are listed in Table 41.2.

A brief discussion of autoregulatory mechanisms may allow a better understanding of the development of the

Table 41.2 Conditions Associated with the Development of Hypertensive Emergencies

System	Underlying disorder
General	
Hypertension	Essential hypertension (accelerated)
Kidney	
Renal disease	Acute glomerulonephritis, tubulointerstitial nephritis, vasculitis (including Takayasu's arteritis and polyarteritis nodosa), hemolytic uremic syndrome, thrombotic microangiopathy, renovascular hypertension (atherosclerotic), renovascular disease (fibromuscular dysplasia), advanced chronic kidney disease or end-stage renal disease with volume overload, systemic lupus erythematous, systemic sclerosis
Cardiovascular	
Aorta	Acute dissection, coarctation of the aorta
Heart	Congestive heart failure, ischemic cardiac disease
Obstetrical/gynecology	
Pregnancy	Preeclampsia/eclampsia
Endocrine	
Catecholamine system	Pheochromocytoma
Glucocorticoids	Cushing's syndrome
Renin–angiotensin–aldosterone axis	Renin secreting tumor (rare) with subsequent hyperreninemic–hyperaldosteronism Aldosterone secreting tumors (rare) with hyperaldosteronism
Neurologic systems	
Autonomic hyperreactivity	Guillain–Barré syndrome, acute intermittent porphyria
Central nervous system	Acute head injury, stroke, brain tumor
Exogenous agents	
Drugs	Antihypertensive medication withdrawal (e.g., clonidine withdrawal), sympathomimetics, cocaine use, phencyclidine use, ingestion of tyramine-containing foods in a patient on a monamine-oxidase inhibitor, cyclosporin (rare), oral contraceptive medication (rare), erythropoietin (rare)
Other	
Situational	Severe postoperative hypertension

Note: In select cases, the clinical presentation and recommendations for further evaluation are noted (2,7).

hypertensive emergency, as well as the logic behind the treatment goals. In all mammalian organisms, there exists a multitude of factors which impact upon blood pressure on a moment-to-moment basis and which threaten to disrupt blood flow. To attenuate this possibility, autoregulatory mechanisms have developed and act to stabilize the pressure/flow relationship within different organ systems. The premier example of this is the autoregulation of cerebral blood flow (9). The brain is an organ with a high, fixed metabolic rate which requires a constant stable blood flow for optimum function. Thus, the vasculature supplying the brain must continuously adjust to deviations in systemic blood flow in order to deliver this required constant cerebral perfusion. In normotensive individuals, this is accomplished by variable regulation in the tone of cerebral resistance vessels: during periods of relative systemic hypotension these resistance vessels dilate to increase blood flow, whereas during period of relative systemic hypertension these same vessels constrict to decrease blood flow (10). In this manner, cerebral blood flow is maintained across the spectrum of blood pressures observed daily in a normal individual. The extremes beyond which this mechanism fails are not exactly known; however, it seems adequate for the 50–150 mmHg range of blood pressures. Lower systemic pressures result in a fall in cerebral blood flow, whereas higher pressures exceed the ability of autoregulatory-

mediated dampening and can precipitate hypertensive crises (11–13).

This situation is somewhat modified in the hypertensive patient population. Exposure to chronically elevated blood pressure seems to result in structural changes in resistance vessels, resulting in an increased media–lumen ratio (14–16). These changes may be compensatory mechanisms, which reduce wall stress and otherwise allow the small vessels to affect a higher net resistance, in keeping with the higher systemic pressures over which autoregulation must be effective in this population (14). Primate models suggest this results in improved preservation of cerebral blood flow at higher systemic pressures (17). Chronic hypertension, by priming the body's auto regulatory system to function better at higher pressures, also tends to raise the threshold for the development of a hypertensive emergency (9,11,12,18). As a result, the chronically hypertensive patient can tolerate higher blood pressures, upward of a mean arterial pressure of 180 mmHg (19), before autoregulation fails. The cost for this adaptation is that these morphologically altered blood vessels are less able to dilate in response to sudden drops in systemic pressure, and the entire range over which cerebral blood flow can be maintained by autoregulation is shifted in this circumstance (14).

This can be represented graphically by plotting blood pressure vs. blood flow relationships in normal patients and in hypertensive patients as shown in Fig. 41.1.

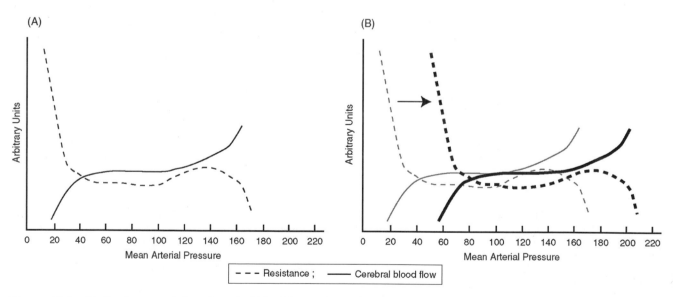

Figure 41.1 Idealized autoregulation of cerebral blood flow and vascular bed resistance in normotensive and chronically hypertensive patients. (A) Autoregulation in normotensive patients. The lower limit of autoregulation occurs at mean blood pressures <70–80 mmHg (12,18). (B) Autoregulation in chronic hypertensive patients. The lower limit of autoregulation occurs at mean blood pressures below ~115–120 mmHg in uncontrolled hypertensives, and below ~100 mmHg in patients with improved hypertension control (12,18). Note the shift rightward in mean arterial blood pressures over which autoregulation functions in the setting of chronic hypertension. As a result, patients with chronic underlying hypertension are more resistant to developing hypertensive emergencies. However, by virtue of this shift in autoregulation, these same patients are more susceptible to the adverse effect of cerebral hypoperfusion, as a result of rapid reduction in blood pressure. Adapted from Strandgaard et al. (12), Strandgaard et al. (17), Strandgaard et al. (18), Gao et al. (20).

In either case, an extreme deviation in blood pressure above the upper limits of the autoregulatory process results in a dramatic increase in blood flow which overwhelms the ability of the vascular bed to constrict. This surge of flow is transmitted directly to the vascular and organ tissues and is thought to be the mechanical origin of the damage seen in hypertensive encephalopathies (8,11,21). It then follows that although there is no minimal threshold with regard to the level of blood pressure for the diagnosis of hypertensive emergency, it is unusual for this condition to develop in any individual patient without a severe increase in blood pressure above the normal resting blood pressure for that patient. Further, the maintenance of a hypertensive emergency presumably requires that the elevation in blood pressure be maintained at a level which overwhelms the normal autoregulatory mechanisms present in the patient.

The exact pathophysiology surrounding the failure of autoregulatory mechanisms during a hypertensive emergency is complex and poorly understood. One important factor involves the vascular endothelium, which functions as a mediator of normal blood pressure regulation in the mammal (2). The endothelium is known to produce factors which can constrict resistance vessels, and data suggests removal of vascular endothelium impairs vasoconstrictor-mediated autoregulation in animal models (22,23). Intact endothelium is also able to secrete substances such as nitric oxide, a potent vasodilator, in response to mechanical stress or hormonal or paracrine substances (2,24–26). This process is partially disrupted in the microvasculature of hypertensive patients (26), and animal data suggests that high arterial pressure itself induces oxidative stress in the endothelium and elicits production of reactive oxidative species which interfere with nitric oxide-mediated vasodilation (27). Taken together, these findings suggest that endothelial dysfunction may play a central part in disorders of impaired autoregulation; in some instances this dysfunction may permit hyperperfusion in the setting of high blood pressure, whereas in other cases this results in a deficiency of vasorelaxation as pressures are acutely reduced.

The precipitating event for the development of a hypertensive emergency seems to be an abrupt rise in blood pressure. This may be mediated by a number of factors working in isolated or additive combinations including release of catecholamines, vasopressin, or endothelin or thromboxane. In addition, abundant data suggests that over-activation of the renin–angiotensin–aldosterone system alone or in conjunction with the earlier-mentioned factors seems to be a key component in the initiation, maintenance, and progression of hypertensive crises (2,28). In cases of hypertensive emergency, the endothelium is either abnormally activated or overwhelmed; this leads to inadequate dampening of blood flow with

the resulting hyperperfusion of target organs. In addition to the mechanical impact implied in the earlier construct, there exists mounting evidence that as elevations in hypertension approach more extreme values, endothelial damage and a prothrombotic state ensue. The endothelium itself becomes increasingly permeable with the development of perivascular edema and endothelial cell dysfunction, with resultant exposure of the intima-media layers of blood vessels to clotting factors (2,19). A recent study found a stepwise increase in fibrinogen, soluble p-selectin, and von Willebrand factor when measured in normal, hypertensive, and severely hypertensive patients (29). Some of these changes were favorably altered with antihypertensive treatment. These alterations may help explain why many of the major complications of hypertensive emergencies center around microangiopathic hemolysis and intravascular thrombotic events, rather than purely hyperperfusion-mediated mechanical damage.

As these mechanisms of injury progress, there is compromise of blood flow and resultant target-organ hypoperfusion. This leads to release of cytokines and proinflammatory agents and further activation of the renin–angiotensin–aldosterone system. These effectively promote vasoconstriction and fluid retention and lead to further aggravation of the injury to the endothelium; ultimately, the situation becomes cyclical as blood pressure rises and target-organ damage worsens (2,19,28).

A. Initial Evaluation

Particular areas of the history, physical examination, and laboratory work-up must be carefully addressed when evaluating a patient for a hypertensive emergency. Presented here is a general approach to the evaluation of any patient presenting with extreme elevations in blood pressure; a more specific approach to select hypertensive emergencies follows. However, it must be remembered that patients presenting with hypertensive emergency are in need of immediate therapy; therefore, the desire to completely explore all areas of the history and physical examination must often be delayed until after initial treatment based upon a presumptive diagnosis has been initiated. The prime duty of the clinician caring for any patient presenting with severe hypertension is to perform a concise, targeted assessment of those portions of the history, examination, and laboratory work-up sufficient to diagnose target-organ damage and, if present, embark immediately upon treatment of the hypertension.

B. The History

The vast majority of patients presenting to the emergency room with a hypertensive emergency carry a known diagnosis of hypertension; it is therefore important in the patient presenting with severe hypertension to inquire about this diagnosis and, if positive, the cause, duration, intensity, and previous treatment efforts with regard to the hypertension. If the patient is not known to have hypertension, it is insightful to inquire as to the last time the patient was known to have had a normal recorded blood pressure.

Background demographics of patients with malignant hypertension is helpful in determining the etiology of the underlying disorder. In white subjects, essential hypertension is the cause of malignant hypertension in only ~30% of cases, and secondary causes are almost always discovered in white patients presenting with malignant hypertension under age 30. On the other hand, >80% of black patients presenting with malignant hypertension have underlying essential hypertension, and these patients may present at a younger age (5).

A detailed history of drug therapy with a specific focus on prescription drug medication, particularly antihypertensive medications, is mandated. Many antihypertensives can result in significant rebound hypertension when noncompliance with the prescribed dosage and/or schedule occurs. This possibility must be sought. Abrupt discontinuation of clonidine is a common situation in which extreme hypertension occurs as a result of drug withdrawal. A number of nonprescription or illicit drugs can cause significant hypertension; this includes over-the-counter sympathomimetics, cocaine, amphetamines, and other illicit substances. Extreme hypertension can be seen in withdrawal states of patients with a history of heavy alcohol or benzodiazepines use. Finally, foodstuffs and seemingly unrelated drugs may have interactions with other conditions or medications which can result in severe hypertension; example include the use of erythropoietin, interactions with monamine-oxidase inhibitors and tyramine, haloperidol and other neuroleptics, and others (2). These possibilities should be explored.

Female patients should have a detailed documentation of obstetrical history, including information on previous pregnancies and oral contraception usage. A history of previous hypertension during pregnancy is a known risk factor for the development of hypertensive emergency (30).

Renal disease, whether renal vascular disease or parenchymal injury, accounts for the majority of secondary causes of hypertension in all patient populations (5). Patients with known chronic kidney disease and particularly end-stage renal disease must be questioned regarding their compliance with diet and medications, changes in weight, and any change or alterations in dialysis therapy if applicable.

The clinician must also determine the presence of symptoms which may be related to the hypertension, particularly those which may represent ongoing organ damage. Important are symptoms of neurologic compromise such as seizures, confusion, or headaches, which

may represent hypertensive encephalopathy; chest pain or pressure, which may represent acute myocardial infarction; severe neck, chest, or back pain, which may represent carotid or aortic dissection; dyspnea, orthopnea, cough, or hemoptysis, which may represent pulmonary edema from congestive heart failure; hematuria or alteration in voiding character or frequency, which may represent renal compromise.

C. The Physical Examination

Key areas of the physical examination center around the evaluation and stratification of the blood pressure, as well as the identification of the end-organ effects seen in hypertensive emergencies.

The vital signs should include a blood pressure taken by the clinician in each arm, as previously outlined, in both the sitting and the standing position to aid in assessing intravascular volume status. Blood pressure should be compared between the two arms, and any significant differences should immediately raise suspicion for aortic dissection or coarctation of the aorta. If possible, the presenting blood pressure should be compared with previously recorded values in the patient to establish the degree of change from baseline. The heart rate and rhythm should be noted and extremes in either direction must be incorporated into the decision on therapeutics, as many antihypertensives will influence heart rate.

Physical examination should start with a neurologic assessment to exclude signs of stroke, meningeal irritation, and encephalopathy, and to gage the level of consciousness. A fundoscopic examination with visualization and grading of the fundi is crucial. This allows direct inspection of the effects of the blood pressure on a vascular bed and is necessary to exclude papilledema, hemorrhage, or exudates. Any of these, if new, are diagnostic of hypertensive emergency. Cardiovascular exam should focus on assessment of the intravascular volume status with estimation of the jugular venous pressure and should seek to determine any negative effect of the hypertension on cardiac function as indicated by the presence of a third or fourth heart sound, a cardiac murmur, or the presence of pulmonary rales. A peripheral vascular examination should be performed to assess intactness of the vasculature and exclude the presence of bruits or discordant pulse characteristics which may indicate vascular dissection. Careful assessment of the abdominal area may disclose the presence of a pulsatile mass consistent with an abdominal aortic aneurysm or the bruit of a renovascular lesion.

D. The Laboratory Investigation

The minimum laboratory investigation will include a complete blood count and peripheral smear to exclude schistocytes, determination of the serum chemistries and blood urea and creatinine, urinalysis with careful inspection of the urinary sediment, chest radiograph, and electrocardiogram. It is reasonable to include markers of cardiac ischemia, including creatinine kinase and troponin, particularly if the history is suggestive or the electrocardiogram reveals any abnormalities. In addition, reproductive age females should have pregnancy confirmed or excluded by laboratory means during the initial evaluation.

E. Diagnostic Stratification

The aforementioned information will allow the clinician to assess the end-organ impact of the elevated blood pressure and allow a risk stratification of patients. Those patients in whom signs or symptoms suggest progressive end-organ damage should be classified as true hypertensive emergencies. These patients may require further evaluation centered upon the organ system at risk and will require immediate treatment in the hospital, preferably in the intensive care unit, using parenteral agents. Specific recommendations depending upon the specific organ system in jeopardy follows. Patients in whom there is no sign of imminent organ damage should be considered to have hypertensive urgency, and the treatment of this follows in the subsequent section.

F. Secondary Causes of Hypertension

If the history, physical examination, or initial laboratory testing is suggestive, investigations should be undertaken to exclude underlying disorders which may be causing the severe hypertension. Again, it must be emphasized that the prime duty of the physician assessing a patient with severe hypertension is to assess for target-organ damage and to treat immediately, if detected. However, once blood pressure has been appropriately treated, an investigation into possible causes of the hypertension may be helpful in guiding future therapy.

IV. PHARMACOLOGY OF THE TREATMENT OF HYPERTENSIVE EMERGENCIES

It would be helpful to have a strong evidence base to dictate to the treating clinician the exact reduction in blood pressure, optimal agents, and precise time course over which the reduction in pressure should occur, which lead to optimal outcomes in hypertensive emergencies. Unfortunately, as noted in a recent review of the literature, there is no such evidence base upon which to build a standard algorithm to fulfill all these requirements (7). The authors of this review suggest the guidelines of a reduction in mean blood pressure of <25% in 2 h and a goal of 160/

100 mmHg by 6 h of treatment, subject to modification based upon clinical context and frequent ongoing assessment of the patient's course. We agree that these are reasonable benchmarks to keep in mind when reviewing the specific therapeutic agents and types of emergencies, with a strong emphasis on the point that the clinician should feel comfortable customizing the treatment program to the individual patient's circumstance.

A. Agents Used in the Treatment of Hypertensive Emergency

Select preferred agents used for the acute treatment of hypertensive emergencies are listed in Table 41.3. Hypertensive emergencies require treatment in the hospital, preferably within the intensive care unit, where adequate nursing care and continuous blood pressure monitoring are available. In these situations, the goals of treatment include an immediate and sustained reduction in blood pressure, not necessarily to normal values. Because most patients presenting with hypertensive emergency either have known previous hypertension or have unclear history regarding hypertension, it is prudent in the acute setting to attempt to immediately lower blood pressure to a level below which target-organ damage occurs yet within the potentially higher range at which autoregulatory function can reasonably be expected to operate. These requirements mandate the use of parenteral agents with a short onset of action, as well as a short half-life, in order that precise control of the timing and magnitude of antihypertensive therapy remain in the hands of the treating physician. However, other circumstances may dictate the use of oral therapeutic agents even in emergencies; these are covered in a subsequent portion of the text (see Section E).

B. Specific Agents for Discussion

1. Sodium Nitroprusside

Nitroprusside is a lipophilic, hydrated nitrosylpentacyanofcrate which acts as a nonselective vasodilator. It is metabolized by sulfhydryl groups found in blood vessels and red cells into cyanogen as well as nitric oxide. Its ultimate mechanism of action is identical to that of endogenous nitric oxide; specifically it mediates vascular relaxation through the generation of cyclic GMP and intracellular calcium modulation (33). It causes vasodilation of both arterial and venous vessels and is effective in reducing hypertension of any etiology. Nitroprusside has an immediate onset of action and is rapidly titratable to desired effect.

Nitroprusside-induced vasodilation generally results in a decrease in cardiac output as a result of decreased venous return to the heart. However, it is effective in decreasing

Table 41.3 Preferred Agents Used for the Acute Treatment of Hypertensive Emergencies

Drug	Dose/route	Onset of action	Duration of action	Side effects	Cautions
Direct vasodilators					
Sodium nitroprusside	0.25–10 µg/kg per min Constant intravenous infusion	Instantaneous	2 min	Nausea, vomiting, muscle twitching, thiocyanate (fatigue, disorientation, psychosis), and cyanide (metabolic acidosis) poisoning	Toxic metabolites accumulate in renal failure Thiocyanate levels should be monitored in patients requiring prolonged (days) treatment Drug is susceptible to photodegredation Avoid prolonged administration at high doses (10 µg/kg per min), if possible
Fenoldopam	0.01–1.6 µg/kg per min Constant intravenous infusion	15 min	15 min	Headache, nausea, vomiting, sweating, hypokalemia	Seems to maintain renal perfusion despite reduction in overall blood pressure
Hydralazine	10–40 mg dose Injection, repeat at 4–6 h intervals	2 h	2–8 h	Tachycardia, angina pectoris, dizziness, paroxysmal hypertension, peripheral edema, increased intracranial pressure, lupus-like syndrome, intracranial strokes- or ischemia	Use in caution with patients with azotemia Dilution with sugar-containing solutions should be avoided Generally considered safe in pregnancy
Nitroglycerin	5–100 µg/min Constant intravenous infusion	2 min	3–5 min	Headache, lightheadedness, tachycardia	Ergot alkaloids may increase blood pressure with concomitant use Overdose can result in methemoglobinemia; this is treated with methylene blue Potency best preserved by glass containers
Nicardipine	5–15 mg/h Constant intravenous infusion	5–10 min	30 min–4 h	Flushing, palpitations, peripheral edema, headache, dizziness, weakness	Use with caution in acute coronary syndromes Increases level of metoprolol, if used concomitantly
Enalaprilat	0.625–1.25 mg Injection, repeat at 6 h intervals	30 min–1 h	12–24 h	Hypotension, chest pain, headache, syncope, increased creatinine	Starting dose: use 0.625 mg, if patient is receiving concomitant diuretics; if not, start with 1.25 mg Use with caution in situations of suspected volume depletion, in patients with chronic kidney disease, or in acute renal failure Contraindicated in patient suspected of having bilateral renal artery stenosis

	Dose	Onset	Duration	Adverse effects	Special indications
Diazoxide	50–150 mg IV bolus Injection, repeat at 15–30 min intervals until blood pressure goal achieved, then re-administer at 4–24 h intervals May also be used as slow infusion 15–30 mg/min (30).	5 min	3–12 h	Hypotension, dizziness, nausea, vomiting, reflex tachycardia, weakness	Do not use in patients suspected of having coronary ischemia or aortic dissection Use with caution in patients with renal impairment (long duration of action) Larger boluses (300 mg) associated with hypotension
Antiadrenergic agents					
Labetalol	20–80 mg injection, repeat every 10 min as indicated, up to 300 mg total dose 2 mg/min Constant intravenous infusion Titrate up to 300 mg total dose	2–5 min	2 h	Dizziness, nausea, edema, hypotension, bradycardia, fatigue, paresthesias, elevated liver enzymes, mental depression	Use with caution in patients with asthma, bronchospastic disease, or congestive heart failure
Esmolol	Bolus 500–1000 μg/kg over 30 s followed by a 25–150 μg/kg per min constant intravenous infusion Titrate infusion up to 300 μg/kg per min	2 min	10–30 min	Hypotension, diaphoresis, dizziness, nausea	Use with caution in patients with asthma, bronchospastic disease, or congestive heart failure
Phentolamine	5–20 mg injection, repeat every 1–4 h as indicated	Immediate	15–20 min	Hypotension, tachycardia, flushing, weakness, dizziness	Give 1–2 h prior to surgery for pheochromocytoma and repeat as needed Not recommended for patients with renal impairment, cardiac disease, or gastric ulcer

Source: Adapted from Vaughan and Delanty (2) and Kaplan (31).

both pulmonary capillary wedge pressures and reducing myocardial oxygen demands and can increase cardiac output in patients with heart failure. These actions make it an excellent choice for postoperative hypertension in patients with impaired left ventricular function and in patients with heart failure and pulmonary edema.

Its effects on patients with cardiac disease have been compared principally against nitroglycerin. Nitroprusside is an effective antihypertensive in these patients; however, nitroglycerin may be preferable in situations in which ongoing myocardial ischemia is suspected, as it seems to improve electrocardiographic abnormalities and cause a greater reduction in myocardial oxygen requirements than nitroprusside (34,35).

Specific to instances of neurologic hypertensive emergency, there is some concern that nitroprusside decreases cerebral perfusion and increases intracranial pressure, and its use in patients at risk for cerebral perfusion impairment requires attention to this possibility (36,37). Primate models show that nitroprusside augments cerebral blood flow in situations of experimental vasospasm, although it does not appear to affect cerebral blood flow in healthy animals (38,39). Implications of this discrepancy in the treatment of human disease are unclear, although some evidence suggests that the drug does relieve cerebral vasospasm in subarachnoid hemorrhage.

The cyanogen metabolite of nitroprusside is ultimately metabolized by rhodanese in the liver to thiocyanate, and subsequently, thiocyanate is excreted by the kidneys. Thiocyanate can accumulate in renal impairment and has been implicated in causing symptoms such as fatigue, hallucination, nausea, and psychosis. In addition, cyanide toxicity itself, suggested by resistant metabolic acidosis with venous hyperoxemia, can occur with high rates of infusion or in situations in which metabolism of the drug is impaired (19). These occurrences are relatively uncommon; however, high dose nitroprusside (≥ 10 μg/kg per min) for >10 min or situations of prolonged therapy (≥ 48 h infusion) require extreme care. Thiocyanate toxicity can be prevented or treated with hydroxocobalamin crystalline, whereas cyanide toxicity is improved with the use of sodium thiosulfate.

2. Fenoldopam

Fenoldopam mesylate is a vasodilator that predominantly acts as an agonist which binds selectively to the dopamine-1 receptor site at therapeutic dosages and has activity in coronary, renal, mesenteric, and peripheral arteries. This results in a decrease in peripheral vascular resistance and pulmonary capillary wedge pressure, with an increase in heart rate but seemingly without significant impact on cardiac index (40). It has been shown to be an effective parenteral antihypertensive agent in patients

with severe hypertension, with a dose-dependent magnitude of blood pressure reduction observed with titration and a time to maintenance infusion of 1.5 h, similar to nitroprusside (41). Fenoldopam is metabolized by conjugation, with most metabolites excreted by the kidneys.

The mechanism of action of fenoldopam is similar to that postulated for low dose dopamine, and experimental studies on the regional effects of fenoldopam have demonstrated that mesenteric and renal blood flow is increased during infusion, apparently through dopamine-1 receptor-mediated stimulation (42,43). This appears to have clinical implications in the treatment of hypertensive emergencies, and increases in urinary flow rates, natriuresis, and creatinine clearance have been observed in severely hypertensive patients treated with fenoldopam when compared with a similar group treated with nitroprusside (44). In this study, the improvement in these surrogates for renal flow occurred with equivalent hemodynamic impact upon blood pressure and heart rate between the two agents and without significant differences in side effects.

3. Hydralazine

Hydralazine has the principal effect of direct vasodilation at arterioles, with almost no vasoactive effects on veins. It undergoes extensive first pass metabolism by hepatic acetylation into inactive metabolites; the metabolites are excreted by the kidneys and renal failure results in extended half-life.

It is an effective agent and is considered safe in pregnancy. Hydralazine has long been advocated as the agent of choice in suspected preeclampsia, as it may better preserve intrauterine blood flow during systemic blood pressure reduction (45,46). However, a recent meta-analysis did not find firm evidence to support the use of hydralazine over other agents as first line therapy for the treatment of severe hypertension in pregnancy (47).

The use of hydralazine is associated with significant reflex tachycardia, making it unsuitable for situations such as acute coronary syndromes or suspected aortic dissection, unless concomitant rate controlling agents are used. In addition, the use of hydralazine is associated with increases in intracranial pressure, making it unsuitable for patients with hypertensive encephalopathy, stroke, or subarachnoid hemorrhage.

4. Nitroglycerin

Nitroglycerin is a nitric oxide donor with variable, dose-dependent activity. At low doses (5–10 μg/min), nitroglycerin acts predominantly to dilate capacitance vessels, whereas at higher doses some arterial vasodilation occurs. Nitroglycerin has a rapid onset of action and short half-life, allowing for rapid titration to the desired effect. However, it is neither as potent nor as predictable an antihypertensive agent as nitroprusside. In addition, the use of nitroglycerin is associated with tachyphylaxis and, perhaps more importantly, significant tolerance to the antihypertensive effects develops in patients over several hours to days of therapy. Metabolism is hepatic with a significant first pass effect, and metabolites are excreted by the kidneys.

Nitroglycerin is indicated in patients with elevated blood pressure in the setting of an acute coronary syndrome, as nitroglycerin has proven benefits in the treatment of coronary ischemia through a preferential vasodilation of coronary vessels and their collaterals. It diminishes preload and decreases left ventricular volume and wall tension, which reduces myocardial oxygen demand. It is also useful in pulmonary hypertension and in other hypertensive emergencies, particularly in combination with agents such as labetalol, which help to mitigate tachycardia. Nitroglycerin has been used in pregnant patients with hypertension as well.

Of some concern, nitroglycerin has been implicated in increasing intracranial pressure which may increase the transmural pressure on cerebral vasculature; as this can negatively impact upon cerebral blood flow, it should be used only with great caution in patients with neurologic compromise related to hypertension (37).

5. Nicardipine

Nicardipine is a dihydropyridine calcium channel antagonist available for intravenous delivery. Nicardipine has a primary site of action on slow calcium channels, where it inhibits calcium ion entry and produces relaxation of vascular and myocardial smooth muscle cells. Metabolism is hepatic, with a significant first pass effect, and metabolites are excreted by the kidneys.

Nicardipine has a rapid onset of action and is easily titratable without requiring adjustment for weight. Its mode of action may make it useful in vasospastic coronary syndromes, although nitroglycerin is preferable in ischemic coronary disease.

A potential drawback to nicardipine is that it has a relatively long duration of action, and over-titration can result in relative or absolute hypotension and bradycardia. 4-Aminopyridine is an antidote, but is not available in the United States; persistent hypotension may be improved with adrenergic agents, glucagon, or amrinone.

6. Diazoxide

Diazoxide is a benzothiadiazine derivative with a potent direct effect upon the smooth muscle of arterioles which causes smooth muscle relaxation and vasodilation. This results in decreased peripheral resistance with a reflex tachycardia and increased cardiac output. It is also an inhibitor of insulin release from the pancreas.

Approximately 50% of the drug is excreted unchanged by the kidneys.

Diazoxide is rarely used for hypertensive emergencies today. It has numerous potential side effects including tachycardia, significant hypotension, hyperglycemia, and rarely, extrapyramidal effects. It can cause maternal and fetal hyperglycemia and arrest of labor through relaxation of uterine muscles, and so is best avoided in the pregnant female. It is contraindicated in acute coronary syndromes and aortic dissection, and its mode of delivery does not allow for the flexibility of titration afforded by other agents.

7. Enalaprilat

Enalaprilat, the active metabolite of the oral drug Enalapril, is a competitive inhibitor of converting enzyme which is available for intravenous delivery. Enalaprilat prevents the conversion of angiotensin I to the potent vasopressor agent, angiotensin II.

The use of enalaprilat is particularly appropriate in patients with congestive heart failure and hypertension, in whom angiotensin converting enzyme (ACE) inhibitors are a primary treatment.

Caution must be exercised when using enalaprilat in patients with renal insufficiency, as renal blood flow may be dependent upon an intact renin–angiotensin–aldosterone system. Its use is contraindicated in the cases of suspected renal artery stenosis, as ACE inhibition can precipitate acute renal failure in these settings. In addition, there is evidence for teratogenicity when ACE inhibitors are administered to pregnant patients in the second or third trimester; so care must be exercised when enalaprilat is given to reproductive age females.

8. Labetalol

Labetalol is an antiadrenergic agent with predominant nonselective β-receptor blocking activity, which also exhibits α-1 receptor blocking ability. It is principally metabolized by the liver via glucuronide conjugation.

Labetalol has a rapid onset of action and is usable both as an injection and as a continuous infusion for the treatment of hypertensive emergencies. It has significant negative inotropic and chronotropic effects and is an excellent agent for decreasing heart rate and myocardial oxygen consumption in the setting of acute coronary syndrome or suspected aortic dissection. Its α blocking abilities probably help preserve renal blood flow despite systemic reductions in blood pressure by relaxing preglomerular vessels.

Labetalol can cause or exacerbate bradycardia and is contraindicated in heart block greater than first degree (unless a concomitant electronic pacing device is in use). It should be used only with great caution in compensated congestive heart failure and should be avoided in decompensated failure. β-receptor blockade should be avoided in patients with a history of bronchospasm. Although the β-antagonist effects are more potent than the α-agonist effects, the possibility of developing a relative unopposed α-adrenergic stimulation demands extreme caution when labetalol is considered for use in patients with adrenergic crisis, pheochromocytoma, or severe hypertension in the setting of cocaine use (48).

9. Esmolol

Esmolol is a selective competitive β-1 receptor antagonist with almost no effect at the β-2 site. Esmolol is metabolized in the blood by serum esterases and is excreted in the urine predominantly as metabolites.

Esmolol has a rapid onset of action and the shortest half-life of the adrenergic blocking agents in use today. These properties allow for rapid titration of infusions and make it a good choice for hypertension, particularly in patients in whom decreasing the heart rate is desirable (myocardial ischemia or aortic dissection). Esmolol is also useful in perioperative control of severe hypertension.

Similar to labetalol, esmolol is contraindicated in heart block greater than first degree unless a pacing device is in place. It should also be avoided in patients with decompensated congestive heart failure or a history of bronchospasm.

10. Phentolamine

Phentolamine is a competitive α-1 receptor antagonist with some positive inotrophic and chronotrophic effects on the heart. It has a rapid onset of action and is available for intravenous injection. It is metabolized by the liver and metabolites are excreted through the urine.

Phentolamine has a particular role in the diagnosis and management of patients suspected of having a catecholamine excess state driving their hypertension, such as pheochromocytoma. In these settings, phentolamine produces acute and effective lowering of the blood pressure. Phentolamine may also be useful in reversing myocardial ischemia due to cocaine-induced coronary vasospasm (48). It is otherwise somewhat difficult to titrate and, because its use increases myocardial oxygen consumption, it is not suitable in other acute coronary syndrome states.

It is worth remembering that in the event phentolamine causes persistent or severe hypotension, treatment with agents possessing only α-adrenergic agonist action (so as to avoid unopposed β-agonist effects) is appropriate.

C. Specific Hypertensive Emergencies

There are a select number of common situations in which end-organ damage occurs as a result of hypertensive emergencies. These situations are usually apparent after routine history, physical examination, and laboratory work-up. The common situations for each are presented here, along with comments specific to the pathophysiology, diagnosis, and management.

1. Neurologic Emergencies

A patient can be diagnosed with a neurologic hypertensive emergency when any one of the following is present in the setting of severe hypertension: papilledema, exudate or hemorrhage on fundoscopic exam (otherwise unexplained), new focal neurologic finding, or diminished or altered level of consciousness. In addition, patients who present with severe hypertension and new or unexplained neurologic symptoms such as headache, paresthesias, weakness, new onset seizures, or sensory deficits should undergo further work-up to exclude a neurologic hypertensive emergency (Table 41.4).

Neurological hypertensive emergencies result in hemorrhage, thrombotic or ischemic stroke, or pressure-induced extravasation of fluid into the perivascular tissue, and the development of hypertensive encephalopathy. Distinguishing between these potential mechanisms of injury is often difficult clinically, yet the distinction does impact upon management. The best approach is to utilize one of the imaging methods presented in Table 41.4. Stroke or hemorrhage usually presents with a more acute course, and often the clinical signs correlate with the areas of injury identified by imaging. Hypertensive encephalopathy typically follows a more subacute time course; this may be a diagnosis of exclusion once the other possibilities are ruled out by imaging studies.

There is some controversy as to the optimal management of patients suffering from stroke in the setting of hypertension. Stroke or subarachnoid hemorrhages may result from hypertension, or hypertension may be a consequence of the event itself (49). A stroke may result in the creation of watershed areas of tissue which are not truly ischemic and remain viable as long as perfusion is maintained. These areas may depend upon the higher perfusion pressure conferred by systemic hypertension, and thus acute reductions in blood pressure may result in extension of the ischemic damage to these areas. In addition, one study suggests no significant relationship between hypertension at presentation and subsequent outcome in stroke patients, and in fact found a spontaneous decrease in blood pressure in the first 5 days following a stroke to be a poor prognostic sign (49). These results seem to call into question the utility of aggressive treatment of hypertension in this setting. In a recent review, no evidence was found to support the treatment of hypertension *per se* in the setting of ischemic stroke (50). The same authors suggest that antihypertensive therapy be reserved for patients with compelling comorbid conditions (such

Table 41.4 Further Work-up in Patients Presenting with Neurologic Symptoms in the Setting of Severe Hypertension

Test	Results
Computerized axial tomography (CT) or magnetic resonance imaging (MRI) of central nervous system (CNS)	Useful in patients with an array of neurologic signs or symptoms. Imaging of the CNS may reveal a new stroke or cerebral hemorrhage which can be diagnostic of hypertensive emergency and impacts upon treatment; CT is test of choice for evaluation of blood in the subarachnoid space and is 95% positive (Forbes and Jackson, 1997); imaging may reveal tissue edema or posterior leukoencephalopathy consistent with elevated intracranial pressure which may be diagnostic of encephalopathy, a common hypertensive emergency (2); imaging may be needed to exclude evidence of raised intracranial pressure before attempting lumbar puncture
Lumbar puncture	May be indicated in patients with neurologic symptoms, particularly headache, neck pain, or altered consciousness, particularly, if imaging studies are not diagnostic. Uniform blood in the cerebrospinal fluid (CSF) (in first 24 h) or xanthochromia suggest subarachnoid hemorrhage Forbes and Jackson, 1997. CSF is usually under increased pressure in hypertensive encephalopathy

as acute coronary syndrome, acute aortic dissection, or hypertensive encephalopathy) and patients with severe hypertension who require thrombolytic therapy, with a consensus goal of gradual reduction in blood pressure not to exceed a 20 mmHg reduction in mean arterial pressure (8).

Hypertensive encephalopathy is typically treated with sodium nitroprusside to reduce the systemic mean pressure by ~20–25% over 1–3 h or to a diastolic blood pressure of 100 mmHg (whichever is less) (2,37). Other agents which may be used include fenoldopam or labetalol. Certain data suggests that agents which target the renin–angiotensin system may improve cerebral blood flow autoregulation in hypertension, and this benefit should be exploited in the setting of hypertensive encephalopathy by treating with β-blockers or ACE inhibitors (28,51,52). There is some concern regarding the use of hydralazine or nitroglycerin in patients with neurologic compromise related to hypertension, and so these agents are best avoided. As noted previously, the goals of treatment are to reduce blood pressure to a level just below that at which autoregulatory mechanisms can be re-established, and to do so without dropping the blood pressure at too rapid a rate or below a level which would compromise cerebral perfusion. This requires the use of parenteral agents with short half-lives and the frequent assessment of the patient's neurologic status. Reductions in blood pressure usually result in the improvement of neurologic status; consideration for alternative diagnoses and further work-up are required in patients who do not improve despite appropriate treatment.

If treatment of elevated blood pressure in the setting of stroke or subarachnoid hemorrhage is pursued, we recommend not >20% reduction over 1–3 h, while keeping the diastolic blood pressure >100 mmHg. First line agents in this scenario include fenoldopam, nicardipine,

or labetalol. Nitroprusside is also a useful agent in this circumstance, although there is some concern that it can increase intracranial pressure. Calcium channel antagonists have benefit in the setting of subarachnoid hemorrhage; hydralazine and diazoxide should be avoided in patients with stroke or hemorrhage (37).

2. Cardiovascular Emergencies

A patient should be diagnosed with, and immediately treated for, a cardiovascular hypertensive emergency when any one of the following is present in the setting of severe hypertension: new onset chest pain, signs of congestive failure, electrocardiograph or serum chemistry evidence for myocardial ischemia, or evidence of acute aortic dissection (Table 41.5).

Acute coronary syndrome includes patients presenting with unstable angina or myocardial infarction. In this setting, hypertension is often a result of adrenergic stimulation. Hypertension increases myocardial oxygen demands, a direct ongoing threat in a patient with compromised coronary circulation. Effective management of blood pressure will help alleviate this increase in myocardial oxygen demand and should proceed with a goal of 20–25% reduction over 1–3 h. Specific agents that confer advantages in this situation are nitroglycerin, which improves collateral circulation and labetalol, which reduces heart rate and oxygen consumption. Nitroprusside and fenoldopam are also appropriate agents in this setting. Blood pressure control is an important adjuvant to the medical management of acute coronary syndromes and is perhaps the most important step to establish prior to consideration of thrombolytic therapy.

Acute aortic dissection is an extremely dangerous condition which presents almost invariably with severe chest pain and hypertension. The presence of severe

Table 41.5 Further Work-up in Patients Presenting with Cardiovascular Symptoms in the Setting of Severe Hypertension

Test	Results
Electrocardiogram	Evaluate for Q/ST/T wave changes consistent with myocardial infarction or ischemia
Creatinine kinase/ troponin	If positive, these are markers of myocardial cell injury
Chest radiograph	Evaluate for cardiomegaly or pulmonary edema suggestive of congestive failure; evaluate mediastinal shadow for evidence of widening (aortic dissection)
CT or MRI of chest	Useful to evaluate for aortic dissection
Angiography	Useful to evaluate for coronary thrombosis or aortic dissection

hypertension and tachycardia contributes to the pathophysiology by increasing intravascular pressure and shear stress on the already dissecting vessel. This can result in propagation of the dissection or overt rupture of the vessel. Management requires emergent reductions in blood pressure and heart rate, essentially to the lowest tolerable levels, in an effort to reduce the contributions these make toward the aortic pulse wave (28). This typically requires combination therapy using direct vasodilators in concert with antiadrenergic agents, such as the combination of nitroprusside and labetalol. Once blood pressure control is established, confirmatory studies should be undertaken as proximal aortic dissections may require urgent surgical management.

Congestive heart failure with severe hypertension often results in pulmonary edema and reduction in effective circulating volume. In this setting, agents which reduce preload and left ventricular volume are indicated. The most effective agents in this regard are nitroprusside and fenoldopam, although nitroglycerin can also be effective. In addition, appropriate and timely use of diuretics is usually necessary in these cases.

3. Renal Emergencies

It is important to attempt to distinguish between chronic abnormalities in estimated glomerular filtration rate (GFR) or urinalysis and new findings in the patient presenting with severe hypertension, as chronic kidney disease is commonly associated with hypertension. A patient should be diagnosed with, and immediately treated for, a nephrologic hypertensive emergency when any one of the following is present in the setting of severe hypertension: new or acutely worsening azotemia or presence of dysmorphic red cells or red cell casts in the urine (Table 41.6).

The general goal in treating hypertensive emergencies with renal organ damage remains a reduction in blood pressure of 20–25% over 1–3 h, although some authors advocate a more stepwise reduction in mean pressure of 10–20% over the first 1–2 h followed by a further decrease of 10–15% during the subsequent 6–12 h (8). Nitroprusside, labetalol, and nicardipine are all effective in this setting; however, strong consideration should be given to fenoldopam as the agent of choice, as it is both effective in reducing blood pressure and has the additional advantage of increasing mesenteric and renal blood flow (41).

A temporary reduction in GFR may accompany acute treatment of severe hypertension of any cause, in spite of a careful and appropriate approach to lowering the blood pressure. This may culminate in a need for renal replacement therapy. Fortunately, these occurrences are usually reversible with continued appropriate treatment.

D. Other Select Emergencies

1. Adrenergic Crises

The typical background for hypertensive emergency due to catecholamine excess states includes presence of pheochromocytoma, dietary noncompliance in a patient taking monamine-oxidase inhibitors, and cocaine or amphetamine intoxication (8). In these settings, a careful history and physical examination, and selection of appropriate laboratory tests, can usually distinguish between the three. This is a clinically relevant diagnosis to make, as in all three cases care must be taken to select antihypertensive treatments that will not result in unopposed α-adrenergic stimulation which could worsen hypertension. Phentolamine may be a useful agent in this setting. β-Blockers are generally avoided; if they are

Table 41.6 Further Work-up in Patients Presenting with Nephrologic Symptoms in the Setting of Severe Hypertension

Test	Results
Urinalysis	Screen for proteinuria, hematuria, or both; if present, these are indicative of renal injury
Urine sediment	Evaluate for dysmorphic red blood cells, red blood cell casts, or both; if present, these are indicative of glomerular injury
BUN, creatinine	These are useful as surrogate markers for changes in GFR; an acute decline in GFR may be seen in nephrologic emergencies
Renal ultrasound	Useful to determine the size and echogenicity of the kidneys. Duplex ultrasound is useful to evaluate for renovascular disease

required, they should be used only after appropriate α-receptor blockade has occurred. Labetalol may be useful as a parenteral agent with both α- and β-blocking characteristics.

2. Pregnancy

Hypertensive emergencies occurring during pregnancy constitute a particular problem for the clinician. Most often these occur as part of the syndrome of preeclampsia, defined as the onset of gestational hypertension (systolic blood pressure of >140 mmHg or diastolic blood pressure of >90 mmHg in a patient normotensive before 20 weeks), edema, and proteinuria or as part of the syndrome of eclampsia which includes seizures secondary to hypertensive encephalopathy (28). In addition, patients with chronic hypertension may present with an escalation in blood pressure during pregnancy, a condition distinct from the aforementioned syndromes.

The treatment of hypertensive emergency in the pregnant patient requires particular attention to the use of agents considered safe for both mother and fetus. Hydralazine has traditionally been the drug of choice in this setting, although there is little consensus evidence that it is superior to alternative agents such as parenteral labetalol, nicardipine, and fenoldopam (47). Enalaprilat, other ACE-inhibitors or angiotensin receptor blockers, nitroprusside, and oral or sublingual nifedipine are not recommended in this setting.

Eclampsia can be effectively treated with magnesium sulfate, which is considered preferable to antiepileptic mediations in preventing seizures (53). Of note, the risk of seizures remains high in the early postpartum period and treatment should continue in this period. Concomitant use of magnesium sulfate and calcium channel blockers increases the risk of significant hypotension and requires particular caution (54). In situations of preeclampsia and eclampsia, the syndromes should rapidly resolve following delivery of the fetus.

E. The Hypertensive Urgencies

The hypertensive urgency is a situation in which severe elevations in blood pressure are not accompanied by ongoing or impending end-organ dysfunction. This is a diagnosis of exclusion with important treatment ramifications. The difference between hypertensive emergencies and urgencies is clear: hypertensive emergencies are distinguished by progressive target-organ damage and the requirement of a need for immediate treatment in a hospital setting. As urgencies have neither of these characteristics, the need to distinguish between a hypertensive urgency and simply hypertension (newly diagnosed or chronic) is less clear. There is little evidence to suggest

that patients presenting with hypertensive urgency are at immediate risk for a target-organ event. In fact, it has been demonstrated that patients presenting with severe but uncomplicated hypertension derive no benefit in terms of sustained control of blood pressure when given rapid loading doses of antihypertensive medications when compared with similar patients treated with a single dose of medication and discharged (55). The term "hypertensive urgency" is therefore of questionable value; it may promote an emphasis on the need to acutely lower the presenting blood pressure, which is of uncertain value in this setting, rather than emphasizing the need for appropriate follow-up and long-term treatment of the hypertension.

In light of the lack of evidence favoring acute reductions in blood pressure in patients presenting with uncomplicated hypertension, we suggest that patients with a hypertensive urgency do not require immediate lowering of the blood pressure and do not require parenteral agents for the same. Instead, these patients should be managed with an appropriate regimen of oral medications. This process should start in a supervised setting, such as in the outpatient clinic or within the emergency room; however, the willing and capable patient can then be transitioned to home care with appropriate scheduled follow-up within 48–72 h.

Oral agents which have been studied in the acute setting to treat hypertensive urgencies are presented in Table 41.7. Although these agents are effective in reducing blood pressure within a timely fashion, they are all not necessarily ideal drugs for long-term treatment and do have associated side effects (7). In light of the earlier discussion, many have wondered whether there is any advantage in using these specific drugs over simply starting a more traditional maintenance antihypertensive regimen (56,57). In addition, it is unlikely that severe hypertension will be adequately treated with a single agent; consideration for starting two agents (perhaps with the second a diuretic) should be given. These decisions should be made on a case by case basis. Regardless of the starting regimen, caution should be exercised to avoid overly aggressive initial reductions in blood pressure. A goal of pressure in the range of 160/100 mmHg is an appropriate target. Care should also be taken to place the patient in a quiet room, free of distractions, to avoid anxiety-driven increases in the blood pressure which could be mistaken for resistance to therapy.

It should be kept in mind that patients presenting with uncomplicated hypertension will ultimately require supervised care for the rest of their lives. Multiple studies have documented that attempts to treat such patients without attention to prompt follow-up result in unacceptably high failure rates. Therefore, the best use of time spent treating such patients is in devising arrangements for continuity of

Table 41.7 Preferred Agents Used for the Acute Treatment of Hypertensive Urgencies

Drug	Dose/route	Onset of action	Duration of action	Side effects	Cautions
Calcium channel blockers					
Isradipine	2.5 mg; 5 mg capsules 5 mg; 10 mg controlled release tablets Starting dose 2.5 mg twice daily	2 h	8–16 h	Edema, palpitations, dizziness, fatigue	Little evidence to support efficacy of increasing doses above 10 mg/day
Felodipine	2.5 mg; 5 mg; 10 mg extended release tablets Starting dose 5–10 mg once daily	2 h	16–24 h	Edema, palpitations, dizziness, fatigue	Use with caution in hepatic failure
Nifedipine	30 mg; 60 mg; 90 mg extended release tablets Initial dose 30 mg extended release tablet once daily	20 min	2–5 h	Flushing, edema, dizziness, headache, weakness, palpitations, hypotension	Use of oral or sublingual short acting nifedipine has been associated with severe adverse outcomes (stroke, acute myocardial infarction, severe hypotension) and is to be considered unsafe
Angiotensin-converting Enzyme inhibitors					
Captopril	12.5 mg; 25 mg; 50 mg; 100 mg tablets Starting dose 12.5–25 mg p.o., repeat as needed; once effect obtained give three times daily (may be administered sublingually; no clear benefit of this route)	15 min–1 h	6–8 h, but dose-related	Rash, hypotension, dizziness, hyperkalemia, worsening of renal function, hypersensitivity reaction, cough	Case reports of Stevens–Johnson's syndrome in association with allopurinol Use at lower dose and 12 h intervals in patients with renal impairment Use with caution in patients at risk for hyperkalemia or in association with potassium sparing diuretics
Adrenergic blockers					
Clonidine	0.1 mg; 0.2 mg tablets Initial 0.1–0.2 mg p.o., repeat hourly, maximum total dose 0.6 mg	30–60 min	4–8 h	Dry mouth, drowsiness, rebound hypertension	Clonidine should not be abruptly discontinued as significant rebound hypertension may occur
Labetalol	100 mg; 200 mg; 300 mg tablets Initial 200–400 mg p.o., repeat 2–3 h	30–60 min	2–12 h	Dizziness, nausea, edema, hypotension, bradycardia, fatigue, paresthesias, transaminitis, mental depression	Use with caution in patients with asthma, bronchospastic disease, or congestive heart failure

care, rather than the search for an "optimal" primary treatment agent.

F. Other Agents

Urapidil is a peripheral α-1 blocker with central 5-hydroxytriptamene$_{1a}$ receptor antagonist activity, which has been widely studied and seems effective in the treatment of hypertensive urgencies and emergencies. Most studies have used intravenous doses of 12.5–25 mg, repeating, if needed. This agent has been shown to be safe and efficacious and perhaps particularly useful in the setting of intracranial pathology; however, it is not yet approved in the United States (58–60).

V. PITFALLS, DANGERS AND SIDE EFFECTS

Unquestionably, the major risk involved with patients with a hypertensive emergency involves either the failure to recognize the condition or the failure to ensure appropriate and immediate treatment of the blood pressure.

Beyond this, it is worth repeating that the hypertensive emergency represents a process in which normal autoregulatory mechanisms have failed, and that this usually occurs in the context of chronic underlying hypertension which may have altered the range over which autoregulation occurs. Extreme high blood pressure in this setting should be viewed more as a process than as a measurement, with the goal of treatment to reduce blood pressure to a level at which target-organ damage is minimized, but also to prevent a drop in blood pressure below which autoregulation cannot function in the individual under treatment. The use of potent modern antihypertensive drugs can usually achieve a rapid and dramatic reduction in the level of the blood pressure; however, ongoing clinical assessment is mandatory to confirm resolution of target-organ damage as well as to exclude the development of new signs or symptoms of hypoperfusion possibly related to treatment itself. This requires intensive supervision by nursing staff as well as physicians, best guided by invasive arterial blood pressure monitoring. Just as a hypertensive emergency is not defined by a level of blood pressure, successful management of a hypertensive emergency occurs only after a patient has been transitioned from parenteral medications to a stable oral medicine regimen which maintains blood pressure at a level below which target-organ damage occurs and above which symptoms related to hypotension or hypoperfusion develop.

VI. CONCLUSIONS AND OUTLOOK

Coincident with the development of improved antihypertensive agents and increasing awareness of the importance of controlling high blood pressure, there has been remarkable progress in the prevention and the treatment of hypertensive emergencies. Current estimates of the prevalence of hypertensive emergencies among patients with hypertension are at 1%, a great improvement over previous reported rates of 7% (61,62). Similarly, prior to the modern era of antihypertensives, patients who presented with hypertension and grade IV retinopathy had exceedingly high short-term mortality rates (63). More recent analysis now shows these same patients, treated appropriately, have survival rates nearly equivalent to those seen in patients with uncomplicated hypertension (64). In this respect, modern medicine has made considerable progress in treating this formerly terminal condition.

However, there exists pause for concern. Studies have suggested that in the modern era of medicine, 93% of patients admitted to the hospital with severe hypertension were previously diagnosed with hypertension (2,65). Indeed, the most common history obtained in patients presenting with a hypertensive emergency is that of a patient diagnosed with chronic hypertension who has been noncompliant with treatment or who has been undertreated (8). Similarly, a previous trial identified the absence of access to a primary care provider as the single most important risk factor present in patient seen at an inner-city emergency room for severe hypertension (66). Conversely, persistence in the treatment of hypertensive patients and adherence to an antihypertensive regimen have been conclusively demonstrated to significantly reduce progression to levels of severe hypertension (8,67).

In spite of the tremendous improvements witnessed in the treatment of hypertensive emergencies, they still represent potentially lethal complications of high blood pressure. The earlier-mentioned data suggests that those at highest risk for the development of this complication are easily identified with noninvasive screening tests. Further, hypertension remains an eminently treatable condition and those patients who are continuously and persistently treated are at much less risk to develop a hypertensive emergency, whereas those in whom treatment failure occurs represent the group at highest risk. It stands to reason then that further efforts to make improvements in this arena should focus upon early diagnosis, aggressive treatment, and meticulous follow-up to prevent the progression of hypertension and the resulting presentation with a hypertensive emergency or urgency. Fortunately, the data suggest this is an achievable goal for virtually all communities and populations. In fact, this may require no more, and no less, than a renewed focus on the initial identification, aggressive treatment to goal blood pressures, and routine follow-up of the uncomplicated hypertensive patient in the ambulatory setting by either the primary care doctor or the hypertension specialist.

REFERENCES

1. Vidt DG. Emergency room management of hypertensive urgencies and emergencies. J Clin Hypertens (Greenwich) 2001; 3:158–164.
2. Vaughan CJ, Delanty N. Hypertensive emergencies. Lancet 2000; 356:411–417.
3. Elliot WJ. Clinical features and management of selected hypertensive emergencies. J Clin Hypertens (Greenwich). 2004; 6:587–592.
4. Zampaglione B, Pascale C, Marchisio M, Cavallo-Perin P. Hypertensive urgencies and emergencies. Prevalence and clinical presentation. Hypertension 1996; 27:144–147.
5. Kitiyakara C, Guzman NJ. Malignant hypertension and hypertensive emergencies. J Am Soc Nephrol 1998; 9:133–142.
6. Preston RA, Baltodano NM, Cienki J, Materson BJ. Clinical presentation and management of patients with uncontrolled, severe hypertension: results from a public teaching hospital. J Hum Hypertens 1999; 13:249–255.
7. Cherney D, Straus S. Management of patients with hypertensive urgencies and emergencies: a systematic review of the literature. J Gen Intern Med 2002; 17:937–945.
8. Elliott WJ. Hypertensive emergencies. Crit Care Clin 2001; 17:435–451.
9. Barry DI, Lassen NA. Cerebral blood flow autoregulation in hypertension and effects of antihypertensive drugs. J Hypertens 1984; 2(suppl 3):519–526.
10. Kontos HA, Wei EP, Navari RM, Levasseur JE, Rosenblum WI, Patterson JL Jr. Responses of cerebral arteries and arterioles to acute hypotension and hypertension. Am J Physiol 1978; 234:H371–H383.
11. Skinhøj E, Strandgaard S. Pathogenesis of hypertensive encephalopathy. Lancet 1973; 1:461–462.
12. Strandgaard S, Olesen J, Skinhøj E, Lassen NA. Autoregulation of brain circulation in severe arterial hypertension. BMJ 1973; 3:507–510.
13. McHenry LC Jr, West JW, Cooper ES, Goldberg HI, Jaffe ME. Cerebral autoregulation in man. Stroke 1974; 5:695–706.
14. Folkow B. "Structural factor" in primary and secondary hypertension. Hypertension 1990; 16:89–101.
15. Korsgaard N, Aalkjaer C, Heagerty AM, Izzard AS, Mulvany MJ. Histology of subcutaneous small arteries from patients with essential hypertension. Hypertension 1993; 22:523–526.
16. Ito T, Yamakawa H, Bregonzio C, Terron JA, Falcon-Neri A, Saavedra JM. Protection against ischemia and improvement of cerebral blood flow in genetically hypertensive rats by chronic pretreatment with an angiotensin II AT1 antagonist. Stroke 2002; 33:2297–2303.
17. Strandgaard S, Jones JV, MacKenzie ET, Harper AM. Upper limit of cerebral blood flow autoregulation in experimental renovascular hypertension in the baboon. Circ Res 1975; 37:164–167.
18. Strandgaard S. Autoregulation of cerebral blood flow in hypertensive patients. The modifying influence of prolonged antihypertensive treatment on the tolerance to acute, drug-induced hypotension. Circulation 1976; 53:720–727.
19. Prisant LM, Carr AA, Hawkins DW. Treating hypertensive emergencies. Controlled reduction of blood pressure and protection of target-organs. Postgrad Med 1993; 93:92–94, 101–104, 108–110.
20. Gao E, Young WL, Pile-Spellman J, Ornstein E, Ma Q. Mathematical considerations for modeling cerebral blood flow autoregulation to systemic arterial pressure. Am J Physiol 1998; 274:H1023–H1031.
21. Strandgaard S, MacKenzie ET, Sengupta D, Rowan JO, Lassen NA, Harper AM. Upper limit of autoregulation of cerebral blood flow in the baboon. Circ Res 1974; 34:435–440.
22. Harder DR. Pressure-induced myogenic activation of cat cerebral arteries is dependent on intact endothelium. Circ Res 1987; 60:102–107.
23. Strandgaard S, Paulson OB. Regulation of cerebral blood flow in health and disease. J Cardiovasc Pharmacol 1992; 19(suppl 6):S89–S93.
24. Furchgott RF, Zawadzki JV. The obligatory role of endothelial cells in the relaxation of arterial smooth muscle by acetylcholine. Nature 1980; 288:373–376.
25. Kuchan MJ, Jo H, Frangos JA. Role of G proteins in shear stress-mediated nitric oxide production by endothelial cells. Am J Physiol 1994; 267:C753–C758.
26. Paniagua OA, Bryant MB, Panza JA. Role of endothelial nitric oxide in shear stress-induced vasodilation of human microvasculature: diminished activity in hypertensive and hypercholesterolemic patients. Circulation 2001; 103:1752–1758.
27. Huang A, Sun D, Kaley G, Koller A. Superoxide released to high intra-arteriolar pressure reduces nitric oxide-mediated shear stress- and agonist-induced dilations. Circ Res 1998; 83:960–965.
28. Blumenfeld JD, Laragh JH. Management of hypertensive crises: the scientific basis for treatment decisions. Am J Hypertens 2001; 14:1154–1167.
29. Lip GY, Edmunds E, Hee FL, Blann AD, Beevers DG. A cross-sectional, diurnal, and follow-up study of platelet activation and endothelial dysfunction in malignant phase hypertension. Am J Hypertens 2001; 14:823–828.
30. Lip GY, Beevers M, Beevers DG. Malignant hypertension in young women is related to previous hypertension in pregnancy, not oral contraception. QJM 1997; 90:571–575.
31. Garrett BN, Kaplan NM. Efficacy of slow infusion of diazoxide in the treatment of severe hypertension without organ hypoperfusion. Am Heart J 1982; 103:390–394.
32. Kaplan NM. Management of hypertensive emergencies. Lancet 1994; 344:1335–1338.
33. Schulz V. Clinical pharmacokinetics of nitroprusside, cyanide, thiosulphate and thiocyanate. Clin Pharmacokinet 1984; 9:239–251.
34. Kaplan JA, Jones EL. Vasodilator therapy during coronary artery surgery. Comparison of nitroglycerin and nitroprusside. J Thorac Cardiovasc Surg 1979; 77:301–309.
35. Fremes SE, Weisel RD, Mickle DA, Teasdale SJ, Aylmer AP, Christakis GT, Madonik MM, Ivanov J, Houle S, McLaughlin PR. A comparison of nitroglycerin and nitroprusside: I. Treatment of postoperative hypertension. Ann Thorac Surg 1985; 39:53–60.

36. Henriksen L, Paulson OB. The effects of sodium nitroprusside on cerebral blood flow and cerebral venous blood gases. II. Observations in awake man during successive blood pressure reduction. Eur J Clin Invest 1982; 12:389–393.

37. Tietjen CS, Hurn PD, Ulatowski JA, Kirsch JR. Treatment modalities for hypertensive patients with intracranial pathology: options and risks. Crit Care Med 1996; 24:311–322.

38. Pluta RM, Oldfield EH, Boock RJ. Reversal and prevention of cerebral vasospasm by intracarotid infusions of nitric oxide donors in a primate model of subarachnoid hemorrhage. J Neurosurg 1997; 87:746–751.

39. Joshi S, Hartl R, Sun LS, Libow AD, Wang M, Pile-Spellman J, Young WL, Connolly ES, Hirshman CA. Despite in vitro increase in cyclic guanosine monophosphate concentrations, intracarotid nitroprusside fails to augment cerebral blood flow of healthy baboons. Anesthesiology 2003; 98:412–419.

40. Bodmann KF, Troster S, Clemens R, Schuster HP. Hemodynamic profile of intravenous fenoldopam in patients with hypertensive crisis. Clin Investig 1993; 72:60–64.

41. Murphy MB, Murray C, Shorten GD. Fenoldopam: a selective peripheral dopamine-receptor agonist for the treatment of severe hypertension. N Engl J Med 2001; 345:1548–1557.

42. Lappe RW, Todt JA, Wendt RL. Effects of fenoldopam on regional vascular resistance in conscious spontaneously hypertensive rats. J Pharmacol Exp Ther 1986; 236:187–191.

43. Clark KL, Hilditch A, Robertson MJ, Drew GM. Effects of dopamine DA1-receptor blockade and angiotensin converting enzyme inhibition on the renal actions of fenoldopam in the anaesthetized dog. J Hypertens 1991; 9:1143–1150.

44. Elliott WJ, Weber RR, Nelson KS, Oliner CM, Fumo MT, Gretler DD, McCray GR, Murphy MB. Renal and hemodynamic effects of intravenous fenoldopam versus nitroprusside in severe hypertension. Circulation 1990; 81:970–977.

45. Lunell NO, Lewander R, Nylund L, Sarby B, Thornstrom S. Acute effect of dihydralazine on uteroplacental blood flow in hypertension during pregnancy. Gynecol Obstet Invest 1983; 16:274–282.

46. Paterson-Brown S, Robson SC, Redfern N, Walkinshaw SA, de Swiet M. Hydralazine boluses for the treatment of severe hypertension in pre-eclampsia. Br J Obstet Gynaecol 1994; 101:409–413.

47. Magee LA, Cham C, Waterman EJ, Ohlsson A, von Dadelszen P. Hydralazine for treatment of severe hypertension in pregnancy: meta-analysis. BMJ 2003; 327:955–960.

48. Hollander JE. The management of cocaine-associated myocardial ischemia. N Engl J Med 1995; 333:1267–1272.

49. Boreas AM, Lodder J, Kessels F, de Leeuw PW, Troost J. Prognostic value of blood pressure in acute stroke. J Hum Hypertens 2002; 16:111–116.

50. Brott T, Bogousslavsky J. Treatment of acute ischemic stroke. N Engl J Med 2000; 343:710–722.

51. Squire IB. Actions of angiotensin II on cerebral blood flow autoregulation in health and disease. J Hypertens 1994; 12:1203–1208.

52. Vacher E, Richer C, Giudicelli JF. Effects of losartan on cerebral arteries in stroke-prone spontaneously hypertensive rats. J Hypertens 1996; 14:1341–1348.

53. Lucas MJ, Leveno KJ, Cunningham FG. A comparison of magnesium sulfate with phenytoin for the prevention of eclampsia. N Engl J Med 1995; 333:201–205.

54. Carbonne B, Jannet D, Touboul C, Khelifati Y, Milliez J. Nicardipine treatment of hypertension during pregnancy. Obstet Gynecol 1993; 81:908–914.

55. Zeller KR, Von Kuhnert L, Matthews C. Rapid reduction of severe asymptomatic hypertension. A prospective, controlled trial. Arch Intern Med 1989; 149:2186–2189.

56. Fagan TC. Acute reduction of blood pressure in asymptomatic patients with severe hypertension. An idea whose time has come—and gone [editorial]. Arch Intern Med 1989; 149:2169–2170.

57. Ferguson RK, Vlasses PH. How urgent is 'urgent' hypertension? [editorial]. Arch Intern Med 1989; 149:257–258.

58. Malbrain ML, Wyffels E, Lins RL, Daelemans R. Treating hypertensive patients with intracranial pathology. Crit Care Med 1996; 24:2072–2074.

59. Dooley M, Goa KL. Urapidil. A reappraisal of its use in the management of hypertension. Drugs 1998; 56:929–955.

60. Alijotas-Reig J, Bove-Farre I, Cabo-Frances F, Angles-Coll R. Effectiveness and safety of prehospital urapidil for hypertensive emergencies. Am J Emerg Med 2001; 19:130–133.

61. Calhoun DA, Oparil S. Hypertensive crisis since FDR—a partial victory. N Engl J Med 1995; 332:1029–1030.

62. Calhoun DA. Hypertensive crisis. In: Oparil S, Weber MA, eds. Hypertension: A Companion to Brenner and Rector's The Kidney. Philadelphia: W.B. Saunders Co., 2000:715–718.

63. Keith NM, Wagener HP, Barker ND. Some different types of essential hypertension: their course and prognosis. Am J Med Sci 1939; 197:332–343.

64. Webster J, Petrie JC, Jeffers TA, Lovell HG. Accelerated hypertension—patterns of mortality and clinical factors affecting outcome in treated patients. Q J Med 1993; 86:485–493.

65. Bennett NM, Shea S. Hypertensive emergency: case criteria, sociodemographic profile, and previous care of 100 cases. Am J Public Health 1988; 78:636–640.

66. Shea S, Misra D, Ehrlich MH, Field L, Francis CK. Predisposing factors for severe, uncontrolled hypertension in an inner-city minority population. N Engl J Med 1992; 327c:776–781.

67. Moser M, Hebert PR. Prevention of disease progression, left ventricular hypertrophy and congestive heart failure in hypertension treatment trials. J Am Coll Cardiol 1996; 27(5):1214–1218.

42

Pregnancy and Hypertension

JASON G. UMANS

Georgetown University Medical Center and MedStar Research Institute, Washington, District of Columbia, USA

KEYPOINTS

- Hypertension is a common medical complication of pregnancy with morbid consequences to mother and fetus and may be not only due to essential or secondary hypertension, but also due to two pregnancy-specific conditions, preeclampsia and gestational hypertension.

- While hypertension is defined as BP > 140 systolic or 90 diastolic, these values are based on auscultation, as oscillometric measurements are often incorrect. There is disagreement regarding appropriate treatment targets for BP during pregnancy.

- The clinical diagnosis of preeclampsia or "superimposed preeclampsia" is often uncertain, especially in parous women or those with underlying hypertension or renal disease; one should err towards overdiagnosis and careful clinical evaluation.

- Gestational vasodilation often obviates the need for antihypertensive drugs early in pregnancy. ACE inhibitors and ARBs are contraindicated in the latter half of pregnancy.

- Magnesium prevents and treats eclamptic convulsions. It remains unclear whether specific groups of preeclamptic women benefit from this therapy and how long it should be administered.

SUMMARY

Evaluation and treatment of hypertension in pregnancy is more the subject of consensus statements, meta-analyses, and often-thoughtful reviews than it is of well-designed and adequately-powered clinical studies or treatment trials. Care of these women depends on some understanding of the normal hemodynamic adaptations to pregnancy, on the differing pathophysiology of specific hypertensive disorders in pregnancy, and on pregnancy-specific concerns in blood pressure measurement. Choice of antihypertensive agents and blood pressure targets remain as important subjects for research, though guidelines are available. Importantly, blood pressure control in hypertensive gravidas should be but part of a multidisciplinary attempt to assure maternal well-being and optimize pregnancy outcome. This chapter attempts to provide the clinician with practical guidance regarding the evaluation and management of these high-risk pregnant women, with reference to the latest research and clinical information.

I. INTRODUCTION

Hypertension complicates 10–15% of all pregnancies, is the second leading cause of maternal death and increases risk of other morbid outcomes to mother and fetus, including those of preterm birth, intrauterine growth restriction (IUGR), placental abruption, and perinatal mortality. Hypertension in pregnancy may be due to underlying chronic essential or secondary hypertension, to gestational hypertension, or to preeclampsia; the latter two disorders are unique to human pregnancy. Importantly, each of these causes of hypertension may have distinct hemodynamics, molecular mechanisms, risks to mother and fetus, and long-term sequelae. The cardiovascular adaptations which attend normal pregnancy make it surprisingly difficult to diagnose underlying hypertension in many women and it is often difficult to distinguish preeclampsia from the other disorders, particularly from gestational hypertension. There are no data to guide treatment goals or blood pressure targets in hypertensive gravidas. Defining blood pressure targets is even more difficult as most automated oscillometric blood pressure devices give erroneous results in hypertensive pregnant women. In most women without target organ damage, there appears to be no benefit of tight blood pressure control, but, since cerebrovascular catastrophe may occur in women with blood pressure of 170 systolic or 110 diastolic, efforts focus on avoiding these high levels and on early recognition of preeclampsia, which may evolve rapidly and unpredictably towards multisystem failure and life-threatening complications. Antihypertensive therapy is limited by contraindications to the use of

angiotensin-converting enzyme (ACE) inhibitors and AT1 receptor blockers late in pregnancy, by concerns regarding fetal safety of other agents, and by a paucity of well-designed and adequately powered studies, all of which have not limited a profusion of meta-analyses and consensus treatment guidelines.

II. BLOOD PRESSURE MEASUREMENT AND DEFINITION OF HYPERTENSION

Hypertension in pregnancy is defined as a blood pressure >140 systolic or >90 diastolic, occurring at any time during pregnancy (1). In the past, many had also used a case definition of an increase in blood pressure of >30 systolic or >15 diastolic over values noted prior to conception or early in the first trimester. Although outcomes data have not supported the latter definition, women with increasing blood pressure should be considered high risk and demanding of close antenatal monitoring.

Blood pressure measurement during pregnancy is best performed in the sitting position, with the arm supported, using an appropriately sized cuff, a mercury sphygmomanometer, and defining diastolic blood pressure as the fifth Korotkoff sound (2). In some women, blood pressure may be increased late in pregnancy because of mass effect of the gravid uterus when supine. This has led to an unfortunate folklore favoring blood pressure measurement in the left lateral decubitus position; when blood pressure is recorded from the right arm (inadvertently elevated relative to the heart), it is then artifactually low and falsely reassuring. In contrast, it is not unreasonable to record blood pressure from the left arm with a patient in the left lateral decubitus position when it is impractical for her to sit. Most of the oscillometric devices now used routinely for blood pressure measurement in hospital clinics and even in labor and delivery units have not been validated in hypertensive pregnant women; nearly all provide erroneous calculations of diastolic blood pressure, so all automated readings should be confirmed by auscultation when they might impact on the need for urgent antihypertensive therapy.

Despite the difficulties that attend use of automated oscillometric devices, there seems to be great utility in home blood pressure monitoring by women at high risk for preeclampsia or with more severe underlying hypertension (3). This is based not on their accuracy, but rather on their ability to detect significant changes in systolic pressure, leading to early evaluation of preeclampsia or to more careful titration of antihypertensive medications. An evolving literature suggests some promise in the use of ambulatory blood pressure monitoring for risk assessment in pregnancy, though confirmatory and outcomes data remain lacking (4).

III. RISKS OF HYPERTENSION IN PREGNANCY AND GUIDELINES FOR EVALUATION AND MANAGEMENT

There have been many reviews describing the increased risk of morbid outcomes in hypertensive pregnancy, including superimposed preeclampsia, preterm birth, IUGR, placental abruption, perinatal death, and accelerated hypertension threatening the mother, which result from hypertension in pregnancy (5–7). Recognition of these risks has led to recent consensus guidelines for the evaluation and management of hypertensive gravidas by groups in the United States, Canada, and Australia (2,8,9). Unfortunately, antihypertensive treatment fails to prevent any of these outcomes, save for the occurrence of more severe hypertension later in pregnancy. This may, however, be of considerable importance because adverse perinatal outcomes seem closely related to severity of maternal hypertension and because severe hypertension may be a major cause of both hospitalization and early delivery.

Even without clear outcomes data, it is well established that blood pressures as low as 170/110 mmHg can lead to cerebrovascular hemorrhage during pregnancy, making treatment of such pressures a medical emergency. At the opposite extreme, it has been suggested that tight blood pressure control may impair fetal growth (10). The Australasian Society for the Study of Hypertension in Pregnancy suggests maintaining blood pressures <140/90 mmHg (8). Similarly, the Canadian Hypertension Society suggests tight control only for some groups of women (9). In contrast, the NHBPEP Working Group on Hypertension in Pregnancy suggests (re)instituting drug therapy at pressures of 150–160/100–110, targeting lower pressures in selected patients with end organ damage or underlying renal disease (2). A recent survey of Canadian practitioners highlighted the lack of consensus regarding blood pressure targets in hypertensive pregnant women (11) and serves as justification for adequately powered prospective trials, which would be more informative than our current collection of consensus guidelines.

A. Hemodynamic Adaptation to Pregnancy

An understanding of hypertension in pregnancy depends on appreciation of the striking hemodynamic and renal adaptations that characterize normotensive pregnancy, is reviewed briefly in subsequent sections. Pregnancy is characterized by systemic vasodilation so striking that, despite an increase in cardiac output (CO) of nearly 50%, blood pressure falls early in the first trimester (12,13). Paradoxically, this gestational hypotension is even more striking in women with chronic hypertension,

so that blood pressure may fall by 30/15 mmHg, masking the recognition of underlying hypertension when the patient is examined at her first prenatal visit (14). In this respect, careful history, review of records, funduscopic exam, and evidence of target organ damage may be the only good clues to chronic hypertension and blood pressure of 120/80 should lead to suspicion of underlying hypertension. The mechanisms of gestational vasodilation remain uncertain, but appear not to depend upon either vasodilator prostaglandins or nitric oxide (NO).

Pregnancy leads to striking changes in the renin–angiotensin–aldosterone system (15). Levels of angiotensinogen, plasma renin activity, angiotensin II, Ang 1–7, and aldosterone are all increased markedly in normal pregnancy. However, there is a specific refractoriness to the vascular AT1 receptor-mediated effects of angiotensin, leading to impaired constriction of isolated human resistance arteries and to a decreased pressor response to infused angiotensin II.

In addition to generalized systemic vasodilation, pregnancy leads to specific renal vasodilation with balanced afferent and efferent arteriolar vasodilation and parallel increments of renal plasma flow and glomerular filtration rate (GFR) (13). As in the case of underlying essential hypertension, these normal changes may obscure underlying renal insufficiency (chronic kidney disease); a serum creatinine ≥0.8 mg/dL early in pregnancy should be viewed with suspicion. Careful animal experimentation has suggested a mechanistic cascade leading to renal vasodilation in rat pregnancy. The ovarian hormone relaxin appears to act via gelatinase to cleave big endothelin (ET), leading to ET_B receptor-mediated activation of NO synthase (16). Whether similar mechanisms occur in women is yet to be determined.

IV. CLASSIFICATION AND DIAGNOSIS OF HYPERTENSION IN PREGNANCY

In accord with the recommendations of the International Society for the Study of Hypertension in Pregnancy (ISSHP), along with several national and international obstetrics groups, and the National High Blood Pressure Education Program (NHBPEP) Working Group, we currently recognize four diagnostic categories for hypertensive disorders of pregnancy (1,2). Chronic hypertension (antedating pregnancy) may be either essential or secondary. Two hypertensive disorders occur only in pregnancy: gestational hypertension and preeclampsia. Finally, preeclampsia may be superimposed upon underlying chronic hypertension. Older terms such as pregnancy-induced hypertension usually include a mix of disorders, with differing pathophysiology and risks; both the literature and our patients are ill-served by their continued use.

A. Chronic Hypertension

With an epidemic of obesity, insulin-resistance, and early onset of essential hypertension, this appears to be the most rapidly growing cause of hypertension in pregnancy. Most chronic hypertension is essential in nature, though young women may certainly suffer from secondary forms of hypertension. Three of these are worthy of specific mention: pheochromocytoma, renovascular hypertension, and primary hyperaldosteronism (14). Although extraordinarily rare, physicians should have a low threshold for suspecting pheochromocytoma when hypertension is associated with classic symptoms and signs, as it may lead to hypertensive crisis during labor. Suspicion of pheochromocytoma should lead to α-adrenoreceptor blockade and confirmatory measurements of catecholamines and their metabolites; there are several case reports of life-saving surgical management with proper pharmacologic blockade during pregnancy. Renovascular hypertension, as may most commonly result from fibromuscular dysplasia in women of childbearing age, carries such a high risk of superimposed preeclampsia and poor outcome that it also should be corrected prior to or even during pregnancy if diagnosed. Unfortunately, diagnosis is difficult because usual measurements of circulating elements of the renin–angiotensin system are of no diagnostic utility during pregnancy, doppler ultrasound measurements are often misleading, and radionuclide renal scans are avoided in pregnancy. There are, however, case reports of diagnosis by magnetic resonance angiography and of correction by angioplasty during pregnancy with good outcome. Finally, hypertension due to hyperaldosteronism may have a variable and often surprisingly benign course during pregnancy. This is because progesterone may act in part as an aldosterone receptor antagonist (15,17). In these cases, both hypertension and hypokalemia may be unmasked following delivery.

Importantly, the lack of routine medical care for apparently healthy young women conspires with the normal hemodynamic changes of early pregnancy to make it difficult to diagnose underlying chronic hypertension, which may then only be recognized later in pregnancy and mistaken either for gestational hypertension or for preeclampsia.

B. Gestational Hypertension

Gestational hypertension is hypertension occurring *de novo*, usually during the latter half of pregnancy in the absence of proteinuria and other signs or symptoms suggestive of preeclampsia and resolving postpartum. Although it may result in severe hypertension-requiring treatment, its course is usually more benign than that of preeclampsia. It may recur in subsequent pregnancies and often predicts essential hypertension and increased cardiovascular risk later in life.

C. Preeclampsia

Preeclampsia is a multisystem disorder characterized by *de novo* hypertension, usually during the latter half of pregnancy, though cases have been reported as early as 16 weeks, associated with proteinuria (>300 mg/day) and resolving postpartum. It occurs in $\sim6\%$ of (usually primigravid) pregnancies. Risk factors, listed in Table 42.1, include a family history of preeclampsia, multifetal gestation, diabetes mellitus, renal or collagen vascular diseases, and obesity with insulin resistance. In addition, a variety of unrelated genetic abnormalities seem to increase the risk of preeclampsia in some populations, including mutations of angiotensinogen or NO synthase genes. Although clinically evident target organ damage characterizes more severe disease, subtle symptoms or laboratory evidence of target organ damage is common, including hyperuricemia and sometimes thrombocytopenia or abnormalities of liver function or coagulation tests. As preeclampsia can have a variable course and explosive clinical evolution (18), with real risks of maternal morbidity and mortality, one should err towards diagnosing preeclampsia, even in the absence of proteinuria (which can occur later in the evolution of the disorder), when hypertension is accompanied by abdominal pain, neurologic symptoms including headache or blurred vision, or any evidence of thrombocytopenia or liver function or coagulation abnormalities (2). Preeclampsia can evolve rapidly to a convulsive and life-threatening phase, termed eclampsia. An especially threatening variant of preeclampsia is the HELLP (Hemolysis, Elevated Liver enzymes, Low Platelets) syndrome, which may seem mild in its initial presentation, then evolve over hours to microangiopathic hemolysis, severe thrombocytopenia, and hepatic necrosis with rupture.

Table 42.1   Risk Factors for Preeclampsia

Primigravida
First pregnancy with this partner
Family history of preeclampsia
Multifetal pregnancy
Preeclampsia in prior pregnancy
IUGR, placental abruption, or fetal demise in prior pregnancy
Obesity
Renal disease of any cause or severity (including microhematuria or microproteinuria without specific etiologic diagnosis)
Diabetes mellitus
Chronic hypertension
Connective tissue disease

It would seem easy to distinguish preeclampsia from gestational hypertension by the detection of proteinuria and, perhaps by hemodynamic assessment; unfortunately, this is often not the case. Obstetricians in the United States typically screen for proteinuria using urine dipsticks, confirming positive (1+) results by 24 h urine collection. The sensitivity of urine dipsticks and their prediction of 24 h urine protein are poor (19), due in large part to variations in urine concentration, which might be overcome by efforts to standardize screening techniques on the basis of measurement of albumin:creatinine ratios (20). Moreover, although proteinuria may occur in synchrony with hypertension, it may be delayed, by many weeks in some cases (21). This important observation explains why the diagnosis of preeclampsia can only now be made with any certainty in retrospect and also may explain the common misconception that gestational hypertension may "evolve into preeclampsia". It is hoped that markers such as soluble fomesin-like tyrosine kinase-1 (sFLT-1) or AT1 receptor autoantibodies (see in the following section) or convenient noninvasive hemodynamic measurements may, in the future, allow for more certain differential diagnosis during pregnancy.

D. Superimposed Preeclampsia

Although "pure" preeclampsia occurs in ~6% of (usually primigravid) pregnancies, it can be superimposed on up to 20–40% of underlying cases of chronic hypertension, or other predisposing medical diseases including (even minor) renal disease of any cause, such as early diabetic nephropathy or microscopic hematuria (22,23), or collagen vascular disease. Superimposed preeclampsia is apt to be more severe, with greater risks to mother and fetus than preeclampsia absent an underlying medical predisposition; as well, it is more apt to recur in subsequent pregnancies. Superimposed preeclampsia, along with progression to more severe hypertension, represent the two major risks of chronic hypertension in pregnancy. It is often difficult to decide when an already-hypertensive or already-proteinuric woman's course has worsened due to the onset of superimposed preeclampsia. Indeed, in a careful study which used renal biopsies to verify diagnosis, a nephrologist and obstetrician correctly diagnosed preeclampsia and distinguished it from competing disorders in only 58% of cases (24). Underlying proteinuria can be expected to worsen during pregnancy, often to nephrotic levels, in any woman with underlying glomerular disease. Because of these diagnostic uncertainties, we advocate a strategy of close monitoring, repeatedly re-establishing baseline data in order to detect interval changes in blood pressure, proteinuria, symptoms, or blood test results, which might suggest superimposed preeclampsia.

V. PATHOPHYSIOLOGY OF PREECLAMPSIA AND ECLAMPSIA

Elegant invasive hemodynamic studies of untreated preeclamptic women demonstrate that hypertension in this disorder is due to systemic vasoconstriction, associated with decreased CO and left ventricular filling pressures (25). Interestingly, early in pregnancy, CO is increased more in women who subsequently develop either gestational hypertension or preeclampsia than in women who progress to uneventful normotensive pregnancies, although not so reliably as to provide a premorbid diagnosis of these disorders. Hemodynamics diverge when hypertension becomes manifest, with further increments of CO [and low systemic vascular resistance (SVR)] in women with gestational hypertension and a "switch" to high SVR and low CO in women with preeclampsia (26). Preeclampsia is characterized not only by vasoconstrictor hypertension but also by widespread endothelial dysfunction and by evidence of increased oxidative stress.

Preeclampsia decreases GFR more so than ERPF, consistent with selective afferent arteriolar renal vasoconstriction, and usually decreases renal uric acid clearance, elevating serum levels above the norms for pregnancy (2.8–3.2 mg/dL) (13). Proteinuria is nonselective, with increased excretion of albumin and nonalbumin proteins. Preeclampsia is the major cause of nephrotic range proteinuria during pregnancy. The occurrence of edema (which is common even in normal pregnancy) is quite variable in preeclampsia; indeed, many women who present with eclamptic seizures may be free of edema.

There has been persisting controversy regarding the mechanisms which lead to CNS complications in preeclampsia and which may result in eclamptic seizures. Some have viewed these complications as a form of hypertensive encephalopathy, whereas others have suggested that brain injury is due to ischemia resulting from local vasoconstriction. The latter view seems best supported by the classic autopsy series of Sheehan and Lynch (27) noting hemorrhage and petechiae, likely the result of focal ischemia. In contrast, several recent studies have used noninvasive Doppler techniques to suggest a role for increased cerebral perfusion pressure in most, but not all, cases (28). If confirmed, this may have significant implications for the choice of antihypertensive agents in preeclamptic women, as labetalol and magnesium (but not vasodilators) appear to decrease elevated cerebral perfusion pressure in hypertensive gravidas (29).

As preeclampsia may occur in molar pregnancy (i.e., without a fetus), tends to resolve following delivery of the placenta, and seems uniformly associated with typical defects in placentation, much attention has been focused on a pathophysiologic role of the placenta. It is currently held that early abnormalities in trophoblastic invasion and remodeling of spiral arteries may fail to decrease placental resistance appropriately, leading to focal ischemia in the placenta and elaboration of factors which may act on the maternal vasculature to result in preeclampsia. A large literature seems to support this construct by demonstrating that experimental uteroplacental hypoperfusion leads to hypertension in pregnant laboratory animals (30). Indeed, in preeclamptic women, the placenta elaborates sFLT-1, a soluble receptor for (and functional antagonist of) the growth factors VEGF and PlGF (16,31). Decreased availability of these growth factors may increase blood pressure and almost certainly leads to proteinuria and to the renal biopsy lesion of "glomerular endotheliosis", which is typical of preeclampsia.

Sympathetic outflow is increased in women with preeclampsia, perhaps contributing to hypertension (32). More recently, several studies have demonstrated changes in angiotensin receptor expression and activity (33) or the occurrence of autoantibodies which activate AT1 receptors in women with preeclampsia (16,34). These autoantibodies, which clear following delivery, may underlie not only vasoconstriction and hypertension, but also oxidative stress (via AT1 receptor activation of superoxide synthesis by NAD(P)H oxidase) and endothelial dysfunction. Unfortunately, even though the effect of these autoantibodies is inhibited *in vitro* by angiotensin receptor blockers (ARBs), their use, along with use of ACE inhibitors, is contraindicated in late pregnancy because of fetal toxicity.

VI. STRATEGIES TO PREVENT PREECLAMPSIA

Several meta-analyses of antihypertensive use in pregnant women with chronic hypertension suggest that blood pressure control *per se* fails to prevent preeclampsia (35,36). Likewise, neither salt restriction nor prophylactic diuretics prevent preeclampsia; earlier claims to the contrary were wrong, due to misdiagnosis of gravidas with misdiagnosis of gravidas with nonproteinuric hypertension (37). Despite observations of hypocalciuria in preeclamptic women, several large studies of calcium supplementation failed to demonstrate any significant prevention of proteinuric hypertension (38). There remains the possibility of some benefit to women with extremely low dietary calcium, the subject of a recently completed trial in developing countries.

Among many studies of circulating vasoconstrictor factors in women with preeclampsia, several suggested an imbalance in arachidonic acid metabolism, favoring vasoconstrictor thromboxanes over prostacylcin and leading to many studies of low dose (60–100 mg/day) aspirin. Unfortunately, extraordinarily promising results of many early small studies have not been confirmed in subsequent

well-designed large trials including more than 25,000 women and demonstrating only trivial effects on maternal or fetal outcome or on the occurrence of preeclampsia (39,40). Additional studies of women at high risk for recurrent or superimposed preeclampsia (as described in the following sections) also failed to demonstrate meaningful prevention of proteinuric hypertension. Although meta-analyses of trials including more than 36,000 women have suggested some benefit (RR 0.81 [0.75–0.88]) of aspirin prophylaxis, it is striking that this conclusion is not supported by any of the larger well-designed trials included within the meta-analysis and has failed to identify any aspirin-sensitive subgroups of women at risk (41). For example, in women at moderate risk for preeclampsia, aspirin was without significant effect in any of the eight trials with more than 400 women/study arm. Similarly, a single negative study accounted for 2503 of the 4222 women included in the meta-analysis of 19 aspirin trials in women at high risk for preeclampsia. It remains possible that increased dose or altered dosing schedule might reveal benefits of antiplatelet therapy, though further large studies seem unlikely (42).

More recently, on the basis of the increased oxidative stress which characterizes preeclampsia and could account for its vascular abnormalities, a small study of vitamins C and E supplementation in women at high risk for preeclampsia appeared to decrease proteinuria (and thus the diagnosis of preeclampsia) but not hypertension (43). Of concern, the incidence of low birthweight seemed to increase in the treatment group. On the basis of these early results, two large and hopefully definitive, trials are currently underway (44).

VII. EVALUATION AND MANAGEMENT OF HYPERTENSION IN PREGNANCY

Evaluation of women with chronic hypertension or with a history of hypertension in a previous pregnancy should ideally begin prior to conception. Evaluation should focus on the possibility of secondary hypertension, on assessment of renal function and hypertensive target organ damage, on detection of underlying diabetes or renal disease, and on family history of pregnancy complications. Proteinuria, *per se*, appears to increase pregnancy risk in hypertensive women. In addition, the obstetric history should focus on both maternal and neonatal outcome, including premature birth, IUGR leading to small-for-gestational-age infants, placental abruption, fetal demise, neonatal morbidity and mortality, and the severity and timing of superimposed preeclampsia.

Early in pregnancy it is reasonable to discontinue all antihypertensive drugs in women whose hypertension was reasonably well controlled using two or fewer agents. Owing to gestational vasodilation, most of these women will require no antihypertensives, at least until later in pregnancy, and will avoid any concerns regarding antihypertensive safety during the first trimester. Women should have a baseline laboratory evaluation, including urinalysis and urine culture, 24 h urine for evaluation of creatinine clearance, protein and albumin excretion, comprehensive chemistry panel including measurement of transaminases, uric acid and electrolytes, and CBC with platelets. Most would repeat these studies each trimester in order to establish a new baseline to aid in the recognition of superimposed preeclampsia. Women will then be seen every 2–3 weeks for measurement of blood pressure, urine protein, and for fetal assessment as indicated.

Higher risk chronic hypertensive women include those with advanced maternal age, longstanding hypertension or any evidence of target organ damage, diabetes mellitus, renal disease of any cause or severity, any connective tissue disease, cardiomyopathy, vascular malformation, previous history of fetal or perinatal loss, or worsened hypertension early in pregnancy. These women require closer observation, collaborative care with appropriate subspecialists, and probably tighter blood pressure control to avoid progressive target organ damage during the course of pregnancy. Worsened hypertension or suspicion of superimposed preeclampsia will commonly lead to inpatient evaluation in order to assure maternal and fetal well-being, titrate antihypertensive therapy, and to decide whether pregnancy may be prolonged safely with close monitoring.

VIII. ANTIHYPERTENSIVE THERAPY REMOTE FROM DELIVERY

With some small differences, the American, Canadian, and Australia–New Zealand consensus statements recognize methyldopa as a preferred antihypertensive with the greatest experience in pregnancy (2,8,9). It is well tolerated by pregnant women, does not alter uteroplacental or fetal hemodynamics, and has the best long-term follow-up of childhood development following exposure *in utero*, albeit in an underpowered study (45). Methyldopa-induced hepatitis is a rare adverse effect; Coombs positive hemolytic anemia is rare with short-term treatment, though many women will be unable to tolerate its common adverse effects of drowsiness or dry mouth. Of note, a recent meta-analysis along with a large retrospective single-center report suggested that other antihypertensive drugs might be superior to methyldopa in limiting perinatal morbidity and mortality (36,46). Adequately powered prospective comparative trials are entirely lacking and should be required before we would be comfortable abandoning the long clinical experience and consensus support for use of methyldopa.

β-blockers are near to methyldopa in their wide use in pregnancy, have been assessed in several randomized trials, and are the subject of a Cochrane meta-analysis (35). Early preclinical and clinical observations raised concerns of impaired uteroplacental perfusion, fetal growth restriction, and harmful cardiovascular effects on the fetus. However, most prospective studies, focusing on β-blocker use in the third trimester, have shown effective blood pressure control, prevention of more severe hypertension, and an absence of significant adverse effects on the fetus. In contrast, early use of atenolol in one trial led to striking fetal growth restriction, a conclusion supported by several reviews, retrospective series, and meta-analyses (47–49). More recently, a large nonrandomized single-center series noted improved perinatal outcome with β-blockers (primarily atenolol) compared with other agents (primarily nifedipine or methyldopa) (46). Finally, there was a suggestion in one recent meta-analysis of several small trials that β-blockers might decrease (and calcium channel blockers increase) the incidence of proteinuria or superimposed preeclampsia; this preliminary observation should provoke further study rather than a change in practice (36). Although many older studies focused on agents such as atenolol, the NHBPEP Working Group advocates labetalol (a combined α- and β blocker) as an alternative to methyldopa, and the Australasian group advocates use of β-blockers with intrinsic sympathomimetic activity, such as oxprenolol (not available in the USA) or pindolol (8).

Calcium channel blockers, principally extended-release nifedipine, are widely used, apparently safe and effective in pregnancy (2). Although data are limited, nifedipine is widely viewed as an acceptable alternative to methyldopa or β-blockers for chronic use during pregnancy.

Hydralazine is the most commonly used second-line agent (following combinations of those discussed previously); it is used in combination with either a β-blocker or methyldopa to limit reflex tachycardia. There seems little basis for use of α-adrenergic blockers other than in the setting of suspected pheochromocytoma. Diuretic use during pregnancy is quite controversial. Diuretics will limit normal gestational volume expansion, can decrease amniotic fluid volume, and lead to electrolyte abnormalities. However, they do not seem to impair fetal outcome, may be continued if they were crucial to blood pressure control prior to conception, and may be combined with other agents, especially in patients with renal insufficiency, heart disease, or when clinical volume overload is a problem. Diuretics are not used when preeclampsia is suspected, as its hemodynamics are characterized by decreased CO and primary systemic vasoconstriction (12,25).

Increased circulating elements of the renin–angiotensin system during pregnancy and evidence for AT1 receptor activation in preeclampsia might seem to support use of

Table 42.2 Oral Antihypertensives Used Commonly in Pregnancy

Drug (FDA risk[a,b])	Dose	Concerns or comments
Most commonly used first-line agents		
Methyldopa (B)	0.5–3.0 g/day in 2–3 divided doses	Preferred agent of the NHBPEP working group; maternal side effects sometimes limit use.
Labetalol (C) or other β-receptor antagonists	200–2400 mg/day in 2–3 divided doses	Labetalol is preferred by NHBPEP working group as alternative to methlydopa. Atenolol most commonly used in Canada and β-blockers with intrinsic sympathomimetic activity are preferred by some in Australia. May cause fetal growth restriction when started early.
Nifedipine (C)	30–120 mg/day of a slow-release preparation	Less experience with other calcium entry blockers.
Adjunctive agents		
Hydralazine (C)	50–300 mg/day in 2–4 divided doses	Few controlled trials, long experience; used only in combination with sympatholytic agent (e.g., methyldopa or a β-blocker) to prevent reflex tachycardia.
Thiazide diuretics (C)	Depends on specific agent	Most studies in normotensive gravidas.
Contraindicated		
ACE inhibitors and AT1 receptor antagonists (D)		Leads to fetal loss in animals; human use associated with fetopathy, oligohydramnios, growth retardation, and neonatal anuric renal failure, which may be fatal.

[a]No antihypertensive has been proven safe for use during the first trimester (i.e., FDA Category A).
[b]US Food and Drug Administration classifies risk for most agents as C: "Either studies in animals have revealed adverse effects on the fetus (teratogenic or embryocidal effects or other) and there are no controlled studies in women, or studies in women and animals are not available. Drugs should only be given if the potential benefit justifies the potential risk to the fetus". This nearly useless classification unfortunately still applies to most drugs used during pregnancy.

ACE inhibitors or AT1 receptor blockers in hypertensive gravidas. Indeed, these drugs are now widely used for "renal protection" in young women of childbearing age with underlying diabetic nephropathy or proteinuric renal disease. Unfortunately, they are contraindicated during the latter half of pregnancy, because of a specific fetopathy (including renal dysgenesis and calvarial hypoplasia) and the risk of (fatal) neonatal acute renal failure (50). These drugs are often discontinued when pregnancy is planned but, as they are not teratogenic and all adverse outcomes appear because of fetal exposure in the second or third trimester (51), reliable patients who are followed closely can continue these drugs through conception, discontinuing them in the first trimester if pregnancy is detected early. Table 42.2 summarizes those agents most commonly used for chronic blood pressure control in pregnancy.

IX. ANTIHYPERTENSIVE THERAPY OF MORE SEVERE HYPERTENSION

Table 42.3 lists the antihypertensives most commonly used for urgent control of severe hypertension late in pregnancy. Hydralazine is used either in small (5–10 mg) repeated doses or as a continuous infusion, because larger doses or frequent dosing may lead to precipitous maternal hypotension and fetal distress. Parenteral labetalol, by continuous intravenous infusion or in repeated boluses, has replaced hydralazine at many centers and appears to have similar safety and efficacy, though comparative studies are few and it may result in less effective blood pressure control (52,53). Despite its lack of approval by the US Food and Drug Administration for the treatment of hypertension, the NHBPEP Working Group, along with many workers, advocated oral (or sublingual) nifedipine as an acceptable alternative to hydralazine or labetalol for urgent blood pressure control during pregnancy (2). Its efficacy and safety appear similar to the other agents, whereas diazoxide and ketanserin seem inferior (52). Although most studies have suggested little difference in outcome among patients treated with these three agents, a recent meta-analysis has suggested that hydralazine may be inferior to labetalol or calcium channel blockers because it more often leads to excessive hypotension, fetal distress, oliguria or renal dysfunction, maternal side effects, placental abruption, and caesarian delivery, clearly suggesting the need for further studies (53). Sodium nitroprusside remains a relatively contraindicated agent of last resort, usually reserved for urgent blood pressure control in the minutes leading up to delivery (54). Finally, although there have been reports of ACE inhibitor use as "salvage therapy" during pregnancy (55),

Table 42.3 Antihypertensives Used Commonly for Urgent Blood Pressure Control

Drug (FDA risk[a])	Dose and route	Concerns or comments[b]
Hydralazine (C)	5 mg, iv or im, then 5–10 mg every 20–40 min; or constant infusion of 0.5–10 mg/h	Preferred by NHBPEP working group. Higher doses or more frequent administration often precipitate maternal or fetal distress, which appear more common than with other agents.
Labetalol (C)	20 mg iv, then 20–80 mg every 20–30 min, up to maximum of 300 mg; or constant infusion of 1–2 mg/min	Probably less risk of tachycardia and arrhythmia than with other vasodilators, likely less blood pressure control than hydralazine.
Nifedipine (C)	5–10 mg po, repeat in 30 min if needed, then 10–20 mg every 2–6 h	Parenteral calcium channel blockers seem reasonable alternatives, but less data.

[a]US Food and Drug Administration Class C, as noted in footnote to Table 42.2.
[b]Adverse effects for all agents, except as noted, may include headache flushing, nausea, and tachycardia (primarily because of precipitous hypotension and reflex sympathetic activation).

there seems to be no justification for use of these agents or of ARBs during the second or third trimester.

X. CLINICAL AND ADJUNCTIVE MANAGEMENT OF PREECLAMPSIA

Suspicion of preeclampsia should lead to hospitalization and inpatient evaluation. Near to term (>34 weeks), if fetal maturity can be assured, delivery is the definitive treatment of choice for preeclampsia. Earlier in pregnancy, it may seem desirable to temporize, attempting to control blood pressure, administer glucocorticoids to hasten fetal lung maturation, and monitor laboratory and clinical status closely so as to prolong pregnancy. The obstetric literature on such temporizing strategies often appears confusing and contradictory, but seems to agree that such approaches may result in days to weeks of additional fetal maturation; however, they are best reserved to tertiary centers and, regardless of gestational age, any of the ominous signs or symptoms noted in Table 42.4 should lead to delivery. As noted earlier, accelerated hypertension should be treated at systolic levels of >160 or diastolic levels of >105, to avoid the intracerebral bleeds which can occur at pressures of ≥170/110. We

Table 42.4 Ominous Signs and Symptoms in Preeclampsia Suggesting Prompt Delivery

Inability to control blood pressure (systolic <160 mmHg or diastolic <105 mmHg)
Any evidence of acute renal failure or progressive oliguria
Falling platelets or thrombocytopenia <10^5/mm^3
Any evidence of microangiopathic hemolysis or coagulopathy
Upper abdominal (epigastric or right upper quadrant) pain
Headache, visual disturbance, or any CNS signs
Retinal hemorrhage or papilledema
Acute congestive heart failure or pulmonary edema

advocate treatment at these somewhat lower pressures because of increased blood pressure lability and uncertainty in blood pressure measurement in women with preeclampsia. Central nervous system signs or symptoms (including even headache or blurred vision) should provoke treatment at even lower pressures.

Parenteral magnesium sulfate has long been favored by North American clinicians for prevention or treatment of eclamptic seizures. It has been proven more effective than either phenytoin or diazepam in preventing recurrent seizures in women with eclampsia (56,57). More recently, a placebo-controlled, double-blind study demonstrated the efficacy of 24 h of magnesium therapy for primary prevention of eclamptic seizures in women with preeclampsia (58). This study of over 10,000 women was without significant short-term adverse effects to mother or baby, and was conducted without monitoring of serum magnesium levels. Interestingly, there was a strong trend towards decreased maternal death, apparently unrelated to the effect on convulsions. It remains unclear, however, which women with preeclampsia should be offered magnesium and for how long. In most centers, treatment usually entails a loading dose of 4–6 g MgSO$_4$ (infused >10 min, never as a bolus), followed by continuous infusion of 1–2 g/h to achieve plasma levels of 5–9 mg/dL. Magnesium is then usually continued until the patient stabilizes or for 24 h following delivery. Lower doses should be used without continuous infusion, guided by serum levels, in women with any degree of renal insufficiency, as magnesium is excreted renally. Finally, a vial of calcium gluconate should always be kept at the patient's bedside to treat magnesium toxicity, should it occur.

Overall, our clinical approach to evaluation, management, and treatment of pregnant women with underlying hypertension is in accord with recommendations made by the NHBPEP Working Group (2). Our key objectives, to be carried out in close coordination with experienced high-risk obstetric colleagues, are to achieve blood pressure control adequate to assure maternal safety, to carefully and serially monitor maternal blood pressure, well-being, and laboratory data in order to facilitate early recognition of superimposed preeclampsia, and to proceed to expeditious delivery ($\pm$ magnesium prophylaxis) in the face of preeclampsia or accelerated hypertension when it presents a threat to maternal safety.

XI. POSTPARTUM ANTIHYPERTENSIVE THERAPY IN NURSING MOTHERS

Although the pharmacokinetic principles which govern drug distribution to milk and delivery to the infant are well understood (59), there are few well-designed studies assessing neonatal effects of maternally administered antihypertensive drugs delivered via breast milk, though this literature was the subject of a comprehensive and thoughtful recent review (60). Factors which favor drug passage into milk are a small maternal volume of distribution, low plasma protein binding, high lipid solubility, and lack of charge at physiologic pH. Even when drugs are ingested by nursing infants, effective infant exposure depends on the volume of milk ingested, intervals between drug administration and nursing, oral bioavailability (in the infant), and the capacity of the infant to clear the drug.

Neonatal exposure to methyldopa appears low and it is considered safe. Similarly, calcium channel blockers, while transferred into milk, appear safe to nursing infants. Exposure to either labetalol or propranolol likewise seems low, while atenolol and metoprolol are concentrated in breast milk. Diuretics may decrease milk production significantly, though studies are limited. Because of concerns regarding effects of ACE inhibitors and AT1 receptor antagonists on neonatal renal function, these drugs are usually avoided, especially in very premature infants; however, milk concentrations of captopril are undetectable, suggesting use of this agent when an ACE inhibitor is required (61).

XII. CONCLUSIONS

Medical treatment of hypertension in pregnancy or of preeclampsia may seem to have changed little over the past three decades. While basic and translational research on these disorders have made tremendous leaps forward, this has not yet resulted in answers to simple questions regarding choice of antihypertensive agents or treatment targets, strategies for clinical monitoring, or early diagnosis of preeclampsia. In the meantime, careful attention to appropriate blood pressure measurement, understanding of expected hemodynamic changes during pregnancy,

vigilance for subtle signs and symptoms of target organ damage, collaborative management with obstetric colleagues, and familiarity with drugs commonly used during pregnancy will all aid us in optimizing care and improving pregnancy outcome.

REFERENCES

1. Brown MA, Lindheimer MD, de Swiet M, Van Assche A, Moutquin JM. The classification and diagnosis of the hypertensive disorders of pregnancy: statement from the International Society for the Study of Hypertension in Pregnancy, Hypertens Pregnancy 2001; 20:IX–XIV.
2. Report of the National High Blood Pressure Education Project Working Group on High Blood Pressure in Pregnancy, NIH Publication No. 00–3029, July 2000, 38pp (available online at http://www.nhlbi.nih.gov/health/prof/heart/hbp_preg.htm).
3. Waugh J, Habiba MA, Bosio P, Boyce T, Shennan A, Halligan AW. Patient initiated home blood pressure recordings are accurate in hypertensive pregnant women. Hypertens Pregnancy 2003; 22:93–97.
4. Hermida RC, Ayala DE. Prognostic value of office and ambulatory blood pressure measurements in pregnancy. Hypertension 2002; 40:298–303.
5. Rey E, Couturier A. The prognosis of pregnancy in women with chronic hypertension. Am J Obstet Gynecol 1994; 171:410–416.
6. Ferrer RL, Sibai BM, Mulrow CD, Chiquette E, Stevens KR, Cornell J. Management of mild chronic hypertension during pregnancy: a review. Obstet Gynecol 2000; 96:849–860. Available at (http://www.ahcpr.gov/clinic/evrptfiles.htm).
7. Sibai BM, Lindheimer M, Hauth J, Caritis S, VanDorsten P, Klebanoff M, MacPherson C, Landon M, Miodovnik M, Paul R, Meis P, Dombrowski M. Risk factors for preeclampsia, abruptio placentae, and adverse neonatal outcomes among women with chronic hypertension. N Engl J Med 1998; 339:667–671.
8. Brown MA, Hague WM, Higgins J, Lowe S, McCowan L, Oats J, Peek MJ, Rowan JA, Walters BN. Austalasian Society of the Study of Hypertension in Pregnancy. The detection, investigation and management of hypertension in pregnancy: full consensus statement. Aust NZ J Obstet Gyn 2000; 40:139–155.
9. Rey E, LeLorier J, Burgess E, Lange IR, Leduc L. Report of the Canadian Hypertension Society consensus conference. 3. Pharmacologic treatment of hypertensive disorders in pregnancy. Can Med Assoc J 1997; 157:1245–1254.
10. von Dadelszen P, Ornstein MP, Bull SB, Logan AG, Koren G, Magee LA. Fall in mean arterial pressure and fetal growth restriction in pregnancy hypertension: a meta-analysis. Lancet 2000; 355:87–92.
11. Caetano M, Ornstein MP, Von Dadelszen P, Hannah ME, Logan AG, Gruslin A, Willan A, Magee LA. A survey of Canadian practitioners regarding the management of the hypertensive disorders of pregnancy. Hypertens Pregnancy. 2004; 23:61–74.

12. McLaughlin MK, Roberts JM. Hemodynamic Changes. In: Lindheimer MD, Roberts JM, Cunningham FG, eds. Chesley's Hypertensive Disorders in Pregnancy, 2d ed., Chapter 3. Stamford: Appleton & Lange, 1999:69–102.

13. Conrad KP, Lindheimer MD. Renal and Cardiovascular Alterations. In: Lindheimer MD, Roberts JM, Cunningham FG, eds. Chesley's Hypertensive Disorders in Pregnancy, 2d ed., Chapter 8, Stamford: Appleton & Lange, 1999:263–326.

14. August P, Lindheimer MD. Chronic hypertension. In: Lindheimer MD, Roberts JM, Cunningham FG, eds. Chesley's Hypertensive Disorders in Pregnancy, 2d ed. Stamford: Appleton & Lange, 1999:605–633.

15. August PA, Seeley JE. The renin angiotensin system in normal and hypertensive pregnancy and in ovarian function. In: Laragh JH, Brenner BM, eds. Hypertension: Pathophysiology, Diagnosis, and Management, 2nd ed. New York: Raven Press, 1995:2225–2244.

16. Davison JM, Homuth V, Jeyabalan A, Conrad KP, Karumanchi SA, Quaggin S, Dechend R, Luft FC. New aspects in the pathophysiology of preeclampsia. J Am Soc Nephrol 2004; 15:2440–2448.

17. Lindheimer MD, Richardson DA, Ehrlich EM, Katz AI. Potassium homeostasis in pregnancy. J Reprod Med 1987; 32:517–532.

18. Hauth JC, Cunningham FG. Preeclampsia-Eclampsia. In: Lindheimer MD, Roberts JM, Cunningham FG, eds. Chesley's Hypertensive Disorders in Pregnancy, 2d ed., Chapter 5, Stamford: Appleton & Lange, 1999:169–199.

19. Meyer NL, Mercer BM, Friedman SA, Sibai BM. Urinary dipstick protein: a poor predictor of absent or severe proteinuria. Am J Obstet Gynecol 1994; 170(1 Pt 1):137–141.

20. Waugh J, Kilby M, Lambert P, Bell SC, Blackwell CN, Shennan A, Halligan A. Validation of the DCA 2000 microalbumin:creatinine ratio urinanalyzer for its use in pregnancy and preeclampsia. Hypertens Pregnancy 2003; 22(1):77–92.

21. Wolf M, Shah A, Jimenez-Kimble R, Sauk J, Ecker JL, Thadhani R. Differential risk of hypertensive disorders of pregnancy among Hispanic women. J Am Soc Nephrol 2004; 15:1330–1338.

22. Ekbom P, Damm P, Nogaard K, Clausen P, Feldt-Rasmussen U, Feldt-Rasmussen B, Nielsen LH, Molsted-Pedersen L, Mathiesen ER. Urinary albumin excretion and 24-hour blood pressure as predictors of preeclampsia in Type I diabetes. Diabetologia 2000; 43:927–931.

23. Stehman-Breen CO, Levine RJ, Qian C, Morris CD, Catalano PM, Curet LB, Sibai BM. Increased risk of preeclampsia among nulliparous pregnant women with idiopathic hematuria. Am J Obstet Gynecol 2002; 187:703–708.

24. Fisher KA, Luger A, Spargo BH, Lindheimer MD. Hypertension in pregnancy: clinical–pathological correlations and remote prognosis. Medicine 1981; 60:267–276.

25. Visser W, Wallenburg HCS. Central hemodynamic observations in untreated preeeclamptic patients. Hypertension 1991; 17:1072–1077.

26. Bosio PM, McKenna PJ, Conroy R, O'Herlihy C. Maternal central hemodynamics in hypertensive disorders of pregnancy. Obstet Gynecol 1999; 94:978–984.

27. Sheehan H, Lynch JB. Pathology of Toxemia of Pregnancy. London: Churchill, 1973.

28. Belfort MA, Varner MW, Dizon-Townson DS, Grunewald C, Nisell H. Cerebral perfusion pressure, and not cerebral blood flow, may be the critical determinant of intracranial injury in preeclampsia: a new hypothesis. Am J Obstet Gynecol 2002; 187:626–634.

29. Belfort MA, Tooke-Miller C, Allen JC Jr, Dizon-Townson D, Varner MA. Labetalol decreases cerebral perfusion pressure without negatively affecting cerebral blood flow in hypertensive gravidas. Hypertens Pregnancy 2002; 21:185–197.

30. Khalil RA, Granger JP. Vascular mechanisms of increased arterial pressure in preeclampsia: lessons from animal models. Am J Physiol 2002; 283:R29–R45.

31. Maynard SE, Min JY, Merchan J, Lim KH, Li J, Mondal S, Libermann TA, Morgan JP, Sellke FW, Stillman IE, Epstein FH, Sukhatme VP, Karumanchi SA. Excess placental soluble fms-like tyrosine kinase 1 (sFlt1) may contribute to endothelial dysfunction, hypertension, and proteinuria in preeclampsia. J Clin Invest 2003; 111:649–658.

32. Schobel HP, Fischer T, Heuszer K, Geiger H, Schmieder RE. Preeclampsia—a state of sympathetic overactivity. N Engl J Med 1996; 335:1480–1485.

33. AbdAlla S, Lother H, el Massiery A, Quitterer U. Increased AT(1) receptor heterodimers in preeclampsia mediate enhanced angiotensin II responsiveness. Nat Med 2001; 7:1003–1009.

34. Wallukat G, Homuth V, Fischer T, Lindschau C, Horstkamp B, Jupner A, Baur E, Nissen E, Vetter K, Neichel D, Dudenhausen JW, Haller H, Luft FC. Patients with preeclampsia develop agonistic autoantibodies against the angiotensin AT1 receptor. J Clin Invest 1999; 103:945–952.

35. Magee LA, Duley L. Oral β blockers for mild to moderate hypertension during pregnancy. Cochrane Database Syst Rev 2003;(3):CD002863

36. Abalos E, Dulcy L, Steyn DW, Henderson-Smart DJ, Antihypertensive drug therapy for mild to moderate hypertension during pregnancy. Cochrane Database Syst Rev 2001; 2:CD002252

37. Collins R, Yusuf S, Peto R. Overview of randomised trials of diuretics in pregnancy. Brit Med J 1985; 290:17–23.

38. Levine RJ, Hauth JC, Curet LB, Sibai BM, Catalano PM, Morris CD, DerSimonian R, Esterlitz JR, Raymond EG, Bild DE, Clemens JD, Cutler JA. Trial of calcium to prevent preeclampsia. N Engl J Med 1997; 337:69–76.

39. Sibai BM, Caritis SN, Thom E, Klebanoff M, McNellis D, Rocco L, Paul RH, Romero R, Witter F, Rosen M. Prevention of preeclampsia with low-dose aspirin in healthy, nulliparous pregnant women. N Engl J Med 1993; 329:1213–1218.

40. CLASP (Collaborative Low-dose Aspirin Study in Pregnancy) Collaborative Group, CLASP: a randomised trial of low-dose aspirin for the prevention and treatment of

preeclampsia among 9364 pregnant women. Lancet 1994; 343:619–629.

41. Duley L, Henderson-Smart DJ, Knight M, King JF. Antiplatelet agents for preventing pre-eclampsia and its complications. Cochrane Database Syst Rev 2004; (1):CD004659.

42. Hermida RC, Ayala DE, Fernandez JR. Administration time-dependent effects of aspirin in women at differing risk for preeclampsia. Hypertension 1999; 34:1016–1023.

43. Chappell LC, Seed PT, Briley AL, Kelly FJ, Lee R, Hunt BJ, Parmar K, Bewley SJ, Shennan AH, Steer PJ, Poston L. Effect of antioxidants on the occurrence of pre-eclampsia in women at increased risk: a randomised trial. Lancet 1999; 354:810–816.

44. Raijmakers MT, Dechend R, Poston L. Oxidative Stress and Preeclampsia. Rationale for Antioxidant Clinical Trials. Hypertension. Epub Hypertension 2004, doi:10.1161/01.HYP.0000141085.98320.01

45. Cockburn J, Moar VA, Ounsted M, Redman CW. Final report of study on hypertension during pregnancy: the effects of specific treatment on the growth and development of the children. Lancet 1982; 1(8273):647–649 (Earlier followup papers from this trial were by Mutch, Moar, Ounsted, and Redman, appearing in Early Hum Dev 1977; 1:47–57 and 1:59–67).

46. Ray JG, Vermeulen MJ, Burrows EA, Burrows RF. Use of antihypertensive medications in pregnancy and the risk of adverse perinatal outcomes: McMaster outcome study of hypertension in pregnancy 2 (MOS HIP 2). BMC Pregnancy Childbirth 2001; 1:6.

47. Butters L, Kennedy S, Rubin PC. Atenolol in essential hypertension during pregnancy. Brit Med J 1990; 301:587–589.

48. Lip GY, Beevers M, Churchill D, Shaffer LM, Beevers DG. Effect of atenolol on birthweight. Am J Cardiol 1997; 79:1436–1438.

49. Bayliss H, Churchill D, Beevers M, Beevers DG. Antihypertensive drugs in pregnancy and fetal growth: evidence for "pharmacological programming" in the first trimester? Hypertens Pregnancy 2002; 21:161–174.

50. Sedman AB, Kershaw DB, Bunchman TE. Recognition and management of angiotensin converting enzyme inhibitor fetopathy. Pediatr Nephrol 1995; 9:382–385.

51. Postmarketing surveillance for angiotensin-converting enzyme inhibitor use during the first trimester of pregnancy—United States, Canada, and Israel, 1987–1995, MMWR Morb Mortal Wkly Rep 1997; 46:240–242.

52. Duley L, Henderson-Smart DJ. Drugs for treatment of very high blood pressure during pregnancy. Cochrane Database Syst Rev 2002; (4):CD001449.

53. Magee LA, Cham C, Waterman EJ, Ohlsson A, von Dadelszen P. Hydralazine for treatment of severe hypertension in pregnancy: meta-analysis. Brit Med J 2003; 327(7421):955–960.

54. Shoemaker CT, Meyers M. Sodium nitroprusside for control of severe hypertensive disease of pregnancy: a case report and discussion of potential toxicity. Am J Obstet Gynecol 1984; 149:171–173.

55. Easterling TR, Carr DB, Davis C, Diederichs C, Brateng DA, Schmucker B. Low-dose, short-acting, angiotensin-converting enzyme inhibitors as rescue therapy in pregnancy. Obstet Gynecol 2000; 96:956–961.

56. The Eclampsia Collaborative Group. Which anticonvulsant for women with eclampsia? Evidence from the collaborative eclampsia trial. Lancet 1995; 345:1455–1463.

57. Lucas MJ, Leveno KJ, Cunningham FG. A comparison of magnesium sulfate with phenytoin for the prevention of eclampsia. N Engl J Med 1995; 333:201–205.

58. The Magpie Trial Collaborative Group. Do women with pre-eclampsia, and their babies, benefit from magnesium sulphate? The Magpie Trial: a randomised placebo-controlled trial. Lancet 2002; 359(9321):1877–1879.

59. Atkinson HC, Begg EJ, Darlow BA. Drugs in human milk: clinical pharmacokinetic considerations. Clin Pharmacokinet 1988; 14:217–240.

60. Beardmore KS, Morris JM, Gallery EDM. Excretion of antihypertensive medication into human breast milk: a systematic review. Hypertens Pregnancy 2002; 21:85–95.

61. Devlin RG, Fleiss PM. Captopril in human blood and breast milk. J Clin Pharmacol 1981; 21:110–113.

43

Childhood Hypertension

BONITA FALKNER

Thomas Jefferson University, Philadelphia, Pennsylvania, USA

KEYPOINTS

- Hypertension occurs in 1 to 3% of children.
- Secondary causes of hypertension can be identified more frequently in younger children.
- Children with hypertension should receive treatment to lower blood pressure.

SUMMARY

Essential or primary hypertension can occur in childhood. Because of the rising rates of childhood obesity, the expression of essential hypertension in childhood will increase. Despite this trend, the possibility of secondary hypertension should be considered in a child with documented hypertension. Children with suspected secondary hypertension may require a more extensive when evaluation when compared with children and adolescents expressing characteristics of essential hypertension.

I. INTRODUCTION

The literature on hypertension has generally regarded hypertension in children and adolescents as a "special population" problem. Certain aspects of childhood hypertension are unique with the young. Compared with hypertension in adults, childhood hypertension is defined differently and occurs less frequently. Secondary causes of hypertension are detected more frequently in children than in adults, often requiring a different approach in the evaluation of the hypertension. But childhood hypertension also has some striking similarities to hypertension in adults. Severe untreated hypertension in children has as poor an outcome as it does in adults (1). Children with essential hypertension can express the same risk factors as adults for cardiovascular disease, and children with hypertension can benefit from interventions to control blood pressure.

Hypertension may occur at any phase of childhood, from the newborn period through adolescence. An important aspect of blood pressure surveillance in the young is to determine when elevated blood pressure in a child is a symptom of an underlying disease, that is, secondary hypertension, or an early expression of primary (essential) hypertension.

II. DEFINITION OF HYPERTENSION IN CHILDHOOD

The definition of hypertension in children and adolescents is based on the upper portion of the normal blood pressure distribution for children. The definition of hypertension in adults is based on the level of blood pressure that is linked with an increase in risk for cardiovascular events. Although the risk for cardiovascular events increases as blood pressure rises >120 mmHg (2), hypertension continues to be defined as blood pressure that exceeds 140/90 mmHg, regardless of adult age or gender. However, in children, with the exception of extreme hypertension noted earlier, there is not yet data that definitively links a level of blood pressure with subsequent cardiovascular events. In the absence of such data, childhood hypertension is defined statistically. The results of several large epidemiologic studies that measured blood pressure in healthy children and adolescents (3–9) provide data on blood pressure pattern and distribution. There is a progressive increase in blood pressure level with increasing age throughout childhood concurrent with the normal age-related increase in height and weight. Thus, there is a consistent relationship of blood pressure to body size in childhood, with a normal upward shift in blood pressure with growth. A gender difference in blood pressure distribution emerges in adolescence that is consistent with a gender difference in height.

The current definition of hypertension in children and adolescents is systolic or diastolic blood pressure that is equal to or greater than the 95th percentile for age, gender, and height (5). This definition delineates the top segment of the normal blood pressure distribution at each phase of childhood. prehypertension is systolic blood pressure or diastolic blood pressure that is between the 90th and 95th percentile for age, gender, and height. Normal blood pressure is systolic and diastolic blood pressure that is less than the 90th percentile for age, gender, and height. Table 43.1 provides the level of blood pressure for the 95th and 90th percentile for age, gender, and height percentile for boys, and Table 43.2 provides the same percentile levels for girls (5).

Although it is limited, there is some data on the normal range of blood pressure in newborns and very young infants (6,7,10). When blood pressure is measured at birth and then daily in healthy newborns, there is a rapid and consistent increase in blood pressure from day of birth through the first 5 days of life (11). This upward shift in blood pressure, over the first few days following birth, reflects the normal hemodynamic transition from intrauterine to extrauterine life. Similar observations were made in a larger study on newborn infants that included a broad range of birth weight and gestational age (12). There is a direct relationship of blood pressure with both birth weight and gestational age at birth. Regardless of birth weight or gestational age at birth, there is a transition, reflected by a progressive increase in blood pressure that occurs during the first 5 days of postnatal life. Subsequently, blood pressure is directly related to body weight and age in terms of gestation or postconception age. The upper 95th percentile confidence limit for systolic blood pressure in a term infant (40 weeks postconception) is 90 mmHg. Blood pressure levels that exceed 90 mmHg are considered to be hypertensive in a term infant; by 4–6 weeks of age (44–46 weeks postconception), a systolic blood pressure that exceeds 100 mmHg is hypertension.

III. MEASUREMENT OF BLOOD PRESSURE IN THE YOUNG

Measurement of blood pressure in children and adolescents should be performed in a standardized manner that is similar to the methods that were used in the development of the blood pressure tables. In an outpatient office or clinic setting, the preferred method for blood pressure measurement in children aged ≥3 years is by auscultation with a standard sphygmomanometer. The recommended instrument is mercury column manometers. However, access to mercury-containing instruments is becoming restricted at many clinical sites because of concern about the environmental hazards of accidental mercury spills. When mercury-containing devices for blood pressure measurement are not available, auscultation with an aneroid instrument is an acceptable alternative.

Correct blood pressure measurement in children requires the use of a cuff that is appropriate for the size of the child's upper arm (13). A technique that can be used to select a blood pressure, cuff size of appropriate size is to select a cuff that has a bladder width ~40–50% of the arm circumference midway between the olecranon and the acromion. This usually will be a cuff bladder that will cover 80–100% of the circumference of the arm. The equipment that is necessary to measure

Table 43.1 BP Levels for Boys by Age and Height Percentile

Age (years)	BP Percentile	SBP (mmHg) Percentile of height							DBP (mmHg) Percentile of height						
		5th	10th	25th	50th	75th	90th	95th	5th	10th	25th	50th	75th	90th	95th
1	50th	80	81	83	85	87	88	89	34	35	36	37	38	39	39
	90th	94	95	97	99	100	102	103	49	50	51	52	53	53	54
	95th	98	99	101	103	104	106	106	54	54	55	56	57	58	58
	99th	105	106	108	110	112	113	114	61	62	63	64	65	66	66
2	50th	84	85	87	88	90	92	92	39	40	41	42	43	44	44
	90th	97	99	100	102	104	105	106	54	55	56	57	58	58	59
	95th	101	102	104	106	108	109	110	59	59	60	61	62	63	63
	99th	109	110	111	113	115	117	117	66	67	68	69	70	71	71
3	50th	86	87	89	91	93	94	95	44	44	45	46	47	48	48
	90th	100	101	103	105	107	108	109	59	59	60	61	62	63	63
	95th	104	105	107	109	110	112	113	63	63	64	65	66	67	67
	99th	111	112	114	116	118	119	120	71	71	72	73	74	75	75
4	50th	88	89	91	93	95	96	97	47	48	49	50	51	51	52
	90th	102	103	105	107	109	110	111	62	63	64	65	66	66	67
	95th	106	107	109	111	112	114	115	66	67	68	69	70	71	71
	99th	113	114	116	118	120	121	122	74	75	76	77	78	78	79
5	50th	90	91	93	95	96	98	98	50	51	52	53	54	55	55
	90th	104	105	106	108	110	111	112	65	66	67	68	69	69	70
	95th	108	109	110	112	114	115	116	69	70	71	72	73	74	74
	99th	115	116	118	120	121	123	123	77	78	79	80	81	81	82
6	50th	91	92	94	96	98	99	100	53	53	54	55	56	57	57
	90th	105	106	108	110	111	113	113	68	68	69	70	71	72	72
	95th	109	110	112	114	115	117	117	72	72	73	74	75	76	76
	99th	116	117	119	121	123	124	125	80	80	81	82	83	84	84
7	50th	92	94	95	97	99	100	101	55	55	56	57	58	59	59
	90th	106	107	109	111	113	114	115	70	70	71	72	73	74	74
	95th	110	111	113	115	117	118	119	74	74	75	76	77	78	78
	99th	117	118	120	122	124	125	126	82	82	83	84	85	86	86
8	50th	94	95	97	99	100	102	102	56	57	58	59	60	60	61
	90th	107	109	110	112	114	115	116	71	72	72	73	74	75	76
	95th	111	112	114	116	118	119	120	75	76	77	78	79	79	80
	99th	119	120	122	123	125	127	127	83	84	85	86	87	87	88
9	50th	95	96	98	100	102	103	104	57	58	59	60	61	61	62
	90th	109	110	112	114	115	117	118	72	73	74	75	76	76	77
	95th	113	114	116	118	119	121	121	76	77	78	79	80	81	81
	99th	120	121	123	125	127	128	129	84	85	86	87	88	88	89
10	50th	97	98	100	102	103	105	106	58	59	60	61	61	62	63
	90th	111	112	114	115	117	119	119	73	73	74	75	76	77	78
	95th	115	116	117	119	121	122	123	77	78	79	80	81	81	82
	99th	122	123	125	127	128	130	130	85	86	86	88	88	89	90
11	50th	99	100	102	104	105	107	107	59	59	60	61	62	63	63
	90th	113	114	115	117	119	120	121	74	74	75	76	77	78	78
	95th	117	118	119	121	123	124	125	78	78	79	80	81	82	82
	99th	124	125	127	129	130	132	132	86	86	87	88	89	90	90
12	50th	101	102	104	106	108	109	110	59	60	61	62	63	63	64
	90th	115	116	118	120	121	123	123	74	75	75	76	77	78	79
	95th	119	120	122	123	125	127	127	78	79	80	81	82	82	83
	99th	126	127	129	131	133	134	135	86	87	88	89	90	90	91
13	50th	104	105	106	108	110	111	112	60	60	61	62	63	64	64
	90th	117	118	120	122	124	125	126	75	75	76	77	78	79	79

(*continued*)

Table 43.1 *Continued*

Age (years)	BP Percentile	SBP (mmHg) Percentile of height							DBP (mmHg) Percentile of height						
		5th	10th	25th	50th	75th	90th	95th	5th	10th	25th	50th	75th	90th	95th
	95th	121	122	124	126	128	129	130	79	79	80	81	82	83	83
	99th	128	130	131	133	135	136	137	87	87	88	89	90	91	91
14	50th	106	107	109	111	113	114	115	60	61	62	63	64	65	65
	90th	120	121	123	125	126	128	128	75	76	77	78	79	79	80
	95th	124	125	127	128	130	132	132	80	80	81	82	83	84	84
	99th	131	132	134	136	138	139	140	87	88	89	90	91	92	92
15	50th	109	110	112	113	115	117	117	61	62	63	64	65	66	66
	90th	122	124	125	127	129	130	131	76	77	78	79	80	80	81
	95th	126	127	129	131	133	134	135	81	81	82	83	84	85	85
	99th	134	135	136	138	140	142	142	88	89	90	91	92	93	93
16	50th	111	112	114	116	118	119	120	63	63	64	65	66	67	67
	90th	125	126	128	130	131	133	134	78	78	79	80	81	82	82
	95th	129	130	132	134	135	137	137	82	83	83	84	85	86	87
	99th	136	137	139	141	143	144	145	90	90	91	92	93	94	94
17	50th	114	115	116	118	120	121	122	65	66	66	67	68	69	70
	90th	127	128	130	132	134	135	136	80	80	81	82	83	84	84
	95th	131	132	134	136	138	139	140	84	85	86	87	87	88	89
	99th	139	140	141	143	145	146	147	92	93	93	94	95	96	97

blood pressure in children 3 years of age through adolescence includes three pediatric cuffs of different sizes, as well as a standard adult cuff and an oversized cuff, and a thigh cuff for leg blood pressure measurement. The latter two cuffs may be needed for use in obese adolescents.

Blood pressure measurement in children should be conducted in a quiet and comfortable environment after 3–5 min of rest. With the exception of situations of acute illness, the blood pressure should be measured with the child in a seated position, with the cubital fossa supported at heart level. It is preferable that the child has their feet on the floor while the blood pressure is measured, rather than having the feet dangling from an exam table. Overinflation of the cuff should be avoided because of the discomfort it causes, particularly in younger children. The blood pressure should be measured and recorded at least twice on each measurement occasion.

Systolic blood pressure is determined by the onset of the auscultated pulsation—the first Korotkoff sound. The last Korotkoff sound that is heard, or fifth Korotkoff sound (K5), is the definition of diastolic pressure in adults. In children, particularly preadolescents, a difference of several millimeters of mercury is frequently present among the fourth Korotkoff sound, the muffling of Korotkoff sounds, and K5 (14). The substantial body of normative blood pressure data in children indicates that K5 can be used as the measure of diastolic blood pressure in children as well as in adults. At least two blood pressure measurements should be taken and the average of these two measurements used as the blood pressure measurement.

The measured blood pressure level in a child is interpreted by comparing the child's blood pressure to the blood pressure tables. Precise interpretation requires plotting the blood pressure according to the child's height percentile as well as to age and gender. The child's height is measured and plotted on the standard child growth curves. The height percentile is used in the tables, wherein the blood pressure level for the 90th and 95th percentile at the child's age, gender, and height percentile are compared with the child's measured blood pressure.

Elevated blood pressure measurements in a child or adolescent must be confirmed on repeated visits before characterizing a child as having hypertension. A more accurate characterization of an individual's blood pressure level is an average of multiple blood pressure measurements taken for weeks or months. A notable exception to this general guideline would be situations in which the child is symptomatic or has profoundly elevated blood pressure. Children with elevated blood pressure on repeat measurements also should have their blood pressure measured in the leg as a screen for coarctation of the aorta. To measure the blood pressure in the leg, a thigh cuff, or an oversized cuff should be placed on the thigh and the blood pressure measured by auscultation over the popliteal fossa. Coarctation is suspected if the systolic blood pressure measured in the thigh is ≤10 mmHg than the systolic blood pressure measured in the arm.

Table 43.2 BP Levels for Girls by Age and Height Percentile

Age (years)	BP Percentile	SBP (mmHg)							DBP (mmHg)						
		Percentile of height							Percentile of height						
		5th	10th	25th	50th	75th	90th	95th	5th	10th	25th	50th	75th	90th	95th
1	50th	83	84	85	86	88	89	90	38	39	39	40	41	41	42
	90th	97	97	98	100	101	102	103	52	53	53	54	55	55	56
	95th	100	101	102	104	105	106	107	56	57	57	58	59	59	60
	99th	108	108	109	111	112	113	114	64	64	65	65	66	67	67
2	50th	85	85	87	88	89	91	91	43	44	44	45	46	46	47
	90th	98	99	100	101	103	104	105	57	58	58	59	60	61	61
	95th	102	103	104	105	107	108	109	61	62	62	63	64	65	65
	99th	109	110	111	112	114	115	116	69	69	70	70	71	72	72
3	50th	86	87	88	89	91	92	93	47	48	48	49	50	50	51
	90th	100	100	102	103	104	106	106	61	62	62	63	64	64	65
	95th	104	104	105	107	108	109	110	65	66	66	67	68	68	69
	99th	111	111	113	114	115	116	117	73	73	74	74	75	76	76
4	50th	88	88	90	91	92	94	94	50	50	51	52	52	53	54
	90th	101	102	103	104	106	107	108	64	64	65	66	67	67	68
	95th	105	106	107	108	110	111	112	68	68	69	70	71	71	72
	99th	112	113	114	115	117	118	119	76	76	76	77	78	79	79
5	50th	89	90	91	93	94	95	96	52	53	53	54	55	55	56
	90th	103	103	105	106	107	109	109	66	67	67	68	69	69	70
	95th	107	107	108	110	111	112	113	70	71	71	72	73	73	74
	99th	114	114	116	117	118	120	120	78	78	79	79	80	81	81
6	50th	91	92	93	94	96	97	98	54	54	55	56	56	57	58
	90th	104	105	106	108	109	110	111	68	68	69	70	70	71	72
	95th	108	109	110	111	113	114	115	72	72	73	74	74	75	76
	99th	115	116	117	119	120	121	122	80	80	80	81	82	83	83
7	50th	93	93	95	96	97	99	99	55	56	56	57	58	58	59
	90th	106	107	108	109	111	112	113	69	70	70	71	72	72	73
	95th	110	111	112	113	115	116	116	73	74	74	75	76	76	77
	99th	117	118	119	120	122	123	124	81	81	82	82	83	84	84
8	50th	95	95	96	98	99	100	101	57	57	57	58	59	60	60
	90th	108	109	110	111	113	114	114	71	71	71	72	73	74	74
	95th	112	112	114	115	116	118	118	75	75	75	76	77	78	78
	99th	119	120	121	122	123	125	125	82	82	83	83	84	85	86
9	50th	96	97	98	100	101	102	103	58	58	58	59	60	61	61
	90th	110	110	112	113	114	116	116	72	72	72	73	74	75	75
	95th	114	114	115	117	118	119	120	76	76	76	77	78	79	79
	99th	121	121	123	124	125	127	127	83	83	84	84	85	86	87
10	50th	98	99	100	102	103	104	105	59	59	59	60	61	62	62
	90th	112	112	114	115	116	118	118	73	73	73	74	75	76	76
	95th	116	116	117	119	120	121	122	77	77	77	78	79	80	80
	99th	123	123	125	126	127	129	129	84	84	85	86	86	87	88
11	50th	100	101	102	103	105	106	107	60	60	60	61	62	63	63
	90th	114	114	116	117	118	119	120	74	74	74	75	76	77	77
	95th	118	118	119	121	122	123	124	78	78	78	79	80	81	81
	99th	125	125	126	128	129	130	131	85	85	86	87	87	88	89
12	50th	102	103	104	105	107	108	109	61	61	61	62	63	64	64
	90th	116	116	117	119	120	121	122	75	75	75	76	77	78	78
	95th	119	120	121	123	124	125	126	79	79	79	80	81	82	82
	99th	127	127	128	130	131	132	133	86	86	87	88	88	89	90
13	50th	104	105	106	107	109	110	110	62	62	62	63	64	65	65
	90th	117	118	119	121	122	123	124	76	76	76	77	78	79	79

(continued)

Table 43.2 *Continued*

Age (years)	BP Percentile	SBP (mmHg)							DBP (mmHg)						
		Percentile of height							Percentile of height						
		5th	10th	25th	50th	75th	90th	95th	5th	10th	25th	50th	75th	90th	95th
	95th	121	122	123	124	126	127	128	80	80	80	81	82	83	83
	99th	128	129	130	132	133	134	135	87	87	88	89	89	90	91
14	50th	106	106	107	109	110	111	112	63	63	63	64	65	66	66
	90th	119	120	121	122	124	125	125	77	77	77	78	79	80	80
	95th	123	123	125	126	127	129	129	81	81	81	82	83	84	84
	99th	130	131	132	133	135	136	136	88	88	89	90	90	91	92
15	50th	107	108	109	110	111	113	113	64	64	64	65	66	67	67
	90th	120	121	122	123	125	126	127	78	78	78	79	80	81	81
	95th	124	125	126	127	129	130	131	82	82	82	83	84	85	85
	99th	131	132	133	134	136	137	138	89	89	90	91	91	92	93
16	50th	108	108	110	111	112	114	114	64	64	65	66	66	67	68
	90th	121	122	123	124	126	127	128	78	78	79	80	81	81	82
	95th	125	126	127	128	130	131	132	82	82	83	84	85	85	86
	99th	132	133	134	135	137	138	139	90	90	90	91	92	93	93
17	50th	108	109	110	111	113	114	115	64	65	65	66	67	67	68
	90th	122	122	123	125	126	127	128	78	79	79	80	81	81	82
	95th	125	126	127	129	130	131	132	82	83	83	84	85	85	86
	99th	133	133	134	136	137	138	139	90	90	91	91	92	93	93

There continues to be an increase in the use of automated devices to measure blood pressure in children. Because of concerns about the reliability of the various instruments, lack of established reference standards, and the difficulty in obtaining regular recalibration of these devices, auscultation continues to be the recommended method for measurement of blood pressure in the young. However, situations in which use of an automated device are acceptable include blood pressure measurement in newborn and young infants in whom auscultation is difficult, as well as in an intensive care setting, where frequent blood pressure measurement is necessary.

IV. CAUSES OF SECONDARY HYPERTENSION IN THE YOUNG

Prior to the development of normative data on blood pressure levels in children, blood pressure was measured infrequently. When elevated blood pressure was detected in children, the hypertension was, by current standards, quite severe. Because secondary hypertension is generally characterized by marked blood pressure elevation, this lead to the belief that hypertension in children is always secondary. This concept has now changed, largely because of a better understanding of normal levels of blood pressure in the young and the practice of regularly measuring the blood pressure in children as part of health maintenance. However, in comparing children with hypertension to adults with hypertension, underlying causes of hypertension, or secondary hypertension due to renal or endocrine disorders, occur more frequently among children. The portion of children with hypertension who have a secondary cause of hypertension varies according to the age of the child and the severity of the hypertension. Hanna et al. (15) identified a secondary cause of hypertension in 90% of children who were <10 years of age, and only 10% of these young children were considered to have essential hypertension. Another report on a series that included both children and adolescents with hypertension, describes secondary hypertension in 65% of the adolescents, with 35% of the adolescents having essential hypertension (16).

Young children, <12 years of age, with sustained hypertension are more likely to have a secondary cause for the hypertension. Also, the degree of hypertension is an important clue because severe blood pressure elevation in a young child is most likely to be a result of an underlying abnormality. In general, a child that has either a systolic or a diastolic blood pressure that is consistently 8–10 mmHg above the 95th percentile has significant hypertension, and a child that has either a systolic or a diastolic blood pressure that is consistently 15 mmHg or more above the 95th percentile has severe hypertension. Children and adolescents with this degree of hypertension should have a careful evaluation for the possible cause of the hypertension and also for evidence of target damage from the hypertension. Although the list of conditions that can cause hypertension in the young is quite long, the majority of the identifiable causes of hypertension in the young are related to renal disorders. Table 43.3 provides a list of underlying causes for chronic hypertension in the young, as well as the conditions associated with acute hypertension in the young.

Hypertension is uncommon in healthy newborn infants. However, certain neonatal conditions increase the risk for hypertension. Some severely ill newborn infants require treatment in intensive care units where umbilical artery catheterization may be required for vascular access. The umbilical artery catheters are a risk for thromboembolic events (17,18), and a thrombus in a renal vessel can cause acute hypertension. Low birth weight infants, with respiratory distress syndrome, can progress to bronchopulmonary dysplasia, a chronic lung condition. The chronic steroid therapy used to treat bronchopulmonary dysplasia can cause sodium retention and subsequent blood pressure elevation (19). The most commonly identified causes of hypertension in the newborn infant are renal artery thrombosis, renal artery stenosis, congenital renal malformations, coarctation of the aorta, and bronchopulmonary

dysplasia (4). In some critically ill newborn infants with hypertension, an underlying cause may not be identified. Regardless of whether an etiology for the hypertension is determined, blood pressure control and monitoring in these infants are important.

Leading causes of hypertension in children up to 10 years of age are renal parenchymal diseases, coarctation of the aorta, and renal artery stenosis. Coarctation of the aorta, a congenital cardiac anomaly that can be missed in infants and toddlers, should be considered in a hypertensive child (20–22). In the clinic or office, measurement of the blood pressure in the leg is an effective way to screen for coarctation. In later childhood, essential hypertension also can be detected. The acute childhood illness hemolytic uremic syndrome may cause permanent renal scaring that results in chronic hypertension.

During the adolescent years, the most common cause of hypertension is essential hypertension. The secondary causes of hypertension that are detected most frequently in adolescents are renal parenchymal diseases such as chronic pyelonephritis and chronic glomerulonephritis. Some toxic adolescent behaviors that may contribute to high blood pressure are illicit substance use, especially

Table 43.3 Secondary Causes of Hypertension

Chronic hypertension

Renal
  Chronic glomerulonephritis
  Interstitial nephritis
  Chronic pyelonephritis
  Collagen vascular diseases
  Reflux nephropathy
  Polycystic kidney disease
  Medullary cystic disease
  Hydronephrosis
  Hypoplastic/dysplastic kidney
Cardiac and Vascular
  Coarctation of aorta
  Renal artery stenosis
  Takayasu arteritis
Endocrine
  Hyperthyroidism
  Pheochromocytoma
  Primary aldosteronism

Drugs
  Corticosteroids
  Alcohol
  Appetite suppressants
  Anabolic steroids
  Oral contraceptive
  Nicotine
Syndromes
  Alport syndrome (renal parenchymal)
  Williams (renovascular lesions)
  Turner (coarctation or renovascular)
  Tuberous sclerosis (cystic renal)
  Neurofibromatosis (renovascular)
  Nail patellar syndrome (renal parenchymal)
  Adrenogenital syndromes
  Little syndrome

Acute hypertension

Renal
  Acute postinfectious glomerulonephritis
  Schönlein-Henoch purpura
  Hemolytic uremic syndrome
  Acute tubular necrosis
Vascular
  Renal or renal vascular trauma
Neurogenic
  Increased intracranial pressure
  Guillain–Barré syndrome

Drugs
  Cocaine
  Phencyclidine
  Amphetamines
  Jimson weed
Miscellaneous
  Burns
  Orthopedic surgery
  Urologic surgery

cocaine and amphetamine-related compounds (23,24). Other substances that have been associated with high blood pressure in adolescents include appetite suppressants (both prescription and over the counter remedies), oral contraceptives, excessive alcohol intake, and use of anabolic steroids for body building (25).

V. CAUSES OF ESSENTIAL HYPERTENSION IN THE YOUNG

Essential hypertension had been considered to be a disorder that occurred only in adulthood. The concept that essential hypertension has its origins in childhood can be inferred from blood pressure tracking data that demonstrates that children with elevated blood pressure will continue to have elevated blood pressure as adults (5). Classic risk factors for hypertension, such as overweight and a positive family history of hypertension or cardiovascular disease, may be present in childhood. The combination of higher blood pressure and typical risk factors had been considered to be a risk for future hypertension. However, recent reports indicate that this condition is more than a risk for future problems. Effects of high blood pressure on left ventricular mass have been investigated. Using echocardiography and appropriate childhood reference values for cardiac structure, left ventricular hypertrophy has been reported in 30–40% of children and adolescents with hypertension (26,27). Longitudinal data is now becoming available that demonstrates a direct link between risk factors in childhood (including blood pressure level) with evidence of target-organ injury in young adulthood (including greater intima-media thickness of carotid arteries and stiffening of the aorta) (26,28,29). Essential hypertension in childhood should now be considered an early phase of a chronic disease.

Children and adolescents with essential hypertension generally demonstrate several clinical characteristics or associated risk factors. The degree of blood pressure elevation is generally mild, approximating the 95th percentile, and there is often considerable variability in blood pressure level over time. Laboratory and observational studies have demonstrated a marked cardiovascular response to stress, characterized by large heart rate and blood pressure responses to stimuli (30–33). A positive history of hypertension in parents or grandparents is a consistent clinical observation in children with mild essential hypertension (30,34,35).

In both children and adults, greater body weight and increases in body weight correlate with higher blood pressure (36,37). Essential hypertension in children is frequently associated with obesity, which appears to be a contributory factor because even a modest reduction in excess adiposity is associated with a reduction in blood pressure (38,39). The cluster of mild blood pressure elevation, a positive family history of hypertension, and obesity is a typical pattern in children and adolescents with essential hypertension (40).

Currently, the prevalence of childhood obesity is increasing (41) and has more than doubled in the past 20 years (42). Obesity augments the risk for cardiovascular disease and warrants attention for both prevention of chronic disease and for health promotion. In a study by Daniels et al. (27), cardiac structure was examined by echocardiography in young adolescents with essential hypertension. The echocardiographic data in these youngsters with even mild blood pressure elevation, demonstrated a 30% incidence of left ventricular hypertrophy. The adolescents who had echo criteria of cardiac hypertrophy, despite mild blood pressure elevation, were all obese. Rocchini et al. (38,39) have demonstrated augmented blood pressure sensitivity to sodium intake in obese adolescents and a significant dampening in the blood pressure response to sodium following weight reduction.

Over the past two decades, the literature on hypertension and cardiovascular disease in adults has focused on the overlap of hypertension, noninsulin-dependent diabetes mellitus, atherosclerosis, and obesity. This constellation within individuals and within populations has been described as the *insulin-resistance syndrome* (43–45). Children as well as adults may exhibit characteristics of the insulin-resistance syndrome (39,46,47). Some investigators have detected the insulin-resistance syndrome in nonobese offspring of hypertensive parents (48,49), which indicates a hereditary component to the syndrome. The characteristics of the insulin-resistance syndrome also are congruent with the overweight child who has a strong family history of hypertension or early heart disease. These children often have high blood pressure (50). Although these children are not at risk for immediate adverse effects of the higher than normal blood pressure, they should be considered at risk for future cardiovascular disease (51). These children can benefit from health behavior changes that improve insulin action, including an increase in physical activity, diet modifications, and control of excess adiposity.

The cause of essential hypertension is believed to be multifactorial and the outcome of an interplay of genetic and environmental factors. Barker et al. (52) have proposed an alternative cause of hypertension based on observations of an association of hypertension and ischemic heart disease in adults with a low recorded birth weight. These investigators propose that lower birth weight is a consequence of abnormalities in the intrauterine nutritional environment. Impaired fetal growth affects an alteration in organ structure and impairment in organ function in later life (52,53). Higher blood pressure is the link between compromised intrauterine growth and the long-term risk for cardiovascular disease (52). Despite the reports, based on retrospective data, which support the low birth weight–high blood pressure hypothesis (52–55), this concept is in conflict with the body of data for hypertension in childhood as well as in adulthood, which consistently demonstrates a direct relationship between body weight and blood pressure (56–59). Longitudinal data that demonstrates blood pressure tracking in childhood (34,60–65) also is in conflict with the birth weight concept. Studies on small cohorts have failed to detect a significant relationship between low birth weight and later elevations in blood pressure (58,59). When the reports on the association of birth weight with future blood pressure are examined, the effect of birth weight on future blood pressure level is in the range of 2–3 mmHg blood pressure reduction for each 1 kg increase in birth weight. When the current child weight or adult weight is taken into consideration, the birth weight effect is minimal (66). Although the birth weight hypothesis has some appeal, clinical investigations have not yet firmly demonstrated that birth weight has a substantial effect on future blood pressure level.

VI. EVALUATION OF HYPERTENSION IN CHILDREN AND ADOLESCENTS

When sustained hypertension is established in a child by repeated blood pressure measurements that are at or above the 95th percentile, additional evaluation is needed. The extent of the diagnostic evaluation is determined by the type of hypertension that is suspected. When a secondary cause is considered, a more extensive evaluation may be necessary. On the other hand, when the patient's elevated blood pressure is more likely to be an early expression of essential hypertension, a few screening studies may be sufficient. The medical history and physical examination are key in determining if the patient's presentation is characteristic of essential hypertension or if the patient's presentation is indicative of a secondary, and potentially correctable, cause. Children or adolescents with severe hypertension, in particular very young children, generally have an identifiable underlying cause. As noted previously, the higher the blood pressure and the younger the child, the more likely a secondary cause is present.

A particular symptom complex revealed in the history or findings upon physical examination also may prompt a thorough investigation. In these patients, the direction of the evaluation is dictated by the particular symptom or physical examination findings. Any pediatric patient who is hypertensive and is not growing normally also should undergo an evaluation for secondary causes. A sudden onset of elevated blood pressure in a previously normotensive child should always prompt a search for secondary causes. Absence of a positive family history of hypertension should increase the level of suspicion for an underlying disorder.

Another set of findings characterize children and adolescents with essential hypertension. These characteristics include the following: slight to mild elevations in blood pressure, a strong family history of essential hypertension, an elevated resting heart rate, variable blood pressure readings upon repeat measurements, and obesity. If no other abnormalities are found in the medical history or on physical examination, these children require less extensive evaluations than those in whom secondary causes are suspected.

A. Medical History

The medical history and physical examination are used to detect clues to determine whether the blood pressure elevation is secondary or essential. It is also helpful to determine whether the hypertension is long-standing or of acute onset. The family history is particularly important. In both first-degree and second-degree relatives, the family history of essential hypertension, myocardial infarction, stroke, renal disease, diabetes, and obesity should be obtained. It can be relevant to the diagnosis in a hypertensive child if relatives had an early onset of any of the earlier conditions. Parents should also be asked about those conditions in family members that are inheritable and have hypertension as a component (e.g., polycystic kidney disease, neurofibromatosis, and pheochromocytoma). Another familial type of hypertension is glucocorticoid-remediable aldosteronism, an autosomal dominant condition, which should be considered when multiple family members have childhood-onset hypertension associated with hypokalemia or stroke (67,68).

Details about previous health problems, such as history of urinary tract infections, are important because there may be associated reflux nephropathy, renal scarring, and resultant hypertension. A history of both prescribed medications and over-the-counter medications can be helpful (69,70). Information should be obtained about health-related behaviors such as the child's usual diet, amount of physical activity, or athletic participation. Other adverse lifestyles to consider in adolescents are the use of "street" drugs, smokeless tobacco, oral contraceptive pills, cigarette smoking, diet aids, ethanol, and anabolic steroids.

B. Physical Examination

The physical examination of a hypertensive child should be comprehensive. An assessment of the child's general growth rate and growth pattern should be made. Weight, height, and body mass index (BMI) should be plotted according to age and gender on the child growth charts. Abnormalities in growth that are associated with hypertension can be seen with chronic renal disease, hyperthyroidism (causing primarily systolic hypertension), pheochromocytoma, adrenal disorders, or certain genetic abnormalities, such as Turner syndrome.

To rule out coarctation of the aorta, the evaluation of every child for hypertension should include upper- and lower-extremity blood pressure measurements taken with appropriately-sized cuffs. Normally, the leg blood pressure levels are slightly higher than the arm blood pressure levels. A child with coarctation will have systolic hypertension in an upper extremity, sometimes absent or decreased femoral pulses, and a blood pressure level in the lower leg that is >10 mmHg lower when compared with the blood pressure level in the arm (20,22).

There are other physical exam clues that could suggest a secondary etiology for child hypertension (71). Abnormal facies or dysmorphic features may suggest one of the syndromes that are associated with specific lesions causing hypertension. For example, both Turner and Williams syndromes are associated with renovascular or cardiac lesions, which cause hypertension. Renal vascular lesions may sometimes have an audible abdominal bruit that is detectable by auscultation of the abdomen. Skin lesions are sometimes the first manifestation of disorders such as tuberous sclerosis and systemic lupus erythematosus.

C. Diagnostic Testing

When the medical history and physical examination provide clues for a specific underlying cause for the hypertension, such as an endocrine or cardiac disorder, the testing should be directed to the area of clinical suspicion. Other important historical information, such as a history of urinary tract infections, might dictate studies to evaluate vesicoureteral reflux and renal scarring. However, in the absence of clues, renal parenchymal disease should be considered a likely etiology because this diagnosis is the most frequent cause of secondary hypertension in the pediatric population. The initial studies to screen for renal abnormalities include a full urinalysis, electrolytes, creatinine, complete blood count, urine culture, and renal ultrasound.

The other component of the evaluation includes an assessment of target-organ injury. The presence of target-organ injury provides a measure of chronicity and severity (characteristics sometimes difficult to ascertain from the medical history) and will aid in determining whether pharmacologic therapy should be initiated. Echocardiography is a sensitive means to detect interventricular septal and posterior ventricular wall thickening (72–75). Chest X-ray and ECG are much less sensitive measures of left ventricular hypertrophy in children. An

ophthalmologic examination can also be helpful. In a study of 97 children and adolescents with essential hypertension, Daniels et al. (76) found that 51% displayed retinal abnormalities. The usefulness of microalbuminuria, sometimes used as a marker for renal injury in adults (77), has not been determined for children. The remainder of the evaluation should be directed by specific findings in the medical history and physical examination as well as by the results of initial screening studies.

The use of 24 h ambulatory blood pressure monitoring has become used increasingly in the evaluation of adults with hypertension (78). Some population standards for ambulatory blood pressure values in children and adolescents are now available (79), and there are some situations in which this information can be quite helpful (80). Ambulatory blood pressure monitoring can be used to determine how consistently blood pressure readings are elevated over a 24 h period. If <25% of the ambulatory blood pressure measurements are above the 95th percentile, the child or adolescent may have white coat hypertension. The degree of blood pressure elevation and the frequency of abnormal blood pressure measurements also are helpful in assessing the need for implementing pharmacologic therapy. The following summarizes a method for applying diagnostic studies in hypertensive children:

Blood pressure is above 90th percentile, but below 95th percentile
 Counseling on lifestyle changes and monitoring of blood pressure
Blood pressure is above 95th percentile
 Detailed medical history and physical examination
 Complete blood count, electrolytes, creatinine, urinalysis
If <12 years of age and blood pressure above 95th percentile
 Additional diagnostic tests based on screening results
 Renal ultrasound, echocardiogram, endocrine studies, and treatment to lower blood pressure (below 90th percentile)
If >12 years of age and blood pressure above 95th percentile (mild) and with risk factors for essential hypertension plus negative screening
 Treat with lifestyle changes.
 If no response, consider renal ultrasound, echocardiogram, and drug treatment.
If >12 years of age and blood pressure above 95th percentile (mild) and with no risk factors or with positive screening tests
 Do additional diagnostic tests based on screening results (renal ultrasound, echocardiogram, endocrine studies) and use drug treatment to lower blood pressure (below 90th percentile).

If >12 years of age and blood pressure above 95th percentile (significant or severe)

Do additional diagnostic tests based on screening results (renal ultrasound, echocardiogram, endocrine studies, and renal vessel imaging studies) and use drug treatment to lower blood pressure (below 90th percentile).

VII. TREATMENT OF HYPERTENSION IN CHILDREN AND ADOLESCENTS

In adults with mild essential hypertension, changes in health-related behaviors, including diet patterns, physical activity, and weight control may facilitate blood pressure control. Children may also benefit in these lifestyle changes. Children and adolescents with a mild elevation of blood pressure and without end-organ damage, should begin treatment with nonpharmacologic interventions that include weight reduction if overweight, aerobic exercise (particularly if sedentary), and diet modification.

Obesity, as discussed earlier, is often associated with mild hypertension in childhood. When weight reduction can be achieved, there is often a reduction in blood pressure in obese children. Brownell et al. (81) showed that weight loss in obese adolescents, achieved by a program of both behavior modification and parental involvement, was associated with a significant decrease in blood pressure. There is also evidence that exercise training lowers blood pressure in both school aged children and adolescents (82–84). Rocchini et al. (38) demonstrated that a program that included both caloric restriction and exercise produced a decrease in blood pressure as well as a reversal of structural changes in forearm resistance vessels. Weight reduction can be extremely difficult and generally requires multiple strategies that include the input of a nutritionist, dietary education, emotional support, information about exercise, and family involvement. Power weight-lifting should be discouraged in hypertensive adolescents because of its potential to induce marked blood pressure elevation. Participation in other sports should be encouraged as long as blood pressure is under reasonable control, regular monitoring of blood pressure occurs, and a thorough examination has been conducted to exclude cardiac conditions (25).

The guidelines for dietary modifications in the pediatric population are less clear than in adults. Information about the effects of salt on blood pressure in children are not as definitive as in adults. There does seem to be a subset of adolescents, particularly those who are obese, who demonstrate blood pressure sensitivity to salt as well as other risk factors for hypertension (38). Because the usual dietary intake of sodium for most children and adolescents in the United States far exceeds nutrient requirements, it is reasonable to restrict sodium intake to <4 g/day by decreasing fast-food consumption and refraining from adding salt to cooked foods (85).

Current information about the effects of potassium and calcium intake on blood pressure in children are even less definitive. Some reports suggest that a diet high in potassium and calcium may help to lower blood pressure (86), yet no study has definitively shown this effect in children or adolescents. The dietary intervention clinical trial, Dietary Approaches to Stop Hypertension (DASH) reported results that could be relevant to diet benefits in children. This study, which was conducted on adults with mild hypertension, demonstrated a significant reduction in both systolic and diastolic blood pressure in subjects who consumed a diet high in fruits, vegetables, and low-fat dairy products compared with subjects who consumed the usual diet. These results indicate that a benefit on blood pressure occurs from diets that are high in potassium, calcium, magnesium, and other vitamins (87). A similar approach may be of benefit for children and adolescents, although investigations to test this effect in children or adolescents with hypertension have not yet been conducted.

Pharmacologic therapy is indicated if nonpharmacologic approaches are unsuccessful, or when a child is symptomatic, has severe hypertension, or has end-organ damage. Children with diabetes mellitus or chronic renal disease may achieve renal protective benefits from blood pressure reduction. For children with these disorders, it is reasonable to use pharmacologic therapy to lower blood pressure to a level that is below the 90th percentile for age, gender, and height.

Most of the medications used for adults can be used for children. However, efficacy data, as well as long-term safety data, are limited for the pediatric population. The choice of antihypertensive medication must be individualized and depends on the child's age, the etiology of the hypertension, the degree of blood pressure elevation, adverse effects, and concomitant medical conditions. In most patients, therapy is begun with a single agent. The dose is titrated upward until control of the blood pressure is attained. Blood pressure control, in most instances, is defined as maintaining systolic and diastolic pressure below the 90th percentile. If control cannot be achieved by using the maximum dose of a single agent, a second medication can be added or, alternatively, another agent from a different class selected. The more commonly used medications for chronic antihypertensive therapy in children are listed in Table 43.4; those more commonly used in acute, hypertensive emergencies are listed in Table 43.5. Presently, the dosing recommendations for children have been largely based upon practitioner experience, not on large, multicenter trials. Some clinical trial work is now being conducted on the

Table 43.4   Treatment of Chronic Hypertension in Children

Drug	Dose	Frequency	Available preparations
Diuretics			
Chlorothiazide	20–30 mg/kg per day Max: 2 g per day	q12–24 h	Tablets: 250, 500 mg Solution: 250 mg/5 mL
Hydrochlorothiazide	1–4 mg/kg per day Max: 200 mg/day	q12–24 h	Tablets: 25, 50, 100 mg
Metolazone	0.1–0.5 mg/kg per day Max: 20 mg/day (Zaroxolyn) 0.5–1 mg/day (Mykrox)	q24 h q24 h	Tablets: 2.5, 5, 10 mg (Zaroxolyn) Tablets: 0.5, 1.0 mg (Mykrox)
Furosemide	0.5–4 mg/kg per day Max: 80 mg/dose	q6–24 h	Tablets: 20, 40, 80 mg Solution: 10 mg/mL, 40 mg/5 mL, 80 mg/10 mL
Spironolactone	1–3.0 mg/kg per day Max: 200 mg/day for hypertension	q8–24 h	Tablets: 25, 50, 100 mg
β-adrenergic antagonists			
Nonselective			
Propranolol	0.5–5 mg/kg per day Max: 480 mg/day	q6–12 h	Tablets: 10, 20, 40, 60, 80 mg Long-acting capsules: 60, 80, 120, 160 mg Solution: 20, 40 mg/5 mL
Nadolol[a]	40–240 mg/day	q24 h	Tablets: 20, 40, 80, 120, 160 mg
Selective			
Atenolol	0.5–2 mg/kg per day Max: 100 mg/day	q24 h	Tablets: 25, 50, 100 mg
Metoprolol	1–6 mg/kg per day Max: 450 mg/day	q12–24 h	Tablets: 50, 100 mg
Bisoprolol/HCTZ	2.5–6.25 mg/day Max: 10–6.25 mg/day	q24 h	Tablets: 2.5/6.25, 5/6.25, 10/6.25 mg
α-adrenergic antagonists			
Prazosin	0.02–0.5 mg/kg per day Max: 20 mg/day	q6–12 h	Tablets: 1, 2, 5 mg
Complex adrenergic antagonists			
Labetalol	2–3 mg/kg per day initially Max: 20 mg/kg per day	q8–12 h	Tablets: 100, 200, 300 mg
Central α agonists			
Clonidine	0.05–0.1 mg/dose Max: 0.6 mg/day	q6–12 h	Tablets: 0.1, 0.2, 0.3 mg Patches: 0.1, 0.2, 0.3 mg/week
Methyldopa	10–65 mg/kg per day Max: 3 g/day	q6–12 h	Tablets: 125, 250, 500 mg Solution: 250 mg/5 mL
Angiotensin-converting enzyme inhibitors			
Captopril	0.05–6 mg/kg per day Max: 200 mg/day	q8–12 h	Tablets: 12.5, 25, 50, 100 mg
Enalapril	0.1–0.6 mg/kg per day Max: 40 mg/day	q12–24 h	Tablets: 2.5, 5.0, 10, 20 mg
Lisinopril[a]	0.07–0.6 mg/kg per day Max: 40 mg/day	q24 h	Tablets: 5, 10, 20 mg
Quinapril[a]	5–80 mg/day	q24 h	Tablets: 5, 10, 20 mg
Ramipril[a]	1.25–20 mg/day	q12–24 h	Capsules: 1.25, 2.5, 5, 10 mg
Fosinopril	0.1–0.6 mg/kg per day Max: 40 mg/day	q24 h	Tablets: 10, 20, 40 mg
Benazepril	0.2–0.6 mg/kg per day Max: 40 mg/day	q24 h	Tablets: 5, 10, 20, 40 mg

(continued)

Table 43.4 *Continued*

Drug	Dose	Frequency	Available preparations
Vasodilators			
Hydralazine	1–8 mg/kg per day Max: 200 mg/day	q12–24 h	Tablets: 10, 25, 50, 100 mg
Calcium antagonists			
Nifedipine	0.25–3 mg/kg per day Max: 180 mg/day	q6–24 h	Capsules: 10, 20 mg Extended release: 30, 60, 90 mg
Isradipine	0.15–0.8 mg/kg per day	q8–12 h	Capsules: 2.5, 5, 10 mg
Amlodipine[a]	0.06–0.34 mg/kg per day Max: 10 mg/day	q24 h	Tablets: 2.5, 5, 10 mg
Felodipine ER	2.5–20 mg/day	q24 h	Tablets: 2.5, 5, 10 mg
Angiotensin II receptor blocking agents			
Losartan	0.75–1.44 mg/kg per day Max: 100 mg/day	q24 h	Tablets: 25, 50, 100 mg
Irbesartan[a]	75–300 mg/day	q24 h	Tablets: 75, 150, 300 mg
Telmisartan[a]	20–80 mg/day	q24 h	Tablets: 40, 80 mg
Candesartan[a]	2–32 mg/day	q24 h	Tablets: 4, 8, 16, 32 mg
Valsartan	80–160 mg/day	q24 h	Tablets: 80, 160 mg

[a]The pediatric dose is under investigation.

Table 43.5 Treatment of Hypertensive Emergencies in Children

Drug	Dose	Route	Comments
Furosemide	1–4 mg/kg per dose Max: 160 mg/dose	IV, IM, or PO	Nephrotoxic, ototoxic When administered in IV, infuse slowly to avoid ototoxicity Onset: 5–20 min
Hydralazine	0.1–0.5 mg/kg per dose Max: 50 mg/dose	IV, IM	Tachycardia, flushing, salt retention Onset: 10–20 min
Diazoxide	1–5 mg/kg per dose q5–15 min Max: 150 mg/dose	IV	Pain at injected vein, sodium retention Onset: 2 min
Sodium nitroprusside	0.3–10 µg/kg per min by continuous infusion	IV	Cyanide poisoning in patients with renal failure Onset: seconds
Nifedipine	0.2–0.5 mg/kg per dose Max: 10 mg/dose	PO, sublingual, bite, and swallow	Headaches, edema Onset: 2–3 min
Nicardipine	0.1–5.0 µg/kg per min	IV	Dizziness, flushing
Labetalol	0.2–1 mg/kg per dose by bolus >2 min period or 0.4–3 mg/kg per h Max: 80 mg/dose or 300 mg/total dose	IV q10 min Continuous IV infusion	Contraindicated in congestive heart failure, diabetes mellitus, and asthma Onset: 5–10 min
Enalapril	15 µg/kg per dose Max: 1.25 mg/dose	IV bolus	Cough, angioedema, renal failure, hyperkalemia Onset: 15 min

Note: Onset, usual time to reduction in blood pressure.

medications that have been tested on adults in large clinical trials and are prescribed for hypertension in adults. This information, as it becomes available, will provide more information about efficacy, safety, and dosing in children.

β-Adrenergic blockers, such as propranolol, metoprolol, and atenolol, are good choices in some non-asthmatic children, but they may not be tolerated well by athletes in whom exercise capacity could be decreased. More frequently, first-line medications are either angiotensin-converting enzyme (ACE) inhibitors or calcium channel blockers. ACE inhibitors rarely cause side effects (e.g., cough, rash, and neutropenia) in children and are usually well tolerated, and many formulations have the advantage of once-a-day dosing. Not only are they effective at controlling blood pressure, but also they may have beneficial effects on renal function, peripheral vasculature, and cardiac function (88). What is most important is that children with diabetes and those with chronic renal disease may be at special risk for progressive renal deterioration and may benefit from ACE inhibitors (89,90). Because of their vasodilator effects on the efferent arteriole, ACE inhibitors can severely reduce glomerular filtration and should therefore be used with caution in patients with renal artery stenosis, a solitary kidney, or a transplanted kidney (91). ACE inhibitors are contraindicated during pregnancy because of teratogenic effects upon the lungs, kidneys, and brain of the fetus (92). Therefore, these drugs should be used with special caution in adolescent females. Angiotensin receptor blockers also interact with the renin–angiotensin system and have benefits similar to the ACE inhibitors. Some experience is now being gained with these agents in treatment of children with hypertension.

Several of the calcium channel blockers are being used in children. In children, the calcium channel blockers can be used as initial therapy, or as the second or third medication when more than one drug is needed to control blood pressure. As with most of the oral antihypertensive preparations, the appropriate dose for small children is often lower than the strength of available tablets, which makes initial dose determinations challenging. Use of short-acting calcium channel blockers should be limited to children with acute hypertension, such as occurs with acute glomerulonephritis. When calcium channel blockers are needed for blood pressure control in chronic hypertension, long-acting preparations are preferred, provided that the correct dosage preparation can be used.

Diuretics are generally recommended as initial drug therapy for uncomplicated hypertension in adults. This recommendation is based on a vast amount of clinical trial data in adults. No such information is available to guide recommendations for pharmacological management of hypertension in children and adolescents. Unless there is clinical evidence of fluid retention in a hypertensive child, such as may occur when the elevated blood pressure is related to chronic steroid use, diuretics are usually not the preferred first step in drug treatment. Although some hypertensive children may achieve adequate blood pressure control with a thiazide diuretic alone, most will not. Children receiving thiazide diuretics often will develop hypokalemia and require potassium supplements; for children, taking the potassium supplements are extremely unpleasant. The necessity of taking potassium supplements in turn can lead to compliance problems. Although low-dose diuretics are not favored as an initial drug for treating hypertension in children, they can be very useful as a second or third drug in those children who require multiple drugs to achieve blood pressure control.

VIII. CONCLUSIONS

Whether the hypertension is determined to be secondary hypertension or essential hypertension, these children require careful monitoring as well as interventions to control their blood pressure. Long-term follow-up, which includes education on the benefits of blood pressure control, is important. Considering the long-term morbidity and mortality associated with essential hypertension, interventions, including preventive interventions, which focus on blood pressure control beginning in the young are needed. Essential hypertension may be found to encompass several distinct pathophysiological entities, each with its own genetic basis and management approach. As new information develops, improved management strategies can be created for hypertension in the young as well as in adults.

REFERENCES

1. Still JL, Cottom D. Severe hypertension in childhood. Arch Dis Child 1967; 42:34–39.
2. The Seventh Report of the Joint National Committee on Prevention, Detection, Evaluation, and Treatment of high blood pressure. J Am Med Assoc 2003; 289:2560–2572.
3. National Heart, Lung, and Blood Institute. Report of the Task Force on Blood Pressure Control in Children. Pediatrics 1977; 59:797–820.
4. Task Force on Blood Pressure Control in Children: Report of the Second Task Force on Blood Pressure Control in Children, 1988. Pediatrics 1987; 79:1–25.
5. National High Blood Pressure Education Program Working Group Report on Hypertension Control in Children and Adolescents. The Update on the 1987 Task Force Report on High Blood Pressure in Children and Adolescents: A Working Group Report from the National High Blood Pressure Education Program. Pediatrics 1996; 98:649–658.

6. de Swiet M, Fayers P, Shinebourne EA. Blood pressure survey in a population of newborn infants. Br Med J 1976; 2:9–11.

7. Schachter J, Kuller LH, Perfetti C. Blood pressure during the first five years of life: relation to ethnic group (black or white) and to parental hypertension. Am J Epidemiol 1984; 119:541–553.

8. Menghetti E, Virdis R, Strambi M, Patriarca V, Riccioni MA, Fossali E, Spagnolo A, on behalf of the 'Study Group on Hypertension' of the Italian Society of Pediatrics'. Blood pressure in childhood and adolescence: the Italian normal standards. J Hypertens 1999; 17:1363–1372.

9. Pall D, Katona E, Fulesdi B, Zrinyi M, Zatik J, Bereczki D, Polgar P, Kakuk G. Blood pressure distribution in a Hungarian adolescent population: comparison with normal values in the USA. J Hypertens 2003; 21:41–47.

10. Zinner SH, Rosner B, Oh WO. Significance of blood pressure in infancy. Hypertension 1985; 7:411–416.

11. Hulman S, Edwards R, Chen YQ, Polansky M, Falkner B. Blood pressure patterns in the first three days of life. J Perinatol 1991; 11:231–234.

12. Zubrow AB, Hulman S, Kushner H, Falkner B. Determinants of blood pressure in infants admitted to neonatal intensive care units: a prospective multicenter study. J Perinatol 1995; 15:470–479.

13. Prineas RJ, Elkwiry ZM. Epidemiology and measurement of high blood pressure in children and adolescents. In: Loggie JMH, ed. Pediatric and Adolescent Hypertension. Boston, MA: Blackwell Scientific Publications, 1992: 91–103.

14. Sinaiko AR, Gomez-Martin O, Prineas RJ. Diastolic fourth and fifth phase blood pressure in 10–15 year old children: The Children and Adolescent Blood Pressure Program. Am J Epidemiol 1990; 132:647–655.

15. Hanna JD, Chan JCM, Gill JR Jr. Hypertension and the kidney. J Pediatr 1991; 118:327–340.

16. Arar MY, Hogg RI, Arant BS Jr, Seikaly MG. Etiology of sustained hypertension in children in the southwestern United States. Pediatr Nephrol 1994; 8:186.

17. Plumer LB, Kaplan GW, Mendoza SA. Hypertension in infants—a complication of umbilical arterial catheterization. J Pediatr 1976; 89:802–805.

18. Vailas GN, Brouillette RT, Scott JP, Shkolnik A, Conway J, Wiringa K. Neonatal aortic thrombosis: recent experience. J Pediatr 1986; 109:101–108.

19. Abman SH, Warady BA, Lum GM, Koops BL. Systemic hypertension in infants with bronchopulmonary dysplasia. J Pediatr 1984; 104:928–931.

20. Ing FF, Starc TJ, Griffiths SP, Gersony WM. Early diagnosis of coarctation of the aorta in children: a continuing dilemma. Pediatrics 1996; 98:378–382.

21. Stafford MA, Griffiths SP, Gersony WM. Coarctation of the aorta: a study in delayed detection. Pediatrics 1982; 69:159–163.

22. Thoele DG, Muster AJ, Paul MH. Recognition of coarctation of the aorta. Am J Dis Child 1987; 141:1201–1204.

23. Adelman RD. Smokeless tobacco and hypertension in an adolescent. Pediatrics 1987; 79:837–838.

24. Blachley JD, Knochel JP. Tobacco chewer's hypokalemia: Licorice revisited. N Engl J Med 1980; 302:784–785.

25. Committee on Sports Medicine and Fitness. Athletic participation by children and adolescents who have systemic hypertension. Pediatrics 1997; 99:637–638.

26. Sorof JM, Alexandrov AV, Dardwell G, Portman JR. Carotid artery intimal-medial thickness and left ventricular hypertrophy in children with elevated blood pressure. Pediatrics 2003; 111:61–66.

27. Daniels SR, Loggie JM, Hhoury P, Kimball TR. Left ventricular geometry and severe left ventricular hypertrophy in children and adolescents with essential hypertension. Circulation 1998; 97:1907–1911.

28. Li S, Chen W, Srinivasan SR, Bond MG, Tang R, Urbina EM, Berenson GS. Childhood cardiovascular risk factors and carotid vascular changes in adulthood. The Bogalusa Heart Study. J Am Med Assoc 2003; 290:2271–2276.

29. Raitakari OT, Juonala M, Kahonen M, Taittonen L, Maki-Torkko N, Jarvisalo M, Uhari M, Jokinen E, Ronnemaa T, Akerblom HK, Viikari JSA. Cardiovascular risk factors in childhood and carotid artery intima-media thickness in adulthood. The Cardiovascular Risk in Young Finns Study. J Am Med Assoc 2003; 290:2277–2283.

30. Falkner B, Onesti G, Angelakos ET, Fernandes M, Langman C. Cardiovascular response to mental stress in normal adolescents with hypertensive parents. Hypertension 1979; 1:23–30.

31. Warren P, Fischbein C. Identification of labile hypertension in children and hypertensive parents. Conn Med 1980; 44:77–79.

32. Matthews KA, Manuck SB, Saab PG. Cardiovascular responses of adolescents during a naturally occurring stressor and their behavioral and psychophysiological predictors. Psychophysiology 1984; 23:198.

33. Falkner B, Kushner H. Racial differences in stress induced reactivity in young adults. Health Psychol 1989; 8:613–617.

34. Shear CL, Burke GL, Freedman DS, Berenson GS. Value of childhood blood pressure measurements and family history in predicting future blood pressure status: results from 8 years of follow-up in the Bogalusa Heart Study. Pediatrics 1986; 77:862–869.

35. Munger R, Prineas R, Gornez-Marin O. Persistent elevation of blood pressure among children with a family history of hypertension: the Minneapolis children's blood pressure study. J Hypertension 1988; 6:647–653.

36. Himes JH, Dietz WH. Guidelines for overweight in adolescent preventive services: recommendations from an expert committee. Am J Clin Nutr 1994; 59:307–316.

37. Havlik R, Hubert H, Fabsity R, Feinleib M. Weight and hypertension. Ann Intern Med 1983; 98:855–859.

38. Rocchini AP, Katch V, Anderson J, Hinderliter J, Becque D, Martin M, Marks C. Blood pressure in obese adolescents: effect of weight loss. Pediatrics 1988; 82:16–23.

39. Rocchini AP, Key J, Bondie D, Chico R, Moorehead C, Katch V, Martin M. The effect of weight loss on the sensitivity of blood pressure to sodium in obese adolescents. N Eng J Med 1989; 321:580–585.

40. Sinaiko AR. Hypertension in children. N Engl J Med 1996; 35:1968–1973.

41. Troiano RP, Flegal KM, Kuczmarski RJ, Campbell SM, Johnson CL. Overweight prevalence and trends for children and adolescents. Arch Pediatr Adolesc Med 1995; 149:1085–1091.

42. Ogden CL, Flegal KM, Carroll MD, Johnson CL. Prevalence and trends in overweight among US children and adolescents, 1999–2000. J Am Med Assoc 2002; 288:1728–1732.

43. DeFronzo RA, Tobin JD, Andres R. Glucose clamp technique: a method for quantifying insulin secretion and resistance. Am J Physiol 1979; 237:E214–E223.

44. Ferrannini E, Buzzigoli G, Bonadonna R, Giorico MA, Oleggini M, Graziadei L, Pedrinelli R, Brandi L, Bevilacqua S. Insulin resistance in essential hypertension. N Eng J Med 1987; 317:350–357.

45. Reaven GM. Role of insulin resistance in human disease. Diabetes 1988; 37:1595–1607.

46. Berenson GS, Wattigney WA, Bao W, Nicklas TA, Jiang X, Rush JA. Epidemiology of early primary hypertension and implication for prevention: the Bogalusa Heart Study. J Hum Hypertens 1994; 8:303–311.

47. Falkner B, Hulman S, Tannenbaum J, Kushner H. Insulin resistance and blood pressure in young Black men. Hypertension 1990; 16:706–711.

48. Ferrari P, Weidmann P, Shaw S, Giachino D, Riesen W, Allemann Y, Heynen G. Altered insulin sensitivity, hyperinsulinemia, and dyslipidemia in individuals with a hypertensive parent. Am J Med 1991; 91:589–596.

49. Grunfeld B, Balzareti M, Romo M, Gimenez M, Gutman R. Hyperinsulinemia in normotensive offspring of hypertensive parents. Hypertension 1994; 23:12–15.

50. Sorof J, Daniels S. Obesity hypertension in children. Hypertension 2002; 40:441–455.

51. Bao W, Srinivasan SR, Wattigney WA, Berenson GS. Persistence of multiple cardiovascular risk clustering related to syndrome X from childhood to young adulthood. Arch Intern Med 1994; 154:1842–1847.

52. Barker DJ, Osmond C, Golding J, Kuh D, Wadsworth ME. Growth *in utero*, blood pressure in childhood and adult life, and mortality from cardiovascular disease. Br Med J 1989; 298:564–567.

53. Law CM, Shiell AW. Is blood pressure inversely related to birth weight? The strength of evidence from a systematic review of the literature. J Hypertens 1996;14:935–941.

54. Barker DJ, Gluckman PD, Godfrey KM, Harding JE, Owens JA, Robinson JS. Fetal nutrition and cardiovascular disease in adult life. Lancet 1993; 341:938–941.

55. Osmond C, Barker DJ, Winter PD, Fall CH, Simmonds SJ. Early growth and death from cardiovascular disease in women. Br Med J 1993; 307:1519–1524.

56. Harlan WR, Cornoni Huntley J, Leaverton PE. Blood pressure in childhood. National Health Examination Survey. Hypertension 1979; 1:566–571.

57. Katz SH, Hediger ML, Schall JI, Bowers EJ, Barker WF, Aurand S, Eveleth PB, Gruskin AB, Parks JS. Blood pressure, growth and maturation from childhood to adolescence. Hypertension 1980; 2:55–69.

58. Falkner B, Hulman S, Kushner H. Birth weight vs childhood growth as determinants of adult blood pressure. Hypertension 1998; 31:145–150.

59. Hulman S, Kushner H, Katz S, Falkner B. Can cardiovascular risk be predicted by newborn, childhood, and adolescent body size? An examination of longitudinal data in urban African Americans. J Pediatr 1998; 132:90–97.

60. Lauer RM, Clarke WR, Beaglehole R. Level, trend, and variability of blood pressure during childhood. The Muscatine Study. Circulation 1984; 69:242–249.

61. Michels VV, Bergstralh EJ, Hoverman VR, O'Fallon WM, Weidman WH. Tracking and prediction of blood pressure in children. Mayo Clin Proc 1987; 62:875–881.

62. Julius S, Jamerson K, Mejia A, Krause L, Schork N, Jones K. The association of borderline hypertension with target organ changes and higher coronary risk. Tecumseh Blood Pressure Study. J Am Med Assoc 1990; 264:354–358.

63. Mahoney LT, Clarke WR, Burns TL, Lauer RM. Childhood predictors of high blood pressure. Am J Hypertens 1991; 4:60–85.

64. Nelson M, Ragland D, Syme S. Longitudinal prediction of adult blood pressure from juvenile blood pressure levels. Am J Epidemiol 1992; 136:633–645.

65. Lauer RM, Clarke WR, Maloney LT, Witt J. Childhood predictors for high adult blood pressure: the Muscatine Study. Pediatr Clin N Am 1993; 40:23–40.

66. Huxley R, Neil A, Collins R. Unraveling the fetal origins hypothesis: is there really an inverse association between birthweight and subsequent blood pressure? Lancet 2002; 360:659–665.

67. Rich GM, Ulick S, Cook S, Wang JZ, Lifton RP, Dluhy RG. Glucocorticoid-remediable aldosteronism in a large kindred: clinical spectrum and diagnosis using a characteristic biochemical phenotype. Ann Intern Med 1992; 116:813–820.

68. Lifton RP, Dluhy RG, Powers M, Rich GM, Gutkin M, Fallo F, Gill JR Jr, Feld L, Ganguly A, Laidlaw JC. Hereditary hypertension caused by chimeric gene duplications and ectopic expression of aldosterone synthase. Nat Genet 1992; 2:66–74.

69. Kroenke K, Omori DM, Simmons JO, Wood DR, Meier NJ. The safety of phenylpropanolamine in patients with stable hypertension. Ann Intern Med 1989; 111:1043–1044.

70. Lake CR, Gallant S, Masson E, Miller P. Adverse drug effects attributed to phenylpropanolamine: a review of 142 case reports. Am J Med 1990; 89:195–208.

71. Hurley JK. A pediatrician's approach to the evaluation of hypertension. Pediatr Ann 1989; 18:542, 544–546, 548–549.

72. Laird WP, Fixler DE. Left ventricular hypertrophy in adolescents with elevated blood pressure: assessment by chest roentgenography, electrocardiography, and echocardiography. Pediatrics 1981; 67:255–259.

73. Shieken RM, Clark WR, Lauer RM. Left ventricular hypertrophy in children with blood pressures in the upper quintile of the distribution: the Muscatine Study. Hypertension 1981; 3:669–675.

74. Zahka KG, Neill CA, Kidd L, Cutilletta MA, Cutilletta AF. Cardiac involvement in adolescent hypertension. Hypertension 1981; 3:664–668.

75. Culpepper WS III, Sodt PC, Messerli FH, Ruschhaupt DG, Arcilla RA. Cardiac status in juvenile borderline hypertension. Ann Intern Med 1983; 98:1–7.

76. Daniels SR, Lipman MJ, Burke MJ, Loggie JM. The prevalence of retinal vascular abnormalities in children and adolescents with essential hypertension. Am J Ophthalmol 1991; 111:205–208.

77. Yudkin JS, Forrest RD, Jackson CA. Microalbuminuria as predictor of vascular disease in non-diabetic subjects. Lancet 1988; 2:530–533.

78. Townsend RR, Ford V. Ambulatory blood pressure monitoring: coming of age in nephrology. J Am Soc Nephrol 1996; 7:2279–2287.

79. Soergel M, Kirschstein M, Busch C, Danne T, Gellermann J, Holl R, Krull F, Reichert H, Reusz GS, Rascher W. Oscillometric 24 h ambulatory blood pressure values in healthy children and adolescents: a multicenter trial including 1141 subjects. J Pediatr 1997; 130:178–184.

80. Harshfield GA, Alpert BS, Pulliam DA, Somes GW, Wilson DK. Ambulatory blood pressure recordings in children and adolescents. Pediatrics 1994; 94:180–184.

81. Brownell KD, Kelman JH, Stunkard AJ. Treatment of obese children with and without their mothers: changes in weight and blood pressure. Pediatrics 1983; 71:515–523.

82. Hagberg JM, Goldring D, Ehsani AA, Heath GW, Hernandez A, Schechtman K, Holloszy JO. Effect of exercise training on the blood pressure and hemodynamic features of hypertensive adolescents. Am J Cardiol 1983; 52:763–768.

83. Hansen HS, Froberg K, Hyldebrandt N, Nielson JR. A controlled study of eight months of physical training and reduction of blood pressure in children: the Odense Schoolchild Study. Br Med J 1991; 303:682–685.

84. Shea S, Basch CE, Gutin B, Stein AD, Contento IR, Irigoyen M, Zybert P. The rate of increase in blood pressure in children 5 years of age is related to changes in aerobic fitness and body mass index. Pediatrics 1994; 94:465–470.

85. Falkner B, Michel S. Blood pressure response to sodium in children and adolescents. Am J Clin Nutr 1997; 65:618S–621S.

86. Sinaiko AR, Gomez-Marin O, Prineas RJ. Effect of low sodium diet or potassium supplementation on adolescent blood pressure. Hypertension 1993; 21:989–994.

87. Appel LJ, Moore TJ, Obarzanek E, Vollmer WM, Svetkey LP, Sacks FM, Bray GA, Vogt TM, Cutler JA, Windhauser MM, Lin PH, Karanja N. For the DASH Collaborative Research Group. A clinical trial of the effects of dietary patterns on blood pressure. N Engl J Med 1997; 336:1117–1124.

88. Doyle AK. Angiotensin-converting enzyme (ACE) inhibition: benefits beyond blood pressure control. Am J Med 1992; 92:1S–107S.

89. Krolewski AS, Canessa M, Warram JH, Laffel LM, Christlieb AR, Knowler WC, Rand LI. Predisposition to hypertension and susceptibility to renal disease in insulin-dependent diabetes mellitus. N Engl J Med 1988; 318:140–145.

90. National High Blood Pressure Education Program. Working group report on hypertension and diabetes. Hypertension 1994; 23:145–158.

91. Hricik DE, Dunn MJ. Angiotensin-converting enzyme inhibitor-induced renal failure: causes, consequences, and diagnostic uses. J Am Soc Nephrol 1990; 1:845–858.

92. Pryde PG, Sedman AB, Nugent CE, Barr M. Angiotensin-converting enzyme inhibitor fetopathy. J Am Soc Nephrol 1993; 3:1575–1582.

44

Blood Pressure and Aging

TIM NAWROT, ELLY DEN HOND, LUTGARDE THIJS, JAN A. STAESSEN

Katholieke Universiteit Leuven, Leuven, Belgium

KEYPOINTS

- Isolated systolic hypertension is the predominant type of hypertension in the elderly and is associated with an increased cardiovascular risk. Isolated systolic hypertension is characterized by an increase in pulse pressure.
- Increased pulse pressure is a late manifestation of increased arterial stiffness, which is generally recognized as an important factor underlying cardiovascular complications in the elderly.
- Placebo-controlled intervention trials have clearly shown that pharmacological treatment of isolated systolic hypertension improves outcome in the elderly.

SUMMARY

Isolated systolic hypertension is the predominant type of hypertension in the elderly and is associated with cardiovascular complications such as stroke, coronary heart disease, and heart failure. In this chapter, the role of arterial stiffness, endothelial function, atherosclerosis, and oxidative stress in the pathogenesis of isolated systolic hypertension is extensively discussed. Placebo-controlled intervention trials such as the Systolic Hypertension in Europe Trial and the Systolic Hypertension in the Elderly Program have clearly shown that pharmacological treatment of isolated systolic hypertension improves outcome in the elderly. Nevertheless, isolated systolic hypertension remains the major subtype of untreated and uncontrolled hypertension.

I. INTRODUCTION

Hypertension refers to a lasting elevation of blood pressure with heterogeneous genetic and environmental causation. The increasing prevalence of hypertension with aging has been noted in numerous epidemiological studies. The process of vascular aging is characterized by a wider pulse pressure. In cross-sectional and longitudinal population studies, systolic blood pressure increase with age until the eighth decade of life (Fig. 44.1) (1). In contrast, diastolic blood pressure rises only until 50 years of age, after which it either becomes constant or even decreases slightly. Isolated systolic hypertension in older patients is a separate disease entity due to stiffening of the large arteries with advancing age. This chapter gives an overview of the epidemiological and pathophysiolocal consequences of the blood pressure–age relationship and the clinical consequences in the elderly.

II. EPIDEMIOLOGY

In the Framingham Heart Study, diastolic pressure was the strongest predictor below age 50, all three blood pressure indexes were comparable predictors at age 50–59, and from 60 years on, diastolic pressure was negatively related to risk of coronary events, so that pulse pressure

became superior to systolic pressure (2). The predictive role of pulse pressure in the elderly is consistent in men and women, in treated and untreated hypertensive subjects (3), and in patients with a history of myocardial infarction (4) or renal failure (5). Furthermore, in older patients with isolated systolic hypertension, pulse pressure (6), and especially ambulatory pulse pressure (7), are a stronger predictor of cardiovascular risk than mean pressure.

According to guidelines proposed by the ESH/ESC, hypertension is defined as a systolic blood pressure $\geq$140 mmHg, a diastolic blood pressure $\geq$90 mmHg, or taking antihypertensive drug treatment. The prevalence of hypertension is ~25% in the general adult population and increases to 60–70% in the age group >60 years (1). In the general US population, studied in the National Health and Nutrition Examination Survey III (NHANES III), men had a higher prevalence of hypertension than women up to 59 years, whereas the reverse was true from 60 years on (1).

In a random Belgian population sample of 2241 men and 2362 women with a median age (IQR) of 41 (29–56), systolic blood pressure averaged 119 mmHg in subjects below the age of 41 and 131 mmHg in subjects above the age of 41 (8). The corresponding mean values for diastolic blood pressure were 71 and 78 mmHg. The distribution of blood pressure according to the WHO criteria in the Belgian population is given in Table 44.1. The prevalence of hypertension in the Belgian population was 25.6% of whom, 52.5% was treated. Blood pressure

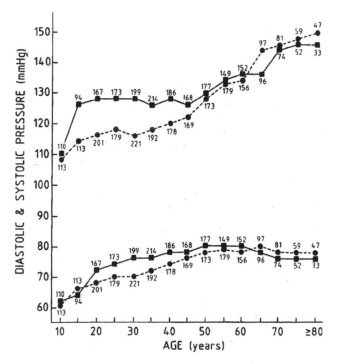

Figure 44.1 Systolic and diastolic blood pressure in 5 year age classes in a representative sample ($n = 4202$) of the population of five Belgian districts. ● represents women; ■ represents men. [From Burt et al. (1).]

Table 44.1 Classification of Blood Pressure Levels (mmHg) Based on Conventional Blood Pressure Measurement in Adults Aged 10 and Older in a Random Population Sample by Median Age

	Age $\leq$42 ($n = 2241$)	Age >42 ($n = 2362$)
Normotension		
Optimal (SBP <120 and DBP <80)	1573 (49.8%)	591 (19.5%)
Normal (SBP <130 and DBP <85)	828 (26.2%)	600 (19.8%)
High-normal (SBP 130–139 or DBP 85–89)	425 (13.5%)	478 (15.8%)
Hypertension		
Controlled on medication	59 (1.9%)	356 (11.8%)
Fase 1 (SBP 140–159 or DBP 90–99)	245 (7.8%)	739 (24.4%)
Fase 2 (SBP 160–179 or DBP 100–109)	20 (0.6%)	195 (6.4%)
Fase 3 (SBP $\geq$180 or DBP $\geq$110)	8 (0.3%)	66 (2.2%)

was well controlled in half of the treated subjects (8). Above the age of 41, only 20% of the subjects had an optimal blood pressure (systolic pressure <120 mmHg and diastolic pressure <80 mmHg).

Isolated systolic hypertension, defined as a systolic blood pressure ≥140 mmHg and a diastolic blood pressure <90 mmHg, is the predominant type of hypertension in the elderly. The NHANES III data demonstrated that below the age of 50, isolated diastolic hypertension (SBP <140 mmHg and DBP ≥90 mmHg) was most common (46.9%) among untreated hypertensives, whereas combined systolic/diastolic hypertension (SBP ≥140 mmHg and DBP ≥90 mmHg) was most common (45.1%) among inadequately treated individuals. In both untreated and inadequately treated groups, isolated systolic hypertension became the primary hypertensive subtype for subjects after the age of 50.

Few studies provide information on the incidence of hypertension in the general population. In the Framingham Heart Study, 5.3% of participants with optimal blood pressure, 17.6% with normal, and 37.3% with high-normal blood pressure below the age of 65 developed hypertension over a period of 4 years (9).

III. PATHOPHYSIOLOGY

Pulse pressure, the difference between systolic and diastolic blood pressure, is determined by the compliance of the arterial vascular bed and the stroke volume, and to a lesser extent by the ejection rate of the left ventricle. Mean arterial pressure, a weighted average of systolic and diastolic blood pressure, is dependent on cardiac output and total peripheral resistance.

A. Arterial Stiffness as Determinant of Systolic Hypertension

Arterial stiffness is emerging as the most important determinant of primary isolated hypertension in our aging community. Arterial distensibility and pulse wave velocity reflect the elasticity of an artery. Aortic pulse wave velocity doubles while distensibility coefficients halve between 20 and 70 years of age [Fig. 44.2(A) and (B)]. The arterial pressure wave consists of a forward component generated by the heart and reflected waves returning to heart form peripheral sites (5). In healthy young adults, the reflected waves coincide with diastole, raise diastolic pressure, and boost coronary perfusion. With arterial stiffening, the reflected waves move faster, reach the proximal aorta during systole, and cause an augmentation of late systolic pressure, whereas diastolic pressure decreases. The early return of the reflected pulse wave to the aorta during systole is the primary mechanism

accounting for the rise in systolic blood pressure and the decline in diastolic blood pressure that occurs with arterial stiffening. Lowered diastolic pressure may impair coronary blood flow and predispose to myocardial ischemia. The higher systolic pressure augments cardiac work and may lead to heart failure (5). Histopathologic examination of the aorta of the elderly reveals thickening of the media because of the accumulation of collagenous fibers as well as calcium deposition (10). A functional component may be superimposed on these structural changes. Indeed, the vasoconstrictor tone in the large arteries may well rise with age, when the number of β_2-adrenoreceptors that mediate vasodilatation decreases (11).

B. Endothelial Function and Arterial Stiffness

Endothelial function estimated as flow-mediated vasodilatation apparently starts to deteriorate at about 50 years [Fig. 44.2 (C)], that is, when pulse pressure begins to rise. Endothelial function is more per formant in premenopausal women than in men. This observation suggests that estrogens might enhance endothelial function [Fig. 44.2 (C)]. Indeed, estrogens activate endothelium-dependent vascular relaxation mechanisms, including the nitric oxide-cGMP and prostacyclin-cAMP pathways (12).

The endothelium generates a variety of biological mediators which influence the tone and structure of the blood vessel and determine the susceptibility of the vessel wall to atherogenesis. One of these mediators is nitric oxide, which is synthesized from the amino acid L-arginine via the action of the enzyme nitric oxide synthase.

Endothelin-1 is an important vasoconstrictor released by the endothelium and may also increase arterial stiffness. Indeed, plasma endothelin-1 concentration, shows a significant positive correlation with aortic stiffness in patients with coronary artery disease (13). This observation illustrates that endothelial function affects the function of large arteries. Thus large arteries are more than simply passive conduits.

C. Atherosclerosis in Hypertension

Many of the histological alterations that occur in the vessel wall with aging resemble those that come with artherosclerosis. Figure 44.2 (D) shows the increase in carotid intima media thickness, a sign of early atherosclerosis associated with advancing age. Nevertheless, the role of atherosclerosis in the pathogenesis of isolated systolic hypertension remains debatable. In autopsy specimens of human aorta, compliance decreases with age, but the relative contributions of aging and atherosclerosis remain unknown (14). Moreover, clinical experience shows that many patients with severe generalized atherosclerosis

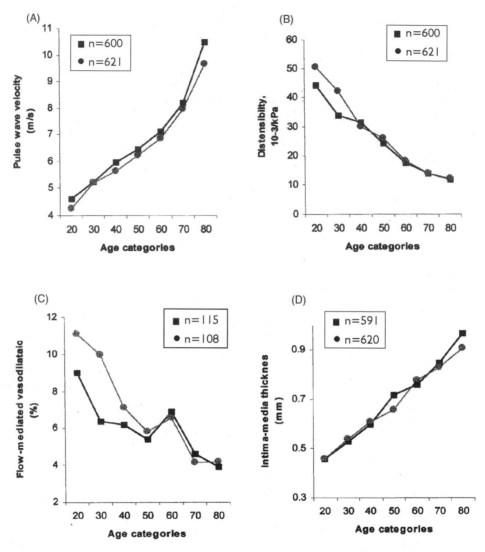

Figure 44.2 Wall characteristics by gender and age in a sample of the general population. ■ represents men and ● represents women. (A) Pulse wave velocity; (B) carotid artery distensibility; (C) endothelial function; (D) Intima-media thickness of the carotid artery. Data are mean for each age group.

maintain a normal central complaince. In contrast, in some populations with a low prevalence of atherosclerosis, systolic pressure does rise with age and isolated systolic hypertension is observed (15).

D. Hypertension Cause or Effect of Arterial Stiffness?

Whether the acceleration of the aging process occurs through an increase in arterial stiffness or through hypertension-associated changes in large artery structure has been debated. Liao et al. (16) evaluated the prospective relation between the baseline arterial elasticity and the development of hypertension in a population sample. After 6 years of follow-up, one standard deviation

decrease in arterial elasticity was associated with a 15% greater risk of hypertension, independent of established risk factors for hypertension, and the level of baseline blood pressure. These results suggest that lower arterial elasticity is causally related to the development of systolic hypertension.

E. Chronological and Biological Aging in Arterial Hemodynamics

The age-related changes in cardiac function, circulatory hemodynamics, lipid metabolism, and detoxification of reactive oxygen species all contribute to morbidity and mortality in the elderly. Although age is an outstanding risk factor for high blood pressure, stroke, and coronary artery disease, the precise pathophysiological mechanisms underlying these observations are presently unknown.

Telomeres are long stretches of characteristic DNA repeat sequences and associated proteins at the ends of chromosomes. These structures are essential to the life of the cell—they cap the ends of the chromosomes and therefore protect them from degradation and fusion. Recent experimental data support the concept that telomere length might serve as a biological clock not only at the cellular level but also probably at the systemic level (17,18). Telomerase is an enzyme that compensates for telomere shortening during DNA replication by adding telomere repeat sequences to the 5′ ends of the DNA strands. Its expression decreases with aging. Consequently, telomeres shorten each time DNA in a somatic cell replicates. The progressive loss of telomere length during life might contribute to cellular aging.

Evidence in support of this hypothesis comes from several observations:

- telomeres are shorter in somatic than in germline cells (17);
- fibroblasts from children suffering from progeria (a congenital disease characterized by accelerated aging) have shorter telomeres (18);
- telomere length in white blood cells decreases with age at a faster rate in men than women (19).

Of interest is the fact that homocysteine, a known risk factor for atherosclerosis (20), enhances the rate of telomere attrition per replicative cycle in cultured human vascular endothelial cells (21). To a large extent, this effect appears to be mediated by reactive oxygen species. Recently, it was shown that both pulse pressure and pulse wave velocity are inversely correlated with telomere length independent of chronological age (22). These observations suggest that pulse pressure and pulse wave velocity might be markers of the biological age of the vascular system.

F. Established Cardiovascular Risk Factors and Arterial Stiffness

Obesity is associated with decreased aortic elasticity. The rise in blood pressure following gain in body-weight is associated with profound changes in cardiovascular–renal physiology, including increased plasma volume, enhanced tubular sodium reabsorption, an initial decrease in total peripheral resistance, increased heart rate, activation of the sympathetic nervous system, and activation of the systemic renin–angiotensin–aldosterone axis (23). Adipose tissue secretes the hormone leptin, which increases sympathetic activity (23).

Adults with familial hypercholesterolemia have a significantly lower aortic distensibility than control subjects (24). The changes in vessel wall properties due to hypercholesterolemia may due to (1) impaired responses to endothelial relaxing factors (such as nitric oxide); (2) an increased content of collagen and calcium subsequent to deposition of cholesterol in the vessel wall; (3) a toxic effect of oxidized lipoproteins on the endothelium (25).

Even in the young, cigarette smoking increases arterial stiffness (26), aortic blood pressure (26), and plasma von Willebrand factor (a marker of endothelial damage) (27). More than 3800 chemicals present in tobacco smoke cause oxidative stress either directly or via biotransformation of these compounds. Smoking acutely increases sympathetic tone (28). Furthermore, smoking decreases nitric oxide production, the primary vasodilator produced by endothelial cells (26).

Diabetes is associated with increase arterial stiffness and decreased endothelial function (29). Glycation of proteins due to alterations in cellular metabolism remain a reasonable pathophysiological link between the hyperglycemia and the development of complication in diabetes. These chemically modified proteins may interact with cells in the vascular wall, inducing expression of cytokines and growth factors, which cause cross-linking of collagen molecules to each other (30), leading to an enhanced loss of collagen elasticity with a subsequent reduction in arterial distensibility.

Homocysteine a sulfur containing amino acid, which is formed in the metabolism of methionine to cysteine, behaves as an independent risk factor for cardiovascular disease. The two most important determinants of the plasma homocysteine concentration are folate status and renal function. From *in vitro* and animal models, there is evidence that high homocysteine concentrations are associated with endothelial toxicity attributed to oxidative stress that results from auto-oxidation of homocysteine (31). During this process, hydrogen peroxide and superoxide are formed that may increase low-density lipoprotein oxidation, and decrease the bioavailability of nitric oxide (31). The decrease in nitric oxide leads to vasoconstriction. In hypertensive patients, plasma homocysteine is positively correlated with aortic stiffness as assessed by carotid–femoral pulse wave velocity, independent of sex, age, blood pressure, and renal function (32). However, homocysteine lowering therapy had no beneficial effect on carotid distensibility in patients with end-stage renal disease (33), nor in healthy siblings of patients with premature atherosclerosis (34).

G. Risk Factors Tracking During Aging

Traditionally, research on aging deals with processes that begin late in life, but many of these processes may have origins at young age. Hypertension, hypercholesterolaemia, and overweight are usually well tolerated at younger age and are therefore barely perceived as harmful, but over time they may track and lead to excess morbidity and mortality from cardiovascular causes in middle-aged people (35–37). Findings from the Bogalusa Heart Study in the USA demonstrated that childhood blood pressure levels at or above the 80th percentile, not necessarily in hypertensive ranges, were associated with an increased prevalence of elevated blood pressure during adulthood (36). A follow-up study (35), showed that blood pressure in a group of male students at the age of 20.5, was associated with the incidence of cardiovascular diseases in the following 41.3 years. These findings suggest that elevated blood pressure during youth may have later clinical significance. Moreover, epidemiological studies have shown that cardiovascular risk factors tend to cluster within young persons (38) and that clustering of cardiovascular risk factors increases the risk of coronary heart disease. From the public health point of view, prevention is better than cure. Among 17-year-old Flemish adolescents, we recently found that 4.5% had hypertension, 9.0% were overweight (body mass index >25 kg/m^2), and 13.5% had a serum cholesterol concentration of 200 mg/dL or higher (38). Girls on oral contraceptive pills had a 4.6 mmHg higher blood pressure and an increase of 4.27 in the odds of not having an optimal blood pressure (systolic blood pressure <120 mmHg and diastolic blood pressure <80 mmHg) (39). If smoking and excessive alcohol intake were considered, 41.0% of the youngsters had one cardiovascular risk factor and 8% combined two or more risk factors. Prevention should therefore start at a young age. In Belgium, school attendance is compulsory until 18 years. Trained physicians examine the students at regular intervals. Unfortunately, the physical examination does not include blood sampling for the measurement of cholesterol and new directives are being implemented which place less emphasis on physical health.

IV. OUTCOME TRIALS

A. Placebo-Controlled Trials

The ultimate goal of treating patients with hypertension is not only to reduce blood pressure, but also to prevent the cardiovascular and renal complications of an elevated blood pressure, so that survival is prolonged and the quality of life is improved. Since 1991, three outcome trials have been published, which addressed the question whether in the elderly the cardiovascular risk conferred by hypertension is reversible by antihypertensive drug treatment. In all trials and subgroups combined (40), among 7757 control patients, 734 deaths and 835 major cardiovascular complications occurred; in 7936 patients allocated active treatment, these numbers were 656 and

647, respectively. Median follow-up amounted 3.8 years. Overall, active treatment reduced total mortality by 13%, cardiovascular mortality by 18%, all cardiovascular complications by 26%, stroke by 30%, and coronary events by 23% (40).

In the Systolic Hypertension in Europe (Syst-Eur) trial, patients (≥60 years) with isolated systolic hypertension were randomized to active treatment ($n = 2398$), that is, nitrendipine, with the possible addition of enalapril and hydrochlorothiazide, or to matching placebos ($n = 2297$) (41). The between-group difference in blood pressure amounted to 10.1/4.5 mmHg ($P < 0.001$). Active treatment reduced the incidence of fatal and nonfatal stroke by 42% and that of major cardiovascular complications by 30%. Cardiovascular mortality tended to be lower on active treatment (-26%, $P = 0.08$), but all-cause mortality was not significantly influenced (-13%, $P = 0.28$) (41,42). Furthermore, active treatment reduced the incidence of mild renal dysfunction (serum creatinine ≥176.8 μmol/L) by 64% (13 vs. 5 cases, $P = 0.04$) (43). The relative benefits of active treatment were evenly distributed across the two sexes and across patients with and without a history of cardiovascular complications (44). Further analysis also suggested similar benefit in patients who remained on nitrendipine monotherapy (45).

At randomization into the Syst-Eur trial, 492 patients (10.5%) had diabetes mellitus. In these patients, with adjustments for possible confounders, active treatment reduced all-cause mortality by 55%, cardiovascular mortality by 76%, all cardiovascular endpoints by 69%, fatal and nonfatal strokes by 73%, and all cardiac endpoints by 63%. The reductions in total mortality ($P = 0.04$), cardiovascular mortality ($P = 0.02$), and all cardiovascular endpoints ($P = 0.01$) were significantly larger in diabetic than in nondiabetic patients (Fig. 44.3) (46). Furthermore, active treatment reduced the risk of proteinuria more ($P = 0.04$) in diabetic than in nondiabetic patients (71 vs. 20%).

The Syst-Eur Vascular Dementia Substudy (47) investigated whether antihypertensive treatment could reduce the incidence of dementia. In total, 2418 patients were enrolled. After a median follow-up of 2 years in the double-blind trial, active treatment reduced the incidence of dementia by 50% ($P = 0.05$) from 7.7 to 3.8 cases per 1000 patient years (11 vs. 21 patients). Active treatment prevented mainly Alzheimer's dementia (8 vs. 15 cases). These results were confirmed in the open-label follow-up study (48). During extended follow-up, the number of incident cases of dementia increased from 32 to 64. Long-term active treatment ($n = 1485$), compared with control ($n = 1417$), reduced the incidence of dementia by 55%, from 7.4 to 3.3 cases per 1000 patient-years (43 vs. 21 patients) (48). Several reports suggest that calcium channel blockers, which cross the blood–brain barrier

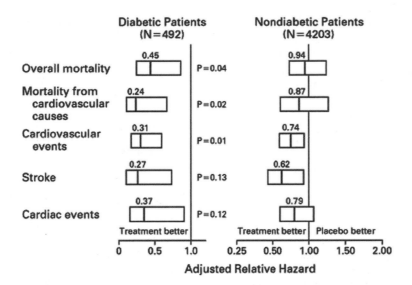

Figure 44.3 Adjusted relative hazard rates associated with active treatment as compared with placebo in diabetic and nondiabetic patients participating in the Syst-Eur trial. The relative hazard rates were adjusted for sex, age, previous cardiovascular complications, systolic blood pressure at enrolment, smoking status, and residence in eastern or western Europe. The P-values are for the interaction between treatment and diabetes and indicate whether the treatment effect was significantly associated with the presence or absence of diabetes at enrolment. Cardiovascular events, stroke, and cardiac events included fatal and nonfatal events. The bars indicate the 95% confidence intervals. The numbers above the bars indicate the benefit of the active treatment when compared with placebo. [From Tuomilehto et al. (46).]

and bind to brain receptors located in areas affected by Alzheimer's disease, may confer specific neuroprotection (49). However, the concept that antihypertensive therapy with long-acting dihydropyridines might protect against dementia needs further testing in controlled clinical trials.

The double-blind Syst-Eur trial ($P = 0.009$) (44) showed an interaction between treatment allocation and age. Randomization to active treatment was associated with a decreased relative risk of death in subjects aged 60–69 (59%) and 70–79 (58%), but with a slightly increased risk of death in patients aged ≥ 80 (11%). Similarly, a meta-analysis of the results of controlled trials in hypertensive patients over the age of 80 showed a nonsignificant of 6% excess death from all causes (50). In view of the remaining uncertainty, the Hypertension in the Very Elderly Trial (HYVET) is currently investigating the potential benefit of antihypertensive drug treatment on stroke and other cardiovascular endpoints in the very elderly (51). This trial will include a subgroup of patients with isolated systolic hypertension.

B. Guidelines for Antihypertensive Drug Therapy

Most experts recommend an integrated approach of risk management to prevent the complications of raised blood pressure. Accordingly, the need to start treatment increases in the presence of other cardiovascular risk factors or when absolute risk reaches a specified threshold

(e.g., in the British population, a 10 year risk of coronary heart disease $\geq 15\%$).

On the basis of evidence from trials, most but not all guidelines suggest that low-dose thiazides might be the most cost-effective way to start pharmacological treatment in most patients. However, for each class of antihypertensive drugs, compelling indications or contraindications exist. For instance, β-blockers or calcium channel blockers can be used in patients with angina pectoris. Stable heart failure is an indication for thiazides, aldosterone receptor blockers, β-blockers, or ACE inhibitors, but not for angiotensin receptor blockers (52). A history of myocardial infarction favors the use of β-blockers or ACE inhibitors. Renal impairment, microalbuminuria, or proteinuria is an indication for ACE inhibitors and/or angiotensin receptor blockers. Systolic hypertension warrants the use of thiazides or long-acting dihydropyridines. In black people, hypertension responds better to thiazides or calcium channel blockers than to inhibitors of the renin system, in terms of both blood pressure reduction and prevention of complications. In the absence of renal impairment at the initiation of antihypertensive treatment, all major drug classes equally prevent end-stage renal disease (52).

V. CONCLUSIONS

Since age and blood pressure are continuous variables with no discernible transition points where there is a sudden increase in morbidity and mortality, arbitrary definitions must be used for classification. Unlike diastolic blood pressure, systolic blood pressure increases progressively with age. The characteristic changes of systolic and diastolic blood pressure with age lead to an increase in pulse pressure, which has emerged as a new and potentially independent risk factor reflecting the biological aging of the vascular system. Arterial stiffness increasingly recognized as an important factor underlying cardiovascular complications in the elderly.

REFERENCES

1. Burt VL, Cutler JA, Higgins M, Horan MJ, Labarthe D, Whelton P et al. Trends in the prevalence, awareness, treatment, and control of hypertension in the adult US population. Data from the Health Examination Surveys, 1960 to 1991. Hypertension 1995; 26:60–69.
2. Franklin SS, Larson MG, Khan SA, Wong ND, Leip EP, Kannel WB et al. Does the relation of blood pressure to coronary heart disease change with aging? The Framingham Heart Study. Circulation 2001; 103:1245–1249.
3. Birkenhäger WH, Staessen JA, Gasowski J, de Leeuw PW. Effects of antihypertensive treatment on endpoints in the diabetic patients randomized in the Systolic Hypertension in Europe (Syst-Eur) trial. J Nephrol 2000; 13:232–237.
4. Mitchel GF, Moyé LA, Braunwald E, Rouleau JL, Bernstein V, Geltman EM et al. Sphygmomanometrically determined pulse pressure is a powerful independent predictor of recurrent events after myocardial infarction in patients with impaired left ventricular function. Circulation 1997; 96:4254–4260.
5. Safar ME, Blacher J, Pannier B, Guerin AP, Marchais SJ, Guyonvarc'h PM et al. Central pulse pressure and mortality in end-stage renal disease. Hypertension 2002; 39(3):735–738.
6. Blacher J, Staessen JA, Girerd X, Gasowski J, Thijs L, Liu L et al. Pulse pressure not mean pressure determines cardiovascular risk in older hypertensive patients. Arch Intern Med 2000; 160:1085–1089.
7. Birkenhäger WH, Forette F, Seux ML, Thijs L, Staessen JA. Increased blood pressure variability may be associated with cognitive decline in hypertensive elderly subjects with no dementia [in reply to Bellelli G, Pezzini A, Bianchetti A, Trabucchi M]. Arch Intern Med 2002; 162:483–484.
8. Nawrot T, Thijs L, Fagard RH, Staessen JA. Blood pressure classification according to the new WHO criteria in a Belgian population sample. J Hypertens 2002; 20:S318.
9. Vasan RS, Larson MG, Leip EP, Evans JC, O'Donnell CJ, Kannel WB et al. Impact of high-normal blood pressure on the risk of cardiovascular disease. N Engl J Med 2001; 345:1291–1297.
10. Asmar R, Safavian A, Tual JL, Safar ME. Arterial and cardiac changes in hypertension in the elderly. Blood Press Suppl 1995; 3:31–37.
11. Schocken DD, Roth GS. Reduced beta–adrenergic receptor concentrations in ageing man. Nature 1977; 267(5614):856–858.
12. Thompson J, Khalil RA. Gender differences in the regulation of vascular tone. Clin Exp Pharmacol Physiol 2003; 30(1–2):1–15.
13. Heintz B, Dorr R, Gillessen T, Walkenhorst F, Krebs W, Hanrath P et al. Do arterial endothelin 1 levels affect local arterial stiffness? Am Heart J 1993; 126(4):987–989.
14. Hallock P, Benson IC. Studies on the elastic properties of human isolated aorta. J Clin Invest 1937; 16:595–602.
15. M'Buyamba-Kabangu JR, Fagard R, Lijnen P, Mbuy wa MR, Staessen J, Amery A. Blood pressure and urinary cations in urban Bantu of Zaire. Am J Epidemiol 1986; 124(6):957–968.
16. Liao D, Arnett DK, Tyroler HA, Riley WA, Chambless LE, Szklo M et al. Arterial stiffness and the development of hypertension. The ARIC study. Hypertension 1999; 34(2):201–206.
17. Delange T, Shiue L, Myers RM, Cox DR, Naylor SL, Killery AM et al. Structure and variability of human-chromosome ends. Mol Cell Biol 1990; 10(2):518–527.
18. Allsopp RC, Vaziri H, Patterson C, Goldstein S, Younglai EV, Futcher AB et al. Telomere length predicts replicative capacity of human fibroblasts. Proc Natl Acad Sci USA 1992; 89(21):10114–10118.
19. Aviv A. Pulse pressue and human longevity. Hypertension 2001; 37:1060–1066.
20. Stein JH, McBride PE. Hyperhomocysteinemia and atherosclerotic vascular disease. Pathophysiology, screening and treatment. Arch Intern Med 1998; 158:1301–1306.
21. Xu D, Neville R, Finkel T. Homocysteine accelerates endothelial cell senescence. FEBS Lett 2000; 470:20–24.
22. Benetos A, Okuda K, Lajemi M, Kimura M, Thomas F, Skurnick J et al. Telomere length as an indicator of biological aging: the gender effect and relation with pulse pressure and pulse wave velocity. Hypertension 2001; 37(2 Part 2):381–385.
23. Mark AL, Correia M, Morgan DA, Shaffer RA, Haynes WG. State-of-the-art-lecture: Obesity-induced hypertension: new concepts from the emerging biology of obesity. Hypertension 1999; 33(1 Pt 2):537–541.
24. Lehmann ED, Hopkins KD, Gosling RG. Aortic compliance measurements using Doppler ultrasound: *in vivo* biochemical correlates. Ultrasound Med Biol 1993; 19(9):683–710.
25. Farrar DJ, Bond MG, Riley WA, Sawyer JK. Anatomic correlates of aortic pulse wave velocity and carotid artery elasticity during atherosclerosis progression and regression in monkeys. Circulation 1991; 83(5):1754–1763.
26. Mahmud A, Feely J. Effect of smoking on arterial stiffness and pulse pressure amplification. Hypertension 2003; 41(1):183–187.
27. Prisco D, Fedi S, Brunelli T, Chiarugi L, Lombardi A, Gianni R et al. The influence of smoking on von Willebrand factor is already manifest in healthy adolescent females: the Floren-teen (Florence Teenager) Study. Int J Clin Lab Res 1999; 29(4):150–154.

28. Winniford MD. Smoking and cardiovascular function. J Hypertens Suppl 1990; 8(5):S17–S23.

29. Wiltshire EJ, Gent R, Hirte C, Pena A, Thomas DW, Couper JJ. Endothelial dysfunction relates to folate status in children and adolescents with type 1 diabetes. Diabetes 2002; 51(7):2282–2286.

30. Larsen ML, Horder M, Mogensen EF. Effect of long-term monitoring of glycosylated hemoglobin levels in insulin-dependent diabetes mellitus. N Engl J Med 1990; 323(15):1021–1025.

31. Welch GN, Loscalzo J. Homocysteine and atherothrombosis. N Engl J Med 1998; 338(15):1042–1050.

32. Bortolotto LA, Safar ME, Billaud E, Lacroix C, Asmar R, London GM et al. Plasma homocysteine, aortic stiffness, and renal function in hypertensive patients. Hypertension 1999; 34(4 Pt 2):837–842.

33. van Guldener C, Lambert J, ter Wee PM, Donker AJ, Stehouwer CD. Carotid artery stiffness in patients with end-stage renal disease: no effect of long-term homocysteine-lowering therapy. Clin Nephrol 2000; 53(1):33–41.

34. van Dijk RA, Rauwerda JA, Steyn M, Twisk JW, Stehouwer CD. Long-term homocysteine-lowering treatment with folic acid plus pyridoxine is associated with decreased blood pressure but not with improved brachial artery endothelium-dependent vasodilation or carotid artery stiffness: a 2-year, randomized, placebo-controlled trial. Arterioscler Thromb Vasc Biol 2001; 21(12):2072–2079.

35. McCarron P, Smith GD, Okasha M, McEwen J. Blood pressure in young adulthood and mortality from cardiovascular disease. Lancet 2000; 355(9213):1430–1431.

36. Bao WH, Threefoot SA, Srinivasan SR, Berenson GS. Essential-hypertension predicted by tracking of elevated blood-pressure from childhood to adulthood—the Bogalusa Heart-Study. Am J Hypertens 1995; 8(7):657–665

37. Klag MJ, Ford DE, Mead LA, He J, Whelton PK, Liang KY et al. Serum-cholesterol in young men and subsequent cardiovascular-disease. N Engl J Med 1993; 328(5):313–318.

38. Nawrot TS, Hoppenbrouwers K, Den Hond E, Fagard RH, Staessen JA. Prevalence of hypertension, hypercholesterolemia, smoking and overweight in older Belgian adolescents. Eur J Public Health 2004; 14(4):361–365.

39. Nawrot TS, Hond ED, Fagard RH, Hoppenbrouwers K, Staessen JA. Blood pressure, serum total cholesterol and contraceptive pill use in 17-year-old girls. J Cardiovasc Risk 2003; 10(6):438–442.

40. Staessen JA, Gasowski J, Wang JG, Thijs L, Den Hond E, Boissel JP et al. Risks of untreated and treated isolated systolic hypertension in the elderly: meta-analysis of outcome trials. Lancet 2000; 355:865–872.

41. Staessen JA, Thijs L, Birkenhäger WH, Bulpitt CJ, Fagard R, on behalf of the Syst-Eur Investigators. Update on the Systolic Hypertension in Europe (Syst-Eur) Trial. Hypertension 1999; 33:1476–1477.

42. Staessen JA, Fagard R, Thijs L, Celis H, Arabidze GG, Birkenhäger WH et al. Randomised double-blind comparison of placebo and active treatment for older patients with isolated systolic hypertension [correction published in The Lancet 1997, volume 350, November 29, p 1636]. Lancet 1997; 350:757–764.

43. Voyaki SM, Staessen JA, Thijs L, Wang JG, Efstratopoulos AD, Birkenhäger WH et al. Follow-up of renal function in treated and untreated older patients with isolated systolic hypertension. J Hypertens 2001; 19:511–519.

44. Staessen JA, Fagard R, Thijs L, Celis H, Birkenhäger WH, Bulpitt CJ et al. Subgroup and per-protocol analysis of the randomized European trial on isolated systolic hypertension in the elderly. Arch Intern Med 1998; 158:1681–1691.

45. Staessen JA, Thijs L, Fagard RH, Birkenhäger WH, Arabidze G, Babeanu S et al. Calcium channel blockade and cardiovascular prognosis in the European trial on isolated systolic hypertension. Hypertension 1998; 32:410–416.

46. Tuomilehto J, Rastenyte D, Birkenhäger WH, Thijs L, Antikainen R, Bulpitt CJ et al. Effects of calcium-channel blockade in older patients with diabetes and systolic hypertension. N Engl J Med 1999; 340:677–684.

47. Forette F, Seux ML, Staessen JA, Thijs L, Birkenhäger WH, Babarskiene MR et al. Prevention of dementia in randomised double-blind placebo-controlled Systolic Hypertension in Europe (Syst-Eur) trial. Lancet 1998; 352:1347–1351.

48. Forette F, Seux ML, Staessen JA, Thijs L, Babarskiene MR, Babeanu S et al. The prevention of dementia with anti-hypertensive treatment. New evidence from the Systolic Hypertension in Europe (Syst-Eur) Study. Arch Intern Med 2002; 162:2046–2052.

49. Parnetti L, Senin U, Mecocci P. Cognitive enhancement therapy for Alzheimer's disease. The way forward. Drugs 1997; 53:752–768.

50. Gueyffier F, Bulpitt C, Boissel JP, Schron E, Ekbom T, Fagard R et al. Antihypertensive drugs in very old people: a subgroup meta-analysis of randomised controlled trials. Lancet 1999; 353:793–796.

51. Beckett NS, Connor M, Sadler JD, Fletcher AE, Bulpitt CJ, on behalf of the HYVET Investigators. Orthostatic fall in blood pressure in the very elderly hypertensive: results from the Hypertension in the Very Elderly Trial (HYVET)—pilot. J Hum Hypertens 1999; 13:839–840.

52. Staessen JA, Wang J, Bianchi G, Birkenhager WH. Essential hypertension. Lancet 2003; 361:1629–1641.

Part E: Secondary Hypertension

45

Renal Parenchymal Hypertension, Post-Transplant Hypertension, Renovascular Hypertension

JULIÁN SEGURA, LUIS MIGUEL RUILOPE

Hypertension Unit, Hospital 12 de Octubre, Madrid, Spain

KEYPOINTS

- Chronic kidney disease, whether manifest by albuminuria or reduced glomerular filtration rate, leads to hypertension and increased cardiovascular risk.
- Hypertension in the framework of chronic kidney disease requires aggressive blood pressure-lowering. ACE inhibitors and angiotensin receptor blockers retard worsening of nephropathy in different types of kidney disease in addition to their antihypertensive action.
- Hypertension after kidney transplantation is due to immunosuppressive drugs, renal dysfunction in the transplanted kidney, the native kidneys, transplant renal stenosis and other reasons.
- Renovascular hypertension is most often caused by renal artery stenosis due to fibromuscular hyperplasia or atherosclerosis. The unambiguous diagnosis is difficult, and renovascular hypertension can only be established in a part of the patients with renal artery stenosis.

SUMMARY

The kidney and arterial hypertension are closely related. In fact, renal disease is the most common cause of secondary hypertension. This chapter will review the relationship between hypertension and parenchymal and renovascular disease, their clinical evaluation and management, with special consideration for patients with end-stage renal disease receiving chronic dialysis therapy or following kidney transplantation.

I.   INTRODUCTION

The kidney is an important organ in most forms of arterial hypertension. Renal disease is by far the most common cause of secondary hypertension and hypertension is present in >80% of patients with chronic renal failure. Increasing data support the significance of chronic kidney disease as an important risk factor for cardiovascular disease.

Through its role in body fluid and electrolyte homeostasis, the kidney plays an important role in long-term arterial pressure regulation. If the kidneys cannot balance the intake of water and electrolytes with an appropriate excretion at a given arterial pressure level, extracellular (including intravascular) volume increases and arterial

pressure rises. Under chronic conditions, this may lead to arterial hypertension.

The term *renal parenchymal hypertension* includes a variety of renal diseases that are often associated with impaired renal function and hypertension. In addition to hypertension in association with chronic renal disease, we will examine specific varieties of renal diseases and how they relate to hypertension, including hypertension after kidney transplantation and elevated blood pressure in chronic dialysis patients. Finally, we will review renovascular hypertension and cardiovascular disease that are associated with chronic kidney disease.

II.   HYPERTENSION IN CHRONIC RENAL DISEASE

Hypertension is common in patients with overt renal insufficiency, as defined by a glomerular filtration rate <60 mL/min or a serum creatinine >1.5 mg/dL. Overall, hypertension is found in ~85% of patients with chronic renal disease. The prevalence is inversely correlated to the glomerular filtration rate, but it varies considerably in various forms of renal disease and even within the category of chronic glomerulonephritis (1). On the other hand, hypertension is associated with a more rapid progression of renal damage regardless of the underlying renal disease (2).

A.   Pathogenic Factors

Several factors have been implicated in the pathophysiology of hypertension in patients with renal disease:

- sodium retention and excessive intravascular volume;
- activation of the renin–angiotensin–aldosterone system (RAAS)
- sympathetic nervous system overactivity;
- endothelial dysfunction;
- oxidative stress;
- insulin resistance and other hormonal mechanism (cortisol, parathyroid hormones);
- Exogenous erythropoietin.

1.   Sodium Retention and Excessive Intravascular Volume

The mechanisms by which sodium excess could lead to arterial hypertension in the uremic patient are complex. In early phases, sodium excess leads to volume expansion, increased cardiac preload, and increased cardiac output. Later, hypertension is usually sustained by increased peripheral vascular resistance.

2. Activation of the RAAS

There is an abnormal relationship between exchangeable sodium or blood volume and plasma renin activity or plasma angiotensin II. Therefore, even "normal" plasma concentrations of renin are inappropriately high in relation to the state of sodium and volume balance.

3. Sympathetic Nervous System Overactivity

In animal models, acute renal injury caused by an intrarenal injection of phenol increases the secretion of norepinephrine, stimulates renal efferent sympathetic nerves, and raises blood pressure. Among patients with renal failure, plasma norepinephrine levels are usually increased. On the other hand, rate of sympathetic nerve discharge is much higher among dialysis patients with their native kidneys than among those who have undergone bilateral nephrectomy or in controls. There are two main functional types of renal sensory receptors and afferent nerves in the kidney: renal baroreceptors, which respond to changes in renal perfusion and intrarenal pressure and renal chemoreceptors, which are stimulated by ischemic metabolites and uremic toxins. Other mechanisms potentially responsible for the increase in sympathetic nerve activity in uremic patients include reduced central dopaminergic tone, reduced baroreceptor sensitivity, abnormal vagal function, increased calcium concentration, and increased plasma β-endorphin and β-lipotropin.

4. Endothelial Dysfunction

A low nitric oxide production and a diminished nitric oxide excretion was reported both in rats and in humans with chronic renal failure. Daily urinary nitric oxide excretion was lower among patients with moderate and severe renal failure compared with those with mild renal failure and normal controls. The 24 h urinary nitric oxide excretion and the nitric oxide clearance directly correlated with the creatinine clearance and inversely correlated with the serum creatinine level. On the other hand, asymmetric dimethylarginine concentrations, an endogenous inhibitor of endothelial nitric oxide synthase, were elevated in patients with end-stage renal disease, in part, because it is excreted via the kidneys (3). It has been well demonstrated that asymmetric dimethylarginine accumulates during chronic renal failure. Although there is controversy concerning the absolute concentration of asymmetric dimethylarginine, all authors found a twofold to sixfold increase in asymmetric dimethylarginine levels in patients with chronic renal failure when compared with controls.

Different dialysis treatment strategies differentially affect asymmetric dimethylarginine levels. The presence of atherosclerosis is associated with higher asymmetric dimethylarginine levels in patients with normal renal function as well as in dialysis patients, but this phenomenon may be unrelated to renal handling of asymmetric dimethylarginine. Reduced nitric oxide elaboration secondary to accumulation of asymmetric dimethylarginine may be an important pathogenic factor for atherosclerosis in chronic renal failure (4). Thus, the early increase of asymmetric dimethylarginine levels may be of relevance for the excess cardiovascular morbidity and mortality due to arterio- and atherosclerotic complications experienced by patients with renal disease (5).

5. Oxidative Stress

Renal toxicity, ischemia/reperfusion, and immunological disorders of the kidney result in an elevated formation of reactive oxygen species active in the pathogenesis of kidney disease. Treatment procedures are also shown to induce oxidative stress. Increased formation of free radicals leads to an accelerated lipid peroxidation. Furthermore, secondary aldehydic lipid peroxidation products, for example, malondialdehyde and 4-hydroxynonenal, are formed. They are shown to deplete antioxidants, inhibit protein syntheses, mitochondrial respiration, and enzyme functions. F2-isoprostanes, also metabolites of polyunsaturated fatty acids represent an additional *in vivo* marker of oxidative stress. Both isoprostanes and aldehydic lipid peroxidation products can be removed by hemodialysis. Protein carbonyls are products of such interventions. Oxysterols, another form of free radical initiated oxidation products, are shown to initiate atherosclerosis and plaque formation and thus increase dramatically the risk of coronary heart disease (6).

6. Insulin Resistance and Other Hormonal Mechanism (Cortisol, Parathyroid Hormones)

Even in patients with glomerular filtration rate within the normal range, insulin resistance and hyperinsulinemia are present early in the course of renal disease (7). This observation may have potential implications with respect to the high cardiovascular morbidity and mortality in patients with renal disease.

7. Exogenous Erythropoietin

Recombinant human erythropoietin (rHu-EPO), which is used to treat anemia in patients with chronic renal failure, can worsen hypertension and increase the need to use antihypertensive drugs. The increase in blood pressure during treatment with rHu-EPO was not observed in patients who were taking it for other reasons and that suggests that renal disease may confer a particular susceptibility to the hypertensive action of rHu-EPO. The rise in blood pressure during rHu-EPO administration occurs within weeks to months. Patients with severe anemia, with preexisting conditions, or those whose anemia is corrected rapidly are at greater risk for developing hypertension.

B. Evaluation of the Hypertensive Patient for Renal Parenchymal Disease

Evaluation for renal parenchymal hypertension includes a history and a physical examination seeking appropriate clues (Table 45.1).

1. Microalbuminuria and Proteinuria

Microalbuminuria is an important clinical finding in patients with renal disease. In patients with diabetes, it has a well-recognized association with progressive renal disease. However, microalbuminuria is becoming increasingly recognized as an independent risk factor for cardiovascular disease in patients with and without diabetes (8). Microalbuminuria is defined as a subclinical increase in urinary albumin excretion that is below the detection of traditional dipstick techniques. Standard urinary reagent dipsticks detect albumin when it is present at concentrations >150 mg%. By definition, microalbuminuria corresponds to the finding of an albumin excretion rate between 20 and 200 µg/min (30–300 mg/day), or an urinary albumin to creatinine ratio (mg/mmol) of 2.5–25 in males and 3.5–35 in females. Even below the

Table 45.1 Clinical Clues That Indicate Renal Parenchymal Disease

Clues from the medical history
  Recurrent urinary tract infections, particularly in young
    patients, which suggests congenial bladder abnormalities
    or reflux nephropathy
  A history of excessive proprietary analgesics; use of any
    potential nephrotoxin
  Previous renal failure
  Diabetic retinopathy, which suggests a diagnosis of diabetic
    nephropathy
  Proteinuria, which indicates glomerular disease
  Red cell casts, which indicate glomerular inflammation
Clues from the physical examination
  Periorbital edema
  Lower back and leg edema
  Rales
  Pallor
  Systolic or diastolic murmur
  Pericardial rub
  Decreased tactile sense
  Loss of muscle mass

traditional microalbuminuria thresholds, urinary albumin levels correlate with renal and cardiovascular events, and all-cause mortality. Reducing proteinuria is renoprotective, particularly in nephrotic patients. It has been recently reported that regardless of blood pressure control, 3 month changes in proteinuria and residual proteinuria predict long-term disease progression (9). Therefore, proteinuria should be a specific target for renoprotective treatment.

2. Microscopic Examination of the Urine

Cells and cellular casts are hallmarks of glomerular diseases. Red blood cell casts represent blood and proteins derived from the glomerulus and are always indicative of glomerulonephritis. White blood cell casts or mixed cellular casts may also be present.

3. Ultrasonography

It is useful to estimate renal size, identify cysts, and screen for obstructive uropathy. Small dense echogenic kidneys may indicate diffuse renal parenchymal disease, except in cases of diabetes and amyloidosis where renal size is often increased.

4. Renal Biopsy

Percutaneous renal biopsy should be performed only when the information will contribute to the treatment of the patient. Indications for renal biopsy are limited:

- to establish a diagnosis in patients with idiopathic nephrotic syndrome or nonpostinfectious glomerulonephritis;
- to establish the severity or prognosis of a renal parenchymal disease such as lupus nephritis;
- to determine the etiology of acute renal failure;
- to determine the primary renal parenchymal disease in potential renal transplant recipients.

Some glomerular diseases, such as diabetes mellitus, lupus, dyslipoproteinemias, and antinuclear cytoplasmic antibody glomerulonephritis, can be diagnosed from blood studies, and a biopsy is not necessary.

C. Management of Renal Disease Treatment

The main objective of treatment is to slow the progress to end-stage renal disease. In addition to control of hypertension, control of hyperlipidemia, reduction in the degree of proteinuria, and restriction of phosphorus intake also may be helpful. Both proteinuria and arterial hypertension often coexist in the same patient, and therapy must be directed at decreasing protein excretion in the urine as well as lowering the blood pressure (10). The optimal level of blood pressure and proteinuria has been amply recognized by guidelines (<130/80 mmHg or >125/75 mmHg if proteinuria >1 g/day is present).

The feasibility of this control is still under debate. Recent clinical trials clearly demonstrate that patients with renal disease and hypertension, should have their blood pressure lowered intensively. For renoprotection, target blood pressure depends on the severity of proteinuria before treatment. For proteinuria of 1–3 g/day, a mean arterial pressure of 98 mmHg provides additional benefit, whereas the target should be as low as 92 mmHg if proteinuria exceeds 3 g/day. The antiproteinuric effect of antihypertensive intervention predicts renoprotection; therefore, it is recommended that therapy should be titrated not only by blood pressure but also by reduction of proteinuria (11).

1. Sodium Restriction

The importance of dietary sodium restriction in proteinuric hypertensive patients goes beyond its ability to enhance the antihypertensive effect of all drugs. It is recommended a sodium intake between 44 and 88 mEq/day.

2. Diuretics

Patients with chronic renal disease are resistant to acidic diuretics, such as thiazides and loop diuretics, both because of their reduced renal blood flow and because of the accumulation of organic acid end products of metabolism that compete for the secretory pump. Thus, higher doses can be needed until a ceiling dose is reached. Once the ceiling dose is reached that dose should be given as often as needed as a maintenance dose. Spironolactone, triamtirene, and amiloride should be avoided in most patients with severe chronic renal disease because they may induce hyperkalemia.

3. Angiotensin-Converting Enzyme Inhibitors and Angiotensin II Receptor Blockers

Apart from its physiological role in the regulation of glomerular filtration rate and sodium excretion, the renal effects of angiotensin II are also crucially involved in the development and maintenance of hypertension. On the other hand, several experimental and clinical studies indicate that the renin system may play a pivotal role in the progression of renal disease (12).

Independent of their effect on systemic blood pressure (13), angiotensin-converting enzyme (ACE) inhibitors reduce blood pressure and decrease glomerular proteinuria by specific effects on the glomerulus. By blocking intrarenal angiotensin II, ACE inhibitors provide greater efferent arteriolar vasodilation. By relieving this efferent vasoconstriction to a greater degree than the reduction of afferent resistance, ACE inhibitors reduce pressure within the glomeruli and thereby provide protection against progressive sclerosis. In addition, they also block other angiotensin II-mediated adverse renal effects. In hypertensive nephrosclerosis, therapy containing an ACE inhibitor alone or in combination significantly reduces the incidence of renal events. This effect is independent of blood pressure control (14).

Renoprotective effects of ACE inhibitors were shown in The Ramipril Efficacy in Nephropathy (REIN) study. Among 352 patients with chronic nondiabetic nephropathies associated with at least 1 g/day proteinuria, ramipril effectively decreased proteinuria, glomerular filtration rate decline, and incidence of end-stage renal disease. Greater blood pressure and degree of proteinuria were the strongest determinants of faster glomerular filtration rate decline. The renoprotective effect of ramipril was similar in patients with normotension and hypertension. Hypertensive patients and those with proteinuria of 2 g/24 h or greater, primary glomerular disease, or nephrosclerosis gained the most from ACE inhibitor treatment (15). The REIN study investigators also reported that ramipril was much more effective in women than in men, regardless of their ACE polymorphism. In men, only those with DD genotype benefited (16).

Angiotensin receptor blockers (ARBs) have also been shown to retard the progression of albuminuria and the development and progression of nephropathy. In the Japanese Losartan Therapy Intended for Global Renal Protection (JLIGHT) Study, losartan reduced blood pressure in similar degrees to that of amlodipine in patients with chronic kidney disease. However, there was a significant reduction in 24 h urinary protein excretion in the losartan group, suggesting a renoprotective effect independent of its antihypertensive action (17).

ARBs produce similar antihypertensive effects and a comparable short-term effect on creatinine clearance and lipid profiles as those of ACE inhibitors. Both drug classes have a dose-response relationship for intermediate renal and cardiovascular parameters. Moreover, combined treatment with ACE inhibition and angiotensin receptor blockade is not only safe and well tolerated in patients with moderate chronic renal failure (18), but also seems to provide better long-term renoprotection than monotherapy (19).

On the other hand, recent evidence implicates aldosterone as an important pathogenic factor in progressive renal disease. Several lines of experimental evidence demonstrate that selective blockade of aldosterone, independent of renin–angiotensin blockade, reduces proteinuria and glomerulosclerosis in rat models. Aldosterone may promote fibrosis by several mechanisms: plasminogen activator inhibitor-1 expression and consequent alterations of vascular fibrinolysis, by stimulation of transforming growth factor-β_1 (TGF-β_1) and by stimulation of reactive oxygen species. Randomized clinical studies with aldosterone receptor blockade are warranted (12).

4. Calcium Channel Blockers

Through membrane-bound voltage-dependent calcium channels, calcium channel blockers inhibit calcium influx and subsequently result in decreased intracellular calcium levels and vasodilation. The family of calcium channel blockers is subdivided into three subclasses. The dihydropyridine group (dihydropyridine calcium channel blockers) has mainly vasodilatory effects and relatively small effects on cardiac inotropism or atrioventricular conduction. Reflex tachycardia can be seen, and edema is the most common side effect. The second group, the benzothiazepines (dilatiazem), has moderate vasodilatory effects and moderate negative inotropic and chronotropic effects. The third group, the phenylalkylamines (verapamil), has similar vascular and cardiac effects as diltiazem. The benzothiazepine diltiazem and the phenylalkylamine verapamil are referred to as NDCCBs (nondihydropyridine calcium channel blockers).

Calcium channel blockers may dilate afferent arterioles as much or more than efferent arterioles. Therefore, glomerular pressure could increase. However, if the calcium channel blocker lowers systemic blood pressure sufficiently, it will also lower intraglomerular pressure and provide renoprotection. In most studies, dihydropyridine calcium channel blockers did not reduce proteinuria, whereas NDCCBs did.

The effects of dihydropyridine calcium channel blockers on 24 h urinary protein excretion rate and glomerular filtration rate decline were evaluated in 117 nondiabetic patients with chronic, proteinuric nephropathies enrolled in the Ramipril Efficacy in Nephropathy study. The effects of dihydropyridine calcium channel blocker on 24 h urinary excretion of protein were dependent on the degree of blood pressure reduction. Among the patients who achieved a mean arterial pressure of 117 mmHg or 105 mmHg, 24 h proteinuria was greater in patients receiving dihydropyridin calcium channel blockers when compared with those subjects receiving other drugs. However, this adverse effect was no longer present in patients achieving lower mean arterial pressure. The combination of an ACE inhibitor and calcium channel blocker resulted in significantly less proteinuria when compared with patients on a calcium channel blocker alone. Thus, in nondiabetic proteinuric nephropathies, dihydropyridine calcium channel blocker may have an adverse effect on renal protein handling; it depends on the severity of hypertension and is minimized by ACE inhibitor therapy or tight blood pressure control (20).

III. DIABETIC NEPHROPATHY

Diabetes is now the most common cause of end-stage renal disease in adults. Approximately 20–30% of patients with type 1 diabetes and 10–20% with type 2 diabetes will develop end-stage renal disease (21). However, because patients with type 2 diabetes compose ~90% of the diabetic population, they make up the largest proportion of diabetics with end-stage renal disease. Among African-Americans, the incidence of end-stage renal disease is five times higher than that of whites; native Americans and Asians also have high rates of end-stage renal disease. In some ethnic groups, like the Pima Indians, diabetic nephropathy is the primary determinant of hypertension in type 2 diabetes (22). Familial and genetic factors play an important role in the development of this complication.

A. Pathophysiology

Glomerulosclerosis in diabetic patients is preceded by membrane thickening, mesangial expansion, and podocyte loss. It is usually associated with microalbuminuria.

In addition to the hyperglycemia, hypertension, and the renin–angiotensin system have been consistently implicated in the pathogenesis of diabetic nephropathy. By a common intracellular signaling pathway, the activation of protein kinase C (PKC) β, each of these pathogenic factors may induce changes in cellular function. Cytokines, in particular TGF-β_1, seem to be important agents in the initiation and progression of nephropathy. In vivo, the inhibition of PKC β led to a reduction in albuminuria, structural injury, and TGF-β expression, despite continued hypertension and hyperglycemia. On the other hand, part of the protective effect of ACE inhibitors may involve their inhibition of TGF-β_1.

Clinical clues in diabetic nephropathy include hyperglycemia, hypertension, and microalbuminuria in patients who have been diabetic for >15 years. In these patients, retinal capillary microaneurysms are usually present. Microalbuminuria is usually the earliest manifestation of nephropathy. The presence of even a minimally elevated albumin–creatinin ratio in morning first-voided samples beyond 30 μg/mg creatinine is an early indicator of the risk of nephropathy. In the presence of nephropathy, extracellular fluid volume, and total body sodium levels are increased. The activity of the RAAS is reduced in these patients, and the hypertension is volume-dependent, similar to other nephropathies (23).

B. Management of Diabetic Neuropathy

In addition to a tight control of blood pressure, measures to prevent progression of overt nephropathy in patients with diabetes include (Table 45.2): the reduction of proteinuria, control of hyperglycemia, the cessation of smoking, and the restriction of dietary protein intake to ~0.9 g/kg of body weight/day.

Table 45.2 Actions to Prevent Progession of Overt Nephropathy in Patients with Type 2 Diabetes

Achieve glycemic control (HbA1C concentration to normal); avoid hypoglycemia
Maintain blood pressure as close to 125/75 mmHg as possible, preferably with the use of an ACE inhibitor or ARB
Reduce the level of proteinuria
Stop smoking
Restrict dietary protein intake to ~0.8 g/kg body weight per day
Control associated risk factors

1. Glycemic Control

Several studies have shown the benefits of hyperglycemic control to slow the progress of nephropathy both in insulin-dependent and in noninsulin-dependent diabetic patients.

2. Antihypertensive Therapy

The purpose of antihypertensive treatment in diabetic patients is not only to slow progress of nephropathy, but also to reduce the morbidity and mortality from cardiovascular complications (congestive heart failure, coronary artery disease, and stroke). The Seventh Report of the Joint National Committee on the Detection, Evaluation, and Treatment of High Blood Pressure (JNC7) recommendations are consistent with guidelines from the American Diabetes Association (ADA) (24), which has also recommended that blood pressure in diabetics should be controlled to levels of $\leq130/80$ mmHg. Whatever the goal level, rigorous control of blood pressure is paramount for reducing the progression of diabetic nephropathy to end-stage renal disease. Combinations of agents are often required. Systolic blood pressure correlates better than diastolic blood pressure with renal disease progression in diabetics. The rate of decline in renal function among patients with diabetic nephropathy has been reported to be a continuous function of arterial pressure until ~125–130 mmHg systolic blood pressure and 70–75 mmHg diastolic blood pressure (24).

Randomized controlled trials that have included large diabetic populations, including the UK Prospective Diabetes Study (UKPDS), Hypertension Optimal Treatment (HOT) Trial, Systolic Hypertension in the Elderly Program study (SHEP), Systolic Hypertension in Europe Study (Syst-EUR), Heart Outcomes Prevention Evaluation Study (HOPE), Losartan Intervention For Endpoint Reduction in Hypertension Study (LIFE), and ALLHAT have demonstrated that adequate blood pressure control improves cardiovascular disease outcomes, especially stroke, when aggressive blood pressure targets are achieved.

Several studies investigated the impact of antihypertensive treatment on diabetic nephropathy both in type 1 or type 2 diabetic patients. In type 2 diabetic patients, a multicenter randomized study, UKPDS Study–Hypertension in Diabetes Study (HDS) (25), evaluated the effects of different levels of blood pressure control on diabetic complications. After a median of 8.4 years, "tight blood pressure control" (goal: blood pressure <150/85 mmHg) was associated with a reduction of 24% in diabetes-related endpoints, 32% in deaths related to diabetes, and 37% in microvascular endpoints (nephropathy and advanced retinopathy). Patients assigned to the tight control group had a 29% reduction in the risk of developing urinary albumin levels >50 mg/L at 6 years, but no significant changes were observed in the development of overt proteinuria or the increase in plasma creatinine levels between the two groups.

In subjects with type 1 diabetes and overt proteinuria (urinary albumin levels >500 mg/24 h), a large placebo-controlled clinical trial using the ACE inhibitor captopril (Collaborative Study Group Trial) showed a significant decrease in the progression of diabetic nephropathy (26). The rate of decline in renal function in this study was 11% per year in the captopril group and 17% per year in the placebo group. The endpoints of death, end-stage renal disease, or doubling the serum creatinine were reduced by 50% in the captopril group compared with standard antihypertensive treatment. The differences in systolic and diastolic blood pressure levels between the two groups (placebo and captopril) studied were small and suggest that ACE inhibitors have a renal protective effect independent of their antihypertensive effect.

Also, in studies of type 1 patients with microalbuminuria without a clinical diagnosis of hypertension, several small clinical trials suggest that ACE inhibitors may be beneficial in delaying or preventing the progression of nephropathy (27). A recent meta-analysis of raw data obtained for 698 type 1 diabetic patients enrolled in several small trials has shown a statistically significant decrease in progression to macroalbuminuria and in regression of albuminuria with ACE inhibition (28).

Which is the best medication for the treatment of the diabetic patients with chronic kidney disease? Both ACE inhibitors and ARBs have been recommended for use in diabetic patients with chronic kidney disease because these agents delay the deterioration in glomerular filtration rate and the worsening of albuminuria (24). In addition, ACE inhibitors have beneficial effects on other diabetic complications such as retinopathy and neuropathy and have been shown to reduce cardiovascular disease in diabetics with and without nephropathy. A recent meta-analysis on studies evaluating the effect of ACE inhibitors on diabetic nephropathy in patients with type 2 diabetes mellitus concluded that ACE inhibitors produce statistically significant reductions in albuminuria and reduce the progression of nephropathy in patients with type 2 diabetes mellitus (29). ACE inhibitors have been shown to preserve renal function in type 1 diabetics with nephropathy, in addition. In normotensive patients with type 1 diabetes mellitus and microalbuminuria, ACE inhibitors reduce the progression to macroalbuminuria and increase the chances of regression. Changes in blood pressure cannot entirely explain the antiproteinuric effect of ACE inhibitors (30).

Excellent protection against the progression of albuminuria and the development and progression of nephropathy in type 2 diabetics has been reported with angiotensin II receptor blockers, in addition. Losartan, ibesartan, telmesartan, candesartan, eprosartan, and valsartan are effective antihypertensive agents (31,32). Angiotensin II receptor blockers have been shown to decrease proteinuria both in type 1 and type 2 diabetic patients (33,34) and several trials reported renoprotective effects of ARBs in hypertensive patients with type 2 diabetes. These trials legitimatize the use of the angiotensin receptor blocker class in forestalling the deterioration in renal function.

Parving et al. (35) studied 590 hypertensive patients with microalbuminuria, comparing irbesartan (at two different doses) vs. placebo. After a 2-year follow-up, the primary outcome (time to onset of diabetic nephropathy, defined by persistent albuminuria, with an urinary albumin excretion rate >200 $\mu g/min$ and $>30\%$ higher than baseline) was found in 5.2% of the 300 mg irbsesartan group, 9.7% of the 150 mg irbesartan group, and 14.9% of the placebo group. They concluded that irbesartan had a renoprotective effect independent of any blood pressure-lowering effect.

Lewis et al. (36) studied 1715 hypertensive patients with nephropathy given irbesartan, amlodipine, or placebo. Treatment with irbesartan (300 mg), after a 2.6 year follow-up, was associated with a reduction of the risk of 20% of the primary composite endpoint (doubling of serum creatinine, development of end-stage renal disease, or death) compared with the placebo group and 23% compared with the amlodipine group after. The risk of doubling serum creatinine was 33% lower compared with the placebo group and 37% compared with the amlodipine group. The relative risk of end-stage renal disease was 23% lower in the irbesartan group than in the placebo or amlodipine groups. These differences were not explained by the blood pressure reduction achieved.

Brenner et al. (37) studied 1513 hypertensive patients with established nephropathy, comparing losartan (100 mg) with placebo. The mean follow-up was 3.4 years. Patients in the losartan group had a 16% risk reduction in the composite primary endpoint (doubling of serum creatinine, end-stage renal disease, or death), a 25% risk reduction in the doubling of serum creatinine, and a 28% reduction in end-stage renal disease. There was no effect seen for the death rate. The composite of mortality and morbidity from cardiovascular causes was similar between the two groups. The benefits exceeded those attributable to changes in blood pressure.

The Reduction in Endpoints in NIDDM with the Angiotensin II Antagonist Losartan (RENAAL) study and the Irbesartan Diabetic Nephropathy Trial (IDNT) are two recently reported trials conducted with patients in the advanced stages of diabetic nephropathy. Both trials showed a significant reduction in the primary pre-specified endpoint of death or worsening of renal function (doubling of serum creatinine) or the development of end-stage renal disease. This effect goes beyond the reduction in blood pressure, and makes of ARBs one of the important tools in the treatment of type 2 diabetic nephropathy.

Two other studies-the Irbesartan Microalbuminuria Study (IRMA)-2 and the Microalbuminuria Reduction with Valsartan study (MARVAL) were trials conducted in patients with type 2 diabetes with microalbuminuria. These trials legitimatize the use of the angiotensin receptor blocker class in forestalling the deterioration in renal function, which is almost inevitable in the patient with untreated diabetic nephropathy (38).

Nevertheless, data from several major prospective trials demonstrate that attainment of goal blood pressures in diabetic patients is virtually impossible to achieve with monotherapy. Antihypertensive therapy for diabetic patients with chronic kidney disease should include ACE inhibitors or ARBs, or both, because these agents delay the deterioration in glomerular filtration rate and the worsening of albuminuria. Furthermore, dual blockade of the renin–angiotensin system with both an ACE inhibitor and an angiotensin II receptor blocker has been superior to maximal recommended dose of ACE inhibitor with regard to lowering of albuminuria and blood pressure in type 1 patients with diabetic nephropathy (39). Multiple antihypertensive medications may be necessary in most cases. Furthermore, a target-driven, long-term, intensified intervention aimed at multiple risk factors (hyperglycemia, hypertension, dyslipidemia, and microalbuminuria) in patients with type 2 diabetes and microalbuminuria reduces the risk of cardiovascular and microvascular events by $\sim50\%$ (40).

IV. HYPERTENSION AFTER KIDNEY TRANSPLANTATION

Hypertension is extremely common in renal transplant patients. It occurs in $\sim75-90\%$ of adults and in $65-75\%$ of pediatric recipients. With the introduction of cyclosporine A, the graft survival rate after renal transplantation has improved. However, the use of cyclosporine A is associated with an increased incidence of hypertension. Tacrolimus is associated with a lower prevalence of hypertension compared with cyclosporine A.

In addition to calcineurin inhibitors, corticosteroids, renal artery stenosis, primary hypertension in the kidney donor or graft recipient, acute and chronic rejection episodes, recurrence or *de novo* renal disease, and obesity have been implicated as causing post-transplant hypertension (Table 45.3). Hypertension may be a significant risk factor for allograft survival (41) and for cardiovascular disease. In renal transplant patients on cyclosporine A, hypertension is characterized by sodium and water retention, enhanced sympathetic nervous system activity, and increased peripheral vascular resistance (42).

The long-term goal in patients with post-transplant hypertension is similar to that of nontransplant patients (43): reduced morbidity and mortality by control blood pressure, hyperglycemia, dyslipidemia, and cigarette smoking. Goal blood pressures should be similar to those in the nontransplant setting. However, the lowering of blood pressure even within the normotensive range attenuates the progression of kidney injury. Hypertensive transplant recipients with diabetes mellitus, dyslipidemia, or cardiac or renal disease may require lower goals ($\leq 130/80$ mmHg).

Pharmacological therapy is appropriate for the majority of patients with post-transplant hypertension. In general, hypertensive transplant recipients require two or more medications.

Animal experiments have shown that endothelin-induced vasoconstriction of cyclosporine A depends on the activation of L-type calcium channels, which are the main target for calcium channel blocking agents. In addition, calcium channel blockers have been shown to antagonize the effects of several of the putative cyclosporine A-stimulated hormonal factors, such as angiotensin II and norepinephrine. On the other hand, calcium antagonists have been shown to be useful in the case of acute toxicity because they allow faster renal function recovery and shorter hospitalization time. The mechanisms by which this class reduces cyclosporin toxicity may be related to a reduction in the calcium influx into cells during ischemic and reperfusion periods. This reduction would reduce the generation of oxygen-free radicals and perhaps reduce thromboxane production (44).

As reviewed by Remuzzi et al. (42), several studies reported benefits of calcium channel blockers in patients with post-transplant hypertension. In fact, calcium channel blockers have been considered for years the antihypertensive agents of choice for renal transplantation. However, the fact that some calcium channel blockers may cause a worsening of proteinuria, which might be detrimental to graft function in the long-term and the higher incidence of myocardial infarction with short acting dihydropyridines compared with patients given diuretics and β-blockers, raises concerns about the safety of these agents in transplant patients. On the other hand, since some calcium channel blockers (verapamil, diltiazem, and nicardipine) interfere with the degradation of calcineurin inhibitors, it is prudent to monitor the cyclosporine or tacrolimus blood levels during the initiation of calcium channel blocker therapy.

ACE inhibitors and ARBs are usually effective in reducing blood pressure in renal transplant recipients (45). Their beneficial kidney effects derive from their ability to reduce intraglomerular pressure. In addition, they inhibit the expression of TGF-β, cytokine implicated in the pathogenesis of chronic allograft nephropathy, and decrease proteinuria, which is regarded as a powerful predictor of long-term graft outcome. On the other hand, the beneficial effects of ACE inhibitors and ARBs after myocardial infarction and congestive heart failure may also be favorable for renal transplant recipients. Furthermore, both agents can be used to counteract the erythrocytosis after transplantation. A point of concern is that renal dysfunction may occur early after the initiation of the therapy with ACE inhibitors or ARBs. This is the consequence of a reduction of the glomerular perfusion pressure and a fall in glomerular filtration due to the ACE inhibitor/angiotensin receptor blocker induced dilatation of the efferent arterioles together with a simultaneous cyclosporin-related constriction of the afferent arterioles. In the majority of cases, only a small and transient increase in serum creatinine occurs.

β-Blockers are also effective in post-transplant hypertension and are also recommended for those with coronary disease.

Table 45.3 Causes of Post-Transplant Hypertension

Use of immunosuppressive drugs
Cyclosporine
Tacrolimus
Corticosteroids
Renal dysfunction
Perioperative ischemic damage
Drug induced nephrotoxicity
Chronic allograft rejection
Recurrence of original renal disease
Native kidneys
Transplant renal artery stemosis
Donor-kidney associated hypertension
Other causes
Obesity
Use of alcohol
Obstructive sleep apnea

V. HYPERTENSION IN CHRONIC DIALYSIS PATIENTS

By the time chronic renal failure progresses to end-stage renal disease, hypertension is present in 80–90% of patients. It is one of the major risk factors that contributes to the development of cardiovascular disease in patients undergoing dialysis (46). Cardiovascular disease mortality is 5–30 times higher in dialysis patients than in subjects of the same age, race, and gender from the general population. The relative risk is higher at younger ages and lower at older ages.

A weight gain as small as 2.5 kg between dialysis sessions is associated with a significant rise in blood pressure. There is a significant correlation between blood pressure and interdialytic weight gain in hypertensive patients. Despite the use of multiple antihypertensive drugs, control of blood pressure may not be possible if dry weight is not achieved by ultrafiltration and dietary sodium restriction.

Systolic hypertension and age are determinants of complex ventricular arrhythmia in hemodialysis patients after adjustment for other associated factors (47). The arrhythmogenic effect of hypertension possibly involves the promotion of myocardial ischemia aggravated by concomitant left ventricular hypertrophy.

VI. RENOVASCULAR HYPERTENSION

Renovascular hypertension refers to hypertension that is caused by renal hypoperfusion due to stenosis, constriction, or lesion of the renal arteries involving one or both kidneys. However, it is important to note that the mere demonstration of a renal artery stenosis in a patient with hypertension does not necessarily constitute renovascular hypertension. Often, clinically nonsignificant (asymptomatic) renal artery lesions are found in patients with essential hypertension, renal failure of other etiology (chronic hypertension for example), or even those with normal blood pressure. Renovascular hypertension must be distinguished from the much more prevalent condition of renovascular disease.

Renovascular disease is a complex disorder with various causes and presentations. The most common causes of renovascular disease are fibromuscular dysplasia and atherosclerosis. Patients with fibromuscular dysplasia may be quite hypertensive; they generally do not develop renal insufficiency. There is usually a good clinical response to interventions like percutaneous renal artery angioplasty (PTRA). In contrast, atherosclerotic disease can be difficult to evaluate and manage. These patients often have coexistent essential hypertension; progressive loss of renal function is common; and response to surgical or percutaneous intervention is often suboptimal. Angiographic data confirm that patients with atherosclerotic vascular disease tend to have atherosclerosis in multiple arteries (especially in elderly patients), and thus are prone to complications, such as stroke, myocardial infarction, and cardiovascular death.

Because fibromuscular dysplasia and atherosclerosis are two distinct diseases, their diagnostic and treatment strategies differ considerably. If identified, renovascular hypertension is a potentially curable disease. If left undiagnosed and untreated, it may lead to permanent end-stage renal disease, heart disease, retinopathy, and cerebrovascular disease.

A. Mechanisms of Hypertension in Animal Models

Animals' models allow an understanding of the local paracrine and systemic endocrine role of the renin–angiotensin system. Whatever the method used to induce renovascular hypertension, the model goes through an initial stage of renin–angiotensin activation, which is followed sooner or later by retention of salt and water (48).

There are two main subtypes of renovascular hypertension: unilateral and bilateral renal artery stenosis. In animals, these conditions are represented by two models: the two-kidney, one-clip model where a constricting clip is applied to one or both renal arteries, and the two-kidney, two-clip model. In latter model, although there is an inappropriate increase in the activity of the RAAS, impaired salt and water excretion is the main mechanism of chronic hypertension. The difference between hypertension caused by unilateral vs. bilateral renal arterial stenosis is the persistent angiotensin II-dependency in unilateral stenosis.

Renovascular hypertension appears to evolve over three distinct phases: the early or acute phase, a transitional phase, and a chronic or sustained late phase. The early phase depends primarily on the renin–angiotensin system. Through the renal receptor mechanism, reduced renal perfusion stimulates renin secretion and leads to an increase in plasma angiotensin II, which provokes systemic hypertension. Plasma renin activity in the early phase typically may become 3–10 times higher than normal.

In the second or transitional phase, angiotensin remains elevated. In addition to its direct vasoconstrictor effect, it may increase blood pressure through activation of secondary vasoconstrictors, such as the endothelium-derived constricting factor thromboxane-endoperoxide. Angiotensin II stimulation of aldostrone secretion also results in sodium and water retention and increased extracellular volume, which may sustain hypertension and secondarily suppress renin release. Thus, the transitional phase is characterized by changes away from the predominant angiotensin dependence of the early phase.

The chronic or sustained late phase of renovascular hypertension is characterized by secondary structural damage to the kidneys, vasculature, and other organs. In contrast to the early phase, the influence of angiotensin on maintaining elevated blood pressure in chronic renovascular hypertension is not clear. Plasma renin activity returns toward normal values. Elevated blood pressure no longer completely or consistently responds to short-term treatment with either the ACE inhibitors or the angiotensin II antagonist saralasin. This suggests a diminished role for the renin–angiotensin system in maintaining hypertension (49).

B. Studies in Humans

As in the animal models, renovascular hypertension in humans is caused by increased renin release from the ischemic kidney (50). Experimental evidence indicates that other systems may have a critical role in the long-term maintenance of high blood pressure after renal artery stenosis:

- activation of the sympathetic nervous system;
- increased lipoxygenase and thromboxane pathways;
- vasopressin;
- cellular hypertrophy and thickening of subcutaneous small arteries;
- increased levels of atrial natriuretic factor, kalikrein, vasodilative prostaglandins, and nitric oxide, which may counter the effects of the activated renin–angiotensin system.

Renovascular hypertension is one of the most common causes of secondary hypertension, with reports of its frequency varying from <1% in unselected populations to as high as 30% in highly selected referral populations (e.g., white adults with diastolic blood pressure >120 mmHg and grade III or grade IV retinopathy) (51).

Atherosclerotic renovascular disease is usually seen in patients over 50 years of age with traditional risk factors for atherosclerosis. Recent reports from the Cardiovascular Health Study in North Carolina indicate that among 834 individuals over 65-year-old, important renovascular stenosis (defined as Doppler peak systolic velocities ≥ 1.8 m/s) could be detected in 6.8% of the general population. The mean age of those with renovascular disease was 77.2 years. Predictive variables include age, reduced HDL cholesterol, and increased systolic blood pressure (52).

Fibromuscular dysplasia tends to be present in young women (although many cases are not diagnosed until after age 40). Occasionally, fibromuscular dysplasia and atherosclerotic disease may coexist in older patients.

C. Causes and Clinical Features

Numerous causes can lead to renovascular disease (Table 45.4), but the two most common are atherosclerosis and fibromuscular dysplasia.

As the population ages and mortality due to cerebrovascular and coronary events decreases, advanced atherosclerotic disease is more frequently seen in other vascular beds. Patients with atherosclerotic renovascular

Table 45.4 Types of Lesions Associated with Renovascular Hypertension

Intrinsic lesions
  Atherosclerosis
  Fibrosmuscular dysplasia
  Aneurysm
  Emboli
  Arteritis
Ateriovenous malformation or fistula
  Angioma
  Thrombosis after antihypertensive treatment
  Rejection of renal transplant
  Injury to the renal artery (surgical ligation, trauma, radiation)
  Intrarenal cysts
Extrinsic lesions
  Pheocromocitoma or paraganglioma
  Tumors
  Retroperitoneal fibrosis
Ureteral obstruction

hypertension are older and have higher systolic pressure compared with patients with primary hypertension. They have more extensive renal damage and vascular disease elsewhere. It typically occurs in male smokers aged over 50. Other clinical features (Table 45.5) include malignant or drug resistant hypertension, high-grade retinopathy, abdominal or flank bruits, and absence of family history of hypertension.

Laboratory findings that were more common in the population with renovascular hypertension include: secondary aldosteronism, higher plasma renin, hypokalemia, metabolic alkalosis, proteinuria, elevated serum creatinine, and an elevated blood urea nitrogen level (>20 mg/dL). Proteinuria is now recognized as a clinical feature associated with renal arterial disease. It sometimes reaches nephrotic range and can reverse with nephrectomy of the stenotic kidney, blockade of the renin–angiotensin system, or successful renal revascularization. Nevertheless, with the widespread application of antihypertensive

Table 45.5 Characteristics of Renal Artery Stenosis Atherosclerosis

Patient age usually >50 years
More commonly found in men
More commonly found in patients who smoke
May be associated with vascular disease elsewhere in system
May be associated with malignant or drug-resistant hypertension
Often associated with renal impairement
Fibromuscular dysplasia
  Patient age usually ≤ 50 years
  More commonly found in women
  Presents as hypertension
  Rarely causes renal impairement

drugs that block the renin–angiotensin system, many patients with unilateral renal arterial disease and renovascular hypertension are never detected as long as blood pressures are well controlled and kidney function remains stable. Deterioration of kidney function, reflected by a rapid rise in serum creatinine, can occur with renal arterial disease during blood pressure reduction. This represents a "functional" renal insufficiency produced by reduced transcapillary filtration pressure. Such a change develops most commonly with ACE inhibition and angiotensin receptor blocker therapy.

Through medial fibroplasia of the renal artery, fibromuscular dysplasia leads to renovascular disease and hypertension. It is seen most commonly in young females (Table 45.5) and often involves multiple arteries originating from the aorta, including the carotid and celiac vessels. Some features were reported as more common among patients with medial fibromuscular dysplasia than those with normal renal arteries: cigarette smoking, HLA-DRw6 antigen, and a family history of cardiovascular disease (53). Abdominal bruits have a prevalence of 6.5–31% in the healthy population and a prevalence of 28% in patients with all-cause hypertension. However, in patients with angiographically proven renal artery stenosis, the prevalence ranges from 78% to 87% (54).

D.　Diagnostic Tests for Renal Artery Stenosis

Diagnostic tests for renal artery stenosis are expensive, invasive, and limited by their lack of sensitivity and specificity. Therefore, the selection of patients with hypertension for evaluation of renal artery stenosis can be challenging. Some clinical clues (Table 45.6) may increase one's clinical index of suspicion and direct an appropriate work-up. Mann and Pickering (55) have formulated a diagnostic guide based on a selective approach in which only patients with suggestive clinical clues are tested (Table 45.7).

Table 45.6　Clinical Features and Indicators of Renal Artery Disease

Young hypertensive patient with no family history of hypertension (fibromuscular dysplasia)
Peripheral vascular disease
Resistant hypertension
Deteriorating blood pressure control in compliant, long-standing hypertensive patients
Deterioration in renal function with use of ACE inhibition
Renal impairment, but with minimal proteinuria
"Flash" pulmonary edema
1.5 cm difference in kidney size on ultrasonography
Secondary hyperaldosteronism (low plasma sodium and potassium concentrations)

Table 45.7　Testing for Renovascular Hypertension: Clinical Index of Suspicion

Low index of suspicion (should not be tested)
　Borderline, mild to moderate hypertension
Moderate index of suspicion (non hypertension-invasive tests recommended)
　Severe hypertension (diastolic blood pressure >120 mmHg)
　Hypertension refractory to standard therapy, excluding ACE inhibitor or ARB
　Abrupt onset of sustained, moderate to severe hypertension at age <20 or >50 years
　Hypertension with a suggestive abdominal or flank bruit
　Moderate hypertension (diastolic blood pressure >105 mmHg) in a person who smokes, a patient with evidence of occlusive vascular disease, or a patient with unexplained but stable elevation of serum creatinine
　Normalization of blood pressure in a patient with moderate to severe hypertension who is being treated with an ACE inhibitor or an ARB (particularly if the patient smokes or it is a patient in whom the onset of hypertension is recent)
High index of suspicion (consider proceeding directly to arteriography)
　Severe hypertension (diastolic blood pressure >120 mmHg) with either progressive renal insufficiency or refractory hypertention even with aggressive treatment, particularly in a patient who has been a smoker or who has other evidence of occlusive arterial disease
　Accelelerated or malignant hypertension (grade III or grade IV retinopathy)
　Hypertension with recent elevation of serum creatinine, either unexplained or reversibly induced by an angiotensin-converting enzyme inhibitor or an angiotensin receptor blocker
　Moderate to severe hypertension with incidentally detected asymmetry of renal size

Two classes of diagnostic tests are used to investigate the presence of renal artery stenosis and indirectly renovascular hypertension: tests assessing plasma renin activity and the ones imaging the renal arteries.

1.　Tests Assessing Renin Release

Patients with renovascular hypertension may have elevated plasma renin activity, mainly during early phases because renal hypoperfusion is associated with hypersecretion of renin. However, plasma renin activity is a complex variable affected by medications, volume status, and numerous other variables. Furthermore, the plasma renin activity may decrease over time in patients with renovascular hypertension. Thus, renin levels are generally higher in patients with fibromuscular dysplasia and less useful in elderly patients. Since it lacks specificity, this test is not very helpful. However, a highly suppressed plasma renin activity (<1.0) makes uncomplicated renovascular hypertension less likely, while extremely high values (>10.0) suggests a more careful work-up.

2. Tests Assessing Captopril-Enhanced Peripheral Plasma Renin Activity

In order to improve the sensitivity and specificity of plasma renin activity measurements, investigators have measured plasma renin activity after captopril administration. To perform this test, all patients must discontinue diuretics and ACE inhibitors for 2 weeks before testing. The plasma renin activity level is tested before and 30 min after a captopril dose. A positive test requires three features: a stimulated plasma renin activity >12 ng/mL per hour, an absolute increase in plasma renin activity of at least 10 ng/mL per hour, and an increase in plasma renin activity levels of >150% (or >400% if the baseline plasma renin activity level was <3 ng/mL per hour). This is a highly sensitive test, but a high rate of false-positive captopril renin tests can be seen among patients with high baseline plasma renin activity levels. High unilateral renal vein renin levels with contralateral suppression are seen in the setting of renovascular hypertension secondary to unilateral renal artery stenosis. This test may be particularly helpful in determining the functional significance of a renal artery lesion of "borderline" angiographic appearance and its predictive curability with revascularization. However, this test loses its accuracy in the setting of renal insufficiency, bilateral renal artery stenosis, or with the use of antihypertensive medications.

3. Doppler Ultrasound of the Renal Arteries

Duplex ultrasonography is a noninvasive, which combines direct visualization of the renal arteries (B-mode) with hemodynamic measurements in the renal arteries (Doppler) allowing direct measurement of renal size. The procedure allows identification and measurements of blood velocity in the renal arteries, measurements of the renal parenchymal velocities from the upper, middle, and lower poles of the kidneys, and renal size. The presence of an asymmetric kidney size may be a clue to underlying renal artery stenosis and renal ischemia.

The important Duplex ultrasonography parameter is the ratio of velocity in the renal artery to that of the aorta. A ratio >3.5 may indicate a stenosis >60% (56). If the renal artery velocity is >180 cm/s, this is also considered abnormal. The test is limited by the experience of the operator and is more difficult in obese patients; bowel gas also makes the test more difficult. Thus, Doppler ultrasonography of the kidneys is best performed in the early morning after fasting. Reported sensitivity and specificity range from 90% to 95% and 60% to 90%, respectively (56). Doppler ultrasonography may be useful in predicting

which patients would benefit from revascularization (57). A renal resistive index [RRI = 1 − (end-diastolic velocity/maximal systolic velocity) × 100] > 80 identified patients with renal artery stenosis in whom angioplasty or surgery did not improve blood pressure or renal function (57).

4. Captopril-Augmented Nuclear Renography

Captopril-Augmented Nuclear Renography (also known as ACE-inhibitor augmented scintigraphy) is performed with radioactive agents that are excreted either by glomerular filtration (99Tc-DPTA) or by mainly tubular secretion combined with glomerular filtration (99Tc-MAG3). This latter agent gives a good representation of renal blood flow. ACE inhibitors and diuretics should be discontinued for at least 48 h before the test. During the test, blood pressure must be closely monitored because systolic blood pressures <100 mmHg or mean arterial pressures <70 mmHg can invalidate the test. Both scintigraphic images and time-activity curves are measured after the injection of the tracer. Captopril is used to augment the sensitivity of the scan. Normally, there is a rapid uptake, followed by excretion of the tracer. However, in the presence of renal artery stenosis and captopril, there is delayed uptake and excretion. Studies have documented a sensitivity of ~83% and a specificity of 93% for detecting renal artery stenosis >70% (57). Perhaps, more importantly, the renogram had 93% sensitivity and 100% specificity for predicting blood pressure response to revascularization if the kidney function was normal (58). The sensitivity and specificity of renograms decline considerably in renal impairment. Unfortunately, ACE-inhibitor augmented scintigraphy, like all functional tests for renovascular hypertension, loses its accuracy in the setting of bilateral disease and renal insufficiency.

5. Magnetic Resonance Angiography

This relatively new magnetic resonance angiography technique shows great promise for the diagnosis of proximal atherosclerotic renal artery stenosis. Gadolinium, which has a low degree of nephrotoxicity and can thus be utilized in patients with renal insufficiency, is used as a contrast agent. Various small trials have reported sensitivities ranging from 83% to 100% and specificities of 92–97% (59). In a meta-analysis (60) in which more than 4000 patients had conventional contrast angiography, both gadolinium-enhanced magnetic resonance angiography and computed tomographic angiography (CTA) (as described subsequently) performed significantly better than duplex ultrasonography, ACE-inhibitor augmented scintigraphy, or the plasma renin captopril test for diagnosing. However, among patients with fibromuscular dysplasia accuracy was reported to be lower. Therefore, magnetic resonance angiography is not an ideal test for patients with suspected fibromuscular dysplasia. Other limitations of this method include the high cost, limited availability, and substantial expertise needed to analyze images. Besides, because this technique requires breath holding, it may be difficult for patients with significant cardiac or pulmonary disease to cooperate and claustrophobia may create a problem. In addition, magnetic resonance angiography is contraindicated in patients with pacemakers, cerebral aneurysm clips, or intraocular metal.

Low false-negative rate in determining global renal ischemia (bilateral renal artery stenosis or renal artery stenosis in the main renal artery to a single kidney) is perhaps the most striking aspect of magnetic resonance angiography. A patient with renal dysfunction, who has normal main renal arteries on magnetic resonance angiography, is unlikely to have significant ischemic nephropathy.

6. Computed Tomographic Angiography

CTA (also referred to as "helical" or "spiral" CT) has emerged as a promising new technique for the identification of patients with renal artery stenosis (RAS). It allows for high-resolution images. When compared with conventional contrast angiography, CTA has been found to have excellent sensitivity (up to 100%) and specificity (98%) for detecting a $>50\%$ main renal artery lesion (61). However, when accessory renal arteries are included in these analyses, sensitivities can fall dramatically.

The principal disadvantage of CTA is the necessity to administer significant amounts of potentially nephrotoxic intravenous iodinated contrast. For this reason, CTA is not optimal for patients with renal insufficiency. In addition, like Duplex ultrasonography and magnetic resonance angiography, CTA currently may not successfully image accessory renal arteries and the distal renal artery. Although accessory renal arteries can often be identified, the extent of disease in these vessels is difficult to assess.

7. Renal Arteriography

This standard diagnostic test has long been considered to be the gold standard in the diagnosis of renovascular hypertension. It has the advantage of allowing for therapeutic intervention at the time of diagnosis. Advantages of contrast angiography include excellent resolution, high accuracy, and the ability to simultaneously measure a pressure gradient across the lesion. In addition, with new digital-subtraction techniques, small volumes of ionic-contrast or gadolinium–carbon dioxide contrast can be used to minimize the risk of contrast nephropathy. However, conventional contrast angiography is invasive, expensive, and associated with a risk of complications. The possible complications include pseudoaneurysm, hematoma, contrast-induced nephropathy, cholesterol

embolization, and anaphylaxis. These risks increase in the presence of diffuse atherosclerosis, severe hypertension, and renal insufficiency all of which may be seen in a patient with suspected atherosclerotic renovascular disease. In high-risk patients, carbon dioxide and gadolinium have been reported to confer less risk of nephrotoxicity than traditional iodinized contrast agents do; however, their use decreases diagnostic resolution.

The greatest limitation of conventional contrast angiography is that while it can detect the anatomic presence of renin–angiotensin system, it does not necessarily provide data with regard to its physiologic, hemodynamic, or clinical significance. Despite these limitations, if the index of suspicion is high, the patient is at relatively low risk, and the results of noninvasive testing would not effectively exclude the possibility of renin–angiotensin system, it may be appropriate to proceed directly to conventional contrast angiography in selected patients.

E. Management of Renovascular Hypertension

The goals of therapy of renovascular hypertension are: effective control of blood pressure and preservation of renal function. Three choices are available for the treatment of renovascular hypertension: medical therapy, percutaneous interventions with or without stenting, and surgical revascularization.

Generally, in patients with fibromuscular disease, the results of surgery and percutaneous approaches appear to be superior. In patients with atherosclerotic disease, the data is less consistent and it appears from some trials that a substantial number of patients can achieve reasonable blood pressure control with medication alone. In the Scottish and Newcastle trial (62), subjects with unilateral renal artery stenosis had no difference in follow-up blood pressure between the medical and PTRA group at either 6 months or the last follow-up. In patients with bilateral disease, there was no difference between groups at 6 months, but an advantage to PTRA at the last follow-up.

In the Essai Multicentrique vs. Angioplastie (EMMA) study, although the angioplasty group required fewer antihypertensive medication on average (63), there was no significant difference in 24 h ambulatory blood pressure after 6 months. Complications were three times more common in the angioplasty group, but early termination due to refractory hypertension was required in seven medically treated patients. In the Dutch Renal Artery Stenosis Intervention Cooperative (DRASTIC) trial (64), the blood pressures were similar among those of the PTRA and medically managed group, although the PTRA subjects were taking significantly less medication. Nearly one-half of the medically managed patients crossed over to PTRA because of uncontrolled hypertension.

In general, percutaneous or surgical intervention for renal artery disease should be limited to patients with physiologic evidence of renovascular hypertension or ischemic nephropathy. It is also preferable to be able to predict whether the clinical manifestations (hypertension or renal dysfunction) are at least partially reversible. In summary, the appropriate management for individual patients with renovascular disease depends on the cause (fibromuscular disease or atherosclerosis) and the clinical presentation.

1. Surgical Revascularization

Surgical procedures include endarterectomy, aortorenal bypass, and extra-anatomic bypass (bypass from the celiac or mesenteric branches). Extra-anatomic bypasses are generally associated with fewer complications. Rates of perioperative mortality range from 1% to 6% and are usually higher with concurrent repair of aortic aneurysms. Other possible complications include bleeding, infection, myocardial infarction, stroke, atheroembolic disease, and acute renal failure.

Most studies of surgical revascularization have shown excellent short- and long-term patency, ~85–95% at 5 years (65). Surgical revascularization has been shown to result in clinical improvement in hypertension and in preservation of renal function. However, due to the associated significant morbidity and mortality, and perhaps, most importantly, patient discomfort, surgical intervention is usually reserved either for patients with concomitant aortic aneurysms requiring repair or complex lesions that are not amenable to percutaneous transluminal revascularization and stenting. Surgical revascularization should also be considered in patients who have failed previous percutaneous procedures.

2. PTRA and Stenting

Numerous publications reported the safety and efficacy of PTRA. Patients with fibromuscular dysplasia usually show a substantial clinical and anatomic responses to PTRA. Due to the high rate of cure and the relatively low risk of complications in these patients (who are less likely to develop atheroembolic disease or acute renal failure), PTRA is generally considered to be the initial procedure of choice for patients with fibromuscular dysplasia. However, reported technical success rates with PTRA in atheromatous renal artery stenosis are >70%, clinical improvement is rare. Most atheromatous renal artery stenosis is due to aortic plaques on the ostium of the renal artery. Angioplasty is less than ideal in this situation because of the elastic recoil of the aortic plaques. To overcome this obstacle, endoluminal stent deployment was developed. Renal artery stenting has been shown to achieve better long-term patency of the atherosclerotic

renal artery. Reported technical success rates are usually >90%. Although there are very few clinical trials directly comparing stenting to PTRA alone, the reported blood pressure responses with stenting are generally better. However, although there are excellent assisted-patency and immediate clinical benefits for most patients, as demonstrated by improved control of hypertension and preservation of renal function, the benefit is not maintained within the 5-year follow-up (66).

The current indications for stenting include: poor angiographic response to routine PTRA, early restenosis after PTRA, and renal artery dissection during PTRA.

F. Potential Complications of PTRA and Stenting

Complications occur in ~10–20% of patients. The complications have been divided into those that involve the puncture site (hematoma or pseudoaneurysm), the renal artery (dissection, thrombosis, bleeding), and systemic complications (e.g., atheroembolism, myocardial infarction, acute renal failure, infection). Patients with atherosclerosis are more likely to have complications than those with fibromuscular disease. The presence of extensive aortic atherosclerosis, significant cardiovascular disease, and chronic renal failure can also lead to increased risk.

G. Medical Management of Renovascular Hypertension

Before the use of ACE inhibitors and ARBs, effective control of blood pressure of patients with renovascular disease was difficult to achieve. In 74% of 188 hypertensive subjects, captopril was effective to control of blood pressure, with no improvement in only 5%. (67). In patients with unilateral renal artery stenosis or other forms of moderate renal artery disease, ACE inhibitors may be effectively used either alone or combined with other antihypertensive agents, particularly diuretics.

In patients with high-grade bilateral renal artery stenosis or stenosis of a solitary kidney, ACE inhibitor therapy should be used with caution. Acute renal failure may appear because of a decrease in blood flow to the kidney beyond the stenosis. It is reversible with discontinuation of the agent. However, there is the potential risk of developing irreversible damage in the affected kidney. ACE inhibition may hasten renal atrophy and fibrosis in the ischemic kidney. These risks must be weighed against the potential long-term benefits of renin–angiotensin system blockade among patients with known atherosclerotic disease.

Calcium antagonists also are quite effective in lowering blood pressure and inducing the overall impairment of renal function in renovascular hypertension. Calcium antagonists maintain renal blood flow and function because of their preferential preglomerular (afferent arteriolar) vasodilatory effect.

The choice of an optimal treatment for renovascular disease includes a careful risk-benefit analysis in each patient, considering not only the patient's blood pressure control and renal function but also an assessment of the patient's overall mortality risk and the potential for morbidity from invasive procedures. In patients with fibromuscular disease and in many patients with uncomplicated atherosclerotic renovascular hypertension, it is usually reasonable to proceed directly to revascularization. Patients at high risk for occlusion, including those with rapidly progressive disease or >95% stenosis, may be good candidates for intervention. In patients with fibromuscular disease and nonostial atherosclerotic disease, an attempt at routine PTRA is appropriate. For patients with ostial lesions or who have a poor response to initial PTRA, stent placement should be considered. Surgical revascularization is usually reserved for those patients who have failed percutaneous attempts, have complicated anatomy, or concomitant aortic aneurysms.

Medical management remains an important adjunct in patients who have undergone either surgical or percutaneous revascularization. In patients with atherosclerotic disease where the likelihood of success is less and the risk of complications is greater, it is reasonable to proceed with medical management. It is essential to carefully monitor for disease progression with serial serum creatinine and renal ultrasound in medically managed patients. In those patients whose blood pressure cannot be adequately controlled or who exhibit progression of clinical renal disease despite aggressive medical management, PTRA with stent placement should be reconsidered (67). In patients with atherosclerotic disease, aggressive medical management requires not only just blood pressure medications, but also antiplatelet agents, lipid-lowering therapy, and smoking cessation. The most common cause of death among patients with atherosclerotic renovascular disease is cardiovascular disease.

VII. CARDIOVASCULAR DISEASE ASSOCIATED TO CHRONIC KIDNEY DISEASE

During the past few years, increasing evidence has shown that chronic kidney disease, whether manifested by elevated serum creatinine, albuminuria, or reduced glomerular filtration rate, is associated with a high risk of cardiovascular disease, independently of its origin. A statement from the councils on Kidney in Cardiovascular Disease, High Blood Pressure Research, Clinical Cardiology and Epidemiology, and Prevention of the American Heart Association (43) has recently summarized the evidence for kidney disease as a risk factor for the development of cardiovascular disease and recommended that patients with chronic kidney disease be considered as memebers of the "highest risk group" for subsequent cardiovascular disease events. As reviewed by Coresh et al. (68), several prospective studies reported the strong association between chronic kidney disease and cardiovascular disease. Data from over 15,000 adults 45–65-year-old at baseline and followed for 5 years in the Atherosclerosis Risk in Communities study showed that reduced kidney function is an independent risk factor for both *de novo* and recurrent cardiovascular disease.

In the Cardiovascular Health Study, elevated serum creatinine level (at least 1.5 mg/dL in men and 1.3 mg/dL in women) was associated with an approximately twofold higher risk of overall and cardiovascular disease mortality. After adjustment for cardiovascular risk factors and subclinical disease measures, elevated serum creatinine remained an independent risk factor for these outcomes as well as those for total cardiovascular disease, congestive heart failure, and claudication. In the Coronary Prevention Project, 1 year mortality after a myocardial infarction increased from 24% to 46% and 66% among patients with serum creatinine <1.5 mg/dL, 1.5–2.4 mg/dL, and 2.5–3.9 mg/dL, respectively. After adjustment for patient and treatment characteristics, elevated serum creatinine was independently associated with a substantially elevated risk of death during the first month following a myocardial infarction.

The predictive capacity of small increases in serum creatinine has been confirmed by the data of the Intervention as a Goal in Hypertension Treatment study (INSIGHT), SYST-EUR study, Systolic Hypertension in China (SYST-China), and SHEP study. In fact, the capacity of serum creatinine was comparable to that of other well established risk factors like diabetes or a previous myocardial infarction in the HOT study. A negative correlation between risk of cardiovascular disease and glomerular filtration rates was reported both in middle aged and in elderly cohorts even after adjustment for a large number of risk factors. Even mildly reduced kidney function (60–89 mL/min per 1.73 m^2) was associated with an increased risk of cardiovascular disease. On the other hand, albuminuria, even at low levels predicted cardiovascular risk among 40,548 adults from Groningen in the Netherlands. Similar findings were reported in the HOPE study.

Mild degrees of renal failure have been shown to be associated to a series of risk factors or markers that are summarized in Table 45.8. Gender differences have been shown to exist in the association between cardiovascular

Table 45.8 Cardiovascular Risk Factors or Markers Associated with a Mild Decrease in Estimated Glomerular Filtration Rate

Disturbed lipoprotein (a) concentrations
Insulin resistance and impaired glucose tolerance
Increased oxidative stress
Increment in pulse wave velocity
Increased serum uric acid levels
Sympathetic overactivity
Accumulation of asymmetric dimethiylarginine
Inflammatory and procoagulant biomarkers (C-reactive protein, fibrinogen, interleukin 6, factor VIIc, factor VIIIc, plasmin–antiplasmin complex, and D-dimmer)
Obesity and body fat distribution
Nondipping pattern of ambulatory blood pressure

risk factors and albuminuria. At higher ages, body mass index and plasma glucose, men are prone to a more elevated urinary albumin excretion than women. Available data points to the association between chronic kidney disease in hypertensive patients and the components of the metabolic syndrome (Fig. 45.1). The presence of minor abnormalities of renal function is mostly related to the presence of metabolic alterations of glucose, together with blood pressure levels among young hypertensive patients with metabolic syndrome (69).

Simultaneous correction or prevention of renal and cardiovascular damages are required. Life-style changes, with particular relevance of diminishing salt intake, avoiding obesity, and refraining from smoking are very important. Treatment of dyslipidemia with statins are consistent with a similar benefit among chronic kidney disease patients to that seen in other populations. A number of clinical trials have been initiated to test therapies for cardiovascular disease risk reduction in chronic kidney disease. These have focused on dyslipidemia, hyperhomocysteinemia, hypertension, and anemia.

Strict blood pressure control (probably <125/75 mmHg) is required. A combination of drugs is needed in most cases. ACE inhibitors and ARBs should be included because they have been shown to improve the long-term renal outcome of patients with nephrosclerosis. Furthermore, dual blockade of the renin–angiotensin system with both an ACE inhibitor and an angiotensin II receptor blocker has been shown to safely retard the progression of nondiabetic renal disease compared with either drug alone (70).

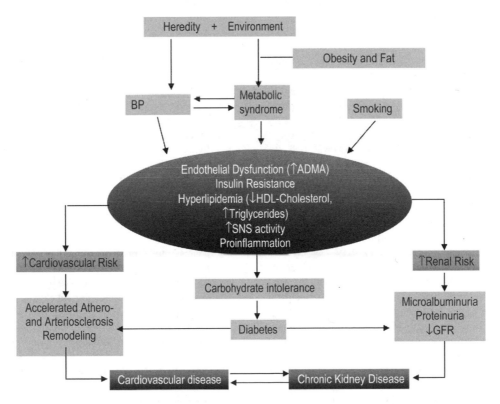

Figure 45.1 Chronic kidney disease, hypertension, and the components of the metabolic syndrome. ADMA, Asymmetric dimethylarginine; BP, Blood pressure; GFR, Glomerular filtration rate; HDL, High-density lipoprotein cholesterol; SNS, Sympathetic nervous system.

VIII. CONCLUSIONS

During the past years, increasing evidence has shown that chronic kidney disease, whether manifest by albuminuria or reduced glomerular filtration rate, is associated with a high risk of cardiovascular disease. Although much of the high risk of cardiovascular disease in chronic kidney disease is the result of elevations in traditional cardiovascular disease risk factors, in several large studies have shown that an independent contribution of chronic kidney disease to cardiovascular disease risk also exists. There may be exceptions, but therapies that have been beneficial at normal levels of kidney function are increasingly being shown beneficial at lower levels of kidney function.

REFERENCES

1. Brown MA, Whitworth JA. Hypertension in human renal disease. J Hypertens 1992; 10:701–712.
2. Lazarus JM, Bougorignie JJ, Buckalew VM, Greene T, Levey AS, Milas NC, Paranandi L, Peterson JC, Porush JG, Rauch S, Soucie JM, Stollar C. Achievement and safety of a low blood pressure goal in chronic renal disease. The Modification of Diet in Renal Disease Study Group. Hypertension 1997; 29:641–650.
3. Blum M, Yachnin T, Wollman Y, Chernihovsky T, Peer G; Grosskopf I, Kaplan E, Silverberg D, Cabili S, Iaina A. Low nitric oxide production in patients with chronic renal failure. Nephron 1998; 79:265–268.
4. Kielstein JT, Bode-Boger SM, Frolich JC, Haller H, Boger RH. Relationship of asymmetric dimethylarginine to dialysis treatment and atherosclerotic disease. Kidney Int 2001; 78:S9–S13.
5. Kielstein JT, Boger RH, Bode-Boger SM, Frolich JC, Haller H, Ritz E, Fliser D. Marked increase of asymmetric dimethylarginine in patients with incipient primary chronic renal disease. J Am Soc Nephrol 2002; 13:170–176.
6. Siems W, Quast S, Carluccio F, Wiswedel I, Hirsch D, Augustin W, Hampi H, Riehle M, Sommerburg O. Oxidative stress in chronic renal failure as a cardiovascular risk factor. Clin Nephrol 2002; 58:S12–S19.
7. Fliser D, Pacini G, Engelleiter R, Kautzky-Willer A, Prager R, Franek E, Ritz E. Insulin resistance and hyperinsulinemia are already present in patients with incipient renal disease. Kidney Int 1998; 53:1343–1347.
8. Segura J, Campo C, Ruilope LM. Proteinuria: an underappreciated risk factor in cardiovascular disease. Curr Cardiol Rep 2002; 4:458–462.
9. Ruggenenti P, Perna A, Remuzzi G, GISEN Group Invesitigators. Retarding progression of chronic renal disease: the neglected issue of residual proteinuria. Kidney Int 2003; 63:2254–2261.
10. Ruilope LM, Campo C, Rodicio JL. Blood pressure control, proteinuria and renal outcome in chronic renal failure. Curr Opin Nephrol Hypertens 1998; 7:145–148.
11. Kocks MJ, de Zeeuw D, Navis GJ. Optimal blood pressure control and antihypertensive regimens in hypertensive renal disease: the potential of exploring the mechanisms of response variability. Curr Opin Nephrol Hypertens 2002; 11:135–140.
12. Epstein M. Aldosterone and the hypertensive kidney: its emerging role as a mediator of progressive renal dysfunction: A paradigm shift. J Hypertens 2001; 19:829–842.
13. Ruilope LM, Miranda B, Oliet A, Millet VG, Rodicio JL, Romero JC, Raij L. Control of hypertension with the angiotensin converting enzyme inhibitor captopril reduces glomerular proteinuria. J Hypertens Suppl 1988; 6:S467–S469.
14. Segura J, Campo C, Rodicio JL, Ruilope LM. ACE inhibitors and appearance of renal events in hypertensive nephrosclerosis. Hypertension 2001; 38:645–649.
15. Ruggenenti P, Perna A, Gherardi G, Benini R, Remuzzi G. Chronic proteinuric nephropathies: outcomes and response to treatment in a prospective cohort of 352 patients with different patterns of renal injury. Am J Kidney Dis 2000; 35:1155–1165.
16. Ruggenenti P, Perna A, Zoccali, Gherardi G, Benini R, Testa A, Remuzzi G. Chronic proteinuric nephropathies. II. Outcomes and response to treatment in a prospective cohort of 352 patients: differences between women and men in relation to the ACE gene polymorphism. Gruppo Italiano di Studi Epidemologici in Nefrologia (Gisen). J Am Soc Nephrol 2000; 11:88–96.
17. Iino Y, Hayashi M, Kawamura T, Shiigai T, Tomino Y, Yamada K, Kitajima T, Ideura T, Koyama A, Sugisaki T, Suzuki H, Umemura S, Kawaguchi Y, Uchida S, Kuwahara M, Yamazaki T. Japanese Lasartan Therapy Intended for the Global Renal Protection in Hypertensive Patients (JLIGHT) Study Investigators. Interim evidence of the renoprotective effect of the angiotensin II receptor antagonist losartan versus the calcium channel blocker amlodipine in patients with chronic kidney disease and hypertension: a report of the Japanese Losartan Therapy Intended for Global Renal Protection in Hypertensive Patients (JLIGHT) Study. Clin Exp Nephrol 2003; 7:221–230.
18. Ruilope LM, Aldigier JC, Ponticelli C, Oddou-Stock P, Botteri F, Mann JF. Safety of the combination of valsartan and benazepril in patients with chronic renal disease. European Group for the Investigation of Valsartan in Chronic Renal Disease. J Hypertens 2000; 18:89–95.
19. Laverman GD, Remuzzi G, Ruggenenti P. ACE Inhibition versus angiotensin receptor blockade: which is better for renal and cardiovascular protection? J Am Soc Nephrol 2004; 15:S64–S70.
20. Ruggenenti P, Perna A, Benini R, Remuzzi G. Effects of dihydropyridine calcium channel blockers, angiotensin-converting enzyme inhibition, and blood pressure control on chronic, nondiabetic nephropathies. Gruppo Italiano di Studi Epidemiologici in Nefrologia (GISEN). J Am Soc Nephrol 1998; 9:2096–2101.
21. Arauz-Pacheco C, Parrott MA, Raskin P. The treatment of hypertension in adult patients with diabetes. Diabetes Care 2002; 25:134–147.

22. Nelson RG, Bennett PH, Beck GJ, Tan M, Knowler WC, Mitch WE, Hirschman GH, Myers BD. Development and progression of renal disease in Pima Indians with non-insulin-dependent diabetes mellitus. N Engl J Med 1996; 335:1636–1642.

23. O'Haare JA, Ferris JB, Brady D, Twomey B, O'Sullivan DJ. Exchangeable sodium and renin in hypertensive diabetic patients with and without nephropathy. Hypertension 1985; 7:S43–S48.

24. Chobanian AV, Bakris GL, Black HR, Cushman WC, Green LA, Izzo JL Jr, Jones DW, Materson BJ, Oparil S, Wright JT Jr, Roccella EJ; the National High Blood Pressure Education Program Coordinating Committee. Seventh Report of the Joint National Committee on Prevention, Detection, Evaluation, and Treatment of High Blood Pressure. Diabetes and Hypertension. Hypertension 2003; 42:1206–1252.

25. UK Prospective Diabetes Study Group: Tight blood pressure control and risk of macrovascular and microvascular complications in type 2 diabetes: UKPDS 38. Br Med J 1998; 317:703–713.

26. Lewis EJ, Hunsicker LG, Bain RP, Rohde RE. The effect of angiotensin-converting enzyme inhibition on diabetic nephropathy. N Engl J Med 1993; 329:1456–1462.

27. Marre M, Chatellier G, LeBlanc II, Guyene TT, Menard J, Passa P. Prevention of diabetic nephropathy with enalapril in normotensive diabetics with microalbuminuria. Br Med J 1998; 297:1092–1095.

28. The ACE Inhibitors in Diabetic Nephropathy Trialist Group: Should all patients with type 1 diabetes mellitus and microalbuminuria receive angiotensin-converting enzyme inhibitors? A meta-analysis of individual patient data. Ann Intern Med 2001; 134:370–379.

29. Hamilton RA, Kane MP, Demers J. Angiotensin-converting enzyme inhibitors and type 2 diabetic nephropathy: a meta-analysis. Pharmacotherapy 2003; 23:909–915.

30. ACEI Inhibitors In Diabetic Nephropathy Trialist Group. Should all patients with type 1 diabetes mellitus and microalbuminuria receive angiotensin-converting enzyme inhibitors? A meta-analysis of individual patient data. Ann Intern Med 2001; 134:370–379.

31. MacKay JH, Areuri KE, Goldberg AI, Snapinn SM, Sweet CS. Losartan and low-dose hydrochlorothiazide in patients with essential hypertension: a double-blind, placebo-controlled trial of concomitant administration compared with individual components. Arch Intern Med 1996; 156:278–285.

32. Ruilope LM, Simpson RL, Toh J, Arcuri KE, Goldberg AL, Sweet CS. Controlled trial of losartan gives concomitantly with different doses of hydrochlorothiazide in hypertensive patients. Blood Press 1996; 5:32–40.

33. Andersen S, Tarnow L, Rossing P, Hansen BV, Parving HH. Renoprotective effects of angiotensin II receptor blockade in type 1 diabetic patients with diabetic nephropathy. Kidney Int 2000; 57:601–606.

34. Lacourcière Y, Bélanger A, Godin C, Hallé J-P, Ross S, Wright N, Marion J. Long-term comparison of losartan and enalapril on kidney function in hypertensive type 2 diabetics with early nephropathy. Kidney Int 2000; 58:762–769.

35. Parving HH, Lehnert H, Brochner-Mortensen J, Gomis R, Andersen S, Arner P. The effect of irbesartan on the development of diabetic nephropathy in patients with type 2 diabetes. N Engl J Med 2001; 345:870–878.

36. Lewis EJ, Hunsicker LG, Clarke WR, Berl T, Pohl MA, Lewis JB, Ritz E, Atkins RC, Rohde R, Raz I. Renoprotective effect of the angiotensin-receptor antagonist irbesartan in patients with nephropathy due to type 2 diabetes. N Engl J Med 2001; 345:851–860.

37. Brenner BM, Cooper ME, de Zeeuw D, Keane WF, Mitch WE, Parving HH, Remuzzi G, Snapinn SM, Zhang Z, Shahinfar S. Effects of losartan on renal and cardiovascular outcomes in patients with type 2 diabetes and nephropathy. N Engl J Med 2001; 345:861–869.

38. Sica DA, Bakris GL. Type 2 diabetes: RENAAL and IDNT—the emergence of new treatment options. J Clin Hypertens 2002; 4:52–57.

39. Jacobsen P, Andersen S, Rossing K, Jensen BR, Parving HH. Dual blockade of the renin–angiotensin system versus maximal recommended dose of ACE inhibition in diabetic nephropathy. Kidney Int 2003; 63:1874–1880.

40. Gaede P, Vedel P, Larsen N, Jensen GV, Parving HH, Pedersen O. Multifactorial intervention and cardiovascular disease in patients with type 2 diabetes. N Engl J Med 2003; 348:383–393.

41. Opelz G, Wujciaz T, Ritz E, for the Colloborative Transplant Study. Association of chronic kidney graft failure with recipient blood pressure. Kidney Int 1998; 53:217–222.

42. Remuzzi G, Perico N. Routine renin–angiotensin system blockade in renal transplantation? Curr Opin Nephrol Hypertens 2002; 11:1–10.

43. Sarnak MJ, Levey AS, Schoolwerth AC, Coresh J, Culleton B, Hamm LL, McCullough PA, Kasiske BL, Kelepouris E, Klag MJ, Parfrey P, Pfeffer M, Raij L, Spinosa DJ, Wilson PW. Kidney Disease as a Risk Factor for Development of Cardiovascular Disease. A Statement From the American Heart Association Councils on Kidney in Cardiovascular Disease, High Blood Pressure Research, Clinical Cardiology, and Epidemiology and Prevention. Hypertension 2003; 42:1050–1065.

44. Rodicio JL, Morales JM, Alcazar JM, Ruilope LM. Calcium antagonists and renal protection. J Hypertens Suppl 1993; 11:S49–S53.

45. Suwelack B, Gerhardt U, Hausberg M, Rahn KH, Hohage H Comparison of quinapril versus atenolol: effects on blood pressure and cardiac mass after renal transplantation. Am J Cardiol 2000; 86:583–584.

46. Chen-Huan Chen, Yao-Ping Lin, Wen-Chung Yu, Wu-Chang Yang, Yu-An Ding. Volume Status and Blood Pressure During Long-Term Hemodialysis. Role of Ventricular Stiffness. Hypertension 2003; 42:257–262.

47. De Lima JJG, Lopes HF, Grupi CJ, Abensur H, Giorgi MCP, Krieger EM, Pileggi P. Blood Pressure Influences the Occurrence of Complex Ventricular Arrhythmia in Hemodialysis Patients. Hypertension 1995; 26:1200–1203.

48. Michel JB. Renal artery obstruction: from experimental models to logical approach to diagnosis and treatment. Rev Prat 1996; 46:1077–1083.

49. Martinez-Maldonado M. Pathophysiology of renovascular hypertension. Hypertension 1991; 17:707–719.

50. Welch WJ. The pathophysiology of renin release in renovascular hypertension. Semin Nephrol 2000; 20:394–401.

51. Davis BA, Crook JE, Vestal RE, Oates JA. Prevalence of renovascular hypertension in patients with grade III or IV hypertensive retinopathy. N Engl J Med 1979; 301:1273–1276.

52. Hansen KJ, Edwards MS, Craven TE, Cherr GS, Jackson SA, Appel RG, Burke GL, Dean RH. Prevalence of renovascular disease in the elderly: a population based study. J Vasc Surg 2002; 36:443–451.

53. Sang CN, Whelton PK, Hamper UM, Connolly M, Kadir, White R, Sanders R, Liang KY, Bias W. Etiologic factors in renovascular fibromuscular dysplasia. a case-control study. Hypertension 1989; 14:472–479.

54. Turnbull JM. Is listening for abdominal bruits useful in the evaluation of hypertension? J Am Med Assoc 1995; 274:1299–1301.

55. Mann SJ, Pickering TG. Detection of renovascular hypertension. State of the art. Ann Intern Med 1992; 117:845–853.

56. Strandness DE Jr. Duplex imaging for the detection of renal artery stenosis. Am J Kidney Dis 1994; 24:674–678.

57. Radermacher J, Chavan A, Bleck J, Vitzthum A, Stoess B, Gebel MJ, Galanski M, Koch KM, Haller H. Use of doppler ultrasonography to predict the outcome of therapy for renal-artery stenosis. N Engl J Med 2001; 344:410–417.

58. Fommei E, Ghione S, Hilson AJ, Mezzasalma L, Oei HY, Piepsz A, Volterrani D. Captopril radionucleotide test in renovascular hypertension: a European multicentre study of the European Multicentre Study Group. Eur J Nucl Med 1993; 20:617–623.

59. Qanadli SD, Soulez G, Therasse E, Nicolet V, Turpin S, Froment D, Courteau M, Guertin MC, Oliva VL. Detection of renal artery stenosis: prospective comparison of captopril-enhanced Doppler sonography, captopril-enhanced scintigraphy, and MR angiography. AJR Am J Roentgenol 2001; 177:1123–1129.

60. Taylor A, Sheppard D, MacLeod MJ. Renal artery stent placement in renal artery stenosis: technical and early clinical results. Clin Radiol 1997; 52:451–457.

61. The Heart Outcomes Prevention Evaluation Study Investigators. Effects of an angiotensin-converting-enzyme inhibitor, ramipril, on cardiovascular events in high-risk patients. N Engl J Med 2000; 342:145–153.

62. Webster J, Marshall F, Abdalla M, Dominiczak A, Edwards R, Isles CG, Loose H, Main J, Padfield P, Russell IT, Walker B, Watson M, Wilkinson R. Randomized comparison of percutaneous angioplasty vs. continued medical therapy for hypertensive patients with atheromatous renal artery stenosis. J Hum Hypertens 1998; 12:329–335.

63. Plouin PF, Chatellier G, Darne B, Raynaud A. Blood pressure outcome of angioplasty in atherosclerotic renal artery stenosis: a randomized trial. Hypertension 1998; 31:823–829.

64. van Jaarsveld BC, Krijnen P, Pieterman H, Derkx FH, Deinum J, Postma CT, Dees A, Woittiez AJ, Bartelink AK, Man in 't Veld AJ, Schalekamp MA. The effect of balloon angioplasty on hypertension in atherosclerotic renal-artery stenosis. Dutch Renal Artery Stenosis Intervention Cooperative Study Group. N Engl J Med 2000; 342:1007–1014.

65. Bloch MJ. The Diagnosis and Management of Renovascular Disease: A Primary Care Perspective. Part II. Issues in Management. J Clin Hypertens 2003; 5:210–218.

66. Yutan E, Glickerman DJ, Caps MT, Hatsukami T, Harley JD, Kohler TR, Davies MG. Percutaneous transluminal revascularization for renal artery stenosis: Veterans Affairs Puget Sound Health Care System experience. J Vasc Surg 2001; 34:685–693.

67. Hollenberg NK. Medical therapy of renovascular hypertension: efficacy and safety of captopril in 269 patients. Cardiovasc Rev Rep 1983; 4:852–876.

68. Coresh J, Astor B, Sarnak M. Evidence for increased cardiovascular disease risk in patient with chronic kidney disease. Hypertension 2004; 13:73–81.

69. Segura J, Campo C, Roldan C, Christiansen H, Vigil L, García-Robles R, Rodicio JL, Ruilope LM. Hypertensive renal damge in metabolic syndrome is associated with glucose metabolism disturbances. J Am Soc Nephrol 2004; 15:S37-S42.

70. Nakao N, Yoshimura A, Morita H, Takada M, Kayano T, Ideura T. Combination treatment of angiotensin-II receptor blocker and angiotensin-converting-enzyme inhibitor in non-diabetic renal disease (COOPERATE): a randomized controlled trial. Lancet 2003; 361:117–124.

46

Endocrine Hypertension

LUKAS ZIMMERLI, BEAT MUELLER

University Hospital, Basel, Switzerland

KEYPOINTS

- In case of suspected endocrine disorder it is important to follow a stepwise diagnostic approach with special focus on clinical and laboratory clues.
- In the diagnostic process of endocrine hypertension biochemical diagnosis always precedes imaging studies.
- In daily clinical practice, hypertensive patients often are under treatment with different medications that may interfere with diagnostic tests.
- The most common causes of endocrine hypertension are excess production of mineralocorticoids, glucocorticoids, and catecholamines.
- Although endocrine hypertension is a rare form of secondary hypertension, a correct and timely diagnosis is important, in view of the available causal treatment and because of the potential harmful complications.

SUMMARY

Endocrine causes of hypertension are relatively rare, but their detection offers a real chance for cure. The combination of the patient's history, physical examination, astute observation, and accurate interpretation of laboratory tests may identify such patients. In practice, it is important to follow a stepwise diagnostic approach with special focus on clinical and laboratory clues, suggesting the possible presence of secondary hypertension.

Important physical findings suggestive for endocrine hypertension include the presence of a low to low-normal circulating serum potassium levels (suggestive of mineralocorticoid hypertension), a metabolic syndrome such as central obesity, striae, and bruising, osteoporosis (suggestive of Cushing syndrome); tremor, sweating, or rapid pulse (suggestive of hyperthyroidism or pheochromocytoma); or pallor and diaphoresis (suggestive of pheochromocytoma).

The most common causes of endocrine hypertension are excess production of mineralocorticoids, glucocorticoids, and catecholamines. The physio-pathological mechanisms of endocrine hypertension encompass hormonal excess secretion by a tumor or hyperplasia, respectively, deficiencies of key enzymes in hormonal synthesis and mutations altering receptor or ion channel function. Although many tests are available for biochemical testing, the diagnostic potential of many tests have not vigorously been examined prospectively in large-scale studies. One should be aware that some of the tests are appropriate for screening purposes, but not for confirming the diagnosis. Furthermore, treatment with different medications may interfere with these tests. As a general rule, in the diagnostic process of endocrine hypertension biochemical diagnosis always precedes imaging studies.

I. INTRODUCTION

Endocrine hypertension is a term assigned to states in which hormonal derangements result in clinically significant hypertension. Hypertension is a feature of a number of endocrine disorders, with the most common forms resulting from excess production of mineralocorticoids [i.e., primary hyperaldosteronism (PA)], glucocorticoids (Cushing's syndrome), and catecholamines (pheochromocytoma and other paragangliomas). Endocrine causes of hypertension are relatively rare (1–3%), although there is evidence that primary aldosteronism may be much more frequent than initially suspected (1). In view of the available causal treatment options and because of the potential harmful complications, a correct and timely diagnosis is important.

Because endocrine causes of hypertension are relatively rare, extensive testing for endocrine hypertension is primarily indicated, if history and physical examination suggest it or if adequate blood pressure control is not achieved (2,3). Taking a careful medical history and a step-wise approach remains mandatory for the differential diagnosis of endocrine hypertension. Secondary hypertension should be suspected in severe and resistant hypertension, ideally confirmed in a 24 h ambulatory blood pressure monitoring, despite appropriate three-drug regimen that

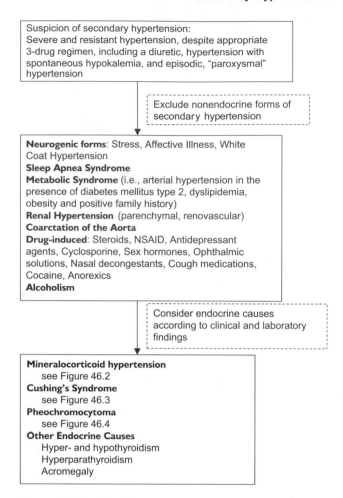

Figure 46.1 Algorithm for the diagnosis of endocrine hypertension. NSAID, nonsteroidal anti-inflammatory drug.

includes a diuretic, hypertension with spontaneous hypokalemia, and episodic, "paroxysmal" hypertension with sweating, tachycardia, and headaches. Thereafter, more frequent, nonendocrine causes of secondary hypertension should be excluded, namely stress factors including "white-coat hypertension," the metabolic syndrome (which can be part of Cushing's syndrome, however), obstructive sleep apnoea syndrome, vascular causes (i.e., renal artery stenosis, coarctation of the aorta), and medication and drugs with hypertensive side effects (e.g., nonsteroidal anti-inflammatory drugs, cycolosporin A, antidepressants, cocaine, and alcohol) (Fig. 46.1).

Important physical findings suggestive for endocrine hypertension include the presence of a metabolic syndrome including central obesity, striae rubrae, and bruising, osteoporosis (suggestive of Cushing syndrome); tremor, sweating, rapid pulse, or pallor and diaphoresis (suggestive of hyperthyroidism or pheochromocytoma).

The mechanisms of endocrine hypertension encompass hormonal excess secretion by a tumor or hyperplasia, respectively, deficiencies of key enzymes in hormonal synthesis and mutations altering receptor or ion channel function.

II. MINERALOCORTICOID HYPERTENSION

Mineralocorticoid hypertension, the most common form of endocrine hypertension, is due to an excess of mineralocorticoid action either by inappropriately high levels of aldosterone or compounds with mineralocorticoid action like deoxycorticosterone. This form of hypertension is caused by increased sodium and water retention by the kidney and by a consecutive expansion of the extracellular fluid compartment, which by feedback suppresses endogenous active plasma renin (aPR) concentrations. However, hypertension cannot solely be ascribed to the increased circulating volume but is also due to an increased peripheral vascular resistance.

Frequently, mineralocorticoid hypertension is associated with hypokalemia, either spontaneous or diuretic-induced and metabolic alkalosis. Evaluation for the presence is recommended under the following circumstances (4):

- Diuretic therapy results in serum potassium <3.0 mmol/L, even if levels normalize after diuretics are withdrawn.
- Oral potassium supplementation and/or potassium-sparing agents fail to maintain serum potassium levels of ≥3.5 mmol/L in a patient on diuretics.
- Serum potassium levels fail to normalize after 4 weeks off diuretics.
- Patients with refractory hypertension with no evidence for another secondary cause (as outlined earlier) and with serum potassium levels of <4 mmol/L in the absence of diuretics.

A. Primary Aldosteronism

The syndrome of PA was first described by Conn (5). It was characterized by salt-sensitive hypertension associated with hypokalemia, metabolic alkalosis, and suppressed renin secretion and an adrenal adenoma. Initially, primary aldosteronism was believed to be a rare form of hypertension with prevalence rates of 0.5–2.0% in unselected patients (6). Many of these studies relied on detection of hypokalemia and an adenoma in the adrenal cortex and underestimated true prevalence rates. Screening of normokalemic patients for an increased aldosterone: renin-ratio, also referred to as "low-renin hypertension," has resulted in the diagnosis of larger number of patients with primary aldosteronism with prevalence rates of 5–12% in selected patients (7,8). It is, however, disputed whether this functional dysregulation

in low-renin hypertension is indeed a relevant pathologic entity and should be treated specifically (9,10). Against a widespread use of spironolactone in patients with an increased aldosterone:renin-ratio, the relatively high rate of side effects can be raised. Possibly, the improved side effect profile of newer aldosterone antagonists (e.g., eplerenone) will change this view in the future.

In about two-thirds of the cases, PA is caused by the classically described aldosterone-producing adenoma (APA) of the adrenal gland (Conn's syndrome). In the remaining one-third in whom no adenoma can be found, bilateral adrenal hyperplasia is suspected. Extremely rare forms (<2%) are glucocorticoid-remediable aldosteronism or adrenal carcinomas.

The clinical features of PA are nondistinctive. Some patients are completely asymptomatic or have minimal symptoms. Most symptoms are related to hypokalemia or water and salt retention and include tiredness, muscle weakness, thirst, polyuria, and nycturia.

The optimal method for screening and establishing the differential diagnosis of PA is controversial. The determination of decreased serum potassium levels is considered to be a possible screening test for the disease (3). However, only ~80% of the patients have hypokalemia (<3.5 mmol/L) in an early phase, and some authorities maintain that hypokalemia may even be absent in severe cases (11,12). Conversely, a circulating potassium level of >4 mmol/L makes the diagnosis of PA extremely unlikely. The next step in evaluation is to document renal potassium wasting. A 24 h urinary potassium excretion >30 mmol in the presence of a serum potassium level of <3.5 mmol/L reflects inappropriate renal potassium wasting. Lower excretion rates suggest extrarenal loss caused by diarrhea, vomiting, or laxative abuse. Interpretation of the rate of potassium excretion requires attention to the patient's volume status and rate of sodium excretion. Low-sodium intake (<4–5 g sodium/day, U_{Na} <100 mmol/L) or hypovolemia can physiologically increase aldosterone levels and, thus, potassium excretion (13).

According to Bravo et al. (14), the single best test for identifying patients with PA is the measurement of 24 h urinary aldosterone excretion during salt loading. An aldosterone excretion rate >54 nmol/24 h keeping to a high-sodium diet (>4–5 g sodium/day) distinguishes most patients with PA from those with essential hypertension; sensitivity and specificity of the test are 96% and 93%, respectively (14).

In the sequential evaluation of a patient with suspected PA, the measurement of the aPR and aldosterone concentration follows. The diagnostic algorithm of PA became complicated recently, as renin activity became replaced by the measurement of the active renin concentrations (Fig. 46.2). Unfortunately, ratios of the aldosterone

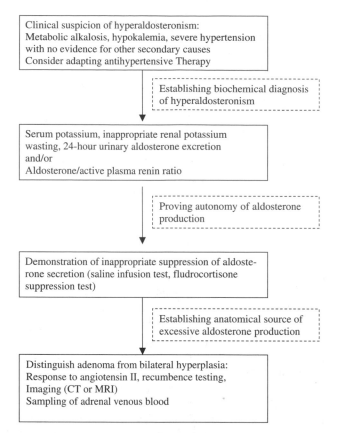

Figure 46.2 Algorithm for the diagnosis of hyperaldosteronism. CT, computed tomography; MRI, magnetic resonance imaging.

concentration to aPR are only in part comparable with the older aldosterone concentration:renin-acitivity ratio. Therefore, the establishment of local cut-offs must be achieved (15). The aPR is typically suppressed to <5 mU/L in patients with PA, but unfortunately it is also low in 25% of patients with essential, so-called "low-renin," hypertension. In the latter patients, a functional disturbance of the renin–angiotensin–aldosterone system is in debate. The simultaneous measurement of plasma aldosterone concentration (PAC) and the aPR permits calculation of the PAC:aPR-ratio in pmol/L:mU/L as a sensitive screening test for PA (16). The mean value for the ratio in patients with essential hypertension is <25 vs. >80 in most patients with primary aldosteronism. According to Weinberger the combination of a PAC/PRA ratio >30 and a PAC >550 pmol/L had sensitivity of 90% and specificity of 91% for PA (17). Measuring an ambulatory paired random PAC and aPR is preferably done in the morning (18). A number of drugs and hormones affect the renin–angiotensin–aldosterone axis. According to Seifarth et al. (19), β-blockers and aldosterone antagonists have the strongest impact on

the renin–angiotensin system. The decrease in active renin concentration by β-blockers leads to an increase in the PAC/aPR ratio, thus decreasing the specificity of the ratio. Patients taking spironolactone should have their medication withheld for 6 weeks prior to blood sampling, as the ratio and thereby sensitivity is decreased. Calcium channel blockers, and probably also ACE inhibitors and ARB alone or in combination, may be continued. Because hypokalemia reduces the biosynthesis of aldosterone, diagnostic studies should be performed in a potassium-repleted state to optimize sensitivity of the ratio.

For the diagnosis of PA, an elevated PAC/aPR ratio warrants confirmation by demonstrating inappropriate suppression of aldosterone secretion. This can be achieved by oral or intravenous sodium chloride challenge. At our institute, we perform the saline infusion test. Plasma aldosterone is measured in the morning after 2 h of upright posture, then 4 h after receiving 2 L of isotonic saline infusion in the supine position. The PAC will fall <170 pmol/L in normal subjects, whereas values >280 pmol/L are consistent with PA (20). Another very sensitive test to demonstrate the inability to suppress plasma aldosterone in PA is the 3 day or 4 day fludrocortisone suppression test (21). Fludrocortisone 0.1 mg qid or 0.2 mg twice a day is given along with supplement sodium chloride (200 mEq/d). Other authors have used a dose of 1 mg/day for 3 days (20). It is often necessary to supplement with potassium to prevent aggravation of hypokalemia. A PAC of >140 pmol/L after 3 days of fludrocortisone confirms the diagnosis (20).

After the biochemical diagnosis of PA has been established, a unilateral adenoma or rarely carcinoma must be distinguished from bilateral hyperplasia. Distinction between adenomas and hyperplasia is crucial because the surgical removal of a unilateral adrenal adenoma results in cure of PA and normalization of hypertension as well as reversal of the biochemical defects in the majority of patients. Importantly, a nonfunctional incidentaloma can be found in 1–5% of patients with hypertension. A functional adenoma can be distinguished from bilateral zona glomerulosa hyperplasia by a variety of tests and techniques. Clinical and laboratory features of classic APA (ACTH-responsive) are typically more severe and can be further differentiated by the aldosterone response to stimulation by angiotensin II or maintaining an upright posture for 2–4 h in the morning. Simultaneous measurement of plasma aldosterone and cortisol is a key requirement in the evaluation of the results of the postural test. In the classical APA, markedly elevated plasma aldosterone levels (recumbent typically >700 nmol/L) declines upon rise, whereas PACs increase typically in patients with idiopathic hyperaldosteronism (IHA). Unfortunately, ~20% of patients with aldosteronoma are responsive to angiotensin II and, thus, plasma aldosterone increase upon rising. Some adjunctive tests can assist in the differential diagnosis. 18-Hydroxycorticosterone is markedly elevated in classic APA. Excretion of 18-hydroxycortisol and 18-oxocortisol may also be elevated in classical ACTH-responsive APA, but these corticosteroids are not elevated in patients with angiotensin II-responsive APA. These corticosteroids are of limited clinical relevance because they are available only in a few centers worldwide. The differentiation between angiotensin II-responsive APA and IHA is more difficult and requires imaging procedures and eventually bilateral adrenal vein catheterization (discussed subsequently) (22).

Imaging should be performed only after establishing the biochemical diagnosis of aldosteronism due to the prevalence of functionally inactive "incidentalomas" in up to 5% of the population. Both high resolution computed tomography (CT) and magnetic resonance imaging (MRI) scanning are the radiological procedures of choice and can detect adrenal mass >5 mm but cannot distinguish between nonfunctional adenoma and an APA. The finding of an adrenal mass >3–5 cm in diameter should raise the possibility that the patient has adrenal carcinoma. An abnormality in both glands suggests adrenal hyperplasia.

Sampling of adrenal venous blood, preferably with corticotropin stimulation, for measurement of aldosterone and cortisol response is invasive but is considered the gold standard test for diagnosis of APA. This procedure requires considerable skill and experience and carries a risk of adrenal hemorrhage. Nuclear scanning with [131]I-6β-idiomethyl-19-norcholesterol in dexamethasone-suppressed patients is helpful when bilateral zona glomerulosa hyperplasia is suspected and CT scan does not detect an adenoma.

If an adenoma is found, laparoscopic adrenalectomy should be performed (23). Patients undergoing surgery should receive drug treatment both to decrease blood pressure and to correct metabolic abnormalities. Spironolactone for 3–4 weeks before surgery may be useful to minimize postoperative hypoaldosteronism and to restore potassium levels in the body to normal. The blood pressure response to spironolactone before surgery can be a predictor of surgical outcome in patients with aldosteronoma. The patient's age at the time of surgery and the duration of the preoperative elevated blood pressure strongly influence the outcome of surgical therapy. Patients aged 50 years or younger with a duration of hypertension of less than 5 years are more likely to become normotensive after adrenalectomy (24). Conversely, a lack of response to spironolactone prior to surgery should provoke second thoughts on the true diagnosis of the hypertension. Long-term medical therapy is indicated in patients with IHA, in those with adenoma who are poor surgical risks, and in those with bilateral adrenal adenomas. Spironolactone

has been the mainstay of medical treatment for many years with dosages varying from 25 to 400 mg/day. Spironolactone is often associated with considerable side effects like gastrointestinal symptoms, fatigue, and gynecomastia. In these cases, the new drug eplerenone should be instituted (50–100 mg/day). The aldosterone receptor antagonists can be used in combination with other antihypertensive agents.

B.　Glucocorticoid-Remediable Hyperaldosteronism

An extremely rare form of hyperaldosteronism is the glucocorticoid-remediable hyperaldosteronism (GRA), inherited in an autosomal dominant trait (25). The cause is a mutation on chromosome 8q24.3, inducing a chimeric gene caused by unequal crossover between the gene coding for the enzyme 11-β-hydroxylase and that for aldosterone synthase. Because of this hybrid gene, the enzyme aldosterone synthase becomes expressed in the zona fasciculata and, thus, under control of ACTH. Consequently, aldosteronism and thus the hypertension can be treated with low doses of a glucocorticoid (e.g., 0.5 mg of dexamethasone daily).

Young hypertensive patients, especially with and without a family history of hypertension, should be tested for glucocorticoid-remediable aldosteronism. Increase or suppression of aldosterone concentrations after ACTH or dexamethasone-testing, respectively, is highly sensitive and specific (26). The genetic mutation can be identified by polymerase chain reaction and sequencing.

C.　Pseudo-Hyperaldosteronism

In the following syndromes that cause mineralocorticoid hypertension, plasma aldosterone and plasma renin are indeed suppressed, yet, they resemble PA in that they also have hypertension and a hypokalemic alkalosis.

1.　HSD Deficiency ("Apparent Mineralocortocoid Excess Syndrome")

Deficiency of the 11-β-hydroxysteroiddehydrogenase (11-β-HSD) causes inhibition of the intrarenal conversion from cortisol to cortisone. In this form of low-renin, low-aldosterone hypertension, the glucocorticoid cortisol acts as a potent mineralocorticoid. This syndrome is inherited as an autosomal recessive trait and most heterozygotes have a normal phenotype (27). A specific cause of acquired 11-β-HSD deficiency is licorice abuse. In these patients, an increase in the ratio of cortisol to cortisone metabolites in their urine (ratio of tetrahydrocortisol to tetrahydrocortisone) can be used to make the diagnosis.

2. *Desoxycorticosterone Excess*

11-β-Hydroxylase and 17α-hydroxylase deficiency are forms of congenital adrenal hyperplasia in which mineralocorticoid excess occurs because of ACTH-driven desoxycorticosterone excess. Especially, female patients with these syndromes also show abnormalities in sexual development.

3. *Primary Cortisol Resistance*

This rare syndrome is inherited as an autosomal recessive or dominant disorder characterized by mutations in the glucocorticoid receptor gene, leading to diminished cortisol action and secondary stimulation of ACTH release (28).

4. *Liddle's Syndrome*

First described by Liddle in 1963, this syndrome is inherited as an autosomal dominant trait in which there is a primary increase in collecting tubule sodium reabsorption and, in most cases, potassium secretion (29,30). So-called "gain of function" mutations in the genes coding for the β-subunit or γ-subunit of the renal epithelial sodium channel, located at chromosome 16p13, lead to constitutive activation of renal sodium resorption and subsequent volume expansion (31). None of the known mineralocorticoids was found to be present in increased amounts, and, more important, neither treatment with spironolactone nor inhibitors of adrenal biosynthesis ameliorates this disorder. It responds well to inhibitors of epithelial sodium transport such as triamterene.

D. Secondary Aldosteronism

This term refers to an appropriately increased production of aldosterone in response to activation of the renin–angiotensin system. It usually occurs in association with the accelerated phase of hypertension or on the basis of an underlying edema disorder. In hypertensive states, this disorder is due either to a primary overproduction of renin or to an overproduction of renin secondary to a decrease in renal blood flow and/or perfusion pressure. Secondary aldosteronism is characterized by hypokalemic alkalosis, increases in plasma renin activity, and increases in aldosterone levels. In some conditions, such as edema disorders, this represents a partially beneficial response to restore volume and sodium at the expense of hypokalemia. Secondary aldosteronism may also occur without edema or hypertension (e.g., Bartter's and Gitelman's syndrome).

III. CUSHING'S SYNDROME

Hypertension is a common finding in Cushing's syndrome, affecting ∼80% of patients, but occurs less frequently with exogenous glucocorticoid therapy (32). Cardiovascular disease, in particular hypertension, is a major cause of morbidity and death in patients with Cushing's syndrome (33).

The causes of Cushing's syndrome include Cushing's disease (68%), ectopic ACTH excess (12%), adrenal adenoma (10%), carcinoma (8%), and hyperplasia (2%) (34). Importantly, the most common etiology of detrimental hypercorticism is treatment with steroids, for example, in the therapy of inflammatory diseases or after

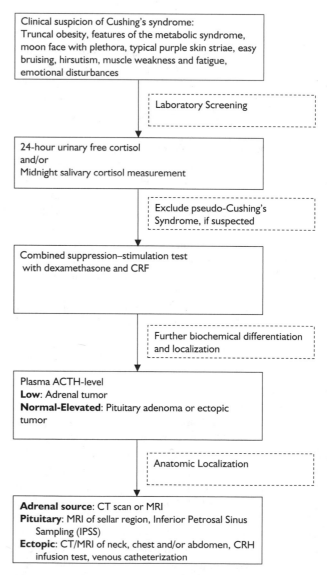

Figure 46.3 Algorithm for the diagnosis of Cushing's syndrome. ACTH, adrenocorticotropic hormone; CT, computed tomography; MRI, magnetic resonance imaging.

transplantations. Regardless of the etiology, all causes of endogenous Cushing's syndrome are characterized by an increased production of cortisol by the adrenal glands. Many of the signs and symptoms of the disease follow logically from the known action of glucocorticoids. The typical clinical presentation includes truncal obesity and features of the metabolic syndrome (i.e., diabetes mellitus type 2, dyslipidemia, obesity, and hypertension), moon facies, plethora, typical purple skin striae, easy bruising, hirsutism, muscle weakness and fatigue, and emotional disturbances. Other symptoms are amenorrhea, loss of libido, and osteoporosis with spontaneous fractures of ribs and vertebrae.

The pathogenesis of hypertension in Cushing's syndrome is multifactorial and the following factors are thought to be relevant: increased peripheral vascular sensitivity to adrenergic agonists, increased hepatic production of angiotensinogen, and activation of renal tubular type 1 (mineralocorticoid) receptors by cortisol excess (35). The last mechanism is mainly seen in patients with severe hypercortisolism, which is usually a result of ectopic ACTH-secretion. These patients often have concurrent hypokalemia. Hypokalemia also can occur as a result of adrenal hypersecretion of mineralocorticoids such as corticosterone and deoxycorticosterone.

The diagnosis of Cushing's syndrome depends on the demonstration of increased cortisol production, the loss of circadian cortisol production and, eventually, failure to suppress cortisol secretion normally when dexamethasone is administered (Fig. 46.3). To document hypercortisolism the determination of 24 h urinary free cortisol is recommended. Reported normal values are <250–500 nmol/24 h, depending on the use of a specific HPLC assay, which results in lower reference ranges. To assess the adequacy of the urine collection, creatinine excretions should also be quantified. As the cortisol production is typically stress dependent in healthy persons, limitations of the 24 h urinary cortisol production can be anticipated. False-positive results, however, may be obtained in several non-Cushing's hypercortisolemic states like major stress (i.e., trauma or infection), psychiatric states, chronic strenuous exercise, glucocorticoid resistance, and malnutrition. Conversely, rare cases of hypophyseal form of Cushing's disease with only a periodic increase in cortical production have been described (36). Thus, 24 h urine measurement should be repeated up to three times in order to exclude or confirm Cushing's syndrome, respectively (37). The loss of circadian rhythm can be assessed measuring "midnight" (i.e., 11:00 p.m. to 12:00 a.m.) serum or salivary cortisol (38). The salivary cortisol measurement has several advantages, namely, it is stable, can be collected in outpatients, and shows less fluctuations when compared with serum cortisol levels (39). At our institution, normal reference ranges are <6 nmol/L, ranging from 1 to 15 nmol/L in the literature. Thus, individual cut-offs have to be defined for each institution. The standard suppression tests designed to identify patients with Cushing's syndrome are the 2 day, low-dose dexamethasone suppression test (0.5 mg every 6 h for eight doses) and the overnight dexamethasone suppression test. The overnight dexamethasone suppression test requires only a blood collection for serum cortisol, the morning after the patient has taken a 1 mg dose of dexamethasone at 11:00 p.m. of the previous day. Reduction of basal plasma cortisol levels at 8:00 a.m. to values <50–130 nmol/L is defined as normal suppression, depending on the center evaluated and the assay used. The suppression tests are useful for confirming a diagnosis of Cushing's syndrome, but should be reserved primarily for patients with mildly increased urinary cortisol excretion and those thought to have pseudo-Cushing's syndrome (34). In latter cases, the combined suppression–stimulation test with dexamethasone and CRF was reported to be more reliable (40). After establishment of hypercortisolism, plasma-ACTH levels determine ACTH-dependence in Cushing's syndrome. In patients with ACTH-independent Cushing's syndrome, ACTH levels are usually suppressed to <5 ng/L. Patients with the ACTH-dependent form tend to have either normal or elevated levels of ACTH, usually >10 ng/L. However, variable ACTH-levels in healthy subjects as well as patients suffering from Cushing's syndrome are in part due to instability of the circulating molecule or pulsatile secretion pattern, respectively. Hence, ACTH levels may overlap in patients with hypothalamic-pituitary dysfunction, pituitary macroadenomas, ectopic CRH production, and ectopic ACTH production. For this reason, several additional tests have been advocated, such as the CRH infusion test, inferior petrosal sinus sampling (IPSS), or venous catheterization, to identify ectopic sources, respectively (37,40).

After the biochemical diagnosis of the etiology of Cushing's syndrome radiographic localization follows, by MRI of the sellar region in suspected Cushing's disease, CT scan or MRI of the adrenals in primary forms of the disease, or imaging of neck, chest and/or abdomen by CT or MRI in the search for an ectopic source. Thereby, the ACTH or CRH source can be very small, less than a few millimeters and, hence, not detectable by any imaging technique.

Treatment should be directed, whenever possible, at the primary cause of the syndrome. Therefore, establishing accurate differential diagnosis is essential. In patients with Cushing's disease, treatment of choice is the resection of the microadenoma by transsphenoidal microadenomectomy, if a clearly circumscribed tumor can be identified. Hemihypophysectomy or subtotal resection of the anterior pituitary might be necessary. Additional therapeutic options are pituitary irradiation and/or bilateral total adrenalectomy. Early evidence for a cure can be an undetectable plasma cortisol concentration in the morning (<1 µg/mL) and an ACTH concentration of <5 pg/mL 24 h after the last 10–15 mg dose of hydrocortisone, 4–7 days after surgery (34). It is important to note that postcure of a patient with Cushing's syndrome, the HPA axis is still insufficient because of the preceding long-term suppression of the nontumorous parts of the HPA axis by the hypercortisolism. Therefore, a cortisol substitution therapy with increasing substitution doses in stressful life events and detailed information of the patient are mandatory.

Some nonpituitary tumors that secrete either ACTH or CRP are not resectable. In these cases, the hypercortisolism can be controlled with adrenal enzyme inhibitors such as metyrapone (250–750 mg tid–qid) or ketoconazole (600–1200 mg qid). Unilateral adenomas of the adrenal are cured with unilateral adrenalectomy. In patients with bilateral micronodular or macronodular adrenal hyperplasia, bilateral total adrenalectomy is required. Mitotane, a specific adrenocorticolytic agent, may be offered to patients with inoperable, residual, or recurrent disease.

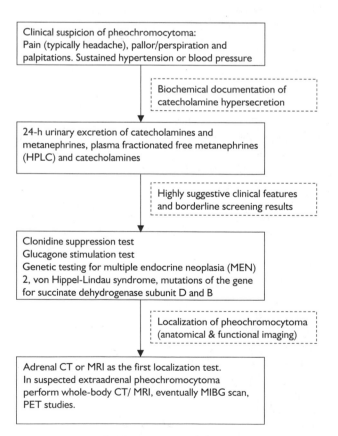

Figure 46.4 Algorithm for the diagnosis of pheochromocytoma. CT, computed tomography; MRI, magnetic resonance imaging.

In children and adolescent with Cushing's syndrome, blood pressure normalized within a year from the correction of hypercortisolism (41). A positive correlation between the systolic blood pressure and the duration of the disease points toward the deleterious effects of prolonged hypercortisolism and the significance of early diagnosis and treatment.

Blocking mineralocorticoid activity with spironolactone may be effective in patients with very high serum cortisol levels, especially those with hypokalemia.

IV. PHEOCHROMOCYTOMA

Tumors of the adrenal medulla are a rare, but eminently curable, form of endocrine hypertension. Pheochromocytoma occurs in $<0.2\%$ of patients with hypertension (42). Because hypertension is one of the key symptoms and because hypertension is highly prevalent in the population, many hypertensive patients undergo testing by clinicians. Nevertheless, the diagnosis is rarely confirmed (Fig. 46.4). These tumors are usually found in the adrenal medulla, but as paragangliomas also occur in other neurone ectoderm-derived tissue. Because the clinical presentation and diagnostic approach are similar, the term pheochromocytoma is used to refer to both adrenal pheochromocytoma and catecholamine-secreting paragangliomas. Most pheochromocytomas (90%) are benign, but a small percentage (10%) is malignant and may metastasize to liver and bone. Histologically and biochemically malignant pheochromocytomas are comparable to benign ones. Clues to the presence of a malignant form are local invasion or distant metastases (43). Ten percent of the adrenal pheochromocytomas arise bilaterally, whereas 90% are unilateral (44,45). In 10%, the pheochromocytomas are familial and these are often multicentric and bilateral. There are several primary familial disorders associated with pheochromocytoma, both of which have autosomal dominant inheritance: von Hippel–Lindau syndrome, glomustumors, neurofibromatosis type I, and MEN-2 (46). The latter is also characterized by medullary carcinoma of the thyroid and, in some cases, hyperparathyroidism due to primary parathyroid hyperplasia. Recently, a higher percentage of genetic causes of pheochromocytoma associated syndromes due to germline mutations has been suggested, with a prevalence ranging up to 25% of pheochromocytoma cases (47). Therefore, the following axioma may no longer be valid as molecular analysis has advanced the knowledge that came from clinical observation (48). Traditionally, the "rule of 10" means 10% is familial, and 10% is bilateral, 10% is malignant, and 10% is extra-adrenal (49).

Patients with catecholamine-secreting tumors may be asymptomatic, at times, or have nonspecific symptoms like weight loss, nausea, or constipation. However, symptoms usually are present and are predominantly due to the release of catecholamines and, to a lesser extent, to the co-secretion of other substances. The classical "triad of symptoms" consists of pain (mostly headache), perspiration/pallor, and palpitations. These symptoms often have an episodic character and even hypertension is paroxysmal in ~50% of the cases. The other 50% have sustained hypertension, although significant blood pressure lability and variability are usually present, and half of patients with sustained hypertension have distinct crises or paroxysms (50). Paroxysms of these signs and symptoms can be elicited by all kinds of physical or chemical stimuli like anesthetics, food, micturition, and some drugs. Typically, psychological stress does not induce these paroxysmal attacks, in contrast to physical manipulation of the tumor. The diagnosis should also be considered in other circumstances: for example, hypertension resistant to conventional agents, when there is marked variability in blood pressure readings, or hypertension where control deteriorates after β-blockade.

Biochemical documentation of catecholamine hypersecretion should precede any form of imaging study. Biochemical tests of catecholamine excess commonly used for diagnosis of pheochromocytoma include measurements of urinary and plasma catecholamines (noradrenaline and adrenaline), urinary metanephrines (normetanephrine and metanephrine), and urinary vanillylmandelic acid. More recent developed tests include measurements of plasma concentrations of the free (i.e., nonconjugated and biologically active), fractionated metanephrines (i.e., measured by HPLC). There is still an ongoing controversy about the diagnostic accuracy of the different tests available (51,52).

According to the ESH, the urinary excretion rates of catecholamines and metanephrines are the test of choice to screen for pheochromocytomas (3). Urine collections may be indexed to time (12 or 24 h) or to creatinine levels. Despite claims for the adequacy of determinations made on random and "postparoxysmal" urine samples, we recommend the analysis of a full 24 h urine sample. To assess the adequacy of the urine collection, creatinine excretions should also be quantified. Before testing, one should be aware that some medications and clinical situations may affect the measurements of catecholamines and metabolites (Table 46.1). At our institution, the upper normal reference limit for total urinary adrenaline is 22 nmol/mmol creatinine (<130 nmol daily) and for noradrenaline 45 nmol/mmol creatinine (<610 nmol daily). For urinary metanephrine, the upper limit of normal is 200 nmol/mmol creatinine (<1500 nmol/24 h) and for normetanephrine 250 nmol/mmol creatinine (<4500 nmol/24 h).

Table 46.1 Drugs and Conditions that may Alter Measured Levels of Catecholamines and Metabolites

Tricyclic antidepressants and antipsychotics
Levodopa
Methyldopa
Labetalol
Sotalol
Drugs that contain catecholamines (e.g., decongestants)
Ethanol
Withdrawal from clonidine
Benzodiazepines
Acetaminophen and phenoxybenzamine
Major physical stress (e.g., surgery, stroke, myocardial ischemia)

The measurement of plasma free metanephrine has a reported sensitivity of nearly 100% (51). However, plasma free, fractionated metanephrines may lack the specifity to recommend it as a first line test in adults (53). The sole reliance on this test must await its transfer to more usual clinical settings and local regional reference laboratories (54). Measurements of free, fractionated plasma normetanephrine and metanephrine may be useful in screening for pheochromocytomas in patients with a familial predisposition to these tumors where a highly sensitive test is required (55).

When clinical features are highly suggestive for pheochromocytoma and the urinary assay results are borderline, functional measurement of plasma catecholamines may be worthwhile. The usefulness of plasma catecholamine determinations may be increased by agents that suppress sympathetic nervous system activity. The clonidine-suppression test is particularly useful in cases with increased levels of catecholamines. A large decrease in plasma noradrenaline after clonidine suggests that increased baseline values are due to sympathoneuronal activation, whereas consistently and highly elevated plasma concentrations of noradrenaline before and after clonidine strongly indicate a pheochromocytoma. A positive clonidine suppression test is indicated by failure of plasma catecholamines (especially norepinephrine) to fall at least 40% from baseline and <2750 pmol/L 3 h after a single oral dose of 0.3 mg clonidine (56). A fall in blood pressure associated with heart rate reduction assures that clonidine has been adequately absorbed. Conversely, the glucagon stimulation test can be useful in patients with normal baseline plasma catecholamine levels. A positive glucagon stimulation test requires a threefold increase in plasma catecholamine (especially norepinephrine) concentration 2 min after a bolus iv administration of 1 mg glucagon (57). An increase in blood pressure is corroborative but not essential, can be marked and potentially dangerous, and may be treated with regitin iv in 5–10 mg boluses.

Radiological evaluation to locate the tumor should not be initiated until biochemical studies have confirmed the diagnosis of catecholamine-secreting tumor. Localization of pheochromocytomas should be attempted using at least two imaging modalities. Anatomical imaging studies (CT and MRI) should be combined with functional imaging studies for optimal results to locate primary, recurrent, or metastatic pheochromocytomas (58). CT or MRI of the adrenal glands and abdomen should be the first localization test. They should always be carried out over the abdomen first, because pheochromocytomas are mostly situated within the adrenal medulla. With CT, there is a slight risk of exacerbation of hypertension if a radiographic contrast agent is given, which can be prevented by pre-treatment with a α-adrenergic blocker (i.e., phenoxybenzamine 10 → 30 mg bid or tid) (59). MRI can distinguish pheochromocytoma from other adrenal masses; on T2-weighted images, as pheochromocytomas appear hyperintense, typically cystic and other adrenal tumors isointense and more homogenous, when compared with the liver. Both techniques have a sensitivity of 90–100%, but the specificity of both is limited to only 70% (54).

In patients in whom anatomic imaging with CT or MRI is negative and in the detection of metastatic lesions, nuclear medicine imaging is important. Pheochromocytomas usually abundantly express specific catecholamine plasma membrane and vesicular transporter systems, enabling imaging with [131]I- and ^{123}I-MIBG, as well as with several PET ligands (58). If both MIBG and PET studies are negative, the patient probably has an unusual type or malignant pheochromocytoma. In these cases, scintigraphy with nonspecific ligands, such as somatostatin receptor scintigraphy with octreotide or FDG-PET, should be carried out (58).

Once a pheochromocytoma is diagnosed, surgical resection of the tumor is the definite therapy. Nowadays, laparoscopic adrenalectomy is the procedure of first choice (60). Because the removal of a catecholamine secreting tumor is a high-risk surgical procedure, adequate medical preparation and an experienced team of surgeons and anesthesiologists are required. One approach is to give the α-blocker phenoxybenzamine, 10 mg once daily, and raise the dose every few days until the patient's symptoms and blood pressure are controlled. However, phenoxybenzamine produces significant orthostatic hypotension and reflex tachycardia. In ~30%, a β-blocker has to be added to overcome tachycardia. A β-blocker should never be started first because blockade of vasodilatory peripheral β-receptors with unopposed α-receptor stimulation can lead to a further elevation in blood pressure. Selective postsynaptic α-1 adrenergic receptor antagonists have been used to circumvent some of the disadvantages of phenoxybenzamine. According to Bravo, calcium channel

blockers have also been effective in controlling blood pressure in pheochromocytoma (54,61). Acute hypertensive crises may occur before or during operation and should be treated with nitroprusside or phentolamine administered intravenously. Postoperative hypotension can be avoided by adequate fluid replacement, already started preoperatively, and hypoglycemia by glucose infusion. After removal of the tumor, catecholamine secretion should fall to normal in ~1 week. About 2 weeks postoperatively, a 24 h urine sample should be obtained for measurement of preoperatively elevated catecholamine levels. Increased levels indicate the presence of residual tumor, a second primary lesion, or occult metastases. Thereafter, 24 h urinary excretion of catecholamines should be checked annually for at least 5 years as surveillance for tumor recurrence in the adrenal bed, metastatic disease, or delayed appearance of multiple primary tumors (62). In one series of 114 patients, pheochromocytoma recurred in 16, and the recurrence was malignant in nine (63). Diagnostic and genetic studies for familial disorders, such as MEN-II, von Hippel–Lindau syndrome, and familial pheochromocytoma, should be considered during the first postoperative visit. Testing to be considered includes RET proto-oncogene or pentagastrin stimulation test with measurement of calcitonin response, ophthalmology consult, head MRI scan, and screening for pheochromocytoma of all immediate family members (64,65).

Because the manifestations of pheochromocytoma can be versatile, the diagnosis must be considered and excluded in many patients with suggestive clinical symptoms. However, it should be recognized that many conditions associated with increased activity of the sympathetic nervous system may mimic a pheochromocytoma. For example, the use of sympathomimetic drugs as appetite suppressants or decongestants or the abrupt discontinuation of a short-acting sympathetic antagonist drug (e.g., clonidine or propranolol) can lead to severe hypertension and coronary ischemia. Increased sympathetic activity also can be found, for example, in autonomic dysfunction, hypoglycemia, panic disorder, migraine, and heart failure. So-called pseudo-pheochromocytoma is a rare cause of paroxysmal hypertension. This disorder may be due to stress or emotional distress, which is only uncovered after careful psychological evaluation (66).

V. OTHER FORMS OF ENDOCRINE HYPERTENSION

The above mentioned endocrine diseases cause hypertension in the majority of patients who have them. There are, however, other endocrine conditions that have been associated with hypertension. The evidence for causality is not equally strong across all of these conditions. While most of them are relatively rare in the evaluation of hypertensive patients, asymptomatic thyroid dysfunctions might be found in ~5% of elderly patients with hypertension (67).

A. Hyperthyroidism and Hypothyroidism

Both hyperthyroidism and hypothyroidism are reportedly associated with hypertension. The prevalence of hypertension in hypothyroidism may be as high as 40% (68). In hypothyroidism, the diastolic blood pressure, in particular, is increased which is associated with an increased vascular resistance (69,70). One of the possible mechanisms is an increased activity of the sympathetic nervous system, as is also demonstrated by increased plasma catecholamine levels (70).

The prevalence of hypertension in hyperthyroidism is ~25%. Systolic hypertension dominates because of the increased cardiac indices and decreased peripheral resistance (71). Adequate treatment of hypo- and hyperthyroidism usually restores blood pressure (68,72).

B. Hyperparathyroidism

Hypertension is frequently associated with primary hyperparathyroidism (10–60%). It is likely that this is merely due to the effect of PTH rather than due to the effect of calcium. PTH can cause hypertension either by increasing total peripheral resistance or by increasing blood volume (73,74).

C. Acromegaly

The majority of cases of acromegaly are caused by GH-producing pituitary adenomas. Approximately half of the patients with acromegaly exhibit high blood pressure (75). Left ventricular hypertrophy or cardiomyopathy is a very frequent finding in acromegaly. Cardiovascular accidents are claimed to be the main cause of the increased mortality in acromegaly (76). The poor prognosis for cardiovascular accidents is not only due to systemic hypertension, coronary artery disease, and arrhythmias, but also due to a specific cardiomyopathy. Sodium retention caused by growth hormone, an increased sympathetic tone and an impaired endothelium-mediated vasodilation may contribute to the development of hypertension. Removal of excess growth hormone can improve the blood pressure level considerably.

VI. CONCLUSION

Both clinical experience and clinical studies have helped to improve the diagnostic approach and to optimize therapeutic options in the past. In the future, larger prospective clinical studies and more experimental research, hopefully, allow to circumscribe the optimal and simplified approach to the individual patient with suspected endocrine hypertension.

REFERENCES

1. Cleland SJ, Connell JM. Endocrine hypertension. J R Coll Physicians Lond 1998; 32:104–108.
2. Chobanian AV, Bakris GL, Black HR, Cushman WC, Green LA, Izzo JL Jr, Jones DW, Materson BJ, Oparil S, Wright JT Jr, Roccella EJ; National Heart, Lung, and Blood Institute Joint National Committee on Prevention, Detection, Evaluation, and Treatment of High Blood Pressure; National High Blood Pressure Education Program Coordinating Committee. The Seventh Report of the Joint National Committee on Prevention, Detection, Evaluation, and Treatment on High Blood Pressure: the JNC 7 report. J Am Med Assoc 2003; 289:2560–2572.
3. European Society of Hypertension–European Society of Cardiology Guidelines Committee. 2003 European Society of Hypertension–European Society of Cardiology guidelines for the management of arterial hypertension. J Hypertens 2003; 21:1011–1053.
4. Bravo EL. Adrenal cortex. In: Oparil S, Weber M, eds. Hypertension—A Companion to Brenner and Rector's. The Kidney. Philadelphia: WB Saunders, 2000:674–685.
5. Conn JW. Primary aldosteronism, a new clinical syndrome. J Lab Clin Med 1955; 45:3–17.
6. Lund JO, Nielsen MD, Giese J. Prevalence of primary aldosteronism. Acta Med Scand Suppl 1981; 646:54–57.
7. Gordon RD, Stowasser M, Tunny TJ, Klemm SA, Rutherford JC. High incidence of primary aldosteronism in 199 patients referred with hypertension. Clin Exp Pharmacol Physiol 1994; 21:315–318.
8. Fardella CE, Mosso L, Gomez-Sanchez C, Cortes P, Soto J, Gomez L, Pinto M, Huete A, Oestreicher E, Foradori A, Montero J. Primary hyperaldosteronism in essential hypertensives: prevalence, biochemical profile, and molecular biology. J Clin Endocrinol Metab 2000; 85:1863–1867.
9. Padfield PL. Prevalence and role of a raised aldosterone to renin ratio in the diagnosis of primary aldosteronism: a debate on the scientific logic of the use of the ratio in practice. Clin Endocrinol 2003; 59:422–426.
10. Lim PO, MacDonald TM. Primary aldosteronism, diagnosed by the aldosterone to renin ratio, is a common cause of hypertension. Clin Endocrinol 2003; 59:427–430.
11. Ganguly A. Primary aldosteronism. N Engl J Med 1998; 339:1828–1834.
12. Gordon RD. Diagnostic investigations in primary aldosteronism. In: Hansen K, Rodicio J, Zanchetti A, eds. Hypertension. London: McGraw Hill International, 2001:101–114.
13. Young DB. Quantitative analysis of aldosterone's role in potassium regulation. Am J Physiol 1988; 255:F811–F822.

14. Bravo EL, Tarazi RC, Dustan HP, Fouad FM, Textor SC, Gifford RW et al. The changing clinical spectrum of primary aldosteronism. Am J Med 1983; 74:641–651.

15. Tanabe A, Naruse M, Takagi S, Tsuchiya K, Imaki T, Takano K. Variability in the renin/aldosterone profile under random and standardized sampling conditions in primary aldosteronism. J Clin Endocrinol Metab 2003; 88:2489–2494.

16. Hiramatsu K, Yamada T, Yukimura Y, Komiya I, Ichikawa K, Ishihara M et al. A screening test to identify aldosterone-producing adenoma by measuring plasma renin activity. Results in hypertensive patients. Arch Intern Med 1981; 141:1589–1593.

17. Weinberger MH, Fineberg NS. The diagnosis of primary aldosteronism and separation of two major subtypes. Arch Intern Med 1993; 153:2125–2129.

18. Tiu SC, Choi CH, Shek CC, Ng YW, Chan FK, Ng CM, Kong AP. The use of aldosterone-renin ratio as a diagnostic test for primary hyperaldosteronism and its test characteristics under different conditions of blood sampling. J Clin Endocrinol Metab 2005; 90:72–78.

19. Seifarth C, Trenkel S, Schobel H, Hahn EG, Hensen J. Influence of antihypertensive medication on aldosterone and renin concentration in the differential diagnosis of essential hypertension and primary aldosteronism. Clin Endocrinol 2002; 57:457–465.

20. Holland OB, Brown H, Kuhnert L, Fairchild C, Risk M, Gomez-Sanchez CE. Further evaluation of saline infusion for the diagnosis of primary aldosteronism. Hypertension 1984; 6:717–723.

21. Gomez-Sanchez CE. Primary aldosteronism and its variants. Cardiovasc Res 1998; 37:8–13.

22. Phillips JL, Walther MM, Pezzullo JC, Rayford W, Choyke PL, Berman AA et al. Predictive value of preoperative tests in discriminating bilateral adrenal hyperplasia from an aldosterone-producing adrenal adenoma. J Clin Endocrinol Metab 2000; 85:4526–4533.

23. Takeda M, Go H, Imai T, Nishiyama T, Morishita H. Laparoscopic adrenalectomy for primary aldosteronism: report of initial ten cases. Surgery 1994; 115:621–625.

24. Meyer A, Brabant G, Behrend M. Long-term follow-up after adrenalectomy for primary aldosteronism. World J Surg 2005 Jan 20; [Epub ahead of print].

25. Lifton RP, Dluhy RG, Powers M, Rich GM, Cook S, Ulick S, Lalouel JM. A chimaeric 11 β-hydroxylase/aldosterone synthase gene causes glucocorticoid-remediable aldosteronism and human hypertension. Nature 1992; 355:262–265.

26. Jonsson JR, Klemm SA, Tunny TJ, Stowasser M, Gordon RD. A new genetic test for familial hyperaldosteronism type I aids in the detection of curable hypertension. Biochem Biophys Res Commun 1995; 207:565–571.

27. White PC, Mune T, Agarwal AK. 11 β-hydroxysteroid dehydrogenase and the syndrome of apparent mineralocorticoid excess. Endocr Rev 1997; 18:135–156.

28. Chrousos GP, Detera-Wadleigh SD, Karl M. Syndromes of glucocorticoid resistance. Ann Intern Med 1993; 119:1113–1124.

29. Liddle GW, Bledsoe T, Coppage WS. A familial renal disorder simulating primary aldosteronism but with negligible aldosterone secretion. Trans Assoc Am Phys 1963; 76:199–213.

30. Palmer BF, Alpern RJ. Liddle's syndrome. Am J Med 1998; 104:301–309.

31. Hansson JH, Nelson-Williams C, Suzuki H, Schild L, Shimkets R, Lu Y, Canessa C, Iwasaki T, Rossier B, Lifton RP. Hypertension caused by a truncated epithelial sodium channel γ subunit: genetic heterogeneity of Liddle syndrome. Nat Genet 1995; 11:76–82.

32. Gomez-Sanchez CE. Cushing's syndrome and hypertension. Hypertension 1986; 8:258–264.

33. Whitworth JA. Studies on the mechanisms of glucocorticoid hypertension in humans. Blood Press 1994; 3:24–32.

34. Orth DN. Cushing's syndrome. N Engl J Med 1995; 332:791–803.

35. Mantero F, Boscaro M. Glucocorticoid-dependent hypertension. J Steroid Biochem Mol Biol 1992; 43:409–413.

36. Loh KC. Cyclical Cushing's syndrome—a trap for the unwary. Singapore Med J 1999; 40:321–324.

37. Arnaldi G, Angeli A, Atkinson AB, Bertagna X, Cavagnini F, Chrousos GP, Fava GA, Findling JW, Gaillard RC, Grossman AB, Kola B, Lacroix A, Mancini T, Mantero F, Newell-Price J, Nieman LK, Sonino N, Vance ML, Giustina A, Boscaro M. Diagnosis and complications of Cushing's syndrome: a consensus statement. J Clin Endocrinol Metab 2003; 88:5593–5602.

38. Papanicolaou DA, Mullen N, Kyrou I, Nieman LK. Nighttime salivary cortisol: a useful test fort he diagnosis of Cushing's syndrome. J Clin Endocrinol Metab 2002; 87:4515–4521.

39. Yaneva M, Mosnier-Pudar H, Dugue MA, Grabar S, Fulla Y, Bertagna X. Midnight salivary cortisol for the initial diagnosis of cushing's syndrome of various causes. J Clin Endocrinol Metab 2004; 89:3345-3351.

40. Yanovski JA, Cutler GB Jr, Chrousos GP, Nieman LK. Corticotropin-releasing hormone stimulation following low-dose dexamethasone administration. A new test to distinguish Cushing's syndrome from pseudo-Cushing's states. J Am Med Assoc 1993; 269:2232–2238.

41. Magiakou MA, Mastorakos G, Zachman K, Chrousos GP. Blood pressure in children and adolescents with Cushing's syndrome before and after surgical care. J Clin Endocrinol Metab 1997; 82:1734–1738.

42. Stein PP, Black HR. A simplified diagnostic approach to pheochromocytoma. A review of the literature and report of one institution's experience. Medicine (Baltimore) 1991; 70:46–66.

43. Pattarino F, Bouloux PM. The diagnosis of malignancy in phaeochromocytoma. Clin Endocrinol 1996; 44:239–241.

44. Bravo EL. Pheochromocytoma: new concepts and future trends. Kidney Int 1991; 40:544–556.

45. Whalen RK, Althausen AF, Daniels GH. Extra-adrenal pheochromocytoma. J Urol 1992; 147:1–10.

46. Neumann HP, Berger DP, Sigmund G, Blum U, Schmidt D, Parmer RJ, Volk B, Kirste G. Pheochromocytomas, multiple endocrine neoplasia type 2, and von Hippel–Lindau disease. N Engl J Med 1993; 329:1531–1538, Erratum in: N Engl J Med 1994; 331:1535.

47. Neumann HP, Bausch B, McWhinney SR, Bender BU, Gimm O, Franke G, Schipper J, Klisch J, Altehoefer C,

Zerres K, Januszewicz A, Eng C, Smith WM, Munk R, Manz T, Glaesker S, Apel TW, Treier M, Reineke M, Walz MK, Hoang-Vu C, Brauckhoff M, Klein-Franke A, Klose P, Schmidt H, Maier-Woelfle M, Peczkowska M, Szmigielski C, Eng C; Freiburg–Warsaw–Columbus Pheochromocytoma Study Group. Germ-line mutations in nonsyndromic pheochromocytoma. N Engl J Med 2002; 346:1459–1466.

48. Dluhy RG. Pheochromocytoma—death of an axiom. N Engl J Med 2002; 346:1486–1488.

49. Bravo EL, Gifford RW Jr. Current concepts. Pheochromocytoma: diagnosis, localization, and management. N Engl J Med 1984; 311:1298–1303.

50. Baguet JP, Hammer L, Mazzuco TL, Chabre O, Mallion JM, Sturm N, Chaffanjon P. Circumstances of discovery of phaeochromocytoma: a retrospective study of 41 consecutive patients. Eur J Endocrinol 2004; 150:681–686.

51. Lenders JW, Pacak K, Walther MM, Linehan WM, Mannelli M, Friberg P, Keiser HR, Goldstein DS, Eisenhofer G. Biochemical diagnosis of pheochromocytoma: which test is best? J Am Med Assoc 2002; 287:1427–1434.

52. Pacak K, Linehan WM, Eisenhofer G, Walther MM, Goldstein DS. Recent advances in genetics, diagnosis, localization, and treatment of pheochromocytoma. Ann Intern Med 2001; 134:315–329.

53. Sawka AM, Jaeschke R, Singh RJ, Young WF Jr. A comparison of biochemical tests for pheochromocytoma: measurement of fractionated plasma metanephrines compared with the combination of 24 h urinary metanephrines and catecholamines. J Clin Endocrinol Metab 2003; 88:553–558.

54. Bravo EL. Pheochromocytoma. Cardiol Rev 2002; 10:44–50.

55. Eisenhofer G, Lenders JW, Linehan WM, Walther MM, Goldstein DS, Keiser HR. Plasma normetanephrine and metanephrine for detecting pheochromocytoma in von Hippel–Lindau disease and multiple endocrine neoplasia type 2. N Engl J Med 1999; 340:1872–1879.

56. Bravo EL, Tarazi RC, Fouad FM, Vidt DG, Gifford RW Jr. Clonidine-suppression test: a useful aid in the diagnosis of pheochromocytoma. N Engl J Med 1981; 305:623–626.

57. Grossman E, Goldstein DS, Hoffman A, Keiser HR. Glucagon and clonidine testing in the diagnosis of pheochromocytoma. Hypertension 1991; 17:733–741.

58. Ilias I, Pacak K. Current approaches and recommended algorithm for the diagnostic localization of pheochromocytoma. J Clin Endocrinol Metab 2004; 89:479–491.

59. Bouloux PG, Fakeeh M. Investigation of pheochromocytoma. Clinical Endocrinology 1995; 43:657–664.

60. Kazaryan AM, Kuznetsov NS, Shulutko AM, Beltsevich DG, Edwin B. Evaluation of endoscopic and traditional open approaches to pheochromocytoma. Surg Endosc 2004; 18:937–941.

61. Bravo EL. Secondary hypertension: adrenal and nervous systems. In: Hollenberg NK, ed. Atlas of Heart Diseases. Philadelphia: Current Medicine, 2001:118–143.

62. van Heerden JA, Roland CF, Carney JA, Sheps SG, Grant CS. Long-term evaluation following resection of apparently benign pheochromocytoma(s)/paragangliomas(s). World J Surg 1990; 14:325–329.

63. Plouin PF, Chatellier G, Fofol I, Corvol P. Tumor recurrence and hypertension persistence after successful pheochromocytoma operation. Hypertension 1997; 29:1133–1139.

64. Ledger GA, Khosla S, Lindor NM, Thibodeau SN, Gharib H. Genetic testing in the diagnosis and management of multiple endocrine neoplasia type II. Ann Intern Med 1995; 122:118–124.

65. Eng C, Clayton D, Schuffenecker I, Lenoir G, Cote G, Gagel RF, van Amstel HK, Lips CJ, Nishisho I, Takai SI, Marsh DJ, Robinson BG, Frank-Raue K, Raue F, Xue F, Noll WW, Romei C, Pacini F, Fink M, Niederle B, Zedenius J, Nordenskjold M, Komminoth P, Hendy GN, Mulligan LM. The relationship between specific RET proto-oncogene mutations and disease phenotype in multiple endocrine neoplasia type 2. International RET mutation consortium analysis. J Am Med Assoc 1996; 276:1575–1579.

66. Mann SJ. Severe paroxysmal hypertension (pseudo-pheochromocytoma): understanding the cause and treatment. Arch Intern Med 1999; 159:670–674.

67. Anderson GH Jr, Blakeman N, Streeten DH. The effect of age on prevalence of secondary forms of hypertension in 4429 consecutively referred patients. J Hypertens 1994; 12:609–615.

68. Streeten DH, Anderson GH Jr, Howland T, Chiang R, Smulyan H. Effects of thyroid function on blood pressure. Recognition of hypothyroid hypertension. Hypertension 1988; 11:78–83.

69. Saito I, Ito K, Saruta T. Hypothyroidism as a cause of hypertension. Hypertension 1983; 5:112–115.

70. Fommei E, Iervasi G. The role of thyroid hormone in blood pressure homeostasis: evidence from short-term hypothyroidism in humans. J Clin Endocrinol Metab 2002; 87:1996–2000.

71. Woeber KA. Thyrotoxicosis and the heart. N Engl J Med 1992; 327:94–98.

72. Klein I. Thyroid hormone and the cardiovascular system. Am J Med 1990; 88:631–637.

73. Nussdorfer GG, Bahçelioglu M, Neri G, Malendowicz LK. Secretin, glucagons, gastric inhibitory polypeptide, parathyroid hormone, and related peptides in the regulation of the hypothalamus–pituitary–adrenal axis. Peptides 2000; 21:309–324.

74. Mazzocchi G, Aragona F, Malendowicz LK, Nussdorfer GG. PTH and PTH-related peptide enhance steroid secretion from human adrenocortical cells. Am J Physiol Endocrinol Metab 2001; 280:E209–E213.

75. Lopez-Velasco R, Escobar-Morreale HF, Vega B, Villa E, Sancho JM, Moya-Mur JL, Garcia-Robles R. Cardiac involvement in acromegaly: specific myocardiopathy or consequence of systemic hypertension? J Clin Endocrinol Metab 1997; 82:1047–1053.

76. Orme SM, McNally RJ, Cartwright RA, Belchetz PE. Mortality and cancer incidence in acromegaly: a retrospective cohort study. United Kingdom Acromegaly Study Group. J Clin Endocrinol Metab 1998; 83:2730–2734.

47

Coarctation of the Aorta

TED LO, GREGORY Y. H. LIP

University Department of Medicine, City Hospital, Birmingham, UK

KEYPOINTS

- Coarctation of the aorta results in upper body hypertension.
- Prenatal diagnosis is possible and early repair must be considered.
- Patients showing symptoms after the age of 1 year should be immediately assessed for repair.
- Patients should be evaluated for the presence of other cardiac malformations.

SUMMARY

Coarctation of the aorta is a congenital vascular abnormality, which results in upper body hypertension. Long-term follow-up of patients with previous coarctectomy reveals the presence of adult hypertension in up to 75% of patients 20–30 years after surgery. Of these patients, about 3–26% have a recurrence of the coarctation, but the remaining patients appear to have developed hypertension despite the anatomical repair.

Prenatal diagnosis is now possible, and once detected, early repair must be considered. The optimal time for elective surgical repair is about 1 year of age. If patients show symptoms after the age of 1 year, repair should be considered immediately to improve long-term prognosis. The patients also are at risk of accelerated coronary artery disease and cerebrovascular accident. Strict control of blood pressure along with appropriate reduction of other cardiovascular and cerebrovascular risks should minimize subsequent morbidity and mortality. Patients should be evaluated for the presence of other cardiac malformations.

I. BRIEF HISTORY

Coarctation of the aorta is a congenital localized narrowing of the aorta. "Coarctation" is derived from the Latin word *coarctatio*, meaning a drawing or pressing together. Meckel first noted such a finding at postmortem in 1750, and Legrand was the first to diagnose coarctation in a living patient in 1835. Bonnet later categorized coarctation into "infantile" and "adult" forms, subsequently revised to "preductal" and "postductal."

The clinical presentation of coarctation of the aorta varies from cardiovascular collapse in the neonate to being a rare finding in an adult during investigation of secondary causes of hypertension. Untreated patients rarely survive >50 years of age and usually die from heart failure, rupture of the aorta, intracranial hemorrhage, hypertension, endocarditis, or coronary artery disease.

Blalock and Park proposed the first surgical repair technique with a bypass from the left subclavian artery to the aorta to circumvent the area of narrowing in 1944. Crafoord and Nylin reported the first coarctation repair in 1945 by performing resection with end-to-end reanastomosis; Gross used homograft to replace the narrowed segments of aorta a few years later. Waldhausen and Nahrwold performed the first subclavian flap aortoplasty in 1966. Coarctation has, therefore, been surgically corrected for >50 years, and multiple large series of postsurgical-correction patients are now available, which allows long-term evaluation of outcomes. Advances in interventional cardiology techniques over the last two decades have led to an ever-increasing interest in percutaneous transluminal aortoplasy, first by plain balloon dilatation and, more recently, with endovascular stent deployment. No long-term data are available at present to evaluate or to compare outcomes with surgical correction.

Even with the complete anatomical repair of coarctation, patients frequently have premature morbidity and even mortality because of a combination of recoarctation, late aneurysm formation, severe late hypertension, and premature cardiovascular and cerebrovascular disease. Ongoing surveillance on an annual basis along with alternate yearly imaging is the minimum requirement in order to improve the survival rate of these patients.

II. EPIDEMIOLOGY

The epidemiological study of congenital heart disease is limited by technical difficulties, and this has led to a lag in our understanding of both the prevalence and the risk factors for cardiac malformation. Changes in screening, particularly the improvement in prenatal echocardiography, have allowed *in utero* detection, but there are no historical comparisons possible.

A. Prevalence

The incidence of coarctation of the aorta is 1–8 per 1000 live births, but the incidence is thought to be as high as 1 in 10 in the case of spontaneous abortions and stillbirths. It accounts for ∼6–8% of congenital heart disease. It is twice as common in males as in females. Using the 10 year data from the Baltimore–Washington Infant Study (BWIS), Ferencz et al. (1) showed that the prevalence of coarctation was 1.39 per 10,000 live births compared with 4 per 1000 live births for all cardiovascular malformations. Siblings of individuals affected by cardiac malformations are more likely to be affected, a phenomenon known as familial aggregation. The overall precurrence risk (chance of a sibling of an affected individual having the same cardiac malformation) for all cardiovascular malformations is 3.1%; but in left-sided obstructive lesions, it is significantly higher. The BWIS showed a precurrence rate of 6.3% for coarctation of the aorta, which was second only to hypoplastic left heart syndrome at 8.0%.

B. Inheritance

The nature of inheritance is unknown, but it is most likely to be polygenic in combination with environmental risks. Autosomal dominant inheritance with incomplete penetrance has been reported in one family, although most mathematical models have favored a simple Mendelian pattern (2). Multiple chromosomal abnormalities are associated with coarctation. For example, the DiGeorge syndrome that results from a microdeletion on the long arm of chromosome 22 (22q11.2) is known to contain abnormalities in conotruncal development. Although the 22q11 region has been mapped entirely, no single gene function has been shown to produce the malformations seen in the DiGeorge syndrome (3).

Some maternal infections or illnesses in early pregnancy have been linked to cardiac malformations but not specifically to coarctation. For example, children with congenital rubella syndrome have a cardiovascular defect, most commonly pulmonary stenosis or patent ductus arteriosus. Preconception maternal diabetes shows the strongest association with early embryonic malformations, including left heart outflow tract abnormalities, although this is thought to be a general risk for all cardiac defects and other serious birth defects (4). Other factors that have been investigated include anti-epileptic medications, maternal fever (particularly influenza), alcohol consumption, and cigarette smoking, although none has been definitely linked to birth defects (5).

A common maternal concern is workplace exposure to paints and organic solvents. Tikkanen and Heinonen (6) reported an association between mineral oil solvents and coarctation of the aorta, and this was supported by

BWIS, which showed an odds ratio of 3.2 (CI = 1.3–7.9) for development of coarctation of the aorta with daily exposure to organic solvents (7). Glutathione-S-transferases are involved in metabolizing organic solvents, and genetic polymorphisms have been shown to mediate the risk of pulmonary valve stenosis and atrial septal defect with solvent exposure, but as yet, the precise mechanism(s) that cause coarctation is unknown.

The only well-studied and accepted method of preventive strategies for reducing risk for cardiac malformations is the consumption of folic acid in the periconception period, although, again, this a heterogeneous effect rather than being specific for coarctation.

III. PATHOPHYSIOLOGY

Development of the heart is a complex process. A detailed description is beyond the scope of this chapter. Nonetheless, a brief description of heart development is relevant, because it is in the early stages of cardiac formation that the likely defects responsible for coarctation are present.

A. Cardiac Embryogenesis

Bilateral cardiac primordia are derived from the cardiac mesoderm, which is predetermined prior to development. These symmetrical regions migrate to the midline where they fuse to form the primitive heart tube by 22 days of gestation. This tube contains five regions: the aortic sac, conotruncus (outflow tract), the right ventricle, the left ventricle, and the bilateral atria. The tube is aligned with an anteroposterior polarity. Via a series of folds and loops, the functioning tube aligns itself into left–right polarity and a four-chambered heart. To produce septation and formation of the aorta and pulmonary arteries, the migration of a population of cells from the neural crest is required. These cells condense in the conotruncus to allow aortic formation. In addition to this migration, blood flow through the developing area is required to drive the process. The entire process is completed by the eighth week of gestation because a functioning cardiovascular system is required for further embryogenesis.

Abnormal migration at the stage where the heart tube forms is thought to be responsible for the formation of coarctation. A family of nuclear transcription factors known as the helix–loop–helix family is known to be required for neural crest migration both in humans and in other species. In fish, it has been shown that a specific gene, gridlock (*grl*), codes for a helix–loop–helix factor that is expressed highly at the stage where the neural crest migrates (8). In addition, *grl* is strongly expressed at a later stage when blood flow begins. Loss of *grl* in zebra fish produces failure of tube formation at the point where the primordia fuse. It is therefore likely that the loss of this gene would account for both stages of incorrect development—failure of migration and the subsequent flow-dependant development. Defects in helix–loop–helix expression may be responsible for the development of aortic coarctation in humans, although this is still unconfirmed.

IV. MORPHOLOGY OF COARCTATION

Coarctation may occur at any point in the thoracic or abdominal aorta. The most common type of coarctation is a discrete narrowing at the insertion of the ductus or ligamentum arteriosum. The presence of an additional membranous structure at this level causes further luminal narrowing. It is thought that the formation of this membrane occurs as the ductus arteriosus shrinks. The other types of coarctation, by definition, do not have this membranous structure and are classified as tubular hypoplasia, or arch interruption. They are diffuse and do not have a structural relationship to the ductus origin. Abdominal coarctation occurs in two morphologies and may be above or below the renal arteries. The first type of morphology is proximal to the renal vessels and is an hourglass type of narrowing; the second type of morphology, called "tubular hypoplasia," occurs distal to this.

V. HEMODYNAMIC CHANGES

The hemodynamic consequences of aortic coarctation depend on three factors: the relationship of the stenotic segment to the ductus arteriosus, the level of prenatal adaptation, and the presence of additional cardiovascular malformations. The majority of discrete coarctations occur proximal to the mouth of the ductus, which allows the right ventricle to supply the systemic circulation *in utero*. Until the ductus closes, the coarctation does not obstruct blood flow significantly within the aortic arch and fetal development continues—a duct-dependant circulation. Hypertrophy of the left ventricle and formation of arterial collaterals do not occur because there is no pressure stimulus. Therefore, as the ductus closes 2–3 days after birth, the aortic arch pressure and afterload to the left ventricle rapidly rise. End diastolic pressure increases, and stroke volume decreases. In the most severe cases, because there has been no prenatal compensation, left ventricular failure ensues; otherwise, adaptation begins. As left atrial pressure increases, the foramen ovale is opened and left-to-right shunting occurs, which increases pulmonary artery pressure. This left-to-right shunting is exacerbated with concurrent ventricular septal defects and leads to severe pulmonary hypertension. If the ductus arteriosus remains patent, which it commonly does, this situation is improved as right-to-left shunting continues and adaptation again takes place. For patients who survive the initial stages of coarctation and go on to have the condition surgically repaired, it is felt that long-term changes in the pulmonary vascular bed may be only mild.

More rarely, the stenotic segment in coarctation occurs after the opening of the ductus, and left ventricular hypertrophy and collateralization take place before birth. Changes in the pulmonary vascular bed usually are rare. If the coarctation is at the level of the ductus, a bidirectional shunt develops that may partially counteract the hemodynamic consequences of the stenosis.

From the hemodynamic changes that occur shortly after birth, it is obvious that higher pressures will be required in the prestenotic aorta to provide a gradient to supply the lower limbs. These early mechanical changes are the catalyst of upper limb hypertension in aortic coarctation. Despite apparent successful early repair, patients are still at substantial risk of developing late hypertension 20–30 years later. The exact etiology is unknown, although two theories have been proposed to explain this phenomenon. The first theory is that hypertension is produced through a generalized increase in vascular tone mediated by a systemic humeral response. The second theory is that as upper limb hypertension becomes established, the upper limb vascular bed alone undergoes changes that propagate hypertension by a combination of paracrine and localized baroreceptor responses; these changes may be only partially reversible. Neither mechanism has been proven, although, as discussed later, the evidence suggests that changes in the upstream vascular bed are likely to be the responsible mechanism.

VI. HYPERTENSION IN COARCTATION OF THE AORTA

Long-term follow-up of patients with previous coarctectomy by Brouwer et al. (9) reported the presence of adult hypertension in up to 75% of patients 20–30 years after surgery to repair coarctation. Of these patients, ~3–26% have a recurrence of their coarctation, but the remaining patients appear to have developed hypertension despite the anatomical repair. Subanalysis has suggested that the high prevalence of hypertension is related to the increased age of the patient at the time of the operation. Certainly, this is partially true, because repair after the age of 10 is associated with increased hypertension in adult life; and, historically, repairs were performed on older individuals. O'Sullivan et al. (10) demonstrated that despite the strategy of early repair, up to 28.5% of children have systolic blood pressures >95th percentile when measured casually 7–16 years later. If the patients included in this analysis are limited to patients on whom the operation was performed in infancy, this number is 26%. Removing those children from the analysis who, the authors felt, had

significant residual obstruction, reduced this number to 21.5%. The 24 h ambulatory blood pressure readings in this group corroborated these findings. This supports previous evidence that suggests that despite the young age at the time of the operation, 19–45% of the patients will be hypertensive at early follow-up (11). The true number of individuals who become hypertensive may be an underestimate because the follow-up interval for such studies is currently 16 years, and it is expected that additional patients will develop hypertension after this time interval.

In an attempt to further predict which individuals would subsequently become hypertensive, investigators have retrospectively analyzed case notes, looking for other postoperative or perioperative factors that are associated with late hypertension. Other variables that have repeatedly been shown to correlate with development of hypertension are resting arm–leg gradient prior to surgery, adult body mass index, postoperative paradoxical hypertension, and hypertension at the first clinic visit (12). Adult body mass index may be considered to be an independent factor, but the remaining measures are all established within days of the operation, although the previously mentioned caveat regarding a delay to surgery will still apply and the role of such variables with the current strategy of early repair awaits long-term follow-up.

The relationship of compensatory left ventricular changes and aortic changes to the subsequent development of hypertension has been investigated. In survivors, there is an increase in left ventricular mass and left ventricular remodeling in response to chronically increased after load. The left ventricular mass has been demonstrated to be hyperdynamic, and despite successful repair of the condition, these changes persist even in normotensive individuals (13). It can be postulated, therefore, that the left ventricle is preconditioned to respond to other stimuli in the development of hypertension.

Assessment of the response of the prestenotic vascular bed to infusions of vasoconstrictors has supported the principal that hypertension is mediated at a local level. This was confirmed by assessing vascular tone following infusion of norepinephrine in normotensive patients who had undergone coarctation repair. Gidding et al. (14) demonstrated that the forearm vasculature responds three times more readily in patients with repaired coarctation than in matched controls. Gardiner et al. (15) also demonstrated the abnormal forearm response, but his investigation showed that there was no difference in calf vessel responses between subjects and controls, which suggests a localized effect. Histologically, this is supported by findings of increased arterial stiffness, decreased smooth muscle, and high levels of collagen in these arteries. Animal studies also have demonstrated a reduced bioavailability of nitric oxide in the upstream vascular bed compared with bioavailability of nitric oxide below the stenosis (16); this also supports the principal that localized vascular changes are responsible for the condition.

A systemic role of the renin–angiotensin system and sympathetic nervous systems also has been investigated. Multiple studies have attempted to link the increased output of the renin–angiotensin system and sympathetic nervous system to hypertension in coarctation. The results of these studies are conflicting, and it is unlikely that generalized changes are responsible. Circulating levels of norepinephrine and renin at rest are normal in both normotensive and hypertensive coarctectomy patients, but these levels have been shown to increase dramatically during exercise when compared with controls, which suggests that responses of the sympathetic and renin–angiotensin system may be hyperreactive (17). It has been postulated that this may be due to early resetting of regulatory control, although again there is little corroborative evidence.

Established changes can therefore be demonstrated at a hemodynamic, vascular, histological, and molecular level at an early stage in patients who have undergone coarctation repair. These changes are restricted to the prestenotic vascular bed, and despite normal circulating levels of renin and sympathetic hormones at rest, hyperreactivity of these systems also may be responsible for propagating hypertension. The mechanisms of hypertension development in coarctation are summarized in Fig. 47.1.

A. Exercise-Induced Hypertension

During exercise, the usual response of the cardiovascular system is to increase systolic blood pressure by a combination of increased cardiac output and vasoconstriction of vascular beds not involved in supplying skeletal muscle mass. Although total vascular resistance decreases, there is a stepwise increment in systolic pressure that correlates to work load. This peaks at maximal exertion and decreases rapidly during recovery.

Numerous studies have demonstrated that normotensive patients with repaired coarctation have a pathological response to exercise testing. There is an excessive increase in the systolic pressure with a delay in recovery. In addition, the arm–leg blood pressure gradient becomes re-established. This phenomenon has been demonstrated in up to 20% of normotensive patients who do not have a significant anatomical cause for a residual gradient (10).

Hypertension in this case is postulated to be a combination of left ventricular hyperkinesis and hyperreactivity of the upper limb vascular beds. Of more importance is the role of exercise testing in predicting subsequent cardiovascular risk. As yet, long-term follow-up in such individuals is not available to link the development of exercise-induced hypertension and the subsequent development of sustained hypertension. But some clinicians advocate considering treatment of exercise-induced hypertension in normotensive individuals if their systolic pressure increase to >200 mmHg (18). Other clinicians, such as Swan et al. (19) believe that exercise-induced hypertension is of limited predictive value in these patients.

VII. CLINICAL FEATURES AND INVESTIGATION

The presentation and subsequent features of coarctation clearly can be divided into two broad stages according to

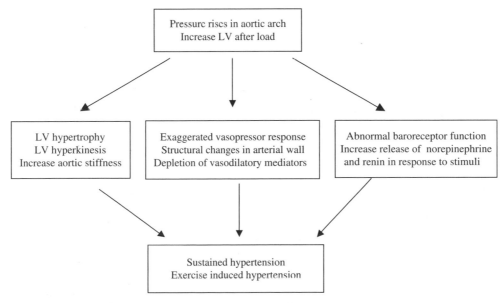

Figure 47.1 Mechanisms of hypertension development in coarctation of the aorta.

the degree of duct dependency in the circulation. Neonates with severe coarctation return to the hospital 2–3 days after birth, in extremis. They will be hypotensive, tachycardic, and cyanosed and have features of left ventricular failure along with absent femoral pulses. The characteristic murmur and other clinical features at this time are generally absent, and these neonates require ventilatory and circulatory support in an intensive care setting prior to correcting the defect as soon as it is possible to do so. A period of stability may be gained by the use of prostaglandin E2 infusions to maintain the ductus arteriosus until definitive correction can take place. The presence of a ventricular- or atrial-septal defect, with left-to-right shunting, exacerbates this situation and leads to pulmonary hypertension and biventricular failure. However, if neonates survive this period, it is suggested that the long-term changes in the pulmonary vascular bed may be only mild-to-moderate.

Infants with less severe, but significant, coarctation usually show symptoms within the first 12 months of life. A similar clinical picture develops, although the onset of left ventricular failure is more insidious in nature. As in the case of more severe coarctation, the management of the condition centers on stabilization prior to surgical correction.

Infants over the age of 1 often remain asymptomatic, although they may develop vague symptoms, particularly during exercise, including headache and lower limb claudication. Other symptoms are often discovered after the discovery of a heart murmur. Clinical examination reveals prominent brachial and radial pulses with diminished, delayed, or absent femoral pulsation. Upper limb hypertension is present, and if coarctation is suspected, blood pressure in the lower limbs should be measured; this pressure in the presence of coarctation is often normal or reduced. A pressure gradient of >20 mmHg is invariably present in significant coarctation, but asymmetry between lower limbs and upper limbs is rarely reported. Auscultation reveals a loud systolic murmur at the second left intercostal space and below the left clavicle. This radiates into the back and to the apex. If the degree of obstruction is mild, the murmur is usually mid-systolic, but as the degree of obstruction becomes worse, the murmur lengthens to be continuous as a high-velocity jet is forced through the constricted aorta.

Coarctation of the aorta is associated with a number of other cardiac and noncardiac abnormalities, which may also be detected. They are summarized in Table 47.1.

Adults in whom the condition remains undetected usually start mentioning vague symptoms, such as headache or exercise-induced claudication, in their third decade. These patients may exhibit complications of coarctation such as aortic dissection, endocarditis, or intracerebral hemorrhage. Otherwise coarctation will be suspected as a secondary cause of hypertension. The clinical findings are the same as the symptoms in the asymptomatic child.

A rare but clinically important consideration is in the pregnant mother who becomes hypertensive. Although pregnancy-induced hypertension is common, first-trimester and second-trimester hypertension should alert the clinician to the possibility of a secondary cause. For example, Lip et al. (21) reported three cases of coarctation that were detected as hypertension in pregnancy; these features should be actively excluded in all pregnant women.

A. Electrocardiographical Features

In the neonate and younger infant, the electrocardiogram (ECG) will show right ventricular hypertrophy and

Table 47.1 Abnormalities Associated with Coarctation of the Aorta in Order of Frequency

Cardiac	Noncardiac: chromosomal	Noncardiac: other
Patent ductus arteriosus	Turner syndrome	Prematurity
Ventricular septal defect	Trisomy 21	Diaphragmatic hernia
Atrial septal defect	Trisomy 13	Tracheo-esophageal hernia
Aortic valve abnormality	Trisomy 18	Hydrops fetalis
Hypoplastic left heart syndrome	Not specified	DiGeorge syndrome
Transposition of the great arteries		
Mitral valve abnormality		
Endocardial cushion defect		
Common ventricle		
Tricuspid atresia		
Pulmonary stenosis		
Tetralogy of Fallot		

Source: Adapted from Gutgesell et al. (20).

strain because of the role of the right ventricle in supplying the systemic circulation until the duct closes. In older patients, the ECG may be normal or show a pattern of left ventricular hypertrophy as left ventricular mass increases. Older patients with coarctation have an increased frequency of conduction defects although this is a nonspecific finding.

B. Radiological Features

On a plain postero-anterior chest radiograph, the characteristic features of coarctation are absent in a child until the age of 4, and there may be only cardiomegaly and engorgement of the pulmonary vasculature up to this time. The other classic features of coarctation develop after the age of 4. These other features include inferior rib notching that is a result of increased blood flow through collateral vessels and a prestenotic and poststenotic dilatation of the aorta that visually looks like a numeral 3 or an inverted letter E sign. This condition is best detected through use of an orally administered barium test. If coarctation is suspected, either computed tomography (CT) or magnetic resonance imaging (MRI) should be performed. Coarctation can be detected by using either CT or MRI, and it has been suggested that magnetic resonance angiography provides a direct equivalent to standard angiography in mapping the lesion (22). Cardiac catheterization and an aortogram will allow assessment of the coarctation gradient and visualization of the stenosis (Fig. 47.2).

C. Echocardiography

This is now the diagnostic test of choice, especially in neonates. Two-dimensional echocardiography can show

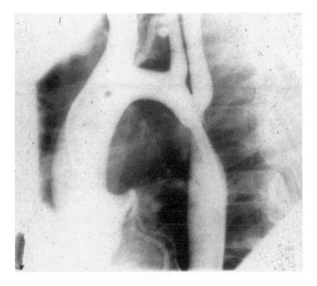

Figure 47.2 Aortogram showing coarctation of the aorta.

the site of coarctation and the presence of other cardiac anomalies. Doppler flow can evaluate the severity of coarctation by measuring the pressure gradients. Transesophageal echocardiography also is widely used and is invaluable intraoperatively.

D. Prenatal Detection

Prenatal detection of coarctation has been possible through the use of a detailed two-dimensional echocardiography for >15 years (23), although it is a difficult diagnosis to make and screening has both a high false-positive rate and a high false-negative rate (24). It has been postulated that prenatal diagnosis allows stabilization prior to surgery; by the time infants are diagnosed postnatally, they tend to be extremely unwell. A recent retrospective analysis of case notes demonstrated that in infants in whom the condition was detected prenatally, there was improved survival and preoperative state when compared with infants who were diagnosed postnatally (25).

VIII.   TREATMENT OPTIONS AND OUTCOME

There are two principal treatment options for correcting coarctation and its effects, and their outcomes vary according to the conditions, timing of the diagnosis, and constraints of the treatment method. The treatment options include surgery and percutaneous intervention.

A.   Surgery

Surgical correction of coarctation of the aorta has been used for >50 years. Common procedures have been resection of the stenosed region with end-to-end anastomosis, resection and extended end-to-end anastomosis, Dacron or polytetrafluoroethylene patch aortoplasty, and subclavian flap repair.

Considering the technical complexity of the surgery, the list of complications is remarkably short. These include perioperative mortality, suboptimal repair, recoarctation, aneurysm formation, and later onset of hypertension. The most feared perioperative complication of coarctectomy is paraplegia that is a result of spinal artery occlusion. The incidence is thought to be 0.1–1.0% with no definitive known predisposing factors. Probable risk factors, however, include poor collaterals, distal hypertension during cross-clamp, anomalies of the origin of the right subclavian artery, and reoperation or relative hyperthermia during surgery. Cunningham et al. (26) and Maeda et al. (27) have demonstrated that the use of somatosensory-evoked potentials can help prevent cord ischemia.

Other perioperative complications include paradoxic hypertension, postcoarctectomy syndrome, and injury to the phrenic and recurrent laryngeal nerves. Paradoxic hypertension is a two-phase phenomenon and was first described by Sealy et al. (28) in 1957. The first phase is a rapid increase in systolic blood pressure within 24 h after the operation that is a result of activation of the sympathetic nervous system with elevation of serum catecholamines. An increase in the diastolic blood pressure occurs ~72 h after surgery and is a result of activation of the renin–angiotensin system. This may lead to postcoarctectomy syndrome with ileus, abdominal pain, mesenteric vasculitis, and even visceral infarction. This syndrome is not encountered if the postoperative diastolic blood pressure is maintained within the normal range. Treatment postoperatively with propranolol appears to minimize occurrence of paradoxic hypertension (29), but its effect on late hypertension remains uncertain.

A large amount of data is now available for evaluating the long-term outcomes of various techniques used in coarctation repair. A few institutes still performed Dacron patch aortoplasty because late aneurysm formation was found to be as high as 51% (30). Individual operator preference, as well as the patient's condition, now underlies the use of resection with end-to-end anastomosis, resection and extended end-to-end anastomosis, or polytetrafluoroethylene patch repair techniques. Walhout et al. (31) compared resection with end-to-end anastomosis and polytetrafluoroethylene patch repair and found no difference between the two techniques in the incidence of recoarctation (21%), although polytetrafluoroethylene patch repair, including coarctation ridge resection, was found to be a risk factor for late aneurysm formation. This compares less favorably with resection and extended end-to-end anastomosis, which is claimed to have a recoractation rate as low as 3.7% (32). In a 40 year review of a single institute's practice, it was found that resection with end-to-end anastomosis and subclavian flap repair, when associated with aortic arch hypoplasia, have a high incidence of restenosis (33); this further supports the use of the resection and extended end-to-end anastomosis technique.

Of more importance have been questions about when to operate and about the relationship to long-term survival and the development of hypertension. These questions pertain to elective patients, because in the case of neonates with compensated coarctation of aorta, it has been standard to proceed to surgery as an emergency as soon as possible after a short period of stabilization.

The ideal time to operate in elective patients remains controversial. Repair during infancy was associated with a higher rate of recurrence than later repair (34,35). Delaying the repair until later in childhood, on the other hand, carries a higher risk of late hypertension (36,37). Data from older studies in the 1970s and 1980s suggested that perioperative mortality was lowest in infants between the age of 1 and 14 and then steadily rose to its peak at a patient age of >30 years (38). Toro-Salazar et al. (12) reported the outcome in 274 patients who underwent coarctation repair between 1948 and 1976 and showed that the lowest perioperative mortality was in the 5–10-year-old group at 1.4% compared with an age of <1 at 2.2%, an age of 1–5 at 4.6%, and an age of >10 at 6.4%, respectively (Fig. 47.3). However, when each group was reviewed at a 20 year follow-up of these patients, the outcomes were reversed, with survival being highest (95.4%) in the original 1–5-year-old group compared with 91.4% in original 5–10-year-old group. At a 40 year follow-up, the survival probability was 91.3% in original <1-year-old group of patients, 95.4% in the original 1–5-year-old group, 87.1% in the original 5–10-year-old group, and 60.5% in the original >10-year-old group (Table 47.2). The overall life expectancy for the group of patients as a whole was 95% at 10 years postrepair, 89% at 20 years postrepair, 82% at 30 years postrepair, and 79% at 40 years postrepair. This data implied that the optimum age for coarctation repair is when the patient is 1–5-year-old. Data from current surgical era by Seirafi et al. (39), suggest that elective coarctation repair should be performed within the first year of life to minimize the risk of late hypertension.

With the improvement in surgical techniques and technology, surgery-related mortality is related almost exclusively to associated cardiac anomalies. The devastating complications of paraplegia and mesenteric ischemia have been eliminated. The focus now is to try to perfect the techniques of coarctation repair to eliminate recoarctation and minimize late postoperative hypertension.

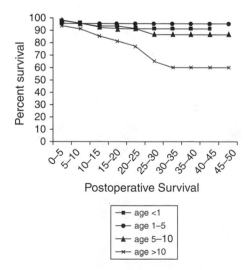

Figure 47.3 Mortality in survivors of coarctation repair with respect to age of patient at the time the operation was performed.

Table 47.2 Survival Probability Stratified by Age at the Time the Operation was Performed

Number of years after surgery	Patient age at time of operation ($n = 252$) (% surviving $\pm$ SE)			
	<1 year (n = 47)	>1 ≤5 years (n = 22)	≥5 ≤10 years (n = 74)	>10 years (n = 109)
0–5	97.8 ± 2.1	95.4 ± 4.4	98.6 ± 1	93.6 ± 2.2
5–10	95.7 ± 2.9	95.4 ± 4.4	95.9 ± 1.4	91.6 ± 2.5
10–15	93.6 ± 3.6	95.4 ± 4.4	93.1 ± 1.8	85.6 ± 3.2[a]
15–20[b]	93.6 ± 3.6	95.4 ± 4.4	91.4 ± 2.1	81.4 ± 3.4[b]
20–25	91.3 ± 4.2	95.4 ± 4.4	91.4 ± 2.4	76.8 ± 3.7[c]
25–30	91.3 ± 4.2	95.4 ± 4.4	87.1 ± 3[d]	65.2 ± 4.4[c]
30–35	91.3 ± 4.2	95.4 ± 4.4	87.1 ± 3[d]	60.5 ± 4.7[c]
35–40	91.3 ± 4.2	95.4 ± 4.4	87.1 ± 3[d]	60.5 ± 4.7[c]
40–45	91.3 ± 4.2	95.4 ± 4.4	87.1 ± 3[d]	60.5 ± 4.7[c]
45–50		95.4 ± 4.4	87.1 ± 3[d]	60.5 ± 4.7[c,d]

[a]$P < 0.05$ for <1 year, >1 ≤5 years, ≥5 ≤10 years >10 years.
[b]$P < 0.01$ for <1 year, >1 ≤5 years, ≥5 ≤10 years >10 years.
[c]$P < 0.001$ for <1 year, >1 ≤5 years, ≥5 ≤10 years >10 years.
[d]$P < 0.05$ for >1 ≤5 years vs. ≥5 ≤10 years.
Note: SE, standard error.
Source: Toro-Salazar et al. (12).

B. Percutaneous Intervention

The first case of balloon angioplasty for coarctation was reported in 1982 (40), and since then it has become the accepted procedure for repairing recoarctation following previous surgery. Its role as the primary treatment modality in native coarctation did not become popular until the 1990s. Early limitations were related to the technique used and the devices that were available and to suboptimal immediate results that were caused by elastic recoil. Earlier studies of balloon angioplasty also reported a significantly high postprocedural aneurysm rate of 5–55% (41), although these aneurysms were now thought to be related to over dilatation. The limitations associated with balloon angioplasty motivated the use of endovascular stenting following the first report on this technique by O'Laughlin et al. (42) in 1991.

Zabal et al. (43) reported their experience comparing balloon angioplasty and primary stenting in adult patients with native coarctation and showed that the procedure was safe, with zero mortality. The event rate (defined in this case as unsuccessful dilatation, aneurysm formation, a residual gradient >20 mmHg, recoarctation, or hypertension) was 14.8% overall, although all but one of these occurred in the balloon angioplasty group. Subanalysis suggests that all such events occurred in patients in whom the intra-aortic gradient failed to drop <10 mmHg and that in these patients the operator should proceed to stent deployment at the same session. In addition, it is suggested that all nondiscrete lesions and all lesions with pre- or poststenotic aneurysm should be stented. A potentially beneficial role for stenting is to function as a bridge to surgery in the duct-dependant neonate.

To date, 369 cases of aortic stenting have been reported in series (44–56) (Table 47.3) with 240 cases in patients with native coarctation, which included both children and adults. Generally excellent results have been achieved with almost complete abolishment of gradient in >95% of the cases. Restenosis has not been a major problem, and further dilatation for residual stenosis also has been effective so far. In adddition, stents are effective in treating coarctation with hypoplasia of the isthmus and transverse arch as well as in cases of long tubular stricture. Blood pressure control usually improved following stenting, and there appears to be a beneficial effect on left ventricular end-diastolic function (47).

Major complications seem to be rare. No deaths have been reported to date, and the need of emergency surgery is in <1% of cases. Late aneurysm formation is reported in 4% of cases, although their true incidence in unknown. The inherent bias in reporting such series is likely to underestimate the incidence of major complications, so the data should be viewed cautiously. Other complications include balloon rupture, malposition of the stent, stent embolization, femoral artery access-site neurovascular complications, myocardial infarction, and stroke. Many of these complications can be avoided with increased experience and improvements in the technology.

The short-term results of transcatheter treatment of aortic coarctation with endovascular stenting appear excellent and encouraging. This is particularly true in the case

Table 47.3   Results of Stent Implantation for Coarctation of Aorta in Studies of Adult Patients

Study	Number of patients	Native/Rec.A	Age in years (range)	Peak systolic gradient mean (mmHg)		Number of complications (major/minor)	FU aneurysm/n (%)
				Preballoon	Poststent		
Bulbul et al. (45)	6	2/4	19.8 + 5.1 (13–34)	36.7 + 16.9	13.3 + 23.2	0/1	—
Ebeid et al. (46)	9	2/7	(14–63)	37 + 7	4 + 1	—	—
Magee et al. (47)	17	6/11	(4.4–45)	26	5	0/5	1/7 (14)
Suarez de Lezo et al. (48)	48	42/6	14 + 12 (0.5–45)	42 + 12	3 + 4	1/6	2/30 (6)
Marshall et al. (49)	33	6/27	(5–60)	25[a]	5[a]	1/2	0/16[b]
Thanopoulos et al. (55)	17	6/9	0.4–15	50 + 24.5	2.1 + 2.4	0	0
Alcibar et al. (51)	14	11/3	20 + 12	43 + 19	2 + 12	0	0/7
Hamdan et al. (50)	33	13/21	16+8 (4–36)	32 + 12	4 + 11	2/4	0/4
Harrison et al. (52)	27	20/7	30.1 + 13 (14–63)	46 + 20	3 + 5	1/0	3/18 (17)
Cheatham (56)	46	25/21	—	—	—	—	—
Ledesma et al. (53)	54	49/5	22+9 (8–49)	50 + 20	5 + 8	0/6	0/1
Duke et al. (54)	22	15/7	23.3 (5.6–65)	20.5	2.5	0/3	0/20
Zabal et al. (43)	22(32)	22/0	25.9 + 7.9	63.9 + 20.8	2.7 + 4.3	0/1	
Tyagi et al. (44)	21	21/0	28.6 + 11.2 (18–61)	68.4 + 22	8.3 + 4.2	0/1	0/19

[a]Median.
[b]Balloon angioplasty followed by stent.
Note: ReCoa, recoarctation.
Source: Adapted from Tyagi et al. (44).

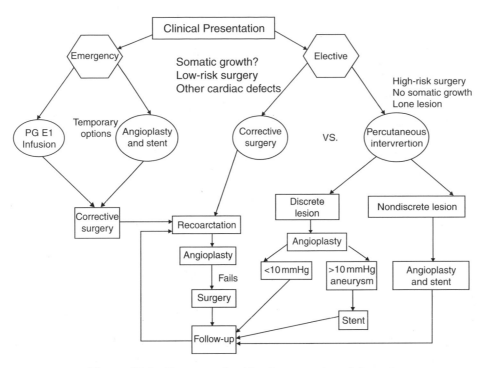

Figure 47.4 Treatment algorithm for coarctation of the aorta.

of adults in whom the operative risk is much higher. However, case numbers are small, and long-term data are needed to evaluate the ultimate outcomes.

Figure 47.4 suggests a possible decision-making flow chart that takes into account patient characteristics and data from the current literature.

IX. CONCLUSIONS

Coarctation of the aorta provides a unique challenge to the physician and surgeon. Prenatal diagnosis is now possible and may help to stabilize the patient prior to intervention. When coarctation is detected, early repair must be considered. The optimal period for elective surgical repair is around 1 year of age. This strategy provides both the lowest perioperative mortality and the best 50 year survival rate. If the condition is detected in patients present after the age of 1, repair should be considered immediately to improve the long-term prognosis. Even when the condition has been anatomically repaired and patients are "cured," up to 30% of individuals will develop late hypertension and another 20% will have exercise-induced hypertension. These patients also are at risk of accelerated coronary artery disease and cerebrovascular events. Strict control of blood pressure along with appropriate reduction of other cardiovascular and cerebrovascular risks should minimize subsequent morbidity and mortality. The clinician also should proactively evaluate the patient for the presence of other cardiac malformations and manage them.

The benefits of angioplasty and stenting over surgery remain to be determined, although these are definitely viable alternative treatment strategies, and the current short-term results are very encouraging. It is anticipated that stenting may become the default option for catheter-based intervention in the future if current trends with respect to results continue. All patients with treated coarctation should have active follow-up with detailed scanning, preferably magnetic resonance angiography, which makes possible an accurate assessment of the aorta, and with exercise testing to predict future risk.

REFERENCES

1. Ferencz C, Rubin JD, McCarter RJ, Brenner JI, Neill CA, Perry LW, Hepner SI, Downing JW. Congenital heart disease: prevalence at livebirth. The Baltimore–Washington Infant Study. Am J Epidemiol 1985; 121:31–36.
2. Maestri NE, Beaty TH, Boughman JA. Etiologic heterogeneity in the familial aggregation of congenital cardiovascular malformations. Am J Hum Genet 1989; 45:556–564.
3. Lund J, Roe B, Chen F, Budarf M, Galili N, Riblet R, Miller RD, Emanuel BS, Reeves RH. Sequence-ready physical map of the mouse chromosome 16 region with conserved synteny to the human velocardiofacial syndrome region on 22q11.2. Mamm Genome 1999; 10:438–443.

4. Loffredo CA, Wilson PD, Ferencz C. Maternal diabetes: an independent risk factor for major cardiovascular malformations with increased mortality of affected infants. Teratology 2001; 64:98–106.

5. Loffredo CA. Epidemiology of cardiovascular malformations: prevalence and risk factors. Am J Med Genet 2000; 97:319–325.

6. Tikkanen J, Heinonen OP. Risk factors for coarctation of the aorta. Teratology 1993; 47:565–572.

7. Wollins DS, Ferencz C, Boughman JA, Loffredo CA. A population-based study of coarctation of the aorta: comparisons of infants with and without associated ventricular septal defect. Teratology 2001; 64:229–236.

8. Weinstein BM, Stemple DL, Driever W, Fishman MC. Gridlock, a localized heritable vascular patterning defect in the zebrafish. Nat Med 1995; 1:1143–1147.

9. Brouwer RM, Erasmus ME, Ebels T, Eijgelaar A. Influence of age on survival, late hypertension, and recoarctation in elective aortic coarctation repair. Including long-term results after elective aortic coarctation repair with a follow-up from 25 to 44 years. J Thorac Cardiovasc Surg 1994; 108:525–531.

10. O'Sullivan JJ, Derrick G, Darnell R. Prevalence of hypertension in children after early repair of coarctation of the aorta: a cohort study using casual and 24 hour blood pressure measurement. Heart 2002; 88:163–166.

11. Cohen M, Fuster V, Steele PM, Driscoll D, McGoon DC. Coarctation of the aorta. Long-term follow-up and prediction of outcome after surgical correction. Circulation 1989; 80:840–845.

12. Toro-Salazar OH, Steinberger J, Thomas W, Rocchini AP, Carpenter B, Moller JH. Long-term follow-up of patients after coarctation of the aorta repair. Am J Cardiol 2002; 89:541–547.

13. Ong CM, Canter CE, Gutierrez FR, Sekarski DR, Goldring DR. Increased stiffness and persistent narrowing of the aorta after successful repair of coarctation of the aorta: relationship to left ventricular mass and blood pressure at rest and with exercise. Am Heart J 1992; 123:1594–1600.

14. Gidding SS, Rocchini AP, Moorehead C, Schork MA, Rosenthal A. Increased forearm vascular reactivity in patients with hypertension after repair of coarctation. Circulation 1985; 71:495–499.

15. Gardiner HM, Celermajer DS, Sorensen KE, Georgakopoulos D, Robinson J, Thomas O, Deanfield JE. Arterial reactivity is significantly impaired in normotensive young adults after successful repair of aortic coarctation in childhood. Circulation 1994; 89:1745–1750.

16. Barton CH, Ni Z, Vaziri ND. Enhanced nitric oxide inactivation in aortic coarctation-induced hypertension. Kidney Int 2001; 60:1083–1087.

17. Ross RD, Clapp SK, Gunther S, Paridon SM, Humes RA, Farooki ZQ, Pinsky WW. Augmented norepinephrine and renin output in response to maximal exercise in hypertensive coarctectomy patients. Am Heart J 1992; 123:1293–1299.

18. Mullen MJ. Coarctation of the aorta in adults: do we need surgeons? Heart 2003; 89:3–5.

19. Swan L, Goyal S, Hsia C, Hechter S, Webb G, Gatzoulis MA. Exercise systolic blood pressures are of questionable value in the assessment of the adult with a previous coarctation repair. Heart 2003; 89:189–192.

20. Gutgesell HP, Barton DM, Elgin KM. Coarctation of the aorta in the neonate: associated conditions, management, and early outcome. Am J Cardiol 2001; 88:457–459.

21. Lip GY. Singh SP, Beevers DG. Aortic coarctation diagnosed after hypertension in pregnancy. Am J Obstet Gynecol 1998; 179:814–815.

22. Godart F, Labrot G, Devos P, McFadden E, Rey C, Beregi JP. Coarctation of the aorta: comparison of aortic dimensions between conventional MR imaging, 3D MR angiography, and conventional angiography. Eur Radiol 2002; 12:2034–2039.

23. Allan LD, Chita SK, Anderson RH, Fagg N, Crawford DC, Tynan MJ. Coarctation of the aorta in prenatal life: an echocardiographic, anatomical, and functional study. Br Heart J 1988; 59:356–360.

24. Sharland GK, Chan KY, Allan LD. Coarctation of the aorta: difficulties in prenatal diagnosis. Br Heart J 1994; 71:70–75.

25. Franklin O, Burch M, Manning N, Sleeman K, Gould S, Archer N. Prenatal diagnosis of coarctation of the aorta improves survival and reduces morbidity. Heart 2002; 87:67–69.

26. Cunningham JN Jr, Laschinger JC, Merkin HA, Nathan IM, Colvin S, Ransohoff J, Spencer FC. Measurement of spinal cord ischemia during operations upon the thoracic aorta: initial clinical experience. Ann Surg 1982; 196:285–296.

27. Maeda S, Miyamoto T, Murata H, Yamashita K, Iwaoka S, Yasuoka T, Hara Y, Ueda T. Prevention of spinal cord ischemia by monitoring spinal cord perfusion pressure and somatosensory evoked potentials. J Cardiovasc Surg (Torino) 1989; 30:565–571.

28. Sealy WC, Harris JS, Young WG Jr, Callaway HA Jr. Paradoxical hypertension following resection of coarctation of aorta. Surgery 1957; 42:135–147.

29. Gidding SS, Rocchini AP, Beekman R, Szpunar CA, Moorehead C, Behrendt D, Rosenthal A. Therapeutic effect of propranolol on paradoxical hypertension after repair of coarctation of the aorta. N Engl J Med 1985; 312:1224–1228.

30. Parks WJ, Ngo TD, Plauth WH Jr, Bank ER, Sheppard SK, Pettigrew RI, Williams WH. Incidence of aneurysm formation after Dacron patch aortoplasty repair for coarctation of the aorta: long-term results and assessment utilizing magnetic resonance angiography with three-dimensional surface rendering. J Am Coll Cardiol 1995; 26:266–271.

31. Walhout RJ, Lekkerkerker JC, Oron GH, Hitchcock FJ, Meijboom EJ, Bennink GB. Comparison of polytetrafluoroethylene patch aortoplasty and end-to-end anastomosis for coarctation of the aorta. J Thorac Cardiovasc Surg 2003; 126:521–528.

32. Backer CL, Mavroudis C, Zias EA, Amin Z, Weigel TJ. Repair of coarctation with resection and extended end-to-end anastomosis. Ann Thorac Surg 1998; 66:1365–1370; discussion 1370–1371.

33. Dodge-Khatami A, Backer CL, Mavroudis C. Risk factors for recoarctation and results of reoperation: a 40-year review. J Card Surg 2000; 15:369–377.

34. Kappetein AP, Zwinderman AH, Bogers AJ, Rohmer J, Huysmans HA. More than thirty-five years of coarctation repair. An unexpected high relapse rate. J Thorac Cardiovasc Surg 1994; 107:87–95.

35. van Heurn LW, Wong CM, Spiegelhalter DJ, Sorensen K, de Leval MR, Stark J, Elliott MJ. Surgical treatment of aortic coarctation in infants younger than three months: 1985 to 1990. Success of extended end-to-end arch aortoplasty. J Thorac Cardiovasc Surg 1994; 107:74–85; discussion 85–86.

36. Koller M, Rothlin M, Senning A. Coarctation of the aorta: review of 362 operated patients. Long-term follow-up and assessment of prognostic variables. Eur Heart J 1987; 8:670–679.

37. Clarkson PM, Nicholson MR, Barratt-Boyes BG, Neutze JM, Whitlock RM. Results after repair of coarctation of the aorta beyond infancy: a 10 to 28 year follow-up with particular reference to late systemic hypertension. Am J Cardiol 1983; 51:1481–1488.

38. Bergdahl L, Bjork VO, Jonasson R. Surgical correction of coarctation of the aorta. Influence of age on late results. J Thorac Cardiovasc Surg 1983; 85:532–526.

39. Seirafi PA, Warner KG, Geggel RL, Payne DD, Cleveland RJ. Repair of coarctation of the aorta during infancy minimizes the risk of late hypertension. Ann Thorac Surg 1998; 66:1378–1382.

40. Singer MI, Rowen M, Dorsey TJ. Transluminal aortic balloon angioplasty for coarctation of the aorta in the newborn. Am Heart J 1982; 103:131–132.

41. Rao PS. Long-term follow-up results after balloon dilatation of pulmonic stenosis, aortic stenosis, and coarctation of the aorta: a review. Prog Cardiovasc Dis 1999; 42:59–74.

42. O'Laughlin MP, Perry SB, Lock JE, Mullins CE. Use of endovascular stents in congenital heart disease. Circulation 1991; 83:1923–1939.

43. Zabal C, Attie F, Rosas M, Buendia-Hernandez A, Garcia-Montes JA. The adult patient with native coarctation of the aorta: balloon angioplasty or primary stenting? Heart 2003; 89:77–83.

44. Tyagi S, Singh S, Mukhopadhyay S, Kaul UA. Self- and balloon expandable stent implantation for severe native coarctation of aorta in adults. Am Heart J 2003; 146:920–928.

45. Bulbul ZR, Bruckheimer E, Love JC, Fahey JT, Hellenbrand WE. Implantation of balloon-expandable stents for coarctation of the aorta: implantation data and short-term results. Cathet Cardiovasc Diagn 1996; 39:36–42.

46. Ebeid MR, Prieto LR, Latson LA. Use of balloon-expandable stents for coarctation of the aorta: initial results and intermediate-term follow-up. J Am Coll Cardiol 1997; 30:1847–1852.

47. Magee AG, Brzezinska-Rajszys G, Qureshi SA, Rosenthal E, Zubrzycka M, Ksiazyk J, Tynan M. Stent implantation for aortic coarctation and recoarctation. Heart 1999; 82:600–606.

48. Suarez de Lezo J, Pan M, Romero M, Medina A, Segura J, Lafuente M, Pavlovic D, Hernandez E, Melian F, Espada J. Immediate and follow-up findings after stent treatment for severe coarctation of aorta. Am J Cardiol 1999; 83:400–406.

49. Marshall AC, Perry SB, Keane JF, Lock JE. Early results and medium-term follow-up of stent implantation for mild residual or recurrent aortic coarctation. Am Heart J 2000; 139:1054–1060.

50. Hamdan MA, Maheshwari S, Fahey JT, Hellenbrand WE. Endovascular stents for coarctation of the aorta: initial results and intermediate-term follow-up. J Am Coll Cardiol 2001; 38:1518–1523.

51. Alcibar J, Pena N, Onate A, Cabrera A, Galdeano JM, Pastor E, Inguanzo R, Vitoria Y, Gomez S, Arana JI, Barrenechea JI. Primary stent implantation in aortic coarctation. Mid-term follow-up. Rev Esp Cardiol 2000; 52:797–804.

52. Harrison DA, McLaughlin PR, Lazzam C, Connelly M, Benson LN. Endovascular stents in the management of coarctation of the aorta in the adolescent and adult: one year follow-up. Heart 2001; 85:561–566.

53. Ledesma M, Alva C, Gomez FD, Sanchez-Soberanis A, Diaz y Diaz E, Benitez-Perez C, Herrera-Franco R, Arguero R, Feldman T. Results of stenting for aortic coarctation. Am J Cardiol 2001; 88:460–462.

54. Duke C, Rosenthal E, Qureshi SA. The efficacy and safety of stent redilatation in congenital heart disease. Heart 2003; 89:905–912.

55. Thanopoulos BD, Hadjinikolaou L, Konstadopoulou GN, Tsaousis GS, Triposkiadis F, Spirou P. Stent treatment for coarctation of the aorta: intermediate term follow-up and technical considerations. Heart 2000; 84:65–70.

56. Cheatham JP. Stenting of coarctation of the aorta. Catheter Cardiovasc Interv 2001; 54:112–125.

48

Central Nervous System Diseases and Hypertension

STEFAN T. ENGELTER
University Hospital Basel, Basel, Switzerland

KEYPOINTS

- Central nervous system disease can be the cause of secondary arterial hypertension, but this is a rare scenario.
- Intracranial tumors, traumatic brain injuries, stroke, dolichoectasia or aneurysms of vertebrobasilar arteries, and high spinal cord injuries are the most common central nervous system diseases that can cause arterial hypertension. They usually have distinct clinical neurological signs.
- Hypertension as the sole manifestation of yet unknown central nervous system disease has been reported, but should be considered extremely rare.
- Unusual presentation, such as paroxysmal hypertension in the absence of a pheochromocytoma or

treatment refractory hypertension starting at a very young age, may point to an underlying central nervous system disease. However, the predictive value of clinical characteristics in order to reveal central nervous system disease-related hypertension has yet to be studied.
- Magnetic resonance imaging (MRI) of the brain covering also the cranio-cervical junction is the diagnostic tool of choice to reveal an underlying central nervous system disease in suspected secondary hypertension.
- Surgical cure of central nervous system disease-related arterial hypertension is possible in selected patients with either hormone-producing tumors or brainstem-compressing lesions.

- In patients with chronic high spinal cord injuries, acute hypertension can occur as a result of autonomic dysreflexia. Lacking supraspinal control, overreaction of the spinal sympathetic nervous system below level T6 triggered by a noxious stimulus can result in hypertensive crises.
- Autonomic dysreflexia is common in patients with chronic high upper spinal cord injuries, with lifetime frequencies ranging from 20% to 70%.

SUMMARY

Central nervous system diseases are a rare cause of secondary hypertension. Intracranial tumors, spinal cord injuries, traumatic brain injuries, ischemic and hemorrhagic stroke, medullary compression by ectactic vertebrobasilar arteries, as well as idiopathic intracranial hypertension, and several other rare diseases can lead to arterial hypertension by multiple mechanisms. No data are available about the discriminative power of clinical characteristics in stratifying, in which hypertensive patients with an underlying central nervous system disease should be searched for. As a rough rule of thumb, paroxysmal hypertension without evidence of pheochromocytoma, treatment refectory hypertension starting at a very young age, and the occurrence of hypertension associated with central neurological signs may point to an underlying central nervous system disease. In such situations, MRI of the brain with covering the cranio-cervical junction is the diagnostic method of choice to reveal central nervous system abnormalities that are possibly responsible for arterial hypertension. Treatment recommendations depend on the nature of the central nervous system disease. Surgical cure has been reported in some space-occupying lesions and brainstem distortion-producing lesions. In patients with injury to the upper end of the spinal cord, autonomic dysreflexia is a common cause of acute hypertension. Removal of the noxious trigger is crucial, followed by applying antihypertensive agents.

I. INTRODUCTION

Hypertension is a major risk factor for several diseases of the central nervous system, such as acute stroke, chronic brain ischemia, vascular dementia, and hypertensive encephalopathy. Chapter 17 has elaborated on how arterial hypertension causes or contributes to these central nervous system diseases. Conversely, central nervous system diseases themselves can be the cause of arterial hypertension. Although epidemiological studies are missing, central nervous system diseases that result

in arterial hypertension should be considered a rare condition estimated to account for <1% of all hypertensive patients.

This chapter provides a brief overview about the mechanisms by which central nervous system disorders can result in arterial hypertension. In addition, possible clinical indicators for underlying central nervous system diseases are discussed. Several central nervous system diseases that can cause arterial hypertension are described and diagnostic procedures and therapeutic options for treating them are discussed.

II. PATHOPHYSIOLOGY AND MECHANISMS OF CENTRAL NERVOUS SYSTEM DISEASE-RELATED ARTERIAL HYPERTENSION

The physiology and pathophysiology of central nervous control of blood pressure are broadly discussed in Chapter 10. The following paragraph provides a brief overview of the most important mechanisms.

First, increased arterial blood pressure can result as a consequence of increased intracranial pressure after a specific threshold is reached. The sense of this pressure response, namely, Cushing response is to maintain a difference between both pressures in order to assure cerebral perfusion. The Cushing response is mediated from the medulla oblongata and operates without higher brainstem or supratentorial regions, as early animal studies have shown.

Secondly, compression or distortion of the brainstem, particularly those of the medulla oblongata, can result in hypertension by compromising medullary pressure regions also in the absence of elevated intracranial pressure.

Thirdly, an increase in catecholamine production (1) or upregulated sympathetic activity (2) can trigger arterial hypertension.

Fourthly, baroreflex dysfunction can occur by injury of pressure regulating medullary sides. As a consequence, the ability of the baroreflex to buffer changes of the vascular tone is impaired, as suggested recently (3).

Fifthly, according to older experimental studies, stimulation of supratentorial lesions has been reported to increase blood pressure, in addition. However, it remains unclear whether these supramedullary mechanisms actually can be considered as independent pathways in generating arterial hypertension as a result of a central nervous system disease.

Sixthly, autonomic dysreflexia, defined as sympathetic overreaction below a high spinal cord lesion, is a mechanism of acute hypertension operative in tetraplegic patients.

III. CLINICAL INDICATORS OF A CENTRAL NERVOUS SYSTEM DISEASE-CAUSING ARTERIAL HYPERTENSION

Central nervous system diseases causing arterial hypertension are rare. In addition, most such patients present with neurological signs and symptoms of the underlying central nervous system disease; arterial hypertension is a subsidiary finding. Furthermore, the presence of arterial hypertension and central nervous system disease in a given patient can reflect a coincidental, rather than a causal relationship. However, there are some reported cases in which hypertension is the presenting symptom of an yet unknown central nervous system disease (4,5). The problem in clinical practice is, therefore, to identify those hypertensive patients in whom a yet to be detected central nervous system disease may be operative. It has been suggested that atypical presentation of hypertension might indicate an underlying central nervous system disease. Hypertension may start abruptly, may be refractory to treatment from the beginning, show a paroxysmal pattern, or may affect children or most elderly. However, such features usually trigger diagnostic workup for a secondary cause of hypertension that is mostly unrevealing. Only 2% of the patients with paroxysmal hypertension, for example, have pheochromocytomas. Interestingly, several case studies of central nervous system disease-related hypertension had the same paroxysmal blood pressure increase (6–9). Others describe a persistent pattern of arterial hypertension (4,5). In terms of the age of the patient, although some patients were children (7) or young adults (4,5), age at hypertension onset was in middle-aged or advanced-aged individuals reported by others (2,6,10). In the absence of any systematic investigations, it remains speculative whether specific blood pressure pattern (e.g., paroxysmal hypertension) and early onset hypertension are useful indicators of an underling central nervous system disease. In fact, the frequent occurrence of these clinical features in case reports of central nervous system disease-related hypertension may simply reflect a selection or publication bias. Thus, the value of distinct clinical characteristics in answering the question of which hypertensive patients should have investigations to reveal a causal central nervous system disease has yet to be studied systematically (11). In the meantime, as a rough rule of thumb, in patients with paroxysmal hypertension in the absence of a pheochromocytoma or treatment refractory hypertension starting at a very young age, a diagnostic search for one of the central nervous system diseases described in the next section might be justified, especially if there are also neurological signs or symptoms.

IV. CENTRAL NERVOUS SYSTEM DISEASES THAT CAUSE ARTERIAL HYPERTENSION

The pathological conditions in the central nervous system that are known to cause arterial hypertension include the following:

- Tumors
- Spinal cord injury
- Traumatic brain injury
- Stroke
- Dolichoectasia and aneurysm of vertebrobasilar arteries
- Idiopathic intracranial hypertension
- Other more rare central nervous system diseases

A. Tumors

Intracranial tumors are associated with arterial hypertension. Specifically, neoplasms in the posterior fossa are assumed to have a significantly higher prevalence of hypertension (9%) when compared with supratentorial tumors ($\sim$1%), as reported in early studies published in 1935 by Ask-Upmark (12). Supratentorially, meningeomas, gliomas, and astrocytomas located in the frontal, temporal, or parietal lobes have been reported. Infratentorially, medulloblastomas, astrocytomas, gliomas, hemangioblastomas located in the cervico-medullary junction, the medulla oblongata, the cerebellum, or the pons have been described (1,5,7,10,12). Catecholamine and catecholamine metabolite levels were elevated during the hypertensive episodes in several patients, but normal in others. Paroxysmal hypertension was a frequent but not an unique finding reported in these case studies.

Tumors of the posterior fossa can cause arterial hypertension by increased intracranial pressure, increased catecholamine production, and direct stimulation or inhibition of cardiovascular centers in the medulla. The nucleus tractus solitarius and the caudal ventrolateral medulla have inhibitory effects; the rostral ventrolateral medulla has excitatory effects on sympathetic outflow (11). In particular, tumors affecting the left side of these medullary areas can cause arterial hypertension.

In many patients with supratentorial tumors, an acute increase in blood pressure indicates brain herniation as a preterminal feature.

About one-third of the patients with hormone secreting tumors, such as pituitary adenomas (e.g., acromegaly), have arterial hypertension. Please see Chapter 46 for further details about endocrinological forms of hypertension.

As diagnostic method of choice, MRI should be performed, if an intracranial tumor responsible for arterial hypertension is suspected. MRI has the advantage of a higher spatial resolution and less artifacts when compared with computed tomography scanning. Furthermore, modern magnetic resonance sequences, such as diffusion and perfusion imaging, provide additional hints regarding the histological type or the grade of malignancy of a brain tumor (13). Removal of the tumor has been shown to cure arterial hypertension in some case reports (1,5). In several cases, sudden and marked drops in blood pressure immediately after surgery have been reported (4,5), which made dopamine infusion necessary. Within a few weeks, blood pressure reached normal values, and there was no need for further antihypertensive medication in most of these patients (4,5).

Patients in whom surgery was not possible, radio and chemotherapies should be considered, depending on the histological findings. In the clinical case study of a 10-year-old boy with astrocytoma Grad 2 adherent to the left side of the brainstem near the floor of the fourth ventricle, such an approach was successful both in improvement of the neurological findings and in better control of his hypertension (7).

Dexamethasone (initially 8–12 mg iv, followed by 4 mg iv every 6 h) could be used to reduce the surrounding vasogenic edema, which is not curative but may relieve the patient's symptoms.

In patients who underwent brainstem surgery for tumor removal, acute arterial hypertension that was not present preoperatively has been described. Autonomic dysreflexia, typically occurring in spinal cord patients, was the underlying mechanism.

B. Spinal Cord Injury

In chronic spinal cord injury, acute hypertension can occur as a result of sympathetic overshooting caused by spinal reflex mechanisms, namely, autonomic dysreflexia. Autonomic dysreflexia can appear in patients with spinal cord lesions at level T6 or higher. In these patients, a considerable portion of the spinal sympathetic nervous system lacks supraspinal control. Thus, a noxious stimulus, mostly from bladder distension (e.g., obstruction of urine catheter), below the level of the lesion generates a spinal cord-mediated sympathetic response that results in arterial hypertension (14). The increase in blood pressure is more pronounced in complete than in incomplete transverse spinal cord lesions. In incomplete cord lesions, some of the descending central inhibitory pathways remain intact, although they are blocked in complete spinal cord injuries.

The clinical picture of autonomic dysreflexia is a sudden increase in blood pressure, which can reach values up to 240/140 mmHg. However, it is important to remember that resting blood pressure declines after a spinal cord injury, often to ~90/60 mmHg. Thus, even a

blood pressure of 120/80 mmHg might be considered elevated (15). Further symptoms are bilateral pounding headaches, along with flushing, sweating, and nasal congestion. These signs reflect the hypertension-mediated parasympathetic output lacking the sympathetic counterpart above the spinal cord lesion. Concerning heart rate, tachycardia, and less often bradycardia are seen (14,15). The diagnosis is based on the mentioned clinical signs and symptoms. Treatment should start immediately. The first step in measurement is to seat a patient upright to provoke an orthostatic decline in blood pressure (15). The next step is to search for and eliminate noxious triggers. Particularly, urinary catheterization should be done. Or if an indwelling catheter is already present, any obstructions should be removed. If symptoms are still present and systolic blood pressure is ≥ 150 mmHg, antihypertensive agents should be given (15). Nifedipine in a dose of 10 mg is often used. Alternatively, transdermal nitrates applied on the skin above the level of the spinal cord lesion can be used. The advantage of this application is that treatment can be stopped readily when normal blood pressures are achieved. This approach reduces the chance for subsequent hypotension. As a caveat, before using nitrates, male patients should be asked whether they take sildenafil for the treatment of erectile dysfunction; the use of sildenafil within the previous 24 h is a contraindication for nitrates because of the risk of profound hypotension (14). If neither of these agents are successful, sodium nitroprusside can be used. Hydralazine, clonidine, and magnesium sulfate (dose of 5 g $>$15 min followed by 1–2 g/h) have been successfully used (15–17).

Autonomic dysreflexia is common among patients who had a spinal cord injury. The wide spectrum of lifetime frequencies, ranging from 20% in more recent studies up to 70% in older studies, may indicate that owing to consequent prophylaxis the prevalence has decreased in recent years (15).

Though well recognized in chronic spinal cord lesions, autonomic dysreflexia also can occur in acute spinal cord injury. The incidence in the acute stage is estimated to be ~5% (18).

C. Traumatic Brain Injury

Hypertension after traumatic brain injury can have several causes. In severe injuries, increased intracranial pressure causes the increase in blood pressure via the Cushing response. Such patients should be monitored in an intensive care unit with intracranial pressure monitoring, optimal body and neck positioning, treatment to relieve pain, elimination of hypoxia, and correction of hyponatremia. Hyperventilation and mannitol administration are the next steps. Propofol, pentobarbital, or hypothermia can be used in selected patients. However, a detailed discussion about the management of traumatic brain injury is outside the scope of this chapter.

Alternative mechanisms of hypertension caused by brain trauma are direct injuries to the centers of blood pressure regulation and high levels of circulating catecholamines from generalized traumas. Treatment with a β-blocker is appropriate in these situations (19). Pheochromocytomas unmasked after trauma and occult spinal cord injuries with autonomic dysreflexia represent alternative, although uncommon, causes of hypertension after brain injury (19).

D. Stroke

Hypertension is a major risk factor for stroke (Chapter 17). Furthermore, most stroke patients present with raised blood pressure. Usually, blood pressure decline occurs without specific therapy. However, in rare occasions stroke itself can be the cause for secondary hypertension (2,9). All mentioned case reports had brainstem strokes and presented with paroxysmal hypertension. In one patient, MRI demonstrated major infarction of the left medulla oblongata in the area of the nucleus tractus solitarius and intermediate reticular zone, where all the baroreceptor afferents enter the brainstem. This infarction led to baroreflex dysfunction over a 20 day period, mimicking pheochromocytoma.

MRI with diffusion-weighted imaging sequences should be performed, if brainstem stroke is clinically suspected. Diffusion-weighted imaging offers a high lesion detection rate in infratentorial strokes and provides hints to the underlying etiology (20).

E. Dolichoectasia and Aneurysm of Vertebrobasilar Arteries

Dilation of vertebrobasilar arteries that results in dolichoectasia or aneurysms of vertebrobasilar arteries have been described to cause arterial hypertension by vascular compression of the brainstem (21–23). Particular attention has been focused on the left ventrolateral medulla oblongata. On the basis of results from animal studies, the assumed mechanism is that vessel ectasia contributes to arterial elongation and looping at the base of the brain. An arterial loop causes pulsatile compression of medullary pressure areas that stimulate sympathetic pathways and results in increased blood pressure. Early case reports, such as that of a patient with basilar artery aneurysm and clinical features mimicking pheochromocytoma who was cured of hypertension after microvascular decompression surgery, seemingly proved the value of surgery in these patients (8). However, after mostly successful and beneficial results of microvascular decompression in earlier case series, more recent studies have raised doubts about the importance or relevance of a left-sided neurovascular

contact in the brainstem as a frequent cause of hypertension (24,25); neurovascular contact or compression of the ventral medulla oblongata on the left or right side was a frequent finding both in hypertensive patients and in normotensive control individuals (26).

F. Idiopathic Intracranial Hypertension

Marked increases in intracranial pressure caused by tumors usually result in arterial hypertension (Cushing response). Such a pressure response is less frequently found in idiopathic intracranial hypertension. Digre and Corbert (27) reported that 42% of their male and 21% of their female patients with idiopathic intracranial hypertension also had arterial hypertension. In some of the patients, the presence of both idiopathic intracranial hypertension and arterial hypertension may be coincidental, considering that $\sim$90% of patients with idiopathic intracranial hypertension are overweight (28). Furthermore, two patients were diagnosed recently with idiopathic intracranial hypertension plus arterial hypertension and primary hyperaldosteronism, which is a result of adrenal adenoma (29). Endocrine extra–central nervous system lesions that mimic central nervous system-related hypertension may be the actual cause of hypertension in these patients.

Idiopathic intracranial hypertension has been attributed to cerebral sinus venous stenosis, vitamin A intoxication, drug side effects, and others (30). The typical patient is young obese women who have complaints about chronic daily headache and, less frequently, about tinnitus or visual disturbances. Neurological evaluation shows only papilledema and, in some cases, diplopia, which is due to sixth nerve palsy. Lumbar puncture shows increased intracranial pressure and is otherwise normal. MRI is normal except for an empty sella and excludes hydrocephalus, intracranial mass, or other structural lesions (33).

Treatment focuses on the decrease of the elevated intracranial pressure. About one-fifth of the patients experience some symptom relief after the first diagnostic lumbar puncture. Repetitive lumbar punctures can be done. Acetazolamide (500 mg two times/day) has been helpful because it depresses the production of cerebrospinal fluid. It can be combined with furosemid (20–80 mg/day). Optic nerve sheath fenestration and lumbar peritoneal shunt are options that should be reserved for patients for whom there is a threat of visual loss despite conservative treatment. Weight loss is recommended as long-term management (2,8,31).

G. Other Uncommon Central Nervous System Diseases that Cause Hypertension

Table 49.1 summarizes other central nervous system diseases that can, in very rare occasions, also cause arterial

Table 48.1 Central Nervous System Diseases that Can Cause Arterial Hypertension

More commonly encountered diseases
    Infratentorial- and supratentorial tumors
    Spinal cord injury (acute and chronic)
    Traumatic brain injury (including brainstem surgery)
    Stroke (including subarachnoidal hemorrhage)
    Dolichoectasia/aneurysm of vertebrobasilar arteries
    Idiopathic intracranial hypertension
Rare diseases
    Syndrome of inappropriate antidiuretic hormone secretion
    Multiple-system atrophy with orthostatic dysfunction
    Arnold Chiari malformation
    Bulbar poliomyelitis
    Tabes dorsalis
    Meningoencephalitis
    Postdiphtheritic paralysis
    Prion diseases (e.g., fatal familial insomnia)
    Leigh's disease

Source: Refs (1–10,12,14,18,19,23,27,29,32–39).

hypertension. Chronic syndrome of inappropriate anti-diuretic hormone secretions (SIADH) causing hypertension have been reported in a patient with olfactory neuroblastoma producing arginine vasopressin, also known as antidiuretic hormone (32). In another patient with SIADH and hypertension, the blood pressure increase was attributed to enlarged vascular volumes. Blood pressure declined with fluid restriction (33). However, Padfield and co-workers (34) found that in patients with SIADH, vasopressin was increased, but blood pressure was neither elevated nor there was a correlation between vasopressin concentration and systolic or diastolic pressure. This data questioned the concept that an excess of vasopressin contributes relevantly to the increased blood pressure.

In multiple system atrophy with prominent dysfunction of the autonomic nervous system (formerly named "Shy–Drager Syndrome"), disabling orthostatic hypotension is the primary problem. Nevertheless, about half of these patients have severe supine hypertension, mostly at night. Supine hypertension can be treated with a bedtime transdermal nitroglycerin (35).

Subacute necrotizing encephalopathy (also known as Leigh's disease) with bilateral loss of function of the tractus solitarius (36) has been treated successfully with clonidine (17).

Arnold Chiari malformation was revealed in a child with chronic hypertension. After posterior fossa surgery, chronic hypertension ceased (37). This case illustrates that cranio-cervical junction abnormalities are another very rare, but treatable cause of arterial hypertension in selected cases.

V. PITFALLS AND DANGERS

The most important danger in secondary hypertension that is a result of central nervous system diseases is a rapid and marked blood pressure decline in the setting of acute stroke, triggered by aggressive antihypertensive treatment (40). Up to 70% of acute stroke patients have hypertensive blood pressures ($\geq 170/100$ mmHg) (41). Some patients, especially those with lacunar infarcts, may have systolic blood pressures ≥ 200 mmHg (41,42). Nevertheless, these high blood pressure values are usually clinically well tolerated. Furthermore, during the first 4–7 days, there is a spontaneous decline in blood pressure (41,42). The optimal strategy for blood pressure management in acute stroke has been debated again recently (43). Nevertheless, the current consensus is to withhold anti-hypertensive agents unless the diastolic blood pressure is >120 mmHg or the systolic blood pressure is >220 mmHg (44). There are situations that might require urgent blood pressure lowering therapy; however, these include aortic dissection, acute pulmonary edema, acute myocardial infarction, and thrombolytic stroke treatment (44,45). When antihypertensive treatment is indicated, blood pressure should be lowered cautiously. Labetalol (10–20 mg iv $>$1–2 min) is recommended because it can easily be titrated with minimal vasodilation of the cerebral blood vessels. Calcium antagonists (e.g., nimodipine) should be avoided because hazardous effects with a worsening of the stroke syndrome have been reported in a randomized controlled trial (46).

REFERENCES

1. Hedderwick SA, Bishop AE, Strong AJ, Ritter JM. Surgical cure of hypertension in a patient with brainstem capillary haemangioblastoma containing neuropeptide Y. Postgrad Med J 1995; 71:371–372.
2. Phillips AM, Jardine DL, Parkin PJ, Hughes T, Ikram H. Brain stem stroke causing baroreflex failure and paroxysmal hypertension. Stroke 2000; 31:1997–2001.
3. Jordan J, Toka HR, Heusser K, Toka O, Shannon JR, Tank J. Severely impaired baroreflex-buffering in patients with monogenic hypertension and neurovascular contact. Circulation 2000; 102:2611–2618.
4. Pallini R, Lauretti L, Fernandez E. Chronic arterial hypertension as unique symptom of brainstem astrocytoma. Lancet 1995; 345:1573.
5. Barzo P, Voros E, Csajbok E, Veres R. Odontoidectomy in the treatment of neurogenic hypertension. Case illustration. J Neurosurg 2003; 99:934.
6. Montgomery BM. The basilar artery hypertensive syndrome. Arch Intern Med 1961; 108:559–569.
7. Evans CH, Westfall V, Atuk NO. Astrocytoma mimicking the features of pheochromocytoma. N Engl J Med 1972; 286:1397–1399.

8. Emanuele MA, Dorsch TR, Scarff TB, Lawrence AM. Basilar artery aneurysm simulating pheochromocytoma. Neurology 1981; 31:1560–1561.

9. Gandhavadi B. Hypertension after brainstem stroke. Arch Phys Med Rehabil 1988; 69:130–131.

10. Cameron SJ, Doig A. Cerebellar tumours presenting with clinical features of phaeochromocytoma. Lancet 1970; 1:492–494.

11. Mann SJ. Neurogenic essential hypertension revisited: the case for increased clinical and research attention. Am J Hypertens 2003; 16:881–888.

12. Bell MB. Intracranial disorders and hypertension. In: Laragh JH, Brenner, BM, eds. Hypertension: Pathophysiology, Diagnosis, and Management. New York: Raven Press Ltd, 1995:2451–2458.

13. Wong JC, Provenzale JM, Petrella JR. Perfusion MR imaging of brain neoplasms. AJR Am J Roentgenol 2000; 174:1147–1157.

14. Karlsson AK. Autonomic dysreflexia. Spinal Cord 1999; 37:383–391.

15. Blackmer J. Rehabilitation medicine: 1. Autonomic dysreflexia. CMAJ 2003; 169:931–935.

16. Jones NA, Jones SD. Management of life-threatening autonomic hyper-reflexia using magnesium sulphate in a patient with a high spinal cord injury in the intensive care unit. Br J Anaesth 2002; 88:434–438.

17. Robertson D, Hollister AS, Biaggioni I, Netterville JL, Mosqueda-Garcia R, Robertson RM. The diagnosis and treatment of baroreflex failure. N Engl J Med 1993; 329:1449–1455.

18. Krassioukov AV, Furlan JC, Fehlings MG. Autonomic dysreflexia in acute spinal cord injury: an under-recognized clinical entity. J Neurotrauma 2003; 20:707–716.

19. Sandel ME, Abrams PL, Horn LJ. Hypertension after brain injury: case report. Arch Phys Med Rehabil 1986; 67:469–472.

20. Engelter ST, Wetzel SG, Radue EW, Rausch M, Steck AJ, Lyrer PA. The clinical significance of diffusion-weighted MR imaging in infratentorial strokes. Neurology 2004; 62:574–580.

21. Levy EI, Clyde B, McLaughlin MR, Jannetta PJ. Microvascular decompression of the left lateral medulla oblongata for severe refractory neurogenic hypertension. Neurosurgery 1998; 43:1–6.

22. Jannetta PJ, Segal R, Wolfson SK Jr, Dujovny M, Semba A, Cook EE. Neurogenic hypertension: etiology and surgical treatment. II. Observations in an experimental nonhuman primate model. Ann Surg 1985; 202:253–261.

23. Jannetta PJ, Segal R, Wolfson SK Jr. Neurogenic hypertension: etiology and surgical treatment. I. Observations in 53 patients. Ann Surg 1985; 201:391–398.

24. Hohenbleicher H, Schmitz SA, Koennecke HC, Offermann J, Offermann R, Wolf KJ. Neurovascular contact and blood pressure response in young, healthy, normotensive men. Am J Hypertens 2002; 15:119–124.

25. Hohenbleicher H, Schmitz SA, Koennecke HC, Offermann R, Offermann J, Zeytountchian H. Neurovascular contact of cranial nerve IX and X root-entry zone in hypertensive patients. Hypertension 2001; 37:176–181.

26. Johnson D, Coley SC, Brown J, Moseley IF. The role of MRI in screening for neurogenic hypertension. Neuroradiology 2000; 42:99–103.

27. Digre KB, Corbett JJ. Pseudotumor cerebri in men. Arch Neurol 1988; 45:866–872.

28. Digre KB. Not so benign intracranial hypertension. BMJ 2003; 326:613–614.

29. Weber KT, Singh KD, Hey JC. Idiopathic intracranial hypertension with primary aldosteronism: report of 2 cases. Am J Med Sci 2002; 324:45–50.

30. Silberstein SD, McKinstry RC III. The death of idiopathic intracranial hypertension? Neurology 2003; 60:1406–1407.

31. Digre KB. Idiopathic intracranial hypertension headache. Curr Pain Headache Rep 2002; 6:217–225.

32. Osterman J, Calhoun A, Dunham M, Cullum UX Jr, Clark RM, Stewart DD. Chronic syndrome of inappropriate antidiuretic hormone secretion and hypertension in a patient with olfactory neuroblastoma. Evidence of ectopic production of arginine vasopressin by the tumor. Arch Intern Med 1986; 146:1731–1735.

33. Whitaker MD, McArthur RG, Corenblum B, Davidman M, Haslam RH. Idiopathic, sustained, inappropriate secretion of ADH with associated hypertension and thirst. Am J Med 1979; 67:511–515.

34. Padfield PL, Brown JJ, Lever AF, Morton JJ, Robertson JI. Blood pressure in acute and chronic vasopressin excess: studies of malignant hypertension and the syndrome of inappropriate antidiuretic hormone secretion. N Engl J Med 1981; 304:1067–1070.

35. Biaggioni I, Robertson RM. Hypertension in orthostatic hypotension and autonomic dysfunction. Cardiol Clin 2002; 20:291–301.

36. Ketch T, Biaggioni I, Robertson R, Robertson D. Four faces of baroreflex failure: hypertensive crisis, volatile hypertension, orthostatic tachycardia, and malignant vagotonia. Circulation 2002; 105:2518–2523.

37. Tubbs RS, Wellons JC III, Blount JP, Oakes WJ, Grabb PA. Cessation of chronic hypertension after posterior fossa decompression in a child with Chiari I malformation. Case report. J Neurosurg 2004; 100:194–196.

38. Kaplan NM. Other forms of secondary hypertension. In: Kaplan NM, ed. Kaplan's Clinical Hypertension. Philadelphia: Lippincott Williams & Williams, 1998:495–511.

39. Montagna P, Cortelli P, Gambetti P, Lugaresi E. Fatal familial insomnia: sleep, neuroendocrine and vegetative alterations. Adv Neuroimmunol 1995; 5:13–21.

40. Britton M, de Faire U, Helmers C. Hazards of therapy for excessive hypertension in acute stroke. Acta Med Scand 1980; 207:253–257.

41. Britton M, Carlsson A, de Faire U. Blood pressure course in patients with acute stroke and matched controls. Stroke 1986; 17:861–864.

42. Morfis L, Schwartz RS, Poulos R, Howes LG. Blood pressure changes in acute cerebral infarction and hemorrhage. Stroke 1997; 28:1401–1405.

43. Hills AE. Systemic blood pressure and stroke outcome and recurrence. Curr Hypertens Rep 2005; 7(1):72–78.

44. Adams HP Jr, Adams RJ, Brott T, del Zoppo GJ, Furlan A, Goldstein LB. Guidelines for the early management of patients with ischemic stroke: A scientific statement from the Stroke Council of the American Stroke Association. Stroke 2003; 34:1056–1083.

45. Ringleb PA, Bertram M, Keller E, Hacke W. Hypertension in patients with cerebrovascular accident. To treat or not to treat? Nephrol Dial Transplant 1998; 13:2179–2181.

46. Ahmed N, Nasman P, Wahlgren NG. Effect of intravenous nimodipine on blood pressure and outcome after acute stroke. Stroke 2000; 31:1250–1255.

49

Affective Illness and Hypertension

THOMAS RUTLEDGE

University of San Diego, San Diego, California, USA

KEYPOINTS

- Affective distress is a common and underappreciated contributor to hypertension.
- Negative emotions may have widespread effects on hypertension development and treatment as well as patients quality of life.
- There exists a significant body of prospective evidence linking chronic negative emotional states such as anger, hostility, and depression with the emergence of hypertension.
- Arguments for psychological "causes" of hypertension are based on both physiological changes documented among individuals reporting high level of affective distress, as well as higher rates in known coronary risk factor behaviors.
- Treatments for affective illness in hypertension vary significantly in scope, and, to date, suggest modest blood pressure reductions for most individuals.

SUMMARY

Evidence from several recent large-scale prospective studies suggests a relationship between chronic negative emotions and the development of hypertension; however, psychological features are not assessed routinely by physicians in hypertension clinics. The psychological characteristics with the strongest epidemiological evidence till date include anger, anxiety, hostility, Type A behavior pattern, and depression. A variety of mechanisms have been hypothesized to explain the relationship between affect and hypertension risk, including heightened cardiovascular responsiveness to stress, impaired diurnal blood pressure regulation, changes in neurohormonal activity, and increases in behavioral risk factors that are associated with hypertension and cardiovascular diseases. Clinical research that investigates the effects of treating mental health problems among patients with established hypertension indicates only modest reductions in blood pressure. However, treatment of psychiatric conditions may also assist in reducing hypertension risk factors such as obesity, high-fat diet, smoking, and low physical activity levels. At present, there exists no data on which to evaluate the treatment effects of modifying negative affect on long-term hypertension risk. This chapter summarizes our current knowledge on this issue, and offers suggestions—based on the latest research—for clinicians seeking to incorporate psychological assessment and treatment options into their service delivery to patients.

I. INTRODUCTION

Hypertension is one of the most common chronic diseases among adults in Europe and North America. Statistics from the Center for Disease Control (CDC) and the National Heart, Lung, and Blood Institute (NHLBI) suggest that high blood pressure affects upwards of 50 million people— nearly one in five over the age of 20—in the United States alone and accounts for >75 billion in estimated healthcare dollars worldwide (1,2). Despite the alarming prevalence of hypertension, however, the cause(s) of most identified cases of high blood pressure are unknown. This is not to suggest that we have a poor understanding of risk factors for developing hypertension, because an enormous and ever growing scientific literature identifies a long list of biological, social, and psychological suspects (3).

The absence of a "smoking gun" equivalent biological cause for hypertension raised the possibility nearly a century ago (4) that psychosocial characteristics could be a primary determinant in blood pressure regulation. At the time, this perspective was strengthened anecdotally from clinical reports made by physicians and psychiatrists that also suggested connections between intense anger, blood pressure, and cardiovascular events.

Our knowledge of hypertension and methods of study have evolved dramatically in the years since these initial speculations, but the interest in emotions and emotional disorders as factors disposing high blood pressure risk remains remarkably consistent. Recent years, in fact, have witnessed some of the most methodologically compelling evidence till date on the issue. This chapter will review this evidence, exploring our current understanding of affective responses with respect to hypertension risk, discussing the possible clinical implications of and state of the art methods for assessing and treating psychiatric symptoms in hypertensive or at-risk patient groups, and highlighting issues in this area that remain problematic for researchers and practicing clinicians.

II. OVERVIEW OF RESEARCH ASSOCIATING PSYCHOLOGICAL FACTORS WITH HYPERTENSION

Prior to 1990, the majority of research investigating psychological factor–blood pressure research was cross-sectional in nature. This research typically comprised two forms; either correlational surveys of emotional characteristics among hypertensive and nonhypertensive groups completed for comparison purposes, or laboratory models in which experimental participants made self-reports about psychological states and traits before they completed one or more experimental exercises. This literature base is extensive and consists of many hundreds of studies carried out over the past 50 years. Fortunately, there exist several high-quality narrative and meta-analytic reviews of this area to summarize the dominant themes (5,6). Generally speaking, the evidence favored a relationship between high blood pressure and chronic negative emotional states, in particular, characteristics such as anxiety, anger, hostility, and Type A behavior—but the conclusions were limited by the inconsistency in measures and methodology. Quantitative summaries also suggested that the magnitude of relationships between affective symptoms and hypertension was small, at least in the metric of correlation coefficients common to behavioral research, and that the clinical importance of psychiatric symptoms was likely small for nurses and physicians practicing with at-risk patients (5). Variations on these research approaches, notably the currently interest in "cardiovascular reactivity" to mental stress, remain till date popular topics of study in both the areas of hypertension and cardiovascular disease.

A critical limitation to this cross-sectional research was related to the inability to know when the affective problems appeared in relation to the emergence of the high blood pressure. Without evidence to show that a proposed symptom, such as an anxiety disorder, actually preceded the onset of hypertension, it was impossible to disprove the very credible argument that affective distress was a consequence of learning that one had a serious chronic illness, and not a cause of the illness itself. Some later studies even provided direct data in support of this perspective, showing, for example, that awareness of a positive hypertension status was associated with increases in self-reported mood symptoms, whereas no such increases were observed among normotensive subjects or patients with undiagnosed hypertension (7). Although methodologically appealing, randomized controlled trials are not a practical solution to the problem, as we are—for obvious ethical reasons—unable to assign chronic mental health symptoms or illness to research participants.

As it turns out, the strongest method available by which to assess possible affective illness and hypertension relationships is the prospective cohort design, in which a normotensive sample can be tracked over a period of years to determine risk in association with baseline or historical psychological symptoms. The advantages of this approach are twofold. First, the cohort study, by design, allows the researcher to disentangle the temporal sequence of affective illness and hypertension. Secondly, the use of epidemiological methods supports the assessment of additional risk factors or covariates and the use of epidemiological statistics, such as risk ratios, by which to draw better estimates of clinical significance. However, cohort studies are vastly more expensive compared with cross-sectional designs, making their completion comparatively rare, and they also suffer from their own problems in the form of maintaining participant follow-up and the inability to randomize important variables (e.g., the risk that low socioeconomic standing may predispose both depression and hypertension risk).

Methodological issues aside, the biggest drawback to cohort studies of psychological factors was that they were simply not enough of them from which to draw any definitive conclusions. But this has begun to change. A recent quantitative review identified 15 longitudinal studies, dating from the mid-1970s to 2001, that investigates psychological factors as predictors of hypertension (8). One additional study, a follow-up from the Coronary Artery Risk Development in Young Adults (CARDIA) in the United States, has appeared since the release of the latest review (9). This new evidence, summarized in Table 49.1, overwhelmingly supports the presence of a statistical relationship between a number of psychological characteristics and the emergence of hypertension across a range of age, gender, and ethnic cohorts. Further, because many of these findings are drawn from relatively large epidemiological studies in which major coronary artery disease risk and hypertension risk factors were also sampled, we are able to evaluate the impact of affective conditions in comparison to more established biomedical predictors. In the majority of cases, not only do

psychological factors remain reliable predictors of hypertension development after controlling for standard risk factors, but the magnitude of the adjusted risk ratio values also rival that of commonly used predictors such as smoking, obesity, and low physical activity (8).

The types of psychological characteristics that are associated with hypertension risk in the prospective studies largely mirror that of the affective factors measured in the previously discussed cross-sectional literature. As Table 49.1 indicates, anger, anxiety, depression, emotional defensiveness, hostility, social isolation, and Type A behavior remain the primary targets of study (10–14). The emphasis on these symptom patterns is grounded in psychological theory that, while still evolving, dates back to the early part of the 20th century. Probably, the most important elements of this theoretical groundwork are the continuing integration of social, psychological, and medical evidence, and the importance placed on identifying biobehavioral pathways by which affective illness may confer an increased risk of hypertension. The identification of mediating pathways, or mechanisms as they are perhaps more frequently described, turns out to be one of the still incomplete pieces of the puzzle in qualifying the relationship between psychological characteristics and hypertension.

III. MECHANISMS

From a medical perspective, several criteria must be met in order to establish that a proposed factor is a cause of disease. The factor must precede the onset of the disease; it must

Table 49.1 Prospective Studies Associating Affective Symptoms with Hypertension Development

Authors	Sample number	Duration (years)	Primary finding(s)
Davidson et al.	3343	5	Depression increases hypertension risk
Everson et al.	537	4	Anger expression predicts hypertension
Everson et al.	616	4	Feelings of hopelessness are associated with hypertension development
Jenkins	231	3	Anger levels predict hypertension
Jonas et al.	2992	9	Anxiety and depression are linked to hypertension risk
Kahn et al.	3829	5	Anger and social isolation predict later hypertension
McClelland	78	20	Inhibition of anger is associated with hypertension
Markovitz et al.	468	3	Anxiety symptoms increase the risk of hypertension
Markovitz et al.	1123	18	Anxiety levels predict hypertension risk
Pernini et al.	121	2.5	Anger and anxiety levels are tied to an increase in hypertension risk
Rutledge et al.	127	3	Emotional defensiveness increases hypertension risk
Siegler et al.	4650	21	There is no relationship between hostility and hypertension
Somova et al.	501	4	Inward-directed anger predicts hypertension development
Spiro et al.	838	17	A neurotic personality is associated with hypertension
Vaillant et al.	193	20	Psychiatric history does not predict hypertension later in life
Yan et al.	3308	15	Type A behavior and hostility are linked to hypertension risk

show a statistical relationship independent of other known causes or contributors; there should exist an established biological process by which the factor produces the disease in question; and finally, the removal or treatment of the factor should result in the remission of the disease or a reduction of symptoms. For a complex, multifactorial condition such as high blood pressure, establishing causal factors is often difficult, thus the common diagnosis of "essential hypertension." On the basis of these criteria, affective conditions make the initial grades of causation largely because of the recent prospective evidence; however, the arguments for biological pathways and the success of treatment remain controversial. Although it is not the purpose here to comprehensively review the quite extensive literatures available in behavioral medicine, psychology, and psychiatry on these subjects, there are a select number of empirically supported theories that may assist both researchers and clinicians in working with hypertension patients.

Figure 49.1 illustrates a typical overview of arguments made to connect psychological characteristics to the development of hypertension. Importantly, these arguments typically take one of the two forms: either they are based on physiological processes with known involvement in blood pressure regulation, or they are based on health behaviors that are established predictors of hypertension. The presence of psychological distress has been linked to a number of pathophysiological mechanisms, including impaired vagal control, decreases in baroreceptor sensitivity, increases in platelet and cortisol release, and exaggerated sympathetic nervous system activity. Sympathetic nervous system responsiveness, often referred to as *reactivity* by researchers, is the topic of hundreds of studies

and has been independently linked to hypertension development in several longitudinal investigations (15,16). Researchers speculate that, over time, a pattern of enhanced reactivity produces changes in baroreceptor regulation and neuroendocrine and neurohormonal responses, and also enduring changes in underlying blood vessels and vascular tissues that may lead to increases in tonic blood pressure levels (17). The status of reactivity itself as a causal agent in the hypertension process—or merely a marker of disease—remains a subject of some debate (18). However, the emerging consensus is that cardiovascular reactivity is a risk factor for both hypertension and cardiovascular disease.

The results of many studies favor the presence of a relationship between psychological factors such as anger, emotional defensiveness, and hostility with increased reactivity responses to mental stressors conducted in the laboratory (15); and newly released research further suggests that emotional stress can produce blood pressure increases under real-life circumstances as measured by ambulatory blood pressure monitors (19). The aggregated consistency of this relationship with reactivity, accompanied by the growing evidence for reactivity as an important mechanism in the cardiovascular disease process, provides by far the most compelling pathophysiological argument for psychological factors as a cause of hypertension. Notably, increased cardiovascular responsiveness is also the primary pathway believed to account for the relationship observed between affective symptoms and stroke in several studies (20,21).

Direct evidence that stress-induced reactivity responses may produce vascular damage or permanent increases in

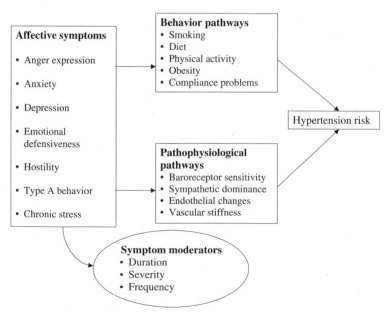

Figure 49.1   Primary pathways associating psychological characteristics with hypertension risk.

blood pressure is limited; the strongest support for this idea comes from primate studies completed in the 1980s by Manuck and coworkers (22). Results from their controlled laboratory studies indicated that exposure to chronic psychosocial stress—in the form of social instability—among male monkeys was associated with significantly larger atherosclerotic lesions compared with lesion size in the low-stress primate groups. Equally compelling was that the introduction of a β-blockers prevented the development of endothelial damage in the high-stress group, which suggests that the atherosclerotic lesions were mediated by an increased sympathetic nervous system response to the social environment (23). Many theorists argue that a similar physiological process may account for the relationship between low socioeconomic status and heart disease rates (24).

A single prospective study of college age adults completing a series of mental stress exercises in the laboratory, as well as a period of ambulatory blood pressure monitoring, also suggested that reactivity responses could explain the relationship between psychological characteristics and 3 year hypertension risk (25). In the latter investigation, reactivity responses documented in the laboratory statistically mediated the relationship between emotional defensiveness and hypertension risk, which means that increased reactivity patterns by participants with higher defensiveness scores functioned as the primary mechanism for hypertension status at follow-up.

In contrast to the large research base assessing reactivity responses, the association between symptoms of affective illness and behavioral risk factors for cardiovascular disease is sometimes overlooked; but this relationship may be the most important pathway connecting psychological health to hypertension development. Anxiety, depression, and hostility are each established predictors of poor health behaviors, including increased smoking and substance abuse rates, obesity, and lower physical activity levels, lower socioeconomic status and unemployment, and social isolation (26,27). Increased affective distress also has been shown to undermine compliance to medical treatments (28), a frequently underappreciated but critical factor influencing patient outcomes. The contention is sometimes raised that affective symptoms may be as much a result of behavioral risk factors as a determinant, a position that has support from several empirical sources, including, for example, data showing that smoking cessation is associated with an increase in self-reported depression symptoms (29). However, the relationship between mental health and behavioral risk factors is a poor example of the classic chicken-and-egg dilemma. On whole, the evidence overwhelmingly shows that the onset of either affective or behavioral symptoms raises the risk of developing additional risk factors and mental health problems in a bidirectional, and potentially synergistic manner.

In a typical epidemiological study, psychological characteristics are associated with hypertension outcomes; the objective is to show that the psychological predictor(s) in question has a statistically independent relationship with hypertension rates after controlling for any number of control variables. The latter usually consists of at least a subset of known coronary risk factors. Many of the prospective studies listed in Table 49.1 reflect this type of multivariate design (30,31). Much less common is the goal of the investigator to examine established risk factors in either the role of a moderator (i.e., an interaction with the predictor) or as explanatory mechanisms in the disease process (32). In the scientific arena, a variable linked to an important health endpoint such as hypertension gains more credibility if it cannot be easily explained by established predictors, although the justification for this approach is sometimes nonsensical and can eventually produce a body of statistically intriguing but poorly understood relationships. The large number of studies showing relationships between affective symptoms and hypertension represents a convenient example of this result, with five decades of emphasis placed on demonstrating quantitative associations, but a comparatively meager collection of findings from which we can derive meaningful, practical interpretations concerning whether or how to incorporate psychological assessment into cardiovascular care settings. The most pronounced casualty of this research approach is the difficulty quantifying the clinical importance of affect-hypertension relationships.

A. Clinical Significance

Even the most consistent collection of statistical relationships does not necessarily imply the presence of a clinically meaningful relationship. The practical impact of a relationship is affected by many variables, including the base rate and severity of the health variable, the populations at risk, effectiveness of treatment options, and the magnitude of the statistical association, among other contingencies (33). Inferences regarding the potential clinical significance of a relationship can also be profoundly affected by the type of statistical analysis employed. In much of the behavioral health literature, for example, correlation and linear regression analyses are the common medium of presentation. However, the use of correlation coefficients with dichotomous health measures such as hypertension status can be misleading because of the typically low base rates of disease incidence and subsequent nonlinearity of the variable distribution. The usual effect of this scenario is that the size of the correlation coefficient is small, often between 0.0 and 0.10, a value most researchers consider to be inconsequential, even in those cases in which it meets the criteria for statistical significance. Well over 90% of the research that describes relationships between affective symptoms and hypertension express their findings as correlation coefficients. Not surprisingly, the conclusion of most experts was that affective illness was probably of small interest to practitioners who are working with hypertension patients.

Rosenthal et al. (33), however, argue that the size of correlation coefficients—large or small—cannot be accurately interpreted in relation to dichotomous health outcomes without additional consideration. Although a number of alternatives are available, probably the most common alternative is the use of odds ratio and risk ratio analyses. The use of epidemiological statistics by behavioral medicine researchers offers the primary advantage of a standard statistical language with which to share findings with biomedical researchers. Risk ratio measures are, of course, not without flaws, not the least being that they are insensitive to base rates. The simple conclusion is that no statistical measure can serve, in isolation, as a metric for quantifying clinical significance. Epidemiological statistics are, however, a superior alternative to correlation and linear regression.

As described earlier, many of the more recent prospective studies have reported outcomes in the preferred epidemiological format, allowing direct comparisons of risk for established risk factors for hypertension and affective symptom predictors. The results of these analyses, at least for proponents of behavioral health research, are encouraging, suggesting on the whole that high levels of anger, hostility, depression, anxiety, and possibly other Type A behavior components more than double the risk of future hypertension. Quantitative reviews of the prospective evidence are equally favorable, showing that the combined published data not only suggest effects on a par with better-known risk factors for hypertension, but

that the findings also are highly robust to any future negative results (8). Because even the combination of all recognized hypertension risk factors account for less than half of all identified cases of hypertension, it is clear that our understanding of dispositional variables remains incomplete. With this new behavioral evidence, demonstrating that the initial statistical significance detailed in many laboratory and cross-sectional studies is consistent with and enhanced by prospective results possessing much stronger implications for clinical significance, this is an important opportunity to advance and clarify the implications of affective illness for hypertension management.

As a final comment on the potential clinical significance of affective symptoms in hypertension, despite the promising evidence reviewed here, there remain several very challenging methodological obstacles. These include, but are not limited to, furthering our understanding of mechanisms involved, establishing criteria for the type, severity, and duration of affective illness sufficient to dispose risk, standardizing measures for the assessment of affective symptoms, and demonstrating that treatments for affective conditions can assist in the prevention or management of hypertension. We look at some of these clinical issues in more detail in the following section.

IV. PSYCHOLOGICAL SYMPTOMS IN THE CLINIC

On the basis of the reviewed evidence, should clinicians incorporate psychological assessments in their examination of patients with hypertension or at risk for hypertension? The best answer to this question ranges from "possibly" to "probably"; but even the most agreeable practitioner

Table 49.2 Primary Emotional States Linked to Hypertension Risk, Clinical Definitions, and Validated Measurement Instruments

Psychological feature (synonyms)	Definition	Scale(s) of measurement
Anger (anger expression, anger-in, anger-out)	Behavior pattern characterized by the frequent experience and displays of anger through verbal or physical means. Anger may also appear as a pattern of frequent anger experience, but with intentional inhibition/repression	Spielberger anger expression scale State-Trait anger scale
Hostility	An attitude characterized by mistrust of others, cynicism, disposition to anger, and a negative orientation toward interpersonal relationships	Cook–Medley hostility scale
Type A behavior pattern	A syndrome characterized by competition, hostility, time urgency, and excessive commitment to work	Framingham Type A questionnaire Jenkins activity survey
Depression (hopelessness, vital exhaustion)	Psychiatric condition characterized by persistent depressed mood, loss of interest in activities, low self-esteem, changes in sleep patterns, excessive guilt, and thoughts of suicide, among other clinical features	Beck depression scale Center for Epidemiological Studies-depression scale
Anxiety	Characterized by excessive, uncontrollable, fears and worries	State-Trait anxiety inventory

should take heed of several qualifying factors. First of all, only a select few affective conditions are linked reliably to hypertension. Table 49.2 summarizes the list of psychological symptoms with the most credible evidence for hypertension impact, along with a brief description of each symptom pattern and a sample of validated measurement questionnaires. The list of questionnaires for each characteristic is not comprehensive, but does include measurement scales used in one or more prospective studies that identify increased hypertension risk. In contrast to this list, we have no compelling evidence that schizophrenia, personality disorders, somatic disorders, hyperactivity, or other psychiatric conditions listed among the hundreds of recognized mental disorders listed in an authoritative manual, such as the DSM-IV, bear any relationship with hypertension risk. What is also noteworthy is that some of the psychological characteristics (e.g., anger, Type A behavior, and hostility) with the most abundant evidence for hypertension associations are not recognized as an official mental illness by any formal classification body.

Another empirically based finding from the research literature is that even among established psychiatric conditions such as anxiety and depression, it is not necessary for a patient to meet clinical criteria for a disorder for their symptoms to predict an elevated risk for hypertension development. In fact, the vast majority of participants in the research base reviewed failed to meet clinical criteria. For the clinician, simply the presence of elevated symptoms is probably enough to dispose risk and to have implications for intervention. This conclusion is further supported by a number of depression studies among post-myocardial infarction patients, in which even subclinical depression levels were associated with higher mortality risk (6). The measurement scales listed for each affective category in Table 49.2, although validated for the assessment of their respective symptoms, are not diagnostic instruments and may not always be appropriate for the particular age, ethnic, or medical population of interest to the clinician.

A third critical implication for the clinician interested in including psychological assessment in their services is that even the presentation of significant symptoms in a given clinical examination or interview are not necessarily a cause for action by the hypertension specialist. On the basis of our current understanding of behavioral and pathophysiological mechanisms, it is *sustained* or *recurrent* episodes of significant affective symptoms over a period of time that are most capable of affecting tonic blood pressure levels for an individual. Short-term or less severe episodes may incur an ethical obligation for the clinician to perform a more in depth assessment, refer the patient to a more qualified mental health colleague, or encourage treatment by the patient, but these shorter or less severe episodes are less likely to have implications for cardiovascular health. This is an important distinction because many presentations of affective distress occur in the aftermath of significant life events or periods of stress in which emotional distress is normal and appropriate, as long as the duration of the symptoms is reasonable. Even in cases of untreated clinical depression, patients frequently experience periods of symptom remission. These clinical modifiers are included in the bottom of the Fig. 49.1 as factors to consider by both researchers and clinicians.

An important final consideration in the clinical arena is that affective symptoms are highly correlated in practice. Scores from depression and anxiety measures, for example, typically correlate near 0.60, a value that represents a high degree of overlap. To a lesser but still significant extent, depression symptoms also are usually more severe among those reporting higher levels of anger and hostility. It is not known whether a combination of two or more affective symptoms affects hypertension risk to greater extent than the presence of only a single symptom category. However, there is evidence from coronary artery disease research that "clusters" of psychological factors can synergistically increase the risk of mortality for patients after a heart attack relative to single symptom presentations (34).

In light of these multiple qualifiers and precautions, how might hypertension clinicians effectively incorporate knowledge of psychological symptoms into their assessment and treatment process? In this era of high patient volumes and ever present budget limitations, the objective of including further testing materials can appear as an unmanageable goal, but these obstacles are not daunting as they may seem to be. Probably, the most efficient route is to include a short set of screening tools to be completed by patients in the course of their routine physical or cardiovascular examinations. Many clinics already include such measures, at this stage most commonly for highly prevalent symptoms such as depression and pain. Screening tools usually consist of only a handful of items, sometimes as short as a single question, and therefore should never serve as the basis for any treatment decision other than to perform a more comprehensive assessment. Nevertheless, screening measures can serve a valuable role by flagging important symptoms to time-strapped clinicians. In cases for which positive scores occur on screening measures, the clinician is encouraged to follow-up either verbally or in questionnaire form with questions that can be helpful in identifying the severity, duration, and quality of life effects of these symptoms and to help make the patient aware of the potential significance of the symptoms on their physical health. Forming a relationship with a locally based and regionally licensed psychologist or psychiatrist is highly recommended because this specialist can offer considerable expertize in developing screening tools for your clinic, aid in the selection of appropriate questionnaires, supervise scoring and administration details, provide guidance or clarification on any ethical issues (e.g., the endorsement of suicidal ideation on a depression measure), and otherwise assist the clinician in making psychological data collection maximally useful and minimally time intrusive. The presence of an accessible mental health specialist is also valuable in circumstances in which significant affective symptoms are identified because many medical practitioners will not have the time or training to conduct interviews for psychiatric symptoms.

A. Treatment of Affective Symptoms

One of the most pressing questions in this field also is one that currently cannot be answered. Given the growing number of findings in support of a relationship between affective symptoms and hypertension risk, the question that follows is, "Can interventions reducing the severity or psychological distress lower a patient's future risk of developing hypertension?" To date, there is not a single study that addresses this issue. Many readers may balk at this statement, recalling that there is a long and methodologically varied history of research assessing the effects of psychological treatments on blood pressure. Although it is true, and also relevant for the purpose of this discussion, the stated question is fundamentally different from the one addressed in earlier studies. From a physiological perspective, affecting the course of a chronic disease after its incidence is almost always less effective than successful prevention efforts. For example, the treatment of coronary artery disease, despite the remarkable progress in treating the disease in the last two decades, is largely resigned to minimizing the risk of future coronary events and improving the quality of life for patients, rather than focused on actually reversing the course of atherosclerosis. Similarly, even the most successful pharmacological interventions for hypertension usually require a lifelong program of medication for individuals in order to maintain blood pressure at healthy levels. An expectation that a short-term (usually 8–12 weeks) program centered on stress-management, anger reduction, or depression can achieve large and permanent blood pressure reductions among patients with hypertension is not realistic, and failure to achieve this goal frequently is cited by those who seek to downplay the role of behavioral treatments for blood pressure (35). However, some of the latest and most rigorously collected data from randomized clinical trials suggests that psychological and stress-management treatments can produce relatively enduring and clinically relevant blood pressure reductions (i.e., >10 mmHg systolic) among hypertension patients when the programs are individually tailored to the needs of the patient (36).

V. CONCLUSIONS

This chapter began with broad aims—to review and summarize an extensive body of cross-sectional, laboratory, and cohort data that assess associations between hypertension and affective symptoms, to critically examine evidence for behavioral and pathophysiological mechanisms by which blood pressure could be affected by psychological factors, to form useful recommendations for clinicians aiming to incorporate psychological assessment and treatment into their services to hypertension and cardiovascular patients, to highlight some of the primary methodological obstacles that remain, and finally, to touch on implications for treatment. The following is a summary statement for each of these topics.

A. Affective Symptoms and Hypertension

In the face of still accumulating prospective data from several large United States studies, the evidence supporting a relationship between high levels of psychological distress and greater hypertension risk has never been stronger. Anger, anxiety, depression, hostility, and Type A behavior (e.g., time urgency) characteristics appear to be the most reliable predictors in these studies, and the results generally hold true for women as well as men, and for African-American as well as Caucasian subsamples.

B. Mechanisms

Theorists have proposed a variety of mechanisms in explaining affect-hypertension relationships. Those with the most empirical support include heightened cardiovascular reactivity among individuals reporting affective symptoms and individuals with a low socioeconomic status and an increase in behavioral risk factors such as smoking, obesity, alcohol use, and low physical activity patterns. For patients with existing hypertension, data also suggest that affective distress can impair adherence to treatment.

C. Recommendations for Clinicians

For practitioners who seek to incorporate psychological measurement in their clinics, the most important goal is to create a streamlined and time-efficient process that provides clinically useful information. The recommendation offered here was to create a tiered system in which a set of brief screening tools could be completed by patients as part of their routine assessments to identify symptoms; only those patients with positive screens would be evaluated with validated measurement tools or interview methods. The clinical emphasis should be on recognizing affective symptoms that are severe, relatively longstanding or recurrent, and inappropriate in light of the patient's recent life circumstances. An alliance with a mental health professional can be invaluable in establishing this addition to clinical service delivery.

D. Remaining Methodological Questions

At the present time, even the best cohort studies fail to address the importance of symptom duration on the risk for hypertension, many use nonstandardized measurement tools for affective symptoms, and mechanism data is sorely lacking. Some studies also based their findings on suspect definitions of hypertension that do not rule out the risk of white-coat hypertension or other methodological problems.

E. Treatment Implications

The possible benefits of hypertension prevention efforts, in which affective symptoms are targeted in high-risk normotensive samples, are unknown because of the absence of research on this issue. The literature examining the blood pressure effects of treating stress, anger, and other affective symptoms among hypertension patients is inconsistent in methodology and results, with the overall effects small by most clinical standards (i.e., <5 mmHg). The majority of these studies, however, were group-based, standardized treatments, whereas newer research is focusing on individualized treatment programs and appears more promising.

REFERENCES

1. Hajjar I, Kotchen TA. Trends in prevalence, awareness, treatment, and control of hypertension in the United States, 1988–2000. J Am Med Assoc 2003; 290:199–206.
2. Wolf-Maier K, Cooper RS, Banegas JR, Giampaoli S, Hense HW, Joffres M, Kastarinen M, Poulter N, Primatesta P, Rodriguez-Artalejo F, Stegmayr B, Thamm M, Tuomilehto J, Vanuzzo D, Vescio F. Hypertension prevalence and blood pressure levels in 6 European countries, Canada, and the United States. J Am Med Assoc 2003; 289:2363–2369.
3. Whelton PK, He J, Appel LJ, Cutler JA, Havas S, Kotchen TA, Roccella EJ, Stout R, Vallbona C, Winston MC, Karimbakas J; National High Blood Pressure Education Program Coordinating Committee. Primary prevention of hypertension: clinical and public health advisory from The National High Blood Pressure Education Program. J Am Med Assoc 2002; 288:1882–1888.
4. Alexander F. Emotional factors in essential hypertension. Psychosom Med 1939; 1:175–179.
5. Jorgensen RS, Johnson BT, Kolodziej ME, Schreer GE. Elevated blood pressure and personality: a meta-analytic review. Psychol Bull 1996; 120:293–320.
6. Rozanski, A, Blumenthal JA, Kaplan J. Impact of psychological factors on the pathogenesis of cardiovascular disease and implications for therapy. Circulation 1999; 99:2192–2217.
7. Irvine MJ, Garner DM, Olmstead MP, Logan AG. Personality differences between hypertensive and normotensive individuals: influence on knowledge of hypertension status. Psychosom Med 1989; 51:537–549.
8. Rutledge T, Hogan BE. A quantitative review of prospective evidence linking psychological factors with hypertension development. Psychosom Med 2002; 64:758–766.
9. Yan LL, Lio K, Matthews KA, Daviglus ML, Ferguson TF, Kiefe CI. Psychosocial factors and risk of hypertension. J Am Med Assoc 2003; 290:2138–2148.
10. Markovitz JH, Matthews KA, Wing RR, Kuller LH, Meilahn EN. Psychological, biological, and health behavior predictors of blood pressure changes in middle-aged women. J Hypertens 1991; 9:399–406.
11. Everson SA, Goldberg DE, Kaplan GA, Julkunen J, Salonen JT. Anger expression and incident hypertension. Psychosom Med 1998; 60:730–735.
12. Davidson K, Jonas BS, Dixon KE, Markovitz JH. Do depression symptoms predict early hypertension incidence in young adults in the CARDIA study? Arch Intern Med 2000; 160:1495–1500.
13. Jonas BS, Lando JF. Negative affect as a prospective risk factor for hypertension. Psychosom Med 2000; 62:188–196.
14. Somova LI, Connolly C, Diara K. Psychosocial predictors of hypertension in black and white Africans. J Hypertens 1995; 13:193–199.
15. Schwartz AR, Gerin W, Davidson KW, Pickering TG, Brosschot JF, Thayer JF, Christenfeld, Linden W. Toward a casual model of cardiovascular responses to stress and the development of cardiovascular disease. Psychosom Med 2003; 65:22–35.
16. Lovallo WR, Gerin W. Psychophysiological reactivity: mechanisms and pathways to cardiovascular disease. Psychosom Med 2003; 65:36–45.
17. Gerin W, Pickering TG, Glynn L, Christenfeld N, Schwartz A, Carroll D, Davidson K. An historical context for behavioral models of hypertension. J Psychosom Res 2000; 48:369–377.
18. Steptoe A. Psychosocial factors in the development of hypertension. Ann Behav Med 2000; 32:371–375.
19. Kamarck TW, Janicki DL, Shiffman S, Polk DE, Muldoon MF, Liebenauer LL, Schwartz JE. Psychosocial demands and ambulatory blood pressure: a field assessment approach. Physiol Behav 2002; 77:699–704.
20. Jonas BS, Mussolino ME. Symptoms of depression as a prospective risk factor for stroke. Psychosom Med 2000; 62:463–471.
21. Williams JE, Nieto FJ, Sanford CP, Couper DJ, Tyroler HA. The association between trait anger and incident stroke risk: the Atherosclerosis Risk in Communities (ARIC) Study. Stroke 2002; 33:13–19.
22. Kaplan JR, Manuck SS, Clarkson TB, Lusson FM, Taub DM, Miller EW. Social stress and atherosclerosis

in normocholesterolemic monkeys. Science 1983; 220:733–735.

23. Kaplan JR, Manuck SB, Adams MR, Weingard KW, Clarkson TB. Inhibition of coronary atherosclerosis by propranolol in behaviorally predisposed monkeys fed an atherogenic diet. Circulation 1987; 76:1365–1372.

24. Gallo LC, Matthews KA. Understanding the association between socioeconomic status and physical health: do negative emotions play a role? Psychol Bull 2003; 129:10–51.

25. Rutledge T, Linden W. Defensiveness and prospective blood pressure increases: the mediating effect of cardiovascular reactivity. Ann Behav Med 2003; 25:34–40.

26. Sielger IC, Peterson BL, Barefoot JC, Williams RB. Hostility during late adolescence predicts coronary risk factors at mid-life. Am J Epidemiol 1992; 136:146–154.

27. Rutledge T, Reis SE, Olson M, Owens J, Kelsey SF, Pepine CJ, Reichek N, Rogers WJ, Merz CN, Sopko G, Cornell CE, Matthews KA. Psychosocial variables are associated with atherosclerosis risk factors among women with chest pain: the WISE study. Psychosom Med 2001; 63:282–288.

28. Zigelstein RC, Bush DE, Fauerbach JA. Depression, adherence behavior, and coronary disease outcomes. Arch Intern Med 1998; 158:808–809.

29. Glassman AH, Covey LS, Stetner F, Rivelli S. Smoking cessation and the course of major depression: a follow-up study. Lancet 2001; 357:1929–1932.

30. Everson SA, Kaplan GA, Goldberg DE, Salonen JT. Hypertension incidence is predicted by high levels of hopelessness in Finnish men. Hypertension 2000; 35:561–567.

31. Jonas BS, Franks P, Ingram DD. Are symptoms of anxiety and depression risk factors for hypertension? Longitudinal evidence from the National Health and Nutrition Examination Survey I epidemiologic follow-up study. Arch Fam Med 1997; 6:43–49.

32. Everson S, Kauhanen J, Kaplan G, Goldberg D, Julkunen J, Tuomilehto J, Salonen JT. Hostility and risk of mortality and acute myocardial infarction: the mediating role of behavioral risk factors. Am J Epidemiol 1997; 146:142–152.

33. Rosenthal R, Rosnow RL, Rubin DB. Contrasts and Effect Sizes in Behavioral Research: a Correlational Approach. UK: Cambridge University Press, 2000.

34. Frasure-Smith N, Lesperance F, Talajic M. The impact of negative emotions on prognosis following myocardial infarction: is it more than depression? Health Psychol 1995; 14:388–398.

35. The sixth report of the Joint National Committee on prevention, detection, evaluation, and treatment of high blood pressure. Arch Intern Med 1997; 157:2413–2446.

36. Linden W, Lenz JW, Con AH. Individualized stress management for primary hypertension. Arch Intern Med 2001; 161:1071–1080.

50

Sleep Apnea and Hypertension

MATTHEW T. NAUGHTON

Monash University, Melbourne, Victoria, Australia

KEYPOINTS

- Obstructive sleep apnea is a cause of systemic hypertension and associated cardiovascular events.
- Hypoxemia, hypercapnia, large negative intra-thoracic pressures, and arousal from sleep with endothelial vascular damage are proposed mechanisms.
- Longstanding loud snoring with witnessed apneas by the bed partner strongly indicate the possibility of obstructive sleep apnea.
- Treatment of obstructive sleep apnea is associated with a reduction in blood pressure.

SUMMARY

Obstructive sleep apnea is a disorder, which occurs in ~10% and 50% of the general healthy and hypertensive populations, respectively, and causes significant cognitive impairment, excessive daytime sleepiness and cardiovascular disease.

Obstructive apneas during sleep, lasting 10–90 s and occurring up to 600 times per night, are associated with acute, brief, elevations in systemic blood pressure. Accordingly, there is sawtooth blood pressure response and, eventually, loss of the normal nocturnal dip in blood pressure (1) (Fig. 50.1).

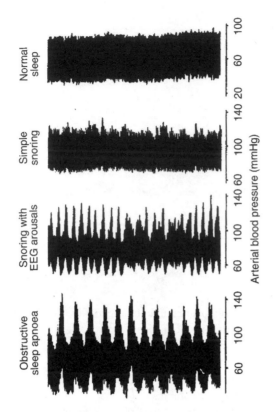

Figure 50.1 Ten minute recordings of continuous blood pressure from four patients. One patient has normal ventilation during sleep; the second patient snores; the third patient snores and awakens from sleep; and the fourth patient has obstructive sleep apnea. [With permission from Davies et al. (1).]

Over the space of weeks to months of recurrent apneas during sleep, blood pressure increases not only during sleep but also during periods of wakefulness. Proposed mechanisms for the rise in 24 h blood pressure include elevated sympathetic activity due to nocturnal hypoxemia, hypercapnia and resetting of baroreflex activity, and vascular endothelial damage. Hypertension associated with obstructive sleep apnea is often refractory to conventional pharmacotherapy.

Reversal of obstructive sleep apnea results in significant reductions in blood pressure and is now recognized as an important, although largely unrecognized, cause of systemic hypertension.

I. INTRODUCTION

Although an association between snoring and hypertension has been known for 25 years (2), coexistent obesity, male gender, sedentary lifestyle, alcohol consumption, and cigarette smoking were put forward as confounding factors to explain the association. However, recent robust cross-sectional (3) and prospective (4)

epidemiological studies and detailed animal (5,6) and human basic physiological (7–9) and interventional (10,11) studies have confirmed that obstructive sleep apnea is a common and reversible cause of systemic hypertension. This causal relationship was recognized recently by the United States National Institutes of Health document which lists obstructive sleep apnea as a cause of hypertension (12).

Given the high prevalence of snoring among the general (13) and hypertensive populations (14,15) and that pharmacological management of hypertension is poorly adhered to (16), consideration of obstructive sleep apnea should be made in all patients with hypertension.

II. DEFINITION

The term *sleep apnea* encompasses an array of breathing disorders during sleep, which can be divided into obstructive and central types. The former group (obstructive) is considered a cause of systemic hypertension, whereas the latter group (central) is considered a consequence of hypertension-related complications (e.g., heart failure and stroke).

A. Obstructive Sleep Apnea

Complete or partial collapse of the upper airway due to physiological (e.g., sleep-related loss of upper airway muscle tone) or anatomical causes (e.g., retrognathia, enlarged tonsils) results in obstructive sleep disordered breathing, an all encompassing term to describe conditions of upper airway obstructed breathing during sleep (as opposed to obstructed lower airways, e.g., asthma).

At the most benign end of the obstructive spectrum, snoring occurs intermittently or only when the patient lies supine or is under the influence of alcohol or muscle relaxing or sedating drugs. With increasing severity, snoring becomes more regular, and then it is associated with partial reductions in airflow for >10 s associated with increased respiratory effort sufficient to cause arousals from sleep.

Thereafter, snoring with hypopneas (reductions in ventilation) sufficient to cause subconscious sleep fragmentation and brief periods of hypoxemia occur. With disease progression, apneas (absence of airflow up to 90 s) associated with futile inspiratory effort, large negative intrathoracic pressure (to $-80\ cmH_2O$) occur with hypoxemia (SpO_2 down to ~50%) and hypercapnia (rise of 1–2 mmHg), and a terminating arousal from sleep (often unrecognized by the patient) accompanied by an acute rise in blood pressure (to ~300/120 mmHg).

In more severe cases, prolonged periods of hypoventilation occur, particularly during rapid eye movement (REM) sleep, associated with awake hypercapnia, hypoxemia, polycythemia, and pulmonary hypertension which is known as the Pickwician Syndrome. Patients with underlying cardiac, pulmonary, or neurological disease are more likely to express hypoventilation earlier in the disease process.

Symptoms of obstructive sleep disordered breathing include excessive daytime sleepiness, nocturnal choking, nocturnal dyspnea, orthopnea, nocturia, unrefreshing sleep, and dry throat. The signs indicative of obstructive sleep apnea are outlined in Table 50.1.

Various physiological metrics are used to measure sleep disordered breathing severity with polysomnography or limited channel monitors. *Polysomnography* refers to monitoring of EEG, EOG, EMG (submental and leg), body position, snoring noise, ECG, and respiratory channels (airflow, respiratory effort, oxygen, and carbon dioxide) and allows details of sleep architecture to be measured. *Limited channel monitoring* generally refers to monitoring of ECG and respiratory channels, without detailed EEG, EOG, or EMG, thus not measuring sleep.

Using polysomnography, the apnea hypopnea index (AHI) can be calculated from the number of apneas and hypopneas per hour of sleep. Alternatively, using limited channel monitoring, the respiratory disturbance index can be calculated as the number of apneas and hypopneas per hour recording time. In either monitoring system, the minimum oxygen saturation and the percent sleep (or recording) time spent with an oxygen saturation <90% are useful markers of sleep disordered breathing severity.

Newer measures of sleep apnea include standardized clinical assessment and indirect markers of autonomic and inflammatory disturbance. A standardized clinical assessment based upon symptoms (cardiovascular risk profile and severity of neurocognitive impairment) and signs (e.g., neck circumference, blood pressure) has been proposed (17) with a sleep specific questionnaire (18). Indirect assessment of autonomic disturbance due to hypoxia and arousal from sleep have been suggested as surrogates of sleep monitoring such as overnight urinary norepinephrine (19), heart rate variability (20), peripheral arterial tonometry (21), pulse transit time (22), and vascular endothelial and inflammatory markers such as C reactive protein (23).

B. Central Sleep Apnea

This category of sleep disordered breathing can be divided into hypercapnic and nonhypercapnic groups. The former are associated with hypoventilation and hypercapnia (e.g., neuromuscular or chest wall disorders), whereas the latter are associated with disorders of ventilatory control and usually hypocapnia.

This latter group have a characteristic ~30 s period of hyperventilation followed by an ~30 s central apnea, recurring cyclically. Common causes of central sleep apnea are congestive heart failure (when the condition is known as Cheyne-Stokes respiration), frontal stroke, high-altitude periodic breathing, narcotic use, and periodic breathing of infancy. Acute elevations in systemic blood pressure have also been shown to transiently pause ventilation through baroreflex activity (24).

Central sleep apnea, associated with Cheyne-Stokes respiration, is seen commonly in patients who have severe congestive heart failure, many with underlying and longstanding systemic hypertension. Such patients have elevated pulmonary capillary wedge pressures (25) and catecholamine activity (19) and may have a reduced survival.

Table 50.1 Symptoms and Signs of Obstructive Sleep Disordered Breathing

Symptoms of Sleep Disorder
  Excessive sleepiness despite getting 8 h of sleep
  Snoring more than two nights per week; audible in other rooms; also in nonsupine position
  Witnessed apneas
  Nocturnal dyspnea
  Nocturnal wheezing
  Personality change
  Nocturia

Physical Signs
  Large neck circumference (>43 cm)
  Difficult to visualize posterior pharyngeal wall
  Retrognathia
  Nasal obstruction
  Systemic hypertension
  Overnight tachy/brady-cardia
  Nocturnal atrial fibrillation
  Nocturnal pulmonary edema
  Pulmonary hypertension
  Hypercapnia
  Difficult to intubate

III. CARDIOVASCULAR PHYSIOLOGY: A SLEEP PERSPECTIVE

Normal sleep is a complex physiological state accompanied by a 1°C fall in body temperature. Darkness, sensed by the suprachiasmic nucleus via the optic nerve, causes the pineal gland to release melatonin, which allows a cascade of hormonal and neuroendocrine and autonomic changes that characterize sleep. Polysomnography allows further staging of sleep into phasic and nonphasic REM and non-REM stages 1, 2, and slow-wave sleep.

Changes from wake to sleep result in muscle hypotonia and specific neurochemical (e.g., melatonin and serotonin release) and endocrine changes (e.g., increase in plasma histamine and growth hormone and falls in cortisol and catecholamines). Skeletal muscle hypotonia, greatest in REM, affects primarily the muscles of posture (thus, the requirement of humans to sleep horizontally) and is under the control of the locus coeruleus nucleus in the brainstem.

During wakefulness, respiration is maintained by a waking neural drive, a cortical drive, and a metabolic-chemical drive (effects of $PaCO_2$, pH, and PaO_2 on chemoreceptors). During non-REM sleep, respiration is controlled primarily by the metabolic-chemical drive. During REM sleep, metabolic and cortical factors are thought to contribute, thus ventilation becomes characteristically erratic.

With sleep onset, the respiratory muscles of the upper airway and respiratory pump are partially inhibited so that upper airway resistance commonly increases and minute ventilation is reduced. Pulmonary functional residual capacity decreases (and thus also the pulmonary oxygen stores) because of a reduction in the balance between chest wall muscle activity (expansive) and elastic recoil of lung parenchyma (restrictive). Mild hypoxemia and hypercapnia may result.

From wakefulness to non-REM sleep, sympathetic activity is reduced and parasympathetic activity is increased. From non-REM to REM sleep, sympathetic activity to the skeletal muscles increases to twice that of waking levels, especially during phasic REM. Low-frequency power, measured by ECG spectral analysis, indicative of cardiac sympathetic activity is reduced with the transition from wakefulness to non-REM sleep and increases in REM sleep. High-frequency power, indicative of parasympathetic activity, is increased with the transition from wakefulness to non-REM sleep and reduced again in REM sleep. Baroreceptor sensitivity is increased in non-REM sleep compared with wakefulness.

Overall, there is a ~10–15% reduction in stroke volume, heart rate, and systemic blood pressure during non-REM sleep compared with wakefulness (30). Regional blood flow is altered such that during REM sleep, blood flow is negligible to peripheral skeletal muscles but greatest to the brain. Blood pressure and heart rate may rise in REM, particularly phasic REM sleep.

IV. EPIDEMIOLOGY

Epidemiological studies of obstructive sleep apnea have focused on the relationship between obstructive sleep apnea and breathing.

A. Obstructive Sleep Disordered Breathing

In 1956, Burwell et al. (26) described the Pickwickian syndrome in an obese male with pulmonary and systemic hypertension who had evidence of hypercapnic respiratory failure and hypersomnolence. In 1966, Gastaut et al. (27) described sleep-related hypoxemia using continuous oximetry in such patients. In 1972, Coccagna et al. (28) described the acute rises pulmonary and systemic blood pressure (measured invasively) that occur during sleep in patients with severe obstructive sleep apnea with mild or nonexistent systemic hypertension awake. By 1975, the association between obstructive sleep apnea, loss of the nocturnal dip in blood pressure, and awake hypertension had been made (2).

On the basis of results from modern surveys in the United States, regular snoring is reported to occur in 44% and 28% of the middle-aged men and women, respectively (13), whereas obstructive sleep apnea, defined as five or more apneas and hypopneas per hour sleep, occurs in 24% of men and 9% of women. The prevalence of symptomatic obstructive sleep apnea (excessive sleepiness and AHI >5 events per hour), also known as the *obstructive sleep apnea hypopnea syndrome*, is 4% in men and 2% in women.

B. Obstructive Sleep Disordered Breathing and Systemic Hypertension

Since the mid-1970s, an association between systemic hypertension and snoring has been observed (2). In one of the first studies, 30% of patients with essential systemic hypertension had sleep apnea (as defined by >30 apneas per night) compared with 24% in a control group matched for age and gender (29). Worsnop et al. (14), in a carefully conducted study that controlled for age, alcohol consumption, and body weight, reported a similar figure of 38% of treated and untreated hypertensives having AHI >5 events per hour compared with 4% in a nonhypertensive population. Patients with refractory hypertension (patients with blood pressure ≥140/90 mmHg on more than three antihypertensive agents) were found to have a 83% prevalence of obstructive sleep apnea (15).

Two large epidemiological studies (3,4) have now confirmed an epidemiological association between obstructive sleep apnea and systemic hypertension.

The first was a large cross-sectional study (3) of 11,053 community participants over 40 years in age with no history of sleep disordered breathing treatment, of whom 6841 (62%) agreed to undergo home polysomnography, detailed general health and sleep questionnaires, and blood pressure measurement. The severity of obstructive sleep disordered breathing (AHI, arousal frequency and hypoxemia) was significantly associated with blood pressure values. When controlled for body mass index, the AHI and hypoxemic time remained significantly associated with blood pressure. The prevalence rates for hypertension were 43% for AHI <1.5 events per hour; 53% for AHI 1.5–4.9 events per hour; 59% for AHI 5.0–14.9 events per hour; 62% for AHI 15.0–29.9 events per hour; and 67% for AHI >30 events per hour. Although this provided an association between severity of obstructive sleep apnea and systemic hypertension, the authors could not claim a causal relationship.

In the second study, known as the Wisconsin Sleep Cohort Study (4), a causal relationship could be made. Detailed sleep monitoring was performed at baseline and again at 4 years on 709 volunteers (and at 8 years on 184 volunteers) along with detailed body mass index, blood pressure, and health history. Compared with no sleep disordered breathing, the odds ratio for developing systemic hypertension was 1.42 (95%CI 1.13–1.78) with an AHI of 0.1–4.9 events per hour; 2.03 (95%CI 1.29–3.17) with an AHI of 5.0–14.9 events per hour; and 2.89 (95%CI 1.46–5.64) with an AHI of >15 events per hour. These odds ratios were made after adjustment for body habitus, age, gender, cigarette use, and alcohol use. This finding that obstructive sleep apnea preceded the diagnosis of hypertension suggests strongly that obstructive sleep apnea plays an important role in the development of hypertension.

V. PHYSIOLOGICAL STUDIES

The primary physiological effects of obstructive sleep apnea are hypoxia with hypercapnia, large negative intrathoracic pressures (with impaired baroreflex control), and arousal from sleep, all of which lead to heightened sympathetic nerve activity (SNA) and alterations to vascular endothelial biology.

A. Hypoxemia and Hypercapnia

Hypoxemia and hypercapnia lead to local tissue vasodilatation. However, hypoxia is also sensed by the peripheral chemoreceptor (carotid body) and hypercapnia is sensed by the central chemoreceptors in the brain stem, which results in an overriding and counteracting stimulus that results in globally heightened central SNA outflow. Vasoconstriction results in most arterial beds apart from the coronary and cerebral vessels. Increased SNA leads to increased ventilation, which results in vagal afferent stimulation and attenuation of the elevated SNA, thus completing a negative feedback physiological loop.

In normal humans who are exposed to episodic hypoxia that is sufficient to cause a drop in SpO_2 to 75–85% for 20 s and then recovery to normoxia (~95%) for 40 s,

SNA to skeletal muscle remains elevated for a prolonged period following resolution of normoxia and normal ventilation (31). Thus, episodic hypoxia causes persistently elevated central SNA outflow activity.

Elevated plasma and urine norepinephrine levels and elevated skeletal muscle SNA (awake and asleep) are observed in untreated obstructive sleep apnea patients compared with normal matched controls. In addition, treatment of obstructive SDB is associated with reductions in markers of SNA (8,32) (Fig. 50.2). Animals exposed to intermittent hypoxemia have increased systemic hypertension mediated via peripheral chemoreflex (6).

Blood pressure and ventilation responses to hypoxia are exaggerated in both hypertensive and obstructive sleep apnea populations compared with appropriate control groups. Young hypertensive patients have a twofold greater SNA response to hypoxia than age- and body mass index-matched controls and a 12-fold greater SNA during a simulated apnea (33). Moreover, patients with obstructive sleep apnea have a significantly greater pressor response to hypoxia than do nonapnea patients (34).

The genetic makeup of neurons of the nucleus tractus solitarius and other brain stem regions involved in regulation of tonic and reflex control of SNA and integration of peripheral input have been observed (using c-Fos techniques) to alter in rats that are exposed to episodic hypoxia for 30 days (35). Thus, episodic hypoxia may cause long-term cellular changes in areas of the brain stem that affect cardiopulmonary control.

B. Arousal from Sleep

In the absence of hypoxemia, arousal from sleep also causes acute rises in mean blood pressure of up to 8 mmHg and 5–6 beats per minute (bpm) heart rate in normal healthy subjects exposed to auditory stimuli (36). Thus, arousal is thought to be a factor, in addition to hypoxemia, in the connection between obstructive sleep apnea and hypertension.

To determine whether arousal or hypoxemia is sufficient to cause an acute increase in blood pressure, supplemental oxygen was provided to abolish hypoxemia during obstructive sleep apnea. Arousals persisted and were associated with acute elevations in blood pressure (37). The authors estimated that ~75% of the increase in blood pressure acutely with obstructive sleep apnea could be attributed to the arousal and ~25% to the hypoxemia. Thus, additional factors to hypoxia, such as arousal, impaired baroreceptor activity, and vascular endothelial factors, are likely to play a role.

A series of canine studies, in which simulated obstructive sleep apnea caused awake hypertension, auditory arousals during sleep and elevated blood pressure during sleep but not during wakefulness (5). Clinical human

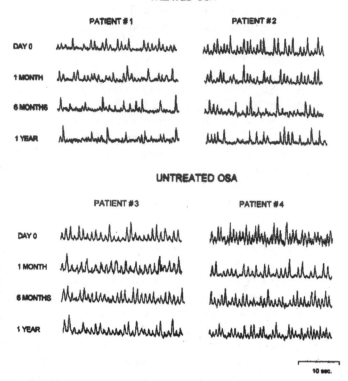

Figure 50.2 Direct sympathetic nerve to skeletal muscle recordings from two patient groups with obstructive sleep apnea. In one of the groups, patients are treated for obstructive sleep apnea, and in the other group, they are not. Note that the first group has a progressive drop in the height and frequency of sympathetic bursts. In the untreated group, there is no change in burst amplitude or in frequency over a period of 6 months. [With permission from Narkiewicz et al. (9).]

trials of sleep-related arousals and their effect on blood pressure (e.g., periodic limb movement disorders) are required to answer the question of whether sleep-related arousals increase blood pressure and cardiovascular risk (37).

C. Negative Intrathoracic Pressure

The negative intrathoracic pressures during the apnea are much greater than during normal inspiration (e.g., -5 vs. -80 cmH$_2$O), which lead to increased venous return, increased left ventricular wall transmural pressure gradient, left ventricular chamber dilatation, and impaired relaxation. In addition, the negative intrathoracic pressures cause stretch of the aortic arch baroreceptors, intermittently inhibiting sympathetic outflow. Evidence exists that baroreflex control is attenuated with recurrent obstructive SDB in humans (38) and dogs (39). In humans, baroreflex activity is normalized with continuous positive airway pressure (CPAP) treatment of obstructive sleep apnea (40).

Whether episodic hypoxia or hypoxia with negative intrathoracic pressure is required to develop awake systemic hypertension has been an area of debate until

recently. In an excellent series of experiments of Fletcher et al. (6), rats exposed to episodic hypoxia (FiO$_2$ 3–5% for 3–6 s followed by normoxia every 30 s for 6–8 h per day for 35 days) developed a 10–20 mmHg increase in mean arterial blood pressure that lasts 1–3 weeks following cessation of hypoxia. Carotid sinus nerve sectioning blocked this effect, suggesting that intermittent hypoxia effects on blood pressure are mediated by peripheral chemoreflex and ultimately sympathetic activity (6).

In a series of experiments in which tracheostomized dogs had intermittent occlusion of tracheostomy during sleep ($\sim$20 per hour for 1 week, then $\sim$55 per hour thereafter) for 1–3 months, awake mean systemic blood pressure rose 16 mmHg, which reversed with discontinuation of apnea (5). Moreover, the authors described a shift in the baroreflex activity curve to the left (39) and reduced systolic and diastolic left ventricular function (41) with the simulated obstructive sleep apnea.

Human observational data suggest that obstructive sleep apnea is also associated with left ventricular hypertrophy and diastolic dysfunction that can occur in childhood (42) as well as in adulthood (43). Children $\sim$9-year-old who have obstructive sleep apnea (AHI $\sim$18 events per hour) have significantly greater chance of having systemic hypertension and a much greater degree of left ventricular hypertrophy and estimated left ventricular mass compared with snoring and nonsnoring body mass index-matched children (42). Similarly in adults, over one-third of all patients with obstructive sleep apnea had evidence of left ventricular hypertrophy and diastolic dysfunction (43). This latter observation may indicate that obstructive sleep apnea takes a period of years before clinically significant structural or physiological changes (i.e., diastolic dysfunction) occur and are recognized.

D. Vascular Biology

The role of vascular biology and function has come under attention of sleep scientists, and an attempt has been made to summarize the role of vascular biology and function in the development of hypertension in obstructive sleep apnea. Although several in number, the precise effect of one peptide over another has not been clarified (Fig. 50.3).

First, vascular wall thickening has been observed in obstructive sleep apnea, indicating the clinical importance of such vascular hormones (44). Arterial diameter is reduced in obstructive sleep apnea patients compared with body mass index-, age-, and gender-matched controls (45).

In one of the earlier experiments, patients with obstructive sleep apnea and systemic hypertension had impaired acute vasodilator response to acetylcholine and sodium nitroprusside (nitric oxide-dependent and nitric oxide-independent, respectively) compared with age- and body mass index-matched controls (46). The same group observed a heightened vasoconstrictor activity to angiotensin II infusion in those with obstructive sleep apnea (47).

In a 2 month longitudinal study, forearm vasodilatation response curves to bradykinin (nitric oxide-independent) and nitroglycerine (nitric oxide-dependent) were impaired in normotensive obstructive sleep apnea patients compared with normal controls and improved to normal following two months of CPAP (48).

Obstructive sleep apnea has been associated with increased baseline levels of the potent vasoconstrictor endothelin-1 (49). Moreover, plasma endothelin-1 levels were significantly elevated ~4 h following sleep onset in a group of patients with severe untreated obstructive sleep apnea, whereas the levels did not change in a normal control group. In the obstructive sleep apnea group, the changes in endothelin-1 paralleled changes in blood pressure and changes in oxygen saturation. Thus, endothelin-1 may be an important factor in the pathogenesis of hypertension in obstructive sleep apnea patients.

Plasma angiotensin II and aldosterone were both elevated in a group of patients with severe obstructive sleep apnea ($n = 24$) compared with age- and body mass index-matched control groups ($n = 18$) (50). The authors did not find altered levels of other vasoactive hormones

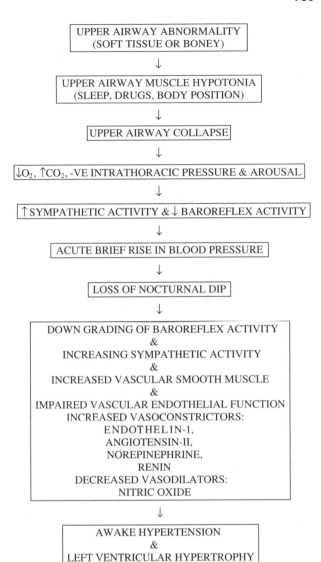

Figure 50.3 A flow diagram of possible mechanisms that connect obstructive sleep apnea with systemic hypertension.

such as atrial natriuretic peptide or brain natriuretic peptide. After 14 months of CPAP therapy, systemic blood pressure and plasma angiotensin II and renin levels decreased toward those levels observed in the control group.

In contrast to vasodilatation induced by smooth muscle relaxation (e.g., nitroglycerine), vasodilatation can occur secondary to endothelial actions. Endothelium-dependent, or "flow-mediated" vasodilatation, is a commonly utilized technique to assess vascular function and has been used in several recent experiments in patients with obstructive sleep apnea. Impaired flow-mediated vasodilatation is associated with known cardiovascular risk factors and improves following antihypertensive therapy.

Two recent reports have added considerable strength to the proposed role that impaired vasodilatation has in patients with obstructive sleep apnea who develop hypertension (45,51). The first comes from cross-sectional epidemiological data of the Sleep Heart Health Study (45). In that study, 1037 volunteers underwent diagnostic sleep studies and assessment of flow-mediated vasodilatation. The authors reported a significant association between sleep-related hypoxemia and both flow-mediated vasodilatation and baseline brachial arterial diameter. Of note, the association with flow-mediated vasodilatation was stronger for hypoxemia than for AHI suggesting that perhaps hypoxemia is a more important factor contributing to vasoconstriction than arousal.

In the second recent study, Ip et al. (51) assessed the endothelium-dependent and endothelium-independent response between 28 obstructive sleep apnea patients and 12 age-, gender-, and body mass index-matched healthy controls. The flow-mediated vasodilatation, but not nitroglycerine-induced vasodilation, was reduced in the obstructive sleep apnea group but not in the control group. Moreover, following 4 weeks randomization process to CPAP or control, CPAP treatment was associated with a significant increase (normalization) in flow-mediated vasodilatation compared with the untreated obstructive sleep apnea group. Finally, the CPAP treated group experienced a drop in flow-mediated vasodilatation following a brief withdrawal of CPAP.

Thus, there is now very good evidence that untreated obstructive sleep apnea patients have impaired endothelium-mediated vasodilation, which can be reversed with obstructive sleep apnea treatment with CPAP.

Elevated plasma leptin levels (49) and insulin resistance (52) were observed to be more common in patients with obstructive sleep apnea compared with weight- and age-matched control subjects without obstructive sleep apnea (49). Treatment with CPAP reduces leptin levels (53), although its effect on insulin sensitivity remains uncertain. A recent study revealed that insulin sensitivity, measured via the hyperinsulinemic euglycemic clamp technique, increased from 5.75 to 6.79 μmol/kg in 40 patients with obstructive sleep apnea treated with CPAP for two nights, an effect that persisted during a 3 month CPAP treatment time (54). The effect was greatest in those who had a body mass index of $<30 \, kg/m^2$, which suggests that obesity had an effect on insulin sensitivity independent of obstructive sleep apnea.

E. Pregnancy-Related Hypertension

An important category of systemic hypertension is that related to pregnancy, which in its most severe form can be associated with preeclampsia. Preeclampsia is characterized by systemic hypertension, proteinuria, and placental insufficiency.

The prevalence of obstructive sleep apnea in pregnancy is not known; however, snoring is three times more common in pregnancy compared with nonpregnant

controls and is thought to be due to increased upper airway edema, preexisting obesity, upper airway anatomical abnormalities, increased nasal resistance, narrow upper airway, and an increased drive to breathe. Approximately 75% of preeclamptic patients snore and have altered sleep architecture (55).

Snoring in pregnancy is associated marked intra-uterine growth retardation and lower APGAR scores (56). In patients with preeclampsia, snoring (often without the clear-cut obstructive apneas and hypopneas) is common and associated with increases in blood pressure during sleep. Preeclamptic women with obstructive sleep apnea had greater pressor responses to obstructive events than pregnant women with obstructive sleep apnea alone (57).

Reversal of snoring or coexistent sleep apnea with CPAP is associated with a drop in systemic blood pressure and a trend towards improved fetal outcome (58). Further studies are required to determine the role obstructive sleep apnea plays in the pathogenesis of pregnancy-related hypertension and preeclampsia.

VI. INTERVENTION STUDIES

Intervention studies have focused on the effects of antihypertension treatment on systolic blood pressure and effects of obstructive sleep apnea on systemic hypertension.

A. Effect of Antihypertensive Drugs on Systolic Blood Pressure

In a study of antihypertensive drugs in obstructive sleep apnea and systemic hypertension, five groups of drugs were studied in 40 males with 6.4 years of systemic hypertension and 2.5 years of sleepiness (59). None of the drugs had a significant effect on sleep disordered breathing. Atenolol caused the greatest fall in 24 h ambulatory mean systemic blood pressure (↓12 mmHg) compared with amlodinine (↓6.8 mmHg), enalapril (↓4.6 mmHg), hydrochlorthiazide (↓7.4 mmHg), and losartan (↓5.2 mmHg). Two conclusions can be drawn: antihypertensive drugs have little effect on obstructive sleep apnea, and β-blockers and, to a lesser extent, the other drug groups have an antihypertensive effect.

B. Effect of Obstructive Sleep Apnea Treatment on Systemic Hypertension

Randomized, controlled studies of the effects of obstructive sleep apnea treatment on systemic hypertension have been limited to CPAP and mandibular advancement splints. Alternative therapies, which include lifestyle modification (weight loss, avoidance of alcohol, upper airway surgery), have unfortunately not undergone controlled trials, let alone with cardiovascular outcomes (Fig. 50.4).

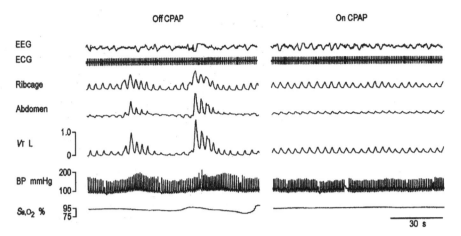

Figure 50.4 A polysomnogram of a patients with obstructive sleep apnea. (The left side of the illustration shows the surges in systemic blood pressure, with each awakening terminating in an apnea. On the right side of the illustration is the same patient with obstructive sleep apnea that is controlled with CPAP. Note the absence of surges in systemic blood pressure.) [With permission from Logan et al. (40).]

In one of the first medium-term, randomized controlled trails, Engleman (60) reported a drop in daytime blood pressure with CPAP compared to treatment with a placebo pill in a small group of patients with nondipping evening blood pressure over a 3 week period.

Thereafter, Dimsdale et al. (61) reported a fall in night time mean systemic blood pressure in 21 patients (14 of whom were normotensive) compared with 19 placebo-treated control subjects over 1 week using ambulatory blood pressure measurements.

Faccenda (62) reported ~3 mmHg decrease (borderline significance) in 24 h systemic blood pressure with CPAP compared with a placebo pill in 68 patients with obstructive sleep apnea, unselected for hypertension, and a mean blood pressure of 127/78 mmHg. Significant reductions in blood pressure were noted from 02:00 to 10:00 h, whereas blood pressure remained unchanged from 10:00 to 02:00 h. In a subgroup that had more severe obstructive sleep apnea (more than twenty and >4% dips in oxygen saturation per hour sleep), a greater drop in blood pressure of ~7 mmHg occurred.

Pepperell (10) reported a 3.3 mmHg drop in mean blood pressure with 1 month of CPAP in a randomized, controlled, and parallel design study involving 118 males, 19% of whom were taking antihypertensive medications. Baseline blood pressure for the group was 134/85 mmHg. Subgroup analysis of this hypertensive group revealed a ~8 mmHg drop in mean blood pressure with CPAP compared with the control group.

Becker (11) reported a ~10 mmHg drop in mean 24 h blood pressure in 32 patients randomized to either CPAP or a placebo CPAP over a 9 week time period without any change in body weight. A greater drop in blood pressure in this study compared with previous studies was thought to be due to greater hypertensive population

(66%), longer duration of treatment, and the method of blood pressure measurement. In contrast to the previous studies in which ambulatory cuff inflation techniques were used, continuous photoplethysmography was used in the current study (11). These studies on the effect of sleep apnea treatment with CPAP on blood pressure are summarized in Table 50.2.

In a rather unusual tack, 24 patients with untreated hypertension, 14 with and 10 without obstructive sleep apnea, underwent a 3 week trial of CPAP during which time 24 h ambulatory blood pressure was monitored (63). The mean nocturnal systolic and diastolic pressures decreased significantly in the obstructive sleep apnea group (−10.4/−5.2 mmHg) compared with the non-obstructive sleep apnea group (+1.9/+0.3 mmHg), findings that were sustained when the two groups were controlled for age and body mass index. There was a "borderline significant" trend towards a drop in daytime blood pressure levels in the obstructive sleep apnea group that was treated with CPAP (−2.7/−2.3 mmHg) compared with the nonobstructive sleep apnea group (+0.4/−1.7 mmHg). Thus, the effect of CPAP treatment on blood pressure is greatest during sleep and depends on treating the underlying obstructive sleep apnea and is not an effect of CPAP per se.

Recently, a group of 25 patients with severe obstructive sleep apnea, of whom 52% were receiving treatment for hypertension, had detailed echocardiography (64). Eighty-five percent had left ventricular hypertrophy, 64% had enlarged left atria, 48% had elevated right atrial size, and 16% had right ventricular hypertrophy. These findings supported the observation by Fung (43). After 6 months of CPAP treatment, there was a significant (~5%) reduction in the interventricular septal wall thickness.

Table 50.2 Effect of Sleep Apnea Treatment with CPAP on Blood Pressure

Author	Study design	Subjects who completed study/ eligible number of subjects	Age	Body mass index	%HT	Baseline blood pressure	AHI/min oxygen	Treatment	Outcome
Engleman et al. (60)	Cross-over, Placebo pill 3 weeks	13/16	51	36	31	139/85	49/71	CPAP	Drop in blood pressure dippers
Dimsdale et al. (61)	Parrallel Sham CPAP 1 week	39/?	48	31	26	125/80	48/	CPAP	Drop in overnight blood pressure
Faccenda et al. (62)	Parallel pill placebo 1 month	68/107	50	30	0	128/79	35/	CPAP	Drop in nocturnal blood pressure in group overall and drop in 24 h blood pressure, if severe OSA (>20 per h)
Pepperell et al. (10)	Parallel Sham CPAP 1 month	95/339	51	35	23	134/85	37/	CPAP 9.8 × 4.9 h	Drop in mean 24 h blood pressure of 3.3 mmHg Drop in mean blood pressure of 6.7 mmHg in HT group
Becker et al. (11)	Parallel Sham CPAP 9 weeks	32/283	51	33	66	136/82	64/72	CPAP ? ×5.5 h	Drop in mean blood pressure of 9.9 mmHg

Adherence to treatment with CPAP can be problematic. In the largest follow-up studies to-date, 1200 patients were contacted several years after initiating CPAP via a dedicated sleep center in Scotland (65). Approximately 70% of the patients continued with CPAP at the 5 year point, with 86% adherence in the patient group with severe obstructive sleep apnea (AHI >30 events per hour).

Whether alternative treatments of obstructive sleep apnea alter blood pressure is not known. In one of the randomized, controlled trials of splints, a small drop in blood pressure was observed in 27 patients who were treated with mandibular advancement splint over 4 weeks (66).

VII. PITFALLS WITH BLOOD PRESSURE MONITORING

During sleep, the automatic cuff inflation of ambulatory blood pressure monitors fragment sleep that causes an arousal-related surge in blood pressure (36). In a carefully conducted study in five normal subjects, with full polysomnography, blood pressure was measured by finger photoplethysmography on one hand and by automatic inflatable cuff on the other. Cuff inflation was associated with an arousal detected on polysomnography and ~30/20 mmHg increase in blood pressure in ~10 s, and a slow return to normal blood pressure over ~30 s. Thus, it would appear that automatic cuff inflation is associated with arousal from sleep, one of the proposed mechanisms of obstructive sleep apnea-related hypertension.

VIII. CONCLUSIONS

Recently, long term (12 year) follow-up studies have shown 3 fold greater fatal and nonfatal cardiovascular event risk in patients with obstructive sleep apnea untreated (67). Treatment of apnea reduced this risk to normal control group (67). The recognition that obstructive sleep apnea is a cause of systemic hypertension has been a significant advance in the knowledge areas of sleep apnea and systemic hypertension. This causal relationship is independent of obesity, diet, level of exercise, and amount of cigarette smoking. The job ahead is to determine to what degree the secondary effects of hypertension reverse and to what extent this reversal depends on how soon obstructive sleep apnea treatment is initiated after the onset of symptom of sleep apnea. Importantly, a large educational process is required for healthcare professionals to incorporate searching symptoms and signs of sleep apnea in their patients with hypertension. Consideration of the new dimension in blood pressure, namely, the sleep–wake dimension is important and should be considered in patients with *idiopathic* hypertension.

REFERENCES

1. Davies RJO, Crosby J, Vardi-Visy K, Clarke M, Stradling JR. Non-invasive beat to beat arterial blood pressure during non-REM sleep in obstructive sleep apnoea and snoring. Thorax 1994; 49:335–339.

2. Lugaresi E, Coccagna G, Faneti P, Mantovani M, Cirignotta F. Snoring. Electroencephalogr Clin Neurophysiol 1975; 39:59–64.

3. Neito FJ, Young TB, Lind BK. Association of sleep disordered breathing, sleep apnea, and hypertension in a large community-based study. J Am Med Assoc 2000; 283:1829–1836.

4. Peppard PE, Young T, Palta M, Skatrud J. Prospective study of the association between sleep-disordered breathing and hypertension. N Engl J Med 2000; 342:1378–1384.

5. Brooks D, Horner RL, Kozar LF, Render-Teixeira CL, Phillipson EA. Obstructive sleep apnoea as a cause of systemic hypertension. Evidence from a canine model. J Clin Invest 1997; 99:106–109.

6. Fletcher EC, Lesske J, Behm R, Miller CC III, Stauss H, Unger T. Carotid chemoreceptors, systemic hypertension, and chronic episodic hypoxia mimicking sleep apnea. J Appl Physiol 1992; 72:1978–1984.

7. Carlson JT, Hedner J, Elam M, Ejnell H, Sellgren J, Wallin BG. Augmented resting sympathetic activity in awake patients with and without obstructive sleep apnea. Chest 1993; 103:1763–1768.

8. Conway J, Boon N, Jones JV, Sleight P. Involvement of the baroreceptor reflexes in the changes in blood pressure with sleep and mental arousal. Hypertension 1983; 5:746–748.

9. Narkiewicz K, Masahiko K, Phillips BG, Pesek CA, Davison DE, Somers VK. Nocturnal CPAP decreases daytime sympathetic traffic in OSA. Circulation 1999; 100:2332–2335.

10. Pepperell JC, Ramdassingh-Dow S, Crosthwaite N, Mullins R, Jenkinson C, Stradling JR, Davies RJ. Ambulatory blood pressure following therapeutic and sub-therapeutic nasal continuous positive airway pressure for obstructive sleep apnoea: a randomised controlled parallel trial. Lancet 2002; 359:204–210.

11. Becker HF, Jerrentrup A, Ploch T, Grote L, Penzel T, Sullivan CE, Peter JH. Effect of nasal continuous positive airway pressure treatment on blood pressure in patients with obstructive sleep apnea. Circulation 2003; 107:68–73.

12. The 7th report of the joint national committee on prevention, detection, evaluation and treatment of high blood pressure. May 2003, NIH Publication no. 03-5233. (http://www.nhbli.nih.gov).

13. Young T, Palta M, Dempsey J, Skatrud J, Weber S, Badr S. The occurrence of sleep disordered breathing among middle aged adults. N Engl J Med 1993; 32:1230–1235.

14. Worsnop CJ, Naughton MT, Barter CE, Morgan TO, Anderson AI, Pierce RJ. The prevalence of obstructive sleep apnea in hypertensives. Am J Respir Crit Care Med 1998; 157:111–115.

15. Logan AG, Perlikowski SM, Mente A, Tisler A, Tkacova R, Niroumand M, Leung RS, Bradley TD. Increased prevalence of unrecognised sleep apnoea in drug resistant hypertension. J Hypertens 2001; 19:2271–2277.

16. Berlowitz DR, Ash AS, Hickey EC, Friedman RH, Glickman M, Kader B, Moskowitz MA. Inadequate management of blood pressure in a hypertensive population. N Engl J Med 1998; 339:1957–63.

17. Flemons WW. Obstructive sleep apnea. N Engl J Med 2002; 347:498–504.

18. Johns MW. A new method for measuring daytime sleepiness: the Epworth sleepiness scale. Sleep 1991; 14:540–545.

19. Solin P, Kaye DM, Little PJ, Bergin P, Richardson M, Naughton MT. Impact of sleep apnea on sympathetic nervous system activity in heart failure. Chest 2003; 123:1119–1126.

20. Roche F, Gaspoz JM, Court-Fortune I, Minini P, Pichot V, Duverney D, Costes F, Lacour JR, Barthelemy JC. Screening of obstructive sleep apnea syndrome by heart rate variability analysis. Circulation 1999; 100:1411–1415.

21. Schall RP, Shlitner A, Sheffy J, Kedar R, Lavie P. Periodic, profound peripheral vasoconstriction—a new marker of obstructive sleep apnea. Sleep 1999; 22:939–946.

22. Argod J, Pepin JL, Levy P. Differentiating obstructive and central sleep respiratory events through pulse transit time. Am J Respir Crit Care Med 1998; 158:1778–1783.

23. Shamsuzzaman AS, Winnicki M, Lanfranchi P, Wolk R, Kara T, Accurso V, Somers VK. Elevated C-reactive protein in patients with obstructive sleep apnea. Circulation 2002; 105:2462–2464.

24. Garpestad E, Basner RC, Ringler R, Lilly J, Schwartzstein R, Weinberger SE, Weiss JW. Phenylephrine-induced hypertension acutely decreases genioglossus EMG activity in awake humans. J Appl Physiol 1992; 72:110–115.

25. Solin P, Bergin P, Richardson M, Kaye DM, Walters EH, Naughton MT. Influence of pulmonary capillary wedge pressure on central apnea in heart failure. Circulation 1999; 99:1574–1579.

26. Burwell CS, Robin ED, Whaley RD, Bickelmann AG. Extreme obesity associated with alveolar hypoventilation—a Pickwician Syndrome. Am J Med 1956; 21:811–817.

27. Gastaut H, Tassinari CA, Duron B. Polygraphic study of the episodic diurnal and nocturnal (hypnic and respiratory) manifestations of the Pickwickian syndrome. Brain Res 1966; 2:167–186.

28. Coccagna G, Mantovani M, Brignani F, Parchi C, Lugarsei E. Continuous recording of the pulmonary and systemic arterial pressure during sleep in syndromes of

hypersomnia with periodic breathing. Bull Physiopathol Respir 1972; 8:1159–1172.

29. Kales A, Bixler EO, Cadieux RJ, Schneck DW, Shaw LC 3rd, Locke TW, Vela-Bueno A, Soldatos CR. Sleep apnea in a hypertensive population. Lancet 1984; ii:1005–1008.

30. Verrier RL, Dickerson LW. Autonomic nervous system and coronary blood flow changes related to emotional activation and sleep. Circulation 1991; 83(suppl II):II-81–II-89.

31. Xie A, Skatrud JB, Crabtree DC, Puleo DS, Goodman BM, Morgan BJ. Neurocirculatory consequences of intermittent asphyxia in humans. J Appl Physiol 2000; 89:1333–1339.

32. Fletcher EC, Miller J, Scharf JW, Fletcher JG. Urinary catecholamines before and after tracheostomy in patients with obstructive sleep apnea and hypertension. Sleep 1987; 10:35–44.

33. Narkiewicz K, Somers VK. The sympathetic nervous system and obstructive sleep apnea: implications for hypertension. J Hypertens 1997; 15:1613–1619.

34. Hedner JA, Wilcox I, Lake L, Grunstein RR, Sullivan CE. A specific and potent pressor effect of hypoxia in patients with sleep apnea. Am Rev Respir Med 1992; 146:1240–1245.

35. Greenberg HE, Sica AL, Scharf SM, Ruggerio DA. Expression of c-fos in the rat brainstem after chronic intermittent hypoxia. Brain Res 1999; 816:638–645.

36. Davies RJO, Belt PJ, Roberts SJ, Ali NJ, Stradling JR. Arterial blood pressure responses to graded transient arousal from sleep in normal humans. J Appl Physiol 1993; 74:1123–1130.

37. Ali NJ, Davies RJO, Fleetham JA, Stradling JR. The acute effects of continuous positive airway pressure and oxygen administration on blood pressure during obstructive sleep apnea. Chest 1992; 101:1526–1532.

38. Carlson JT, Hedner JA, Sellgren J, Elam M, Wallin BG. Depressed baroreflex sensitivity in patients with obstructive sleep apnea. Am J Respir Crit Care Med 1996; 154:1490–1496.

39. Brooks D, Horner RL, Floras JS, Kozar LF, Render-Teixeira CL, Phillipson EA. Baroreflex control of heart rate in a canine model of obstructive sleep apnea. Am J Respir Crit Care Med 1999; 159:1293–1297.

40. Logan AG, Tkacova R, Perlikowski SM, Leung RS, Tisler A, Floras JS, Bradley TD. Refractory hypertension and sleep apnea: effect of CPAP on blood pressure and baroreflex. Eur Respir J 2003; 21:241–247.

41. Parker JD, Brooks D, Kozar LF, Render-Teixeira CL, Horner RL, Douglas Bradley T, Phillipson EA. Acute and chronic effects of airway obstruction on canine left ventricular performance. Am J Respir Crit Care Med 1999; 160:1888–1896.

42. Amin RS, Kimball TR, Bean JA, Jeffries JL, Willging JP, Cotton RT, Witt SA, Glascock BJ, Daniels SR. Left ventricular hypertrophy and abnormal ventricular geometry in children and adolescents with obstructive sleep apnea. Am J Respir Crit Care Med 2002; 165:1395–1399.

43. Fung JW, Li TS, Choy DK, Yip GW, Ko FW, Sanderson JE, Hui DS. Severe obstructive sleep apnea is associated with left ventricular diastolic dysfunction. Chest 2002; 121:422–429.

44. Silvestrini M, Rizzato B, Placidi F, Baruffaldi R, Bianconi A, Diomedi M. Carotid artery wall thickness in patients with obstructive sleep apnea syndrome. Stroke 2002; 33:1782–1785.

45. Neito GJ, Herrington DM, Redline S, Benjamin EJ, Robbins JA. Sleep apnea and markers of vascular endothelial function in a large community sample of older adults. Am J Respir Crit Care Med. In press.

46. Carlson JT, Rangemark C, Hedner JA. Attenuated endothelium-dependent vascular relaxation in patients with sleep apnea. J Hypertens 1996; 14:577–584.

47. Kraiczi H, Hedner J, Peker Y, Carlson J. Increased vasoconstrictor sensitivity in obstructive sleep apnea. J Appl Physiol 2000; 89:493–498.

48. Duchna HW, Guilleminault C, Stoohs RA, Faul JL, Moreno H, Hoffman BB, Blaschke TF. Vascular reactivity in OSA syndrome. Am J Respir Crit Care Med 2000; 161:187–191.

49. Moller DS, Lind P, Strunge B, Pedersen EB. Abnormal vasoactive hormones and 24 h blood pressure in obstructive sleep apnea. Am J Hypertens 2003; 16:274–280.

50. Phillips BG, Kato M, Narkiewicz K, Choe I, Somers VK. Increases in leptin levels, sympathetic drive and weight gain in obstructive sleep apnea. Am J Physiol Heart Circ Physiol 2000; 279:H234–H237.

51. Ip MS, Tse HF, Lam B, Tsang KW, Lam WK. Endothelial function in obstructive sleep apnea and response to treatment. Am J Respir Crit Care Med 2004; 169:348–353.

52. Ip MS, Lam B, Ng MM et al. Obstructive sleep apnea is independently associated with insulin resistance. Am J Respir Crit Care Med 2002; 165:670–676.

53. Chin K, Shimizu K, Nakamura T, Narai N, Masuzaki H, Ogawa Y, Mishima M, Nakamura T, Nakao K, Ohi M. Changes in intra-abdominal visceral fat and serum leptin levels in patients with obstructive sleep apnea syndrome following nasal CPAP therapy. Circulation 1999; 100:706–712.

54. Harsch IA, Schahin SP, Redespiel-Troger M. CPAP treatment rapidly improves insulin sensitivity in patients with OSAS. Am J Respir Crit Care Med 2003; 164:156–162.

55. Izci B, Riha RL, Martin SE, Vennelle M, Liston WA, Dundas KC, Calder AA, Douglas NJ. The upper airway in pregnancy and preeclampsia. Am J Resp Crit Care Med 2003; 167:137–140.

56. Franklin KA, Holmgren PA, Jonsson F, Poromaa N, tenlund H, Svanborg E. Snoring, pregnancy induced hypertension and growth retardation of the fetus. Chest 2000; 117:137–141.

57. Edwards N, Blyton DM, Kirjavainen TT, Sullivan CE. Hemodynamic respiratory events during sleep are augmented in women with preeclampsia. Am J Hypertens 2001; 14:1090–1095.

58. Edwards N, Blyton DM, Kirjavainen TT, Kesby GJ, Sullivan CE. Nasal continuous positive airway pressure reduces sleep-induced blood pressure increments in preeclampsia. Am J Respir Crit Care Med 2000; 162:252–257.

59. Kraiczi H, Hedner JA, Peker Y, Grote L. Comparison of atenolol, amlodipine, enalapril, hydrochlorthiazide and losartin for antihypertensive treatment in patients with obstructive sleep apnea. Am J Respir Crit Care Med 2000; 161:1423–1428.

60. Engleman HM, Gough K, Martin SE, Kingshott RN, Padfield PL, Douglas NJ. Ambulatory blood pressure on and off continuous positive airway pressure therapy for the sleep apnea/hypopnea syndrome: effects in "non-dippers." Sleep 1996; 19:378–381.

61. Dimsdale JE, Loredo JS, Profant J. Effect of continuous positive airway pressure on blood pressure: a placebo trial. Hypertension 2000; 35:144–147.

62. Faccenda JF, Mackay TW, Boon NA, Douglas NJ. Randomized controlled trial of continuous positive airway pressure therapy for the sleep apnoea/hypopnoea syndrome. Am J Respir Crit Care Med 2001; 163:344–348.

63. Hla KM, Skatrud JB, Finn L, Palta M, Young T. The effect of correction of sleep-disordered breathing on blood pressure in untreated hypertension. Chest 2002; 122:1125–1132.

64. Cloward TV, Walker JM, Farney RJ, Anderson JL. Left ventricular hypertrophy is a common echocardiographic abnormality in severe obstructive sleep apnea and reverses with nasal continuous positive airway pressure. Chest 2003; 124:594–601.

65. McArdle N, Devereux G, Heidarnejad H, Engleman HM, Mackay TW, Douglas NJ. Long-term use of CPAP therapy for sleep apnea/hypopnea syndrome. Am J Respir Crit Care Med 1999; 159:1108–1114.

66. Gotsopoulos H, Mowbray J, Lawson L et al. Effect of mandibular advancement splint therapy on blood pressure in obstructive sleep apnea syndrome. Respirology 2001; 6(suppl):A51.

67. Martin JM, Carrizo SJ, Vicente E, Agusti AGN. Long-term cardiovascular outcomes in men with destructive sleep apnoea-hypopnoea with or without treatment with continuous positive airway pressure: an observational study. Lancet 2005; 365:1046–1053.

51

Oral Contraceptive Pills, Hormonal Replacement Therapy, Pre-Eclampsia, and Hypertension

HOSSAM EL-GENDI, GREGORY Y. H. LIP

University Department of Medicine, City Hospital, Birmingham, UK

KEYPOINTS

- The combined oral contraceptives have a small adverse effect on blood pressure—on average, ~5/3 mmHg.
- As the blood pressure response to any combined oral contraceptive preparation is unpredictable, the blood pressure should be measured before starting oral contraceptives use and then every 6 month thereafter.
- Hormone replacement therapy (HRT) use is not usually associated with an increase in blood pressure and can be prescribed safely to hypertensive women, but careful supervision is necessary.
- Cocaine, ecstasy, amphetamines, and LSD are among the many sympathomimetic drugs that can produce severe elevations in blood pressure, and with increasing substance abuse from these agents, clinicians will encounter more patients with drug-induced severe hypertension.

SUMMARY

Hypertension in women can be influenced by many factors, including oral contraceptive use and hormone replacement therapy (HRT), many drugs can have effects on blood pressure. The combined oral contraceptives have a small adverse effect on blood pressure, whereas HRT use is not usually associated with an increase in blood pressure and generally, can be prescribed safely. Many sympathomimetic drugs can produce severe elevations in blood pressure, and cause severe drug-induced hypertension.

I. THE ORAL CONTRACEPTIVE PILL AND HYPERTENSION

Unlike other commonly prescribed drugs, relatively healthy women take oral contraceptive pills for long periods of time. Thus, the challenge over the years have always been to change its formulations in order to enhance its efficacy and reduce its undesirable effects.

The first oral contraceptive pill, introduced in 1960, contained high doses of norethynodrel (progestin) and mestranol (estrogen). The original pills were monophasic with a fixed dose of estrogen and progestin throughout the whole cycle. Second-generation progestin was developed a decade later, in the 1970s. Over the following several decades, the dose of the estrogen component of oral contraceptive pills has been reduced, in addition, multiphasic preparations were developed (1). These changes were made mainly to lower the thrombogenic risk associated with the use of oral contraceptive pills which had gained much publicity at that time (2). Eventually, over the last decade, third-generation progestins from the gonane class were incorporated into oral contraceptive pill formulations to reduce the androgenic and metabolic side effects that occur with older agents (3,4). These oral contraceptive pills containing third-generation pills have several advantages with less side effects, mainly thrombogenic and androgen related effects associated with older progestins and therefore, less adverse lipoprotein and carbohydrate changes, weight gain, acne, hirsutism, mood changes, and anxiety. The third-generation progestins also have minimal effect on both the plasma insulin concentrations and the lipid profile (5).

The use of the combined oral contraceptive pill could affect blood pressure via different mechanisms which include salt and water retention, its effect on the renin–angiotensin system, body mass index, lipid metabolism, thrombotic, and atherogenic effects. Hypertension appears to be two to three times more common in women taking oral contraceptive pills, regardless of their initial blood pressure measurement prior to starting the pill (1). Oral contraceptives induce hypertension in ~5% of users of high-dose pills that contain at least 50 μg estrogen and 1–4 mg progestin. In spite of the change of contraceptive pill constitution and the emergence of modern low-dose formulations, small increases in blood pressure have been reported among users (6). However, neither the responsible hormone in the oral contraceptive nor particular subgroups of women who might be susceptible to the hypertensive effect of oral contraceptives have been clearly identified.

A. Oral Contraception in Normotensive Subjects

Oral contraceptive pills have long been thought to have no effect on the blood pressure when prescribed in normotensive women. However, in a landmark multicenter study conducted in the United States, a prospective cohort of 68,297 female nurses aged 25–42 years and free of diagnosed hypertension, diabetes, ischemic heart disease, cerebrovascular disease, and cancer at baseline were followed up for the duration of 4 years. After adjustments were made for age, body mass index, hormones, cigarette smoking, family history of hypertension, parity, physical activity, alcohol intake, and racial factors, the women taking oral contraceptive pills had an increased risk of development of hypertension when compared with women who had never used contraceptive pills, with a multivariate relative risk for the users of 1.2 (95% CI 1.0–1.4). This study suggested that users of oral contraceptives had a small but significant, moderately increased risk of hypertension. However, the risk may seem negligible as only 41.5 hypertensive cases per 10,000 person-years could be attributed to oral contraceptive use alone. This is to be balanced against the health and socioeconomic risks attached to an unwanted pregnancy. In addition, risk was markedly reduced following cessation of oral contraceptive pills, and past users appeared to have only a slightly increased risk. The increase in blood pressure appears to be idiosyncratic and may occur many months or years after first using a combined oral contraceptive pill. In a small proportion of women (~1%), severe hypertension may be induced.

In summary, the combined oral contraceptives do have a small adverse effect on blood pressure—on average, ~5/3 mmHg. As the blood pressure response to any combined oral contraceptive preparation is unpredictable, the blood pressure should certainly be measured before starting oral contraceptives use and then every 6 month thereafter (Fig. 51.1) (7).

B. Oral Contraception in Hypertensive Women

The use of oral estrogen–progesterone type combined contraceptive pills by women with hypertension on regular antihypertensive medication may have a negative impact on their pressure control, independent of age, weight, and antihypertensive drug treatment (8). Ambulatory blood pressure measurement is an even more sensitive tool to detect such impact. Some studies have shown no difference in blood pressure measurement in hypertensive women using contraceptive pills during outpatient visits; however, with the use of ambulatory blood pressure monitoring, the diurnal and nocturnal systolic blood pressure values were significantly higher in oral contraceptive users (9). These findings support the opinion that alternative methods of contraception should be considered for hypertensive women, rather than oral estrogen–progesterone type contraceptives, especially if blood pressure is difficult to control.

As an alternative, progesterone-only contraceptive pills may have less effect on blood pressure and may be worth considering, but have a higher failure rate than combined

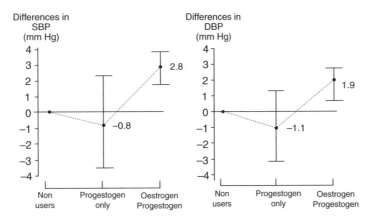

Figure 51.1   Blood Pressure and oral contraceptives, blood pressure differences adjusted for multiple confounding variables. (Adapted from Dong et al. J Hypertens 1997; 15:1063–1068.)

preparations. These oral progestogen-only contraceptive pills do not increase blood pressure, and can be used in women with a previous history of combined oral contraceptive-induced hypertension, or those women with hypertension wishing to use an oral contraceptive. If the blood pressure remains elevated, antihypertensive therapy should be started.

C.   Identification of High-Risk Groups for Hypertension with Oral Contraception

Particular groups of patients are more susceptible to the adverse hypertensive effect of oral contraceptive pill, especially obese and older women (10). Women aged 35 and older who smoke cigarettes should be strongly advised to stop smoking; if they continue to smoke, they should be strongly discouraged from using oral contraceptives and a different contraceptive method should be offered specially if hypertension develops in these women. Blood pressure usually drops to baseline level in most cases within few months of stopping contraceptive pills. If high blood pressure persists, if the risks for pregnancy are considered to be greater than the risks for hypertension, and if other contraceptive methods are not suitable, then oral contraceptives may have to be continued and therapy for hypertension should be started (1).

Oral contraceptive usage increases serum angiotensinogen levels to three to five times the normal and ~5% of these women develop arterial hypertension. Polymorphisms of angiotensin converting enzyme and angiotensinogen gene appear to be more prevalent in the group of women who subsequently developed clinical hypertension. In addition, a subanalysis of the Framingham study has shown that women taking contraceptive pills with a certain estrogen-receptor genotype appear to have a greatly increased risk of myocardial infarction (11).

II.   HORMONAL REPLACEMENT THERAPY

Hormone replacement therapy (HRT) is one of the most commonly prescribed drugs in the developed world, with perceived benefits on a wide range postmenopausal conditions including general wellbeing, osteoporosis, and cardiovascular morbidity and mortality. Furthermore, despite the increased risk of breast cancer with HRT, the early observational studies and meta-analyses actually suggested a reduction in mortality, cardiovascular disease, and osteoporosis risk among users of HRT when compared with nonusers (12,13).

For many years, HRT was considered to be contraindicated in hypertensive postmenopausal women, because of concerns that HRT may have an adverse effect on blood pressure, similar to that seen with the oral contraceptive pill. However, differences exist between the formulation and doses of estrogen preparations used, either as oral contraceptives in premenopausal women (in whom high-dose synthetic estrogens are used) or as HRT in postmenopausal women (in whom low "replacement" doses of natural estrogens are used).

The Heart and Estrogen/Progestin Replacement Study (HERS), published in 1998, was the first randomized controlled trial to show a significant increase in cardiovascular events in HRT users compared with non-HRT users. Similar findings have since been reported in several good studies, most notably the Women's Health Initiative (WHI) study (15)—which was stopped early due to an increase in breast cancer, coronary heart disease events (acute myocardial infarction, silent myocardial infarction, and coronary heart disease death), and stroke.

However, HRT use is not usually associated with an increase in blood pressure (see Fig. 51.2) and can be prescribed safely to hypertensive women, but careful supervision is necessary. Indeed, symptomatic women with hypertension should not be denied access to HRT as

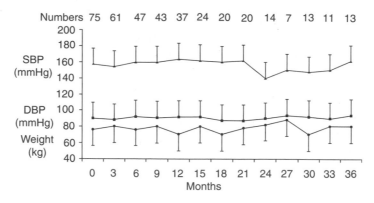

Figure 51.2   HRT in hypertensive women. (Adapted from Lip et al. J Human Hypertens 1994; 8:491–494.)

long as blood pressure levels can be controlled by antihypertensive medication. Suitable guidelines for the management of hypertensive women taking HRT are summarized as follows (12):

- All clinicians should measure blood pressure before starting HRT.
- In a normotensive postmenopausal woman, blood pressure should be measured annually following the start of HRT. One exception may be the use of premarin, where a follow-up blood pressure measurement should probably be made at 3 months (in view of reports of a possible rare idiosyncratic rise in blood pressure).
- In hypertensive menopausal women, blood pressure should at least be measured initially and at intervals of 6-month thereafter. If blood pressure is labile or difficult to control, 3 monthly measurements should be taken. If a hypertensive woman on HRT demonstrates a rise in blood pressure, careful monitoring or observation and perhaps an alteration or increase of their antihypertensive treatment should be considered.

III.   PREGNANCY INDUCED HYPERTENSION

Pregnancy induced hypertension is dealt with in detail in Chapter 43.

One in 10 women would experience a problem related to high blood pressure during pregnancy. It is worth emphasizing here that hypertension is an important cause of both maternal and fetal morbidity and mortality in pregnant women. There are still no definitive guidelines as to when and how patients should be treated, but it is important that appropriate treatment is initiated early in patients at highest risk and they are closely monitored.

Hypertension in pregnancy can be a difficult condition to diagnose and treat because of the numerous and differing classification systems that have been used in the past.

One classification system, which accounts for the multisystem involvement which can occur in pre-eclampsia and eclampsia, divides hypertension in pregnancy into three main groups: pre-eclampsia, gestational hypertension, and chronic hypertension. The pathophysiology, consequences and management of these disorders may differ, but there is an overlap in their presentation and clinical findings. Different metabolic, endocrinal and circulatory changes take place during pregnancy and in the early postnatal period however, the exact pathogenesis of hypertensive disorders in pregnancy is still obscure with much research trying to detect the possible underlying mechanisms. The implication of pregnancy induced hypertension could even extend beyond the duration of gestation, as the development of the relatively life threatening condition as malignant hypertension later in life has been linked to the development of hypertension during pregnancy rather than the past use of oral contraceptive pills (16).

Pre-eclampsia is a pregnancy related condition which is defined as a syndrome of the last trimester of pregnancy, characterized by hypertension, generalized edema with fluid retention and the development of proteinuria; however, the presence of the whole triad may not be necessary to establish the diagnosis of pre-eclampsia. This syndrome can progress unpredictably to a variety of life threatening conditions, including eclamptic seizures and renal failure, and contributes significantly to both maternal and perinatal mortality as well as morbidity (17).

Albeit the overall benefit of using antihypertensive therapy in pregnant women with severe hypertension is not debatable, the use of antihypertensive drugs in pregnant women with mild hypertension continues to be an area of uncertainty that there is hardly any evidence to confidently evaluate the clinical benefits of treating mild hypertension during pregnancy (18). Little benefit to the fetus has been shown from treating gestational and chronic hypertension, but studies in this area have been small and would not have had the power to show a difference in outcome between treated and untreated groups. However, the reduction in morbidity and mortality in the treatment of pre-eclampsia is significant. Therefore, all pregnancies complicated by hypertension require monitoring to detect the possible onset of superimposed pre-eclampsia/eclampsia. Institutions should have a management strategy for those mothers with severe hypertension including a multidisciplinary approach, where the patient is to be monitored and which antihypertensive agents are to be used. It should not be forgotten that the definitive treatment for severe hypertension is delivery of the fetus, despite risks to fetal morbidity and mortality. This will reduce blood pressure, but hypertension *per se* may still persist postpartum requiring short-term therapy, and follow-up of mothers postdelivery is needed.

REFERENCES

1. Pillssylvia L, Cerel-suhl, Bryan F. Update on Oral Contraceptive. 1st ed. American Academy of Family Physicians, 1999.
2. Linn ES. Clinical significance of the androgenicity of progestins in hormonal therapy in women. Clin Ther 1990; 12(5):447–455.
3. Hannaford PC, Webb AM. Evidence-guided prescribing of combined oral contraceptives: consensus statement. Contraception 1996; 54:125–129.
4. Kaplan B. Desogestrel, norgestimate, and gestodene: the newer progestins. Ann Pharmacother 1995; 29:736–742.
5. Darney PD. The androgenicity of progestins. Am J Med 1995; 98(suppl 1A):1A–104S.
6. Sitruk-ware R. Side effects of third generation progestagens. Contracept Fertil Sex (Paris) 1993; 21(4):295–300.
7. Chassan-Taber L, Willett WC, Manson JE, Spiegelman D, Hunter DJ, Curhan G, Colditz GA, Stampfer MJ. Prospective study of oral contraceptives and hypertension among women in the United States. Circulation 1996; 94(3):483–489.
8. Lubianca JN, Faccin CS, Fuchs FD. Oral contraceptives: a risk factor for uncontrolled blood pressure among hypertensive women. Contraception 2003; 67(1):19–24.
9. Narkiewicz K, Graniero GR, D'Este D, Mattarei M, Zonzin P, Palatini P. Ambulatory blood pressure in mildly hypertensive women taking oral contraceptives. A case–control study. Am J Hypertens 1995; 8(3):249–253.
10. Woods JW. Oral contraceptives and hypertension. Hypertension 1988; 11:(suppl II):II-11–II-15.
11. Mulatero P, Rabbia F, di Cella SM, Schiavone D, Plazzotta C, Pascoe L, Veglio F. Angiotensin-converting enzyme and *angiotensinogen* gene polymorphisms are non-randomly distributed in oral contraceptive-induced hypertension. J Hypertens 2001; 19(4):713–719.
12. Edmunds E, Lip GYH. Cardiovascular risk in women: the cardiologist's perspective. Q J Med 2000; 93:135–145.
13. Grady D, Rubin SM, Petitti DB, Fox CS, Black D, Ettinger B, Ernster VL, Cummings SR. Hormone therapy to prevent disease and prolong life in postmenopausal women. Ann Intern Med 1992; 117:1016–1037 [S].
14. Grady D, Herrington D, Bittner V, Blumenthal R, Davidson M, Hlatky M, Hsia J, Hulley S, Herd A, Khan S, Newby LK, Waters D, Vittinghoff E, Wenger N; HERS Research Group. Cardiovascular outcomes during 6.8 years of hormone therapy. JAMA 2002; 288:49–57.
15. Wassertheil-Smoller S, Hendrix SL, Limacher M, Heiss G, Kooperberg C, Baird A, Kotchen T, Curb JD, Black H, Rossouw JE, Aragaki A, Safford M, Stein E, Laowattana S, Mysiw WJ; WHI Investigators. Effect of estrogen plus progestin on stroke in postmenopausal women: the Women's Health Initiative: a randomised trial. J Am Med Assoc 2003; 289(20):2673–2684.
16. Lip GYH, Beevers M, Beevers DG. Malignant hypertension in young women is related to previous hypertension in pregnancy, not oral contraception. QJM 1997; 90(9):571–575.
17. Zamorski MA, Green LA. Preeclampsia and hypertensive disorders of pregnancy. Am Fam Physician 1996; 53(5):1595–1610.
18. Chung NAY, Beevers DG, Lip GYH. Management of hypertension in pregnancy. Am J Cardiovasc Drugs 2001; 1:253–262.

52

Drug Induced Hypertension

RETO NÜESCH

University Hospital Basel, Basel, Switzerland

KEYPOINTS

- Many different drugs, foods, poisons, and stimulants can cause arterial hypertension.
- The response to anti-hypertensive therapy can be impaired by exogenous agents.
- A careful drug history is essential in the assessment of hypertensive patients.

SUMMARY

A huge diversity of drugs, poisons, and stimulants can cause arterial hypertension. Typically, these drugs stimulate pressor responses, increase extracellular volume, and impair vascular compliance. Drugs associated with hypertension include: ergot alkaloids, ketamine, yohimbine, decongestants, metoclopramid, sulpiride, droperidol, monoamine oxidase inhibitors, anti-depressants such as venlafaxine, glucocorticoids, mineralocorticoids, oral contraceptives and estrogens, anabolic steroids, vitamin D and derivatives, lithium, nonsteroidal anti-inflammatory drugs, cyclosporin, tacrolimus, sirolimus, alkylating agents, erythropoietin, linezolid, amphotericin B, bromocryptine, disulfiram, and VEGF antagonists and stimulants such as caffeine, amphetamines, nicotine, alcohol, cocaine, and poisons, for example, heavy metals. Therefore, a meticulous drug history should be standard in assessing patients with arterial hypertension.

I. INTRODUCTION

Hypertension is usually diagnosed after a thorough evaluation of cardiovascular risk factors, causes of secondary hypertension, and hypertension-induced organ damage (1,2). Much less attention is paid to a detailed medical history which should include inquiries concerning foods, medications, poisons, and recreational drugs. Patients often do not consider them to be relevant in the context of arterial hypertension, and therefore often omit these substances from their history. However, identification of such substances is important. First, it may benefit the patient directly by reducing a health hazard. Furthermore, costs can be reduced, if the substance can be omitted and anti-hypertensive treatment withheld. Secondly, it may prevent unnecessary and often extensive investigations for secondary hypertension and hypertension refractory to therapy (3). Several detailed reviews on this topic have been published (4–6). With new therapeutic agents being licensed, the number of drugs potentially causing hypertension increases. A variety of chemical substances can induce a sustained or transient rise in arterial blood pressure (BP). The common feature is that these agents induce arterial pressure either by causing sodium retention, and thus expansion of the extracellular volume, or by direct or indirect activation of the sympathetic nervous system or by direct vasoconstriction. In a few cases, the mechanism of action is still unknown.

II. DRUGS AFFECTING THE SYMPATHETIC SYSTEM

All sympathicomimetic agents have pressor effects via direct or indirect stimulation of vascular α-adrenoreceptors causing vasoconstriction.

Amphetamines and its derivatives produce a dose-related pressor response by releasing noradrenaline from adrenergic nerve endings. Most nonprescription anorectics including dietary supplements contain combinations with adrenergic agonists. Known adverse effects include hypertension, agitation, abnormality of cardiac rhythm, psychosis, and seizures (7–10). Because of these health hazards, the use of such substances has been restricted in many countries.

Many decongestants include substances with structural similarities to amphetamines and ephedrine. They increase BP by raising peripheral vascular resistance as a result of α-adrenergic activity from direct stimulation of the receptors and release of neuronal norepinephrine (11). Hypertensive complications have occurred even with a single dose of such agents (11,12).

There is extensive evidence that caffeine at dietary doses increases BP by increasing peripheral vascular resistance (13,14). Findings from experimental and epidemiological studies show that BP remains reactive to the pressor effects of caffeine in the diet. Overall, its impact on population BP is likely to be in the range of 4–2 mmHg (15).

Nicotine is a well-known ganglionic stimulant and as such can produce hypertension. Further, nicotine impairs endothelial functions (16). Smoking one cigarette containing 1 mg of nicotine increases systolic BP by 10–15 mmHg and diastolic BP by 5–10 mmHg (17,18). Deaths due to hypertension are more common in smokers (19), smoking increases the risk of malignant

hypertension (20), and chronic smoking is associated with impaired efficacy of anti-hypertensive drugs (3).

Ergot alkaloids are (partial) agonists at the α-adrenoreceptor and serotonin receptor, and thus cause contraction of vascular smooth muscle cells and a consecutive rise in BP. Their use has been widespread for the treatment of migraine and management of orthostatic hypotension, but of late they have been replaced by newer drugs such as triptans.

Ketamine hydrochloride is widely used as an anesthetic in children and in developing countries. It can increase arterial BP very severely (21). The mechanism by which ketamine increases BP is not fully understood. However, the fact that clonidine attenuates the hypertensive response to ketamine indicates that sympathetic activity may be important in the hypertensive response to ketamine (22).

Effect of alcohol on BP was first described in the medical literature at the beginning of the last century (23). According to a review of 30 cross-sectional population-based studies, the majority of reports document small but significant increases in BP with alcohol consumption (24). Interestingly, some studies report that the rate of hypertension to be higher in nondrinkers than in those consuming one to two standard drinks per day. However, population-based cohort studies have shown a dose-dependant relationship between the quantity of alcohol consumption and the development of hypertension over time (24,25). Alcohol seems to exert its pressor effect by an increase in sympathetic activity. An increase in plasma adrenalin, noradrenalin, renin, and cortisol levels have been described in heavy drinkers (26–29). Of note, withdrawal from drinking can induce hypertension too.

Yohimbine, a drug formerly used for the treatment of male erectile dysfunction has been found to be relatively free of serious adverse events in short- and long-term studies. It can increase BP, particularly with high doses, by acting on the α-2 adrenoreceptor (30).

III. INDIRECT ACTIVATION OF THE SYMPATHETIC SYSTEM

Metoclopramid, sulpiride, and droperidol administered intraveneously to patients with pheochromocytoma may induce hypertensive crisis. The mechanism of action may not be direct stimulation of catecholamine release from the tumor. More likely, these agents stimulate catecholamine release by their presynaptic dopaminergic blocking effect (31). Anti-dopaminergic drugs such as metoclopramid, alizapride, and prochlorperazine have been reported to increase BP in previously normotensive patients receiving chemotherapy with cisplatine (32).

Cocaine increases BP and produces a variety of cardiovascular events due to adrenergic activation by blocking norepinephrine reuptake at the sympathetic nerve terminal (33,34). Abuse may cause strokes and cardiac damage. Most cardiac deaths were associated with myocadial injury similar to the one seen from catecholamine excess and possibly aggravated by hypertension (35).

Monoamine oxidase inhibitors and other anti-depressants delay the metabolism of sympatheticomimetic amines and 5-hydroxytryptophan and increase the norepinephrine store in the postganglionic sympathetic neurons. In addition, many anti-depressants have anti-cholinergic properties. Thus, hypertensive crises can be induced when these substances are used together with exogenous sympathomimetic amines or overdosed. The interaction of monoamine oxidase inhibitors with food containing tyramine, such as some cheeses, wines, avocado, chocolate, and carrot is well known (36). The proposed mechanism of action is that the uptake of tyramine into the sympathetic nerve ending causes release of noradrenaline which overloads the vesicle stores when intraneuronal monoamine oxidase is inhibited (37). Other types of anti-depressants have been known to produce a variety of cardiovascular effects including hypertension. In placebo-controlled studies with venlafaxine, a clinically significant increase in BP has been observed in 5.5% of patients (38).

Linezolid is a representative of the new class of synthetic antibiotics called oxazolidones. It is a week, reversible monoamine oxidase inhibitor, and thus may cause hypertension by the same mechanisms as other monoamine oxidase inhibitors (39).

IV. INCREASE IN EXTRACELLULAR VOLUME

Adrenocortical steroids increase BP through increasing cardiac output with little change in peripheral vascular resistance. The following mechanisms have been proposed to induce hypertension. Adrenocortical steroids can cause salt and water retention, increased angiotensinogen production with consecutive increase in angiotensin II levels, inhibition of vasodilatating hormones (kalikrein, prostaglandines, nitric oxide), increased vascular responsiveness to catecholamines, and increased number of angiotensin II type I receptor (40). Administration of high doses of glucocortocoids induces hypertension in adults and infants. Hypertension is a prominent feature of Cushing's syndrome and occurs in 20% of patients with iatrogenic Cushing's syndrome (41,42). Of note, hypertension can also be induced by topical application of glucocorticoids (43,44). After cessation of steroid exposure, BP usually normalizes.

Mineralocorticoids produce arterial hypertension by increasing exchangeable sodium and blood volume, hypokalemia with metabolic alkalosis, and suppressing plasma renin and aldosterone levels. Such changes can also be induced by exogenous compounds with mineralocorticoid activity. Interestingly, the active ingredient of a licorice extract and carbenoxolone a semisynthetic hemisuccinate derivative of glycyrrhenetic acid can cause a syndrome of apparent mineralocortcoid excess. Sodium retention, potassium wastage, and hypertension result from the ingestion of glycyrrhetinic acid (45,46).

Oral contraceptives and estrogens induce hypertension with an incidence of ~5% among the users of high-dose pills that contain ~50 mg of estrogens and 1–4 mg of progestogen (47). Some reports even found elevated BP in 18% of women taking oral contraceptives (48). However, the incidence of hypertension may be less with the present-day lower dose formulas containing a substantially lower dose of estrogens and new synthetic progestogens (49).

A more recently introduced method of contraception is contraceptive implants, which have been used by millions of women. Findings from observational studies on the safety of contraceptive implants have been recently reviewed. A more marginal yet significant elevation in BP was observed when compared with oral contraceptives (50). Contraceptive-associated hypertension is more likely to occur in women with a history of hypertension in pregnancy or preexisting primary hypertension, and these women should therefore be carefully monitored for increases in BP (51).

Another issue is the replacement of estrogens and progestogens after menopause. In one report, postmenopausal estrogen replacement therapy increased BP measured with a 24 h ambulatory device in almost one-third of the women given either oral or transdermal estrogen replacement (52). However, large prospective studies have not shown an increase in office BP in women given estrogen replacement (53).

Anabolic steroids produce a small but consistent increase in systolic BP when given for various indications (54,55).

V. IONS

Lithium intoxication has been accompanied by severe hypertension in rare cases (56). A significant increase in lithium levels has also been described after co-administration of ACE inhibitors or angiotensin I inhibitors (57,58).

Hypercalcemia has been identified as a common cause of arterial hypertension. A variety of pressor mechanisms can be affected by calcium, such as direct vasoconstriction of peripheral blood vessels and alterations in vasoactive hormones. In most cases related to hypertension, hypercalcemia was induced iatrogenically. Hypertension due to vitamin D intoxication tends to parallel the degree of hypercalcemia (59), and even topic applications of vitamin D derivatives can lead to hypercalcemia and hypertension (60).

Heavy metals including lead, copper, and cadmium are supposed to elevate BP. Possible mechanisms for lead-induced hypertension comprise changes in calcium metabolism inhibition of NA^+, K^+-ATPase, and alterations of humoral factors such as endothelin and nitric oxide released from endothelium. Epidemiologic studies confirm the high incidence of hypertension among patients exposed to lead, and it has even been speculated that lead may be a major contributor of essential hypertension (61).

VI. MIXED OR UNKNOWN

Nonsteroidal anti-inflammatory drugs may impair renal function and raise BP. They also interact with many anti-hypertensive drugs and reduce their effectiveness (62). In humans, they mainly act by inhibiting prostaglandin-induced vasodilatation although other factors, such as augmented responsiveness to pressor substances, sodium retention, and direct vasoconstrictive effects, are also involved. Clinically, significant increases in BP may occur after treatment with either nonselective or selective cox II inhibiting nonsteroidal anti-inflammatory drugs. All products, however, do not change observed BP to the same extent. Increases in BP seems to be more pronounced with indomethacin, naproxen piroxicam and rofecoxib, and in patients currently receiving antihypertensive treatment (62–64).

The incidence of cyclosporin-associated hypertension varies with the patient population under evaluation. Schorn et al. (65) studied the pre- and posttransplantation incidences of hypertension in two groups of renal transplant recipients which were receiving different immunosuppresive therapy. For the group treated with cyclosporin and prednisolone, the incidence of hypertension increased from 71% before transplantation to 85%, and in the comparative group with azathioprin and prednisolone, it decreased from 68% to 53%. Hypertension has also been found in patients treated with cyclosporin for autoimmune diseases (66). Cyclosporin could increase BP by several potential mechanisms: increased sympathetic nervous activity increased renal proximal tubular resorption, altered synthesis of vasodilatating prostaglandines, changes in the renin angiotensin system, and direct vascular effect (67). Tacrolimus, another calcineurin inhibitor has a similar but not identical mechanism of action and was introduced in the 1990s. Hypertension has also been reported with this drug (67). A newly introduced immunosuppressive agent is sirolimus (rapamycine). Compared with cyclosporin, sirolimus-therapy was associated with a lower incidence of hypertension (68). Calcium channel blockers interfere with the renal and vascular effects of cyclosporin and reverse vasoconstriction. Early administration may delay rejection episodes and improve graft function. Calcium channel blockers may offer some advantages over angiotensin-converting enzyme inhibitors for the treatment of hypertension in stable renal transplant recipient patients treated with cyclosporin. Selection of the most appropriate anti-hypertensive agent should take account of possible pharmacokinetic interactions with immunosuppressive agents (69).

Alkylating agents can increase BP. In patients treated with multiple alkylating agents after autologous bone marrow transplantation, hypertension developed in 15 of 18 subjects, and was not related to plasma renin activity, aldosterone, and catecholamins (70).

From the earliest use of recombinant human erythropoietin, hypertension has been recognized as an adverse effect occurring in some patients (71). The increase in BP induced by recombinant human erythropoietin cannot be fully explained by the improvement of anemia and the rise of blood viscosity alone. Erythropoietin may also increase intracellular calcium concentrations suggesting that it exerts a direct vasopressor effect on vascular smooth muscle cells (72). In large multicenter open trials, hypertension has been reported in 29–48% of patients (73–75).

VII. VARIOUS AGENTS

Amphotericin B is used for the therapy of serious fungal infections. Six cases of severe hypertension have been associated with the use of amphotericin B deoxycholate and one with the use of amphotericin B lipid complex (76). Development of severe hypertension has been described after the use of bromocryptine for suppression of lactation (77). Disulfiram, which is used in the treatment of alcoholism, has been reported to increase BP slightly (78). Although rare, a variety of cardiovascular events including hypertension have been reported with carbamazepine (79). Vascular endothelial growth factor antagonists are a new therapeutic strategy for the successful treatment of many cancers. VEGF induces vasodilation by induction of nitric oxide biosynthesis and is an important angiogenesic molecule. Its inhibition, for example with a monoclonal antibody called bevacizumab, inhibits angiogenesis and therefore tumor growth and also causes hypertension in a very substantial proportion of the treated patients (80–82).

VIII. CONCLUSIONS

Arterial hypertension is variably frequent side effect of a significant number of drugs used in different indications and by many different specialists. Induction of hypertension in response to drugs is owing to various mechanisms of action. Further, certain nutrients, poisons, and stimulants also increase BP. Awareness of these effects can significantly improve the management of patients with arterial hypertension. The list of substances causing drug-induced hypertension will probably increase in the future and will remain a challenge for the physician treating patients with hypertension.

REFERENCES

1. Cifkova R, Erdine S, Fagard R, Farsang C, Heagerty AM, Kiowski W, Kjeldsen S, Luscher T, Mallion JM, Mancia G, Poulter N, Rahn KH, Rodicio JL, Ruilope LM, van Zwieten P, Waeber B, Williams B, Zanchetti A. Practice guidelines for primary care physicians: 2003 ESH/ESC hypertension guidelines. J Hypertens 2003; 21:1779–1786.

2. Majernick TG, Madden N. The JNC 7 hypertension guidelines. J Am Med Assoc 2003; 290:1314; (author reply) 1314–1315.

3. Setaro J, Black H. Refractory Hypertension. N Engl J Med 1992; 327:534–547.

4. Grossman E, Messerli FH. High blood pressure. A side effect of drugs, poisons, and food. Arch Intern Med 1995; 155:450–460.

5. Messerli FH, Frohlich ED, Grossman E, Oren S. High blood pressure. A side effect of drugs, poisons, and food. Arch Intern Med 1979; 139:682–687.

6. Oren S, Grossman E, Messerli FH, Frohlich ED. High blood pressure: side effects of drugs, poisons, and food. Cardiol Clin 1988; 6:467–474.

7. Haller CA, Benowitz NL. Adverse cardiovascular and central nervous system events associated with dietary supplements containing ephedra alkaloids. N Engl J Med 2000; 343:1833–1838.

8. Delorio NM. Cerebral infarcts in a pediatric patient secondary to phenylpropanolamine, a recalled medication. J Emerg Med 2004; 26:305–307.

9. Bravo EL. Phenylpropanolamine and other over-the-counter vasoactive compounds. Hypertension 1988; 11:II7–II10.

10. Pentel P, Bravo EL, Haller CA, Benowitz NL, Delorio NM. Toxicity of over-the-counter stimulants. Phenylpropanolamine and other over-the-counter vasoactive compounds. Adverse cardiovascular and central nervous system events associated with dietary supplements containing ephedra alkaloids. Cerebral infarcts in a pediatric patient secondary to phenylpropanolamine, a recalled medication. J Am Med Assoc 1984; 252:1898–1903.

11. Bravo EL, Haller CA, Benowitz NL. Phenylpropanolamine and other over-the-counter vasoactive compounds. Adverse cardiovascular and central nervous system events associated with dietary supplements containing ephedra alkaloids. Hypertension 1988; 11:II7–II10.

12. Heyman SN, Mevorach D, Ghanem J. Hypertensive crisis from chronic intoxication with nasal decongestant and cough medications. DICP 1991; 25:1068–1070.

13. Robertson D, Frolich JC, Carr RK, Watson JT, Hollifield JW, Shand DG, Oates JA. Effects of caffeine on plasma renin activity, catecholamines and blood pressure. N Engl J Med 1978; 298:181–186.

14. Myers MG, Robertson D, Frolich JC, Carr RK, Watson JT, Hollifield JW, Shand DG, Oates JA, Pincomb GA, Wilson MF, Sung BH, Passey RB, Lovallo WR, James JE, Gregg ME. Effects of caffeine on blood pressure. Effects of caffeine on plasma renin activity, catecholamines and blood pressure. Effects of caffeine on pressor regulation during rest and exercise in men at risk for hypertension. Effects of dietary caffeine on mood when rested and sleep restricted. Arch Intern Med 1988; 148:1189–1193.

15. James JE. Critical review of dietary caffeine and blood pressure: a relationship that should be taken more seriously. Psychosom Med 2004; 66:63–71.

16. Sabha M, Tanus-Santos JE, Toledo JC, Cittadino M, Rocha JC, Moreno H Jr. Transdermal nicotine mimics the smoking-induced endothelial dysfunction. Clin Pharmacol Ther 2000; 68:167–174.

17. Baer L, Radichevich I. Cigarette smoking in hypertensive patients. Blood pressure and endocrine responses. Am J Med 1985; 78:564–568.

18. Cryer PE, Haymond MW, Santiago JV, Shah SD. Norepinephrine and epinephrine release and adrenergic mediation of smoking-associated hemodynamic and metabolic events. N Engl J Med 1976; 295:573–577.

19. Doll R, Peto R. Mortality in relation to smoking: 20 years' observations on male British doctors. Br Med J 1976; 2:1525 1536.

20. Isles C, Brown JJ, Cumming AM, Lever AF, McAreavey D, Robertson JI, Hawthorne VM, Stewart GM, Robertson JW, Wapshaw J. Excess smoking in malignant-phase hypertension. Br Med J 1979; 1:579–581.

21. Marlow R, Reich DL, Neustein S, Silvay G. Haemodynamic response to induction of anaesthesia with ketamine/midazolam. Can J Anaesth 1991; 38:844–848.

22. Tanaka M, Nishikawa T. Oral clonidine premedication attenuates the hypertensive response to ketamine. Br J Anaesth 1994; 73:758–762.

23. Lian C. L'alcoholism, cause d'hypertension arterielle. Bull Acad Med 1915; 74:525–528.

24. MacMahon S. Alcohol consumption and hypertension. Hypertension 1987; 9:111–121.

25. Fuchs FD, Chambless LE, Whelton PK, Nieto FJ, Heiss G. Alcohol consumption and the incidence of hypertension: The Atherosclerosis Risk in Communities Study. Hypertension 2001; 37:1242–1250.

26. Arkwright PD, Beilin LJ, Vandongen R, Rouse IL, Masarei JR. Plasma calcium and cortisol as predisposing factors to alcohol related blood pressure elevation. J Hypertens 1984; 2:387–392.

27. Ibsen H, Christensen NJ, Rasmussen S, Hollnagel H, Damkjaer Nielsen M, Giese J, Potter JF, Beevers DG, Arkwright PD, Beilin LJ, Vandongen R, Rouse IL, Masarei JR. The influence of chronic high alcohol intake

on blood pressure, plasma noradrenaline concentration and plasma renin concentration. Pressor effect of alcohol in hypertension. Plasma calcium and cortisol as predisposing factors to alcohol related blood pressure elevation. Clin Sci (Lond) 1981; 61(Suppl 7):377s–379s.

28. Ireland MA, Vandongen R, Davidson L, Beilin LJ, Rouse IL, Ibsen H, Christensen NJ, Rasmussen S, Hollnagel H, Damkjaer Nielsen M, Giese J, Potter JF, Beevers DG, Arkwright PD, Masarei JR. Acute effects of moderate alcohol consumption on blood pressure and plasma catecholamines concentration and plasma renin concentration. Clin Sci (Lond) 1984; 66:643–648.

29. Potter JF, Beevers DG, Arkwright PD, Beilin LJ, Vandongen R, Rouse IL, Masarei JR. Pressor effect of alcohol in hypertension. Plasma calcium and cortisol as predisposing factors to alcohol related blood pressure elevation. Lancet 1984; 1:119–122.

30. Tam SW, Worcel M, Wyllie M. Yohimbine: a clinical review. Pharmacol Ther 2001; 91:215–243.

31. Abe M, Orita Y, Nakashima Y, Nakamura M. Hypertensive crisis induced by metoclopramide in patient with pheochromocytoma. Angiology 1984; 35:122–128.

32. Roche H, Hyman G, Nahas G. Hypertension and intravenous antidopaminergic drugs. N Engl J Med 1985; 312:1125–1126.

33. Silverstein W, Lewin NA, Goldfrank L. Management of the cocaine-intoxicated patient. Ann Emerg Med 1987; 16:234–235.

34. Ramoska E, Sacchetti AD. Propranolol-induced hypertension in treatment of cocaine intoxication. Ann Emerg Med 1985; 14:1112–1113.

35. Nzerue CM, Hewan-Lowe K, Riley LJ Jr. Cocaine and the kidney: a synthesis of pathophysiologic and clinical perspectives. Am J Kidney Dis 2000; 35:783–795.

36. Simpson GM, White K. Tyramine studies and the safety of MAOI drugs. J Clin Psychiatry 1984; 45:59–61.

37. Brown C, Taniguchi G, Yip K. The monoamine oxidase inhibitor-tyramine interaction. J Clin Pharmacol 1989; 29:529–532.

38. Feighner JP. Cardiovascular safety in depressed patients: focus on venlafaxine. J Clin Psychiatry 1995; 56:574–579.

39. French G. Safety and tolerability of linezolid. J Antimicrob Chemother 2003; 51(suppl 2):ii45–ii53.

40. Saruta T. Mechanism of glucocorticoid-induced hypertension. Hypertens Res 1996; 19:1–8.

41. Smets K, Vanhaesebrouck P. Dexamethasone associated systemic hypertension in low birth weight babies with chronic lung disease. Eur J Pediatr 1996; 155:573–575.

42. Whitworth JA, Schyvens CG, Zhang Y, Mangos GJ, Kelly JJ. Glucocorticoid-induced hypertension: from mouse to man. Clin Exp Pharmacol Physiol 2001; 28:993–996.

43. Marin F, Gonzalez Quintela A, Moya M, Suarez E, de Zarraga M. Pseudohyperaldosteronism due to application of an antihemorrhoid cream. Nephron 1989; 52:281–282.

44. Afandi B, Toumeh MS, Saadi HF. Cushing's syndrome caused by unsupervised use of ocular glucocorticoids. Endocr Pract 2003; 9:526–529.

45. Kageyama Y, Suzuki H, Saruta T. Glycyrrhizin induces mineralocorticoid activity through alterations in cortisol metabolism in the human kidney. J Endocrinol 1992; 135:147–152.

46. Stewart PM, Wallace AM, Atherden SM, Shearing CH, Edwards CR. Mineralocorticoid activity of carbenoxolone: contrasting effects of carbenoxolone and liquorice on 11 beta-hydroxysteroid dehydrogenase activity in man. Clin Sci (Lond) 1990; 78:49–54.

47. Wilson ES, Cruickshank J, McMaster M, Weir RJ. A prospective controlled study of the effect on blood pressure of contraceptive preparations containing different types and dosages of progestogen. Br J Obstet Gynaecol 1984; 91:1254–1260.

48. Clezy TM, Foy BN, Hodge RL, Lumbers ER. Oral contraceptives and hypertension. An epidemiological survey. Br Heart J 1972; 34:1238–1243.

49. Fuchs N, Dusterberg B, Weber-Diehl F, Muhe B. The effect on blood pressure of a monophasic oral contraceptive containing ethinylestradiol and gestodene. Contraception 1995; 51:335–339.

50. Curtis KM. Safety of implantable contraceptives for women: data from observational studies. Contraception 2002; 65:85–96.

51. Khaw KT, Peart WS. Blood pressure and contraceptive use. Br Med J (Clin Res Ed) 1982; 285:403–407.

52. Akkad AA, Halligan AW, Abrams K, al-Azzawi F. Differing responses in blood pressure over 24 h in normotensive women receiving oral or transdermal estrogen replacement therapy. Obstet Gynecol 1997; 89:97–103.

53. August P, Oparil S. Hypertension in women. J Clin Endocrinol Metab 1999; 84:1862–1866.

54. Owens P, Lyons S, O'Brien ET. Body beautiful? J Hum Hypertens 1998; 12:485–487.

55. Graham S, Kennedy M. Recent developments in the toxicology of anabolic steroids. Drug Saf 1990; 5:458–476.

56. Michaeli J, Ben-Ishay D, Kidron R, Dasberg H. Severe hypertension and lithium intoxication. J Am Med Assoc 1984; 251:1680.

57. Teitelbaum M. A significant increase in lithium levels after concomitant ACE inhibitor administration. Psychosomatics 1993; 34:450–453.

58. Zwanzger P, Marcuse A, Boerner RJ, Walther A, Rupprecht R. Lithium intoxication after administration of AT1 blockers. J Clin Psychiatry 2001; 62:208–209.

59. Sica DA, Harford AM, Zawada ET. Hypercalcemic hypertension in hemodialysis. Clin Nephrol 1984; 22:102–104.

60. Kawaguchi M, Mitsuhashi Y, Kondo S. Iatrogenic hypercalcemia due to vitamin D3 ointment (1,24(OH)2D3) combined with thiazide diuretics in a case of psoriasis. J Dermatol 2003; 30:801–804.

61. Gonick HC, Behari JR. Is lead exposure the principal cause of essential hypertension? Med Hypotheses 2002; 59:239–246.

62. Pope JE, Anderson JJ, Felson DT. A meta-analysis of the effects of nonsteroidal anti-inflammatory drugs on blood pressure. Arch Intern Med 1993; 153:477–484.

63. Armstrong EP, Malone DC. The impact of nonsteroidal anti-inflammatory drugs on blood pressure, with an emphasis on newer agents. Clin Ther 2003; 25:1–18.

64. Sowers JR, White WB, Pitt B et al. The effects of cyclo-oxygenase-2 inhibitors and nonsteroidal anti-inflammatory therapy on 24-hour blood pressure in patients with hypertension, osteoarthritis and type 2 diabetes wellitus. Arch Int Medicine 2005; 165:161–168.

65. Schorn T, Frei U, Brackmann H, Lorenz M, Vogt P, Wiese B, Pichlmayr R, Koch KM. Cyclosporine-associated posttransplant hypertension incidence and effect on renal transplant function. Transplant Proc 1988; 20:610–614.

66. Dieterle A, Abeywickrama K, von Graffenried B. Nephrotoxicity and hypertension in patients with autoimmune disease treated with cyclosporine. Transplant Proc 1988; 20:349–355.

67. Miller LW. Cardiovascular toxicities of immunosuppressive agents. Am J Transplant 2002; 2:807–818.

68. Legendre C, Campistol JM, Squifflet JP, Burke JT. Cardiovascular risk factors of sirolimus compared with cyclosporine: early experience from two randomized trials in renal transplantation. Transplant Proc 2003; 35:151S–153S.

69. Koomans HA, Ligtenberg G. Mechanisms and consequences of arterial hypertension after renal transplantation. Transplantation 2001; 72:S9–S12.

70. Graves SW, Eder JP, Schryber SM, Sharma K, Brena A, Antman KH, Peters WP. Endogenous digoxin-like immunoreactive factor and digitalis-like factor associated with the hypertension of patients receiving multiple alkylating agents as part of autologous bone marrow transplantation. Clin Sci (Lond) 1989; 77:501–507.

71. Satoh K, Masuda T, Ikeda Y, Kurokawa S, Kamata K, Kikawada R, Takamoto T, Marumo F. Hemodynamic changes by recombinant erythropoietin therapy in hemodialyzed patients. Hypertension 1990; 15:262–266.

72. Vogel V, Kramer HJ, Backer A, Meyer-Lehnert H, Jelkmann W, Fandrey J. Effects of erythropoietin on endothelin-1 synthesis and the cellular calcium messenger system in vascular endothelial cells. Am J Hypertens 1997; 10:289–296.

73. The US Recombinant Human Erythropoietin Predialysis Study Group. Double-blind, placebo-controlled study of the therapeutic use of recombinant human erythropoietin for anemia associated with chronic renal failure in predialysis patients. Am J Kidney Dis 1991; 18:50–59.

74. Eschbach JW, Abdulhadi MH, Browne JK, Delano BG, Downing MR, Egrie JC, Evans RW, Friedman EA, Graber SE, Haley NR et al. Recombinant human erythropoietin in anemic patients with end-stage renal disease. Results of a phase III multicenter clinical trial. Ann Intern Med 1989; 111:992–1000.

75. Sundal E, Businger J, Kappeler A. Treatment of transfusion-dependent anaemia of chronic renal failure with recombinant human erythropoietin. A European multicentre study in 142 patients to define dose regimen and safety profile. Nephrol Dial Transplant 1991; 6:955–965.

76. Rowles DM, Fraser SL. Amphotericin B lipid complex (ABLC)-associated hypertension: case report and review. Clin Infect Dis 1999; 29:1564–1565.

77. Katz M, Kroll D, Pak I, Osimoni A, Hirsch M. Puerperal hypertension, stroke, and seizures after suppression of lactation with bromocriptine. Obstet Gynecol 1985; 66:822–824.

78. Volicer L, Nelson KL. Development of reversible hypertension during disulfiram therapy. Arch Intern Med 1984; 144:1294–1296.

79. Jette N, Veregin T, Guberman A. Carbamazepine-induced hypertension. Neurology 2002; 59:275–276.

80. Yang JC, Haworth L, Sherry RM, Hwu P, Schwartzentruber DJ, Topalian SL, Steinberg SM, Chen HX, Rosenberg SA. A randomized trial of bevacizumab, an anti-vascular endothelial growth factor antibody, for metastatic renal cancer. N Engl J Med 2003; 349:427–434.

81. Kiefer FN, Neysari S, Humar R, Li W, Munk VC, Battegay EJ. Hypertension and angiogenesis. Curr Pharm Des 2003; 9:1733–1744.

82. Diaz-Rubio E. New chemotherapeutic advances in pancreatic, colorectal, and gastric cancers. Oncologist 2004; 9:282–294.

Index